Pharmacology and Physiology for Anesthesia
FOUNDATIONS AND CLINICAL APPLICATION

Pharmacology and Physiology for Anesthesia

Foundations and Clinical Application

Hugh C. Hemmings, Jr., MD, PhD, FRCA
Distinguished Research Professor of Anesthesiology and Vice Chair of Research
Professor of Pharmacology
Weill Cornell Medical College;
Attending Anesthesiologist
New York-Presbyterian Hospital;
Adjunct Professor
The Rockefeller University
New York, New York

Talmage D. Egan, MD
Professor of Anesthesiology
Adjunct Professor of Pharmaceutics
Adjunct Professor of Bioengineering
Attending Anesthesiologist
Vice Chair for Research
K.C. Wong Presidential Endowed Chair
University of Utah School of Medicine
Salt Lake City, Utah

ELSEVIER
SAUNDERS

1600 John F. Kennedy Blvd.
Ste 1800
Philadelphia, PA 19103-2899

PHARMACOLOGY AND PHYSIOLOGY FOR ANESTHESIA: ISBN: 978-1-4377-1679-5
FOUNDATIONS AND CLINICAL APPLICATION

Library of Congress Cataloging-in-Publication Data

Pharmacology and physiology for anesthesia : foundations and clinical application / [edited by]
Hugh C. Hemmings Jr., Talmage D. Egan.
       p. ; cm.
Includes bibliographical references and index.
ISBN 978-1-4377-1679-5 (hardcover : alk. paper)
I. Hemmings, Hugh C.   II. Egan, Talmage D.
[DNLM: 1. Anesthesia.   2. Pharmacological Processes.   3. Physiological Processes. WO 200]
617.9'6—dc23

                                                            2012037216

Executive Content Strategist: William R. Schmitt
Content Developer: Joan Ryan
Publishing Services Manager: Anne Altepeter
Senior Project Manager: Cheryl A. Abbott
Design Direction: Steven Stave

Printed in China

Last digit is the print number: 9 8 7 6 5 4 3 2 1

To my wife, Katherine, and daughter, Emma, whose support and understanding were essential to the completion of this book; to my mentors Paul Greengard and John Savarese; and to my students, all of whom have taught me so much and from whom I continue to learn

H.C. Hemmings, Jr.

To my wife, Julie, and our children: James, Adam, Ezekiel, Sarajane, and Elizabeth—I am the luckiest; to my mentors Drs. Merritt Egan, Glen Church, K.C. Wong, Mike Cahalan, Don Stanski, and Steve Shafer—you are the wind beneath my wings

T.D. Egan

PREFACE

The successful practice of the art of anesthesia, critical care, and pain medicine demands a sound understanding of core scientific concepts founded in physiology and pharmacology. The importance of physiology and pharmacology to anesthesiology is recognized in postgraduate anesthesia training programs and certification examinations worldwide because a thorough understanding of these disciplines is essential for graduation, certification, and successful clinical practice. Although this scientific foundation is available from a number of sources, the necessary level of detail is often insufficient in introductory texts and perhaps too esoteric in specialized monographs targeted to academics. The goal of *Pharmacology and Physiology for Anesthesia: Foundations and Clinical Application* is to bridge this gap between introductory texts and comprehensive reference books by providing a detailed overview of these fundamental subject areas for anesthesiologists, intensivists, and pain practitioners, both in training and in practice.

Pharmacology and Physiology for Anesthesia: Foundations and Clinical Application is intended to be a definitive source for in-depth coverage of these core basic and clinical sciences in a single text. Focusing on physiology, pharmacology, and molecular-cellular biology, the text's approach is integrated and systems oriented, avoiding the artificial boundaries between the basic and clinical sciences. The book is divided into five sections: Basic Principles of Pharmacology; Nervous System; Cardiovascular and Pulmonary Systems; Gastrointestinal and Endocrine Systems; and Fluid, Electrolyte, and Hematologic Homeostasis.

Recognizing that no single author possesses the necessary breadth and depth of understanding in all the core subject areas, each chapter is authored by an expert representing many of the finest institutions of North America, the United Kingdom, Europe, and Asia. This allows an international presentation of current anesthesia science presented by recognized experts at the cutting edge of anesthesia research and education.

A number of features significantly enhance the use of *Pharmacology and Physiology for Anesthesia: Foundations and Clinical Application* as a tool for learning, teaching, and review. These include access to the online text via the Expert Consult platform, including a complete, downloadable image bank. Recognizing that graphics are often the most expressive and effective way of conveying concepts, full-color illustrations facilitate use of the book as a learning aid and make it enjoyable to read. The text is copiously illustrated; all figures having been drawn or redrawn by the superb artists at Elsevier.

Each chapter stresses the scientific principles necessary for the understanding and management of various situations encountered in anesthesia practice. Detailed explanations of clinical techniques are avoided because this information is available in many comprehensive and subspecialty clinical anesthesia texts and handbooks. This book is not intended to provide a detailed review of specialized research areas for the scientist. Rather, the fundamental information necessary to understand essential concepts and principles is stressed, and basic science concepts are related to relevant clinical anesthesia applications. Chapters are self-contained with minimal repetition and include a short list of key points for review and key references to stimulate further exploration of interesting topics.

The expertise and hard work of the contributing authors is evident in the quality of each chapter. And as a whole, the final text reflects the know-how and skill of the professionals at Elsevier and in particular the contributions of William Schmitt, Joan Ryan, and Cheryl Abbott. We are confident that *Pharmacology and Physiology for Anesthesia: Foundations and Clinical Application* will help solidify your understanding of core anesthesia topics and thereby improve the safety and effectiveness of the care you render to your patients.

Hugh C. Hemmings, Jr.
Talmage D. Egan

CONTRIBUTING AUTHORS

Geoffrey W. Abbott, MSc, PhD
Professor and Vice Chair
Department of Pharmacology
School of Medicine
University of California, Irvine
Irvine, California

Martin S. Angst, MD
Professor of Anesthesia
Stanford University School of Medicine
Stanford, California

Christian C. Apfel, MD, PhD
Adjunct Associate Professor
Departments of Anesthesia and Perioperative Care,
    Epidemiology and Biostatistics
Perioperative Clinical Research Core
University of California, San Francisco
University of California San Francisco Comprehensive
    Cancer Center at Mt. Zion
San Francisco, California;
Founder and CEO
SageMedic, Inc.
Larkspur, California

Edward A. Bittner, MD, PhD
Assistant Professor of Anesthesia
Harvard Medical School;
Program Director, Critical Care Fellowship
Department of Anesthesia, Critical Care, and Pain Medicine
Massachusetts General Hospital
Boston, Massachusetts

Michelle Braunfeld, MD
Clinical Professor, Liver Transplant Anesthesiology
David Geffen School of Medicine
University of California, Los Angeles;
Chief, Anesthesiology Service
Greater Los Angeles VA Medical Center
Los Angeles, California

Shane Brogan, MB, BCh
Associate Professor of Anesthesiology
Pain Management Center
University of Utah School of Medicine
Salt Lake City, Utah

Michael Cahalan, MD
Professor and Chair
Department of Anesthesiology
University of Utah School of Medicine
Salt Lake City, Utah

Charles D. Collard, MD
Professor and Anesthesiologist-in-Chief
St. Luke's Episcopal Hospital
Chief, Division of Cardiovascular Anesthesia
Texas Heart Institute
Houston, Texas

George J. Crystal, PhD, FAHA
Professor of Anesthesiology and Physiology and Biophysics
Advocate Illinois Masonic Medical Center
University of Illinois College of Medicine
Chicago, Illinois

Linda J. Demma, MD, PhD
Department of Anesthesiology
Emory University School of Medicine
Atlanta, Georgia

Daniel A. Drennan, MD
President/CEO
Comprehensive Pain Specialists
Denver, Colorado

John C. Drummond, MD, FRCPC
Professor of Anesthesia
University of California, San Diego;
Staff Anesthesiologist
VA San Diego Healthcare System
San Diego, California

Thomas J. Ebert, MD, PhD
Vice Chair for Education
Professor of Anesthesiology and Residency Program
    Director
Medical College of Wisconsin
Milwaukee, Wisconsin

Talmage D. Egan, MD
Professor of Anesthesiology
Adjunct Professor of Pharmaceutics
Adjunct Professor of Bioengineering
Attending Anesthesiologist
Vice Chair for Research
K.C. Wong Presidential Endowed Chair
University of Utah School of Medicine
Salt Lake City, Utah

Matthias Eikermann, MD, PhD
Assistant Professor
Harvard Medical School;
Director of Research, Critical Care Division
Department of Anesthesiology, Critical Care and Pain
    Medicine
Massachusetts General Hospital
Boston, Massachusetts;
Adjunct Professor of Anesthesia and Intensive Care
Essen-Duisburg University
Germany

Charles W. Emala, Sr., MS, MD
Henrik H. Bendixen Professor of Anesthesiology
Vice Chair for Research
Department of Anesthesiology
Columbia University
New York, New York

T. Miko Enomoto, MD
Assistant Professor of Anesthesiology
Department of Anesthesiology and Perioperative Medicine
Oregon Health and Science University
Portland, Oregon

Paul Garcia, MD, PhD
Assistant Professor of Anesthesiology
Emory University School of Medicine;
Staff Anesthesiologist
Atlanta VA Medical Center
Atlanta, Georgia

Peter Gerner, MD
Professor and Chairman
Department of Anesthesiology, Perioperative Medicine,
    and Intensive Care
Salzburg General Hospital
Paracelsus Medical University
Salzburg, Austria

Jacqueline A. Hannam, BSc(Hons)
Faculty of Medical and Health Sciences
Department of Anaesthesiology
University of Auckland
Auckland, New Zealand

Paul M. Heerdt, MD, PhD, FAHA
Professor of Anesthesiology and Pharmacology
Weill Cornell Medical College;
Member, Memorial Sloan-Kettering Cancer Center
New York, New York

Hugh C. Hemmings, Jr., MD, PhD, FRCA
Distinguished Research Professor of Anesthesiology and
    Vice Chair for Research
Professor of Pharmacology
Weill Cornell Medical College;
Attending Anesthesiologist
New York-Presbyterian Hospital;
Adjunct Professor
The Rockefeller University
New York, New York

Karl F. Herold, MD, PhD
Research Associate
Department of Anesthesiology
Weill Cornell Medical College
New York, New York

Philip M. Hopkins, MB, BS, MD, FRCA
Professor of Anaesthesia
Director, Division of Clinical Sciences
Leeds Institute of Molecular Medicine
University of Leeds;
Honorary Consultant Anaesthetist
Leeds Teaching Hospitals NHS Trust
Leeds Institute of Molecular Medicine
University of Leeds
Leeds, United Kingdom

Deborah Horner, MBChB, BSc, FRCA
Specialist Registrar
Department of Anaesthesia
St. James's University Hospital
Leeds, United Kingdom

Andrew E. Hudson, MD, PhD
Clinical Instructor
Department of Anesthesiology
David Geffen School of Medicine
University of California, Los Angeles
Los Angeles, California

Julie L. Huffmyer, MD
Assistant Professor of Anesthesiology
University of Virginia School of Medicine
Charlottesville, Virginia

Joel O. Johnson, MD, PhD
Professor and Vice Chair for Clinical Affairs
University of Wisconsin Hospital and Clinics
Madison, Wisconsin

Abhinav Kant, MBBS, FRCA, FHEA
Consultant Anaesthetist
Department of Anaesthesia
Leeds General Infirmary
Leeds, United Kingdom

Mark T. Keegan, MB, MRCPI, MSc
Associate Professor of Anesthesiology
Division of Critical Care
Department of Anesthesiology
Mayo Clinic
Rochester, Minnesota

Andreas Koköfer, MD
Resident in Anesthesia
Department of Anesthesiology, Perioperative Medicine,
    and Intensive Care
Salzburg General Hospital
Paracelsus Medical University
Salzburg, Austria

Brian P. Lemkuil, MD
Assistant Clinical Professor of Anesthesia
University of California, San Diego;
Staff Anesthesiologist
VA San Diego Healthcare System
San Diego, California

Roberto Levi, MD, DSc
Professor of Pharmacology
Weill Cornell Medical College
New York, New York

Jerrold H. Levy, MD, FAHA, FCCM
Professor and Deputy Chair for Research
Emory University School of Medicine
Division of Cardiothoracic Anesthesiology and Critical Care
Emory Healthcare
Atlanta, Georgia

Cynthia A. Lien, MD
Professor and Vice Chair for Academic Affairs
Department of Anesthesiology
Weill Cornell Medical College
New York, New York

Andrew B. Lumb, MB, BS, FRCA
Consultant Anaesthetist
Department of Anaesthesia
St. James's University Hospital
Leeds, United Kingdom

Srinand Mandyam, MD
Associate Physician
Oklahoma Pain and Wellness Center
Tulsa, Oklahoma

Robert G. Martindale, MD, PhD
Professor of Surgery
Chief, Division of General Surgery
Director, Hospital Nutrition Service
Oregon Health and Science University
Portland, Oregon

J.A. Jeevendra Martyn, MD, FRCA, FCCM
Professor of Anesthesiology
Harvard Medical School;
Director, Clinical and Biochemical Pharmacology
    Laboratory & Anesthetist
Massachusetts General Hospital;
Anesthetist-in-Chief
Shriners Hospital for Children
Boston, Massachusetts

Mary McCarthy, PhD, RN
Senior Nurse Scientist
Madigan Army Medical Center
Tacoma, Washington

Joseph Meltzer, MD
Medical Director, Cardiothoracic Intensive Care Unit
Program Director, Anesthesiology Critical Care Medicine
    Fellowship Program
Associate Clinical Professor, Division of Critical Care,
    Department of Anesthesiology
David Geffen School of Medicine
University of California, Los Angeles
Los Angeles, California

Edward C. Nemergut, MD
Associate Professor of Anesthesiology and Neurological
    Surgery
Program Director
Department of Anesthesiology
University of Virginia School of Medicine
Charlottesville, Virginia

Shinju Obara, MD, PhD
Assistant Professor of Anesthesiology
Fukushima Medical University, School of Medicine;
Deputy Director, Intensive Care Department
Fukushima Medical University Hospital
Fukushima, Fukushima Prefecture, Japan

Takahiro Ogura, MD, PhD
Research Fellow
Department of Anesthesiology
National Defense Medical College
Tokorozawa, Saitama, Japan;
Japan Maritime Self Defense Force Hospital
Yokosuka, Kanagawa Prefecture, Japan

Einar Ottestad, MD
Clinical Assistant Professor of Anesthesia
Stanford University School of Medicine
Stanford, California

Hahnnah Park
Department of Anesthesiology
David Geffen School of Medicine
University of California, Los Angeles
Los Angeles, California

Piyush M. Patel, MD, FRCPC
Professor of Anesthesia
University of California, San Diego;
Staff Anesthesiologist
VA San Diego Medical Center
San Diego, California

Misha Perouansky, MD
Professor of Anesthesiology
University of Wisconsin
Madison, Wisconsin

Tjorvi E. Perry, MD, MMSc
Assistant Professor of Anesthesiology
Department of Anesthesiology, Perioperative,
    and Pain Medicine
Division of Cardiovascular Anesthesiology
Brigham and Women's Hospital of Harvard Medical School
Boston, Massachusetts

Alex Proekt, MD, PhD
Assistant Professor of Anesthesiology
Weill Cornell Medical College
Assistant Attending Anesthesiologist
New York-Presbyterian Hospital/Weil Cornell Medical
    Center
New York, New York

Kane O. Pryor, MD
Assistant Professor of Anesthesiology
Assistant Professor of Anesthesiology in Psychiatry
Weill Cornell Medical College;
Assistant Attending Anesthesiologist
Memorial Sloan-Kettering Cancer Center
New York, New York

Aeyal Raz, MD, PhD
Department of Anesthesiology
University of Wisconsin
Madison, Wisconsin;
Department of Anesthesiology
Rabin Medical Center
Petah-Tikva, Israel;
Affiliated with Sackler Faculty of Medicine
Tel-Aviv University
Tel-Aviv, Israel

Peter Rodhe, PhD, MSc
Department of Clinical Science and Education
Section of Anaesthesiology and Intensive Care
Karolinska Institutet/Södersjukhuset
Stockholm, Sweden

David Royston, FRCA
Consultant in Cardiothoracic Anaesthesia, Critical Care,
    and Pain Management
Royal Brompton & Harefield NHS Foundation Trust
Harefield Hospital
Harefield, United Kingdom

John W. Sear, MA, BSc, PhD, FFARCS, FANZCA
Emeritus Professor of Anaesthetics
University of Oxford
Oxford, United Kingdom

Peter S. Sebel, MD, PhD, MBA
Professor of Anesthesiology
Department of Anesthesiology
Emory University School of Medicine
Atlanta, Georgia

Timothy G. Short, MB, ChB, MD, FANZCA
Honorary Associate Professor
Department of Adult and Trauma Anaesthesia
Auckland City Hospital
Auckland, New Zealand

Roman M. Sniecinski, MD
Associate Professor of Anesthesiology
Division of Cardiothoracic Anesthesiology
Emory University School of Medicine
Atlanta, Georgia

Randolph H. Steadman, MD
Professor and Vice Chair
Director, Anesthesia for Liver Transplant
Residency Program Director
Department of Anesthesiology
Director, Simulation Center
David Geffen School of Medicine
University of California, Los Angeles
Los Angeles, California

Kingsley P. Storer, MD, PhD
Assistant Professor of Anesthesiology
Weill Cornell Medical College;
Assistant Attending Anesthesiologist
New York-Presbyterian Hospital/Weill Cornell Medical
    Center
New York, New York

Suzuko Suzuki, MD
Clinical Associate in Anesthesiology
Department of Anesthesiology, Perioperative,
    and Pain Medicine
Brigham and Women's Hospital
Harvard Medical School
Boston, Massachusetts

Christer Svensén, MD, PhD, DESA, MSc
Associate Professor
Head, Research and Education
Department of Clinical Science and Education
Section of Anaesthesiology and Intensive Care
Karolinska Institutet/Södersjukhuset
Stockholm, Sweden

Kenichi Tanaka, MD, MSc
Visiting Professor of Anesthesiology
University of Pittsburgh Medical Center
Pittsburgh, Pennsylvania

Matthew Keith Whalin, MD, PhD
Assistant Professor of Anesthesiology
Emory University School of Medicine
Atlanta, Georgia

Rachel Whelan
Perioperative Clinical Research Core
Department of Anesthesia and Perioperative Care
University of California San Francisco Comprehensive
    Cancer Center at Mt. Zion
San Francisco, California

Josh Zimmerman, MD
Associate Professor
Medical Director, Preoperative Clinic
Department of Anesthesiology
University of Utah School of Medicine
Salt Lake City, Utah

CONTENTS

Contents

Chapter 1

MECHANISMS OF DRUG ACTION

Alex Proekt and Hugh C. Hemmings, Jr.

Understanding the basic principles of pharmacology is fundamental to the practice of medicine in general, but is perhaps most relevant to the practice of anesthesiology. It is now widely accepted that cells contain a host of specific receptors that mediate the medicinal properties of drugs. Although the use of plant-derived medicinal compounds dates back to antiquity, the mechanisms by which these drugs act to modify disease processes remained mysterious until recently. As late as 1964, de Jong wrote, "To most of the modern pharmacologists the receptor is like a beautiful but remote lady. He has written her many a letter and quite often she has answered the letters. From these answers the pharmacologist has built himself an image of this fair lady. He cannot, however, truly, claim ever to have seen her, although one day he may do so."[1]

This chapter briefly reviews the history of the receptor concept from the abstract notion alluded to by de Jong to the modern view of receptors as specific, identifiable cellular macromolecules to which drugs must bind in order to initiate their effects. Also introduced and defined are basic concepts that describe drug-receptor interactions such as affinity, efficacy, specificity, agonism, antagonism, and the dose-response curve. Finally, the evolving discipline of molecular pharmacology is discussed as it relates to modern drug development. Mathematical representations of the concepts are included in the form of equations for the reader seeking quantitative understanding, although the explanations of key concepts in the text are intended to be understood without reliance on the mathematics.

THE RECEPTOR CONCEPT

Historical Beginnings

The specificity of drugs for a particular disease has been known since at least the 17th century. The best known example of this is the efficacy of Peruvian bark, the predecessor of quinine, in the treatment of malaria.[2] Sobernheim (1803-1846) first applied the concept of selective affinity to explain the apparent specificity of drugs. He believed, for example, that strychnine had an affinity for spinal cord while digitalis had affinity for the heart.[1] Blake (1814-1893) first demonstrated that inorganic compounds with similar macroscopic crystalline structures exert similar effects when administered intravenously.[3] This triggered a vigorous scientific debate at the turn of the 20th century on whether it was the chemical structure or physical properties of drugs that endow them with medicinal properties.[4] This debate was particularly relevant for the theories of actions of general anesthetics because it was believed until recently that their relatively simple and diverse chemical structures precluded the possibility of a specific drug-receptor interaction.[5]

The term *receptor* was first coined in 1900 by Ehrlich (1854-1915) as a replacement for his original term "side-chain" (*Seitenkette*) that he used to explain the specificity of the antibacterial actions of antitoxins (antibodies).[6] Ehrlich did not originally believe that specific receptors existed for small molecules such as medicinal compounds because they could easily be washed out of the body by solvents. This belief was at odds with the remarkable experimental findings of Langley (1852-1925), who was investigating whether the origin of the automatic activity of the heart resided in the heart muscle itself or was imposed on the heart by the nervous system. He demonstrated that the effect of the plant-derived drug jabonardi—bradycardia—occurred even when innervation was blocked, and that this effect was reversed by applying atropine directly to the heart. He went on to show that the relative abundance of the agonist (jabonardi) over its antagonist (atropine) determined the overall physiologic effect. This observation led Langley to propose that competition of the two drugs for binding to the same substance explained their antagonistic effects on the heart rate. However, the key experiment that led Langley to formulate his receptor concept came 30 years later in 1905 when he showed that the contractile effect of nicotine on skeletal muscle can be antagonized by curare. From the observation that even after application of curare the relaxed muscle contracted following direct application of electric current, he concluded that neither curare nor nicotine acted directly on the contractile machinery. Instead, Langley argued that the drugs interacted with a "receptive substance" that was essential for the initiation of the physiologic actions of the drug.[7]

Modern Development

Langley's concept of "receptive substance" forms the basis of the modern concept of a receptor, but it was not accepted without debate. It took years of work by Clark (1885-1941) and Gaddum (1900-1965) among others to solidify the receptor concept. Clark demonstrated that the relationship between drug concentration and the physiologic response formed a hyperbolic relationship (the familiar sigmoidal dose-response curve; see later). Clark concluded that the relationship arose from equilibration between the drug and its receptor, and argued that the effect was directly proportional to the number of drug-receptor complexes.[8] Ariens (1918-2002) elaborated on Clark's theory and showed that the *affinity* of the drug for the receptor is distinct from the ability of the drug-receptor complex to elicit a physiologic response.[9] This distinction was further elaborated by Stephenson (1925-2004), who mathematically defined and quantified *efficacy*—the propensity of a drug to elicit a response.[10] Through his investigation of sympathomimetic compounds, Ahlquist (1914-1983) found that responses in various tissues occurred with two distinct orders of potency. This led him to propose multiple types of receptors for the same drug (α- and β-adrenergic receptors in this case), and the concept of *specificity*, which was finally published in 1948 after multiple rejections.[11]

Ahlquist's work is the foundation of modern pharmacology including the development of the first and still widely used receptor-specific drugs—beta blockers—by Black (1924-2010), who also developed H_2-histamine receptor blockers used to diminish stomach acid production in the treatment of peptic ulcer disease. Since Black's fundamental discovery, many receptors have been identified, structures of many drug-receptor complexes have been solved using x-ray crystallography and nuclear magnetic resonance (NMR), and the concept of drug-receptor interactions is now universally considered as the basis of physiologic actions of drugs.

PHARMACODYNAMICS

Drug Binding

Pharmacodynamics is broadly defined as the biochemical and physiologic effects of drugs. Proteins constitute the largest class of drug receptors, but other biomolecules can also be targeted. Proteins and other complex macromolecules can exist in a number of different conformational states. For simplicity, assume just two receptor conformations: physiologically active and inactive. In the case of an ion channel, for instance, the active conformation is an open conformation that allows ion permeation across the membrane, and the inactive conformation is the closed ion channel.

The following equation describes the relationship between the active and inactive states of the receptor (R):

$$R^I \underset{k_i}{\overset{k_a}{\rightleftarrows}} R^A \qquad [1]$$

R^I denotes the inactive (closed) ion channel and R^A denotes the active (open) ion channel, and k_a and k_i are rate constants for the forward and reverse conformational changes, respectively. In this example, rate k_i is higher than k_a (shown by arrow thickness) to illustrate a situation in which the channel is mostly closed in the absence of drug. The equilibrium relationship between the active and inactive conformations can be written as the ratio of the rate constants:

$$\frac{[R^A]}{[R^I]} = \frac{k_a}{k_i} \qquad [2]$$

In order to initiate its pharmacologic action, a drug (D) first needs to bind its receptor:

$$R^I \underset{k_i}{\overset{k_a}{\rightleftarrows}} R^A + D \underset{k_2}{\overset{k_1}{\rightleftarrows}} R^A*D \qquad [3]$$

In this example, drug D binds an active form of the receptor (R^A) to form the complex R^A*D. As in the first example, this binding reaction has two rate constants k_1 and k_2 that dictate the rates of drug-receptor complex formation and dissociation, respectively. The equilibrium constant for this binding reaction is therefore the ratio of the rate constants (k_1/k_2). The net effect of drug binding is an increase in active receptors as drug selectively binds the active conformation and thus prevents it from converting to the inactive

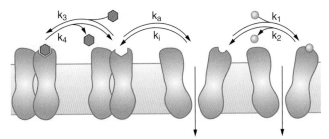

Figure 1-1 Illustration of an ion channel in a lipid bilayer in equilibrium between two conformational states. The abundance of active (open) and inactive (closed) conformations is dictated by the rate constants k_a and k_i. An agonist *(green circle)* selectively binds to the active conformation of the ion channel, while an antagonist *(red hexagon)* selectively binds to the inactive conformation. In both cases, drug binding serves to stabilize the receptor conformation; active in the case of an agonist and inactive in the case of antagonist. The equilibrium for drug binding is dictated by the ratio of the rates k_1/k_2 and k_3/k_4 for the agonist and antagonist, respectively.

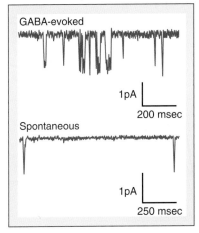

Figure 1-2 An example of agonist elicited and spontaneous formation of the active form of a receptor. A single γ-aminobutyric acid (GABA)$_A$ receptor complex during a voltage clamp experiment. Active (open) GABA$_A$ receptors conduct Cl$^-$ ions; inward flux is seen as downward deflections in the current trace, which reflect the times the channel is open. Even in the absence of GABA (the endogenous ligand at this receptor), the receptor can open spontaneously (trace labeled *Spontaneous*), but these openings occur more frequently and last longer when GABA is present. *(Reproduced from Neelands TR, Fisher JL, Bianchi M, Macdonald RL. Spontaneous and gamma-aminobutyric acid (GABA)-activated GABA(A) receptor channels formed by epsilon subunit-containing isoforms. Mol Pharmacol. 1999;55:168-178.)*

conformation. This type of interaction of drug with a receptor is called *agonism* (discussed later). Figure 1-1 shows a more general case, in which one drug (agonist) binds to an active (open) form of the ion channel while another drug (antagonist) selectively binds the closed form.

Although it might seem at first counterintuitive that even in the absence of agonist a receptor can be found in its active form, modern experimental methods such as single channel patch clamp recordings can show this directly.[12] An example of such a recording is shown in Figure 1-2.[13]

This model of drug stabilizing a receptor in its active conformation nicely explains the actions of GABA on GABA$_A$ receptors (see Figure 1-2), but is a very simplified view in several ways: (1) receptors can have more than two states (e.g., Na channel), (2) different conformational states can have different levels of activity rather than the all-or-none view presented here (e.g., nicotinic acetylcholine receptors), and (3) drugs can bind to more than one state of the receptor or at more than one site.[14-17] However, this model of drug-receptor interactions serves as a foundation for building more sophisticated models. This simplified description is used in the following discussion to derive the basic pharmacologic concepts.

Rearranging the equilibrium expression for drug binding to receptor yields the following expression in which the ratio of the two rate constants is defined as the dissociation constant K_D.

$$\frac{[R][D]}{[R*D]} \approx \frac{k_2}{k_1} \equiv K_D \qquad [4]$$

Note that if K_D is small then $k_1 \gg k_2$ and the complex of drug and its receptor is favored (as illustrated in Equation 3). When the converse is true and K_D is large, the drug-receptor complex is not favored. Thus K_D reflects the propensity of the drug-receptor complex to break down. One can alternatively define *affinity* as the inverse of K_D, which reflects the propensity of the drug to form a complex with the receptor.

$$A \equiv \frac{1}{K_D} = \frac{k_1}{k_2} \qquad [5]$$

To illustrate the importance of the dissociation constant K_D, the parameter f (fraction of receptor occupied by drug) is first defined:

$$f \equiv \frac{[R*D]}{[R]+[R*D]} \qquad [6]$$

and then expressed f as a function of drug concentration and the K_D (or affinity) by substituting Equation 4:

$$f = \frac{[D]}{[D]+K_D} = \frac{[D]}{[D]+\frac{1}{A}} = \frac{A[D]}{A[D]+1} \qquad [7]$$

K_D is a fundamental property of the drug-receptor interaction (given constant conditions such as temperature, pH, etc.), but can be different for different drug-receptor pairs. To illustrate the effect of differences in K_D on the formation of drug-receptor complexes, Equation 7 is plotted for two drugs characterized by different values of K_D (Figure 1-3).

FROM DRUG BINDING TO PHYSIOLOGIC EFFECT

Clark originally proposed that the number of drug-receptor complexes was directly proportional to the physiologic effect of the drug.[8] Although this is not entirely correct, for simplicity, first assume Clark's theory in order to derive the basic concentration (dose)-effect (response) curve and illustrate potency. Then Clark's assumption will be relaxed to arrive at the notion of efficacy.

If a physiologic response is directly proportional to the fraction of bound receptors, one should be able to derive the concentration-response relationship simply from the binding curve illustrated in Figure 1-3. Indeed, the familiar sigmoid concentration-effect curve shown in Figure 1-4 results from plotting the same equation as in Figure 1-3. The only

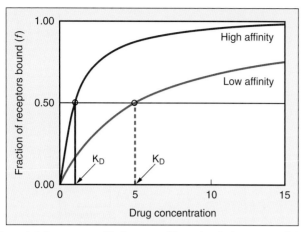

Figure 1-3 Drug-receptor binding curves illustrating the importance of drug affinity for the receptor. As drug concentration increases, the fraction of receptor bound by drug (*f*) increases until all receptors are bound (*f* = 1). Curves are shown for two drugs with $K_D = 1$ (*red*) and for $K_D = 5$ (*blue*). It takes much higher concentrations of drug to occupy the same number of receptors when the K_D is higher (or affinity is lower). When the drug concentration equals K_D, exactly half of the receptors are bound by drug (shown by *circles*).

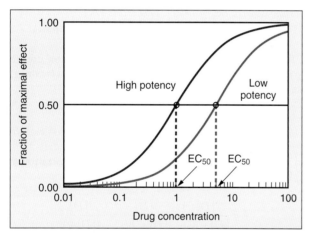

Figure 1-4 Concentration-effect curves illustrating the influence of potency (EC_{50}) on curve position for two drugs of the same class. $EC_{50} = 1$ (*red*) and for $EC_{50} = 5$ (*blue*). EC_{50}, effective concentration for 50% effect.

difference is that drug concentration is plotted on a logarithmic rather than linear scale and the y-axis is labeled as "Fraction of Maximal Effect."

Initially, as drug concentration increases, the increase in effect is rather small. In fact, until a certain concentration threshold is reached, no effect is apparent despite increasing drug concentrations. Further increase in drug concentration causes a steep increase in the effect, until maximal effect is attained. This sigmoid relationship characterizes actions of many different drugs acting at different receptors. The circles in the plot denote drug concentrations at which ½ of the maximal effect is attained. This concentration is termed EC_{50} (effective concentration for 50% effect). Conceptually this is similar to K_D defined earlier. The major difference is that EC_{50} refers to the ½ maximal *effect* while K_D refers to ½ maximal *binding*. The smaller the EC_{50}, the less drug is required to produce the same effect. This is why EC_{50} is

commonly used as a measure of drug *potency* or the ability of the drug to elicit a physiologic response.

The curve in Figure 1-4 is derived from an abstract notion of equilibrium between bound and free receptors. It is totally independent of the chemical identity of the drug or the receptor—it reflects the general property of drug-receptor interactions and is fundamental to the understanding of the action of any drug.

EFFICACY

The concentration-effect curves in Figure 1-4 depend on the important assumption that the effect of the drug is proportional to the amount of receptor bound by the drug. This hypothesis makes very strong predictions: (1) given high enough concentration, all drugs will give the same maximal effect; and (2) the slope of the curve should be similar for all drugs acting on the same receptor. Indeed, the only difference between the red and blue curves in Figure 1-4 is that the blue curve is shifted to the right. However, this is not always true, as shown by Stephenson in 1956 in a landmark study (Figure 1-5).[10]

While investigating the *pharmacodynamics* of tetramethylammonium (TMA) compounds known to elicit muscle contractions, Stephenson observed that different response curves were not simply shifted versions of each other. Specifically it appeared that maximal contraction was not always attainable even at the highest concentration of a drug. For instance, even at the highest concentration octyl-TMA-elicited contraction was only 40% of the maximal attainable, whereas 100-fold smaller concentrations of butyl-TMA elicited near maximal contraction (see Figure 1-5, *A*). This observation alone does not invalidate Clark's theory, however, because of the possibility that octyl-TMA has really low affinity for the receptor and is therefore unable to elicit maximal response in the range of experimental concentrations.

The results in Figure 1-5, *B*, show definitively that binding alone is not sufficient to predict the response. The contraction elicited by butyl-TMA is clearly larger than octyl-TMA. If octyl-TMA is not able to elicit maximal contraction because of its low affinity for the receptor, addition of butyl-TMA should make the contraction maximal. Yet addition of butyl-TMA did very little to the contraction elicited by octyl-TMA alone. Thus, although octyl-TMA is able to bind the receptor, it is unable to elicit maximal contraction.

To explain these observations, Stephenson generalized Clark's theory by proposing that the response *R* is not directly proportional to the fraction of receptor bound by drug, but instead is some function *F* of the stimulus *S*:

$$R = F(S) \qquad [8]$$

where *S* is a product of the efficacy (*e*) and the fraction of the receptors occupied *f*.

$$S = ef \qquad [9]$$

In the case of muscle contraction, *F* can be conceptualized as excitation-contraction coupling and efficacy as the ability of the drug-receptor complex to produce excitation. By substituting Equation 7 into Equation 9, affinity *A*, drug concentration *D*, and efficacy *e* can be combined in the same equation:

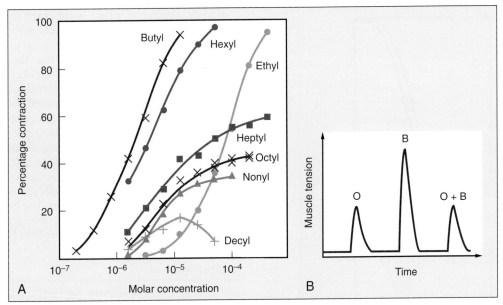

Figure 1-5 Examples of differences in agonist potency and efficacy. **A,** Concentration-effect curves for various tetramethylammonium compounds illustrating that similar molecules can have different potencies (EC$_{50s}$) and different maximal effects (i.e., partial agonists). **B,** Muscle contractions elicited by octyl-TMA *(O)* and butyl-TMA *(B)* applied separately or together *(O + B)*. *(Modified with permission from Stephenson RP. Modification of receptor theory.* Br J Pharmacol Chemother. *1956;11:379-393.)*

$$S = e\left(\frac{A*[D]}{A*[D]+1}\right) \quad [10]$$

For conditions where the fraction of the occupied receptors is small, this simplifies to:

$$S = eAD \quad [11]$$

Accordingly, even when the fraction of the occupied receptors is small, the observed physiologic effect can be quite large if the efficacy is high. Conversely, even if affinity is high but the efficacy is low, the overall effect can be quite low. Therefore the overall drug *potency* for a given system is a function of two variables that characterize drug-receptor interactions: *affinity* and *efficacy*.

Full Agonists, Partial Agonists, and Inverse Agonists

Drugs can be classified based on the features of their concentration-effect relationships. This section focuses on different kinds of agonists and the following section discusses different forms of antagonism. First, features of drug-receptor interactions that make a particular drug an agonist are defined. In schema Equation 3, it is assumed that drug only binds the active conformation of the receptor (see also Figure 1-1). In a more general case (schema Equation 12), drug can bind both active and inactive receptor conformations with different affinities.

$$[12]$$

The higher the affinity for the active conformation, the more equilibrium will be driven to the active receptor

conformation until essentially all receptors are activated. This is called a *full agonist*. If the affinities for both active and inactive conformations of the receptor are comparable, the drug will be unable to convert a significant fraction of the receptor to the active conformation, even at high concentrations (reviewed for glutamate receptors).[18] This drug is called a *partial agonist*.

This is a microscopic level description of the basis of drug agonism, but in most cases, there is no detailed understanding of the molecular events. It is difficult to measure experimentally the differences in affinity for different conformational states of a receptor. Usually this problem is solved by performing molecular dynamics simulations.[19]

There is, however, a way to discover differences between agonists by characterizing their concentration-effect curves on a macroscopic level. Recall that the overall effect of a drug depends on two factors: affinity and efficacy. According to Equation 10, efficacy determines the maximal effect attainable at the limit of high drug concentration, and affinity determines the range of drug concentrations at which the steep portion of the concentration-effect curve occurs. Therefore, the effect of drug affinity can be isolated by scaling the y-axis of the concentration-response curve to the maximal effect attainable for that drug, and differences in efficacy can be characterized by comparing maximal attainable effects.

Figure 1-6, *A,* shows two drugs that are distinguished by their affinity (higher for the red drug) scaled relative to the maximal effect attainable for each drug. When the effect of each drug is plotted relative to the absolute maximal effect (see Figure 1-6, *B*), it becomes evident that although the red drug has higher affinity, it has lower efficacy with a maximal response of ⅓ of that attainable by the blue drug. Therefore the red drug is a *partial agonist* while the blue drug is a *full agonist*. Although the shapes of the plots in Figures 1-6, *A,* and 1-6, *B,* appear quite different, in fact the relationship between their EC$_{50}$ values stays exactly the same regardless of how the data are plotted.

7

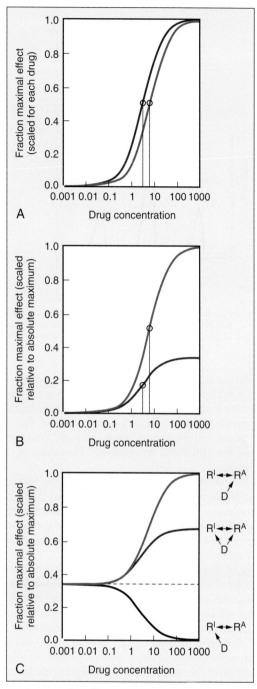

Figure 1-6 Concentration-effect curves illustrating the concepts of EC$_{50}$, agonist, partial agonist, and inverse agonist. **A,** Concentration-effect curves of two drugs. The effect is scaled to the maximal response obtained for each drug. EC$_{50}$ is 3 and 6 for red and blue drug, respectively. **B,** The same data as **A,** but response is scaled to the absolute maximal possible physiologic response. **C,** Concentration-response curve for full agonist *(blue),* partial agonist *(red),* and inverse agonist *(black)* for a receptor with nonnegligible intrinsic activity. Affinity of the drug (D) for the active (R^A) and inactive (R^I) receptor conformations is indicated by the *single arrows.*

In Figure 1-6, *C,* the implicit assumption that curves start at zero effect, which implies that in the absence of drug there is no effect, is relaxed. The plot in Figure 1-6, *C,* shows the behavior of a system exhibiting intrinsic receptor activity, even in the absence of drug. This occurs in systems where

even in the absence of drug a significant number of receptors exist in their active conformations. The blue curve shows a full agonist and the red curve shows a partial agonist. When the black drug is added, it appears that the intrinsic activity of the receptor is diminished. This can occur if the drug has a higher affinity for the inactive conformation of the receptor. This drug-receptor interaction is called *inverse agonism;* an inverse agonist is a drug that has a *negative efficacy.* If the inverse agonist was added after adding the full agonist, the overall effect would be diminished, suggesting that the inverse agonist is an antagonist (see later). In fact, the distinction between an antagonist and an inverse agonist can be subtle and is often evident only in genetically modified systems that express constitutively active receptors. For instance, the commonly used "β-blockers" such as propranolol are in fact inverse agonists at β-adrenergic receptors.[20]

Antagonism

The overall effect of a drug depends on both affinity and efficacy. All agonists have some nonzero value of efficacy and therefore produce an observable biologic effect. Conversely, drugs that have some affinity for the receptor but no efficacy are defined as *antagonists.* Because antagonists do not produce an effect on their own, their actions can only be observed in the context of modification of the effects of an agonist.

The simplest way to conceptualize actions of an antagonist is to consider competition between an agonist and antagonist for binding to the same receptor. When the antagonist binds, no effect is elicited; when the agonist binds, it elicits an effect dictated by its efficacy. At a given concentration of antagonist, the effect elicited by the agonist will be diminished, but if the relative concentration of the agonist is increased the same maximum effect will be eventually attained. Therefore the net effect of *competitive antagonism* is a shift in the agonist concentration-effect curve to the right (Figure 1-7).

This can be expressed mathematically by modifying the previously derived equation for the fraction of receptors bound by agonist as follows:

$$f = \frac{[A]}{[A] + K_{D(A)}\left(1 + \frac{[B]}{K_{D(B)}}\right)} \quad [13]$$

where A is the agonist, $K_{D(A)}$ is its dissociation constant, B is the antagonist and $K_{D(B)}$ is its dissociation constant.[21] The EC_{50} of the agonist can now be expressed as a function of the antagonist concentration and its dissociation constant.

$$EC_{50} = EC_{50}^0\left(1 + \frac{[B]}{K_{D(B)}}\right) \quad [14]$$

If the antagonist concentration is zero then the expression reduces to the EC_{50} of the drug in the absence of antagonist (EC_{50}^0 in Equation 14). The expression $\left(1 + \frac{[B]}{K_{D(B)}}\right)$, known as the *dose ratio,* indicates the fold increase of the agonist needed to achieve the same response at a given concentration of antagonist. The effect of the dissociation constant of a competitive antagonist on the shift in EC$_{50}$ is shown in Figure 1-7, *B.* The shift in EC$_{50}$ is proportional to antagonist

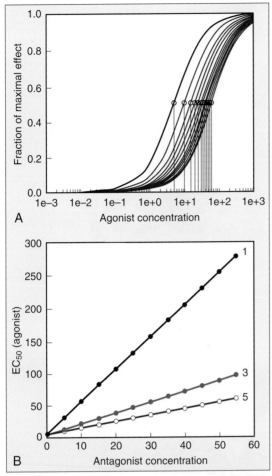

Figure 1-7 Competitive antagonism effect on the EC_{50}. **A,** Effects of increasing concentrations of a competitive antagonist on the concentration-response of a drug. *Black curve* shows curve in the absence of antagonist. EC_{50} for each curve is shown as a circle. **B,** Shift in EC_{50} plotted as a function of antagonist concentration derived using the $K_{D(B)}$ values shown. This plot allows calculation of the dissociation constant of the antagonist from the slope (see text).

concentration, and the proportionality constant (slope) is related to $1/K_{D(B)}$ (the affinity of antagonist for the receptor). The higher the affinity of the antagonist, the less antagonist it takes to shift the concentration-response curve of the agonist.

Another important class of antagonists is *noncompetitive antagonists*. The molecular mechanisms of noncompetitive antagonists are diverse. In the simplest case, irreversible binding of an antagonist takes the receptor out of the available pool to which agonists can bind. If the fraction of these unavailable receptors becomes sufficiently large, the maximal effect of agonist will be partially reduced, even at very high agonist concentrations. Thus a noncompetitive antagonist makes the concentration-effect curve for a full agonist resemble that of a partial agonist.

Allosteric Drug Interactions

The discussion of antagonists in the previous section rests on an idea that both agonist and antagonist compete for binding

to the same receptor site. The notion of what exactly a receptor is has been somewhat abstract, however. As mentioned earlier, most drug receptors are complex biologic macromolecules (example shown in Figure 1-8), and in order to discuss allosteric drug interactions—the subject of this section—a few details about receptor structure are clarified.

MULTIPLE BINDING SITES ON THE SAME RECEPTOR PROTEIN

Proteins constitute the largest class of receptor molecules. Although the amino acid sequence of proteins is encoded in the genetic code, the final three-dimensional structure of the protein is a result of complex interactions among the many amino acids that make up each subunit, interactions between subunits that make up the receptor, post-translational modifications, the cellular milieu, and so on. Only a small part of the resulting large and complex macromolecule is typically directly involved in binding the agonist. For instance, GABA binds the interface between the α and β subunits of the pentameric GABA$_A$ receptor.[22] The specific portion of a receptor molecule that is directly involved in binding drug is called a *binding site*. Identifying the actual binding site is no simple matter and usually requires a combination of experimental approaches. Indirect evidence for the identity of a binding site could be obtained through recombinant DNA techniques aimed at changing the identity of specific amino acids within the overall receptor-protein sequence by site-directed mutagenesis.[22] Direct evidence for the identity of a binding site can be obtained using x-ray crystallography, NMR spectroscopy, and chemical cross-linking, among other techniques.[23-26]

To determine the effect of changing the identity of a particular amino acid on drug binding, a reliable method for estimating drug binding is needed. Drug effect is not necessarily synonymous with drug binding (see earlier), so the concentration-effect curve cannot be directly used to infer the K_D. When a drug binds its receptor, heat is either absorbed (endothermic reaction) or released (exothermic reaction). These changes in heat can be recorded in solution maintained at constant temperature as a function of increasing drug concentration using a technique called *isothermal titration calorimetry* (ITC). In addition to measuring the binding constant, ITC experiments can also yield measurements of changes in entropy, enthalpy, and Gibbs free energy associated with drug binding, and thus provide a complete thermodynamic profile of the binding reaction that can then be used as a guide for molecular dynamic simulations.[27]

The binding site itself typically consists of a very small fraction of the total amino acid sequence of the protein. Yet binding of drug to the binding site induces a set of complex conformational changes in the overall receptor protein. For instance, binding of GABA to its binding site leads to opening a pore, which allows flux of Cl^- ions across the plasma membrane (see Figure 1-2), a process called *gating*.[28]

Competitive antagonists tend to bind to the same binding site as the agonist (GABA in this case); competition for occupancy of the binding site is sufficient to account for the effects of the antagonist. However, other drugs that bind to the same receptor might do so at a site distinct from that occupied by the agonist. The interaction between drugs binding the same molecule at different sites is referred to as *allosteric* ("other site"). For instance, the noncompetitive GABA$_A$ receptor antagonist picrotoxin most likely binds the receptor within the ion pore.[29]

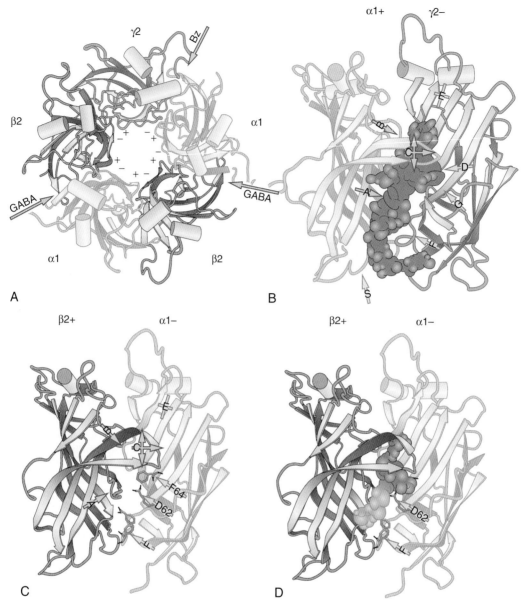

Figure 1-8 Model of the extracellular domains of a pentameric GABA$_A$ receptor. The subtype illustrated consists of two α, two β, and one γ2 subunit. **A,** View from the extracellular space. GABA binds to the interface between the α and β subunits, benzodiazepines bind to the interface between the α and γ2 subunit. **B,** Predicted benzodiazepine-binding pocket between the α and γ2 subunit viewed from the side. The binding site loops are labeled *A* to *G*. **(C)** and **(D)** The α and β subunit viewed from the side. The volume shown in *green* might be occupied in antagonist-bound states. *(Reproduced from Goetz T, Arslan A, Wisden W, Wulff P. GABA(A) receptors: structure and function in the basal ganglia. Progr Brain Res. 2007;160:21-41.)*

ALLOSTERIC BINDING SITES

GABA$_A$ receptors contain a number of distinct binding sites, including those for benzodiazepines, volatile and intravenous anesthetics, and ethanol.[29] Binding of drugs to these allosteric sites can affect GABA affinity, efficacy, and number of spontaneously open ion channels, for example. These kinds of interactions cannot be adequately described as simple agonists and antagonists.

The classic model of allosteric drug interactions was proposed by Ehlert[30] (Figure 1-9). The allosteric nature of drug interactions allows for many more transformations of the concentration-effect curves elicited by two or more drugs binding the same receptor. To quantify the nature of allosteric interactions, a technique called *response surface modeling* is typically applied. A response surface is a generalization of the concentration-effect curve to more than two dimensions. Experimentally this corresponds to determining the effect of different combinations of two or more drugs acting at the same receptor protein (Figure 1-10). This concept will be applied to drug interactions in Chapter 5.

PHARMACOGENETICS

Because most receptors are proteins whose amino acid sequence is encoded in the DNA, the binding sites can vary significantly between individuals. *Pharmacogenetics* refers to the study of how this genetic variability between individuals

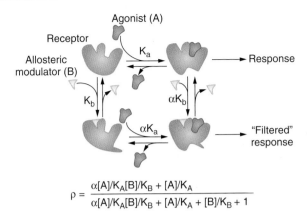

$$\rho = \frac{\alpha[A]/K_A[B]/K_B + [A]/K_A}{\alpha[A]/K_A[B]/K_B + [A]/K_A + [B]/K_B + 1}$$

Figure 1-9 Illustration of allosteric drug-receptor interactions. Agonist *(green)* can bind the receptor *(purple)* with affinity K_a, which leads to a response dictated by the efficacy of the agonist. Alternatively, the receptor can bind an allosteric modulator *(yellow)* with affinity K_b. The receptor-modulator complex can then bind the agonist but not necessarily with the same affinity (thus K_a in this case is multiplied by some modulator-specific constant α). The resulting receptor-agonist-modulator complex can have a different efficacy (expressed as filtered response). This complex can then decay by either dissociation of the agonist or the modulator. The overall fraction of receptor bound by the agonist *p* can be expressed in an equation shown at the bottom. *(Reproduced from Kenakin T. Allosteric modulators: the new generation of receptor antagonist.* Mol Interv. *2004;4:222-229.)*

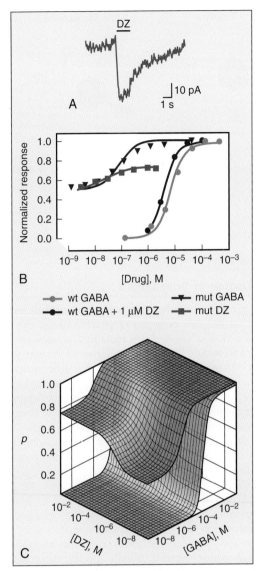

Figure 1-10 Allosteric interaction of GABA and diazepam. **A,** Response of *spontaneously active mutant* GABA$_A$ receptors to 1 μM diazepam (DZ). **B,** Concentration-response dependence of activation of wild-type and mutant receptors by GABA and DZ. **C,** Concentration-response surfaces for GABA and DZ acting at wild-type or α1L263S mutant GABA$_A$ receptors. *(Reproduced from Downing SS, Lee YT, Farb DH, Gibbs TT. Benzodiazepine modulation of partial agonist efficacy and spontaneously active GABA(A) receptors supports an allosteric model of modulation.* Br J Pharmacol. *2005;145:894-906.)*

contributes to differences in drug effects (see Chapter 4). The effect of genetic variability on the pharmacology GABA$_A$ receptor is illustrated in Figure 1-10. Because GABA and diazepam (a benzodiazepine) bind different sites on the GABA$_A$ receptor, it is possible to generate mutant receptor molecules that have different responses to one drug (diazepam), while the responses to the other drug (GABA) are preserved. In the wild-type receptor, diazepam acts as positive modulator of GABA, causing a left shift in the GABA concentration-effect curve. Yet after mutating a single amino acid, diazepam acts as a partial agonist.

The dependence of drug effects on the genotype has profound clinical implications. For instance, specific GABA$_A$ receptor α subunit polymorphisms can predict responses to alcohol such as susceptibility to delirium tremens and withdrawal symptoms; these polymorphisms might even predict a propensity for the development of alcohol addiction.[31] Other examples of genetic factors that contribute to drug responses include genetic variability in enzymes that influence pharmacokinetics (see Chapter 4).[32]

DRUG DISCOVERY

Historically, medicines have been derived from plant extracts used without rigorous testing or validation. Most of these medicines were not single compounds but complex mixtures of compounds, only some of which had the desired physiologic actions. Opium, one of the oldest medicines, is a mixture of a number of alkaloids including morphine which constitutes only ~12% of the total formulation. In the 19th century, major advances in chemistry allowed fractionation of crude plant extracts and isolation of individual compounds, which were then tested to determine which components of the extract were pharmacologically active and had desirable

effects. This development was coupled with the purification and determination of the structure of naturally occurring hormones such as norepinephrine.

Structure-Activity Relationship

In the early to mid-20th century, many new drugs were synthesized as modifications of physiologically active plant and animal-derived compounds yielding new drugs with desirable characteristics. The similarity between the structure of tyramine and epinephrine, for instance (Figure 1-11), suggested the synthesis of many amine compounds that possessed sympathomimetic properties when tested in isolated organ systems such as trachea and heart. One fundamental insight coming from this early work was that even small modifications in the

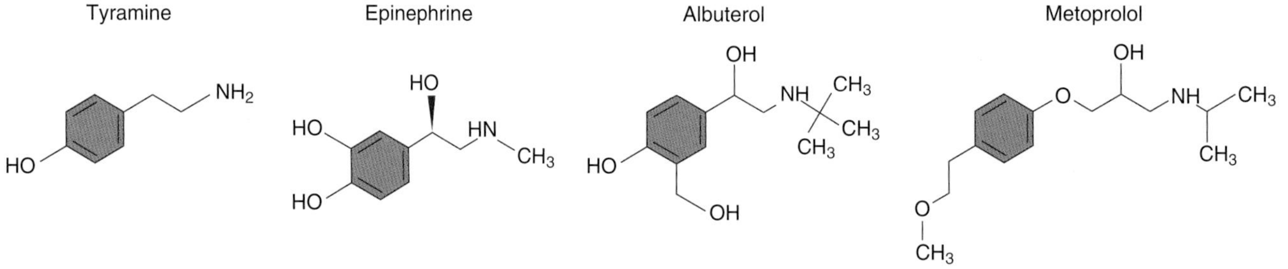

Tyramine   Epinephrine   Albuterol   Metoprolol

Figure 1-11 Similar chemical structures of agonists and antagonists acting on adrenergic receptors. Note the similarity of β agonists such as epinephrine and albuterol with relatively minor modifications needed to generate a β antagonist such as metoprolol.

chemical structure led to the profound changes in physiologic actions.

Identification of Drug Targets

Although many physiologically active compounds were synthesized during this early era of pharmacology, the mechanisms of action of these drugs remained mysterious as their receptors were not known. A fundamental insight was provided by Ahlquist[11] who hypothesized that differences in drug effects might not only be due to differences in drug chemical structure but also to differences in the receptors expressed in different tissues. This led to the development of drugs acting in a tissue-specific manner by Black and colleagues.[33] They used a drug previously known as a bronchoconstrictor to develop the first novel, receptor-selective compounds, the β-blockers.[33]

PURIFICATION OF RECEPTORS

Advances in molecular biology have allowed rapid progress in the identification and molecular characterization of specific receptors for drugs. In the 1980s, receptors were identified using high affinity ligands, usually specific antagonists, that were used as bait in affinity chromatography to isolate the low abundance receptor protein from detergent-solubilized tissue extracts.[34,35] Amino acid sequences of these purified receptors could then be determined, which allowed structural and functional analysis, as well as homology searching.

The advent of molecular cloning of cDNA complementary to cellular messenger RNA (mRNA) species allowed rapid identification of homologous receptors without tedious receptor purification techniques. In the past 20 years, the proteins encoding the receptors for many therapeutic drugs have been identified and most have been expressed at high levels (overexpressed) in other cell types (heterologous expression) to allow more detailed pharmacologic studies of receptors in isolation from other potentially confounding receptors and signaling molecules. It is now possible to express genes coding for a specific receptor protein in cell culture and simultaneously screen many different compounds for their ability to activate or inhibit the receptor using a variety of optical and other high throughput drug screening methods.[36]

DRUG TARGETS

Most drugs act by facilitating or blocking endogenous signaling molecules involved in intercellular and intracellular signaling, most commonly neurotransmitters or hormones.

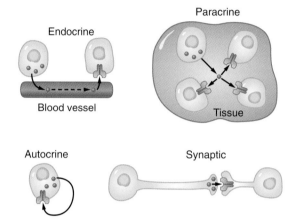

Figure 1-12 Schematic illustration of endocrine, paracrine, autocrine, and synaptic signaling.

Most of these extracellular signaling molecules (ligands) are synthesized and released by one cell to affect another by interacting with a cognate receptor (e.g., endocrine signaling, synaptic transmission), although local effects on adjacent cells (paracrine) or the same cells (autocrine) are also common (Figure 1-12).

Binding sites for hydrophilic extracellular signals typically exist as grooves or pockets on the surface of the extracellular protein domains. Lipophilic compounds (e.g., steroids, retinoids, and thyroxine), in contrast, can traverse membranes to interact with binding sites within the hydrophobic core or intracellular domains of the receptor. Nitric oxide (NO), hydrogen sulfide (HS), and carbon monoxide (CO) are gaseous signaling molecules (gasotransmitters) that can also diffuse across membranes to affect intracellular targets.[37-39] Most transmembrane receptors consist of multiple membrane-spanning segments made up of amphipathic helices that fold to form a complex three-dimensional structure, usually consisting of multiple subunits. In the case of ion channels, these membrane-spanning domains create a gate for ion permeation that is regulated by voltage or ligand binding. In the case of other receptors, the intracellular domain contains protein signaling domains that either directly or indirectly affect signaling pathways. Receptor structures are highly dynamic and can exist in multiple conformations that differ in their activities. Ligands and modulators regulate receptor function by selectively binding to specific conformers to alter these conformational equilibria.

Cell Signaling

Signal transduction refers to the process through which receptors act to mediate their physiologic actions (Figure 1-13). In many cases this process involves molecules that are themselves not involved in binding the original ligand, but act as molecular relays. These molecules are referred to as *second messengers.* Important second messengers include cyclic AMP, cyclic GMP, Ca^{2+}, and inositol phosphates. Changes in concentration and subcellular localization of these molecules are coupled to activity of regulatory enzymes and effectors including ion channels, cyclases, protein kinases, protein phosphatases, and phosphodiesterases. Many second messengers either directly or indirectly regulate protein kinases, which reversibly phosphorylate hydroxylated amino acid residues on key effector molecules in the cell, including receptors, to alter their function and localization.

The interactions between different second messengers form complex molecular signaling networks that allow greater flexibility in how ligand binding affects cellular function and for the coordination between different signals. *Signal amplification* occurs as a result of sequential activation of catalytically active enzymes, each of which can activate multiple downstream targets. *Specificity* is imparted by the receptor itself and its cell- and tissue-specific expression. *Signal integration* occurs as the downstream signaling pathways of different signals interact at multiple levels both positively and negatively (crosstalk).[40] Signals can be graded (i.e., analog) or discrete and bistable.[41] *Feedback*, both positive and negative, can occur when downstream components interact with upstream components of the signaling cascade.[42,43] Many signaling pathways are compartmentalized by protein interaction domains on scaffolding proteins that bring together multiple components of the pathway including receptors and their target effectors to increase their local concentrations.[44] These mechanisms of cell signaling and signal transduction are critical for intercellular communication in multicellular organisms, and provide multiple sites susceptible to modulation by exogenous compounds including drugs and toxins.

The most common types of drug target proteins involved in signal transduction are G protein-coupled receptors (GPCRs), ligand-gated ion channels (ionotropic receptors), which are major targets of general anesthetics, and voltage-gated ion channels, the major targets of local anesthetics and certain antihypertensive drugs.[16,45-47] There are also a number of enzyme-linked cell surface receptors, a heterogenous group of receptors usually coupled to intracellular protein kinase or phosphatase activity. These proteins fall into different classes based on their amino acid sequences and biologic activities. The activation of many receptors leads to transient changes in intracellular second messengers.

GPCRs constitute the largest family of cell surface receptor proteins, and indeed comprise the largest family of membrane proteins in the human genome. They mediate the cellular responses to a diverse array of extracellular signals including hormones and neurotransmitters. GPCRs contain seven transmembrane α helices, and bind their ligands in the extracellular space, as demonstrated by the recent three-dimensional structure determined for several members of this class.[48-51] On the cytoplasmic surface, GPCRs transduce their signals into cells by coupling to intracellular heterotrimeric G proteins that are made up of three subunits (α, β, and γ). Although there are many GPCRs, the number of G proteins is much smaller (21 Gα subunits encoded by 16 genes, 6 Gβ subunits encoded by 5 genes, and 12 Gγ subunits in humans). In the inactive form, G proteins bind GDP. When ligand binds the receptor, GDP is exchanged for GTP, which causes dissociation of the G protein into the α subunit and the $\beta\gamma$ dimer, each of which interacts with specific effectors.[52] This process is terminated once GTP is hydrolyzed to GDP (Figure 1-13) and the G protein subunits reassociate. Some G proteins activate their effectors while others inhibit them. Many endogenous signaling molecules exert their effects through multiple subtypes of GPCRs with distinct downstream targets and/or cellular expression. Examples include multiple receptor subtypes for epinephrine, dopamine, serotonin, and endogenous opioids.[25] Natural ligands for a large fraction of the many GPCRs present in the human genome have yet to be identified (orphan receptors) and represent potential future drug targets.[45]

While the structure of the GPCR determines its ligand recognition, the overall effect is determined by which G protein associates with the receptor and which effectors are coexpressed in the same cell. Some of the well-known effectors of GPCRs are adenylyl cyclases, phospholipases, and various ion channels (Table 1-1). These effector proteins control the concentration of second messenger molecules such as cAMP and phosphatidylinositol bisphosphate (PIP_2) in the case of adenylyl cyclase and phospholipase, respectively. Thus GPCRs are capable of eliciting a diverse range of responses depending on the cellular context in which they are expressed. This feature of G proteins makes them attractive targets for drug development. Furthermore, the effector proteins such as adenylyl cyclases and phosphodiesterases (enzymes that degrade cAMP and cGMP) have themselves been targeted for drug discovery.[53]

Ligand-gated ion channels are involved primarily in fast synaptic transmission between cells (e.g., the nicotinic

Table 1-1. Diversity of G Protein-Coupled Receptor Signal Transduction Pathways

G PROTEIN α SUBUNIT*	REPRESENTATIVE RECEPTORS	EFFECTORS	EFFECT
Gα_s	β_1, β_2, β_3—adrenergic, D_1, D_5-dopamine	Adenylyl cyclase, Ca^{2+} channels	Increased cAMP, increased Ca^{2+} influx
Gα_i	α_2-adrenergic; D_2-dopamine; M_2, M_4 muscarinic; μ, δ, κ opioid	Adenylyl cyclase, phospholipase A_2, K^+ channels	Decreased cAMP, eicosanoid release, hyperpolarization
Gα_t	Rhodopsin	cGMP phosphodiesterase	Decreased cGMP (vision)
Gα_q	M_1, M_3 muscarinic; α_1-adrenergic	Phospholipase Cβ	Increased IP_3, DG, Ca^{2+}
G$\alpha_{12/13}$	Angiotensin II (AT_1), endothelin (ET_A), thromboxane A_2 (TP), and thrombin ($PAR_{1,4}$)	Rho guanine nucleotide exchange factor, others	Rho A activation

*G protein α subunits are encoded by 16 genes classified into four families: Gα_s, Gα_i (Gα_i, Gα_o, Gα_t), Gα_q, and G$\alpha_{12/13}$. See reference 60 for review.

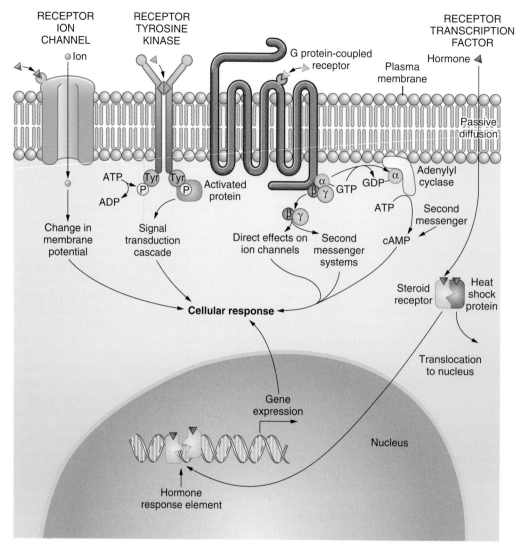

Figure 1-13 Major modes of signal transduction and intracellular signaling. Binding of an agonist to a receptor ion channel (e.g., GABA$_A$ receptor or nicotinic acetylcholine receptor) leads to opening of a transmembrane pore that permits movement of ions across the plasma membrane. This leads to a change in membrane potential that results in the physiologic response (e.g., change in the firing characteristics of a neuron or muscle contraction). Binding of a ligand to a receptor tyrosine kinase results in receptor dimerization and phosphorylation of the intracellular kinase domain. The activated (phosphorylated) kinase domain is then specifically recognized by proteins such as Src and phospholipase C that in turn activate a network of downstream effectors. These signal transduction pathways ultimately lead to changes in physiologic functioning of the cell such as glucose utilization and cell growth. Binding of a ligand to a seven-transmembrane domain G protein-coupled receptor (GPCR) results in the dissociation of the G protein into the membrane α subunit and the soluble βγ dimer. The α subunit then interacts with downstream effectors such as adenylyl cyclase, which converts ATP into cAMP (a second messenger) that then modifies a number of effector proteins. The βγ dimer can also exert direct cellular effects by modulating activity of a number of ion channels, for example. Effects of steroid hormones are mediated by intracellular receptors, which upon binding their ligand dissociate from a heat shock protein and translocate into the nucleus where they serve to modify gene expression by binding to hormone response elements in the promoter regions.

acetylcholine receptor in neuromuscular transmission). GABA$_A$ receptors are ligand-gated Cl$^-$ channels that open in response to binding their principal agonist, γ-aminobutyric acid (GABA) (see Figure 1-2), the major fast inhibitory neurotransmitter in the central nervous system. GABA$_A$ receptors belong to the cys-loop superfamily of ligand-gated ion channels that contains many other neurotransmitter receptors that all share certain structural motifs. Many of the members of this superfamily (Figure 1-14) have been successfully targeted for drug development.

Another large group of drug targets are voltage-gated ion channels (Figure 1-15). Like ligand-gated ion channels, these proteins also form pores that allow permeation of ions across the plasma membrane. However, rather than opening in

response to ligand binding, pores within these proteins open when transmembrane electrical potential reaches a certain value. The voltage and time dependence of pore opening as well as ion selectivity differs widely between these proteins.[54] Many clinically useful drugs such as local anesthetics and several antiarrhythmic drugs target voltage-gated sodium (Na$^+$) channels.

Another prominent family of proteins that has been successfully targeted for drug discovery includes receptor proteins with enzymatic activity. These receptors typically contain a ligand-binding domain, a single transmembrane domain, and the catalytic domain. Of these, the most prominent are the receptor tyrosine kinases, important targets for novel anticancer drugs. Binding of ligand in the extracellular space

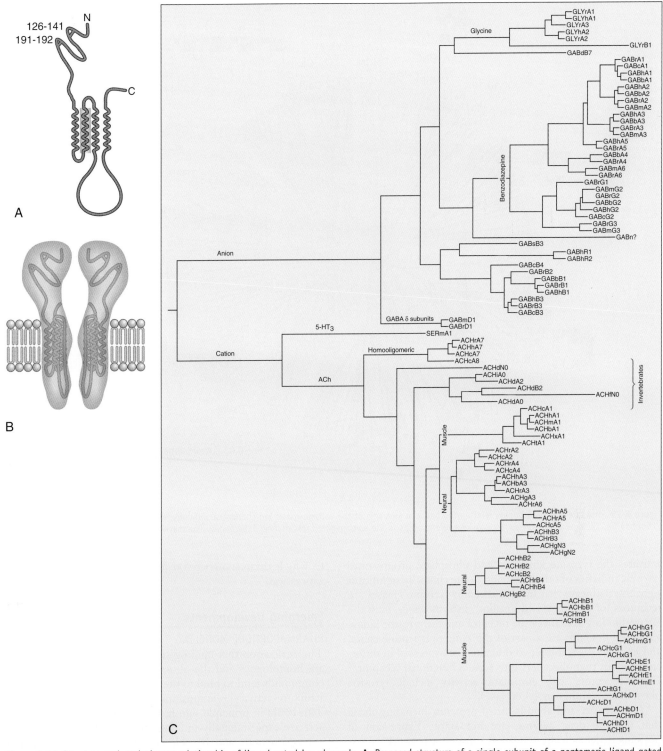

Figure 1-14 Structure and evolutionary relationship of ligand-gated ion channels. **A,** Proposed structure of a single subunit of a pentameric ligand-gated ion channel. **B,** Structure of the whole pentamer viewed from the side (in plane). **C,** Evolutionary relationship between different members of the superfamily based on sequence homology. *(Reproduced from Ortells MO, Lunt GG. Evolutionary history of the ligand-gated ion-channel superfamily of receptors. Trends Neurosci. 1995;18:121-127.)*

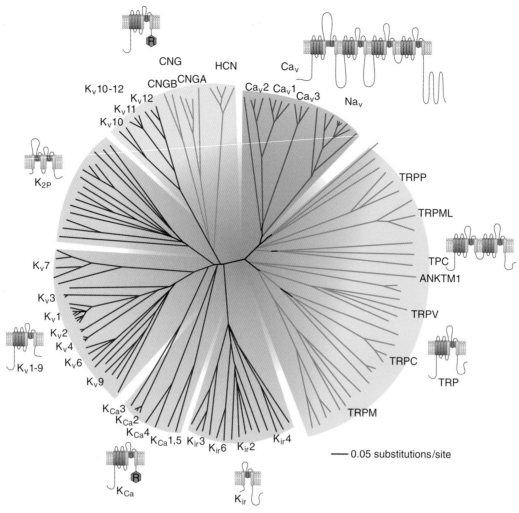

Figure 1-15 Structure and evolutionary relationship between members of the voltage-gated ion channel superfamily. *(Reproduced from Yu FH, Yarov-Yarovoy V, Gutman GA, Catterall WA. Overview of molecular relationships in the voltage-gated ion channel superfamily. Pharmacol Rev. 2005;57:387-395.)*

activates the tyrosine kinase to add phosphate groups onto tyrosine moieties of other proteins. Some clinically significant signaling pathways that involve receptor tyrosine kinases are receptors for cytokines and insulin.[55] In some cases, both the ligand-binding domain of the receptor and the tyrosine kinase structural domains are a part of the same polypeptide chain, and in other cases these two domains are expressed in different proteins that oligomerize to form a functional receptor.[56] Other receptors with enzymatic activity include tyrosine phosphatases and guanylyl cyclases.[57]

The identity and abundance of proteins, including those that mediate drug actions, are not static. Expression of proteins is dynamically regulated through a network of signaling cascades depending on cell type, developmental stage, and environmental demands, for example. These regulatory cascades converge on proteins, known as *transcription factors*, that control transcription of mRNA. Thus, transcription factors play an incredibly important role in controlling the function of the cell and present attractive targets for drug discovery. Various steroid compounds that modulate the endocrine system act on transcription factors to alter gene expression (Figure 1-13). Transcription factors consist of homologous domains that control the specificity of ligand binding and regulatory motifs that determine DNA sequences

to which these transcription factors bind to modulate gene expression.

Emerging Developments

PHARMACOPHORE MODELING
The realization that binding sites of many different proteins are homologous and the observation that chemically similar compounds tend to bind to the same binding site suggest that structure-activity relationships (SARs) can be formalized. This could in principle significantly reduce the need to characterize experimentally binding and efficacy of many different compounds and be able to predict which compounds should have the desirable binding characteristics. In practice, however, it is extremely difficult to develop because at the subatomic level, details of all the different forces that govern noncovalent interactions are extremely complex and analytic solutions exist for only the simplest molecules. Currently each potential drug-receptor pair must be numerically simulated, which is computationally expensive and impractical on a large number of drug candidates.

An exciting development in modern drug design—pharmacophore modeling—provides a way to describe qualitatively drug-receptor interactions to provide an albeit

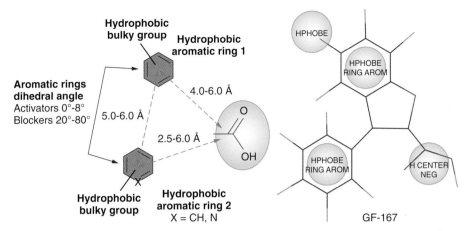

Figure 1-16 Representation of the pharmacophore model illustrating the essential requirements for drug action. For comparison, the stick model and the chemical function descriptors of the master compound GF-167 are shown. *(Reproduced from Liantonio A, Picollo A, Carbonara G, et al. Molecular switch for CLC-K Cl⁻ channel block/activation: optimal pharmacophoric requirements towards high-affinity ligands. Proc Natl Acad Sci USA. 2008;105:1369-1373.)*

imprecise guide for selecting promising drug candidates. Pharmacophore is defined as "an ensemble of steric and electronic features that is necessary to ensure the optimal supramolecular interactions with a specific biologic target and to trigger (or block) its biologic response."[58] Pharmacophore models combine a large number of observations of active and inactive compounds and attempt to extract statistically significant motifs that predict drug activity (Figure 1-16). Pharmacophore modeling has been successful in predicting binding characteristics of many candidate drugs.

PHENOTYPE-BASED DRUG DISCOVERY

Using methodologies like pharmacophore modeling and high-throughput screening, it is now possible to readily synthesize new compounds with high specificity for the desired receptor. This, however, does not guarantee therapeutic efficacy. It has become clear that many of the most prevalent diseases, such as depression and obesity, are mediated by complex changes occurring simultaneously in many biologic macromolecules. Furthermore, these changes are mediated through networks of molecular interactions involved in signal transduction in a cell type-specific manner. It is exceedingly unlikely therefore that specifically targeting a particular receptor, or second messenger system, will guide these molecular networks toward "normal" function. Thus paradoxically it is commonly found that some of the most clinically efficacious compounds are not necessarily the most specific on the molecular level. For instance, tricyclic antidepressants act on adrenergic, cholinergic, serotonergic, histaminergic, and dopaminergic systems. A promising complementary strategy is *phenotype-based* drug discovery. Rather than discovering compounds with the most desirable binding characteristics to a particular receptor, phenotype-based approaches screen compounds based on their ability to produce a desired phenotype in the whole animal. For instance, cholesterol lowering medication ezetimibe (Zetia) was identified based on its ability to lower serum cholesterol level in an animal model, although it was not a successful inhibitor of acyl-coenzyme A cholesterol acetyltransferase (the original target for the target-based drug discovery approach).[59]

KEY POINTS

- A drug must first bind a receptor and form a complex to initiate its physiologic effect. The propensity of the drug-receptor complex to form is described by a constant called *affinity*, whereas its propensity to break down is described by the *dissociation constant*.
- Most drug receptors are proteins in the plasma membrane that are involved in cell signaling, such as G protein-coupled receptors and ion channels.
- Drug binding is not equivalent to *drug effect*. The propensity of the drug-receptor complex to elicit *a physiologic* effect is governed by a characteristic constant called *efficacy*.
- Together, affinity and efficacy give rise to drug *potency*, typically measured as effective concentration for 50% of maximal effect (EC_{50}).
- Depending on their relative efficacies, drugs are characterized as *full, partial,* or *inverse agonists.* Drugs with receptor affinity but no efficacy are referred to as *antagonists.*
- Drugs often bind receptors at multiple distinct binding sites, which can influence receptor actions in complex ways. These interactions are called *allosteric.*
- *Signal transduction* is the process by which receptors transduce signals from extracellular messengers via *second messengers* to regular cellular functions.
- The ability of a drug to bind a particular binding site depends on interactions determined by the chemical structure of the drug and the structure of the binding site. The compatibility between a chemical compound and a binding site can be expressed in a *pharmacophore* model.

Key References

Bean BP, Cohen CJ, Tsien RW. Lidocaine block of cardiac sodium channels. *J Gen Physiol.* 1983;81:613-642. Characterization of the effect of lidocaine on cardiac Na⁺ channels, including use-dependent and use-independent blockade. Mechanisms responsible for antiarrhythmic properties of lidocaine are proposed. (Ref. 16)

Beneski DA, Catteral WA. Covalent labeling of protein components of the sodium channel with a photoactivable derivative of scorpion toxin. *Proc Natl Acad Sci U S A*. 1980;77:639-643. Purification of the sodium channel from neuroblastoma cells and synaptosomes by covalently labeling cells with a toxin. (Ref. 35)

Black JW, Duncan WA, Shanks RG. Comparison of some properties of pronethalol and propranolol. *Br J Pharmacol Chemother*. 1965;25:577-591. Synthesis of the first receptor-specific β-adrenergic antagonist—propranolol, the prototype β-blocker. (Ref. 33)

Cherezov V, Rosenbaum DM, Hanson MA, et al. High-resolution crystal structure of an engineered human beta2-adrenergic G protein-coupled receptor. *Science*. 2007;318:1258-1265. High-resolution crystal structure of human β₂-adrenergic receptor crystallized with a diffusable ligand. This study illustrates the properties of the ligand binding site in a G protein–coupled receptor of major clinical and scientific significance. (Ref. 48)

Gaddum JH, Hameed KA, Hathway DE, Stephens FF. Quantitative studies of antagonists for 5-hydroxytryptamine. *Q J Exp Physiol Cogn Med Sci*. 1955;40:49-74. Derivation of the relationship between antagonist concentration and concentration-effect curve for the agonist. (Ref. 21)

Logothetis DE, Kurachi Y, Galper J, Neer EJ, Clapham DE. The beta gamma subunits of GTP-binding proteins activate the muscarinic K⁺ channel in heart. *Nature* 1987;325:321-326. Direct experimental demonstration that the βγ-subunits of G proteins activate K⁺ channels in the heart as a result of activation of the muscarinic acetylcholine receptor. (Ref. 52)

Stephenson RP. Modification of receptor theory. *Br J Pharmacol Chemother*. 1956;11:379-393. Landmark study where Stephenson modified Clark's receptor theory to account for different efficacies of drugs acting at the same receptor. (Ref. 10)

References

1. Maehle AH. A binding question: the evolution of the receptor concept. *Endeavour*. 2009;33:135-140.
2. Maehle AH. Drugs on trial: experimental pharmacology and therapeutic innovation in the eighteenth century. *Rodopi*; 1999:223-309.
3. Bynum WF. Chemical structure and pharmacological action: a chapter in the history of 19th century molecular pharmacology. *Bull Hist Med*. 1970;44:518-538.
4. Parascandola J. The controversy over structure-activity relationships in the early twentieth century. *Pharm His*. 1974;16/2:54-63.
5. Kaufman RD. Biophysical mechanisms of anesthetic action: historical perspective and review of current concepts. *Anesthesiology*. 1977;46:49-62.
6. Silverstein AM. *Paul Ehrlich's Receptor Immunology: The Magnificent Obsession*. San Diego: Academic Press; 2002.
7. Langley JN. On the reaction of cells and of nerve endings to certain poisons, chiefly as regards the reaction of striated muscle to nicotine and to curari. *J Physiol-London*. 1905:33:374-413.
8. Clark AJ. *The Mode of Action of Drugs on Cells*. Edward Arnold; 1933.
9. Ariens EJ, De Groot WM. Affinity and intrinsic-activity in the theory of competitive inhibition. III. Homologous decamethonium-derivatives and succinyl-choline-esters. *Arch Int Pharmacodyn Ther*. 1954;99:193-205.
10. Stephenson RP. Modification of receptor theory. *Br J Pharmacol Chemother*. 1956;11:379-393.
11. Ahlquist RP. A study of the adrenotropic receptors. *Am J Physiol*. 1948;153:586-600.
12. Hamill OP, Marty A, Neher E, Sakmann B, Sigworth FJ. Improved patch-clamp techniques for high-resolution current recording from cells and cell-free membrane patches. *Pflugers Arch*. 1981;391:85-100.
13. Neelands TR, Fisher JL, Bianchi M, Macdonald RL. Spontaneous and gamma-aminobutyric acid (GABA)-activated GABA(A) receptor channels formed by epsilon subunit-containing isoforms. *Mol Pharmacol*. 1999;55:168-178.
14. Catterall WA. From ionic currents to molecular mechanisms: the structure and function of voltage-gated sodium channels. *Neuron*. 2000;26:13-25.
15. Tank DW, Huganir RL, Greengard P, Webb WW. Patch-recorded single-channel currents of the purified and reconstituted Torpedo acetylcholine receptor. *Proc Natl Acad Sci USA*. 1983;80:5129-5133.
16. Bean BP, Cohen CJ, Tsien RW. Lidocaine block of cardiac sodium channels. *J Gen Physiol*. 1983;81:613-642.
17. Mortensen M, Kristiansen U, Ebert B, et al. Activation of single heteromeric GABA(A) receptor ion channels by full and partial agonists. *J Physiol*. 2004;557:389-413.
18. Chen PE, Wyllie DJ. Pharmacological insights obtained from structure-function studies of ionotropic glutamate receptors. *Br J Pharmacol*. 2006;147:839-853.
19. Swaminath G, Deupi X, Lee TW, et al. Probing the beta2 adrenoceptor binding site with catechol reveals differences in binding and activation by agonists and partial agonists. *The Journal of biological chemistry*. 2005;280:22165-22171.
20. Chidiac P, Hebert TE, Valiquette M, Dennis M, Bouvier M. Inverse agonist activity of beta-adrenergic antagonists. *Mol Pharmacol*. 1994;45:490-499.
21. Gaddum JH, Hameed KA, Hathway DE, Stephens FF. Quantitative studies of antagonists for 5-hydroxytryptamine. *Q J Exp Physiol Cogn Med Sci*. 1955;40:49-74.
22. Boileau AJ, Evers AR, Davis AF, Czajkowski C. Mapping the agonist binding site of the GABAA receptor: evidence for a beta-strand. *J Neurosci*. 1999;19:4847-4854.
23. Pike AC, et al. Structure of the ligand-binding domain of oestrogen receptor beta in the presence of a partial agonist and a full antagonist. *EMBO J*. 1999;18:4608-4618.
24. Armstrong N, Sun Y, Chen GQ, Gouaux E. Structure of a glutamate-receptor ligand-binding core in complex with kainate. *Nature*. 1998;395:913-917.
25. Rosenbaum DM, Rasmussen SG, Kobilka BK. The structure and function of G-protein-coupled receptors. *Nature*. 2009;459:356-363.
26. Herzig MC, Leeb-Lundberg LM. The agonist binding site on the bovine bradykinin B2 receptor is adjacent to a sulfhydryl and is differentiated from the antagonist binding site by chemical cross-linking. *J Biol Chem*. 1995;270:20591-20598.
27. de Azevedo Jr WF, Dias R. Computational methods for calculation of ligand-binding affinity. *Curr Drug Targets*. 2008;9:1031-1039.
28. Kash TL, Jenkins A, Kelley JC, Trudell JR, Harrison NL. Coupling of agonist binding to channel gating in the GABA(A) receptor. *Nature*. 2003;421:272-275.
29. Korpi ER, Grunder G, Luddens H. Drug interactions at GABA(A) receptors. *Prog Neurobiol*. 2002;67:113-159.
30. Ehlert FJ. Estimation of the affinities of allosteric ligands using radioligand binding and pharmacological null methods. *Mol Pharmacol*. 1988;33:187-194.
31. Soyka M, Preuss UW, Hesselbrock W, et al. GABA-A2 receptor subunit gene (GABRA2) polymorphisms and risk for alcohol dependence. *J Psychiatr Res*. 2008;42:184-191.
32. Arranz MJ, de Leon, J. Pharmacogenetics and pharmacogenomics of schizophrenia: a review of last decade of research. *Mol Psychiatry*. 2007;12:707-747.
33. Black JW, Duncan WA, Shanks RG. Comparison of some properties of pronethalol and propranolol. *Br J Pharmacol Chemother*. 1965;25:577-591.
34. Agnew WS, Moore AC, Levinson SR, Raftery MA. Identification of a large molecular weight peptide associated with a tetrodotoxin binding protein from the electroplax of Electrophorus electricus. *Biochem Biophys Res Commun*. 1980;92:860-866.
35. Beneski DA, Catterall WA. Covalent labeling of protein components of the sodium channel with a photoactivable derivative of scorpion toxin. *Proc Natl Acad Sci USA*. 1980;77:639-643.
36. Sundberg SA. High-throughput and ultra-high-throughput screening: solution- and cell-based approaches. *Curr Opin Biotechnol*. 2000;11:47-53.
37. Garthwaite J, Charles SL, Chess-Williams R. Endothelium-derived relaxing factor release on activation of NMDA receptors suggests role as intercellular messenger in the brain. *Nature*. 1988;336:385-388.
38. Garthwaite J, Boulton CL. Nitric oxide signaling in the central nervous system. *Annu Rev Physiol*. 1995;57:683-706.

39. Ryter SW, Otterbein LE, Morse D, Choi AM. Heme oxygenase/carbon monoxide signaling pathways: regulation and functional significance. *Mol Cell Biochem*. 2002;234-235, 249-263.

40. Kaplan DR, Miller FD. Neurotrophin signal transduction in the nervous system. *Curr Opin Neurobiol*. 2000;10:381-391.

41. Ferrell Jr JE. Self-perpetuating states in signal transduction: positive feedback, double-negative feedback and bistability. *Curr Opin Cell Biol*. 2002;14:140-148.

42. Xiong W, Ferrell Jr JE. A positive-feedback-based bistable 'memory module' that governs a cell fate decision. *Nature*. 2003;426:460-465.

43. Kohout TA, Lefkowitz RJ. Regulation of G protein-coupled receptor kinases and arrestins during receptor desensitization. *Mol Pharmacol*. 2003;63:9-18.

44. Whitmarsh AJ, Davis RJ. Structural organization of MAP-kinase signaling modules by scaffold proteins in yeast and mammals. *Trends Biochem Sci*. 1998;23:481-485.

45. Wise A, Gearing K, Rees S. Target validation of G-protein coupled receptors. *Drug Discov Today*. 2002;7:235-246.

46. Alkire MT, Hudetz AG, Tononi G. Consciousness and anesthesia. *Science*. 2008;322:876-880.

47. Braunwald E. Mechanism of action of calcium-channel-blocking agents. *N Engl J Med*. 1982;307:1618-1627.

48. Cherezov V, Rosenbaum DM, Hanson MA, et al. High-resolution crystal structure of an engineered human beta2-adrenergic G protein-coupled receptor. *Science*. 2007;318:1258-1265.

49. Warne T, Serrano-Vega MJ, Baker JG, et al. Structure of a beta1-adrenergic G-protein-coupled receptor. *Nature*. 2008;454:486-491.

50. Palczewski K, Takashi Kumasaka, Tetsuya Hori, et al. Crystal structure of rhodopsin: A G protein-coupled receptor. *Science*. 2000;289:739-745.

51. Kobilka B, Schertler GF. New G-protein-coupled receptor crystal structures: insights and limitations. *Trends Pharmacol Sci*. 2008;29:79-83.

52. Logothetis DE, Kurachi Y, Galper J, Neer EJ, Clapham DE. The beta gamma subunits of GTP-binding proteins activate the muscarinic K+ channel in heart. *Nature*. 1987;325:321-326.

53. Menniti FS, Faraci WS, Schmidt CJ. Phosphodiesterases in the CNS: targets for drug development. *Nat Rev Drug Discov*. 2006;5:660-670.

54. Hille B. *Ionic Channels of Excitable Membranes*. 2nd ed. Sunderland, Mass: Sinauer Associates Inc.; 1992.

55. Avruch J. Insulin signal transduction through protein kinase cascades. *Mol Cell Biochem*. 1998;182:31-48.

56. Hubbard SR, Till JH. Protein tyrosine kinase structure and function. *Annu Rev Biochem*. 2000;69:373-398.

57. Tonks NK, Neel BG. From form to function: signaling by protein tyrosine phosphatases. *Cell*. 1996;87:365-368.

58. Wermuth G, Ganellin CR, Lindberg P, Mitscher LA. Glossary of terms used in medicinal chemistry (IUPAC Recommendations 1998). *Pure Appl Chem*. 1998;70:1129-1143.

59. Clader JW. The discovery of ezetimibe: a view from outside the receptor. *J Med Chem*. 2004;47:1-9.

60. Liantonio A, Picollo A, Carbonara G, et al. Molecular switch for CLC-K Cl- channel block/activation: optimal pharmacophoric requirements towards high-affinity ligands. *Proc Natl Acad Sci U S A*. 2008;105:1369-1373.

Chapter 2

PHARMACOKINETIC AND PHARMACODYNAMIC PRINCIPLES FOR INTRAVENOUS ANESTHETICS

Shinju Obara and Talmage D. Egan

The science broadly referred to as clinical pharmacology is the foundation upon which anesthesiologists base their therapeutic decisions, including the rational selection of anesthetics and the formulation of safe and effective dosage regimens. Focusing exclusively on intravenous anesthetics, this chapter reviews the fundamental theory and practical application of clinical pharmacology in anesthesia, including pharmacokinetics, pharmacodynamics, the "biophase" concept, compartmental models, and pharmacologic simulation. Although clinical pharmacology is grounded in complex mathematics, the chapter avoids excessive reliance on equations by emphasizing a conceptual understanding of the quantitative ideas and highlights the intuitive understanding that comes from computer simulation of pharmacologic models. Understanding what a pharmacologic model is and how such a model is built and applied is therefore an important focus of the chapter.

The ultimate goal of the chapter is to provide the clinician with a solid understanding of the fundamental concepts of clinical pharmacology, thereby enabling practical clinical application of these concepts, primarily through the use of pharmacologic simulation. From a pharmacology perspective, there is perhaps nothing more relevant to day-to-day decision making in anesthesiology than the theories explained here. These concepts are the scientific foundation to answer a very important clinical question: "What are the right drug and the optimal dose for my patient?"

HISTORICAL PERSPECTIVE

From the earliest days of modern anesthesia, anesthesiologists sought to understand the dose-response relationship. Using dose escalation study methods, clinician-scientists quantified the magnitude and duration of anesthetic effect over a spectrum of doses, thereby identifying a dosage range that would produce anesthesia without excessive toxicity. For many decades, modern anesthesia practice relied upon such dose-response studies as the basis for rational drug administration schemes.

With advances in analytic chemistry and the widespread availability of computing technology, new approaches to understanding drug behavior emerged. By measuring blood anesthetic concentrations over time using techniques such as radioimmunoassay or gas chromatography, it became possible to characterize the relationship between drug dose and the time course of drug levels in the bloodstream, a field of study called *pharmacokinetics* (often abbreviated as PKs*). A natural extension of this new discipline of pharmacokinetics was the characterization of the relationship between the concentration of the drug and the magnitude of effect, a branch of pharmacology called *pharmacodynamics* (abbreviated as PDs†). Coherent linkage of these two pharmacologic disciplines, pharmacokinetics and pharmacodynamics, necessitated creation of the "biophase" concept wherein plasma drug concentrations from PK studies are translated into apparent "effect-site" concentrations, which are then related to drug effects measured in PD studies.

The underlying theory of pharmacokinetics was largely developed in therapeutic areas unrelated to anesthesiology.[1-3] However, because the clinical pharmacology of anesthesia is so unique (e.g., the necessity to predict onset and offset of drug effect very accurately), some PK concepts have been developed by anesthesia investigators for specific application in anesthesia.[4-8] Moreover, because of the ease with which profound anesthetic effects can be noninvasively measured in real time (e.g., the twitch monitor for neuromuscular blockers, the electroencephalogram for hypnotics), many important theoretic advances in pharmacodynamics applicable to other fields of medicine have originated from the study of anesthetics. An especially notable example is the conception of the biophase or effect site concept.[9]

Compared to old fashioned dose-response methods, a major advantage of these more sophisticated PK-PD studies is that the analysis results in a quantitative model of drug behavior. Using nonlinear regression techniques, equations are fit to raw PK and PD data, yielding a set of PK-PD parameter estimates (i.e., distribution volumes, clearances, potencies) that constitute a quantitative model.[10] Unlike dose-response studies of the past, these quantitative PK-PD models can be applied to more diverse and clinically relevant circumstances through computer simulation.[11]

The application of modern PK-PD concepts into anesthesia practice has blossomed in unanticipated ways. Automated administration of intravenous anesthetics according to a PK model, a technology known as target-controlled infusion (TCI), is now commonplace.[12] The use of real-time PK-PD simulation to guide anesthetic administration, wherein a PK-PD prediction module is placed alongside a traditional physiologic monitor, is also an emerging technology with promising potential (see Chapter 5).[13]

UNIQUE ASPECTS OF ANESTHETIC PHARMACOLOGY

Anesthesiology versus Other Disciplines

The pharmacology of anesthesia is unique compared with other disciplines within medicine (Table 2-1). Perhaps the most obvious difference relates to the safety of anesthetic drugs. Many drugs within the anesthesia formulary produce profound physiologic alterations (e.g., unresponsiveness, paralysis, ventilatory and hemodynamic depression) and have

*When used as an adjective in this chapter, "pharmacokinetic" is abbreviated as "PK."
†When used as an adjective in this chapter, "pharmacodynamic" is abbreviated as "PD."

Table 2-1. Unique Aspects of Anesthesia Clinical Pharmacology Related to Safety and Efficiency

Safety Issues
Very low therapeutic index drugs
Severe consequences to "under" or "over" dosing
Necessity to adjust the level of drug effect frequently

Efficiency Issues
Necessity to produce onset of drug effect quickly
Necessity to produce offset of drug effect quickly

a very low therapeutic index. There are few therapeutic areas in medicine where two to three times the typical therapeutic dose is often associated with severe adverse or even lethal effects (see Chapter 6). It is perhaps for this reason more than any other that the specialty of anesthesiology evolved. The consequences of "under" or "over" dosing anesthetics can be catastrophic.

Another important difference between anesthesiology and other therapeutic areas relates to efficiency. Most settings in clinical medicine do not require immediate onset and rapid offset of pharmacologic effect. When an internist prescribes an antihypertensive, for example, the fact that a few days may be required for establishment of a therapeutic effect is of little consequence. Similarly, when terminating therapy, the necessity to wait a few days to achieve complete dissipation of drug effect is usually of no clinical importance.

Anesthesiologists, in contrast, must respond to the dynamic needs of patients under anesthesia where the optimal degree of central nervous system depression can vary widely and frequently, requiring continuous adjustment of drug concentrations. In addition, the anesthesiologist must respond to the practical realities of modern medical practice in terms of operating room efficiency and the outpatient revolution; the anesthesiologist must rapidly anesthetize the patient and then quickly reanimate the patient when the surgeons have finished their work, enabling the patient to transition quickly through the recovery process in preparation for going home.

Thus the profound physiologic alterations of the anesthetized state (and their reversal) must be produced on demand in order to ensure the rapid achievement and maintenance of the anesthetic state intraoperatively with return of responsiveness, spontaneous ventilation, and other vital functions at the appropriate time. To achieve this degree of pharmacologic control, anesthesiologists in the modern era increasingly rely on the application of advanced PK-PD concepts and technology to formulate and implement rational dosing schemes.[14,15] In addition, anesthesiologists take advantage of drugs that were specifically developed to address the unique concerns of anesthesia pharmacology (i.e., drugs with rapid onset and predictable offset of effect).[4]

A Surfing Analogy as a Simple Conceptual Framework

A surfing analogy is helpful in simply conceptualizing how PK-PD principles can be applied to the problem of rational drug administration in anesthesia.[16] The anesthesiologist typically targets the upper portion of the steep part of the concentration-effect relationship; that is, the concentration that produces considerable drug effect but from which drug effect will recover quickly once drug administration is

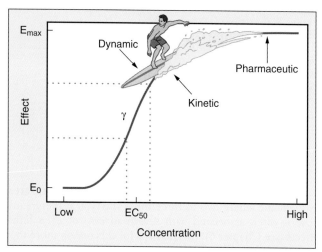

Figure 2-1 A surfing analogy as a graphical explanation of how anesthesiologists use a combination of three approaches (i.e., PK, PD, and pharmaceutic) to administer anesthetics to maintain the anesthetic effect while making rapid recovery possible. See the accompanying text for a detailed explanation. E_0, effect at zero drug concentration; E_{max}, maximal drug effect; EC_{50}, concentration that produces 50% of maximal drug effect; γ, steepness of the curve. *(Reprinted with permission from Egan TD, Shafer SL. Target-controlled infusions for intravenous anesthetics: surfing USA not! Anesthesiology. 2003;99:1039-1041.)*

terminated. This can be visualized as a surfer riding near the crest of a wave as in Figure 2-1. Targeting ("surfing") the steep portion of the concentration-effect relationship makes it possible to achieve large reductions in effect with relatively small decreases in concentration.

In clinical pharmacology terms, there are essentially three approaches to targeting this area of the concentration-effect relationship. Perhaps the most straightforward among them is the PD approach, wherein a drug effect measure is employed as a feedback signal to guide drug administration regardless of the drug concentration achieved. Propofol titrated to a specific processed electroencephalogram (EEG) target or a neuromuscular blocker administered to maintain a specific degree of twitch depression as measured by a peripheral nerve stimulator are examples of this PD approach.

Another common approach in targeting the steep portion of the concentration-effect relationship is the PK approach. Drawing upon knowledge about the concentration-effect relationship (i.e., therapeutic windows), the PK approach targets drug concentrations that are typically appropriate for a given anesthetic application. The use of an agent-specific vaporizer to deliver some fraction or multiple of an inhaled agent's minimum alveolar concentration (MAC), and the use of a TCI device to infuse propofol to a specified concentration (e.g., Diprifusor) are sophisticated examples of this approach. Of course even in situations where an advanced delivery technology is not employed, standard dosage regimens for drugs in anesthesia are devised to achieve concentrations that are within the therapeutic window based on the drug's pharmacokinetics.

A third approach to targeting the steep portion of the concentration-effect relationship can be referred to as the "forgiving drug" or "pharmaceutic" approach. The pharmaceutic approach takes advantage of the responsive pharmacokinetic profiles of modern anesthetic agents. With this approach, within the constraints of acceptable adverse effects

such as hemodynamic depression, it is unnecessary to hit the target with as much precision and accuracy as with the other approaches. Because short acting agent concentrations can be manipulated up or down rapidly, adjustments can be made quickly as suggested by PD feedback. If the empirical dosage scheme is obviously too high or too low, the anesthetist can achieve a more appropriate level of drug effect in short order. Short-acting agents essentially make it unnecessary to hit the target perfectly.

As a practical matter, of course, anesthetists combine all three approaches (i.e., the PD, PK, and pharmaceutic approaches). Pharmacokinetically responsive agents are administered by advanced, target controlled delivery devices according to PD feedback. Adjusting the propofol TCI target based on feedback from a processed EEG brain function monitor is an example of this combined approach to anesthesia drug delivery. The pharmacologic science underpinning this three-pronged approach to rational drug selection and administration for intravenous anesthesia is the focus of this chapter.

CLINICAL PHARMACOLOGY

Posology

Although defining exactly what comprises the field of "clinical pharmacology" is challenging, it consists of numerous branches including pharmacokinetics, pharmacodynamics, toxicology, drug interactions, and clinical drug development.[17] Defined in general terms, *clinical pharmacology* is the branch of pharmacology concerned with the safe and effective use of drugs. Articulated in a more practical way, the ultimate goal of clinical pharmacology is the translation of the relevant pharmacologic science into rational drug selection and dosing strategies.

Posology, although a little used term, is the science of drug dosage and is thus also a branch of clinical pharmacology (or perhaps a synonym). Combining the Greek words *"posos"* (how much) and *"logos"* (science), posology can be thought of more simply as "dosology." In the posology of anesthesia, the fundamental question "What is the optimal dose for my patient?" has numerous, clinically important permutations (Table 2-2). All of these questions have obvious clinical relevance in the day-to-day practice of anesthesia.

The accurate and precise prediction of the time course and magnitude of drug effect is the primary pharmacology-related task of anesthesia. Given the unique challenges of anesthesia pharmacology, one could argue that pharmacokinetics and pharmacodynamics are perhaps more relevant in anesthesia than in any other therapeutic area of medicine. Indeed, despite the conspicuous unpopularity of these mathematically oriented fields among anesthesia practitioners, perhaps without conscious acknowledgement, anesthesiologists are real-time clinical pharmacologists applying PK-PD principles to the optimization of anesthetic posology (and the myriad posologic questions suggested in Table 2-2).

General Schema

A general schema summarizing a framework for understanding clinical pharmacology is presented in Figure 2-2. The topic can be considered clinically from three domains: the dosage, concentration, and effect domains. Similarly, the underlying science can be divided into three areas of study: pharmacokinetics, the biophase, and pharmacodynamics. Before advances in clinical pharmacology, the clinician could only consider the adequacy of intravenous anesthetic therapy in terms of dosage or effect (i.e., without the aid of a computer model, predicted concentrations of plasma and effect site concentrations were not available and thus the concentration domain was unknowable). Likewise, before the development of modern pharmacologic modeling theory, the three distinct disciplines of clinical pharmacology (i.e., pharmacokinetics, the biophase, and pharmacodynamics) were naively lumped together in the study of the dose-response relationship.

Table 2-2. Selected Clinically Important Questions in the Posology of Anesthesia

- What is an appropriate initial dose?
- How soon will the intended effect begin?
- When will the effect peak?
- How long will the effect last?
- Should the drug be given by bolus or infusion or both?
- When will repeat bolus doses or infusion rate changes be necessary?
- When should drug administration stop to promote timely emergence?
- What are the typical therapeutic target concentrations?
- What are the expected consequences of "under" or "over" dosing?
- Will tolerance develop?
- What factors might alter the dosage requirement (e.g., demographic, pathologic, genomic)?
- What is the expected amount of variability in drug response?
- How do I account for the influence of other drugs?
- What clinical sign or surrogate measurement will reflect the magnitude of drug effect?

From the practitioner's standpoint, the adequacy of therapy can be considered in any of the three clinical domains. Is the dosage adequate? Are the predicted concentrations adequate? Is the intended effect adequate? From the scientist's perspective, the answers to these clinically oriented questions are grounded in the principles of pharmacokinetics, pharmacodynamics, and the biophase. For some drugs (now mostly older drugs), because a suitable PK model does not exist, consideration of the concentration domain cannot contribute to therapeutic decisions. Similarly, because for some drugs the measurement of drug effect in real time is difficult (e.g., opioids in unresponsive, mechanically ventilated patients), consideration of the effect domain plays a lesser role in guiding therapy.

Consider the fate of drug molecules as summarized in Figure 2-2. The anesthesiologist administers the desired dose intravenously using a handheld syringe or pump (the dose domain). The drug is then distributed via the circulation to body tissues and eventually eliminated through biotransformation and/or excretion according to the drug's pharmacokinetics. The predicted plasma (or blood) concentration versus time profile can be the basis of therapeutic decisions regarding subsequent doses (the concentration domain), although the plasma concentration is sometimes misleading because it might not be in equilibrium with the site of action. Meanwhile, some very small fraction of the administered drug is distributed from the blood to the target cells in the effect site or biophase according to the drug's biophase behavior. The predicted concentration in the effect site (also the concentration domain) is a more reliable indicator of the adequacy of therapy than is the blood concentration because the target receptors are always in equilibrium with this concentration. Finally, the drug molecules in the biophase interact with the relevant receptors, producing the intended effect (the effect

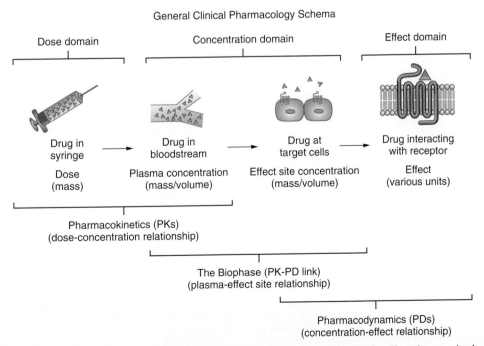

General Clinical Pharmacology Schema

Dose domain   Concentration domain   Effect domain

Drug in syringe   Drug in bloodstream   Drug at target cells   Drug interacting with receptor

Dose (mass)   Plasma concentration (mass/volume)   Effect site concentration (mass/volume)   Effect (various units)

Pharmacokinetics (PKs) (dose-concentration relationship)

The Biophase (PK-PD link) (plasma-effect site relationship)

Pharmacodynamics (PDs) (concentration-effect relationship)

Figure 2-2 A general schema of clinical pharmacology divided into dose, concentration, and effect domains. The science underpinning the field can be divided into the disciplines of pharmacokinetics, pharmacobiophasics, and pharmacodynamics. See the accompanying text for a detailed explanation. Purple triangles represent drug molecules. *PKs,* Pharmacokinetics; *PDs,* pharmacodynamics.

domain). For drugs with easily measurable effects, the dose and concentration domain are obviously less relevant to successful therapy because drug effect is the ultimate goal of therapy; when there is a reliable, real-time effect measurement, the drug can be administered to the targeted level of effect irrespective of what the dose or predicted concentration may be.

Pharmacokinetics

Pharmacokinetics is typically defined in introductory pharmacology courses as "what the body does to the drug." A much better and clinically useful definition is the study of the relationship between the dose of a drug and the resulting concentrations in the body over time (the dose-concentration relationship; see Figure 2-2). In simple terms, pharmacokinetics is the drug's disposition in the body.

Commonly considered PK parameters include distribution volumes, clearances and half-lives; other, less intuitively meaningful PK parameters such as microrate constants are mathematical transformations of these more common parameters.[18] A simple hydraulic model representation of these fundamental parameters for a one compartment model is presented in Figure 2-3. The pharmacokinetics of most anesthetic drugs are described by more complex models with two or three compartments (see also PK-PD Model Building Methods). When conceptualized in terms of a hydraulic model, of course, multicompartment models consist of additional containers (i.e., volumes) connected to the central volume by pipes of varying sizes.

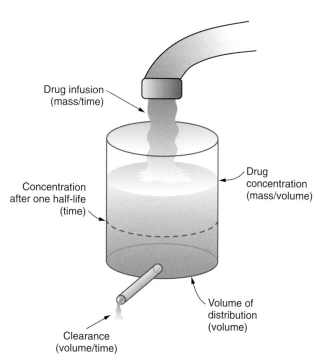

Drug infusion (mass/time)

Concentration after one half-life (time)

Drug concentration (mass/volume)

Volume of distribution (volume)

Clearance (volume/time)

Figure 2-3 A hydraulic representation of a one-compartment PK model simply illustrating the various PK parameters. Water running from the faucet into the container represents an infusion of drug. The size of the container represents the volume into which drug will distribute (i.e., the volume of distribution). The height of the water level is the drug concentration (Cp). The water flowing out of the pipe at the bottom of the container represents drug elimination (i.e., clearance). The concentration after one half-life has elapsed (after stopping the infusion) is also shown.

Distribution volumes, expressed in units of volume such as liters or L/kg, are "apparent" in that they are estimated based on the volume of water into which the drug appears to have distributed; they do not represent any actual volume or anatomic space within the body. Clearance parameters, expressed in units of flow such as L/min or L/kg/min, simply quantify the volume of plasma from which the drug is completely cleared per unit of time. For drugs with a very high hepatic extraction ratio (i.e., the liver biotransforms almost all the drug delivered to it), the central clearance is nearly equal to hepatic blood flow (e.g., about 1 L/min). Half-lives, perhaps the most commonly known PK parameter, are expressed in units of time and represent the time required for the concentration to decrease by 50% after drug administration has ceased. Half-life varies directly with volume of distribution and inversely with clearance; these relationships make intuitive sense given that a larger volume will take longer to clear and that a higher clearance will obviously speed the decline of drug levels.

Pharmacodynamics

Pharmacodynamics is typically defined as "what the drug does to the body." A better definition is the study of the relationship between the concentration of the drug in the body and its effects (i.e., the concentration-effect relationship; see Figure 2-2). In straightforward terms, pharmacodynamics is a description of drug effects, both therapeutic and adverse.

Particularly important PD parameters include potency and the steepness of the concentration-effect relationship (see PK-PD Model Building Methods). Expressed in units of mass per volume (e.g., $\mu g/mL$, ng/mL), potency is usually estimated as the concentration required to produce 50% of maximal effect, often abbreviated as the C_{50} (sometimes called the EC_{50}, the effective concentration producing 50% of maximal effect; see Figure 2-1). The lower the EC_{50}, the more potent is the drug. The EC_{50} is important in determining the range of target concentrations that will be necessary for effective therapy (i.e., the therapeutic window). The steepness of the concentration-effect relationship is typically quantified by a parameter called *gamma*, a unitless number that reflects the verticality of the concentration-effect relationship. A highly vertical concentration-effect relationship (i.e., large gamma) means that small changes in drug concentration are associated with large changes in drug effect; some groups of drugs (e.g., opioids) have steeper concentration-effect relationships than others.[19]

The Biophase

The *biophase* concept is a nuance of clinical pharmacology that is perhaps not as widely covered in pharmacology courses because its clinical application is most relevant to just a few acute care disciplines like anesthesiology. "Pharmacobiophasics," a neologism not in common usage, is the study of drug behavior in the "biophase." The biophase is the site of drug action, often referred to as the "effect site" (e.g., target cells and receptors within the brain, the neuromuscular junction, the spinal cord).

The biophase concept is essential to clinical anesthetic pharmacology because, during non–steady-state conditions (i.e., after a bolus injection or an infusion rate change), the

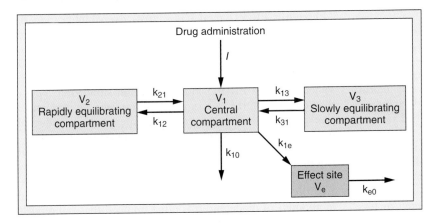

Figure 2-4 A schematic representation of a three-compartment model with an effect compartment attached to the central compartment to account for the equilibration delay between concentration in the central compartment and drug effect. I, drug input; V_1, V_2, etc, compartment volumes; k_{12}, k_{13}, etc, rate constants characterizing drug movement between compartments and out of the system; k_{e0}, rate constant for drug elimination out of the effect compartment. See the accompanying text for a detailed explanation.

concentration of drug in the blood does not correlate well with drug effect. After a bolus injection, compartmental models predict that peak plasma drug concentration occurs immediately (i.e., the "well stirred" model assumption), and yet peak drug effect does not occur immediately. This is because most drugs do not exert their effect in the blood; rather, they must be delivered to the site of action (i.e., the biophase) before they can elicit the desired therapeutic effect. Thus predictions regarding the magnitude of drug effect based on plasma concentrations can be misleading, particularly when plasma drug concentrations are rapidly changing, such as after a bolus injection.

As originally proposed by investigators working with d-tubocurarine and pancuronium, the biophase (effect site) concept has revolutionized the ability to predict the time to maximal drug effect during non–steady-state conditions.[9,20,21] As shown in Figure 2-4, incorporating a theoretic "effect compartment" into a standard compartmental PK model enables characterization of the plasma-biophase equilibration process. It is the central compartment concentration (i.e., the concentration in the arterial blood) that drives the concentration in the effect site.

The key pharmacobiophasics parameter, expressed in units of inverse time, is a rate constant called k_{e0} (see PK-PD Model Building Methods).[9,20,22] The k_{e0} characterizes the rate of equilibration between plasma and effect site concentrations. When k_{e0} is known for a drug, it is possible to predict the time course of "apparent" effect site concentrations based on the time course of plasma concentration. These effect site concentrations correlate directly with drug effect. Thus the biophase can be viewed as the link between drug disposition in the blood (pharmacokinetics) and drug effect at the site of action (pharmacodynamics).

Drug Interactions

In anesthesiology, unlike most medical disciplines, PD drug interactions are frequently produced by design. Anesthesiologists take advantage of the PD synergy that results when two drugs with different mechanisms of action but similar therapeutic effects are combined.[23] These synergistic combinations can be advantageous because the therapeutic goals of the anesthetic can often be achieved with less toxicity and faster recovery than when individual drugs are used alone in higher doses. In fact, except for specific, limited clinical circumstances wherein a volatile agent or propofol alone are acceptable approaches (e.g., a brief procedure in a pediatric patient such as tympanostomy tubes or radiation therapy), modern day anesthesia involves at least a two-drug combination consisting of an analgesic (typically an opioid) and a hypnotic (e.g., an inhaled agent or propofol).[24] Therefore, from a strictly pharmacologic perspective, anesthesiology can be thought of as the practice of PD synergism using central nervous system depressants.

Because anesthetics are rarely administered alone, understanding the interactions between drugs is critical to their safe and effective use.[25,26] Although PK interactions (i.e., where one drug alters the concentration of another) are sometimes observed in select clinical circumstances, PD interactions are an important part of nearly every anesthetic.[27] This topic is of such importance in anesthesia pharmacology that an entire chapter is devoted to it (see Chapter 5); a limited discussion is included here.

The study of drug interactions in anesthesiology has traditionally been approached using the "isobologram" method.[28,29] An isobologram is a curve defining the concentrations of two drugs that, when given together, produce the same effect (the isobole is an "iso" or "equal" effect curve). Perhaps the most common example of an isobole in anesthesiology is a plot showing the reduction in the MAC of an inhaled agent produced by an opioid (see Figure 15-7).[30,31] The main limitation of an isobologram is that the curve applies to only one level of drug effect. This is a problem in anesthesiology because during anesthesia patients experience a spectrum of drug effect ranging from minimal sedation to profound central nervous system depression.

Response surface methods address this shortcoming of the isobologram. The response surface approach creates a three-dimensional plot of the two drug concentrations (e.g., propofol and fentanyl) versus drug effect (e.g., sedation), quantitatively describing the PD interaction of the two drugs (see Chapter 5). The response surface method is an advance because it describes the drug interaction over the entire range of drug effect and thereby enables simulation from one clinical state to another. This is critical in anesthesia pharmacology because anesthesiologists must take the patient from awake to the anesthetized state, and then back to awake again on demand.[4,16] Response surface methods yield a set of parameters that indicate whether the interaction is additive, synergistic, or antagonistic.

PHARMACOLOGIC MODELING

PK-PD Models as Versions of Pharmacologic Reality

Scientific models seek to represent empirical objects, biologic phenomena or physical processes in a coherent and logical way. Models are a way of thinking about and understanding the natural world; models are essentially a simplified version of reality intended to provide scientific insight.

By providing a framework for understanding the natural world, models can also be a means of creating new knowledge. Knowledge from models comes in many forms, each with certain advantages and limitations. In biomedical science, for example, models of physiologic processes conducted in test tube experiments provide *in vitro* knowledge wherein confounding variables can be carefully controlled. Experiments conducted in animal models of disease provide *in vivo* insight that reflects biologic reality at the whole animal level. Since the advent of computational scientific methods, models of natural phenomena are often represented as a mathematical system (an equation or set of equations); these mathematical models provide *in silico* understanding, meaning that experiments that might be practically impossible or too expensive in actual subjects can be conducted by computer simulation.

PK-PD models are examples of this kind of mathematical model applied to clinical pharmacology.[32] Various equations are used to represent the pharmacologic processes of interest.[2]

Although a PK-PD model is a gross oversimplification of reality (e.g., the body is not a set of three containers connected by pipes as suggested in Figure 2-4), considerable insight into drug behavior has come from the application of PK-PD models to important questions in anesthesia pharmacology. When applying PK-PD models through simulation, rather than conducting the experiment in a test tube (*in vitro*) or in an experimental animal (*in vivo*), the experiment is conducted in the computer (*in silico*) on a virtual subject or subjects.

It is axiomatic that the true utility of a pharmacologic model is a function of its performance in the real world. Clinically useful models adequately describe past observations and satisfactorily predict future observations. Among scientists involved in all kinds of modeling, it is often quipped that "all models are wrong, but some models are useful!"[33] There is no question that PK-PD models, despite their limitations, are very useful in refining the posology of anesthesia practice.[14,15]

PK-PD Model Building Methods

A summary of the PK-PD model building process is outlined in Figure 2-5. The process of course begins with the gathering of the raw data in appropriately designed experiments.[34,35] Elements of a well-designed PK-PD modeling experiment for an intravenous anesthetic include careful attention to the administered dose by infusion; frequent, prolonged sampling of arterial blood for concentration measurement; use of a

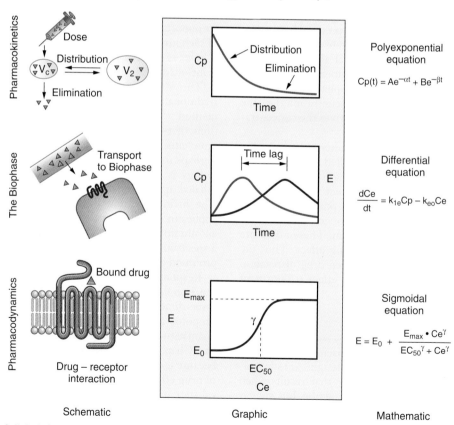

Clinical Pharmacology Modeling Concepts

Polyexponential equation

$$Cp(t) = Ae^{-\alpha t} + Be^{-\beta t}$$

Differential equation

$$\frac{dCe}{dt} = k_{1e}Cp - k_{eo}Ce$$

Sigmoidal equation

$$E = E_0 + \frac{E_{max} \bullet Ce^{\gamma}}{EC_{50}{}^{\gamma} + Ce^{\gamma}}$$

Schematic   Graphic   Mathematic

Figure 2-5 A summary of clinical pharmacology modeling concepts for the disciplines of pharmacokinetics, the biophase, and pharmacodynamics. The modeling foundation for each area is presented schematically, graphically, and mathematically. See the accompanying text for a detailed explanation, including discussion of the equations. *Cp*, Plasma concentration *(blue curves)*; *Ce*, concentration in the effect site; *E*, effect *(purple curves)*; *E₀*, effect at zero drug concentration; *E_max*, maximal drug effect; *EC₅₀*, concentration that produces 50% of maximal drug effect; γ, steepness of the curve.

quality assured, validated drug assay; and administration of sufficient drug to elicit maximal or near maximal effect (but not too rapidly).[15,20,36,37] Without quality raw data it is impossible to characterize the pharmacologic system using modeling techniques.

Because the mathematics involved in PK-PD modeling can be complex, it is perhaps best for the clinician to consider the modeling methods from other perspectives.[38] As shown in Figure 2-5, approaching the modeling process from schematic and graphic perspectives makes the mathematics less intimidating for non-mathematicians. Ultimately the mathematical equations involved are simply quantitative expressions of the ideas and concepts represented by the schematic diagrams and plots.

Schematically, basic PK processes are well represented by a compartmental model (see upper panel of Figure 2-5). After injection into the central compartment, a drug is either distributed to other compartments or is eliminated from the central compartment altogether. Graphing these PK processes reveals the distinct distribution and elimination phases typically observed in plasma concentration decay curves. Curves of this general shape can be represented by polyexponential equations of the form shown in the upper panel of Figure 2-5.[39]

Figure 2-6 summarizes how raw PK data from a single subject might be modeled in a typical PK model building experiment. Using nonlinear regression techniques, a polyexponential equation is fit to the raw concentration versus time data.[40] This is an iterative process in which the nonlinear regression software alters the parameters of the equation repeatedly until the "best model" is obtained, thereby estimating the PK parameters of the model (e.g., distribution volumes, clearances, microrate constants).[41] The best model is one that fits the data well (e.g., minimizes the difference between the measured concentration and the concentration predicted by the model).[42] Typically, hundreds or thousands of models are tested before the final, best model is identified. The PK model enables prediction of the time course of drug concentrations in blood or plasma.

Biophase behavior and pharmacodynamics can be modeled in generally the same way. When the biophase is considered schematically, the delay between peak plasma concentration and peak drug effect is a function of the time required for drug delivery to the site of action (see middle panel of Figure 2-5).[10] This delay (or hysteresis in engineering terms) is represented by a simple plot showing a time lag between peak plasma concentration and peak effect, and can be characterized by a simple differential equation of the general form shown. Using nonlinear regression and other techniques, the biophase modeling process estimates the key biophase model parameter called k_{e0} (see earlier discussion).[9,22] The biophase model enables prediction of effect site concentrations.

These effect site concentration predictions are essential for the PD modeling process. Considered schematically, the PD system is represented by a drug molecule interacting with a target receptor (see bottom panel of Figure 2-5). This drug-receptor interaction is represented graphically by a sigmoidal curve. In the absence of drug, the level of biologic effect is at baseline (E_0). As drug concentration in the effect site (predicted from the biophase model) increases, eventually some drug effect is produced. As the steep portion of the concentration-effect relationship is approached, more pronounced degrees of drug effect are observed. Further increases in drug concentration produce greater and greater effect, eventually reaching the biologic maximum (E_{max}). This sigmoidal curve is represented by equations of the general form shown in the bottom panel of Figure 2-5. Using nonlinear regression techniques like those illustrated in Figure 2-6, the PD modeling process fits the sigmoidal equation to the raw PD data, thereby estimating the parameters of the equation. Combined with the PK and biophase model, the PD modeling process enables prediction of the time course of drug effect.

In summary, PK-PD model building is an exercise in fitting appropriate equations to experimental data using nonlinear regression modeling software and other related techniques.[41] As summarized in Figure 2-7, the mathematical equations simply represent the general shape of the relationships being modeled. A polyexponential equation is typically used to characterize the plasma concentration decay curve. A differential equation is the basis for modeling the delay between equilibration of plasma and effect site concentration. And a sigmoidal equation is used to characterize the concentration-effect relationship. Fitting the equations to the raw data results in a set of PK-PD parameter estimates that constitute the quantitative model.[18] These parameters can then be used to conduct PK-PD simulations to explore the clinical implications of the models. It is important to emphasize that the iterative, non-linear regression process yields only parameter "estimates"; the true values of the parameters are unknowable.*

It is of course possible to fit these equations to an individual subject's data and also to a group of subjects' data. Because a main thrust of PK-PD modeling is to characterize drug behavior in the population for which it is intended, a

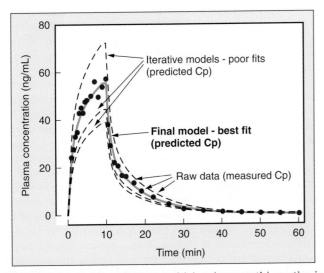

Figure 2-6 An example of fitting a model (a polyexponential equation in this case) to raw PK data from a single experimental subject. The measured plasma concentrations (i.e., the raw data) are represented by the purple circles. Preliminary models (i.e., poor fits) generated during the iterative, nonlinear regression process are shown as dotted lines. The final model (i.e., best fit) is shown as a thick, blue line. The thick, blue line thus represents the predicted concentrations according to the PK model. See the accompanying text for a detailed explanation.

---

*In this chapter, "parameter estimates" are sometimes referred to as just "parameters."

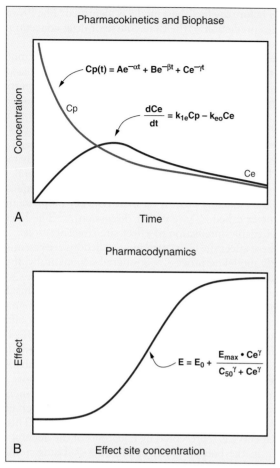

Figure 2-7 Basic equations for modeling drug plasma concentration (Cp), effect site concentration (Ce) in panel A, and drug effect in panel B. These equations (or various transformations of these equations) are the mathematical basis for PK-PD modeling. The equations represent curves of the appropriate shape to characterize the raw data. See text for complete explanation.

primary focus of modeling is to build a model that represents the entire population (not just an individual).[35] Special techniques such as "mixed-effects" modeling (e.g., the NONMEM program) have been developed and refined to estimate typical PK-PD parameter values for an entire population (and also the intersubject variability of the parameters).[43-45] Sophisticated methods to quantify the influence of "covariate" effects (e.g., age, body weight, metabolic organ failure, among others) on the PK-PD system have also been described.[46]

Limitations in Building and Applying PK-PD Models

As simplified versions of reality, PK-PD models fail to account for certain biologic complexities. In selected situations, these complexities make it difficult or impossible to apply PK-PD models in a useful way. Thus, intelligent construction and application of PK-PD models requires awareness of their limitations.

EARLY MODEL MISSPECIFICATION
A major shortcoming of the standard compartmental PK model is a function of model misspecification during the early period after drug injection.[47] Standard compartmental models assume the central volume is "well stirred" and that peak plasma concentration occurs immediately after injection, an

assumption that is obviously invalid. Similarly, standard compartmental models assume that plasma concentration declines monotonically after it reaches a peak; while perhaps less obvious, this assumption is also false.[48] Careful study of the early period after drug injection confirms that standard compartmental models sometimes do not reliably predict drug disposition in the first few minutes after injection.[47] Model misspecification is important because anesthetics are often intended to exert their most profound effects very soon after a bolus is administered.[49]

The reasons underpinning this model misspecification in the period shortly after bolus injection are numerous and include the influence of cardiac output on drug distribution, the appearance of a "recirculatory," second concentration peak (after the first circulation time), and pulmonary uptake of drug, among others.[48,50,51] These limitations of compartmental models can be addressed with more complex "physiologic" and "recirculatory" models, although standard compartmental models are more commonly applied clinically despite their sometimes poor performance.[52-55] These more physiologically based PK modeling approaches have identified factors that influence anesthesia induction doses such as age, cardiac output, and concomitant use of drugs that alter cardiac function.[50,56,57]

STEREOCHEMISTRY
Chirality in molecular structure introduces substantial complexity in characterizing drug behavior with PK-PD models if the chiral drug is studied as a racemate.[58] Taken from the Greek word chier (meaning hand), "chiral" is the term used to designate a molecule that has a center (or centers) of three-dimensional asymmetry. The appropriateness of the term's Greek origin is clear when considering that a pair of human hands are perhaps the most common example of chirality (Figure 2-8). Although they are mirror images of each other, a pair of hands cannot be superimposed. Similarly, chirality in molecular structure results in a set of mirror image molecular twins (i.e., the two enantiomers of a racemic mixture) that cannot be superimposed. This kind of molecular handedness in biologic systems is ubiquitous in nature and is almost always a function of the unique, tetrahedral bonding characteristics of the carbon atom.[59]

Drug chirality is significant because the molecular interactions that are the mechanistic foundation of drug action and disposition occur in three dimensions, and therefore can be altered by stereochemical asymmetry.[60] Thus, pharmacologically, not all enantiomers are created equal. The implications of chirality span the entire PK-PD spectrum. Enantiomers can exhibit differences in absorption and bioavailability, distribution and clearance, potency and toxicology. When a pharmacologic process discriminates in a relative fashion between enantiomers (e.g., one enantiomer being metabolized more rapidly than the other), it is termed *stereoselective*. If the discrimination is absolute (e.g., one enantiomer being completely incapable of producing drug effect), the process is termed *stereospecific*.

The implications of chirality on PK-PD modeling are obvious. A PK-PD model of a racemic mixture is really a model of two drugs with presumably different PK and PD behavior and thus must be interpreted with caution. This "racemate" complexity applies to a surprisingly diverse array of anesthetic drugs, including thiopental, methohexital,

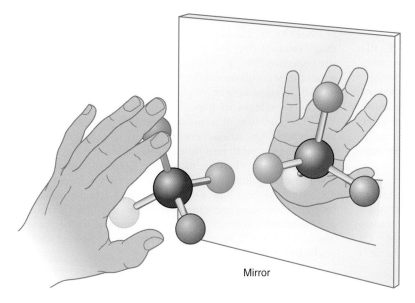

Figure 2-8 The concept of molecular chirality compared to the anatomic asymmetry of a pair of human hands. Like a pair of hands, chiral molecules are identical, mirror images of one another, but they cannot be superimposed. The molecular asymmetry of chirality is a function of the tetrahedral bonding characteristics of the carbon atom (carbon is represented in black; the other colors represent any four different groups of atoms). The two molecules shown are considered enantiomers; when combined together, they constitute a racemic mixture. Chirality has important pharmacologic implications in terms of PK-PD behavior.

Mirror

ketamine, isoflurane, desflurane, mepivacaine, bupivacaine, ibuprofen, ketorolac, and methadone, among others.[61] It is for this reason that novel drug development in anesthesia over the past decade has avoided racemic mixtures (there is considerable pressure from regulatory bodies like the United States Food and Drug Administration to do so).[62,63] Single enantiomer formulations like (S)-ketamine, ropivacaine, cis-atracurium, and levo-bupivacaine are all cases in point; single enantiomer formulations often have some clinical advantage in terms of their PK and/or PD behavior, reflecting the PK-PD differences between enantiomers.[61]

ACTIVE METABOLITES
When a drug has an active metabolite, applying a PK-PD model of the parent compound to predict overall drug effect is obviously problematic. Not only will the metabolite contribute to drug effect, but the metabolite will also have a different rate of concentration decay (i.e., different pharmacokinetics). The PK-PD model of the parent drug does not account for this complexity and thus the model must be applied with awareness of this shortcoming.[64] Therapeutic drug monitoring of parent drugs with active metabolites has long been known to be fraught with similar problems.[65]

This active metabolite issue applies to a number of anesthetic drugs including diazepam, midazolam, codeine, morphine, and ketamine, among others. Particular interest in recent years has been focused on morphine's active metabolite, morphine-6-glucuronide (M6G). Because M6G accumulates in patients with altered renal clearance mechanisms (unlike the parent drug) prolonged administration of morphine in patients with kidney failure can be complicated by severe ventilatory depression.[66-68] PK-PD models for morphine that also include the concentration time course and effect of the M6G metabolite provide a scientific explanation for these clinical observations.[69]

VARIABILITY
Another major shortcoming in applying PK-PD models clinically is that standard simulations using PK-PD model parameters do not typically include an expression of variability in

the PK-PD predictions. As a result, from a statistical perspective, these standard simulations are being applied deterministically rather than probabilistically. Given the well-described and considerable variability in drug behavior in terms of both PK and PD relationships (and that PK-PD model parameters are only estimates), this shortcoming of standard PK-PD model simulation is an important one.[70] Applying advanced statistical methods such as Monte Carlo simulation to standard PK-PD analysis is a means of addressing this problem by providing the clinician with a sense of the expected variability in drug behavior.[71]

PHARMACOLOGIC SIMULATION

Unimportance of Individual PK-PD Model Parameters
In contrast to well-entrenched conventional wisdom, single PK-PD parameter estimates considered in isolation are not very helpful in drawing clinically useful conclusions. PK-PD studies in the anesthesia literature traditionally include a table of values for PK-PD parameters such as in the left column of Table 2-3. In the early days of PK-PD modeling, it was commonplace for investigators to make clinical inference by comparing a particular parameter value for one drug with the corresponding parameter of another drug. For example, certain clinical conclusions might have been drawn depending on how half-lives or clearances for a pair of drugs compared.

The problem with this simplistic approach is that it fails to account for the complexity of the typical PK model. A standard three compartment model as shown in Figure 2-4, for example, has six fundamental parameters (i.e., three clearances and three distribution volumes); these fundamental parameters can be converted to a variety of other parameters (e.g., half-lives, microrate constants).[18] These multiple parameters interact in a complex way over time in determining the predicted drug concentration.[6,72] Thus comparing a single PK parameter value of one drug with that of another drug is of limited value and provides very little clinically relevant intuitive understanding.

Importance of PK-PD Model Simulation

Understanding the clinical implications of a table of PK-PD parameters is best accomplished through *in silico* application of the associated model by computer simulation.[73] Through simulation, the practically oriented clinical questions shown in the right column of Table 2-3 (among many other questions) can be explored and answered. In contrast to a table of parameter values, PK-PD model simulation provides straightforward, clinically oriented information that the practitioner can apply in actual practice.[38]

The PK-PD model simulation process is summarized in Figure 2-9. Using PK-PD model simulation software, the user inputs a dosing scheme of interest. The simulation software predicts the time course and magnitude of drug concentration and effect according to the model. An infinite number of such simulations can be performed *in silico* to gain insight into anesthesia posology. When presented graphically, the results of PK-PD simulations provide a picture of the time course of drug concentration and effect. Most commonly, drug effect site concentrations are simulated. Combined with knowledge about the concentration-effect relationship (i.e., pharmacodynamics), clinical insight into optimal dosing is gained.[74]

The simulation in Figure 2-10 illustrates the power of PK-PD simulation in terms of intuitively understanding the implications of various dosing schemes. The simulation depicts the very different time courses of drug concentration in the biophase when identical total doses of fentanyl (i.e., 300 μg) are administered in three different ways. By providing a simple picture of how a specified dosing scheme translates into effect site concentrations over time (and how the resulting concentration versus time profile compares to therapeutic windows), PK-PD simulation constitutes a powerful tool to study and optimize anesthesia posology.

Table 2-3. Selected Traditional PK-PD Model Parameters versus Practical Model Predictions

TRADITIONAL PARAMETERS (FROM THE MODEL)	PRACTICAL MODEL PREDICTIONS (FROM MODEL SIMULATION)
Pharmacokinetic Distribution volumes Clearances Half-lives	**Front- and Back-End Bolus Behavior** Time to peak effect after a bolus injection? Time to offset of effect after a bolus injection?
Pharmacobiophasic k_{e0}	**Front- and Back-End Infusion Behavior** Time to steady-state after beginning an infusion?
Pharmacodynamic E_0 E_{max} EC_{50} Gamma (γ)	Time to offset of effect after stopping an infusion? **Dosage Domain Issues** Dosage necessary to achieve a specified target concentration? Dosage reduction necessary when combining synergistic drugs? **Concentration Domain Issue** Concentration necessary to achieve specified effect?

k_{e0}, Rate constant for drug elimination out of the effect compartment; E_0, effect at zero drug concentration; E_{max}, maximal drug effect; EC_{50}, concentration that produces 50% of maximal drug effect; gamma (γ), steepness of the curve. See text for complete explanation.

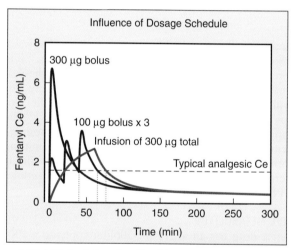

Figure 2-10 A PK simulation of predicted fentanyl effect site concentrations (Ce) resulting from three different regimens to administer 300 μg of fentanyl (a single 300-μg bolus, three 100-μg boluses every 20 minutes, an infusion of 300 μg at a constant rate over 1 hour). The horizontal dotted line indicates a typical analgesic fentanyl level. The colored, vertical dotted lines represent the time at which the fentanyl concentration falls permanently below the typical analgesic level. See the accompanying text for a detailed explanation. The simulations were conducted with PK-PD parameter estimates from the literature.[99]

Pharmacologic Simulation Concept

Figure 2-9 A simple representation of the concept of PK-PD model simulation. Using PK-PD model simulation software, the user inputs a dosing scheme of interest. The simulation software predicts plasma concentrations (Cp), effect site concentrations (Ce), and effect (E) according to the parameters of the PK-PD model. Triangles represent drug molecules in the syringe. See the accompanying text for a detailed explanation.

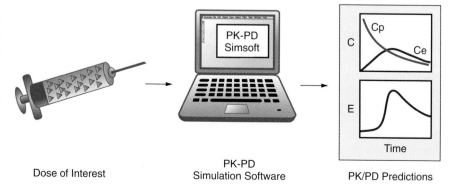

Dose of Interest

PK-PD Simulation Software

PK/PD Predictions

PK-PD MODEL SIMULATION AND ANESTHESIA POSOLOGY

Exploring anesthesia posology through PK-PD simulation equips the practitioner with the knowledge necessary to formulate rational drug selection and administration schemes. Although the possibilities are endless in terms of the number and variety of PK-PD simulations that can be performed, a limited set of straightforward simulations form the foundation upon which the answers to many routine anesthesia posology questions are based.

Among this fundamental set of simulations, perhaps the most important are those that address the front-end and back-end PK behavior of intravenous anesthetics. Because drug behavior is substantially different for bolus injections compared to infusions,[7] the two conditions must be considered separately. Other fundamental simulations include the influence of dose on the onset and offset of effect after bolus injection, the influence of dose on the front- and back-end kinetics of infusions, the influence of special populations on drug behavior, and the influence of a second drug on PD effect.

Bolus Front- and Back-End Kinetics

As noted in Table 2-2, important posologic questions regarding bolus injections include the following: How long will it take to reach peak effect and how long will it take for the effect to dissipate? The simulations plotted in Figure 2-11 explore these questions for a number of commonly used opioids. After bolus injection, remifentanil and alfentanil predicted effect site concentrations reach a peak quickly and then decline significantly before any of the other opioids have even begun to peak. This rapid achievement of peak effect site concentrations for these two highly lipid soluble fentanyl congeners is likely a function of their high "diffusible fractions"

(i.e., the proportion that is un-ionized and unbound). Interestingly, morphine's front-end kinetics are notably different. Morphine does not approach a substantial fraction of the ultimate peak until 20 to 30 minutes have elapsed.

The simulations depicted in Figure 2-11 have obvious clinical implications. When a brief pulse of opioid effect followed by a quick offset is desirable (e.g., a brief period of intense analgesia before injection of local anesthetic during a regional block), remifentanil or alfentanil would be rational choices. In contrast, when the clinical situation calls for a slower onset followed by a more sustained period of opioid effect, one of the other opioids may be more appropriate. Given the lockout period of a typical patient-controlled analgesia (PCA) dosing regimen, it is surprising that morphine has been the mainstay of PCA therapy; fentanyl's latency to peak effect of 4 to 5 minutes is much more favorable for PCA, particularly in terms of avoiding a "dose stacking" problem wherein the patient requests additional doses before the prior doses have reached their peak effect.

Infusion Front-End Kinetics

The relevant questions concerning the posology of anesthetic infusions are similar to those for bolus injections (see Table 2-2). The simulations plotted in Figure 2-12 explore the front-end kinetic behavior of a number of opioids when administered by infusion. With the exception of remifentanil, no opioid comes anywhere near the ultimate steady state level even after many hours of infusion. Remifentanil is the only opioid in common use that can be expected to reach steady state during the time course of typical anesthetic.

Several clinically important points are evident from inspection of the simulations presented in Figure 2-12. Most obviously, although remifentanil is a notable exception, the practitioner must be aware that when an opioid infusion is ongoing, the concentrations will continue to rise for the duration of any conceivable anesthetic (this general rule applies

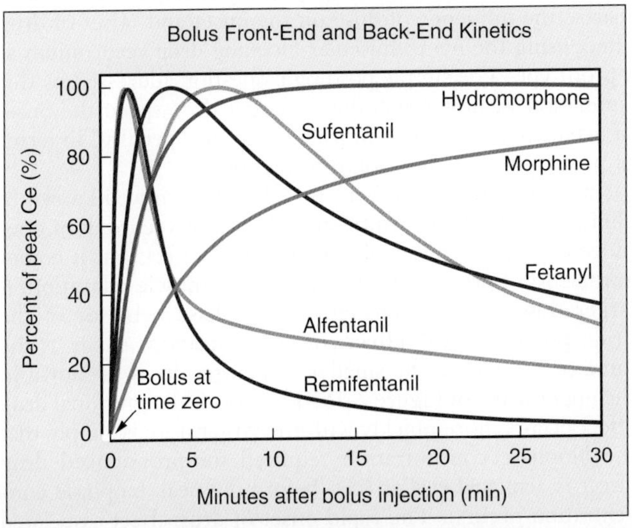

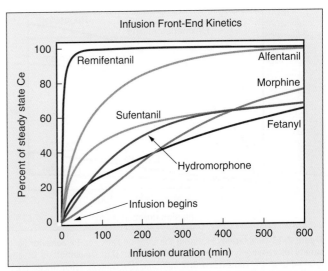

Figure 2-11 A simulation exploring bolus injection front- and back-end PK behavior for a variety of commonly used opioids. For comparison purposes, the effect site concentrations (Ce) are normalized to the percentage of the peak. See the accompanying text for a detailed explanation. The simulations were conducted with PK-PD parameter estimates from the literature.[69,99-106]

Figure 2-12 Simulations exploring infusion front-end PK behavior for a variety of commonly used opioids. For comparison purposes, effect site concentrations (Ce) are normalized to a percentage of the eventual steady state concentration. See the accompanying text for a detailed explanation. The simulations were conducted with PK-PD parameter estimates from the literature.[69,99-106]

less fully to alfentanil). An extension of this observation is that if the level of opioid effect part way through a long anesthetic is appropriate, it would be necessary to decrease the infusion rate somewhat to maintain the existing therapeutic concentration (without the infusion rate decrease, the concentration will continue to rise).

That remifentanil reaches a steady state quickly is at least partially responsible for its popularity as part of a total intravenous anesthetic (TIVA) technique. However, even for remifentanil, it is best to precede an infusion with a bolus injection as a "loading dose" to speed achievement of a steady state drug level (see later). Because they take so long to reach steady-state, the loading dose concept is even more important when using the other opioids in Figure 2-12.

Infusion Back-End Kinetics

The simulations presented graphically in Figure 2-13 summarize the back-end kinetic behavior for a number of commonly used intravenous sedative-hypnotics when administered by infusion. In terms of anesthesia posology, these simulations are valuable in explaining how various sedative-hypnotics exhibit different recovery profiles depending on the duration of the infusion. The simulation also helps guide therapeutic decision making in terms of the best time to turn off a continuous infusion in order to promote a timely emergence from anesthesia.

The simulations in Figure 2-13 predict the time necessary to achieve a 50% decrease in drug concentration after termination of a variable length continuous infusion to a steady state drug level. Using concepts originally developed for opioids, these simulations are an attempt to provide context sensitive half-times (CSHT).[6,7] In this case the "context" is the duration of a continuous infusion. The CSHT has also

been referred to as the 50% decrement time (although the decrement time concept usually refers to simulations of effect site concentrations, not plasma).[8] These simulations illustrate how PK parameters interact in a complex way that can only readily be understood through model simulation.[7,72] The CSHTs also illustrate the utter irrelevance of using terminal half-lives to predict drug offset behavior for intravenous anesthetics described by three compartment models.[72]

Interpreted from a clinical perspective, CSHTs are very instructive. For example, they provide an explanation for why propofol has been so widely embraced as an intravenous anesthetic for TIVA; propofol has a relatively short, time-independent CSHT that is well suited for longer infusions. The CSHTs also explain at least one reason why thiopental and midazolam never emerged as popular anesthetics for infusion (and also why "barbiturate coma" was sometimes complicated by extremely long recovery times). Another interesting clinical correlation from the CSHTs is that when infusion duration is very brief (i.e., less than 15-20 minutes), many of the sedative-hypnotics exhibit similar back-end kinetic behavior.

It is important to emphasize that the shapes of these back-end kinetic curves vary depending on the percentage decrease in concentration simulated; this is why the term *decrement time* was coined (e.g., the 20%, 50%, or 80% decrement times).[8] For most TIVA cases involving propofol, the relevant concentration decrease to promote recovery is closer to 75% than 50% (i.e., the biophase concentration must decline from a therapeutic target of approximately 3-4 µg/mL to 0.5-1 µg/mL for the patient to regain responsiveness). The simulations in Figure 2-14 illustrate this important nuance. For propofol, as for most drugs, the time required for recovery lengthens as the duration of infusion lengthens; the drug input history is clinically important.

Influence of Dose on Bolus Onset and Offset of Effect

The simulations presented graphically in Figure 2-15 summarize the influence of dose on the onset and offset of drug effect using the neuromuscular blocking drug vecuronium as a prototype. The simple posologic question addressed by this simulation is, how much does a larger dose speed the onset of maximal drug effect and what is the PK "penalty" in terms of prolonging the duration of drug effect?

Inspection of Figure 2-15 reveals a pattern well known to clinicians. The larger "intubating" dose of vecuronium does indeed speed the onset of maximal drug effect, but it comes at the cost of prolonging the duration of muscle relaxation. A larger dose does not change the biophase behavior of the drug; predicted peak effect site concentrations occur at the same time for both the smaller and larger doses as shown in the upper panel of Figure 2-15. The reason that maximal drug effect occurs more quickly with the larger dose is simply that the biophase concentration required for pronounced drug effect is achieved earlier (i.e., before the peak biophase concentration occurs). The rapid onset of drug effect associated with the larger dose shown in the middle panel of Figure 2-15 results in the prolonged recovery plotted in the lower panel.

The clinical implications of this simulation are obvious. The clinician must balance the competing clinical imperatives of rapid onset against rapid recovery of neuromuscular

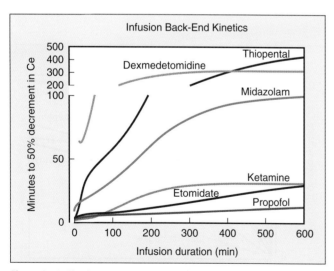

Figure 2-13 Simulations exploring the infusion back-end PK behavior for a variety of commonly used sedative-hypnotics. This simulation is usually referred to as the *context sensitive half-time* (the context being the duration of a continuous, steady-state infusion) or the 50% decrement time (for effect site concentrations). See the accompanying text for a detailed explanation. The upper portion of the vertical axis is shown on a more compressed scale than the lower portion. See the accompanying text for a detailed explanation. The simulations were conducted with PK-PD parameter estimates from the literature.[107-113]

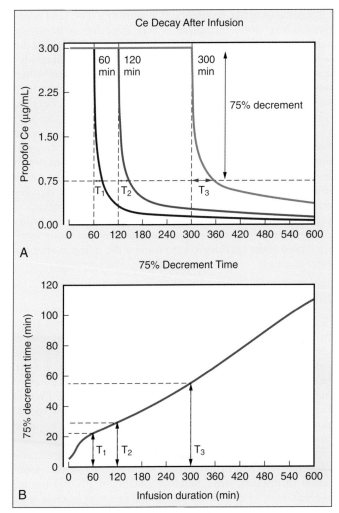

Figure 2-14 A pair of simulations exploring propofol's back-end kinetic behavior. The upper panel simulates the effect site concentration decay curves after continuous, steady state infusions of propofol targeted to 3 µg/mL for infusions lasting 60, 120, and 300 minutes. The lower panel illustrates how the infusions simulated in the upper panel map to a 75% decrement time simulation for propofol. T_1, T_2, and T_3 are the 75% decrement times for the 60-, 120-, and 300-minute infusions respectively. See the accompanying text for a detailed explanation. The simulations were conducted with PK-PD parameter estimates from the literature.[112]

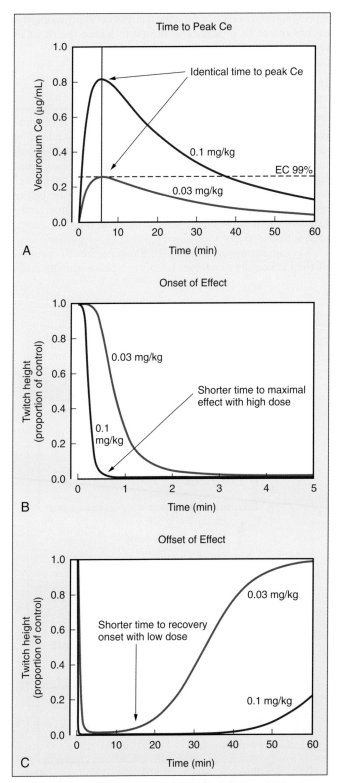

Figure 2-15 A trio of simulations exploring the influence of bolus dosage on the onset and offset of neuromuscular blockade induced by vecuronium. Two doses, one larger (0.1 mg/kg, shown in purple) and the other smaller (0.03 mg/kg, shown in blue) are simulated. The upper panel **(A)** shows the time course of predicted effect site concentrations. The middle panel **(B)** plots the onset of PD effect in the first few minutes in terms of the muscle "twitch" height compared to control. The lower panel **(C)** graphs the drug offset behavior during the first 60 minutes. See the accompanying text for a detailed explanation. The simulations were conducted with PK-PD parameter estimates from the literature.[114] EC_{99}, the effective concentration for 99% of maximal drug effect; Ce, effect site concentration.

blockade. Depending on the duration of the scheduled procedure and other factors (e.g., full stomach considerations or need for postoperative mechanical ventilation), the rapid onset of neuromuscular blockade might be more important than the potential disadvantages of a longer period of muscle relaxation, justifying the selection of a larger initial dose of drug. The advent of shorter acting muscle relaxants and sugammadex has rendered this issue less relevant than in days past, but of course the general concepts involved apply to all intravenous anesthetic classes (not just neuromuscular blockers).

In summary, the time to peak drug effect is a function of not only plasma-biophase concentration equilibration but also pharmacokinetics and potency.[15] If a supramaximal dose is administered, peak clinical effect may be observed before peak effect site concentration is achieved simply because the concentration necessary to produce maximal effect is attained before the effect site concentration peaks (this situation represents an "overshoot" of typical target concentrations; the overshoot can be produced by design to hasten the onset of significant drug effect).

Influence of Loading Dose on Infusion Front- and Back-End Kinetics

The simulations presented graphically in Figure 2-16 illustrate the concept of "loading" doses. A bolus injection loading dose prior to starting an infusion shortens the time to achievement of concentrations nearer the ultimate steady-state. Similarly, while the term is not firmly established, a "negative" loading dose (i.e., briefly stopping an ongoing infusion before reducing the infusion rate) can also be used to hasten establishment of the new steady-state drug concentration associated with the reduced infusion rate.

The simulations in Figure 2-16 illustrate the effectiveness of the loading dose concept. Even for a pharmacokinetically

responsive drug like remifentanil, the loading dose (and negative loading dose) technique is very effective in hastening achievement of steady-state drug concentrations. Without the loading dose (and negative loading dose), the eventual steady-state concentrations are achieved significantly later when considered in the context of the operating room where minute-by-minute adjustments of the level of drug effect are often necessary.

The clinical implications of this loading dose concept are even more important when applied to most other drugs in intravenous anesthesia. As illustrated in the simulations shown in Figure 2-12, for drugs with less favorable PK-PD profiles in terms of the time required to achieve steady-state concentrations (e.g., fentanyl, propofol), the loading dose concept is even more important. It must be emphasized that the utility of the "negative" loading dose may be catastrophically overshadowed if the user neglects to resume the infusion after the brief stoppage.

Influence of Special Populations

A very common posologic issue in everyday anesthesia practice relates to the formulation of rational dosing strategies in special populations. Certain demographic factors (e.g., age, gender), anthropometric measurements (e.g., body weight, height, body mass index), and disease states (e.g., kidney or hepatic failure, hemorrhagic shock) can influence the PK-PD behavior of certain drugs. The doses required in some special populations can be dramatically different from those required in normal patients.

PK-PD modeling techniques can be used to characterize quantitatively how drug behavior is altered in a special population of interest. After building a standard PK-PD model, the influence of the special population factor of interest (e.g., age, body weight, kidney failure), referred to as a *covariate*, can be examined by exploring how the covariate relates to the individual PK-PD model parameters. The covariate can be included in the model to see if it improves model performance. For example, body weight can be related to a distribution volume, or age can be related to drug potency (EC$_{50}$), and so on.

The simulations presented graphically in Figure 2-17 illustrate the important impact that covariate effects can have on PK-PD behavior and thus on rational dosing strategy. According to Figure 2-17 *A*, significantly obese patients require more remifentanil to achieve the same effect site concentration as leaner patients (but not as much as would be suggested by total body weight). Similarly, as depicted in the lower panel of Figure 2-17, older patients require less propofol than younger patients to achieve identical effect site concentrations; in this case, this dosage reduction is a function of both PK and PD factors.

The exploration of covariate effects on PK-PD behavior is perhaps one of the most important aspects of current clinical pharmacology research in anesthesia. Studies examining covariate effects in the form of demographic factors, anthropometric measurements, and disease states now constitute a large part of the anesthesia clinical pharmacology literature. Knowing what factors significantly alter the dosage requirement (and how to implement that knowledge quantitatively) is important in enabling the clinician to "personalize" therapy for each individual patient.

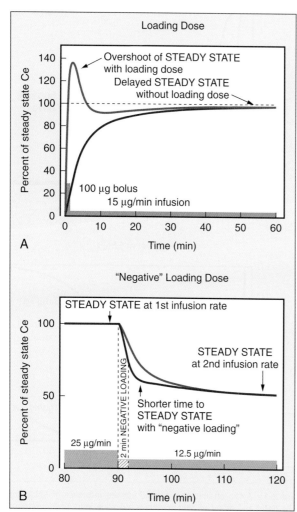

Figure 2-16 A pair of simulations exploring the influence of loading doses on the time to reach steady-state effect site concentrations using remifentanil infusions as an example. The standard loading dose concept, wherein a bolus injection is given before starting a continuous infusion, is illustrated in the upper panel **(A)**. The notion of a "negative" loading dose, wherein the drug infusion is briefly stopped before the existing infusion rate is decreased, is shown in the lower panel **(B)**. See the accompanying text for a detailed explanation. The simulations were conducted with PK-PD parameter estimates from the literature.[102] *Ce,* Effect site concentration.

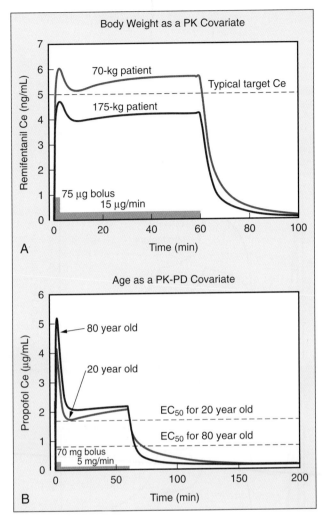

Figure 2-17 A pair of simulations exploring the influence of covariate effects on drug behavior. The upper panel **(A)** plots the predicted effect site concentrations (Ce) of remifentanil when identical doses (i.e., not scaled by weight) are administered to lean and obese adults. The lower panel **(B)** plots the predicted effect site concentrations (Ce) of propofol when identical doses are administered to older and younger patients. See the accompanying text for a detailed explanation. The simulations were conducted with PK-PD parameter estimates from the literature.[115,116] *Ce,* Effect site concentration; *EC$_{50}$,* effective concentration for 50% of maximal drug effect.

Influence of a Second Drug on Effect

Because modern anesthesia is a multidrug process, understanding how anesthetics interact in a quantitative way is critical to formulating optimal dosing strategies. In particular, accounting for the PD synergy of opioids and hypnotics (both intravenous and inhaled) when used in combination is among the most important posologic issues in anesthesia, given the prominent role these combinations play in almost every anesthetic.

The simulations presented graphically in Figure 2-18 illustrate the PD synergy observed when propofol and remifentanil are combined for provision of TIVA. The lower panel *(C)* plots the expected PD effect in terms of the probability of loss of responsiveness. Remifentanil alone at the concentrations predicted from the routine dosing regimen produces zero probability of losing responsiveness. But, when the

remifentanil is added to the propofol regimen, substantial synergy is evident and the likelihood of loss or responsiveness is increased dramatically. This degree of PD synergy is typical of virtually all hypnotic-opioid combinations (i.e., both intravenous and inhaled).

The clinical implications of this PD synergy are enormous. In practical terms, the synergistic interaction decreases the dosage necessary for both drug classes. The main advantage associated with reduced dosage is faster recovery. Viewed in terms of PD theory, the synergistic combinations steepen the concentration-effect relationship and make a faster recovery possible because drug levels need decrease only moderately to promote emergence from anesthesia (see Figure 2-1).

PK-PD MODELS AND TECHNOLOGY

Target Controlled Infusion

Until recently, the most sophisticated delivery system for intravenous anesthetics was the "calculator pump." Combining advances in pharmacologic modeling with modern infusion pump technology has culminated in the development of more sophisticated methods of intravenous drug delivery.[75] By coding a PK model into a computer program and linking it to an electronic pump modified to accept computerized commands, delivery according to a drug's specific PK profile can be achieved.

This concept was first applied to propofol[76]; commercial embodiments of the concept are now available for many commonly used intravenous anesthetics. Called *target controlled infusion* (TCI) systems, the user of a TCI system designates a target concentration rather than specifying an infusion rate as with a traditional calculator pump. The TCI system then calculates the necessary infusion rates to achieve the targeted concentration as shown schematically in Figure 2-19.[12]

Borrowing from inhalation anesthesia concepts, TCI pumps make progress toward the concept of a "vaporizer" for intravenous drugs because they address the fundamental limitation associated with delivering drugs directly into the circulation.[75] Constant rate infusions result in continuous drug uptake. TCI systems, in contrast, gradually decrease the rate of infusion based on the drug's PK behavior.

Known in its general form as the BET method (i.e., bolus, elimination, and transfer), the dosing scheme implemented by a TCI pump accounts for the initial concentration after a bolus dose and the subsequent drug distribution and clearance while an infusion is ongoing.[77] TCI dosing algorithms are essentially functional translations of basic PK equations into operating instructions for the infusion pump.[78] Recognizing the importance of the biophase concept, modern TCI pump algorithms have enabled targeting of effect site concentrations.[79-81]

Delivery of drug via a TCI system requires a different knowledge base of the physician. Rather than setting an infusion rate based on clinical experience and literature recommendations, the physician using a TCI system designates a target concentration and the system determines the infusion rates necessary to achieve that concentration over time. The TCI system changes the infusion rates at frequent intervals, sometimes as often as every 10 seconds. Successful use of a TCI pump thus requires knowledge of the therapeutic concentrations appropriate for the specific clinical application.[12]

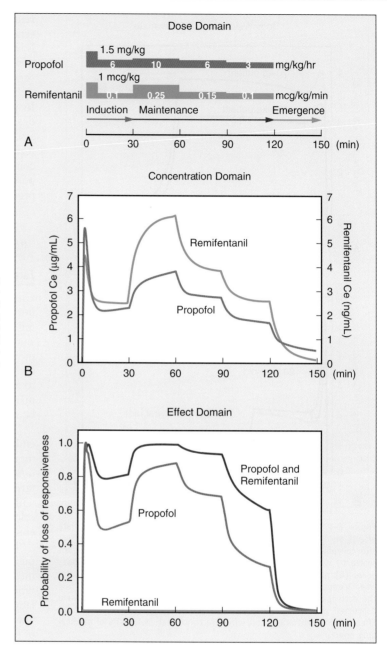

Figure 2-18 Simulations exploring the influence of a second drug using propofol and remifentanil as prototypes. The dose **(A)**, concentration **(B)**, and effect **(C)** domains are presented for an entire anesthetic, from induction to emergence. The effect predictions in the panel **C** are based on a response surface PD drug interaction model. Substantial PD synergy is evident when the opioid is added to the sedative. See the accompanying text for a detailed explanation. The simulations were conducted with PK-PD parameter estimates from the literature.[26,90,112,116] *Ce,* Effect site.

The clinician interfaces with the calculator pump in the dosage domain whereas TCI systems require input in the concentration domain (see Figure 2-2). Successful use of TCI requires knowledge of PK models, the biophase concept, PD models, and the concept of covariate effects for special populations.

Computer-controlled drug delivery in the operating room is now a well-established technique internationally. Although it has not been possible to show an obvious improvement in outcome associated with the technology, its popularity around the world attests to a high level of user satisfaction among clinicians.[82] Sadly, although TCI systems are widely used in North America for research purposes, the systems are not yet commercially available for routine clinical use in the United States (unlike much of the rest of the world), in part because of perceived regulatory barriers.[16] Current research in the area is focused on perfecting drug models used by the TCI

systems, such as expanding the models to include important covariate effects such as body weight, and "personalizing" population models with individualized feedback.[83,84]

EMERGING DEVELOPMENTS

PK-PD Advisory Displays

Research is being conducted to bring anesthetic pharmacology models to the operating room through automated acquisition of the drug administration scheme and real-time display of the predicted pharmacokinetics and pharmacodynamics.[13] Based on high-resolution PK-PD models, including a model of the synergistic PD interaction between sedatives (i.e., propofol and inhaled anesthetics) and opioids, this technology automatically acquires (from pumps and the anesthesia

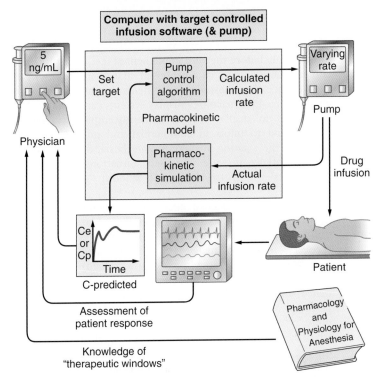

Figure 2-19 A schematic representation of a TCI system for anesthetic drugs. According to knowledge of therapeutic windows, patient response, and the current prediction of drug concentration (C-predicted), the physician sets the anesthetic drug concentration target. Using a pharmacokinetic model for the drug, the computer calculates the appropriate infusion rates over time to achieve and maintain the target concentration and directs the infusion pump to administer the appropriate amount of drug. The pump reports to the computer the amount of drug administered to the patient so that the computer's pharmacokinetic simulation of the current drug concentration can be updated and confirmed (see text for details). (Modified with permission from Egan TD. Target-controlled drug delivery: progress toward an intravenous "vaporizer" and automated anesthetic administration. Anesthesiology. 2003;99:1214-1219.) Ce, Effect site concentration; Cp, plasma concentration; C-predicted, predicted concentration.

machine) the drug doses administered by the clinician and then presents the drug dosing history (bolus doses, infusion rates, and expired concentrations), the predicted drug concentrations in the effect site (past, present, and future), and the predicted drug effects including sedation, analgesia, and neuromuscular blockade.[26,85]

These "advisory" display systems potentially represent an advance compared to "passive" TCI systems in that they include not only PK predictions regarding drug concentrations but also PD predictions regarding the likelihood of certain anesthetic effects. Response surfaces constitute the fundamental basis of these display systems; that is, the information displayed is based on response surface, PD drug interaction models. Existing prototypes of these display systems actually depict two-dimensional, three-dimensional, or topographic views of response surfaces.[86,87]

These display systems can perhaps best be understood as "clinical pharmacology information technology" (IT) at the point of care. In terms of the unmet need that such systems are intended to address, the basic notion is that a great deal of information regarding the behavior of anesthetic drugs exists in the form of PK, PD, and response surface drug interaction models. The information contained within these very numerous pharmacologic models is complex and is by definition mathematically oriented; much of it appears in scientific journals that are not intended for the clinician. The information initially appears in original research publications and then is interpreted and integrated into textbooks, monographs, and reviews. In total, this massive volume of mathematically based information is so large and intimidating that it is very difficult for the clinician to digest and incorporate into daily practice. These pharmacology display systems are meant to bring this sophisticated body of clinical pharmacology information from scientific journals to the bedside by displaying the information in a readily understandable format

in real time.[86-88] That clinicians cannot solve complex polyexponential equations in their heads "on the fly" to guide rational drug administration is a basic assumption of these advisory systems.

There are at least two advisory display systems* currently in development.[86,87] Although quite different in terms of how the information is portrayed, the two systems share in common the tabular and graphic display of predicted drug concentrations and predicted drug effect, including a prediction of the synergism between hypnotics and opioids. The systems include prediction modules that allow the clinician to simulate various dosage regimens in real-time and thereby rationally choose the optimal drug administration scheme to address the dynamic nature of anesthesia and surgery. For example, as illustrated in Figure 2-20, based on information presented by the advisory systems, it is possible to navigate to positions on the drug interaction response surface that optimize the speed of recovery, among other outcomes of interest.

This concept of "navigating" a PD drug interaction response surface is a novel way of conceptualizing how best to adjust drug dosing during an anesthetic.[88] The response surface is "navigated" in the sense that various points on the surface "map" are targeted at different times to achieve the goals of the anesthetic (e.g., immobility, hemodynamic control, rapid emergence, good analgesia upon emergence). Rather than simply thinking about hypnotics and opioids in isolation, the response surface approach enables an in depth, clinically relevant understanding of the significant synergy that results when sedatives and opioids are administered together.

Figure 2-21 presents a graphical example of the concept of navigating the response surface using propofol and remifentanil as prototypes. The simulation illustrates how the clinician

---

*The author TDE has a financial conflict (potential royalties) related to the Navigator system marketed by General Electric Healthcare.

moves to different parts of the surface during different phases of the anesthetic to match drug effect to the prevailing surgical conditions. The notion of integrating PD drug interaction models with PK models to select optimal drug combinations through simulation has been the focus of considerable investigation in recent years. Optimal concentration targets for propofol and remifentanil in combination for the provision of TIVA have been proposed.[25,26,89,90] Similar *in silico* approaches have also been used to identify the optimal combination of opioids and volatile anesthetics using sevoflurane and remifentanil as prototypes.[85,91] Based on the PK-PD models available for other opioids and volatile agents, it appears feasible to develop optimal concentration targets (and dosage schemes)

for nearly any combination of the various opioids and inhalation agents.[92]

The ability to simulate various "navigation" decisions immediately before they are implemented (i.e., to explore the clinical consequences of a proposed change in therapy) is a key advance that these display systems potentially bring to clinical care. Pharmacology display systems can be likened to the "heads-up" display systems frequently employed as a navigational aid to pilots in commercial and military aircraft. Applying the aviation analogy to anesthesia, display systems can potentially provide increased "situational awareness," "waypoints" to fly toward, and a smooth "glide-path" to landing.

There are obvious challenges to be overcome before these display systems can be adopted into clinical practice. Their utility in terms of improved clinical outcomes (e.g., faster recovery, improved analgesia on emergence) and/or user acceptance (e.g., decreased physician workload) must be satisfactorily demonstrated in clinical testing. Preliminary evidence suggests that the models displayed by these systems perform reasonably well, but much work remains to be done.[85,90] An additional barrier to implementation of these advisory systems is the typical clinician's level of understanding regarding these complex models. Education and training will likely be necessary for the clinician to embrace the technology.

Although it is too early to predict what role clinical pharmacology display technology might play in future anesthesia practice, the concept is certainly an exciting area with some potential to bring more sophisticated clinical pharmacology knowledge to the point of care. In the future, real-time display of predicted pharmacokinetics and pharmacodynamics of anesthetic drugs might be found alongside traditional physiologic vital sign monitors.[11,86] The pharmacokinetic component of these systems has already been widely implemented in the form of "passive" TCI systems.

Propofol Measurement in Expired Gas

The ability to measure in real time the concentration of volatile anesthetics in the expired gas of anesthetized patients has

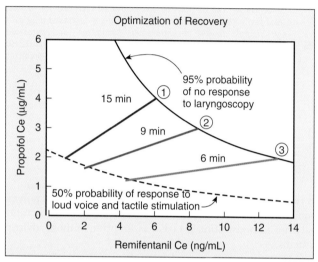

Figure 2-20 A simulation exploring the recovery times associated with different combinations of propofol and remifentanil for a 10-hour intravenous anesthetic. The plot is a topographic view of a PD drug interaction response surface for propofol and remifentanil. The isoboles represent the combinations of the two drugs that produce a 95% probability of no response to laryngoscopy *(solid line)* and a 50% probability of response to "shout and shake" *(dotted line)*. The lines (numbered 1, 2, and 3) between the isoboles show the time required to move from "anesthesia" to "awake" after stopping 10-hour infusions. See the accompanying text for a detailed explanation. The simulations were conducted with PK-PD parameter estimates from the literature.[26,90,112,116]

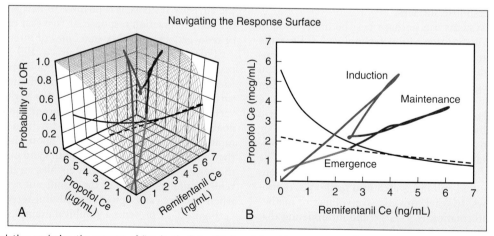

Figure 2-21 A simulation exploring the concept of "navigating" the PD drug interaction response surface. This simulation presents the same information as in Figure 2-18 except that the data are plotted on a three-dimensional response surface **(A)** and a 2-dimensional topographical view of the response surface **(B)**. The three phases of the anesthetic are shown as colored lines. The isoboles represent the combinations of the two drugs that produce a 50% probability of no response to direct laryngoscopy *(solid line)* and "shout and shake" *(dotted line)*. See the accompanying text for a detailed explanation. *LOR,* Loss of responsiveness; *Ce,* effect site.

been viewed as a significant advantage of the inhalation anesthesia approach because it enables drug administration in the concentration domain (see Figure 2-2). Recent work by several laboratories has shown that it might be possible to develop a device that measures the concentration of propofol in expired gas.[93]

The feasibility of the concept was first demonstrated using a variation of mass spectrometry known as proton transfer reaction mass spectrometry that can detect propofol in minute amounts (parts per billion by volume) in the expired breath of anesthetized patients.[94] More recently, several groups have further refined the technology using similar techniques.[95,96] Preliminary results suggest that the overall concept and technique are indeed promising and could have far reaching implications in anesthesia research and practice.[93] For example, real-time measurement of propofol concentration could replace the need for taking arterial blood samples during research studies in which the concentration of propofol must be controlled. Similarly, the online measured propofol concentration could replace or refine the use of TCI systems to deliver propofol. Finally, it is conceivable that real time propofol measurement could be used as the control variable for the closed loop, automated infusion of propofol.

There are many obstacles to be overcome before the technology moves into mainstream clinical practice. For example, the propofol versus time waveform obtained with the current technology is not ideal because it can be difficult to identify the end-tidal portion of the waveform. In addition, there is a significant delay between peak propofol concentration as determined by PK simulation (after a bolus injection) and the detection of peak propofol concentration in expired gas using the current technology.[97,98]

KEY POINTS

- Compared to other therapeutic areas, the pharmacology of anesthesia is unique because of the low therapeutic indices of anesthetic agents (a safety issue), and because anesthesiologists must predict the temporal profile of drug effect with great accuracy and precision (an efficiency issue).
- Clinical pharmacology is the branch of pharmacology concerned with the safe and effective use of drugs and includes pharmacokinetics and pharmacodynamics. Grounded in the principles of clinical pharmacology, posology is the science of drug dosage ("dosology"). The ultimate goal of clinical pharmacology is to provide the scientific foundation for rational posology (i.e., What is the right dose for my patient?).
- Pharmacokinetics, simply described as "what the body does to the drug," is the study of the relationship between drug dose and drug concentrations produced over time (i.e., the dose-concentration relationship).
- Pharmacodynamics, simply described as "what the drug does to the body," is the study of the relationship between drug concentrations and drug effects (i.e., the concentration-effect relationship).
- The "biophase" is the theoretic site of drug action or "effect site" (e.g., target cells and receptors within the brain, neuromuscular junction, spinal cord, and so on). It is important to consider predicted drug concentrations in the biophase (and not just the plasma) because most drugs do not exert their effect in the bloodstream and thus plasma concentrations usually do not correlate well with drug effects, especially during non–steady-state conditions (e.g., after a bolus injection or an infusion rate change).
- Because anesthetics are rarely administered alone (i.e., modern anesthesia usually involves at least a two-drug combination consisting of an hypnotic and an analgesic), the study of drug interactions is an important part of clinical pharmacology. Most anesthetics commonly used in combination, such as remifentanil and propofol, interact in a synergistic way so that much less of each drug is required (compared to doses necessary when the drugs are used alone).
- Pharmacokinetic-pharmacodynamic models are simplified versions of pharmacologic reality. These models are mathematical expressions of the relationship between drug dose and concentration (pharmacokinetics), and drug concentration and effect (pharmacodynamics).
- Pharmacokinetic-pharmacodynamic models are built by fitting appropriately shaped equations to actual experimental data using non-linear regression techniques. Although pharmacologic model building is a mathematical exercise, the models can be readily understood by considering them schematically and graphically.
- The clinical implications of pharmacokinetic-pharmacodynamic models can be easily grasped and conveyed through the use of computer simulation. A proposed dosing scheme can be "input" into a pharmacokinetic-pharmacodynamic model, producing a "picture" of the predicted drug levels and drug effects. These computer simulations (i.e., *in silico* experiments) are intuitively understandable and are readily applied to clinical situations.
- A limited set of straightforward simulations form the foundation upon which the answers to many routine anesthesia posology questions are based. These fundamental simulations explore bolus front- and back-end kinetics, infusion front-end kinetics, infusion back-end kinetics (i.e., the context sensitive half-time), the influence of loading doses, special populations, and a second drug.
- TCI devices represent an important advance in drug delivery technology. By coding a pharmacokinetic model into a computer program and linking it to an electronic pump, drug delivery according to the drug's specific pharmacokinetic profile can be achieved. The TCI user designates a plasma or effect site concentration rather than an infusion rate; the TCI system then computes the appropriate infusion rates based on the kinetic model.
- Response surface models are a sophisticated method to characterize pharmacodynamic drug interactions. When integrated with pharmacokinetic information, response surface models can be used to identify target concentrations that optimize certain outcomes of interest such as the speed of recovery. The concept of "navigating" a pharmacodynamic drug interaction response surface is a novel way of conceptualizing how best to adjust drug dosages during an anesthetic.

Key References

Hughes MA, Glass PS, Jacobs JR. Context-sensitive half-time in multicompartment pharmacokinetic models for intravenous anesthetic drugs. *Anesthesiology.* 1992;76:334-341. This important paper provided the name (i.e., the context sensitive half-time) for the new simulation technique originally put forward by Shafer and Varvel.[7] The simulation study first extended the concept to the sedative-hypnotics. (Ref. 6)

Kern SE, Xie G, White JL, et al. A response surface analysis of propofol-remifentanil pharmacodynamic interaction in volunteers. *Anesthesiology.* 2004;100:1373-1381. This modeling study was an early description of a pharmacodynamic response surface interaction model for propofol and remifentanil that could be used for total intravenous anesthesia dose optimization through simulation. (Ref. 26)

Minto CF, Schnider TW, Shafer SL. Pharmacokinetics and pharmacodynamics of remifentanil. II. Model application. *Anesthesiology.* 1997;86:24-33. This clinical paper illustrated the clinical utility of modern pharmacologic modeling simulation techniques in understanding drug behavior for the new opioid remifentanil. (Ref. 74)

Minto CF, Schnider TW, Short TG, et al. Response surface model for anesthetic drug interactions. *Anesthesiology.* 2000;92:1603-1616. This theoretical paper introduced the concept of response surface modeling to modern anesthesia practice. (Ref. 29)

Shafer SL, Varvel JR. Pharmacokinetics, pharmacodynamics, and rational opioid selection. *Anesthesiology.* 1991;74:53-63. Using the fentanyl congeners as examples, this landmark paper first described the simulation techniques that would ultimately come to be known as the context sensitive half-time and the 20%-80% decrement times. The simulation study also demonstrated the important differences in bolus *versus* infusion kinetic behavior. (Ref. 7)

Shafer SL, Varvel JR, Aziz N, et al. Pharmacokinetics of fentanyl administered by computer-controlled infusion pump. *Anesthesiology.* 1990;73:1091-1102. This paper was one of the first descriptions of the use of target-controlled infusion technology in anesthesia. (Ref. 99)

Sheiner BL, Beal SL. Evaluation of methods for estimating population pharmacokinetic parameters. II. Biexponential model and experimental pharmacokinetic data. *J Pharmacokinet Biopharm.* 1981;9:635-651. This landmark paper was one of the first examples of the use of NONMEM, a mixed-effects pharmacologic modeling software package that eventually emerged as a standard in population pharmacologic modeling. (Ref. 44)

Sheiner LB, Stanski DR, Vozeh S, et al. Simultaneous modeling of pharmacokinetics and pharmacodynamics: application to d-tubocurarine. *Clin Pharmacol Ther.* 1979;25:358-371. This theoretical paper using curare as the prototype example proposed the use of an effect compartment to model non-steady state pharmacodynamic data. The biophase concept revolutionized pharmacologic modeling techniques in anesthesiology and other disciplines. (Ref. 9)

References

1. Wagner JG. History of pharmacokinetics. *Pharmacol Ther.* 1981;12:537-562.
2. Csajka C, Verotta D. Pharmacokinetic-pharmacodynamic modelling: history and perspectives. *J Pharmacokinet Pharmacodyn.* 2006;33:227-279.
3. Atkinson AJ Jr, Lalonde RL. Introduction of quantitative methods in pharmacology and clinical pharmacology: a historical overview. *Clin Pharmacol Ther.* 2007;82:3-6.
4. Egan TD. Is anesthesiology going soft? Trends in fragile pharmacology. *Anesthesiology.* 2009;111:229-230.
5. Fisher DM. (Almost) everything you learned about pharmacokinetics was (somewhat) wrong! [editorial; comment]. *Anesth Analg.* 1996;83:901-903.
6. Hughes MA, Glass PS, Jacobs JR. Context-sensitive half-time in multicompartment pharmacokinetic models for intravenous anesthetic drugs [see comments]. *Anesthesiology.* 1992;76:334-341.
7. Shafer SL, Varvel JR. Pharmacokinetics, pharmacodynamics, and rational opioid selection. *Anesthesiology.* 1991;74:53-63.
8. Youngs EJ, Shafer SL. Pharmacokinetic parameters relevant to recovery from opioids. *Anesthesiology.* 1994;81:833-842.
9. Sheiner LB, Stanski DR, Vozeh S, Miller RD, Ham J. Simultaneous modeling of pharmacokinetics and pharmacodynamics: application to d-tubocurarine. *Clin Pharmacol Ther.* 1979;25:358-371.
10. Holford NH, Sheiner LB. Understanding the dose-effect relationship: clinical application of pharmacokinetic-pharmacodynamic models. *Clin Pharmacokinet.* 1981;6:429-453.
11. Struys MM, De Smet T, Mortier EP. Simulated drug administration: an emerging tool for teaching clinical pharmacology during anesthesiology training. *Clin Pharmacol Ther.* 2008;84:170-174.
12. Egan TD. Target-controlled drug delivery: progress toward an intravenous "vaporizer" and automated anesthetic administration. *Anesthesiology.* 2003;99:1214-1219.
13. Syroid ND, Agutter J, Drews FA, et al. Development and evaluation of a graphical anesthesia drug display. *Anesthesiology.* 2002;96:565-575.
14. Struys MM, Sahinovic M, Lichtenbelt BJ, Vereecke HE, Absalom AR. Optimizing intravenous drug administration by applying pharmacokinetic/pharmacodynamic concepts. *Br J Anaesth.* 2011;107:38-47.
15. Minto CF, Schnider TW. Contributions of PK/PD modeling to intravenous anesthesia. *Clin Pharmacol Ther.* 2008;84:27-38.
16. Egan TD, Shafer SL. Target-controlled infusions for intravenous anesthetics: surfing USA not! *Anesthesiology.* 2003;99:1039-1041.
17. Honig P. The value and future of clinical pharmacology. *Clin Pharmacol Ther.* 2007;81:17-18.
18. Wagner JG. Linear pharmacokinetic equations allowing direct calculation of many needed pharmacokinetic parameters from the coefficients and exponents of polyexponential equations which have been fitted to the data. *J Pharmacokinet Biopharm.* 1976;4:443-467.
19. Austin KL, Stapleton JV, Mather LE. Relationship between blood meperidine concentrations and analgesic response: a preliminary report. *Anesthesiology.* 1980;53:460-466.
20. Stanski DR, Ham J, Miller RD, Sheiner LB. Pharmacokinetics and pharmacodynamics of d-tubocurarine during nitrous oxide-narcotic and halothane anesthesia in man. *Anesthesiology.* 1979;51:235-241.
21. Hull CJ, Van Beem HB, McLeod K, Sibbald A, Watson MJ. A pharmacodynamic model for pancuronium. *Br J Anaesth.* 1978;50:1113-1123.
22. Verotta D, Sheiner LB. Simultaneous modeling of pharmacokinetics and pharmacodynamics: an improved algorithm. *Comput Appl Biosci.* 1987;3:345-349.
23. Hendrickx JF, Eger EI 2nd, Sonner JM, Shafer SL. Is synergy the rule? A review of anesthetic interactions producing hypnosis and immobility. *Anesth Analg.* 2008;107:494-506.
24. Stanski DR, Shafer SL. Quantifying anesthetic drug interaction. Implications for drug dosing [editorial; comment]. *Anesthesiology.* 1995;83:1-5.
25. Bouillon TW, Bruhn J, Radulescu L, et al. Pharmacodynamic interaction between propofol and remifentanil regarding hypnosis, tolerance of laryngoscopy, bispectral index, and electroencephalographic approximate entropy. *Anesthesiology.* 2004;100:1353-1372.
26. Kern SE, Xie G, White JL, Egan TD. A response surface analysis of propofol-remifentanil pharmacodynamic interaction in volunteers. *Anesthesiology.* 2004;100:1373-1381.
27. Bouillon T, Bruhn J, Radu-Radulescu L, Bertaccini E, Park S, Shafer S. Non-steady state analysis of the pharmacokinetic interaction between propofol and remifentanil. *Anesthesiology.* 2002;97:1350-1362.
28. Tallarida RJ. An overview of drug combination analysis with isobolograms. *J Pharmacol Exp Ther.* 2006;319:1-7.
29. Minto CF, Schnider TW, Short TG, Gregg KM, Gentilini A, Shafer SL. Response surface model for anesthetic drug interactions. *Anesthesiology.* 2000;92:1603-1616.
30. Lang E, Kapila A, Shlugman D, Hoke JF, Sebel PS, Glass PS. Reduction of isoflurane minimal alveolar concentration by remifentanil. *Anesthesiology.* 1996;85:721-728.
31. McEwan AI, Smith C, Dyar O, Goodman D, Smith LR, Glass PS. Isoflurane minimum alveolar concentration reduction by fentanyl. *Anesthesiology.* 1993;78:864-869.
32. Boxenbaum H. Pharmacokinetics: philosophy of modeling. *Drug Metab Rev.* 1992;24:89-120.

33. Box GE. Science and statistics. *J Amer Statistical Assoc.* 1976;71: 791-799.
34. Derendorf H, Lesko LJ, Chaikin P, et al. Pharmacokinetic/pharmacodynamic modeling in drug research and development. *J Clin Pharmacol.* 2000;40:1399-1418.
35. Sheiner LB. The population approach to pharmacokinetic data analysis: rationale and standard data analysis methods. *Drug Metab Rev.* 1984;15:153-171.
36. Hermann DJ, Egan TD, Muir KT. Influence of arteriovenous sampling on remifentanil pharmacokinetics and pharmacodynamics. *Clin Pharmacol Ther.* 1999;65:511-518.
37. Chiou WL. The phenomenon and rationale of marked dependence of drug concentration on blood sampling site. Implications in pharmacokinetics, pharmacodynamics, toxicology and therapeutics (Part II). *Clin Pharmacokinet.* 1989;17:275-290.
38. Egan TD. Pharmacokinetics and rational intravenous drug selection and administration in anesthesia. In: Lake CL, Rice LJ, Sperry RJ, eds. *Advances in Anesthesia.* St Louis: Mosby;1995: 363-388.
39. Meibohm B, Derendorf H. Basic concepts of pharmacokinetic/pharmacodynamic (PK/PD) modelling. *Int J Clin Pharmacol Ther.* 1997;35:401-413.
40. Sheiner LB. Analysis of pharmacokinetic data using parametric models–1: regression models. *J Pharmacokinet Biopharm.* 1984;12: 93-117.
41. Motulsky HJ, Ransnas LA. Fitting curves to data using nonlinear regression: a practical and nonmathematical review. *FASEB J.* 1987;1:365-374.
42. Sheiner LB. Analysis of pharmacokinetic data using parametric models. II. Point estimates of an individual's parameters. *J Pharmacokinet Biopharm.* 1985;13:515-540.
43. Sheiner LB, Beal SL. Evaluation of methods for estimating population pharmacokinetics parameters. I. Michaelis-Menten model: routine clinical pharmacokinetic data. *J Pharmacokinet Biopharm.* 1980;8:553-571.
44. Sheiner BL, Beal SL. Evaluation of methods for estimating population pharmacokinetics parameters. II. Biexponential model and experimental pharmacokinetic data. *J Pharmacokinet Biopharm.* 1981;9:635-651.
45. Maitre PO, Vozeh S, Heykants J, Thomson DA, Stanski DR. Population pharmacokinetics of alfentanil: the average dose-plasma concentration relationship and interindividual variability in patients. *Anesthesiology.* 1987;66:3-12.
46. Mandema JW, Verotta D, Sheiner LB. Building population pharmacokinetic–pharmacodynamic models. I. Models for covariate effects. *J Pharmacokinet Biopharm.* 1992;20:511-528.
47. Henthorn TK, Krejcie TC, Avram MJ. Early drug distribution: a generally neglected aspect of pharmacokinetics of particular relevance to intravenously administered anesthetic agents. *Clin Pharmacol Ther.* 2008;84:18-22.
48. Krejcie TC, Henthorn TK, Shanks CA, Avram MJ. A recirculatory pharmacokinetic model describing the circulatory mixing, tissue distribution and elimination of antipyrine in dogs. *J Pharmacol Exp Ther.* 1994;269:609-616.
49. Krejcie TC, Avram MJ. What determines anesthetic induction dose? It's the front-end kinetics, doctor! *Anesth Analg.* 1999;89:541-544.
50. Henthorn TK, Krejcie TC, Avram MJ. The relationship between alfentanil distribution kinetics and cardiac output. *Clin Pharmacol Ther.* 1992;52:190-196.
51. Waters CM, Avram MJ, Krejcie TC, Henthorn TK. Uptake of fentanyl in pulmonary endothelium. *J Pharmacol Exp Ther.* 1999;288: 157-163.
52. Wada DR, Bjorkman S, Ebling WF, Harashima H, Harapat SR, Stanski DR. Computer simulation of the effects of alterations in blood flows and body composition on thiopental pharmacokinetics in humans. *Anesthesiology.* 1997;87:884-899.
53. Bjorkman S, Wada DR, Stanski DR, Ebling WF. Comparative physiological pharmacokinetics of fentanyl and alfentanil in rats and humans based on parametric single-tissue models. *J Pharmacokinet Biopharm.* 1994;22:381-410.
54. Bjorkman S, Wada DR, Stanski DR. Application of physiologic models to predict the influence of changes in body composition and blood flows on the pharmacokinetics of fentanyl and alfentanil in patients. *Anesthesiology.* 1998;88:657-667.
55. Weiss M, Krejcie TC, Avram MJ. A minimal physiological model of thiopental distribution kinetics based on a multiple indicator approach. *Drug Metab Dispos.* 2007;35:1525-1532.
56. Avram MJ, Krejcie TC, Henthorn TK. The relationship of age to the pharmacokinetics of early drug distribution: the concurrent disposition of thiopental and indocyanine green [see comments]. *Anesthesiology.* 1990;72:403-411.
57. Avram MJ, Krejcie TC, Henthorn TK, Niemann CU. Beta-adrenergic blockade affects initial drug distribution due to decreased cardiac output and altered blood flow distribution. *J Pharmacol Exp Ther.* 2004;311:617-624.
58. Ariens EJ. Stereochemistry, a basis for sophisticated nonsense in pharmacokinetics and clinical pharmacology. *Eur J Clin Pharmacol.* 1984;26:663-668.
59. Garay AS. Molecular chirality of life and intrinsic chirality of matter. *Nature.* 1978;271:186.
60. Lee EJ, Williams KM. Chirality. Clinical pharmacokinetic and pharmacodynamic considerations. *Clin Pharmacokinet.* 1990;18:339-345.
61. Egan TD. Stereochemistry and anesthetic pharmacology: joining hands with the medicinal chemists. *Anesth Analg.* 1996;83: 447-450.
62. Nation RL. Chirality in new drug development. Clinical pharmacokinetic considerations. *Clin Pharmacokinet.* 1994;27: 249-255.
63. Ariens EJ. Racemic therapeutics—ethical and regulatory aspects. *Eur J Clin Pharmacol.* 1991;41:89-93.
64. Lotsch J, Geisslinger G. Misestimating the role of an active metabolite when modeling the effects after administration of the parent compound only. *Clin Pharmacol Ther.* 2006;80: 95-97.
65. Atkinson AJ Jr, Strong JM. Effect of active drug metabolites on plasma level-response correlations. *J Pharmacokinet Biopharm.* 1977; 5:95-109.
66. Osborne R, Joel S, Grebenik K, Trew D, Slevin M. The pharmacokinetics of morphine and morphine glucuronides in kidney failure. *Clin Pharmacol Ther.* 1993;54:158-167.
67. Portenoy RK, Foley KM, Stulman J, et al. Plasma morphine and morphine-6-glucuronide during chronic morphine therapy for cancer pain: plasma profiles, steady-state concentrations and the consequences of renal failure. *Pain.* 1991;47:13-19.
68. Angst MS, Buhrer M, Lotsch J. Insidious intoxication after morphine treatment in renal failure: delayed onset of morphine-6-glucuronide action. *Anesthesiology.* 2000;92:1473-1476.
69. Lotsch J, Skarke C, Schmidt H, Liefhold J, Geisslinger G. Pharmacokinetic modeling to predict morphine and morphine-6-glucuronide plasma concentrations in healthy young volunteers. *Clin Pharmacol Ther.* 2002;72:151-162.
70. Levy G. Predicting effective drug concentrations for individual patients. Determinants of pharmacodynamic variability. *Clin Pharmacokinet.* 1998;34:323-333.
71. Bradley JS, Garonzik SM, Forrest A, Bhavnani SM. Pharmacokinetics, pharmacodynamics, and Monte Carlo simulation: selecting the best antimicrobial dose to treat an infection. *Pediatr Infect Dis J.* 2010;29:1043-1046.
72. Shafer SL, Stanski DR. Improving the clinical utility of anesthetic drug pharmacokinetics [editorial; comment]. *Anesthesiology.* 1992;76: 327-330.
73. Ebling WF, Lee EN, Stanski DR. Understanding pharmacokinetics and pharmacodynamics through computer stimulation: I. The comparative clinical profiles of fentanyl and alfentanil. *Anesthesiology.* 1990;72:650-658.
74. Minto CF, Schnider TW, Shafer SL. Pharmacokinetics and pharmacodynamics of remifentanil. II. Model application. *Anesthesiology.* 1997;86:24-33.
75. Egan TD. Intravenous drug delivery systems: toward an intravenous "vaporizer". *J Clin Anesth.* 1996;8:(Suppl 3)8S-14S.
76. Kenny GN. Target-controlled anaesthesia: concepts and first clinical experiences. *Eur J Anaesthesiol Suppl.* 1997;15:29-31.
77. Schwilden H. A general method for calculating the dosage scheme in linear pharmacokinetics. *Eur J Clin Pharmacol.* 1981;20:379-386.
78. Jacobs JR. Algorithm for optimal linear model-based control with application to pharmacokinetic model-driven drug delivery. *IEEE Trans Biomed Eng.* 1990;37:107-109.

79. Jacobs JR, Williams EA. Algorithm to control "effect compartment" drug concentrations in pharmacokinetic model-driven drug delivery. *IEEE Trans Biomed Eng*. 1993;40:993-999.

80. Shafer SL, Gregg KM. Algorithms to rapidly achieve and maintain stable drug concentrations at the site of drug effect with a computer-controlled infusion pump. *J Pharmacokinet Biopharm*. 1992;20:147-169.

81. Van Poucke GE, Bravo LJ, Shafer SL. Target controlled infusions: targeting the effect site while limiting peak plasma concentration. *IEEE Trans Biomed Eng*. 2004;51:1869-1875.

82. Leslie K, Clavisi O, Hargrove J. Target-controlled infusion versus manually-controlled infusion of propofol for general anaesthesia or sedation in adults. *Cochrane Database Syst Rev*. 2008:CD006059.

83. Absalom AR, Mani V, De Smet T, Struys MM. Pharmacokinetic models for propofol–defining and illuminating the devil in the detail. *Br J Anaesth*. 2009;103:26-37.

84. Motamed C, Devys JM, Debaene B, Billard V. Influence of real-time Bayesian forecasting of pharmacokinetic parameters on the precision of a rocuronium target-controlled infusion. *Eur J Clin Pharmacol*. 2012; 68:1025-1031.

85. Johnson KB, Syroid ND, Gupta DK, et al. An evaluation of remifentanil-sevoflurane response surface models in patients emerging from anesthesia: model improvement using effect-site sevoflurane concentrations. *Anesth Analg*. 2010;111:387-394.

86. Gin T. Clinical pharmacology on display. *Anesth Analg*. 2010;111: 256-258.

87. Kennedy RR. Seeing the future of anesthesia drug dosing: moving the art of anesthesia from impressionism to realism. *Anesth Analg*. 2010;111:252-255.

88. Egan TD, Minto CF. Pharmacodynamic drug interactions in anesthesia. In: Evers AS, Maze M, Kharasch ED, eds. *Anesthetic Pharmacology: Basic Principles and Clinical Practice*. 2nd ed. Cambridge: Cambridge University Press; 2011:147-165.

89. Vuyk J, Mertens MJ, Olofsen E, Burm AG, Bovill JG. Propofol anesthesia and rational opioid selection: determination of optimal EC50-EC95 propofol-opioid concentrations that assure adequate anesthesia and a rapid return of consciousness. *Anesthesiology*. 1997; 87:1549-1562.

90. Johnson KB, Syroid ND, Gupta DK, et al. An evaluation of remifentanil propofol response surfaces for loss of responsiveness, loss of response to surrogates of painful stimuli and laryngoscopy in patients undergoing elective surgery. *Anesth Analg*. 2008;106: 471-479.

91. Manyam SC, Gupta DK, Johnson KB, et al. Opioid-volatile anesthetic synergy: a response surface model with remifentanil and sevoflurane as prototypes. *Anesthesiology*. 2006;105:267-278.

92. Syroid ND, Johnson KB, Pace NL, et al. Response surface model predictions of emergence and response to pain in the recovery room: an evaluation of patients emerging from an isoflurane and fentanyl anesthetic. *Anesth Analg*. 2010;111:380-386.

93. Kharasch ED. Every breath you take, we'll be watching you. *Anesthesiology*. 2007;106:652-654.

94. Harrison GR, Critchley AD, Mayhew CA, Thompson JM. Real-time breath monitoring of propofol and its volatile metabolites during surgery using a novel mass spectrometric technique: a feasibility study. *Br J Anaesth*. 2003;91:797-799.

95. Hornuss C, Praun S, Villinger J, et al. Real-time monitoring of propofol in expired air in humans undergoing total intravenous anesthesia. *Anesthesiology*. 2007;106:665-674.

96. Takita A, Masui K, Kazama T. On-line monitoring of end-tidal propofol concentration in anesthetized patients. *Anesthesiology*. 2007;106:659-664.

97. Grossherr M, Hengstenberg A, Meier T, et al. Propofol concentration in exhaled air and arterial plasma in mechanically ventilated patients undergoing cardiac surgery. *Br J Anaesth*. 2009;102:608-613.

98. Miekisch W, Fuchs P, Kamysek S, Neumann C, Schubert JK. Assessment of propofol concentrations in human breath and blood by means of HS-SPME-GC-MS. *Clin Chim Acta*. 2008; 395:32-37.

99. Shafer SL, Varvel JR, Aziz N, Scott JC. Pharmacokinetics of fentanyl administered by computer-controlled infusion pump. *Anesthesiology*. 1990;73:1091-1102.

100. Scott JC, Stanski DR. Decreased fentanyl and alfentanil dose requirements with age. A simultaneous pharmacokinetic and pharmacodynamic evaluation. *J Pharmacol Exp Ther*. 1987; 240:159-166.

101. Drover DR, Angst MS, Valle M, et al. Input characteristics and bioavailability after administration of immediate and a new extended-release formulation of hydromorphone in healthy volunteers. *Anesthesiology*. 2002;97:827-836.

102. Egan TD, Minto CF, Hermann DJ, Barr J, Muir KT, Shafer SL. Remifentanil versus alfentanil: comparative pharmacokinetics and pharmacodynamics in healthy adult male volunteers [published erratum appears in Anesthesiology 1996 Sep;85(3):695]. *Anesthesiology*. 1996;84:821-833.

103. Gepts E, Shafer SL, Camu F, et al. Linearity of pharmacokinetics and model estimation of sufentanil. *Anesthesiology*. 1995;83:1194-1204.

104. Hill JL, Zacny JP. Comparing the subjective, psychomotor, and physiological effects of intravenous hydromorphone and morphine in healthy volunteers. *Psychopharmacology (Berl)*. 2000;152:31-39.

105. Lotsch J, Skarke C, Schmidt H, Grosch S, Geisslinger G. The transfer half-life of morphine-6-glucuronide from plasma to effect site assessed by pupil size measurement in healthy volunteers. *Anesthesiology*. 2001;95:1329-1338.

106. Scott JC, Cooke JE, Stanski DR. Electroencephalographic quantitation of opioid effect: comparative pharmacodynamics of fentanyl and sufentanil. *Anesthesiology*. 1991;74:34-42.

107. Arden JR, Holley FO, Stanski DR. Increased sensitivity to etomidate in the elderly: initial distribution versus altered brain response. *Anesthesiology*. 1986;65:19-27.

108. Buhrer M, Maitre PO, Crevoisier C, Stanski DR. Electroencephalographic effects of benzodiazepines. II. Pharmacodynamic modeling of the electroencephalographic effects of midazolam and diazepam. *Clin Pharmacol Ther*. 1990;48:555-567.

109. Domino EF, Domino SE, Smith RE, et al. Ketamine kinetics in unmedicated and diazepam-premedicated subjects. *Clin Pharmacol Ther*. 1984;36:645-653.

110. Dyck JB, Maze M, Haack C, Vuorilehto L, Shafer SL. The pharmacokinetics and hemodynamic effects of intravenous and intramuscular dexmedetomidine hydrochloride in adult human volunteers. *Anesthesiology*. 1993;78:813-820.

111. Greenblatt DJ, Ehrenberg BL, Gunderman J, et al. Pharmacokinetic and electroencephalographic study of intravenous diazepam, midazolam, and placebo. *Clin Pharmacol Ther*. 1989;45:356-365.

112. Schnider TW, Minto CF, Gambus PL, et al. The influence of method of administration and covariates on the pharmacokinetics of propofol in adult volunteers. *Anesthesiology*. 1998;88:1170-1182.

113. Stanski DR, Maitre PO. Population pharmacokinetics and pharmacodynamics of thiopental: the effect of age revisited. *Anesthesiology*. 1990;72:412-422.

114. Wright PM, McCarthy G, Szenohradszky J, Sharma ML, Caldwell JE. Influence of chronic phenytoin administration on the pharmacokinetics and pharmacodynamics of vecuronium. *Anesthesiology*. 2004;100:626-633.

115. Egan TD, Huizinga B, Gupta SK, et al. Remifentanil pharmacokinetics in obese versus lean patients [see comments]. *Anesthesiology*. 1998;89:562-573.

116. Minto CF, Schnider TW, Egan TD, et al. Influence of age and gender on the pharmacokinetics and pharmacodynamics of remifentanil. I. Model development. *Anesthesiology*. 1997;86:10-23.

Chapter 3

PHARMACOKINETICS OF INHALED ANESTHETICS

Andrew E. Hudson and Hugh C. Hemmings, Jr.

HISTORICAL PERSPECTIVE

The discovery of drugs with anesthetic properties was a landmark event in the history of pharmacology, medicine, and even civilization, in that it made otherwise painful surgical treatments of disease possible. Without a means of providing anesthesia, it was impossible for the modern discipline of surgery to develop. Before the discovery of anesthetic drugs, surgical intervention was limited to simple operations that could be completed quickly. Inhaled anesthetics have had an immense impact on modern medicine and history.

The first anesthetics were administered by inhalation, before the evolution of techniques for intravenous drug administration, and anesthetics remain the most important class of inhaled drugs (barring oxygen of course). Diethyl ether was first used as a general anesthetic by Long in 1842 and was independently discovered by Morton in 1846. Morton's public demonstration of the anesthetic properties of ether at the Massachusetts General Hospital on October 16, 1846 is one of the most important moments in the history of medicine and is now commemorated as Ether Day in Boston; Long's contribution is honored as National Doctor's Day in the United States, marking the day that he administered the first ether anesthetic for surgery (March 30, 1842).

Ether remains in clinical use in developing countries given its low cost and relatively high therapeutic index, but its high volatility and explosivity limit its general use. Nitrous oxide was first used for dental analgesia by Wells in 1844, and in 1847 Simpson introduced chloroform (trichloromethane) as a nonexplosive alternative to ether. The first century of anesthesia was dominated by these drugs, of which only nitrous oxide is still widely used.[1]

Since its early origins, the practice of anesthesia has been driven by the development of techniques for the safe delivery of inhaled anesthetics, and these concepts remain important. Administration of drugs by inhalation has a number of unique and important attributes primarily due to special pharmacokinetic and chemical properties that guide the safe and effective use of inhaled anesthetics.

CLASSES OF INHALED ANESTHETICS

General anesthetics include a range of structurally diverse inhaled and injectable compounds that are defined by their ability to induce a reversible comatose state characterized by unconsciousness, amnesia, and immobility. The inhaled anesthetic drugs belong to three broad classes: ethers, alkanes, and gases (Figure 3-1). The latter classification is somewhat arbitrary as all inhaled anesthetics are delivered as gases, but gaseous anesthetics are those that normally exist as gases at standard temperature and pressure (nitrous oxide, cyclopropane, noble gases). The ethers and alkanes are volatile liquids

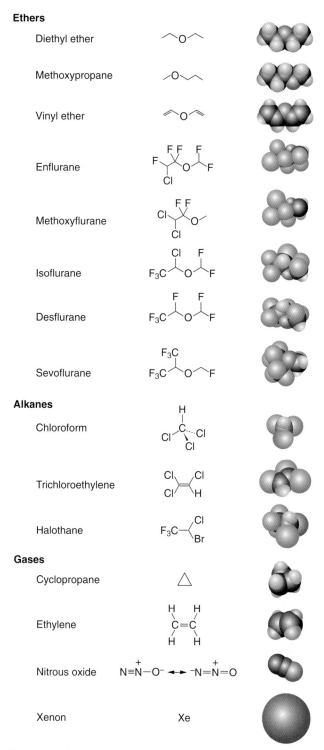

Ethers

Diethyl ether

Methoxypropane

Vinyl ether

Enflurane

Methoxyflurane

Isoflurane

Desflurane

Sevoflurane

Alkanes

Chloroform

Trichloroethylene

Halothane

Gases

Cyclopropane

Ethylene

Nitrous oxide

Xenon

Figure 3-1 Inhaled anesthetic agents by class, with chemical structure and space-filling model drawn to scale.

(i.e., they have a vapor pressure that is less than atmospheric pressure at room temperature; see later) and are delivered as vapors (the gas phase in equilibrium with the liquid phase at a given temperature; a condensable gas). The modern era of volatile anesthetics—those halogenated with fluorine—began with the synthesis of halothane (2-bromo-2-chloro-1,1,1-trifluoroethane) by Suckling in 1951, which was successfully introduced as an anesthetic in clinical trials in 1956. Subsequent attempts to minimize the adverse effects of halothane (particularly the propensity to develop hepatitis, rare but often fatal, or ventricular arrhythmias) led to the development in the 1960s by Terrell and others of a series of halogenated methyl ethyl ethers, including methoxyflurane (2,2-dichloro-1,1-difluoro-1-methoxyethane), enflurane (2-chloro-1-[difluoromethyl]-1,1,2-trifluoro-ethane), isoflurane (2-chloro-2-[difluoromethoxy]-1,1,1-trifluoro-ethane), and subsequently in the 1990s, desflurane (2-[difluoromethoxy]-1,1,1,2-tetrafluoro-ethane) and sevoflurane (1,1,1,3,3,3-hexafluoro-2-[fluoromethoxy]propane).[1]

PHYSICAL PROPERTIES

Inhaled drugs differ from intravenous drugs in that their delivery depends upon uptake into the blood by the lungs, followed by delivery to their effect sites, in the central nervous system in the case of anesthetics. The delivery of inhaled drugs to the lungs depends upon the physical properties of the drugs themselves, in particular their solubility in blood and their vapor pressure (Table 3-1).

Vapor pressure is the partial pressure of a vapor in thermodynamic equilibrium with a liquid, that is, the partial pressure at which the rate of liquid evaporation into the gaseous phase equals the rate of gaseous condensation into liquid. Vapor pressure varies nonlinearly with temperature according to the Clausius-Clapeyron relationship (Figure 3-2). The boiling point is the temperature at which the vapor pressure equals ambient atmospheric pressure. Substances that have high vapor pressures at room temperature (e.g., many of the inhaled anesthetics) are volatile. Partial pressure is the portion of the total pressure of a gaseous mixture supplied by a particular gas; for an ideal gas, this is the mole fraction of the mixture multiplied times the total pressure of the gas. Inhaled anesthetic partial pressures are commonly expressed as volume percent (vol%), which is the percent of the total volume contributed by a particular gas, or for a gas, the mole percent. At standard temperature and pressure, the volume percent times total pressure equals the partial pressure, but partial pressure changes with temperature.

The *solubility* of a gas is the amount of gas that can be dissolved homogenously into a solvent at equilibrium; it is a function of the partial pressure of the gas above the liquid solvent and the ambient temperature. Solubility depends upon the solvent; for example, polar substances tend to be more soluble in polar solvents. According to Henry's law, for a given solvent at a given temperature the amount of gas dissolved in solution is directly proportional to the partial pressure of the gas. Relative solubilities can be described according to the partition ratio (also known as the partition coefficient), defined as the ratio at equilibrium of the concentration of the dissolved gas in one solvent to the concentration of the dissolved gas in the other solvent (or in the gaseous phase). At

Table 3-1. Properties of Inhaled Anesthetics

AGENT	BOILING POINT (°C) AT 1 ATM	VAPOR PRESSURE (mmHg) AT 20°C	MAC FOR 40 YR OLD IN O$_2$	BLOOD:GAS PARTITION RATIO AT 37°C	OIL:GAS PARTITION RATIO AT 37°C
Halothane	50.2	243	0.75%	2.4	224
Enflurane	56.5	172	1.7%	1.8	97
Isoflurane	48.5	240	1.2%	1.4	98
Sevoflurane	58.5	160	2%	0.65	47
Desflurane	22.8	669	6%	0.45	19
Nitrous Oxide	−88.5	39,000	104%	0.47	1.4
Xenon	−108.1	—	60%-70%	0.14	1.9

Modified from Eger EI 2nd, Eisenkraft JB, Weiskopf RB. Metabolism of potent inhaled anesthetics. In: Eger EI 2nd, Eisenkraft JB, Weiskopf RB, eds. *The Pharmacology of Inhaled Anesthetics.* Chicago: Healthcare Press; 2003:167-176.

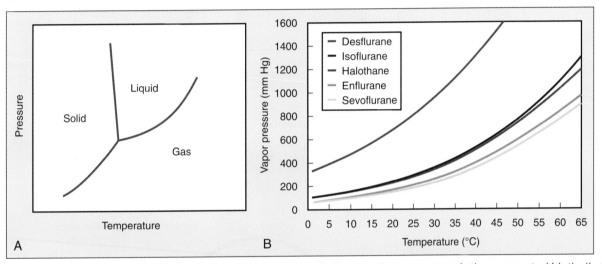

Figure 3-2 Pressure and temperature relationships. **A,** A qualitative state diagram for water. The vapor pressure is the pressure at which the liquid and gaseous phases are in equilibrium for a given temperature, as indicated by the line between the liquid and gaseous phases in the state diagram. **B,** Vapor pressure data for a number of common anesthetics. Note that the vapor pressure of desflurane is much higher at a given temperature than the vapor pressure of the other agents, and that the vapor pressure of desflurane reaches 760 mm Hg (or 1 atm) at approximately 22.8°C (its boiling point), indicating that it will boil in a warm room.

equilibrium the partial pressure of the dissolved gas in the two solvents is equal, even though the concentrations are not (Figure 3-3). The concentration of a gas in a liquid is derived by multiplying the gas partial pressure times its solubility expressed as its solvent:gas partition ratio (at standard temperature and pressure). For inhaled anesthetics, the blood:gas partition ratio is critically important to alveolar uptake. More soluble agents, such as ether or halothane, have high blood gas partition ratios and take longer to reach an equilibrium between the amount inhaled and exhaled due to their greater uptake into blood, and tissues. Conversely, less soluble agents, such as nitrous oxide and desflurane, are dissolved in lower quantities and approach equilibrium more rapidly (see later). Following Henry's law, the solubility of gases such as inhaled anesthetics in aqueous liquids increases at lower temperatures. Various tissues also have tissue-specific partition ratios that depend largely on their biochemical composition. This determines relative anesthetic uptake and concentrations in each tissue. Because of differing partition ratios, the actual concentrations can be very different between various tissues at equilibrium even though the partial pressure will eventually be the same. Figure 3-4 demonstrates that even after a 10-minute wash-in period the differences in partial pressure are pronounced.

MEASURING POTENCY (MAC)

The potency of inhaled anesthetics is commonly expressed using the concept of minimum alveolar concentration (MAC) as described by Eger and colleagues.[2] The MAC of an anesthetic vapor is the steady-state concentration at which 50% of normal (healthy, nonpregnant, adult) human subjects under standard conditions (normal body temperature, 1 atm, no other drugs) do not move in response to a defined stimulus (surgical incision; laboratory studies often substitute application of a tail clamp to rodents). Although MAC is defined in terms of a gas concentration in vol% or fractional atm at 1 atm ambient pressure, it is the partial pressure and resultant concentration at the effect site that is critical to the pharmacologic response (immobility). Thus anesthetic potency expressed in terms of alveolar partial pressure or tissue concentration is constant for a given physiologic state. MAC is expressed as a gas concentration at 1 atm ambient pressure and the vaporizer setting in volume percent that delivers an equivalent alveolar partial pressure varies with atmospheric pressure; this is significant at high altitudes where higher inspired concentrations are required to produce a given tissue partial pressure/concentration. The MAC of an inhaled agent

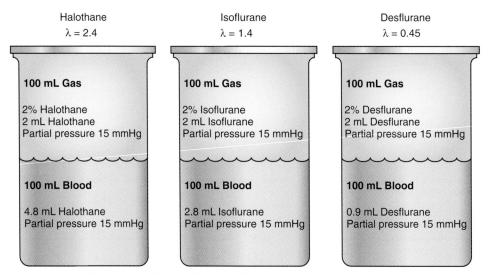

Figure 3-3 Blood:gas partitioning of inhaled anesthetics at 37°C. At equilibrium, the partial pressures of the anesthetics in the gas and liquid (blood) phases (100 mL of each) are equal (15 mmHg for 2 vol% at standard atmospheric pressure of 760 mm Hg). In contrast, blood concentrations differ depending on the drug specific blood:gas partition ratios (λ). Note that λ increases ~4% per 1°C decrease in temperature.

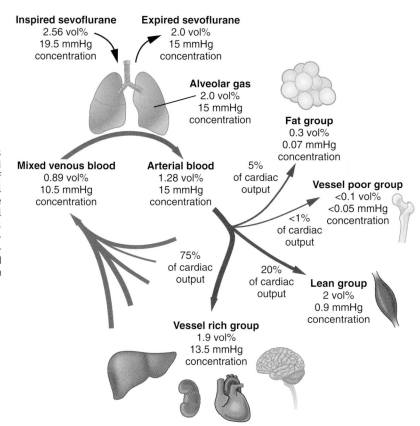

Figure 3-4 Tissue partial pressures of anesthetics. Results of a GAS-MAN simulation of a 70-kg patient administered sevoflurane for 10 minutes at 2.56 vol% in 8 L/min of 100% O_2. The delivered inspiratory and measured end-tidal concentrations of sevoflurane are shown, together with the partial pressure and concentration of anesthetic in arterial blood, mixed venous blood, the vessel rich, vessel poor, lean, and fat groups. If allowed to run until full equilibration between compartments, the partial pressures of anesthetic would equalize, while the concentrations measured as vol% will differ according to the tissue:gas partition ratios.

is analogous to the EC_{50} of intravenous agents; hence, more potent agents have lower MAC values. MAC is defined using only one behavioral component of anesthesia—the lack of a motor response (immobilization) to a painful stimulus—and reflects primarily spinal effect sites (see Chapter 10). The MAC concept has been extended to other endpoints including MAC awake (for emergence),[3] MAC BAR (blunted autonomic response), and so on.

Although MAC was originally developed as a simple method of comparing the potency of inhaled anesthetics, it has emerged as an important clinical tool. Anesthesiologists often formulate an anesthetic plan by targeting a certain MAC multiple for a given patient, procedure, and anesthetic technique (although strictly speaking MAC is a single point on a nonlinear curve, so there are limitations to this approach). The pervasive influence of MAC in the daily practice of anesthesia makes it one of the most important unifying concepts in anesthetic pharmacology. Further consideration of the factors that influence MAC (e.g., age, body temperature, adjuvant drugs, genetics) is provided in Chapter 10.

MONITORING DRUG DELIVERY

Differences Between Inhalational and Intravenous Anesthetic Delivery

Administering volatile anesthetics by inhalation using a calibrated vaporizer affords several fundamental advantages compared to intravenous delivery (Figure 3-5). Because uptake of inhaled anesthetic diminishes as equilibrium between alveolar and pulmonary venous partial pressures is approached, the vaporizer setting reflects the anesthetic concentration in blood and therefore at the site of drug action due to rapid uptake in well perfused tissues (like the central nervous system). This enables accurate administration of the inhaled drug to a target concentration (with an upper limit above which the partial pressure cannot rise). Moreover, the end-expired concentration can be measured and confirmed by respiratory gas monitoring, ensuring that the targeted concentration has been achieved (pharmacokinetic exactness). The pharmacodynamic significance of the measured concentration is standardized in terms of MAC, providing pharmacodynamic exactness.

In contrast, direct access to the circulation as required in intravenous anesthesia delivery does not prevent indefinite uptake of drug (see Figure 3-5, lower panel). Without the aid of a computer model, the infusion rate of an intravenous anesthetic does not reveal much about the resulting concentration in blood, preventing accurate administration targeted to a known concentration. There is currently no commercially available device to measure the concentration of intravenous anesthetics in real time, preventing equivalent pharmacokinetic exactness (delivering a targeted concentration). Even if concentrations of intravenous drugs were

measurable in the clinical setting, the meaning of a given concentration is not yet fully defined. A validated and accepted analog of MAC for intravenous anesthetics in not available, so that pharmacodynamic exactness equivalent to the volatile anesthetics is not yet possible. (Though experimental paradigms developed to determine MAC have been used to determine an intravenous concentration of, for example, propofol required to produce immobility in 50% of patients.[4] Available computer controlled pumps, although accurate and sophisticated, fall short of the theoretical appeal and practical convenience associated with the delivery of volatile anesthetic via the lung. Target controlled infusion technology (see Chapter 2) partly addresses these shortcomings.

Agent Analysis

A number of technologies can be employed to analyze the amount of agent being delivered to the patient. These are usually implemented in a sidestream, or diverting, system that takes a sample of gas from as close to the patient as feasible. In contrast, mainstream systems require attaching the analyzer hardware directly to the end of the endotracheal tube. Delivered volatile anesthetic concentration can be determined using mass spectrometry, Raman spectral analysis, infrared spectrometry, refractometry, or oscillating crystal technology. Nitrous oxide can be detected with mass spectrometry, Raman analysis, or infrared spectrometry.[5] Monitoring of delivered anesthetic concentration allows detection of volatile anesthetic uptake and elimination, vaporizer malfunctions, and estimation of anesthetic depth based on MAC values and age-derived nomograms. Additionally, low flow anesthesia can be more easily implemented if the delivered anesthetic concentration is being monitored. That said, prediction of

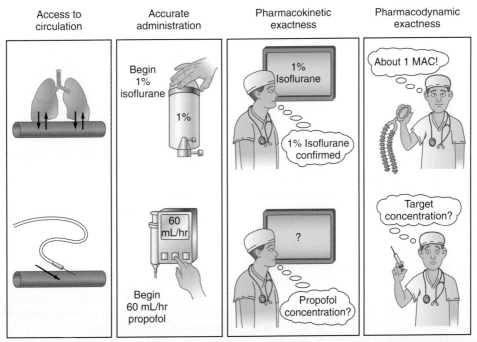

Figure 3-5 Comparison of delivery of anesthetics by inhalation *(upper panel)* or intravenous infusion *(lower panel)*. Inhalational delivery provides both pharmacokinetic and pharmacodynamic accuracy since known concentrations can be titrated by adjusting the vaporizer to known target concentrations (MAC) without accumulation and usually with minimal metabolism. *(Egan TD. Intravenous drug delivery systems: toward an intravenous "vaporizer". J Clin Anesth. 1996;8(3 Suppl):8S-14S.)*

arterial/effect site levels of anesthetic from end-tidal concentrations is difficult, and subject to inaccuracies due to dead space ventilation, for example.[6]

Monitoring Neurophysiologic Effect

While hemodynamic stability under anesthesia is relatively straightforward to monitor, it is surprisingly difficult to monitor the neurophysiologic effect of a given end-tidal concentration of an inhaled anesthetic. This is of particular concern in patients given neuromuscular blockers, who could potentially be aware but unable to move. Monitoring methods focus on the complexity of the electroencephalogram (EEG), which transitions from rapid disorganized activity during wakefulness to slow coherent activity with decreasing levels of arousal. A number of measures of the complexity of EEG, such as dimensional complexity, spectral edge, and spectral entropy, have all been proposed as valuable measures of arousal or awareness. The most frequently used commercial system currently is the BIS (Aspect Medical Systems) which uses a proprietary algorithm to measure EMG and correlations in power between different frequency bands of the EEG to develop an index that the manufacturer claims can predict awareness under anesthesia. Initial reports suggested that use of the BIS within an anesthetic protocol leads to an absolute risk reduction of awareness under anesthesia of 0.74% compared to anesthesia care outside of the protocol.[7] Subsequent studies that did not use BIS within an anesthetic protocol failed to reproduce this result.[8] Another randomized clinical trial that compared a structured anesthetic protocol based on the BIS with an anesthetic protocol based on end-tidal anesthetic gas concentration found that BIS neither lowered the incidence of anesthesia awareness nor reduced the administration of volatile anesthetic gas.[9] This conclusion was then confirmed in a separate study using patients at high risk of awareness.[10] This led the study group to discourage anesthesiologists from attempting to use BIS values to titrate anesthetics.[11] Intriguingly, however, the data suggest that cumulative time spent with very low BIS scores predicts mortality after cardiac, but not noncardiac, surgeries.[12,13]

METABOLISM AND DEGRADATION

Metabolism

Metabolism of volatile anesthetics, the extent of which varies 1000-fold between specific agents, is chiefly via cytochrome P450 enzymes in the liver (Table 3-2), primarily by CYP 2E1.[13,14] Hence patients exposed to agents that induce this enzyme (e.g., ethanol, barbiturates) can have increased metabolism (see Chapter 4). Metabolism is inhibited by the agents themselves at the higher concentrations present during anesthesia, but is enhanced during the elimination of residual anesthetic during the recovery phase, which is more prolonged and extensive for the soluble agents.[16]

Halothane is the most extensively metabolized of the modern agents; its extensive metabolism (up to 40%) has a significant impact on its elimination kinetics, in contrast to other agents.[17] It is also unique among volatile agents in undergoing significant reductive metabolism by CYP 2A6 and

Table 3-2. Degree of Metabolism, Metabolites, and Enzymes Involved for Various Agents

AGENT	DEGREE OF IN VIVO METABOLISM	METABOLITES	ENZYMES CATALYZING METABOLISM
Halothane	15%-40%	Inorganic bromide, fluoride	CYP 2E1 and, to a lesser extent, CYP 3A4 and CYP 2A6
Enflurane	2.4%	Inorganic fluoride	CYP 2E1
Isoflurane	0.2%	Trifluoroacetic acid, inorganic fluoride	CYP 2E1
Sevoflurane	2%-5%	Inorganic fluoride	CYP 2E1
Desflurane	0.02%	Inorganic fluoride	CYP 2E1

Modified from Kharasch ED, Thummel KE. Identification of cytochrome P450 2E1 as the predominant enzyme catalyzing human liver microsomal defluorination of sevoflurane, isoflurane, and methoxyflurane. *Anesthesiology*. 1993;9:795-807; Restrepo JG, Garcia-Martín E, Martínez C, et al. Polymorphic drug metabolism in anaesthesia. *Curr Drug Metab*. 2009;10:236-246.
CYP, Cytochrome P450.

3A4, although this is minor compared to oxidative metabolism.[18] Nitrous oxide and xenon are not metabolized.

Although the agents themselves have certain adverse effects (e.g., cardiac depression), a number of other adverse reactions to anesthesia, particularly hepatic and renal toxicity, are mediated by their metabolites. As a result, agents that undergo little metabolism have become more popular, while agents that undergo more metabolism, such as halothane and methoxyflurane, have fallen into disuse. Discussion of specific metabolites and their organ toxicity is found in Chapter 10.

Chemical Degradation

At temperatures exceeding 50°C in the presence of soda lime carbon dioxide absorbant, and somewhat even at 40°C as often exists in absorbents, sevoflurane undergoes base catalyzed degradation to produce the vinyl ether compound A (fluoromethyl-2,2-difluoro-1-(trifluoromethyl), or FDVE) and trace amounts of compound B (2-(fluoromethoxy)-3-methoxy-1,1,1,3,3-pentafluoropropane).[19] FDVE causes renal tubular necrosis in rats, but toxicity is species-dependent. Human exposure has no clinically significant effects even with low flow sevoflurane generating FDVE exposures of more than 400 ppm hours, although biochemical markers of renal injury have been reported with high compound A exposure in some studies.[20-23] More modern carbon dioxide absorbants have been designed to minimize production of compound A during normal use.[24]

Carbon Monoxide Production

The passage of volatile anesthetics through dry carbon dioxide absorbants can produce potentially life-threatening concentrations of carbon monoxide.[25,26] Severe carbon monoxide poisoning with carboxyhemoglobin levels approaching 40% has been reported in association with desflurane.[27] Carbon monoxide production is insignificant with sevoflurane and halothane, intermediate with isoflurane, and highest with desflurane and enflurane.[28] The quantity of carbon monoxide produced depends upon fresh gas flow, the quantity of dry absorbant, and the water content of the absorbant; barium hydroxide containing absorbant (Baralyme) produces more carbon monoxide than soda lime. No carbon monoxide is produced when the water content of soda lime exceeds approximately 4.8%, or the water content of Baralyme exceeds 9.7%. Baralyme has been removed from the market. With modern absorbants, this concern is largely obviated, with only small amounts of carbon monoxide production (peak concentrations <116 ppm) with desiccated Drägersorb, Medisorb, and Spherasorb, and no appreciable formation with Amsorb, LofloSorb, Superia, or lithium hydroxide.[29] The reaction by which carbon monoxide is produced is unclear; for desflurane the cascade probably begins with base-catalyzed extraction of a proton from the difluoromethyl ethyl group. The absence of this moiety in sevoflurane, methoxyflurane, and halothane thus explains the insignificant production of carbon monoxide by these agents.[30]

UPTAKE AND DISTRIBUTION

General Principles

During the wash-in period, the partial pressure of an inhaled gas in the alveoli increases exponentially to approach that of the inspired fresh gas concentration. This ratio reflects the uptake of anesthetic from the inhaled gas into the blood as well as from blood into the tissues. Assuming no uptake of gas, the alveolar concentration (F_A) approaches the fresh gas concentration (F_I) with first order kinetics:

$$\frac{d}{dt}\left(\frac{F_A}{F_I}\right) = -\frac{t}{\tau} \qquad [1]$$

where τ is the wash-in time constant, which is the ratio of the capacity of the reservoir into which the gas is delivered (the circuit volume plus the lung volume of the patient) to the flow rate at which it is delivered. Thus, τ is the time it takes to fill the system once at the current fresh gas flow. If the circuit starts with no anesthetic at time zero and the fresh gas concentration does not change, then

$$\frac{F_A}{F_I} = 1 - e^{-t/\tau} \qquad [2]$$

After a single time constant has elapsed (when $t = \tau$), F_A is $0.63\,F_I$; at time $t = 2\tau$, $F_A = 0.86\,F_I$; at $t = 3\tau$, $F_A = 0.95F_I$; and at $t = 4\tau$, $F_A = 0.98F_I$ (Figure 3-6).

The response to a drug depends upon the concentration of the drug at its effect site (e.g., a receptor expressed in brain or spinal cord), and is usually not the plasma (see Chapter 1). This is typically modeled by considering the human body as being made up of multiple compartments, one of which contains the effect site. At equilibrium, the concentration of an inhaled anesthetic in brain, for example, depends upon the relative solubilities of the drug in brain and plasma, which depends on the partial pressure of the anesthetic in the alveoli measured as the end-tidal concentration. Assuming

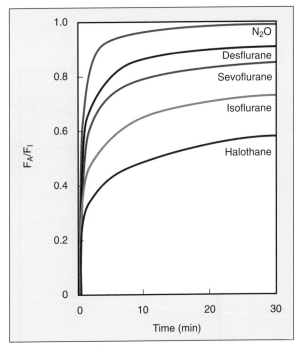

Figure 3-6 Wash-in of nitrous oxide, desflurane, sevoflurane, isoflurane, halothane, and diethyl ether. The rate at which the alveolar concentration (F_A) approaches the inhaled concentration (F_I) for a fixed minute ventilation and cardiac output reflects the solubility of the drug in blood, with wash-in of the least soluble (nitrous oxide and desflurane) being the fastest. (*Modified from Yasuda N, Lockhart SH, Eger EI 2nd, et al. Comparison of kinetics of sevoflurane and isoflurane in humans.* Anesth Analg. *1991;72:316-324.*)

steady-state, the end-tidal anesthetic concentration reflects the concentration of anesthetic in the plasma, and for these highly lipid soluble drugs that easily cross membranes, at the effect site. The effect of an inhaled anesthetic thus depends upon its concentration at its effect site and not on total absorbed mass of drug. The total absorbed dose is a significant determinant of the kinetics of uptake and elimination, however.

Determinants of Wash-in

The rate of wash-in of the anesthetic is determined by the rate of delivery to the alveoli and the rate of removal from the lungs. Factors that affect the rate of delivery to the alveoli include the inspired concentration, the time constant of the delivery system (which is determined by fresh gas flow and circuit volume), anatomical dead space, alveolar minute ventilation, and functional residual capacity (FRC). Factors affecting the rate at which anesthetic is removed from the lungs include the solubility of anesthetic in the blood, cardiac output, and the partial pressure gradient between alveolar gas and mixed venous blood. These concepts are illustrated in the classic uptake curves shown in Figure 3-7.

The gradient between inspired and alveolar anesthetic concentrations drives the increase in alveolar concentration of inhaled drugs. Alveolar ventilation determines the rate at which alveolar gas concentration equilibrates with the concentration in the circuit. A change in FRC changes the total volume of the system and thereby alters τ. As a result, an obese patient with reduced FRC will have faster wash-in

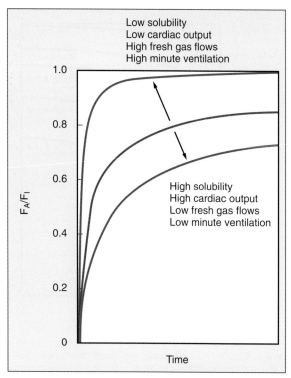

Figure 3-7 Factors affecting the rate of anesthetic wash-in (equilibration between the inspired fraction and the expired fraction) include solubility, cardiac output, fresh gas flow, and minute ventilation.

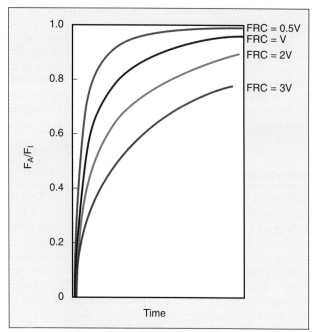

Figure 3-8 Effect of functional residual capacity (FRC) on wash-in for a fixed minute ventilation (V) and cardiac output. Patients with lower FRCs relative to their minute ventilation have more rapid wash-in.

(Figure 3-8). The early rapid increase in F_A/F_I represents the equilibration of anesthetic with the circuit and airways unopposed by alveolar uptake. The rate of change in F_A/F_I slows as alveolar concentrations increase and uptake into blood and tissues lead to increased venous concentration, which reduces the alveolar-to-venous concentration gradient and slows

uptake. For more soluble agents with greater uptake, the knee in the curve occurs at lower F_A/F_I ratios.

Special Factors

For a fixed cardiac output, a left-to-right shunt (which recycles blood through the lungs) does not affect wash-in unless it alters the ventilation to the perfused lung. A right-to-left shunt (where systemic venous blood bypasses the lungs), however, can significantly slow the rate of wash-in. Right-to-left shunt effects are much more prominent with poorly soluble anesthetics (i.e., nitrous oxide and desflurane).

A number of differences contributes to the faster wash-in observed in infants and children compared to adults. Volatile anesthetics are less soluble in neonates, likely secondary to lower serum protein and lipid concentrations. Tissue solubilities, particularly in the muscle group, are also lower in children than in adults. Finally, the cardiac output in neonates is disproportionately distributed to the vessel rich group compared to adults, enhancing drug delivery to the CNS.

Tissue Uptake

Initially during wash-in, anesthetic is avidly taken up by the tissues and anesthetic partial pressure of venous blood returning to the lungs is low. As anesthetic partial pressure in the tissues approaches the alveolar partial pressure, venous anesthetic partial pressure increases to approach alveolar partial pressure. As a result, the anesthetic partial pressure gradient between alveolar gas and venous blood decreases, diminishing the rate of uptake.

Factors that govern the tissue uptake of anesthetics are analogous to those that govern uptake from the lungs: tissue solubility, tissue blood flow and the arterial blood:tissue partial pressure gradient. Tissues can be classified into four groups based upon their relative blood flow: vessel rich group (brain, heart, kidney, and liver; contributing 10% to body mass and 75% to cardiac output), lean group (muscle and skin; contributing 50% to body mass and 20% to cardiac output), vessel poor group (bones and connective tissue; contributing 20% to body mass and <1% to cardiac output), and fat (contributing 20% to body mass and 5% to cardiac output). The time constant (τ) for wash-in of each group is defined as follows:

$$\tau = \frac{V\lambda}{Q} \qquad [3]$$

where V is the volume of tissue, Q is the tissue blood flow, and λ is the tissue:blood partition ratio. Based on tissue-specific differences in each of these factors, equilibration times from shortest to longest are vessel rich group, lean tissue group, vessel poor group, and fat (which has such low blood flow that it usually fails to equilibrate on a clinical time scale). The large mass of the lean tissue group makes it the largest tissue reservoir, and its lower blood flow relative to the vessel rich group (VRG) means that it continues to take up anesthetic long after the VRG approaches equilibrium. Again, more soluble agents have longer time constants. The slower rate of rise in the second phase of uptake evident in the F_A/F_I relationship reflects saturation of the VRG and slower equilibration of other (mainly lean) tissue groups.

Recovery and Elimination

Recovery from anesthesia follows elimination of the inhaled anesthetic agent from the effect site. Most anesthetic is eliminated from the blood via exhalation from the lungs; other routes include transcutaneous and visceral losses (both minor) and a more significant agent-specific metabolic component. Biodegradation has a significant effect on the elimination of the most extensively metabolized agents (in decreasing order of biodegradation: methoxyflurane, halothane, sevoflurane, enflurane, isoflurane, desflurane).[31] The extensive metabolism of methoxyflurane (~75% of absorbed drug) and halothane (~40% of absorbed drug) contributes to the faster decay in alveolar concentration for these drugs compared to less metabolized drugs such as isoflurane and desflurane.[32]

Washout of inhaled anesthetics follows a multiexponential decay. As with wash-in, the lower the solubility, the faster is elimination due to the increased efficacy of ventilation in eliminating anesthetic from the blood. In contrast to wash-in, wherein the inhaled concentration can be raised above the desired target (overpressure) to speed induction by overcoming the effect of solubility to hinder the rise in alveolar concentrations, during washout the alveolar concentration of anesthetic can never be less than zero, limiting the gradient for elimination. Additionally, washout is affected by the differential elimination from the four tissue compartments discussed earlier for uptake. Anesthetics can also redistribute between various tissue groups. For anesthetics with low solubility, duration of anesthesia has relatively little effect on rate of elimination. But for anesthetics with greater solubilities, washout rate is proportional to duration of anesthesia due to accumulation in tissues with longer time constants. This can be expressed as context-sensitive decrement times (Figure 3-9).[33] Evidence for a fifth compartment during washout has been suggested to involve diffusion from highly perfused tissues to adjacent fat that has a much longer time constant than muscle but 10 times faster than bulk fat.[16,34] Compartments with longer time constants (e.g., fat) do not equilibrate during short (<1 hour; longer with desflurane) procedures such that they can continue to take up anesthetic until alveolar elimination reduces arterial anesthetic partial pressure below tissue level. This can accelerate elimination early in recovery, but eventually slows recovery as they continue to unload anesthetic into blood. Complete elimination after a long anesthetic exposure can take days.

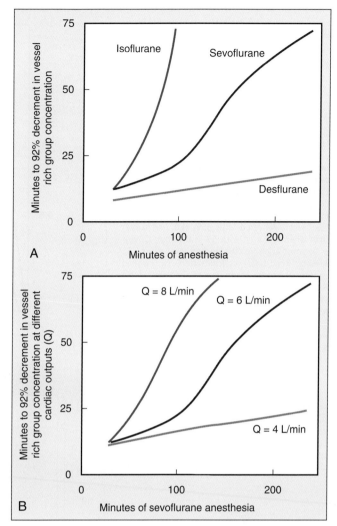

Figure 3-9 Context-sensitive decrement time as a function of total anesthetic time, agent, and cardiac output. **A,** Time required for the vessel rich group (VRG) concentration to decrease 92% from baseline as a function of the duration of the anesthetic. Note that the washout time increases with increasing solubility, as desflurane (the least soluble agent) is the fastest to washout, while isoflurane (the most soluble agent) is the slowest to washout for all anesthetic durations. **B,** Increasing cardiac output (Q) decreases the time to washout; all curves in this panel are for sevoflurane. (Modified from Eger EI 2nd, Shafer SL. Tutorial: context-sensitive decrement times for inhaled anesthetics. Anesth Analg. 2005;101:688-696.)

Nitrous Oxide: Concentration Effect, Second Gas Effect, Diffusion Hypoxia, and Effects on Closed Gas Spaces

The higher the concentration of an inhaled anesthetic, the faster the alveolar concentration approaches the inhaled concentration.[35] This is termed the *concentration effect* and is only of clinical relevance with gases administered at high concentrations such as nitrous oxide and xenon. When an inhaled anesthetic, such as nitrous oxide, is administered in high concentrations, the gas is rapidly taken up into blood (for nitrous oxide, the rate is on the order of 1 L/min). Assuming that the amount of oxygen uptake is approximately balanced by the amount of carbon dioxide eliminated, anesthetic uptake results in reduced alveolar volume. The absorbed nitrous oxide is replaced by a volume of gas with proportions similar to the initial inhaled mixture, resulting in a more rapid rise in the alveolar concentration of nitrous oxide (the so-called concentration effect). The concentration effect is due to both a concentrating of residual gases and an effective increase in alveolar ventilation due to the large volume of anesthetic gas absorbed, which is replaced by additional inspired gas minimizing the fall in alveolar anesthetic concentration (Figure 3-10).[36] At the extreme of 100% inspired anesthetic gas, the effects of dilution of alveolar gas during uptake is completely eliminated and uptake is limited only by alveolar ventilation (other factors staying constant).

The concentration effect also impacts other gases present in the inspired gas, including the more potent volatile agents. If a second gas is administered at the same time as a low potency gas that is taken up in large volumes like nitrous oxide, the concentration of the second gas rises faster than it

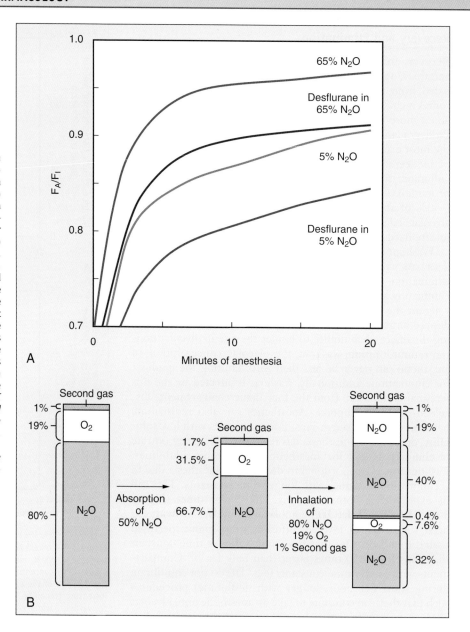

Figure 3-10 Second gas and concentration effects. **A,** The F_A/F_I of nitrous oxide (N_2O) increases to a higher level when delivered at a concentration of 65% (*blue* curve, upper panel) than at a concentration of 5% (*green* curve), a demonstration of the concentration effect. Similarly, the F_A/F_I of desflurane increases to a higher level when delivered with 65% N_2O (*red* curve) than when delivered with 5% N_2O (*brown* curve), a demonstration of the second gas effect. F_A, Alveolar (end-tidal) concentration, F_I, inspired concentration. **B,** Absorption of the very soluble N_2O increases the relative concentration of the second gas. Uptake of 50% of the N_2O does not reduce its concentration by half because the reduction in volume increases its concentration as well as that of the second gases (oxygen and the second gas). A subsequent breath diminishes this effect by mixing the concentrated mixture with the delivered gas, yet the second gas is still more concentrated. (**A,** *Modified from Taheri S, Eger EI 2nd. A demonstration of the concentration and second gas effects in humans anesthetized with nitrous oxide and desflurane. Anesth Analg. 1999;89:774-780.* **B,** *Modified from Stoelting RK, Eger EI 2nd. An additional explanation for the second gas effect: a concentrating effect. Anesthesiology. 1969;30:273-277.*)

would in the absence of the high concentration gas. This is termed the second gas effect, and is due to the uptake of significant volumes of alveolar nitrous oxide that serves to concentrate the residual gases in the inspired mixture and to increased alveolar ventilation (second gas effect).[36,37] This process can speed induction of inhalational anesthesia.

Analogous to the second gas effect during induction, when a low potency gas like nitrous oxide is discontinued, it diffuses rapidly into the alveoli, contributing to second gas removal of more potent volatile anesthetics. Nitrous oxide elimination falls exponentially to low rates after about 5 minutes. The large volumes of dissolved nitrous oxide can also cause diffusion hypoxia by diluting alveolar oxygen. Up to 30 L of nitrous oxide can accumulate in the body within 2 hours, and this volume is added to the expired volumes.[38] This eliminated nitrous oxide mixes with alveolar gas, reducing the concentration of oxygen and potentially generating a hypoxic mixture (diffusion hypoxia); this can be minimized by increasing inhaled oxygen during initial recovery. The large volumes of nitrous oxide can also dilute alveolar carbon dioxide leading

to arterial hypocarbia and reduced respiratory drive.[39] The second gas effect has also been shown to occur in reverse during emergence, where the rapid elimination of nitrous oxide dilutes alveolar partial pressure of the potent volatile anesthetic to speed emergence.[40]

Nitrous oxide (blood:gas partition ratio of 0.47) is roughly 30 times as soluble in blood as nitrogen (blood:gas partition ratio of 0.015). As a result, nitrous oxide accumulates in closed gas spaces that contain nitrogen faster than the nitrogen can diffuse out. This can lead to distention of closed air-containing spaces such as the middle ear, bowel, pneumothorax, air emboli, or tracheal tube cuff. The volume of distensible spaces increases to the extent that the nitrous oxide concentration is equal to the alveolar, and, in turn, blood nitrous oxide concentration in volume percent. Hence, the extent of this increase is proportional to the concentration of alveolar nitrous oxide at low (i.e., single digit concentrations), but is about 2-fold for 50% nitrous oxide and 3-fold for 75% nitrous oxide. Expansion is time-dependent, but can be rapid for air emboli. For poorly compliant spaces like the middle ear, diffusion of nitrous oxide can cause a potentially deleterious increase in pressure proportional to its alveolar concentration.

Gas Delivery Systems

Inhaled anesthetics are delivered to the lungs using an anesthesia circuit. This serves several functions: delivering oxygen and inhaled drugs to the patient, maintaining temperature and humidity of inhaled gases, removing exhaled carbon dioxide, and ultimately removing drugs from the patient. Three broad classes of circuits are in use: rebreathing circuits where inspired and exhaled gases mix (Bain circuit), non-rebreathing circuits in which one-way valves separate inhaled from expired gases (self-inflating resuscitation bag-valve system), and circuits that use a carbon dioxide absorbant (circle systems with both inspiratory and expiratory valves). The most common inhaled drug delivery system used in modern anesthesia machines is a circle system (Figure 3-11).

Circle systems consist of inspiratory and expiratory limbs, a reservoir bag, a canister of CO_2 absorbent (e.g., soda lime), one-way valves to direct gas flows (one each on the inspiratory and expiratory limbs), a Y-piece that attaches the inspiratory and expiratory limbs to the respiratory tract via a mask or tracheal tube, a fresh gas inlet, and a relief valve. The CO_2 absorbent removes CO_2 in an exothermic reaction by producing water and a carbonate:

REACTION OF CARBON DIOXIDE WITH BARIUM HYDROXIDE LIME (BARALYME, OBSOLETE)

$$Ba(OH)_2 + 8\ H_2O + CO_2 \leftrightarrow BaCO_3 + 9\ H_2O + heat$$

$$9\ H_2O + 9\ CO_2 \leftrightarrow 9\ H_2CO_3$$

$$9\ H_2CO_3 + 9\ Ba(OH)_2 \leftrightarrow 9\ BaCO_3 + 9\ H_2O + heat$$

REACTION OF CARBON DIOXIDE WITH SODA LIME (IN CURRENT USE)

$$H_2O + CO_2 \leftrightarrow H_2CO_3$$

$$H_2CO_3 + 2\ NaOH(KOH) \leftrightarrow Na_2CO_3(K_2CO_3)$$
$$+ 2\ H_2O + heat$$

$$Na_2CO_3(K_2CO_3) + Ca(OH)_2 \leftrightarrow CaCO_3 + 2\ NaOH(KOH)$$

The CO_2 absorbent can degrade inhaled anesthetics to potentially harmful breakdown products. Desiccated soda lime and barium hydroxide–based absorbents degrade sevoflurane (see earlier); this can be avoided by eliminating monovalent bases from soda lime. Additionally, the heat produced by desiccated absorbent can be sufficient to ignite combustible degradation products, leading to absorbent canister explosion.[41,42] A number of proprietary absorbents (e.g., Amsorb, Drägersorb) have been developed that do not contain monovalent bases in order to minimize degradation of sevoflurane and desflurane.

Vaporizers are devices that add desired anesthetic concentrations to the fresh gas flow and ultimately to the anesthetic circuit and patient. Most modern vaporizer designs, with the notable exception of one type of desflurane vaporizer, use temperature-compensated variable bypass manifolds that are concentration calibrated for use with a single anesthetic agent (Figure 3-12). These devices function by diverting a portion of the fresh gas flow through a vaporizing chamber where the flow is saturated with volatile anesthetic; the amount of flow that bypasses the chamber is determined by the ambient temperature and the desired concentration (in volume percent) of anesthetic in the vaporizer output. Desflurane vaporizers compensate for the very high vapor pressure of desflurane at room temperature by using an electric heater to warm and pressurize the desflurane into a vapor that is injected into the fresh gas flow at a rate to deliver the set desflurane concentration in the vaporizer output.

The anesthetic circuit has significant effects on the kinetics of inhaled drug delivery and elimination by determining inspired gas concentrations (F_I). Rebreathing allows mixing of inspired and expired gases (with depleted anesthetic concentration due to uptake), and thus reduces delivered anesthetic concentration below that delivered by the vaporizer. This is minimized when the fresh gas flow exceeds minute ventilation. The circuit itself has a time constant (τ) for equilibration with the gas delivered from the machine (τ = volume of the breathing system/fresh gas flow). This determines the wash-in kinetics of the circuit. If the delivered gases immediately mix with the circuit gases, the anesthetic concentration in the breathing system reaches 95% of the delivered concentration in 3τ; however more efficient circuit designs are commonly employed.[43] Increased gas flow or reducing circuit volume accelerates this equilibration, and speeds the rate of induction.

Low Flow Anesthesia

The choice of fresh gas flow in the circuit can dramatically affect the amount of agent used, and hence the cost of anesthetic drugs, particularly for long cases. The lowest cost approach is to use a closed circuit, where there are no leaks in the circuit, the pressure limiting valve is closed, and the fresh gas flow uses 100% FiO_2 to exactly offset the uptake/consumption of oxygen by the patient (roughly 2.5-3 mL O_2/kg/min for adults, or approximately 200 mL/min for a typical 70-kg adult). Closed circuit administration minimizes the cooling and drying effects of the fresh gas flow for the patient, but leaves little margin for error; any change in anesthetic concentration requires temporarily increasing the gas flow to speed equilibration. With slightly higher flow rates, small leaks in the circuit can be overcome and gradual changes in the anesthetic concentration are possible while still keeping costs down. As the fresh gas flow increases, times to equilibration of changes in inhaled anesthetic concentration are faster, but the patient is exposed to cooler and drier gasses potentially compromising their pulmonary function, and more agent and inhaled gases are wasted.[44] Anesthetic agents have substantial greenhouse gas and ozone depletion potential, so minimizing venting to the atmosphere is appropriate.[45] Sevoflurane is usually used at gas flows greater than 2 L/min out of concern for Compound A production, but as discussed earlier there is minimal evidence of clinically significant nephrotoxicity in humans.[20]

Pharmacoeconomic Considerations

The cost of inhaled anesthetic consumed during an anesthetic is determined by four principle factors: the cost of liquid anesthetic per milliliter, the volume of vapor that results from each milliliter of liquid, the volume percent of anesthetic delivered (determined largely by the potency), and the

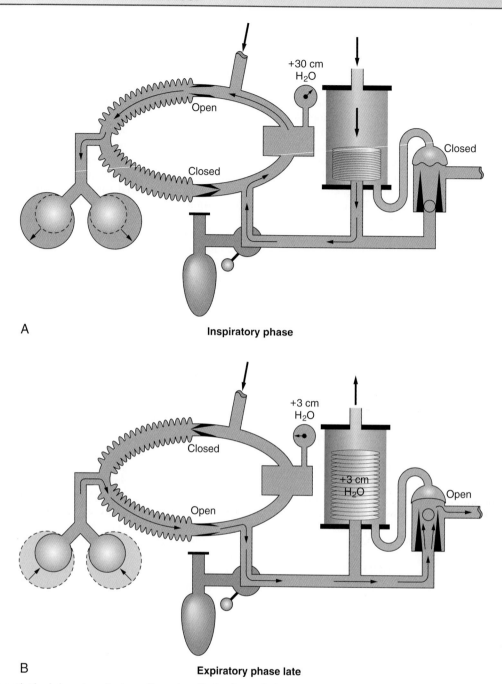

Figure 3-11 The anesthetic circle system. Fresh gas flow enters the inspiratory limb, which has a one-way valve that allows flow toward the patient. The inspiratory limb meets the expiratory limb at the T-piece. The circuit dead space is determined by the volume of everything between the patient and the T-piece. A second one-way valve in the expiratory limb limits flow away from the patient. The bag and ventilator bellows affect circuit pressure on the expiratory side of the circuit. A switch valve gives the user choice between manual and mechanical ventilation. When manual ventilation is selected, an adjustable pressure limiting valve vents excessive pressure to the scavenging system. When the ventilator is in operation, the scavenger system is cyclically opened. Arrows indicate direction of gas flow. During inspiration, oxygen compresses the ventilator bellows and seals the scavenger system. As a result of the one-way valves in the circuit, the increased pressure forces gas into the lungs. Release of the pressure in the ventilator bellows opens the scavenger system and allows gas to return from the patient.

chosen fresh gas flow rate.[46] The volume percent delivered is determined by two factors, anesthetic potency and solubility. While potency determines the vaporizer setting at steady state (when $F_A = F_I$), solubility impacts vaporizer setting during wash-in as some degree of overpressure might be required to speed induction before equilibration to steady state occurs. The significance of the solubility issue is illustrated by a study that used a 10-minute wash-in period before

initiating controlled fresh gas flows for delivery of anesthetic. Desflurane consumption was governed by fresh gas flow, and while there was a trend toward increased consumption of sevoflurane and isoflurane at higher fresh gas flows, halothane consumption was totally independent of the fresh gas flow.[47]

For most institutions in the United States, isoflurane is the least expensive anesthetic on a per milliliter basis and desflurane the most expensive, with sevoflurane being slightly less

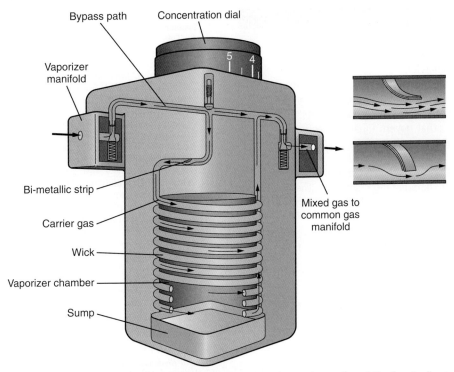

Figure 3-12 A variable bypass anesthetic vaporizer. Fresh gas flows through the vaporizer and a portion of the flow is diverted through the vaporizer chamber. This carrier gas flows over a wick that ensures equilibration of the anesthetic with the carrier gas. The carrier flow, saturated with anesthetic, is then mixed back with the fresh gas that bypasses the reservoir to achieve the desired anesthetic concentration (volume %). A temperature compensating valve adjusts the amount of gas flow that is diverted to ensure stable temperature because vapor pressure is temperature dependent. Note that the portion of flow diverted through the vaporizer chamber, as well as the temperature compensation valve, must both be calibrated for each individual agent. Filling a variable bypass vaporizer with an agent other than the one for which it is calibrated can lead to delivery of a dangerous concentration of anesthetic. *(Adapted from Morgan GE, Mikhail MS, Murray MJ. Clinical Anesthesiology. 4th ed. New York: McGraw-Hill; 2006.)*

expensive than desflurane. However, the lesser potency of desflurane (with a MAC of 6% compared to a MAC of 2% for sevoflurane) means that at steady state significantly more desflurane is consumed per hour for a given anesthetic depth at the same flow rates. Because most anesthesiologists are comfortable with using low flow rates for desflurane, but not sevoflurane, the cost differential for longer cases favors desflurane if low flows are used.

EMERGING DEVELOPMENTS

Intravenous Delivery of Volatile Anesthetics

Early reports suggested that intravenous delivery of liquid volatile agents incurs significant morbidity with risk of pulmonary damage or death.[48-51] Subsequently, several groups have reported that volatile anesthetics, including halothane, isoflurane, and sevoflurane, can be successfully delivered intravenously as a lipid emulsion.[51-55] Initial reports of nonlethal intravenous delivery of anesthetics used lipid emulsion as the carrier vehicle, but ongoing research to increase anesthetic concentrations in the emulsion has led to the development of fluoropolymer based vehicles.[56] Volatile anesthetic emulsions can be delivered by bolus or continuous infusions, and preserve respiratory drive while causing a rapid loss of consciousness in animals. Intravenous delivery appears to preserve most properties of volatile agents, including early and late cardiac preconditioning.[55,57] The principle advantage of these preparations is the rapid onset, because there is no need

to wait for uptake through the lungs and the resultant slow rise in alveolar concentration. However, intravenous delivery gives up the advantages of inhalational delivery. For example, inhalational anesthetic delivery results from equilibration with a (measurable) delivered concentration of anesthetic, and there is no accumulation of agent beyond the inhaled concentration or need for continuous adjustment of delivery rate to ensure a given blood/tissue concentration. As a result, a large amount of research has gone into developing target controlled infusions for intravenous agents to make their use more akin to using a vaporizer for an inhaled agent (see earlier).[58] Adverse effects of the accumulating vehicle are also potentially problematic.

KEY POINTS

- The effects of inhaled anesthetics depend upon the anesthetic concentration at their effect sites. This parallels the alveolar anesthetic concentration and not the total amount of absorbed anesthetic.
- The potency of different agents can be compared using MAC, the minimum alveolar concentration of anesthetic required to prevent movement (immobilize) in 50% of subjects in response to a standardized surgical stimulus.
- Blood and tissue concentration of a gas is determined by the partial pressure of the gas and its blood:gas or tissue:gas partition ratio (an index of its solubility).

Continued

Key References

Eger EI 2nd. *Anesthetic Uptake and Action*. Baltimore: Williams & Wilkins; 1974. The definitive review of the pharmacokinetics of inhaled anesthetics, including an overview of this investigator's immense contributions. This book provides an excellent general review of many of the topics covered in this chapter. (Ref. 59)

Eger EI 2nd, Saidman LJ, Brandstater B. Minimum alveolar anesthetic concentration: a standard of anesthetic potency. *Anesthesiology*. 1965;26:756-763. This landmark paper proposed the minimum alveolar concentration (MAC) of anesthetic that inhibited a movement response in 50% of subjects to a standard surgical stimulus as a standard to compare potency of inhaled agents. The MAC concept later emerged as a clinically useful tool. (Ref. 2)

Kharasch ED, Thummel KE. Identification of cytochrome P450 2E1 as the predominant enzyme catalyzing human liver microsomal defluorination of sevoflurane, isoflurane, and methoxyflurane. *Anesthesiology*. 1993;79:795-807. Describes an ex-vivo assay with human liver microsomes to determine the CYP isoform responsible for volatile anesthetic metabolism. (Ref. 15)

Taheri S, Eger EI 2nd. A demonstration of the concentration and second gas effects in humans anesthetized with nitrous oxide and desflurane. *Anesth Analg*. 1999;89:774-780. An elegant demonstration of the concentration and second gas effects. (Ref. 35)

References

1. Hemmings HC Jr. General anaesthetic agents. In: Webster NR, Galley HF, eds. Landmark Papers in Anaesthesia. Oxford: Oxford University Press; in press.
2. Eger EI 2nd, Saidman LJ, Brandstater B. Minimum alveolar anesthetic concentration: a standard of anesthetic potency. *Anesthesiology*. 1965;26:756-763.
3. Eger EI. Age, minimum alveolar anesthetic concentration, and minimum alveolar anesthetic concentration-awake. *Anesth Analg*. 2001;93:947-953.
4. Hammer GB, Litalien C, Wellis V, et al. Determination of the median effective concentration (EC50) of propofol during oesophagogastroduodenoscopy in children. *Paediatr Anaesth*. 2001;11:549-553.
5. Dorsch JA, Dorsch SE. *Gas Monitoring. Understanding anesthesia equipment*. Philadelphia: Lippincott Williams & Wilkins; 2008.
6. Frei FJ, Zbinden AM, Thomson DA, et al. Is the end-tidal partial pressure of isoflurane a good predictor of its arterial partial pressure? *Br J Anaesth*. 1991;66:331-339.
7. Myles PS, Leslie K, McNeil J, et al. Bispectral index monitoring to prevent awareness during anaesthesia: the B-Aware randomised controlled trial. *Lancet*. 2004;363:1757-1763.
8. Sebel PS, Bowdle TA, Ghoneim MM, et al. The incidence of awareness during anesthesia: a multicenter United States study. *Anesth Analg*. 2004;99:833-839.
9. Avidan MS, Zhang L, Burnside BA, et al. Anesthesia awareness and the bispectral index. *N Engl J Med*. 2008;358:1097-1108.
10. Avidan MS, Jacobsohn E, Glick D, et al. BAG-RECALL Research Group. Prevention of intraoperative awareness in a high-risk surgical population. *N Engl J Med*. 2011;365:591-600.
11. Whitlock EL, Villafranca AJ, Lin N, et al. Relationship between bispectral index values and volatile anesthetic concentrations during the maintenance phase of anesthesia in the B-Unaware trial. *Anesthesiology*. 2011;115:1209-1218.
12. Kertai MD, Pal N, Palanca BJ, et al. B-Unaware Study Group. Association of perioperative risk factors and cumulative duration of low bispectral index with intermediate-term mortality after cardiac surgery in the B-Unaware Trial. *Anesthesiology*. 2010;112:1116-1127.
13. Kertai MD, Palanca BJ, Pal N, et al. B-Unaware Study Group. Bispectral index monitoring, duration of bispectral index below 45, patient risk factors, and intermediate-term mortality after noncardiac surgery in the B-Unaware Trial. *Anesthesiology*. 2011;114:545-556.
14. Kharasch ED. Adverse drug reactions with halogenated anesthetics. *Clin Pharmacol Ther*. 2008;84:158-162.
15. Kharasch ED, Thummel KE. Identification of cytochrome P450 2E1 as the predominant enzyme catalyzing human liver microsomal defluorination of sevoflurane, isoflurane, and methoxyflurane. *Anesthesiology*. 1993;79:795-807.
16. Cahalan MK, Johnson BH, Eger EI 2nd. A noninvasive in vivo method of assessing the kinetics of halothane metabolism in humans. *Anesthesiology*. 1982;57(4):298-302.
17. Yasuda N, Lockhart SH, Eger EI 2nd, et al. Kinetics of desflurane, isoflurane, and halothane in humans. *Anesthesiology*. 1991;74(3):489-498.
18. Spracklin DK, Thummel KE, Kharasch ED. Human reductive halothane metabolism in vitro is catalyzed by cytochrome P450 2A6 and 3A4. *Drug Metab Dispos*. 1996;24(9):976-983.
19. Morio M, Fujii K, Satoh N, et al. Reaction of sevoflurane and its degradation products with soda lime. Toxicity of the byproducts. *Anesthesiology*. 1992;77:1155-1164.
20. Kharasch ED, Frink EJ Jr, Artru A, et al. Long-duration low-flow sevoflurane and isoflurane effects on postoperative renal and hepatic function. *Anesth Analg*. 2001;93:1511-1520.
21. Eger EI 2nd, Gong D, Koblin DD, et al. Dose-related biochemical markers of renal injury after sevoflurane versus desflurane anesthesia in volunteers. *Anesth Analg*. 1997;85:1154-1163.
22. Goldberg ME, Cantillo J, Gratz I, et al. Dose of compound A, not sevoflurane, determines changes in the biochemical markers of renal injury in healthy volunteers. *Anesth Analg*. 1999;88:437-445.
23. Obata R, Bito H, Ohmura M, et al. The effects of prolonged low-flow sevoflurane anesthesia on renal and hepatic function. *Anesth Analg*. 2000;91:1262-1268.
24. Keijzer C, Perez RS, de Lange JJ. Compound A and carbon monoxide production from sevoflurane and seven different types of carbon dioxide absorbent in a patient model. *Acta Anaesthesiol Scand*. 2007;51:31-37.
25. Fang ZX, Eger EI 2nd, Laster MJ, et al. Carbon monoxide production from degradation of desflurane, enflurane, isoflurane, halothane, and sevoflurane by soda lime and Baralyme. *Anesth Analg*. 1995;80:1187-1193.
26. Wissing H, Kuhn I, Warnken U, et al. Carbon monoxide production from desflurane, enflurane, halothane, isoflurane, and sevoflurane with dry soda lime. *Anesthesiology*. 2001;95:1205-1212.
27. Berry PD, Sessler DI, Larson MD. Severe carbon monoxide poisoning during desflurane anesthesia. *Anesthesiology*. 1999;90(2):613-616.
28. Keijzer C, Perez RS, de Lange JJ. Detection of carbon monoxide production as a result of the interaction of five volatile anesthetics and desiccated sodalime with an electrochemical carbon monoxide

sensor in an anesthetic circuit compared to gas chromatography. *J Clin Monit Comput.* 2007;21:257-264.

29. Keijzer C, Perez RS, de Lange JJ. Compound A and carbon monoxide production from sevoflurane and seven different types of carbon dioxide absorbent in a patient model. *Acta Anaesthesiol Scand.* 2007; 51:31-37.

30. Baxter PJ, Garton K, Kharasch ED. Mechanistic aspects of carbon monoxide formation from volatile anesthetics. *Anesthesiology.* 1998; 89(4):929-941.

31. Eger EI 2nd, Eisenkraft JB, Weiskopf RB. Metabolism of potent inhaled anesthetics. In: Eger EI 2nd, Eisenkraft JB, Weiskopf RB, eds. *The Pharmacology of Inhaled Anesthetics.* Chicago: Healthcare Press; 2003:167-176.

32. Carpenter RL, Eger EI 2nd, Johnson BH, et al. The extent of metabolism of inhaled anesthetics in humans. *Anesthesiology.* 1986;65(2): 201-205.

33. Eger EI 2nd, Shafer SL. Tutorial: context-sensitive decrement times for inhaled anesthetics. *Anesth Analg.* 2005;101(3):688-696.

34. Yasuda N, Lockhart SH, Eger EI 2nd, et al. Comparison of kinetics of sevoflurane and isoflurane in humans. *Anesth Analg.* 1991;72(3): 316-324.

35. Taheri S, Eger EI 2nd. A demonstration of the concentration and second gas effects in humans anesthetized with nitrous oxide and desflurane. *Anesth Analg.* 1999;89:774-780.

36. Stoelting RK, Eger EI 2nd. An additional explanation for the second gas effect: a concentrating effect. *Anesthesiology.* 1969;30(3): 273-277.

37. Epstein RM, Rackow H, Salanitre E, et al. Influence of the concentration effect on the uptake of anesthetic mixtures: the second gas effect. *Anesthesiology.* 1964;25:364-371.

38. Severinghaus JW. The rate of uptake of nitrous oxide in man. *J Clin Invest.* 1954;33(9):1183-1189.

39. Rackow H, Salanitre E, Frumin MJ. Dilution of alveolar gases during nitrous oxide excretion in man. *J Appl Physiol.* 1961;16:723-728.

40. Peyton PJ, Chao I, Weinberg L, et al. Nitrous oxide diffusion and the second gas effect on emergence from anesthesia. *Anesthesiology.* 2011;114(3):596-602.

41. Castro BA, Freedman LA, Craig WL, et al. Explosion within an anesthesia machine: Baralyme, high fresh gas flows and sevoflurane concentration. *Anesthesiology.* 2004;101(2):537-539.

42. Wu J, Previte JP, Adler E, et al. Spontaneous ignition, explosion, and fire with sevoflurane and barium hydroxide lime. *Anesthesiology.* 2004; 101(2):534-537.

43. Eger EI 2nd, Ethans CT. The effects of inflow, overflow and valve placement on economy of the circle system. *Anesthesiology.* 1968;29(1): 93-100.

44. Bilgi M, Goksu S, Mizrak A, et al. Comparison of the effects of low-flow and high-flow inhalational anaesthesia with nitrous oxide and desflurane on mucociliary activity and pulmonary function tests. *Eur J Anaesthesiol.* 2011;28(4):279-283.

45. Sherman JD, Ryan S. Ecological responsibility in anesthesia practice. *Int Anesthesiol Clin.* 2010;48(3):139-151.

46. Weiskopf RB, Eger EI 2nd. Comparing the costs of inhaled anesthetics. *Anesthesiology.* 1993;79(6):1413-1418.

47. Coetzee JF, Stewart LJ. Fresh gas flow is not the only determinant of volatile agent consumption: a multi-centre study of low-flow anaesthesia. *Br J Anaesth.* 2002;88(1):46-55.

48. Kopriva CJ, Lowenstein E. An anesthetic accident: cardiovascular collapse from liquid halothane delivery. *Anesthesiology.* 1969;30(2): 246-247.

49. Dwyer R, Coppel DL. Intravenous injection of liquid halothane. *Anesth Analg.* 1989;69(2):250-255.

50. Kawamoto M, Suzuki N, Takasaki M. Acute pulmonary edema after intravenous liquid halothane in dogs. *Anesth Analg.* 1992;74(5):747-752.

51. Biber B, Martner J, Werner O. Halothane by the I.V. route in experimental animals. *Acta Anaesthesiol Scand.* 1982;26(6):658-659.

52. Johannesson G, Alm P, Biber B, et al. Halothane dissolved in fat as an intravenous anaesthetic to rats. *Acta Anaesthesiol Scand.* 1984; 28(4):381-384.

53. Biber B, Johannesson G, Lennander O, et al. Intravenous infusion of halothane dissolved in fat. Haemodynamic effects in dogs. *Acta Anaesthesiol Scand.* 1984;28(4):385-389.

54. Eger RP, MacLeod BA. Anaesthesia by intravenous emulsified isoflurane in mice. *Can J Anaesth.* 1995;42(2):173-176.

55. Chiari PC, Pagel PS, Tanaka K, et al. Intravenous emulsified halogenated anesthetics produce acute and delayed preconditioning against myocardial infarction in rabbits. *Anesthesiology.* 2004;101: 1160-1166.

56. Fast JP, Perkins MG, Pearce RA, et al. Fluoropolymer-based emulsions for the intravenous delivery of sevoflurane. *Anesthesiology.* 2008;109(4):651-656.

57. Rao Y, Wang YL, Zhang WS, et al. Emulsified isoflurane produces cardiac protection after ischemia-reperfusion injury in rabbits. *Anesth Analg.* 2008;106(5):1353-1359.

58. Egan TD. Target-controlled drug delivery: progress toward an intravenous "vaporizer" and automated anesthetic administration. *Anesthesiology.* 2003;99(5):1214-1219.

59. Eger EI 2nd. *Anesthetic Uptake and Action.* Baltimore: Williams & Wilkins; 1974.

Chapter 4

DRUG METABOLISM AND PHARMACOGENETICS

Tjorvi E. Perry and Charles D. Collard

Despite tremendous advances in drug development, patients are still at considerable risk for suffering adverse drug events due to individual variability in their responses to drugs.[1] *Pharmacokinetics* is the branch of pharmacology related to defining how administered drugs are absorbed, distributed, metabolized, and excreted by the body (i.e., the relationship between drug dose and effective drug concentration), while *pharmacodynamics* concerns the relationship between drug concentration and drug effect. In contrast, *pharmacogenetics* is the study of how individuals respond to drugs based on their genetic makeup.[2,3]

Traditionally, human drug dosing regimens have been developed through preclinical studies in animals, followed by clinical trials in humans. However, in individuals with atypical responses to standard dosing regimens, adequate dosing is often determined by trial and error, placing the patient at considerable risk for an adverse drug event. For example, administration of standard opioid doses for postoperative pain control can lead to either *underdosing*, resulting in inadequate analgesia, or *overdosing*, in which the patient is vulnerable to excessive ventilatory depression, perhaps resulting in prolonged mechanical ventilation or even respiratory arrest in an unmonitored setting (Figure 4-1). Such drug reactions, not including adverse reactions as a result of drug administration errors or dosing errors (see Chapter 6), can be associated with prolonged length of hospital stay (1-4 days) and increased cost ($2300-$5600 per patient).[4,5] Thus, over the last decade, the traditional approach to pharmacology has been enhanced by improved understanding of how genotypic variability can influence drug transport, target responses, and metabolism.

BASICS OF GENETICS

Chromosomes, Genes, and Alleles

Nearly 30,000 human *genes* encode the amino acid structure of all proteins.[6] Genes are comprised of linear polymers of deoxyribonucleotide bases, with each base consisting of one of two purines (adenine [A] or guanine [G]) or pyrimidines (cytosine [C] or thymidine [T]). These nucleotide base pair sequences serve as templates for *transcription* of DNA to RNA, and subsequently *translation* from RNA to protein.

Variation in nucleotide base sequence can result in altered protein function or expression. The most commonly

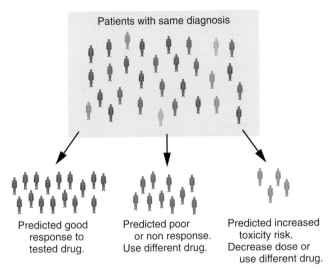

Figure 4-1 Clinical potential of pharmacogenetics. Patients with similar clinical diagnoses are commonly treated with the same medications and same doses. While the majority of patients will have a satisfactory clinical response, some can have a poor or no response, requiring a different medication, while still others can have an adverse response requiring a different dose of the same medication. *(Adapted with permission from Johnson JA. Pharmacogenetics: potential for individualized drug therapy through genetics. Trends Genet. 2003;19:660-666.)*

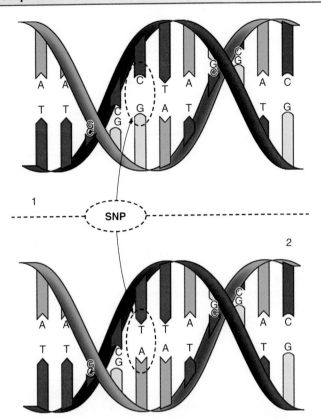

Figure 4-2 A schematic of a single nucleotide polymorphism (SNP). An SNP occurs when a single DNA base pair in the coding sequence of a gene is substituted for another, and occurs with a population frequency of greater than 1%. If its frequency is less than 1%, it is considered a mutation.

recognized genetic variant is a *single nucleotide polymorphism* (SNP), defined as occurring in more than 1% of the general population. SNPs occur when a fragment of DNA differs between individuals by one specific nucleotide in the DNA sequence (Figure 4-2). Over 13 million SNPs have been identified to date, many of which are associated with disease states or altered phenotypes. When a single nucleotide base change occurs with a population frequency of less than 1%, it is referred to as a *mutation*. However, the terms *mutation* and *SNP* are often used interchangeably. Genetic mutations of larger segments of DNA also occur, and include insertions or deletions (also called *indels*) of anywhere from two to several hundred nucleotides, translocations, or inversions of DNA segments.

Genotype and Phenotype

All organisms have a unique, inherited sequence of nucleotide base pairs known as their *genotype*. This genetic blueprint serves as a template for genetic regulation and protein production, which in turn is ultimately responsible for the form, function, and outward appearance of the organism, also known as the *phenotype*. The term *allele* is used to describe the variant forms of a DNA sequence within a specific gene. For example, while most individuals might have the sequence AA**G**TA within a given gene, others might have the sequence AA**C**TA at the same location, differing by only one base pair. In this case, the more common G allele is said to be the *wild type* or common allele, while the C allele is said to be the risk or *minor* allele. Fortunately, due to the redundancy of the genetic coding system, altered protein production rarely occurs with minor allelic variation. For example, phenylalanine is coded for by either a TT**T** or a TT**C** sequence. This type of allelic variation is termed *synonymous* or "silent"

mutation. However, *nonsynonymous* allelic variation within a DNA sequence can result in altered protein production or phenotype.

Phenotype is influenced by both the genotype (the two sets of alleles inherited from the parents) and environmental factors. Individuals can be either *homozygous* for a particular allele, meaning identical alleles are present on both chromosomes, or *heterozygous*, meaning the alleles differ. An individual is homozygous *dominant* if carrying two copies of a dominant allele, and homozygous *recessive* if carrying two copies of a recessive allele. Homozygous dominant individuals express the dominant trait, while homozygous recessive individuals do not. Individuals who are heterozygous carry one dominant allele and one recessive allele, and express the dominant phenotype.

More than 4000 diseases are caused by single gene mutations or monogenic mutations, regardless of environmental influence. Huntington disease and Marfan syndrome, for example, have a dominant inheritance pattern, meaning that inheritance of only one risk allele is necessary for the disease to manifest. Others, such as sickle cell disease or cystic fibrosis, have a recessive inheritance pattern. Recent attention is being directed at defining the molecular basis for *complex* disorders, such as asthma or diabetes mellitus, wherein one or more genes, as well as multiple environmental influences, can play a role. Studying the inheritance pattern for these diseases poses a formidable challenge in that the degree to which different genes and/or environmental influences contribute is highly variable.

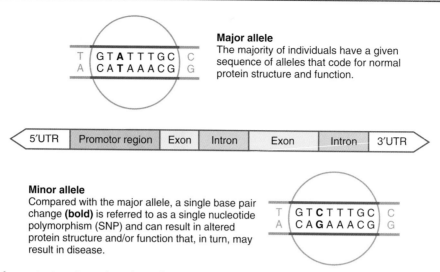

Major allele
The majority of individuals have a given sequence of alleles that code for normal protein structure and function.

Minor allele
Compared with the major allele, a single base pair change **(bold)** is referred to as a single nucleotide polymorphism (SNP) and can result in altered protein structure and/or function that, in turn, may result in disease.

Figure 4-3 Schematic of gene structure. A gene is made up of a promotor region, introns, exons, and 5′ and 3′ untranslated regions on either side. Nucleotides and their respective bases (adenine, thymine, guanine, and cytosine) make up the genomic sequence that ultimately regulates gene expression. *(Adapted with permission from Perry TE, Muehlschlegel JD, Body SC. Genomics: risk and outcomes in cardiac surgery.* Anesthesiol Clin. *2008;26:399-417.)*

Genetic Mutations

All eukaryotic genes have a similar structural makeup, including a 5′ region (which includes the promotor for that particular gene), introns, exons, and a 3′ untranslated region (Figure 4-3). Intronic regions, also referred to as *intervening sequence*, are nucleotide sequences located between exonic regions. Traditionally thought to have little to do with protein coding, intronic regions are spliced out of the final mature messenger RNA (mRNA) after transcription. A main focus of current genomic investigation is on the regulatory role of intergenic nucleotide sequences known as microRNA (miRNA), which are posttranscriptional regulators that bind to complementary sequences on target mRNA transcripts.[7,8] Exonic regions are spliced together to form mRNA following removal of the intronic regions. mRNA is subsequently translated into protein, which can also undergo posttranslational modification. Genetic variation can occur within any of these DNA regions, and knowing the exact site can often help determine the result of a mutation. For example, genetic variation that occurs within promotors or exons can result in a functional change in protein concentration or production. In contrast, genetic variation within an intron often results in no change in protein production or function (i.e., synonymous mutations).

More recently, epigenetic modification has become the focus of intense investigation. Epigenetic research seeks to understand how seemingly heritable changes in gene expression lead to altered phenotypes without changes in the underlying DNA sequence. The mechanisms underlying altered gene expression without changes in DNA sequences can be grouped into three categories: DNA methylation, histone modification, and nucleosome positioning[9] (Figure 4-4). Although DNA methylation is essential for normal cellular development, hypomethylation or hypermethylation can result in altered regulation of gene transcription. Histones are proteins found in the nucleus of eukaryotic cells that package DNA into nucleosomes. Posttranslational modification of histones plays an important role in transcriptional regulation,

DNA repair and replication, and RNA splicing.[10-12] Finally, promotor regions located at the 5′ or 3′ regions of a gene have nucleosome-free regions designated for assembly and disassembly of transcriptional machinery. Changes in the position of nucleosomes can interfere with transcriptional proteins; the result can be altered gene transcription. Altered gene transcription resulting in defective protein production can lead to human disease.

Pharmacogenetic Approach

Phenotypic variability can result from genetic inheritance and/or environmental factors. Pharmacogenetics uses recognized study designs (http://www.oege.org/) to measure the portion of phenotypic variability that can be ascribed to genetic variation. *Familial aggregation* studies determine whether or not there is a significant genetic component to a particular disease. *Familial segregation* studies aim to quantify the pattern of disease inheritance (e.g., whether a disease phenotype is inherited in a dominant or recessive manner). *Linkage studies* aim to determine the relative location of a "disease" gene, while *gene association* studies go one step further, aiming to pinpoint a specific allele or set of alleles associated with the disease phenotype.

While these study designs are valuable for determining the degree to which genetic variability influences phenotype, they are not without limitations. Of major importance in designing genetic association studies is determining a strict phenotype definition that can be used consistently across subsequent studies. A large sample size, not uncommonly in the thousands, is usually required depending on the disease incidence and risk allele frequency (i.e., minor allele frequency) within the study population. Allele frequencies also differ significantly amongst ethnic groups. Population stratification, also referred to as *genetic admixture*, can thus be a source of false-positive findings in gene association studies because the results are linked to the underlying genetic structure of the study population, and not the gene of interest per se, particularly when the study population is composed of two or more ethnic

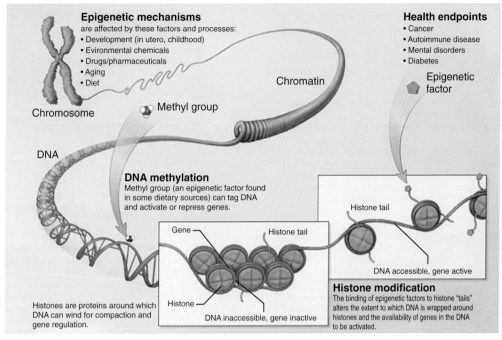

Epigenetic mechanisms
are affected by these factors and processes:
• Development (in utero, childhood)
• Evironmental chemicals
• Drugs/pharmaceuticals
• Aging
• Diet

Health endpoints
• Cancer
• Autoimmune disease
• Mental disorders
• Diabetes

Chromosome

Methyl group

DNA

Chromatin

Epigenetic factor

DNA methylation
Methyl group (an epigenetic factor found in some dietary sources) can tag DNA and activate or repress genes.

Gene

Histone tail

Histone tail

DNA accessible, gene active

Histones are proteins around which DNA can wind for compaction and gene regulation.

Histone

DNA inaccessible, gene inactive

Histone modification
The binding of epigenetic factors to histone "tails" alters the extent to which DNA is wrapped around histones and the availability of genes in the DNA to be activated.

Figure 4-4 Epigenetic modification through DNA methylation or histone modification can result in disease without changes in DNA sequence.

groups. When identifying an association between genetic variability and disease, it is often necessary to compare multiple risk alleles with the phenotype in question. This is especially true in genome-wide association studies (GWAS) where often more than 500,000 alleles are being examined, and therefore more than 500,000 comparisons are being made. Avoidance of false-positive findings requires use of complex multivariate statistical analyses that include controls for multiple genetic comparisons (e.g., permutation testing).

HISTORY OF PHARMACOGENETICS

The underlying concepts of pharmacogenetics were born from clinical observations that standard doses of medications result in varying plasma concentrations and varying clinical responses between individuals. Prolonged muscle paralysis after a standard intubating dose of succinylcholine is an often-cited example of an early pharmacogenetic discovery. Investigators discovered individuals who remained paralyzed for prolonged periods of time had an atypical form of the enzyme responsible for metabolizing succinylcholine, butyrylcholinesterase (BCHE), also called plasma or serum cholinesterase (see Chapter 19).[13-15]

With advances in genotyping, investigators discovered a nonsynonymous or coding SNP associated with the most common atypical form of BCHE. The identified *BCHE* SNP, G209>A, resulted in a change in amino acid sequence (Asp70>Gly) at the active site, rendering the enzyme much less active in catalyzing succinylcholine hydrolysis. Thus recovery from a typical "intubating dose" in a patient heterozygous for the BCHE polymorphism might take 3 to 8 times longer than in an individual expressing the wild type allele. Patients homozygous for the *BCHE* SNP have even more pronounced delay in recovery.[16] More than 20 variants of the serum cholinesterase gene have been identified that are associated with either varying plasma enzyme concentrations or function.[17] The number of BCHE DNA sequence variants and the range in phenotypes with which these variants are associated illustrate the complexity of pharmacogenomic science.

Another early example of the impact of pharmacogenetics was the description of the *CYP2D6* gene polymorphism. Studying metabolism of the antihypertensive drug debrisoquine in more than 1000 Swedish subjects, investigators defined poor metabolizers, extensive metabolizers, and ultrarapid metabolizers.[18] The variability in frequency distribution of debrisoquine metabolism in the general population was later associated with functional *CYP2D6* gene polymorphisms and copy number variations (see later discussion).[19-21]

Since these initial discoveries, individuals with multiple copies of the *CYP2D6* gene are ultrarapid metabolizers of multiple drugs, including nortriptyline and metoprolol, making these drugs largely ineffective in individuals expressing this polymorphism, and putting them at risk of underdosing with traditional dosing regimens.[22-24] Alternatively, individuals with functional polymorphisms or deletions of the *CYP2D6* gene show no or impaired metabolism of various prodrugs, including codeine and tamoxifen, to their active metabolites.[25-28] *CYP2D6* ultrarapid metabolizers are at greater risk for codeine toxicity (see later discussion).[29,30]

The association of volatile anesthetic administration and malignant hyperthermia (MH) is another well-known example of anesthesia pharmacogenetics (see Chapter 6). Although originally thought to be autosomal dominant, evidence now suggests that MH is a complex molecular trait associated with more than 200 ryanodine receptor 1 (*RYR1*) gene polymorphisms.[31-33] Investigators have sequenced all 106 exons of the large *RYR1* gene in 192 individuals susceptible to MH, and found no mutations in 50 of those individuals, which suggests either that genomic information contained

Table 4-1. Recent Pharmacogenetic Discoveries Related to Anesthesia and Pain Medicine Practice

GENE	ASSOCIATED PHENOTYPE AND REFERENCE
Angiotensin converting enzyme (ACE) gene indel	Increased vascular reactivity to phenylephrine in patients with the D allele[102]
Melanocortin-1 receptor (MC1R) gene polymorphisms	Variable in response to volatile anesthetics[103-105]
Mu-opioid receptor (OPRM1) gene polymorphism	Variable response to neuraxial fentanyl in obstetric patients[106]
5, 10-Methylene tetrahydrofolate reductase (MTHFR) gene polymorphism	Acute demyelization in children exposed to nitrous oxide,[107,108] and raised plasma homocysteine levels after nitrous oxide exposure
CYP2C19 gene polymorphism	Patients with variants in the CYP2C19 gene can have lower levels of the active metabolite of clopidogrel and subsequently less inhibition of platelets resulting in a greater risk for death, heart attack, and stroke[109-111]

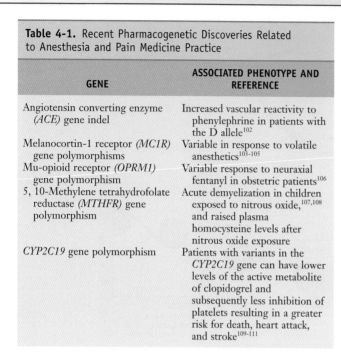

Figure 4-5 The focus of pharmacogenetic research has been to identify variability in drug targets, drug transporters and drug metabolizing enzymes. Genetic variability is responsible for some of the interindividual differences in pharmacodynamic and pharmacokinetic behavior, providing the scientific foundation for whether a medication is effective and safe for a given genotype. The broken line indicates that drug transporters are also occasionally the drug target, in addition to affecting pharmacokinetics. *(Adapted with permission from Johnson JA. Pharmacogenetics: potential for individualized drug therapy through genetics.* Trends Genet. *2003;19:660-666.)*

outside exonic regions (promotor region or introns, most likely) plays a larger role than traditionally thought, or that additional susceptibility loci exist outside the *RYR1* gene that are either directly associated with MH or modify the effects of the *RYR1* gene.[34-40]

There are multiple clinically relevant examples of genetic variation associated with differential drug response between individuals. For example, more than 30 genes have now been associated with mechanisms of warfarin and clopidogrel-mediated anticoagulation, most notably *CYP2C9* and *VKORC1*.[41,42] β-adrenergic receptor (*β-AR*) gene variants have been associated with increased mortality in acute coronary syndrome patients,[43] while other *β-AR* gene variants have been associated with variable response to bronchodilators.[44,45] Other recent pharmacogenetic discoveries are summarized in Table 4-1.

PHARMACOGENETICS AND DRUG METABOLISM

Traditionally, investigators separated the various phases of pharmacokinetics into distinct categories such as absorption, distribution, metabolism, and elimination (ADME). Variability in drug response between individuals is due in part to variability in pharmacokinetic behavior between individuals. Although variability in drug response has been attributed to differences in transporter proteins, cellular receptors or targets, and metabolic enzymes (Figure 4-5), more recent investigation suggests that such variability has important genetic underpinnings.

Phase I Drug Metabolism

CYTOCHROME 450 ENZYME FAMILY
Before elimination, many lipophilic drugs are converted from an active hydrophobic form to a hydrophilic form through a

series of enzymatic reactions that include oxidation, reduction, or hydrolysis. This often results in a more polar molecule in what has been termed *phase I drug metabolism*. Oxidation of drugs during phase I metabolism is mediated primarily by the cytochrome P450 (CYP) enzyme family, which are present in all tissues, with the highest concentration in the liver (Figure 4-6). Genes encoding for CYP enzymes are indicated by an Arabic numeral, followed by a capital letter indicating the subfamily, and then a number indicating the specific gene.[46] Therefore, the gene that codes for isozyme 6 of the cytochrome P450 isoenzyme CYP2B is denoted *CYP2B6*.

Of the CYP enzymes, CYP families 1, 2, and 3 play the most important role in phase I drug metabolism. Within these families, the CYP3A subfamily is responsible for as much as 50% of all CYP-mediated metabolism of clinically relevant drugs (Figure 4-7).[17,47-49] Most pharmacogenetic research has focused on identifying SNPs associated with either altered concentration or function of these specific CYP isoenzymes.

As early as the 1970s, investigators described differential metabolism of the probe antihypertensive drug debrisoquine, including poor metabolizers and ultrarapid metabolizers.[50,51] The majority of people metabolized debrisoquine at a "normal" rate, identified as extensive metabolizers. On sequencing the *CYP2D6* gene, specific genetic variants were associated with each of these three phenotypes as well as an additional group known as intermediate metabolizers (see comprehensive description of all known CYP gene variants at www.imm.ki.se/CYPalleles, and Table 4-2). Poor metabolizers were noted to be homozygous at a given variant, meaning they carried a genetic mutation at both alleles[52]; this phenotype is estimated to occur in approximately 7% to 10% of Caucasians.[53] Intermediate metabolizers were noted to be heterozygous at a given variant, meaning they carried one copy of the polymorphisms, while ultrarapid metabolizers were noted to have gene duplication.[53,54] Gene duplication resulting in ultrarapid phenotype can result in failed analgesic or exaggerated side effects,

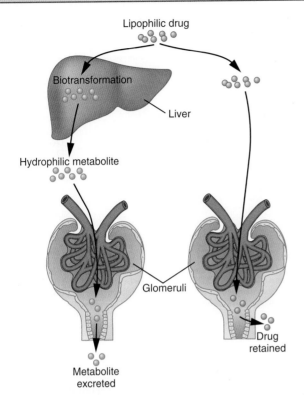

Figure 4-6 Metabolism of lipophilic drugs. Phase I drug metabolism is mediated primarily by the cytochrome P450 enzyme family. The more hydrophilic metabolites are more easily excreted by the kidney. *(Adapted with permission from Weinshilboum R. Inheritance and drug response. N Engl J Med. 2003;348:529-537.)*

Table 4-2. Common Cytochrome P450 (CYP) and Flavin-Containing Monooxygenase (FMO) Gene Variants Associated with Altered Phase I Metabolism

PHASE I GENE	GENE VARIANT	EFFECT ON ENZYME ACTIVITY
CYP1A2	-3860G>A	Decreased
	-163C>A	Increased
CYP 2A6	L160H	Absent
	G479V	Absent
	R128Q	Decreased
	1471T	Decreased
	S224P	Decreased
	V365M	Decreased
	Y392F	Decreased
	K476R	Decreased
	R203C	Decreased
	V110L, N438Y	Decreased
	F118L, R128L, S131A	Decreased
CYP 2B6	785A>G	Increased
	516G>T, 785A>G	Decreased
	983T>C	Decreased
CYP 2C8	805A>T	Increased
	416G>A, 1196A>G	Decreased
CYP 2C9	430C>T	Decreased
	1075A>C	Decreased
	1080C>G	Decreased
CYP 2E1	R76H	Decreased
CYP 2C19	99C>T, 991A>G	Increased
CYP 2D6	100C>T, 1661G>C, 4180G>C	Decreased
CYP 3A4	F189S	Decreased
CYP 3A5	6986A>G	Decreased
CYP 3A7	-314G>A	Increased
FMO3	472G>A, 923A>G	Decreased
	1079T>C	Increased

Modified from Crettol S, Petrovic N, Murray M. Pharmacogenetics of phase I and phase II drug metabolism. *Curr Pharm Des.* 2010;16:204-219; Restrepo JG, Garcia-Martin E, Martinez C, Agundez JA. Polymorphic drug metabolism in anaesthesia. *Curr Drug Metab.* 2009;10:236-246.

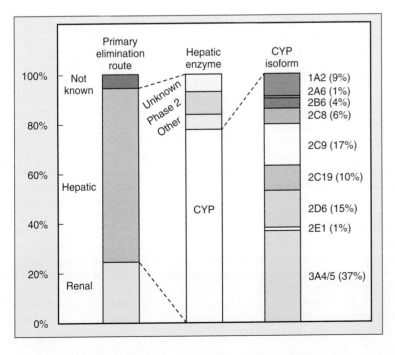

Figure 4-7 Organs and enzymes of drug elimination. Data are shown for the top 200 prescription drugs in the United States, according to RXList data for April 2008 (www.rxlist.com). Phase I drug metabolism is mediated primarily by hepatic cytochrome P450, the most common isoform being CYP3A. *(Adapted with permission from Zanger UM, Turpeinen M, Klein K, Schwab M. Functional pharmacogenetics/genomics of human cytochromes P450 involved in drug biotransformation. Anal Bioanal Chem. 2008;392:1093-1108.)*

depending on whether the prodrug or the metabolite is more active. For example, a patient with renal dysfunction and the *CYP2D6* ultrarapid genotype might experience respiratory depression after receiving tramadol, or a patient with the *CYP2D6* ultrarapid metabolizer genotype may have higher plasma levels of OD-T (active metabolite of tramadol), but more postoperative nausea compared with patients with the extensive metabolizer genotype.[54,55] This holds true for patients receiving codeine (codeine is a prodrug of morphine, the active molecule; see Chapter 15); patients with ultrarapid metabolizer genotype have higher plasma morphine levels, and more analgesia and sedation.[29] The spectrum of *CYP2D6* gene polymorphisms are an example of genetic variation associated with either extreme; ineffective codeine dosing in patients with poor metabolism, and exaggerated effects in patients with ultrarapid metabolism (see later).[56,57] These genetically mediated extreme responses are relevant in as many as 10% to 20% of Caucasians.[57]

FLAVIN-CONTAINING MONOOXYGENASE ENZYMES

To a much lesser extent, flavin-containing monooxygenases (FMO) play a role in phase I drug elimination by oxidizing a wide range of drugs, which usually results in a more polar and therefore less active metabolite compared with CYP enzyme metabolism. Additionally, FMO-catalyzed reactions are less likely to be induced or inhibited by other drugs, making adverse drug-drug reactions rare.[58] Investigators have identified five *FMO* genes all located on chromosome 1. The most well characterized *FMO* gene is *FMO3* (see Table 4-2). Loss of function mutations of the *FMO3* gene, a gene expressed in the liver, is associated with trimethylaminuria. Many SNPs have been identified, but none have been directly associated with altered metabolism of anesthesia-related drugs.[58-62]

Phase II Drug Metabolism

Phase II drug metabolism involves conjugation of a drug or drug metabolite and an endogenous hydrophilic molecule to make a more water-soluble compound easier to eliminate. Compared with phase I drug metabolism, phase II metabolism is mediated by a larger number of enzymes, including N-acetyltransferases (NAT), UDP-glucuronosyltransferases (UGTs), glutathione S-transferases (GSTs), and sulfotransferase (SULT), to name a few.[63] Fewer genetic variations have been associated with altered drug metabolism primarily because phase II enzymes do not play a primary role in the rate-limiting steps of drug metabolism (Table 4-3). As such, a clinical phenotype secondary to altered phase II metabolism is rare, and without a well-defined phenotype, genetic association studies yield very little useful information.

NAT and *UGT* gene variations provide two examples of how phase II gene variation is associated with altered drug metabolism. Two clinical phenotypes have been associated with polymorphisms identified on the *NAT1* and *NAT2* genes. Acetylation polymorphisms of the *NAT* genes are associated with either rapid or slow acetylation. These phenotypes were first identified in tuberculosis patients treated with isoniazid. Rapid acetylators had normal isoniazid levels, while slow acetylators had elevated serum concentrations.[64] While more than 25 SNPs have been identified on the *NAT* genes, the null alleles of the *NAT2* gene have most often been associated with defective acetylation phenotype. The *NAT2* null allele is

Table 4-3. Common Gene Variants Associated with Altered Phase II Metabolism

PHASE II GENE	GENE VARIANT	EFFECT ON ENZYME ACTIVITY
NAT1	R187Q	Decreased
	R64W	Decreased
NAT2	1114T	Decreased
	R197Q	Decreased
	G286E	Decreased
	E167K	Decreased
	R64Q	Decreased
UGT1A1	G71R	Decreased
	1294T	Decreased
	M310V	Decreased
GSTA1	-567T>G, -69C>T, -52G>A	Decreased
GSTP1	1104V, A113V	Decreased
SULT1A1	R213H	Decreased

Modified from Crettol S, Petrovic N, Murray M. Pharmacogenetics of phase I and phase II drug metabolism. *Curr Pharm Des.* 2010;16:204-219.
NAT, N-Acetyltransferase; *UGT,* UDP-glucuronosyltransferase; *GST,* glutathione S-transferase; *SULT,* sulfotransferase.

associated with development of lupus erythematosus in patients who receive hydralazine and procainamide, and hemolytic anemia and inflammatory bowel disease in patients who receive sulfasalazine.[65]

Genetic variants that code for the UGTs are associated with altered glucuronidation. Polymorphisms of the *UGT2B7* gene are associated with altered glucuronidation in which administration of diclofenac, a commonly used nonsteroidal antiinflammatory drug (NSAID), leads to accumulation of hepatotoxic metabolites.[66] There are numerous compensatory glucuronidation pathways that ultimately mitigate the risks associated with *UTG* gene polymorphisms, however.

PHARMACOGENETICS OF ANESTHETIC DRUGS

Opioids

Weaker opioids, including codeine, dihydrocodeine, tramadol, hydrocodone, and oxycodone, are metabolized to more potent opioids such as morphine, hydromorphone, and oxymorphone largely by the CYP enzyme *CYP2D6*.[67] More than 100 SNPs have been identified in the *CYP2D6* gene that result in four different clinical phenotypes: poor (5%-10% of Caucasians), intermediate (10%-15% of Caucasians), extensive (65%-80% of Caucasians), and ultrarapid (5%-10% of Caucasians) metabolizers of opioids.[47,67,68] There are significant differences in plasma morphine concentrations between patients who are poor and extensive (normal) metabolizers of codeine.[69-72] Ultrarapid metabolizers of codeine have as much as 50% higher plasma morphine concentrations compared with extensive codeine metabolizers.[29] While these studies clearly show a difference in intermediate phenotypes such as drug metabolite concentrations, well-designed clinical studies have not been powered to show a difference in opioid efficacy or side effect profile between the varying opioid phenotypes.[73-75] There is also considerable ethnic variability in frequency of phenotypes. For example, 0.5% of Chinese are ultrarapid metabolizers, while 29% of Ethiopians are ultrarapid metabolizers.[48] *COMT* gene variants have also been associated with magnified effects of opioids.[76-78]

Tramadol is a prodrug that undergoes O-demethylation to the opioid agonist M1 by *CYP2D6*. Studies have shown a significantly lower plasma M1 concentration and reduced analgesic effects of tramadol in poor metabolizers compared with extensive metabolizers.[79,80] In 300 patients undergoing abdominal surgery, poor metabolizers received more tramadol postoperatively and were more likely to require additional opioid medication for postoperative pain control compared with extensive metabolizers.[81] These findings have since been corroborated in several small studies, suggesting an association between *CYP2D6* gene polymorphisms and hypoanalgesic effects of tramadol in patients who carry the poor metabolizer phenotype.[52,82,83]

Oxycodone is a potent semisynthetic opioid prodrug that is oxidized to oxymorphone by *CYP2D6* and N-demethylated by CYP3A. Significant differences in the time course of plasma concentrations of oxycodone metabolites occur depending on the *CYP2D6* genotype. Individuals with a *CYP2D6* polymorphism that results in *CYP2D6* deficiency have lower oxymorphone levels compared with individuals with genotypes associated with either normal or ultrarapid metabolism.[84] Individuals with genotype-mediated *CYP2D6* deficiency still have low but measurable levels of oxymorphone such that other metabolic pathways must be involved when *CYP2D6* is either deficient or nonfunctional.

Methadone is a racemic mixture of R- and S-methadone; its metabolism is highly dependent on *CYP2D6*.[85] The *CYP2D6 *6/*6* genotype is associated with higher plasma S-methadone levels compared with the wild type, but there is no significant association between genotype and clinical response to methadone in that R-methadone accounts for most of the opioid effect.[86,87] Variability in plasma methadone concentrations depend on *CYP2D6* genotypes, further supporting CYP enzyme polymorphisms in mediating opioid metabolism. Of 256 subjects genotyped in one study, 228 were extensive metabolizers (metabolized at a normal rate), 18 patients were poor metabolizers, and 10 were ultrarapid metabolizers, with significant differences in methadone concentrations between groups.[88] Although *CYP1A2* and *CYP2C19* gene polymorphisms have been implicated in methadone metabolism, clinical significance has not been demonstrated. While metabolism of alfentanil, fentanyl, and sufentanil can be affected by *CYP3A4* activity, *CYP3A4* gene polymorphisms have not been associated with differences in clinical effects for these opioids.[89]

Inhalation and Intravenous Anesthetic Agents

Biotransformation of inhalation and intravenously administered anesthetic agents are mediated to a large extent by the phase I CYP enzymes.[90] Only a limited number of animal studies have suggested gene-mediated variability in metabolism of these drugs.[91-96] Although many CYP gene polymorphisms have been identified, studies examining an association between these polymorphisms and altered metabolism of either inhalation and intravenous anesthetic agents and associated clinical implications are extremely limited. Two small studies demonstrated an association between the *CYP2C19* gene *G681A* polymorphism and impaired metabolism of diazepam.[97,98] As genotyping becomes more cost effective, larger clinical trials investigating genetic-mediated variability of inhalation and intravenously administered anesthetic agents between individuals should result.

Nonsteroidal Antiinflammatory Drugs

An association between a *CYP2C9* genotype and the risk of gastrointestinal bleeding after NSAID use was suggested by a retrospective study of 2918 patients.[99] In this study, the odds ratio for heterozygous and homozygous carriers of the *CYP2C9* risk allele was 2.5 and 3.7 compared with carriers of the wild type allele.[99] A recent study replicated these findings by showing an association between *CYP2C9* risk alleles and endoscopically confirmed NSAID-related gastrointestinal bleeding.[100] Presumably, *CYP2C9* polymorphisms associated with these adverse effects following NSAID administration can be explained by altered metabolism. Along these lines, there is a three-fold higher 4'-OH diclofenac urinary ratio in carriers of the *CYP2C9 *3/*3* risk allele compared with the wild-type carriers.[101]

EMERGING DEVELOPMENTS

Pharmacogenetics refers to genetic differences in metabolic pathways that can affect individual responses to drugs, including both therapeutic effects and adverse effects. Because the genotype of an individual is essentially invariable and largely remains unaffected by the treatment itself, pharmacogenetic approaches help delineate what is due to genetic rather than environmental factors. The ease of accessibility to genotype information through peripheral blood or saliva sampling, combined with advances in molecular techniques, has increased the feasibility of DNA collection and genotyping in large-scale clinical trials (e.g., genome-wide association study screening). Through such an approach, it should be possible to advance clinical medicine by better targeting drugs to the right populations, reducing adverse outcomes, and minimizing socioeconomic cost. In the future, it is conceivable that routine testing characterizing a patient's pharmacogenomic profile will guide therapeutic decisions prior to the initiation of therapy (Figure 4-8).

KEY POINTS

- Traditional approaches to pharmacology have been challenged by recognition that genotypic variability can influence drug metabolism and response.
- *Pharmacogenetics* attempts to define how individuals respond to a given drug based on their inherited genetic makeup.
- Variability in drug responses between individuals is due in part to differences in pharmacokinetic and pharmacodynamic properties between individuals.
- All organisms have a unique, inherited sequence of nucleotide base pairings known as their *genotype*. This genetic blueprint serves as a template for protein production, which in turn is ultimately responsible for the form, function, and outward appearance of the organism, or its *phenotype*.

Continued

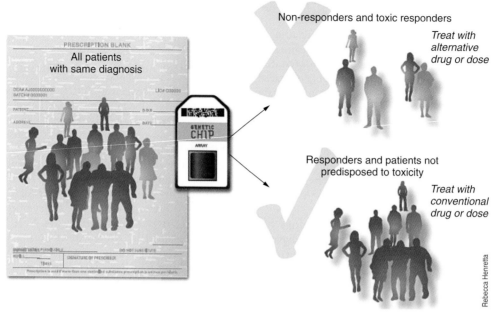

Figure 4-8 In the future, genetic variability contributing to altered drug response will become more easily identifiable through advancing technology. These advances will in turn become the basis for personalized medicine; responders and non-responders will be identified before drug administration by individual genotyping. *(Adapted with permission from Piquette-Miller M, Grant DM. The art and science of personalized medicine.* Clin Pharmacol Ther. *2007;81: 311-315.)*

KEY POINTS—cont'd

- Because the genotype of an individual is essentially invariable and remains unaffected by drug treatment, pharmacogenetic investigations can help differentiate genetic vs. environmental factors in drug responses.
- Prolonged muscle paralysis after a standard dose of succinylcholine is a classic example of a pharmacogenetic effect on drug metabolism (i.e., a pharmacokinetic alteration) in anesthesia.
- Malignant hyperthermia after exposure to succinylcholine or volatile anesthetics is another prototype example of a pharmacogenetic influence on drug response (i.e., a pharmacodynamic alteration) in anesthesia.
- Before elimination, many drugs are converted from an active hydrophobic (lipophilic) form to a hydrophilic form through a series of enzymatic reactions that include oxidation, reduction, and/or hydrolysis to result in a more polar molecule. These *phase I drug metabolism* reactions are catalyzed by the cytochrome P450 (CYP) enzymes, with CYP1, 2, and 3 being most important.
- *Phase II drug metabolism* involves conjugation between the drug and an endogenous hydrophilic molecule to make a more water-soluble compound that is easier to eliminate.
- Independent genetic variants associated with poor, intermediate, or ultrarapid metabolism of administered drugs have been identified. The case of codeine is a prototype example in anesthesia practice.
- Pharmacogenetic approaches will facilitate targeting drugs to the right populations (personalized medicine), reducing adverse outcomes, and minimizing socioeconomic cost.

Key References

Crettol S, Petrovic N, Murray M. Pharmacogenetics of phase I and phase II drug metabolism. *Curr Pharm Des.* 2010;16:204-219. This recent review details the important Phase I and II gene variants associated with altered drug metabolism, including the cytochrome P450 enzyme gene variants, flavin-containing mono-oxygenase gene variants, and NAT, UGT, GST, and SULT gene variants. (Ref. 63)

Gasche Y, Daali Y, Fathi M, et al. Codeine intoxication associated with ultrarapid *CYP2D6* metabolism. *N Engl J Med.* 2004;351:2827-2831. Report of a case of life-threatening codeine intoxication in a patient who received an antitussive dose of codeine. On further investigation, the patient was found to carry at least three functional alleles of the *CYP2D6* gene, the gene responsible for producing the enzyme that activates codeine to morphine. (Ref. 30)

Iohom G, Fitzgerald D, Cunningham AJ. Principles of pharmacogenetics—implications for the anaesthetist. *Br J Anaesth.* 2004;93:440-450. A practical approach to understanding and applying the principles of pharmacogenetics in the current clinical arena. (Ref. 17)

Lehmann H, Ryan E. The familial incidence of low pseudocholinesterase level. *Lancet.* 1956;271(6934):124. A landmark report of a markedly decreased level of pseudocholinesterase levels in seemingly normal family members of patients suffering prolonged wake-up after succinylcholine. From this article was borne the notion that pseudocholinesterase levels might be genetically determined; homozygous individuals had low or missing enzyme, while heterozygous individuals had markedly decreased levels. (Ref. 15)

Restrepo JG, Garcia-Martin E, Martinez C, Agundez JA. Polymorphic drug metabolism in anaesthesia. *Curr Drug Metab.* Mar 2009;10:236-246. Review of the association between altered metabolism of volatile and intravenous anesthetics, and gene variants of phase I and II enzymes. (Ref. 90)

Wang L. Pharmacogenomics: a systems approach. *Wiley Interdiscip Rev Syst Biol Med.* 2010;2:3-22. This recently published review chronicles the history of modern pharmacogenetics and underscores the impact pharmacogenetics will have on how we manage patients on an individualized basis. (Ref. 1)

References

1. Wang L. Pharmacogenomics: a systems approach. *Wiley Interdiscip Rev Syst Biol Med*. 2010;2(1):3-22.
2. Nebert DW. Pharmacogenetics and pharmacogenomics: why is this relevant to the clinical geneticist? *Clin Genet*. 1999;56(4):247-258.
3. West WL, Knight EM, Pradhan S, et al. Interpatient variability: genetic predisposition and other genetic factors. *J Clin Pharmacol*. 1997;37(7):635-648.
4. Lazarou J, Pomeranz BH, Corey PN. Incidence of adverse drug reactions in hospitalized patients: a meta-analysis of prospective studies. *JAMA*. 1998;279(15):1200-1205.
5. Rodriguez-Monguio R, Otero MJ, Rovira J. Assessing the economic impact of adverse drug effects. *Pharmacoeconomics*. 2003;21(9):623-650.
6. Pennisi E. Bioinformatics. Gene counters struggle to get the right answer. *Science*. 2003;301(5636):1040-1041.
7. Pauli A, Rinn JL, Schier AF. Non-coding RNAs as regulators of embryogenesis. *Nat Rev Genet*. 2011;12(2):136-149.
8. Huntzinger E, Izaurralde E. Gene silencing by microRNAs: contributions of translational repression and mRNA decay. *Nat Rev Genet*. 2011;12(2):99-110.
9. Portela A, Esteller M. Epigenetic modifications and human disease. *Nat Biotechnol*. 2010;28(10):1057-1068.
10. Kouzarides T. Chromatin modifications and their function. *Cell*. 2007;128(4):693-705.
11. Huertas D, Sendra R, Munoz P. Chromatin dynamics coupled to DNA repair. *Epigenetics*. 2009;4(1):31-42.
12. Luco RF, Pan Q, Tominaga K, et al. Regulation of alternative splicing by histone modifications. *Science*. 2010;327(5968):996-1000.
13. Kalow W, Gunn DR. Some statistical data on atypical cholinesterase of human serum. *Ann Hum Genet*. 1959;23:239-250.
14. Kalow W, Gunn DR. The relation between dose of succinylcholine and duration of apnea in man. *J Pharmacol Exp Ther*. 1957;120(2):203-214.
15. Lehmann H, Ryan E. The familial incidence of low pseudocholinesterase level. *Lancet*. 1956;271(6934):124.
16. Jensen FS, Viby-Mogensen J. Plasma cholinesterase and abnormal reaction to succinylcholine: twenty years' experience with the Danish Cholinesterase Research Unit. *Acta Anaesthesiol Scand*. 1995;39(2):150-156.
17. Iohom G, Fitzgerald D, Cunningham AJ. Principles of pharmacogenetics—implications for the anaesthetist. *Br J Anaesth*. 2004;93:440-450.
18. Bertilsson L, Lou YQ, Du YL, et al. Pronounced differences between native Chinese and Swedish populations in the polymorphic hydroxylations of debrisoquine and S-mephenytoin. *Clin Pharmacol Ther*. 1992;51(4):388-397.
19. Johansson I, Lundqvist E, Bertilsson L, et al. Inherited amplification of an active gene in the cytochrome P450 CYP2D locus as a cause of ultrarapid metabolism of debrisoquine. *Proc Natl Acad Sci U S A*. 1993;90(24):11825-11829.
20. Gonzalez FJ, Vilbois F, Hardwick JP, et al. Human debrisoquine 4-hydroxylase (P450IID1): cDNA and deduced amino acid sequence and assignment of the CYP2D locus to chromosome 22. *Genomics*. 1988;2(2):174-179.
21. Kimura S, Umeno M, Skoda RC, et al. The human debrisoquine 4-hydroxylase (CYP2D) locus: sequence and identification of the polymorphic CYP2D6 gene, a related gene, and a pseudogene. *Am J Hum Genet*. 1989;45(6):889-904.
22. Dalen P, Dahl ML, Bernal Ruiz ML, et al. 10-Hydroxylation of nortriptyline in white persons with 0, 1, 2, 3, and 13 functional CYP2D6 genes. *Clin Pharmacol Ther*. 1998;63(4):444-452.
23. Kroemer HK, Eichelbaum M. "It's the genes, stupid." Molecular bases and clinical consequences of genetic cytochrome P450 2D6 polymorphism. *Life Sci*. 1995;56(26):2285-2298.
24. Lennard MS, Silas JH, Freestone S, et al. Oxidation phenotype—a major determinant of metoprolol metabolism and response. *N Engl J Med*. Dec 16 1982;307(25):1558-1560.
25. Mortimer O, Persson K, Ladona MG, et al. Polymorphic formation of morphine from codeine in poor and extensive metabolizers of dextromethorphan: relationship to the presence of immunoidentified cytochrome P-450IID1. *Clin Pharmacol Ther*. 1990;47(1):27-35.
26. Sindrup SH, Brosen K. The pharmacogenetics of codeine hypoalgesia. *Pharmacogenetics*. 1995;5(6):335-346.
27. Jin Y, Desta Z, Stearns V, et al. CYP2D6 genotype, antidepressant use, and tamoxifen metabolism during adjuvant breast cancer treatment. *J Natl Cancer Inst*. 2005;97(1):30-39.
28. Stearns V, Johnson MD, Rae JM, et al. Active tamoxifen metabolite plasma concentrations after coadministration of tamoxifen and the selective serotonin reuptake inhibitor paroxetine. *J Natl Cancer Inst*. 2003;95(23):1758-1764.
29. Kirchheiner J, Schmidt H, Tzvetkov M, et al. Pharmacokinetics of codeine and its metabolite morphine in ultra-rapid metabolizers due to CYP2D6 duplication. *Pharmacogenomics J*. 2007;7(4):257-265.
30. Gasche Y, Daali Y, Fathi M, et al. Codeine intoxication associated with ultrarapid CYP2D6 metabolism. *N Engl J Med*. 2004;351:2827-2831.
31. Monnier N, Krivosic-Horber R, Payen JF, et al. Presence of two different genetic traits in malignant hyperthermia families: implication for genetic analysis, diagnosis, and incidence of malignant hyperthermia susceptibility. *Anesthesiology*. 2002;97(5):1067-1074.
32. Urwyler A, Deufel T, McCarthy T, et al. Guidelines for molecular genetic detection of susceptibility to malignant hyperthermia. *Br J Anaesth*. 2001;86(2):283-287.
33. Robinson R, Carpenter D, Shaw MA, et al. Mutations in RYR1 in malignant hyperthermia and central core disease. *Hum Mutat*. 2006;27(10):977-989.
34. Iles DE, Lehmann-Horn F, Scherer SW, et al. Localization of the gene encoding the alpha 2/delta-subunits of the L-type voltage-dependent calcium channel to chromosome 7q and analysis of the segregation of flanking markers in malignant hyperthermia susceptible families. *Hum Mol Genet*. 1994;3(6):969-975.
35. Levitt RC, Olckers A, Meyers S, et al. Evidence for the localization of a malignant hyperthermia susceptibility locus (MHS2) to human chromosome 17q. *Genomics*. 1992;14(3):562-566.
36. Monnier N, Procaccio V, Stieglitz P, et al. Malignant-hyperthermia susceptibility is associated with a mutation of the alpha 1-subunit of the human dihydropyridine-sensitive L-type voltage-dependent calcium-channel receptor in skeletal muscle. *Am J Hum Genet*. 1997;60(6):1316-1325.
37. Robinson RL, Monnier N, Wolz W, et al. A genome wide search for susceptibility loci in three European malignant hyperthermia pedigrees. *Hum Mol Genet*. 1997;6(6):953-961.
38. Robinson RL, Anetseder MJ, Brancadoro V, et al. Recent advances in the diagnosis of malignant hyperthermia susceptibility: how confident can we be of genetic testing? *Eur J Hum Genet*. 2003;11(4):342-348.
39. Robinson RL, Curran JL, Ellis FR, et al. Multiple interacting gene products may influence susceptibility to malignant hyperthermia. *Ann Hum Genet*. 2000;64:307-320.
40. Robinson R, Hopkins P, Carsana A, et al. Several interacting genes influence the malignant hyperthermia phenotype. *Hum Genet*. 2003;112(2):217-218.
41. Sconce EA, Khan TI, Wynne HA, et al. The impact of CYP2C9 and VKORC1 genetic polymorphism and patient characteristics upon warfarin dose requirements: proposal for a new dosing regimen. *Blood*. 2005;106(7):2329-2333.
42. Mega JL, Simon T, Collet JP, et al. Reduced-function CYP2C19 genotype and risk of adverse clinical outcomes among patients treated with clopidogrel predominantly for PCI: a meta-analysis. *JAMA*. 2010;304(16):1821-1830.
43. Lanfear DE, Jones PG, Marsh S, et al. Beta2-adrenergic receptor genotype and survival among patients receiving beta-blocker therapy after an acute coronary syndrome. *JAMA*. 2005;294(12):1526-1533.
44. Israel E, Chinchilli VM, Ford JG, et al. Use of regularly scheduled albuterol treatment in asthma: genotype-stratified, randomised, placebo-controlled cross-over trial. *Lancet*. 2004;364(9444):1505-1512.
45. Wechsler ME, Lehman E, Lazarus SC, et al. Beta-adrenergic receptor polymorphisms and response to salmeterol. *Am J Respir Crit Care Med*. 2006;173(5):519-526.
46. Nelson DR, Kamataki T, Waxman DJ, et al. The P450 superfamily: update on new sequences, gene mapping, accession numbers, early trivial names of enzymes, and nomenclature. *DNA Cell Biol*. 1993;12(1):1-51.

47. Zanger UM, Raimundo S, Eichelbaum M. Cytochrome P450 2D6: overview and update on pharmacology, genetics, biochemistry. *Naunyn Schmiedebergs Arch Pharmacol*. 2004;369(1):23-37.

48. Ingelman-Sundberg M. Duplication, multiduplication, and amplification of genes encoding drug-metabolizing enzymes: evolutionary, toxicological, and clinical pharmacological aspects. *Drug Metab Rev*. 1999;31(2):449-459.

49. Kirchheiner J, Brockmoller J. Clinical consequences of cytochrome P450 2C9 polymorphisms. *Clin Pharmacol Ther*. 2005;77(1):1-16.

50. Eichelbaum M, Spannbrucker N, Steincke B, et al. Defective N-oxidation of sparteine in man: a new pharmacogenetic defect. *Eur J Clin Pharmacol*. 1979;16(3):183-187.

51. Mahgoub A, Idle JR, Dring LG, et al. Polymorphic hydroxylation of Debrisoquine in man. *Lancet*. 1977;2(8038):584-586.

52. Foster A, Mobley E, Wang Z. Complicated pain management in a CYP450 2D6 poor metabolizer. *Pain Pract*. 2007;7(4):352-356.

53. Stamer UM, Stuber F. Genetic factors in pain and its treatment. *Curr Opin Anaesthesiol*. 2007;20(5):478-484.

54. Stamer UM, Stuber F, Muders T, et al. Respiratory depression with tramadol in a patient with renal impairment and CYP2D6 gene duplication. *Anesth Analg*. 2008;107(3):926-929.

55. Kirchheiner J, Keulen JT, Bauer S, et al. Effects of the CYP2D6 gene duplication on the pharmacokinetics and pharmacodynamics of tramadol. *J Clin Psychopharmacol*. 2008;28(1):78-83.

56. Caraco Y, Sheller J, Wood AJ. Pharmacogenetic determination of the effects of codeine and prediction of drug interactions. *J Pharmacol Exp Ther*. 1996;278(3):1165-1174.

57. Caraco Y. Genes and the response to drugs. *N Engl J Med*. 2004;351(27):2867-2869.

58. Phillips IR, Shephard EA. Flavin-containing monooxygenases: mutations, disease and drug response. *Trends Pharmacol Sci*. 2008;29(6):294-301.

59. Lang DH, Yeung CK, Peter RM, et al. Isoform specificity of trimethylamine N-oxygenation by human flavin-containing monooxygenase (FMO) and P450 enzymes: selective catalysis by FMO3. *Biochem Pharmacol*. 1998;56(8):1005-1012.

60. Lattard V, Zhang J, Tran Q, et al. Two new polymorphisms of the FMO3 gene in Caucasian and African-American populations: comparative genetic and functional studies. *Drug Metab Dispos*. 2003;31(7):854-860.

61. Murphy HC, Dolphin CT, Janmohamed A, et al. A novel mutation in the flavin-containing monooxygenase 3 gene, FM03, that causes fish-odour syndrome: activity of the mutant enzyme assessed by proton NMR spectroscopy. *Pharmacogenetics*. 2000;10(5):439-451.

62. Cashman JR, Bi YA, Lin J, et al. Human flavin-containing monooxygenase form 3: cDNA expression of the enzymes containing amino acid substitutions observed in individuals with trimethylaminuria. *Chem Res Toxicol*. 1997;10(8):837-841.

63. Crettol S, Petrovic N, Murray M. Pharmacogenetics of phase I and phase II drug metabolism. *Curr Pharm Des*. 2010;16(2):204-219.

64. Evans DA, White TA. Human acetylation polymorphism. *J Lab Clin Med*. 1964;63:394-403.

65. Chen M, Xia B, Chen B, et al. N-acetyltransferase 2 slow acetylator genotype associated with adverse effects of sulphasalazine in the treatment of inflammatory bowel disease. *Can J Gastroenterol*. 2007;21(3):155-158.

66. Daly AK, Aithal GP, Leathart JB, et al. Genetic susceptibility to diclofenac-induced hepatotoxicity: contribution of UGT2B7, CYP2C8, and ABCC2 genotypes. *Gastroenterology*. 2007;132(1):272-281.

67. Somogyi AA, Barratt DT, Coller JK. Pharmacogenetics of opioids. *Clin Pharmacol Ther*. 2007;81(3):429-444.

68. Lovlie R, Daly AK, Matre GE, et al. Polymorphisms in CYP2D6 duplication-negative individuals with the ultrarapid metabolizer phenotype: a role for the CYP2D6*35 allele in ultrarapid metabolism? *Pharmacogenetics*. 2001;11(1):45-55.

69. Poulsen L, Brosen K, Arendt-Nielsen L, et al. Codeine and morphine in extensive and poor metabolizers of sparteine: pharmacokinetics, analgesic effect and side effects. *Eur J Clin Pharmacol*. 1996;51(3-4):289-295.

70. Chen ZR, Somogyi AA, Bochner F. Polymorphic O-demethylation of codeine. *Lancet*. 1988;2(8616):914-915.

71. Chen ZR, Somogyi AA, Reynolds G, et al. Disposition and metabolism of codeine after single and chronic doses in one poor and seven extensive metabolisers. *Br J Clin Pharmacol*. 1991;31(4):381-390.

72. Yue QY, Svensson JO, Alm C, et al. Codeine O-demethylation co-segregates with polymorphic debrisoquine hydroxylation. *Br J Clin Pharmacol*. 1989;28(6):639-645.

73. Persson K, Sjostrom S, Sigurdardottir I, et al. Patient-controlled analgesia (PCA) with codeine for postoperative pain relief in ten extensive metabolisers and one poor metaboliser of dextromethorphan. *Br J Clin Pharmacol*. 1995;39(2):182-186.

74. Poulsen L, Riishede L, Brosen K, et al. Codeine in post-operative pain. Study of the influence of sparteine phenotype and serum concentrations of morphine and morphine-6-glucuronide. *Eur J Clin Pharmacol*. 1998;54(6):451-454.

75. Williams DG, Patel A, Howard RF. Pharmacogenetics of codeine metabolism in an urban population of children and its implications for analgesic reliability. *Br J Anaesth*. 2002;89(6):839-845.

76. Ross JR, Riley J, Taegetmeyer AB, et al. Genetic variation and response to morphine in cancer patients: catechol-O-methyltransferase and multidrug resistance-1 gene polymorphisms are associated with central side effects. *Cancer*. 2008;112(6):1390-1403.

77. Rakvag TT, Ross JR, Sato H, et al. Genetic variation in the catechol-O-methyltransferase (COMT) gene and morphine requirements in cancer patients with pain. *Mol Pain*. 2008;4:64.

78. Reyes-Gibby CC, Shete S, Rakvag T, et al. Exploring joint effects of genes and the clinical efficacy of morphine for cancer pain: OPRM1 and COMT gene. *Pain*. 2007;130(1-2):25-30.

79. Enggaard TP, Poulsen L, Arendt-Nielsen L, et al. The analgesic effect of tramadol after intravenous injection in healthy volunteers in relation to CYP2D6. *Anesth Analg*. 2006;102(1):146-150.

80. Poulsen L, Arendt-Nielsen L, Brosen K, et al. The hypoalgesic effect of tramadol in relation to CYP2D6. *Clin Pharmacol Ther*. 1996;60(6):636-644.

81. Stamer UM, Lehnen K, Hothker F, et al. Impact of CYP2D6 genotype on postoperative tramadol analgesia. *Pain*. 2003;105(1-2):231-238.

82. Stamer UM, Musshoff F, Kobilay M, et al. Concentrations of tramadol and O-desmethyltramadol enantiomers in different CYP2D6 genotypes. *Clin Pharmacol Ther*. 2007;82(1):41-47.

83. Wang G, Zhang H, He F, et al. Effect of the CYP2D6*10 C188T polymorphism on postoperative tramadol analgesia in a Chinese population. *Eur J Clin Pharmacol*. 2006;62(11):927-931.

84. Samer CF, Daali Y, Wagner M, et al. Genetic polymorphisms and drug interactions modulating CYP2D6 and CYP3A activities have a major effect on oxycodone analgesic efficacy and safety. *Br J Pharmacol*. 2010;160(4):919-930.

85. Kharasch ED, Hoffer C, Whittington D, et al. Role of hepatic and intestinal cytochrome P450 3A and 2B6 in the metabolism, disposition, and miotic effects of methadone. *Clin Pharmacol Ther*. 2004;76(3):250-269.

86. Crettol S, Deglon JJ, Besson J, et al. ABCB1 and cytochrome P450 genotypes and phenotypes: influence on methadone plasma levels and response to treatment. *Clin Pharmacol Ther*. 2006;80(6):668-681.

87. Crettol S, Deglon JJ, Besson J, et al. Methadone enantiomer plasma levels, CYP2B6, CYP2C19, and CYP2C9 genotypes, and response to treatment. *Clin Pharmacol Ther*. 2005;78(6):593-604.

88. Eap CB, Broly F, Mino A, et al. Cytochrome P450 2D6 genotype and methadone steady-state concentrations. *J Clin Psychopharmacol*. 2001;21(2):229-234.

89. Rollason V, Samer C, Piguet V, et al. Pharmacogenetics of analgesics: toward the individualization of prescription. *Pharmacogenomics*. 2008;9(7):905-933.

90. Restrepo JG, Garcia-Martin E, Martinez C, et al. Polymorphic drug metabolism in anaesthesia. *Curr Drug Metab*. 2009;10:236-246.

91. Sato Y, Seo N, Kobayashi E. Genetic background differences between FVB and C57BL/6 mice affect hypnotic susceptibility to pentobarbital, ketamine and nitrous oxide, but not isoflurane. *Acta Anaesthesiol Scand*. 2006;50(5):553-556.

92. Sonner JM, Gong D, Eger II EI. Naturally occurring variability in anesthetic potency among inbred mouse strains. *Anesth Analg*. 2000;91(3):720-726.

93. Stekiel TA, Weber CA, Contney SJ, et al. Differences in cardiovascular sensitivity to propofol in a chromosome substitution rat model. *Croat Med J*. 2007;48(3):312-318.

94. Stekiel TA, Contney SJ, Bosnjak ZJ, et al. Chromosomal substitution-dependent differences in cardiovascular responses to sodium pentobarbital. *Anesth Analg*. 2006;102(3):799-805.

95. Stekiel TA, Contney J, Stephen MS, et al. Reversal of minimum alveolar concentrations of volatile anesthetics by chromosomal substitution. *Anesthesiology.* 2004;101(3):796-798.

96. Cascio M, Xing Y, Gong D, et al. Mouse chromosome 7 harbors a quantitative trait locus for isoflurane minimum alveolar concentration. *Anesth Analg.* 2007;105(2):381-385.

97. Qin XP, Xie HG, Wang W, et al. Effect of the gene dosage of CgammaP2C19 on diazepam metabolism in Chinese subjects. *Clin Pharmacol Ther.* 1999;66(6):642-646.

98. Kosuge K, Jun Y, Watanabe H, et al. Effects of CYP3A4 inhibition by diltiazem on pharmacokinetics and dynamics of diazepam in relation to CYP2C19 genotype status. *Drug Metab Dispos.* 2001;29(10):1284-1289.

99. Martinez C, Blanco G, Ladero JM, et al. Genetic predisposition to acute gastrointestinal bleeding after NSAIDs use. *Br J Pharmacol.* 2004;141(2):205-208.

100. Pilotto A, Seripa D, Franceschi M, et al. Genetic susceptibility to nonsteroidal anti-inflammatory drug-related gastroduodenal bleeding: role of cytochrome P450 2C9 polymorphisms. *Gastroenterology.* 2007;133(2):465-471.

101. Dorado P, Berecz R, Norberto MJ, et al. CYP2C9 genotypes and diclofenac metabolism in Spanish healthy volunteers. *Eur J Clin Pharmacol.* 2003;59(3):221-225.

102. Lasocki S, Iglarz M, Seince PF, et al. Involvement of renin-angiotensin system in pressure-flow relationship: role of angiotensin-converting enzyme gene polymorphism. *Anesthesiology.* 2002;96(2):271-275.

103. Liem EB, Lin CM, Suleman MI, et al. Anesthetic requirement is increased in redheads. *Anesthesiology.* 2004;101(2):279-283.

104. Liem EB, Joiner TV, Tsueda K, et al. Increased sensitivity to thermal pain and reduced subcutaneous lidocaine efficacy in redheads. *Anesthesiology.* 2005;102(3):509-514.

105. Mogil JS, Wilson SG, Chesler EJ, et al. The melanocortin-1 receptor gene mediates female-specific mechanisms of analgesia in mice and humans. *Proc Natl Acad Sci U S A.* 2003;100(8):4867-4872.

106. Landau R, Kern C, Columb MO, et al. Genetic variability of the μ-opioid receptor influences intrathecal fentanyl analgesia requirements in laboring women. *Pain.* 2008;139(1):5-14.

107. Lacassie HJ, Nazar C, Yonish B, et al. Reversible nitrous oxide myelopathy and a polymorphism in the gene encoding 5,10-methylenetetrahydrofolate reductase. *Br J Anaesth.* 2006;96(2):222-225.

108. Selzer RR, Rosenblatt DS, Laxova R, et al. Adverse effect of nitrous oxide in a child with 5,10-methylenetetrahydrofolate reductase deficiency. *N Engl J Med.* 2003;349(1):45-50.

109. Simon T, Verstuyft C, Mary-Krause M, et al. Genetic determinants of response to clopidogrel and cardiovascular events. *N Engl J Med.* 2009;360(4):363-375.

110. Mega JL, Close SL, Wiviott SD, et al. Cytochrome p-450 polymorphisms and response to clopidogrel. *N Engl J Med.* 2009;360(4):354-362.

111. Gladding P, White H, Voss J, et al. Pharmacogenetic testing for clopidogrel using the rapid INFINITI analyzer: a dose-escalation study. *JACC Cardiovasc Interv.* 2009;2(11):1095-1101.

Chapter 5

PHARMACODYNAMIC DRUG INTERACTIONS

Timothy G. Short and Jacqueline A. Hannam

HISTORY

Pharmacology is characterized by detailed descriptions of the actions of individual drugs. In the case of anesthesia, no single drug has been found to be universally satisfactory and indeed general anesthesia is now regarded as a set of desirable clinical endpoints rather than a discrete phenomenon of its own. Useful endpoints include lack of awareness and a pleasant induction and recovery; lack of movement, adequate muscle relaxation, reasonable blood pressure control; and maintenance of homeostasis by suppressing autonomic reflexes whilst balancing the narrow therapeutic index of many of the drugs to ensure positive outcomes. Consequently, multiple drugs are used for all but the simplest of procedures.

This concept of multiple drug use was first described by Lundy in 1926, who used the term *balanced anesthesia*.[1] His concept included the liberal use of local or regional anesthesia as well as hypnotics, volatile anesthetics, and opioids. At the time, use of volatile agents as a sole anesthetic was common, but unacceptable cardiovascular and respiratory depression frequently accompanied the high doses required to suppress movement to noxious stimuli—a finding still true of the volatile anesthetics in use today.[2]

The theory behind balanced anesthesia is that using desirable drug combinations reduces dose requirements of individual drugs, minimizing the incidence of unwanted side effects in those with a narrow therapeutic index and so improving the quality of anesthesia. A review of the contribution of anesthesia to perioperative mortality found evidence to support this notion with the relative risk of dying within 7 days of surgery, being 2.9 times greater if one or two anesthetic drugs were used, as compared to the use of three or more.[3] Today, balanced anesthesia is the standard approach to general anesthesia.

Many drugs used in anesthesia have overlapping actions and, when given in combination, can be used to produce effects distinct from those they create individually. To maximize the clinical utility of any drug, it is important to understand its effects when used alone, and in combination. The interaction between propofol and fentanyl is a notable example. Propofol alone is effective at causing unconsciousness without intolerable adverse effects. The much larger doses required to prevent movement in response to surgical pain also suppress respiration and can unacceptably reduce blood pressure. On the other hand, fentanyl is incapable of reliably causing unconsciousness and even in very high doses does not reliably suppress movement to pain. When these two drugs are used in combination there is only a modest reduction in the dose of propofol required to cause unconsciousness, but a dramatic reduction in the dose required to suppress movement to pain with less reduction in blood pressure. The relative dosage of the combination of propofol and opioids also allows a degree of independent control of two critical variables—unconsciousness and lack of movement in response to pain.

Early studies of drug interactions include that by Fraser in 1872,[4] who described pharmacologic antagonism between physostigmine and atropine, and by Frei in 1913,[5] who used isobolographic analysis to demonstrate increased effectiveness of combinations of disinfectants for killing bacteria when compared to individual agents. The response surface method that is now used to describe the entire dose response relationship of two drugs was first proposed by Loewe in 1928,[6] who described synergy as an "inflated sail" and additivity as a "tense sail." The concept was introduced into modern anesthetic clinical pharmacology analysis by Minto in 2000.[7] The seemingly daunting task of describing an entire response surface for the interaction between two drugs was found to be tractable and as few as 20 intensively studied subjects are needed to adequately describe the interaction between two drugs.[8] The tedious calculations are easily performed on a modern computer, something Loewe clearly lacked. Response surface methodology is now the basis of many studies of commonly used drug combinations. Although outwardly complex, the models increase the accuracy with which anesthetic effects in patients can be predicted, and they have been incorporated into some anesthetic monitors for real-time display. They can be used to optimize drug titration promoting outcomes such as reduced wake-up times or increased cardiovascular stability without increasing hypnotic depth.

This chapter introduces terminology used to describe drug interactions, the methodology used to study drug interactions, and the important interactions between commonly used anesthetic drugs. Some of these interactions are dealt with in other chapters of this text in more detail (see Chapters 2, 9, 10, and 15). Interactions among combinations of analgesics or antiemetics as used postoperatively are not reviewed in this chapter; however similar methodologies and rules can be applied when considering their use in combination.

STUDY OF DRUG INTERACTIONS

Terminology

Drug interactions are usually considered in the dose or concentration domain. A simple experiment that illustrates interactions between two drugs takes half the *dose* of each that alone causes a certain level of effect. Assume that level of effect is equal to 1. If the drugs are additive, one would expect these two half doses given together to produce the same effect as giving the whole dose of either drug alone (i.e., 0.5 + 0.5 = 1). This expected effect for a dose combination becomes the null hypothesis against which one can assess the presence (or absence) of a positive or negative interaction. If the observed effect is greater than expected (<0.5 + <0.5 = 1), synergy exists. A commonly used drug combination in which this occurs is

$$Interaction\ Index = \frac{da}{DA} + \frac{db}{DB}$$

Figure 5-1 General equation for additivity as defined by Loewe. *DA* and *DB* are the doses of drugs *A* and *B*, respectively, that create a given effect alone, while *da* and *db* are the doses of drugs *A* and *B*, respectively, that create that same effect when given in combination. ED_{50} or EC_{50} are the most commonly used values for *DA* and *DB*. An interaction index of 1 = additivity, <1 = synergy, and >1 = infra-additivity. *(Reprinted with permission from Loewe S. The problem of synergism and antagonism of combined drugs. Arzneimittelforschung. 1953;3:285-290.)*

propofol and midazolam. Together, the individual doses are reduced by about one third so that 0.33 + 0.33 ≡ 1. If the observed effect was less than expected (>0.5 + >0.5 = 1), infra-additivity exists (Figure 5-1). If instead one combines half the *effect* of two drugs, the answer would be very different. This is because the sigmoid log-dose effect relationship is highly nonlinear, meaning drug effects cannot be simply added.

The term *infra-additive* is used when less effect than that expected from simple additivity is observed. The combination of midazolam and ketamine exemplifies the effect of infra-additivity. Midazolam has only a moderate effect on the ketamine dose required to suppress response to verbal command and no effect on the ketamine dose required to suppress movement to a noxious stimulus.

The term *antagonism* is reserved for interactions in which there is an absolute reduction in the effect of one drug in the presence of the other. For instance the analgesic effect of fentanyl is reduced in the presence of naloxone. In this example, naloxone is incapable of causing analgesia when given alone. An underlying assumption of this definition of additivity is that a drug cannot interact with itself, so two half doses of the same drug must be additive.

Shift in Dose-Response Curve

The dose-response relationship for most anesthetic drugs can be described using the standard *sigmoid E_{max}* model. Its characteristics include (1) a threshold drug concentration that must be surpassed before any effect is seen, (2) an increase in effect proportional to logarithmic increases in drug concentration, and (3) saturation after which additional increases in drug concentration no longer produce an increase in effect (Figure 5-2).

When a second drug is introduced, the simplest model of an interaction describes its influence, at a single fixed dose, on the dose-response relationship of the first drug. Using the previous example, intravenous fentanyl 1 μg/kg, administered immediately before intravenous propofol, shifts the propofol dose-response curve for unconsciousness to the left. This equates to a 20% reduction in dose for that endpoint. Likewise, the curve for suppression of movement to a noxious stimulus shifts to the left by 50%. This model demonstrates that fentanyl affects the noxious endpoint more than the hypnotic endpoint, which is expected from our knowledge of the individual drugs.

This approach to studying interactions accounts for the dose requirements for the two drugs when given together, but describes the interaction at only one dose of fentanyl. It does not describe whether the interaction with the second drug is additive or synergistic or whether there is a therapeutic advantage to using the combination. To quantitate the

Shift in dose-response curve
The standard dose response curve for a single drug is shifted to the left along the horizontal axis by the presence of a second drug.

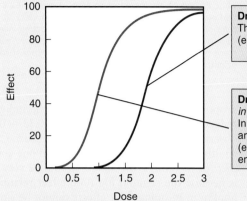

Drug A alone, for example: ED$_{50}$ Drug A = 1.9
This is a standard *sigmoid E$_{max}$* dose-response curve.
(e.g., Propofol for immobility)

Drug A + Drug B e.g., ED$_{50}$ Drug A = 1.0
in presence of drug B
In the presence of Drug B, dose requirements of Drug A are reduced.
(e.g., Propofol in the presence of fentanyl 1 mcg/kg at an endpoint of immobility)

The isobologram
An isobologram is an iso-effect line whereby all the combinations of each drug along the line give the same observed effect. Multiple isobolograms can be drawn for different effect levels such as ED$_{50}$ or ED$_{95}$. The doses required of each drug individually are on the X and Y axes respectively.

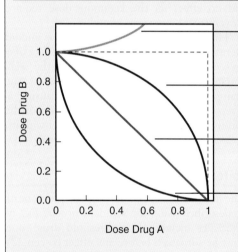

Antagonistic
Drug A increases dose of drug B to achieve the same effect
(e.g., naloxone and fentanyl for analgesia)

Infra-additive e.g., >0.5 + >0.5 = 1
Together the individual doses of each drug are slightly reduced to achieve the same effect
(e.g., ketamine and midazolam for sedation)

Additive e.g., 0.5 + 0.5 = 1
Together, half the dose of each drug will achieve the same effect
(e.g., Isoflurane and nitrous oxide for immobility)

Synergistic e.g., <0.5 + <0.5 = 1
Together, less than half the expected dose of each drug is required to achieve same effect
(e.g., Propofol and midazolam for hypnosis)

The response surface
The response surface is a three dimensional graph with drugs A and B on the horizontal axes and effect on the vertical axis. The concept embraces shift in dose-response curves and the isobologram, and describes effects for the complete set of doses for the endpoint in question. Responses may be either continuous such as bispectral index and blood pressure, or quantal such as a sedation scale, awake/sleep and movement/immobility.

The response surface

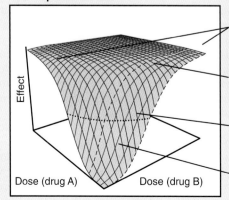

Dose-response curve
Drug A alone is on one axis and drug B in the other axis

Shift in dose response
Drug B in the presence of a constant concentration of Drug A

Isobologram
The 50% effect isobole is shown.
Outward bowing of the surface indicates synergy

Response surface
All doses of drug A and B and their responses are shown
(e.g., Sevoflurane and remifentanil for immobility)

Figure 5-2 Common methods for studying drug interactions using shift in dose response-curve, isobolograms, and response surfaces.

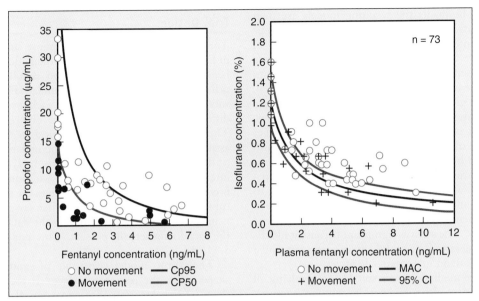

Figure 5-3 Isobolograms for propofol-remifentanil interaction and isoflurane-remifentanil interaction for an endpoint of no movement to surgical incision. Note that not all patients can be immobilized with fentanyl alone even in high doses. Fentanyl 1 ng/mL is equivalent to the peak effect of a bolus of fentanyl 3 µg/kg in a young adult. *(Modified from Smith C, McEwan AI, Jhaveri R, et al. The interaction of fentanyl on the Cp50 of propofol for loss of consciousness and skin incision.* Anesthesiology. *1993;78:864-869; and McEwan AI, Smith C, Dyar O, Goodman D, Smith LR, Glass PS. Isoflurane minimum alveolar concentration reduction by fentanyl.* Anesthesiology. *1994;81:820-828.)*

interaction, and to decide whether synergy exists, a description is needed of the drug's effects when given individually as well as when given together, and for a range of doses. Use of isobolograms is an alternative drugs' approach to interaction analysis that partly addresses these limitations.

ISOBOLOGRAMS

The traditional approach to quantitating a drug interaction for two drugs is to construct graphs of the dose pairs that together produce a single level of effect. These isoeffect lines are called *isoboles*. Comparison of an isobole with a line of additivity signals the interaction type: a straight line indicates additivity; inward bowing indicates synergy; outward bowing indicates infra-additivity or antagonism (see Figure 5-2).

Isobolograms are easy to construct and analyze when both drugs are individually capable of producing the endpoint in question. Numerous studies use this methodology in the literature and their conclusions are comparable to those of studies using more complex methodologies. Typically a departure from additivity of less than 10% has been regarded as additive on the basis that even if statistically significant, it is clinically irrelevant. When one drug cannot achieve the endpoint in question, it is still possible to determine whether synergy exists, but the exact degree of departure from additivity cannot be accurately determined.[9] A limitation of using isobolograms is that the result is only applicable to the effect level investigated. To gain a full understanding of the interaction between two drugs for all effect levels, it is possible to overlay a series of isoboles ranging from minimal effects to the maximal effect attainable[10] (E_{max}).

Analysis of isobolograms involves determining the dose-response relationship for each drug individually and then exploring the dose-response relationship of the drugs in combination. Simple experiments investigate dose pairs that maintain a fixed dose ratio of the individual drugs. It is also possible to combine any number of dose combinations and responses

and to calculate an isoeffect line using nonlinear regression—this is now the preferred method[11,12] (Figure 5-3). The standard isobologram assumes that the potency ratio of the two drugs remains constant for all dose pairs. In some instances this assumption does not hold true, such as when individual dose-response curves reach different levels of maximum effect. These cases require special consideration in that the line of additivity may in fact be curved.[13] Consequently this can lead to false identification of synergistic relationships. Although isobolographic methodology is appropriate for studying interactions of these types, they are better described by more sophisticated analyses.

RESPONSE SURFACE MODELS

Response surface methodology allows one to create a complete description of the dose-response relationship between two drugs for all levels of effect for a given endpoint. That response surfaces characterize the entire spectrum of drug effect is an important advantage of this approach in anesthesia clinical pharmacology. Anesthesia practice is unique in that anesthetists must target profound drug effects during an operation and then reverse the effect rapidly when the operation is finished. Thus, to study anesthetic clinical pharmacology fully, it is necessary to understand the entire concentration-effect relationship and how to transition from full effect to recovery efficiently.

These models all assume that the interaction is constant over time (i.e., stationary). In creating response surfaces, it is also assumed that the surface is smooth and that individuals in the study population show a similar degree of drug interaction. The latter is important because it is not practical to study more than a small part of the entire dose-response surface in each patient. Response surface models are typically built in carefully controlled volunteer studies in which multiple measurements can be made; the resulting models are then validated in patients. The concept embraces previous approaches to drug interaction analysis, including the shift in dose-response curve and the isobologram. It also provides a strong visual representation of the interaction that is easy to remember given the complexity of the mathematics involved. Response surfaces give a mathematical description of the magnitude of an interaction for all dose pairs of two drugs, which enables these models to be used in real time to predict the likely response of patients to the drugs used. They also allow identification of optimal drug dose combinations. For example, a recent study found remifentanil 0.8 ng/mL:propofol 2 to 3 μg/mL was the optimal concentration pairing to prevent movement and blood pressure changes in response to esophageal instrumentation without causing intolerable ventilatory depression.[14] The study is significant because it identifies the optimal dose ratio for a useful clinical endpoint whilst minimizing the risk of an unwanted side effect.

Response surface methodology is suitable for studying all the common types of drug interactions among agonists, partial agonists, antagonists, and inverse agonists (Figure 5-4).

Trial Design

The basic steps to deriving a response surface are described in Figure 5-5. Three different mathematical approaches have been chosen—Greco, Minto, and Bouillon—but the basic principles underlying them are similar. There are also other valid approaches.[7,10,15-20] Although each model draws a slightly different shape for the surface, the differences are not large. The three approaches are empirical in that they make no assumption about the nature of the underlying interaction.

The Greco model is simple to apply and uses a single interaction parameter.[10] In doing so it assumes the interaction is constant for all drug pairs and gives the surface a symmetrical shape. This is an advantage when coverage of the surface is uneven but may lead to forcing the data to fit a shape that the data do not actually possess. (This model is used in Figures 5-11 and 5-12.)

The Minto model is capable of capturing virtually any shape across the response surface.[7] It preserves the sigmoid shape of the dose-response curve for all drug combinations and is suitable for describing all commonly encountered drug

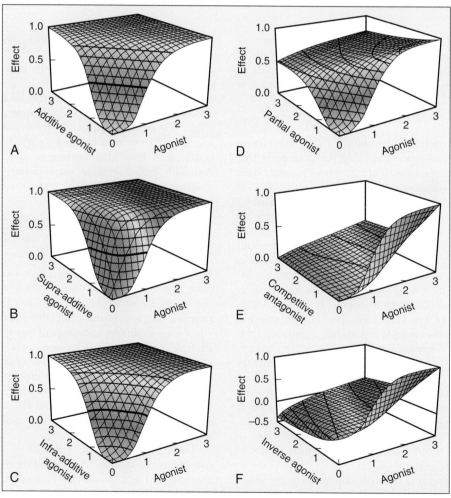

Figure 5-4 Response surfaces for a variety of drug interactions. All drugs have an initial effect = 0. **A** is an additive interaction between two agonists; **B** is a synergistic interaction between two agonists; **C** is an infra-additive interaction between two agonists; **D** is the interaction between a partial agonist and a full agonist; **E** is the interaction between an agonist and antagonist; **F** is the interaction between an inverse agonist and a full agonist. *(Reprinted with permission from Minto CF, Schnider TW, Short TG, Gregg K, Gentilini A, Shafer SL. Response surface model for anesthetic drug interactions. Anesthesiology. 2000;92:1603-1616.)*

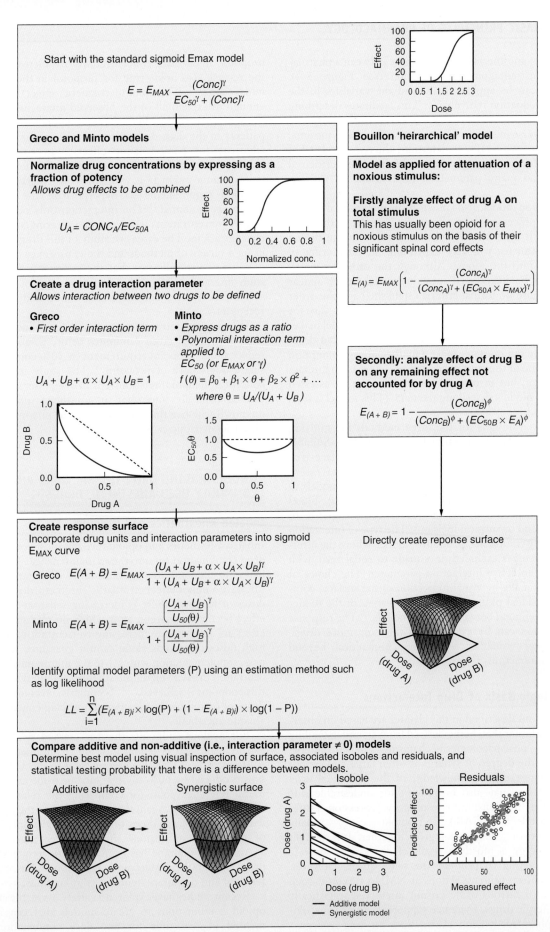

Figure 5-5 Three mathematical approaches to creating a response surface model for a pair of anesthetic drugs. *(Modified from Minto CF, Schnider TW, Short TG, Gregg K, Gentilini A, Shafer SL. Response surface model for anesthetic drug interactions. Anesthesiology. 2000;92:1603-1616; Greco WR, Bravo G, Parsons JC. The search for synergy: a critical review from a response surface perspective. Pharmacol Rev. 1995;47:331-385; and Bouillon TW, Bruhn J, Radulescu L, Andresen C, Shafer TJ, Cohane C, Shafer SL. Pharmacodynamic interaction between propofol and remifentanil regarding hypnosis, tolerance of laryngoscopy, bispectral index, and electroencephalographic approximate entropy. Anesthesiology. 2004;100:1353-1372.)*

interactions in anesthesia, including those between a pharmacologic agonist-antagonist combination (see Figure 5-4). Interactions can be applied to each of the variables in the sigmoid E_{max} equation individually. This facilitates describing interactions between those drugs whose individual response curves are diverse in terms of curve shape, slope, and maxima, and allows the investigator to determine the required level of model complexity, although the model has been criticized for having too many parameters. (This model is used in Figure 5-7.)

The Bouillon model, also known as the hierarchical model, sequentially processes drug effects for one drug, then the other drug.[19] It is simple to implement but has the quirk that parameter estimates will vary depending on their order of introduction into the model. Although the order by which drugs should be introduced into the model might appear logical, there are no formal criteria established and the order of analysis that results in the best fit to the data can vary for different endpoints within the same dataset. The model makes the assumption that the relationship follows a sigmoid dose-response curve but does not make a mathematical assumption about the shape of the combined surface. There is no interaction parameter, but instead goodness-of-fit can be assessed against other models describing the data. (This model is used in Figure 5-9.)

Generic trial designs for the three methods for studying drug interaction are summarized in Figure 5-6. Suitable methodology and power analysis for response surface trial design has been determined by simulation analysis. It is essential that trials cover most of the surface for robust models to be derived.[8] Endpoints can be either continuous (e.g., blood pressure or bispectral index) or quantal (e.g., response to verbal command or surgical incision). The type of interaction is identified by comparing an additive model, where the interaction parameter is excluded or is made to equal zero, with one that has an active interaction parameter. The choice of best model is made by visual inspection of the surface, comparison of residual plots, and statistical testing of the reduction in log likelihood between related models.[7,8] The response surface method can be extended to three or more drugs, although clear visualization becomes impractical beyond three drug interactions (Figure 5-7).

Pharmacologic Basis of Drug Interactions

The interactions described in this chapter are based on observational data rather than being derived from an understanding of underlying pharmacologic mechanisms. They are important because the degree of synergy is often large and cannot usually be inferred from knowledge of the individual drug actions. Synergy may also be present for undesirable side effects such as hypotension or respiratory depression. Drugs with known effects at $GABA_A$ and opioid receptors usually show additivity or synergy when given together.[9] It is thought that this synergy is mostly a result of drugs with separate mechanisms acting to produce the same effect. However, drugs with known primary actions at NMDA receptors such as ketamine or nitrous oxide do not interact synergistically with GABAergic drugs. Evidence supports both pharmacokinetic and pharmacodynamic explanations for drug synergy.

The most extensive research into the mechanisms for synergy is for propofol and midazolam. In the presence of propofol, midazolam concentrations are increased by 25%; the reverse also holds true for propofol in the presence of midazolam.[21,22] This pharmacokinetic effect is not large enough to explain all of the observed interactions. Observations of sedative and hemodynamic endpoints in the same patients in the dose domain found synergy for sedation and additivity for hemodynamic effects.[20] In vitro studies of $GABA_A$ receptors have also shown a similar degree of pharmacodynamic interaction, with midazolam markedly reducing propofol requirements to hyperpolarize the postsynaptic membrane potential.[23] The interaction only occurred when GABA concentrations were low, disappearing at high GABA concentrations. The extensive study of this drug combination using a variety of methods and the consistency of the finding of synergy also indicates that the various methods used to study interactions are robust. In vitro testing of propofol and sevoflurane in combination has also found additivity at $GABA_A$ receptors.[24]

When using intravenous propofol for induction, a small dose of propofol given 2 minutes before a subsequent dose reduced total propofol requirement by 30% compared with a single bolus dose of propofol.[25] The study introduces the concept of temporal relationships in drug interactions, which can be clinically important at anesthetic induction. It is unknown whether this effect was due to pharmacokinetic or pharmacodynamic causes.

UNDERSTANDING DRUG INTERACTIONS AMONG COMMONLY USED ANESTHETIC DRUGS

Inhaled Anesthetics and Opioids

Inhaled anesthetics and opioids are the most commonly used drug combination for anesthesia maintenance. As stated, at a hypnotic endpoint, low concentrations of fentanyl 1 to 2 ng/mL have a minor effect on volatile anesthetic dose.[12] At larger doses of fentanyl, there is increasing sedation and a ceiling effect becomes apparent, after which no further increases in effect are seen despite increasing concentration. In that even high doses of opioids alone cannot guarantee unconsciousness, supplementation with 0.1 to 0.2 minimum alveolar concentration (MAC) volatile anesthetic is required to ensure that this endpoint is achieved.[12,26-29] Similarly, on emergence, small doses of opioid have little effect on waking concentrations of volatile anesthetic.[30]

For noxious endpoints there is marked synergy. This is usually expressed as opioid infusion requirements to reduce MAC by 50%. This value is equivalent to the MAC suppression produced by 60% to 70% nitrous oxide and provides a useful reference point for comparing the relative analgesic effects of opioids.[31] Again there is a ceiling to the opioid effect with even very large doses of opioid not guaranteeing a lack of movement to noxious stimulus when given as a sole agent.[12,26,27] Isoflurane has been the most frequently studied drug, but similar results have been found for sevoflurane-fentanyl and desflurane-fentanyl combinations.

Recent studies have explored a variety of volatile anesthetic-opioid combinations to create models that can be implemented in real time for any dose combination and to make predictions of optimal dose pairings. There are therapeutic benefits to the combination in terms of reduced volatile

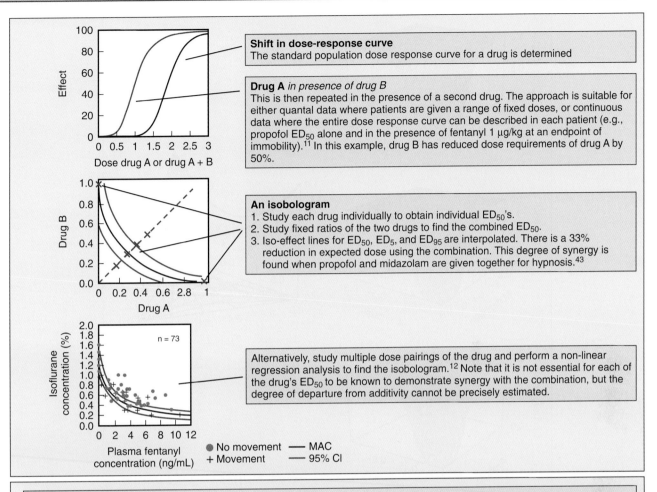

Shift in dose-response curve
The standard population dose response curve for a drug is determined

Drug A *in presence of drug B*
This is then repeated in the presence of a second drug. The approach is suitable for either quantal data where patients are given a range of fixed doses, or continuous data where the entire dose response curve can be described in each patient (e.g., propofol ED_{50} alone and in the presence of fentanyl 1 µg/kg at an endpoint of immobility).[11] In this example, drug B has reduced dose requirements of drug A by 50%.

An isobologram
1. Study each drug individually to obtain individual ED_{50}'s.
2. Study fixed ratios of the two drugs to find the combined ED_{50}.
3. Iso-effect lines for ED_{50}, ED_5, and ED_{95} are interpolated. There is a 33% reduction in expected dose using the combination. This degree of synergy is found when propofol and midazolam are given together for hypnosis.[43]

Alternatively, study multiple dose pairings of the drug and perform a non-linear regression analysis to find the isobologram.[12] Note that it is not essential for each of the drug's ED_{50} to be known to demonstrate synergy with the combination, but the degree of departure from additivity cannot be precisely estimated.

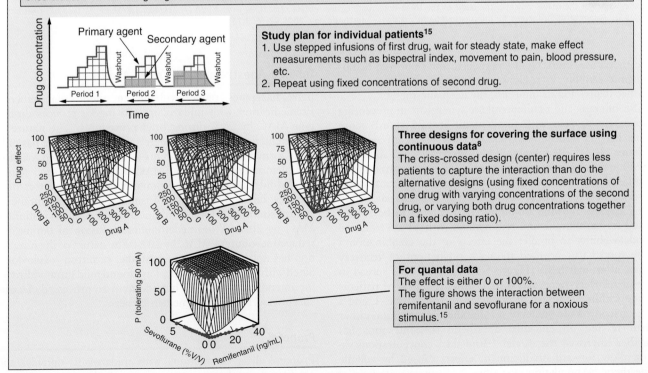

A response surface
These can be created for quantal or continuous data. Studying just 20 patients has been found adequate to characterize response surfaces using a continuous measure such as bispectral index. It is essential to cover most of the surface. The optimal design criss-crosses the surface giving the most robust result.

Study plan for individual patients[15]
1. Use stepped infusions of first drug, wait for steady state, make effect measurements such as bispectral index, movement to pain, blood pressure, etc.
2. Repeat using fixed concentrations of second drug.

Three designs for covering the surface using continuous data[8]
The criss-crossed design (center) requires less patients to capture the interaction than do the alternative designs (using fixed concentrations of one drug with varying concentrations of the second drug, or varying both drug concentrations together in a fixed dosing ratio).

For quantal data
The effect is either 0 or 100%.
The figure shows the interaction between remifentanil and sevoflurane for a noxious stimulus.[15]

Figure 5-6 Trial design for studying drug interactions.

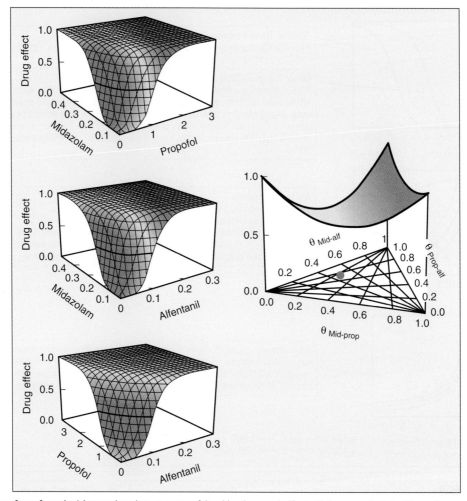

Figure 5-7 Response surfaces for paired interactions between propofol, midazolam, and alfentanil for an endpoint of loss of response to verbal command; the paired combinations all showed synergy. The figure on the right shows the ED_{50} isoboles for each of the paired interactions. The three-drug combination caused no more synergy than expected from the paired interactions but would appear as a deeper hollow in the parameter surface if it existed. The *dot* on the "floor" of the graph indicates the nadir of the three-drug combination surface. *(Modified from Minto CF, Schnider TW, Short TG, Gregg K, Gentilini A, Shafer SL. Response surface model for anesthetic drug interactions. Anesthesiology. 2000;92:1603-1616.)*

anesthetic use, more rapid emergence, and improved hemo-dynamic stability in response to surgery without excessive cardiac depression or unnecessarily deep anesthesia.

Sevoflurane and remifentanil are synergistic in preventing movement to pain with remifentanil at 1.25 ng/mL more than halving sevoflurane requirements when given alone (Figure 5-8).[32] Remifentanil also decreases variability in sevoflurane requirements with increasing concentrations of remifentanil, reflected by much steeper population dose-response curves. These results can be generalized within drug classes, allowing isoflurane and fentanyl to be substi-tuted for sevoflurane and remifentanil without affecting the model's ability to predict the effects of the combination.[33] The model can be used to make predictions of recovery times after anesthesia (Figure 5-9). Although the spread in actual recovery times was 6 to 15 minutes, 50% of patients woke within 2 minutes of predicted recovery time. Using a pharmacodynamic model of sevoflurane concentration rather than relying on end-tidal anesthetic concentrations has further improved the model.[34] End-tidal concentrations do not allow forward prediction of effects caused by volatile anesthetic accumulation over time.

Inhaled Anesthetics and Other Agents

Benzodiazepines reduce volatile anesthetic requirements. Premedication with midazolam 0.05 mg/kg reduces desflu-rane MAC by 20% during brief procedures. The nature of the interaction has not been determined.[35] Ketamine has only been formally studied in animals, wherein marked synergy was demonstrated in the MAC of isoflurane in dogs.[36] The α_2-adrenergic agonists clonidine and dexmedetomidine decrease dose requirements of isoflurane and sevoflurane in clinical studies.[37-40] Oral clonidine 5 µg/kg reduced isoflurane MAC by 20%. A dexmedetomidine infusion of 0.6 ng/mL reduced sevoflurane MAC by 20%. The nature of the interac-tion has not been determined. Studies of nitrous oxide com-bined with volatile anesthetics have found mild infra-additivity for an endpoint of MAC, but additivity in processed electro-encephalogram (EEG) (median power).[41,42]

Propofol

Propofol drug interactions with midazolam, opioids, and volatiles have been extensively studied at a variety of

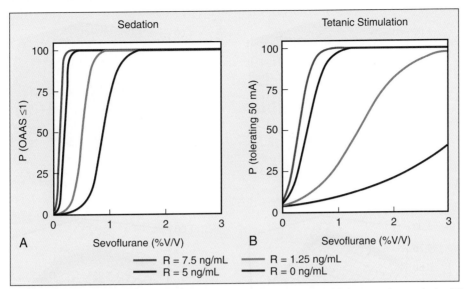

Figure 5-8 Dose-response curves for sevoflurane-remifentanil combinations for a sedative endpoint (**A**) and a noxious endpoint (**B**). Remifentanil markedly reduces dose requirements and also steepens the dose-response curve, making dosage more predictable. *OASS,* Observer assessment of alertness-sedation; *P,* probability; 1 = no response to moderate prodding or shaking; 50 mA is a tetanic stimulus of 50 mA applied for 5 seconds, a noxious stimulus similar to surgical incision. *(Reprinted with permission from Manyam SC, Gupta DK, Johnson KB, et al. Opioid-volatile synergy: a response surface model with remifentanil and sevoflurane as prototypes. Anesthesiology. 2006;105:267-278.)*

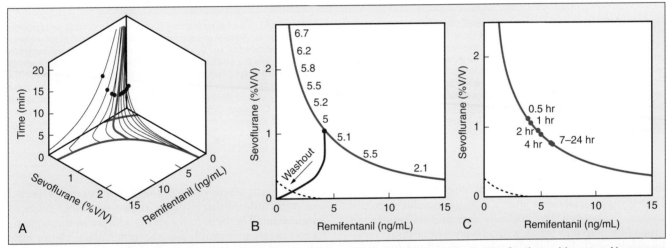

Figure 5-9 Modeling of sevoflurane-remifentanil combinations that suppress response to a noxious stimulus in 95% of patients with most rapid emergence after a 1-hour procedure. Graph **A** shows the predicted decline in effect site and alveolar concentrations for remifentanil and sevoflurane after stopping drug administration regimens targeted to reach the EC_{95} isobole for tetanic stimulation for 1 hour. The EC_{95} isobole is on the "floor" of the cube; the vertical axis represents time elapsed since stopping the administration of the drugs. The isobole representing an 80% probability of the return of responsiveness (Observer's Assessment of Alertness/Sedation score >4) is shown by dots superimposed on the concentration decay curves. The *highlighted curve* is the sevoflurane and remifentanil target concentration pair that resulted in the fastest return of responsiveness. In graph **B,** the numbers on the isobole are wakeup times (in minutes) for a variety of dose pairs; the minimum wakeup time in 50% of patients was 5 minutes. The effect of increasing duration of infusion is shown in graph **C,** wherein a small increase in the ratio of remifentanil to sevoflurane is required for earliest wake-up due to greater accumulation of sevoflurane after prolonged use. *(Reprinted with permission from Manyam SC, Gupta DK, Johnson KB, et al. Opioid-volatile synergy: a response surface model with remifentanil and sevoflurane as prototypes. Anesthesiology. 2006;105:267-278.)*

endpoints including light sedation, lack of movement to a noxious stimulus, and changs in blood pressure.

Propofol and Midazolam

This combination acts synergistically at an endpoint of hypnosis, causing a 37% decrease in expected dose at anesthesia induction (see Figure 5-7).[43] The effect is present both following bolus doses and during infusions and does not depend on the order of administration of the drugs.[20,21] A recent infusion study constructed a response surface for the combination, finding the optimal ratio for hypnotic synergy to be propofol 4.7 ng/mL : midazolam 1 ng/mL.[22] The hemodynamic effects of the combination were additive, with propofol depressing blood pressure 3.1 times more than an equihypnotic dose of midazolam. Because of the hypnotic synergy, this meant that the combination caused less hemodynamic depression than propofol did as a sole agent,

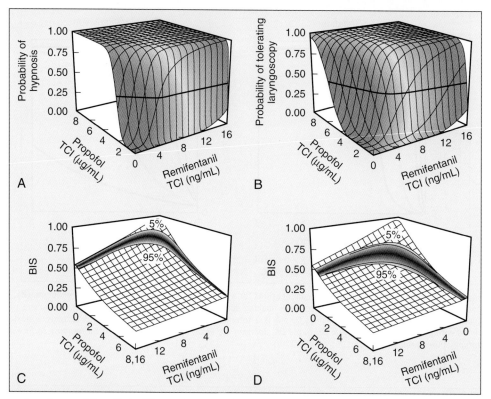

Figure 5-10 Response surfaces for propofol-remifentanil interaction at an endpoint of hypnosis **(A)** defined as no response to shouting and shaking, and response to a noxious endpoint **(B)** defined as no response to laryngoscopy. The isoboles for the two endpoints have been superimposed on the bispectral index response (BIS) surface in **C** and **D**, respectively. The authors have reversed the orientation of the response surface in **C** and **D**, with maximum dose at the back and maximum effect at the bottom of the graph. The study shows a high degree of synergy at both endpoints and the inability of remifentanil when given as a sole agent to reliably achieve either endpoint, even at high doses. The synergy seen in the hypnotic and noxious endpoints does not extend to the bispectral index, where the interaction is additive. This is possibly due to remifentanil having little effect on the electroencephalogram in the clinical dose range used. Overlaying these two clinical endpoints on the bispectral index surface demonstrates the difference between synergy at the noxious endpoint and additivity in the bispectral index. *(Reprinted with permission from Bouillon TW, Bruhn J, Radulescu L, Andresen C, Shafer TJ, Cohane C, Shafer SL. Pharmacodynamic interaction between propofol and remifentanil regarding hypnosis, tolerance of laryngoscopy, bispectral index, and electroencephalographic approximate entropy. Anesthesiology. 2004;100:1353-1372.)*

indicating a therapeutic benefit from use of the combination. Hemodynamic responses after a noxious stimulus were not studied. Midazolam also markedly decreases the amount of propofol required to produce immobility to a noxious stimulus, whilst not being able to produce immobility when given as a sole agent, even at the high dose of 1 mg/kg.[43] This interaction can be used to reduce total propofol dose during prolonged procedures and might also provide a cost benefit.

Propofol and Opioids

This is the most commonly used drug combination for intravenous induction of anesthesia and total intravenous anesthesia (TIVA); it is also used in low doses for procedural sedation. At anesthesia induction, small doses of opioids, such as fentanyl 1 µg/kg, have a small effect on the hypnotic dose of propofol reducing dose requirements by 20%, but a large effect on propofol dose to suppress movement to pain, reducing dose requirements by 50%. There have been four detailed studies of combined propofol and remifentanil infusion using response surface models.[19,44-46] The combination is synergistic at all clinical endpoints and is strongest at concentrations of remifentanil up to 4 ng/mL (equivalent to the effect of a steady-state infusion rate of approximately 0.15 µg/kg/min in

a young adult) where there is a 66% reduction in expected dose with little further synergy shown by higher doses of remifentanil. The bispectral index is additive in this concentration range, presumably because remifentanil causes little sedation when used as a sole agent in low doses; studies using very high concentrations of remifentanil have shown synergy (Figures 5-10 and 5-11).[45]

Response surface models have been used to optimize drug dose ratios for useful clinical endpoints.[46] Optimal combinations for early wakeup times show that using relatively more remifentanil to propofol is advantageous when compared with using fentanyl with propofol. Equipotent optimal dose ratios were approximately propofol 2 µg/mL : remifentanil 5 ng/mL compared with propofol 3.5 µg/mL : fentanyl 1.5 ng/mL (Figure 5-12). A recent study of respiratory effects showed marked synergy for this undesirable side effect and that it is not possible to reliably suppress response to noxious stimuli with the combination without inducing significant respiratory depression in most patients (Figure 5-13). Note that blood pressure changes in response to sustained noxious stimuli such as surgical incision have not been studied. These recommendations might also need to be modified depending on the degree of hemodynamic suppression allowed. For clinical purposes, equivalent doses of the phenylpiperidine opioids

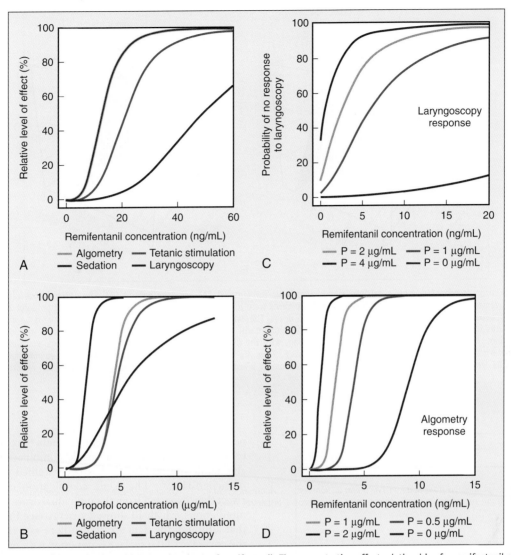

Figure 5-11 Change in propofol requirement with increasing doses of remifentanil. The concentration-effect relationships for remifentanil and propofol alone for various endpoints are shown in **A** and **B** (these represent the far right and far left axes of response surface plots for each endpoint). Plots **C** and **D** are concentration-response curves derived from response surfaces (i.e., these graphs are "cuts" through the surfaces at various propofol concentrations); this representation allows simplified interpretation. Note the very high concentration of remifentanil in graph **A** compared with graphs **C** and **D**; in the standard clinical range up to 10 ng/mL target concentration, remifentanil is only mildly sedative, whereas propofol potently suppresses all but the most painful stimuli. In combination, remifentanil potently decreases the amount of propofol required to suppress noxious stimuli such as laryngoscopy, but there was little additional synergy gained by increasing remifentanil concentrations above 4 ng/mL as illustrated in the study in Figure 5-11. *P,* Steady-state propofol concentration. *(Reprinted with permission from Kern SE, Xie G, White JL, Egan TD. A response surface analysis of propofol-remifentanil pharmacodynamic interaction in volunteers.* Anesthesiology. *2004;100:1373-1381.)*

fentanyl, alfentanil, sufentanil, and remifentanil can be used interchangeably as the degree of interaction with propofol is thought to be the same.[46]

Propofol and Inhaled Anesthetics

This combination is used at non–steady-state at the beginning of all anesthetics where intravenous induction is followed by volatile maintenance. Sevoflurane and propofol have been studied at a variety of endpoints ranging from response to shaking and shouting to response to surgical incision.[47-49] The combination is additive at all endpoints. Additivity was also shown for bispectral index and other processed EEG indices such as spectral entropy and response entropy, both in volunteer studies and in the clinical setting. It is thought that other

volatile agents such as desflurane and isoflurane behave similarly, but they have not been formally studied. Nitrous oxide 67% decreases propofol requirements by 25% to 35% for the endpoint of surgical incision. Two studies of target controlled infusions of propofol in the presence of nitrous oxide 67% have found the ED_{50} of propofol to be 4.5 and 4.9 µg/mL, respectively. This is an example of an infra-additive drug interaction.[50,51]

Midazolam and Opioids

This combination has not been studied in detail using response surface methodology. Basic studies using isobolographic analysis have shown midazolam and fentanyl or alfentanil to act synergistically to produce hypnosis.[52-54] Midazolam also

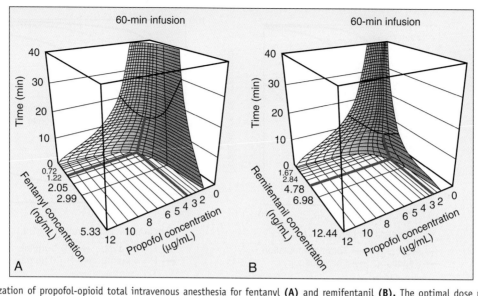

Figure 5-12 Optimization of propofol-opioid total intravenous anesthesia for fentanyl **(A)** and remifentanil **(B)**. The optimal dose ratios to provide 95% probability of no movement to surgical stimulus with earliest wakeup times were propofol 3.4 μg/mL : fentanyl 1.3 ng/mL and propofol 2.5 μg/mL : remifentanil 4.8 ng/mL. The superimposed blue lines indicate these optimal doses. The estimated time to 50% of patients being awake is 12 minutes for propofol-fentanyl and 6 minutes for propofol-remifentanil. The rapid offset of remifentanil compared to fentanyl means a higher ratio of opioid to propofol results in earlier wakeup times. Data are only displayed for a 1-hour infusion, with the differences being smaller after brief infusions and greater with prolonged infusions. *(Reprinted with permission from Vuyk J, Mertens MJ, Olofsen E, Burm AG, Bovill JG. Propofol anesthesia and rational opioid selection: determination of optimal EC50-EC95 propofol-opioid concentrations that assure adequate anesthesia and a rapid return of consciousness. Anesthesiology. 1997;87: 1549-1562.)*

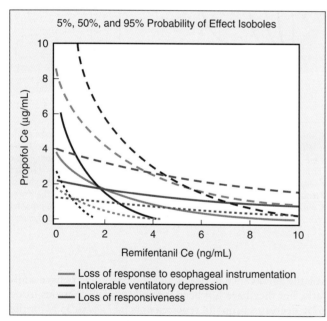

Figure 5-13 Adequate suppression of response to shaking and shouting (given in *blue*) and to a noxious stimulus (esophageal instrumentation, given in *red*) without unacceptable respiratory depression. The latter is defined as a respiratory rate less than five breaths/min (given in *green*). Note that the spread of concentration targets is very wide with the ED_{95} being double the ED_{50}, and the ED_{5} being less than half the ED_{50}. The *solid lines* are for ED_{50}, the *dotted lines* ED_{5}, and the *dashed lines* ED_{95}. *(Reprinted with permission from LaPierre CD, Johnson KB, Randall BR, White JL, Egan TD. An exploration of remifentanil-propofol combinations that lead to loss of response to esophageal instrumentation, a loss of responsiveness, and/or onset of intolerable ventilatory depression. Anesth Analg. 2011;113(3): 490-499.)*

potently suppresses opioid requirements to reduce movement to a noxious stimulus. The triple combination of propofol, alfentanil, and midazolam has been studied for an endpoint of hypnosis.[7,52,53] The triple combination caused no more effect than expected from the individual drugs and their paired interactions, which all showed synergy (see Figure 5-7). Note that although the data are shown here as a response surface, the coverage of the surface is not good with only a single fixed dose ratio having been studied using each combination.

Ketamine and Midazolam or Propofol

Ketamine and propofol are known to have distinctly different modes of action. Midazolam is often used to suppress emergence phenomena due to ketamine and can also be used in combination for sedation or induction of anesthesia. Midazolam has an infra-additive effect on ketamine hypnosis and no effect on the ketamine dose required to suppress movement to a noxious stimulus.[55] The combination of propofol and ketamine has an additive effect for an endpoint of sedation and propofol has only a small influence on ketamine doses required to block movement to a noxious stimulus (i.e., infra-additive).[56] The drugs have opposing effects on hemodynamic variables. At an optimal propofol : ketamine dose ratio of 3 : 1 there is minimal change in both heart rate and blood pressure when used for anesthesia induction.

EMERGING DEVELOPMENTS

Manufacturers have incorporated response surface models of drug action into new anesthesia monitor displays (Navigator Applications Suite, GE Healthcare, Finland; Intelligent

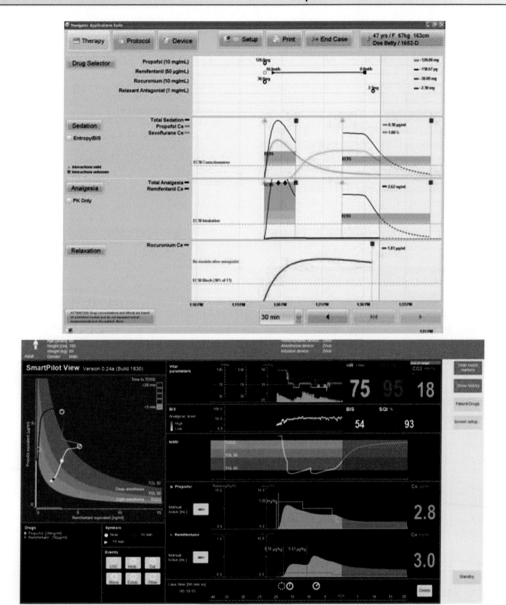

Figure 5-14 Real-time displays of predicted anesthetic drug effects. The top screen shows the interaction between propofol and sevoflurane in a patient induced with propofol for endpoints of sedation and analgesia. Notice the gap in our knowledge soon after induction, because the three-drug interaction between propofol, remifentanil, and sevoflurane has not been studied. The lower display shows propofol-remifentanil anesthesia. The isobologram on the left has shaded scales showing the population ED_{50} for light anesthesia and deep anesthesia and the ED_{95} for deep anesthesia. The line on the isobologram shows the effect course the patient has taken, including a prediction of the future effect course given the current dosage. *(Navigator Applications Suite, GE Healthcare, Finland; and Smart Pilot View, Intelligent Display, Drager Medical AG & Co. KG, Lubeck, Germany.)*

Display, Drager Medical AG & Co. KG, Lubeck, Germany). These systems display probabilities of hypnosis and movement to pain based on population models for the drugs used (Figure 5-14). The models contain adjustments for age, weight, height, and sex and display the influence of opioids on MAC of the volatile anesthetic used and the interaction between propofol and opioid to make predictions of anesthetic effect and time to waking. As well as giving a probability of response, they also display the variation in response expected in a typical patient population with ED_{50} and ED_{95} displayed. The calculations are done in real time with adjustments in dosage being continuously incorporated into the model to predict likely effects. This real time modeling greatly increases the dosing information available to anesthetists and is an improvement on current displays, which are often limited

to a single number for MAC that is not adjusted for age. These prediction modules are intended to bring the detailed knowledge about anesthetic drug behavior found in textbooks and modelling literature to the clinical domain by applying the models in real time in a user friendly display.

Such information can be used to guide a more accurate titration of volatile and opioid dose. The population modelling of the drug interactions also allows prediction of a probability of movement, something that current depth monitors such as bispectral index cannot do.[19,32] The displays provide information at both sedative and noxious endpoints and also provide predictions of recovery time. The inclusion of probabilities of movement and time to waking might appear overly detailed, but they give a more accurate appraisal of the sedative effects of the drugs given and their likely time course than was previously available. They also reduce task load in the operating theatre.[57] The library of drugs incorporated into these displays is currently limited to commonly used opioids, volatile anesthetics, and propofol. A recent study has shown that isoflurane can be substituted for sevoflurane and fentanyl for remifentanil without loss of fidelity of the model, providing further evidence that phenylpiperidine-based opioids behave similarly and can be used interchangeably. Interestingly, the three-drug interaction between propofol, opioid and volatile anesthetic has not been described, and appears as a blank on the "Navigator" display when propofol-opioid induction is followed by a volatile anesthetic for maintenance, until the propofol concentration is negligible. Because balanced anesthesia commonly involves the use of all three drug classes, this represents a gap in our knowledge of pharmacodynamic interactions in anesthesia.

KEY POINTS

- Current anesthetic practice is based on the use of drug combinations, a concept termed *balanced anesthesia* by Lundy in 1926. Study of the pharmacology of common combinations of drugs has greatly increased our knowledge of clinical anesthetic pharmacology.
- Drug interactions can be described by shifts in dose-response curves, where one drug influences the dose-response curve for a second drug; isobolograms, which are isoeffect lines for two drugs both capable of influencing the endpoint in question; and response surfaces, which create models of all possible combinations of two or more drugs for a given effect.
- Drug interaction studies can be used to define optimal dose ratios for desired outcomes such as maximum synergy (or lowest total dose), most rapid emergence, and least respiratory or hemodynamic depression.
- The combinations of propofol with an opioid, and volatile agent with an opioid, show a small effect at hypnotic endpoints and a large degree of synergy in suppression of response to a noxious stimulus. The combination of propofol with a volatile anesthetic such as sevoflurane is additive.
- Response surface models can be used in real time to create predictions of likely anesthetic effect in the operating room. These models have been incorporated into a new generation of monitor displays and are a sophisticated advance on the simple display of a predicted MAC value on most current anesthesia monitors.

Key References

Bouillon TW, Bruhn J, Radulescu L, et al. Pharmacodynamic interaction between propofol and remifentanil regarding hypnosis, tolerance of laryngoscopy, bispectral index, and electroencephalographic approximate entropy. *Anesthesiology.* 2004;100:1353-1372. This study contains a detailed description of propofol-remifentanil interactions on bispectral index and spectral entropy and demonstrates how clinical endpoints such as response to noxious stimuli are not captured by the processed EEG endpoints. The "hierarchical" method of eliciting a response surface that does not rely on use of an interaction parameter is used. (Ref. 19)

Hendrickx JF, Eger II EI, Sonner JM, Shafer SL. Is synergy the rule? A review of anesthetic interactions producing hypnosis and immobility. *Anesth Analg.* 2008;107:494-506. A systematic review of drug interactions in anesthesia. There is an analysis of the likely implications for mechanisms of drug interaction. (Ref. 9)

Lundy JS. Balanced anesthesia. *Minnesota Medical* 1926;9:399-404. The original article describing the idea of balanced anesthesia and its advantages. Lundy's ideas have been refined in the last 85 years with plenty of data to support them, but the concept remains just as true today. (Ref. 1)

Manyam SC, Gupta DK, Johnson KB, et al. Opioid-volatile synergy: a response surface model with remifentanil and sevoflurane as prototypes. *Anesthesiology.* 2006;105:267-278. The first study of volatile anesthetic-opioid interaction that used response surface analysis. It provides a detailed description of the interactions at a variety of relevant clinical endpoints and some modeling of optimal dose combinations. (Ref. 32)

McEwan AI, Smith C, Dyar O, Goodman D, Smith LR, Glass PS. Isoflurane minimum alveolar concentration reduction by fentanyl. *Anesthesiology.* 1994;81:820-828. The first study defining the interaction between a hypnotic and a volatile anesthetic in detail in humans. It demonstrates the strong synergy at a noxious endpoint and the ceiling to opioid effect when used as a sole agent. (Ref. 12)

Mertens MJ, Olofsen E, Engbers FH, Burm AG, Bovill JG, Vuyk J. Propofol reduces perioperative remifentanil requirements in a synergistic manner: response surface modeling of perioperative remifentanil-propofol interactions. *Anesthesiology.* 2003;99:347-359. The first detailed study of propofol-opioid interactions that also includes a response surface showing synergy for respiratory depression caused by the two agents. (Ref. 44)

Minto CF, Schnider TW, Short TG, Gregg K, Gentilini A, Shafer SL. Response surface model for anesthetic drug interactions. *Anesthesiology.* 2000;92:1603-1616. This study introduced the concept of response surfaces to an anesthetic audience, develops a mathematical approach to describing them for two- and three-drug combinations, and provides an example of a three-drug combination. (Ref. 7)

Schumacher PM, Dossche J, Mortier EP, Luginbuehl M, Bouillon TW, Struys MMRF. Response surface modelling of the interaction between propofol and sevoflurane. *Anesthesiology.* 2009;111:790-804. This study provides a description of propofol-volatile anesthetic interaction that is commonly employed but often ignored by anesthetists. It includes a detailed description of the methodology and analysis of a clinical drug interaction study. (Ref. 48)

References

1. Lundy JS. Balanced anesthesia. *Minnesota Medical.* 1926;9:399-404.
2. Zbinden AM, Petersen-Felix S, Thomson D. Anesthetic depth defined using multiple noxious stimuli during isoflurane/oxygen anesthesia. II. Hemodynamic responses. *Anesthesiology.* 1994;80:261-267.
3. Cohen MM, Duncan PG, Tate RB. Does anesthesia contribute to operative mortality? *JAMA.* 1988;260:2859-2863.
4. Fraser TR. The antagonism between the actions of active substances. *Br Med J.* 1872;26:457-459.
5. Frei W. Versuche uber kombination von desinfektionsmitteln. *Zeitschr f Hyg.* 1913;75:433-496.
6. Loewe S. The problem of synergism and antagonism of combined drugs. *Arzneimittelforschung.* 1953;3:285-290.
7. Minto CF, Schnider TW, Short TG, Gregg K, Gentilini A, Shafer SL. Response surface model for anesthetic drug interactions. *Anesthesiology.* 2000;92:1603-1616.
8. Short TG, Ho TY, Minto CF, Schnider TW, Shafer SL. Efficient trial design for eliciting a pharmacokinetic-pharmacodynamic model-based response surface describing the interaction between two intravenous anesthetic drugs. *Anesthesiology.* 2002;96:400-408.
9. Hendrickx JF, Eger II EI, Sonner JM, Shafer SL. Is synergy the rule? A review of anesthetic interactions producing hypnosis and immobility. *Anesth Analg.* 2008;107:494-506.

10. Greco WR, Bravo G, Parsons JC. The search for synergy: a critical review from a response surface perspective. *Pharmacol Rev.* 1995;47:331-385.
11. Smith C, McEwan AI, Jhaveri R, et al. The interaction of fentanyl on the Cp50 of propofol for loss of consciousness and skin incision. *Anesthesiology.* 1993;78:864-869.
12. McEwan AI, Smith C, Dyar O, Goodman D, Smith LR, Glass PS. Isoflurane minimum alveolar concentration reduction by fentanyl. *Anesthesiology.* 1994;81:820-828.
13. Tallarida RJ. An overview of drug combination analysis with isobolograms. *J Pharmacol Exp Ther.* 2006;319:1-7.
14. LaPierre CD, Johnson KB, Randall BR, White JL, Egan TD. An exploration of remifentanil-propofol combinations that lead to loss of response to esophageal instrumentation, a loss of responsiveness, and/or onset of intolerable ventilatory depression. *Anesth Analg.* 2011;113(3):490-499.
15. Manyam SC, Gupta DK, Johnson KB, et al. Opioid-volatile anesthetic synergy: a response surface model with remifentanil and sevoflurane as prototypes. *Anesthesiology.* 2006;105:267-278.
16. Fidler M, Kern SE. Flexible interaction model for complex interactions of multiple anesthetics. *Anesthesiology.* 2006;105:286-296.
17. Kong M, Lee JJ. A generalized response surface model with varying relative potency for assessing drug interaction. *Biometrics.* 2006;62:986-995.
18. Kong M, Lee JJ. A semiparametric response surface model for assessing drug interaction. *Biometrics.* 2008;64:396-405.
19. Bouillon TW, Bruhn J, Radulescu L, et al. Pharmacodynamic interaction between propofol and remifentanil regarding hypnosis, tolerance of laryngoscopy, bispectral index, and electroencephalographic approximate entropy. *Anesthesiology.* 2004;100:1353-1372.
20. Vuyk J, Lichtenbelt BJ, Struys MM, Engbers F, Dahan A, Olofsen E. Response surface modelling of the propofol-midazolam interaction to define the optimal concentration combination that assures unconsciousness and hemodynamic stability. *Anesth Analg.* 2011; in review.
21. Vuyk J, Lichtenbelt BJ, Olofsen E, van Kleef JW, Dahan A. Mixed-effects modeling of the influence of midazolam on propofol pharmacokinetics. *Anesth Analg.* 2009;108:1522-1530.
22. Lichtenbelt BJ, Olofsen E, Dahan A, van Kleef JW, Struys MM, Vuyk J. Propofol reduces the distribution and clearance of midazolam. *Anesth Analg.* 2010;110:1597-1606.
23. McAdam LC, MacDonald JF, Orser BA. Isobolographic analysis of the interactions between midazolam and propofol at GABA_A receptors in embryonic mouse neurons. *Anesthesiology.* 1998;89:1444-1454.
24. Sebel LE, Richardson JE, Singh SP, Shannon BS, Bell V, Jenkins A. Additive effects of sevoflurane and propofol on γ-aminobutyric acid receptor function. *Anesthesiology.* 2006;104:1176-1183.
25. Kataria R, Singhal A, Prakash S, Singh I. A comparative study of efficacy of propofol auto-co-induction versus midazolam propofol co-induction using the priming principle. *Indian J Anaesth.* 2010;54:558-561.
26. Westmoreland CL, Sebel PS, Gropper A. Fentanyl or alfentanil decreases the minimum alveolar anesthetic concentration of isoflurane in surgical patients. *Anesth Analg.* 1994;78:23-78.
27. Lang E, Kapila A, Shlugman D, Hoke JF, Sebel PS, Glass PSA. Reduction of isoflurane minimal alveolar concentration by remifentanil. *Anesthesiology.* 1996;85:721-728.
28. Sebel PS, Glass PS, Fletcher JE, Murphy MR, Gallagher C, Quill T. Reduction of the MAC of desflurane with fentanyl. *Anesthesiology.* 1992;76:52-59.
29. Katoh T, Ikeda K. The effects of fentanyl on sevoflurane requirements for loss of consciousness and skin incision. *Anesthesiology.* 1998;88:18-24.
30. Katoh T, Uchiyama T, Ikeda K. Effect of fentanyl on awakening concentration of sevoflurane. *Br J Anaesth.* 1994;73:322-325.
31. Stevens WD, Dolan WM, Gibbons RT, et al. Minimum alveolar concentrations (MAC) of isoflurane with and without nitrous oxide in patients of various ages. *Anesthesiology.* 1975;42:197-200.
32. Manyam SC, Gupta DK, Johnson KB, et al. Opioid-volatile synergy: a response surface model with remifentanil and sevoflurane as prototypes. *Anesthesiology.* 2006;105:267-278.
33. Syroid ND, Johnson KB, Pace NL, et al. Response surface model predictions of emergence and response to pain in the recovery room: as evaluation of patients emerging from isoflurane and fentanyl anesthetic. *Anesth Analg.* 2010;111:380-386.
34. Johnson KB, Syroid ND, Gupta DK, et al. Evaluation of remifentanil sevoflurane response surface models in patients emerging from anesthesia: model improvement using effect-site sevoflurane concentrations. *Anesth Analg.* 2010;111:387-394.
35. Glosten B, Faure EAM, Lichtor JL, et al. Desflurane MAC is decreased but recovery time is unaltered following premedication with midazolam (0.05 mg/kg). *Anesthesiology.* 1990;73(3A):A346.
36. Solano AM, Pypendop BH, Boscan PL, Ilkiw JE. Effect of intravenous administration of ketamine on the minimum alveolar concentration of isoflurane in anesthetized dogs. *Am J Vet Res.* 2006;67:21-25.
37. Katoh T, Ikeda K. The effect of clonidine on sevoflurane requirements for anaesthesia and hypnosis. *Anaesthesia.* 1997;52:377-381.
38. Goyagi T, Tanaka M, Nishikawa T. Oral clonidine premedication reduces the awakening concentration of isoflurane. *Anesth Analg.* 1998;86:410-413.
39. Aantaa R, Jaakola ML, Kallio A, Kanto J. Reduction of the minimum alveolar concentration of isoflurane by dexmedetomidine. *Anesthesiology.* 1997;86:1055-1060.
40. Fragen RJ, Fitzgerald PC. Effect of dexmedetomidine on the minimum alveolar concentration (MAC) of sevoflurane in adults age 55 to 70 years. *J Clin Anesth.* 1999;11:466-470.
41. Katoh T, Ikeda K, Bito H. Does nitrous oxide antagonise sevoflurane-induced hypnosis? *Br J Anaesth.* 1997;79:465-468.
42. Röpcke H, Wirz S, Bouillon T, Bruhn J, Hoeft A. Pharmacodynamic interaction of nitrous oxide with sevoflurane, desflurane, isoflurane and enflurane in surgical patients: measurements by effects on EEG median power frequency. *Eur J Anaesthesiol.* 2001;18:440-449.
43. Short TG, Chui PT. Propofol and midazolam act synergistically in combination. *Br J Anaesthesia.* 1991;67:539-545.
44. Mertens MJ, Olofsen E, Engbers FH, Burm AG, Bovill JG, Vuyk J. Propofol reduces perioperative remifentanil requirements in a synergistic manner: response surface modeling of perioperative remifentanil-propofol interactions. *Anesthesiology.* 2003;99:347-359.
45. Kern SE, Xie G, White JL, Egan TD. A response surface analysis of propofol-remifentanil pharmacodynamic interaction in volunteers. *Anesthesiology.* 2004;100:1373-1381.
46. Vuyk J, Mertens MJ, Olofsen E, Burm AG, Bovill JG. Propofol anesthesia and rational opioid selection: determination of optimal EC_{50}-EC_{95} propofol-opioid concentrations that assure adequate anesthesia and a rapid return of consciousness. *Anesthesiology.* 1997;87:1549-1562.
47. Harris RS, Lazar O, Johansen JW, Sebel P. Interaction of propofol and sevoflurane on loss of consciousness and movement to skin incision during general anesthesia. *Anesthesiology.* 2006;104:1170-1175.
48. Schumacher PM, Dossche J, Mortier EP, Luginbuehl M, Bouillon TW, Struys MMRF. Response surface modelling of the interaction between propofol and sevoflurane. *Anesthesiology.* 2009;111:790-804.
49. Diz JC, Del Río R, Lamas A, Mendoza M, Durán M, Ferreira LM. Analysis of pharmacodynamic interaction of sevoflurane and propofol on Bispectral Index during general anaesthesia using a response surface model. *Br J Anaesth.* 2010;104(6):733-739.
50. Davidson JA, Macleod AD, Howie JC, White M, Kenny GN. Effective concentration 50 for propofol with and without 67% nitrous oxide. *Acta Anaesthesiol Scand.* 1993;37:458-464.
51. Stuart PC, Stott SM, Millar A, Kenny GN, Russell D. Cp_{50} of propofol with and without nitrous oxide 67%. *Br J Anaesth.* 2000;84:638-639.
52. Short TG, Plummer JL, Chui PT. Hypnotic and anaesthetic interactions between midazolam, propofol and alfentanil. *Br J Anaesth.* 1992;69:162-167.
53. Vinik HR, Bradley Jr EL, Kissin I. Triple anesthetic combination: propofol-midazolam-alfentanil. *Anesth Analg.* 1994;78:354-358.
54. Ben-Shlomo I, abd-el-Khalim H, Ezry J, Zohar S, Tverskoy M. Midazolam acts synergistically with fentanyl for induction of anaesthesia. *Br J Anaesth.* 1990;64:45-47.
55. Hong W, Short TG, Hui TW. Hypnotic and anesthetic interactions between ketamine and midazolam in female patients. *Anesthesiology.* 1993;79:1227-1232.
56. Hui TW, Short TG, Hong W, Suen T, Gin T, Plummer J. Additive interactions between propofol and ketamine when used for anesthesia induction in female patients. *Anesthesiology.* 1995;82:641-648.
57. Syroid ND, Agutter J, Drews FA, et al. Development and evaluation of a graphical anesthesia drug display. *Anesthesiology.* 2002;96:565-574.

Chapter 6

ADVERSE DRUG REACTIONS

Abhinav Kant and Philip M. Hopkins

DEFINITION AND INCIDENCE

No medicine is risk free, yet the definition of an adverse drug reaction may not be straightforward. The World Health Organization states that "harmful, unintended reactions to medicines that occur at doses normally used for treatment are called adverse drug reactions."[1] One particular problem with this vague definition is that it assumes that all individuals are the same and hence the "normal dose" of a drug is to be comparable within a population. It does not consider differences in pathophysiology within individuals, which can alter the way a drug behaves pharmacokinetically or pharmacodynamically. Another problem is that it can be difficult to distinguish an adverse drug reaction from what is commonly known as a side effect. A side effect can occur within or without the normal dosage range of a medication. One particular aspect of a side effect, different than an adverse drug reaction, is that the effect might be beneficial. An example in anesthetic practice is the use of lidocaine as an antiarrhythmic.[2] This drug was originally licensed for use as a local anesthetic yet its cardiotoxic effects can be utilized to treat cardiac rhythm problems in some settings. Further confusion with the definition of an adverse drug reaction results when a drug is being researched or is under surveillance after its initial commercial release. European regulatory guidelines state, "In the preapproval clinical experience with a new medicinal product or its new usages, particularly as the therapeutic dose(s) may not be established: all noxious and unintended responses to a medicinal product related to any dose should be considered adverse drug reactions."[3] In other words, during the drug development process, any and all unintended effects are considered adverse drug reactions that are classified according to severity and the likelihood that the untoward effect is linked to the investigational drug. This usually extensive list of potential adverse effects becomes part of the product label.

Many adverse drug reactions can be attributed to a drug interacting with another or several other drugs. The practice of anesthesia involves the coadministration of several drugs alongside any drugs the patient already takes. The potential for drug interactions perioperatively is therefore very high. The incidence of adverse drug reactions in hospitalized patients in the United States and Canada has been reported to be between 6.7% and 24.1%, and more than 100,000 fatalities per year have been estimated to be attributable. More than 70% were deemed to be preventable.[4,5] A large analysis of more than 11,000 adverse drug reactions in more than 6600 patients receiving anesthetics in the United Kingdom showed a mortality of 9% with the largest proportion attributable to the use of inhalational anesthetics and the smallest proportion (3%) from local anesthetics.[6] The most frequently reported adverse drug reactions were associated with the use of intravenous induction agents and newer drugs such as desflurane and remifentanil.

Historically adverse drug reactions were classified into two distinct categories: type A and type B.[7] Type A reactions were classed as dose-related and included pharmacokinetic and pharmacodynamic variations within populations as well as drug interactions. Type B described reactions that were not dose related but idiosyncratic or allergic and were often in genetically susceptible individuals. This classification has evolved into one described neatly by Edwards and Aronson[8]; a modification is shown in Table 6-1. This chapter focuses on the general principles of the mechanisms of adverse drug reactions that can be applied to a wide range of drugs used in the practice of anesthesia.

Drug Administration Errors

Of course an adverse drug reaction could occur if the drug is incorrectly administered to a patient (e.g., the "syringe swap"). Note that this does not fall into the classification described earlier. Over the past decade, the UK National Patient Safety Agency (NPSA) and the Institute of Medicine in the United States have both compiled massive data highlighting that this is a serious and widespread issue in hospitals. Drug administration errors are the single most preventable cause of patient harm.[9,10] While the majority of these reported errors led to minimal or no harm, in anesthesia they have the potential to cause devastating effects. A UK study of 12,606 reported incidents showed medication errors occurred in 1120 patients.[11] Of these, only 15 (1.3%) resulted in severe harm

or even death. A further 6-month analysis of reports to the NPSA regarding drug errors in intensive care showed that, of the 2428 incidents reported, 355 different drugs were involved, with morphine, gentamicin, and norepinephrine being the most common.[12] A recent review of anesthetic drug errors states that an error can happen as frequently as every 133 anesthetics.[13] Much work is being done to prevent administration error and recent evidence suggests that double checking of drugs with a second person can reduce error.[14,15]

Drug error need not be as late as the administration phase but can occur during prescription. Illegible handwriting, inaccurate medication history, confusion with the drug name, inappropriate use of decimal points, use of abbreviations, and use of verbal orders have all been implicated in prescribing errors.[16]

Inaccurate knowledge of the dosing information amongst prescribers can lead to erroneous dosing.[17] A drug developed in a nonanesthetic context could have its dosing regimen inappropriately applied in the perioperative situation. This applies to some drugs introduced into clinical practice at a time when the regulatory process was less vigorous. A good example is morphine, for which the traditional quoted dose for severe postoperative pain is 0.15 mg/kg given intramuscularly. This dose was deemed the effective dose for battlefield casualties. However, one can now accept that battlefield casualties are an inappropriate model for postoperative pain as their pain tolerance is high as a result of the psychologic and neurohumoral responses.[18]

Another example is antiemetic medication. None of the currently available antiemetics was initially developed primarily for perioperative use. Many were first introduced as treatments for motion sickness, vestibular disorders, migraine, or treatment of side effects of radiation therapy or cytotoxic chemotherapy at doses that are higher than those required for the antiemetic effects. The butyrophenone droperidol, for example, was introduced into anesthetic practice as a

Table 6-1. Classification of Adverse Drug Reactions

MNEMONIC	TYPE OF REACTION	FEATURES	EXAMPLES
A—Augmented	Dose-related	Common Related to pharmacologic action of the drug Predictable Low mortality	Intravenous anesthetics Inhalational anesthetics Local anesthetics
B—Bizarre	Drug idiosyncrasy, non–dose-related	Uncommon Not related to pharmacologic action of the drug Unpredictable High mortality	Penicillin allergy Reduced cytochrome metabolism of warfarin Malignant hyperthermia Isoflurane and hemolytic anemia in G6PD deficiency Barbiturates and porphyria crisis
C—Chronic	Dose-related, time related, direct organ damage	Uncommon Usually dose-related	Bleomycin and lung fibrosis Halothane hepatitis Sevoflurane and renal toxicity
D—Delayed	Time related	Uncommon Usually dose-related Becomes apparent some time after the administration of the drug	Nitrous oxide and megaloblastic anemia Etomidate and adrenal suppression
E—End of use	Withdrawal	Uncommon Occurs soon after withdrawal of the drug	Opioid withdrawal syndrome Nitrous oxide and diffusion hypoxia
F—Failure	Unexpected failure of therapy	Common Dose-related Often caused by drug interactions	Ephedrine and tachyphylaxis

Modified from Edwards R, Aronson JK. Adverse drug reactions: definitions, diagnosis, and management. *Lancet.* 2000;356:1255-1259.

neuroleptic agent in a dose of approximately 0.1 mg/kg.[19] Neurolept anesthesia as a technique is now rarely performed; however, droperidol is still used for its antiemetic properties, sometimes at doses more consistent with the outdated anesthesia technique. Droperidol's antiemetic efficacy is present at doses 10 times lower than those required for the neuroleptic effect. More commonly used antiemetics such as phenothiazines and antihistamines are also sometimes being used in inappropriately high doses in the perioperative setting with potentially avoidable side effects.

Types of Adverse Drug Reactions

A—AUGMENTED—DOSE RELATED

Paracelsus (1493-1541), a founder of toxicology, once noted, "All substances are poisons: there is none which is not a poison. The right dose differentiates a poison and a remedy." Despite the administration of a drug in its intended therapeutic dose range some patients will exhibit an adverse effect. This can occur as a result of variation of an individual's drug response within a unimodal population variation in response.[20] This phenomenon is termed *drug intolerance*. The causes of drug intolerance are invariably multifactorial with environmental and genetic factors involved. Intolerance to the drug is invariably related to the dose administered and there are numerous examples of these in anesthesia. An example is the intrathecal administration of a local anesthetic that can result in either a desired or undesired, low or high block level dependent on patient characteristics.[21-23] The most common dose-related reactions seen from anesthetic agents (inhalational or intravenous) are dampening of normal cardiovascular and respiratory functions; indeed these reactions are sometimes used for clinical benefit.[24,25] This relationship between desired effect and unwanted effect remains at the forefront of toxicology.

Conventionally the propensity for adverse effects of drugs is measured by the *therapeutic index*. In the preclinical testing of new drugs, the therapeutic index provides a ratio of the LD_{50} (dose that causes death of 50% of animals) to the ED_{50} (the dose that produces the desired effect in 50% of animals). The LD_{50} and ED_{50} are calculated from cumulative quantal dose-response curves, illustrated in Figure 6-1.[26] Although

widely established within toxicology, the therapeutic index does have limitations. Consider two drugs—A and B—that have the same ED_{50} value. If the population variability in response to drug B is greater than for drug A (Figure 6-2), there will be a larger ED_{95} (dose that produces the desired effect in 95% of subjects) value for drug B. Clinically the ED_{95} or even the ED_{99} is far more useful than the ED_{50}, because we would want as many patients as possible being treated with a beneficial effective dose, yet the dose must not reach levels that produce important unwanted effects. It also becomes clear that the ED_{50} is not an ideal dose for clinical purposes as one would not want to produce an unwanted effect in 50% of patients. Figure 6-3 further illustrates this principle. A more useful pharmacologic concept revolves around the *certain safety factor*.[27] This is the ratio of the dose to produce an unwanted effect in a defined proportion of the population (usually 1%) to the dose to produce a desired effect in a proportion 100 minus that defined. In other words the certain safety factor is most commonly described as TD_{01}/ED_{99} where TD is the toxic dose. The certain safety factor can be adjusted if the unwanted effect of the drug is particularly serious, for example, $TD_{0.1}/ED_{99.9}$.

The doses used in the calculation of the certain safety factor also define the limits of the *therapeutic window*. Dose-response relationships remain a popular area for anesthetic research.[28-30] Newer drugs, combinations of drugs, and techniques to administer them are slowly being introduced in all areas of anesthetic practice and each will undoubtedly have the ability to cause harm.

B—BIZARRE—DRUG IDIOSYNCRASY, NOT DOSE RELATED

Some adverse drug reactions are not dose related and occur within individuals with genetic susceptibility. Pharmacogenetic variation has been identified in drug metabolism (acetylation, cytochrome P_{450} variants, plasma cholinesterase variants—see Chapter 4 on Drug Metabolism and Pharmacogenetics), inability to compensate for drug effects (glucose 6-phosphate dehydrogenase deficiency, acute porphyrias), in

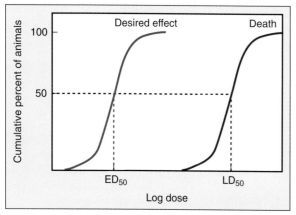

Figure 6-1 Quantal dose response curves to illustrate derivation of the therapeutic index from the ratio of the LD_{50} (dose that causes death of 50% of animals) to the ED_{50} (the dose that produces the desired effect in 50% of animals).

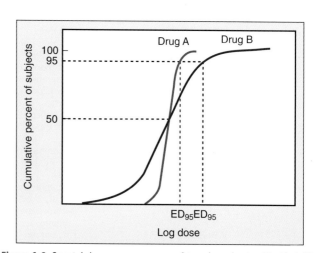

Figure 6-2 Quantal dose response curve of two drugs having identical ED_{50} but different ED_{95} doses. This results from the greater population variability in response to drug B compared with drug A and illustrates how therapeutic effectiveness can vary between two drugs with similar potency when potency is defined on the basis of the ED_{50}.

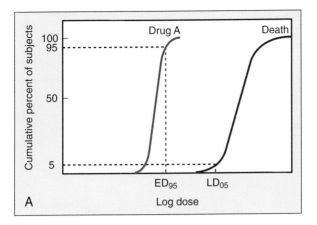

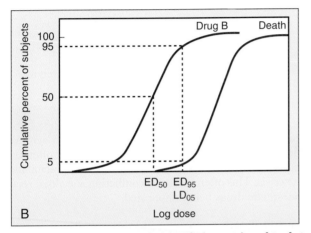

Figure 6-3 Illustration of the principle of the certain safety factor. **A,** Quantal dose response curves for two effects of the same drug, the desirable therapeutic effect and an unwanted effect, in this case death. For the drug in this example, there is good separation between the ED_{95} and LD_{05}. **B,** Illustration of a drug with unfavorable certain safety factor where there is overlap between the ED_{95} and LD_{05}.

drug effects themselves (malignant hyperthermia), or even in immune-mediated responses (allergies). Each of these examples is discussed separately.

Acetylator Status

Drugs such as isoniazid, hydralazine, procainamide, some sulphonamides, sulphasalazine, nitrazepam, and caffeine undergo acetylation. This is a phase 2 non-microsomal conjugation reaction catalyzed by the enzyme N-acetyltransferase, which exists in either a fast or slow form within individuals. The prevalence of slow acetylation can be as high as 60% in Caucasians and 10% to 20% in Asians.[31] Slow acetylation, resulting in a prolonged half-life of the drug, can predispose individuals to a greater risk of side effects such as peripheral neuropathy (isoniazid), lupus syndrome (hydralazine and procainamide), allergic reactions and hemolysis (sulphonamides), and gastrointestinal effects (sulphasalazine).

Cytochrome P450 Variants

The cytochrome P450 (CYP) family of enzymes are responsible for microsomal phase I oxidation reactions. They exist in four classes (CYP1-4), each with several subgroups.[31] Most drugs can be metabolized by one or more of these subgroups. Important polymorphisms exist in four enzymes;

drugs that are metabolized predominately by one of these enzymes could show reduced clearance. Enzymes of particular interest to anesthesiologists include CYP 2D6, CYP 2C9, CYP 2C19, CYP 3A4-5, and CYP 2E1. The CYP 2D6 group is responsible for roughly 25% of drug metabolism, notably of metoprolol, propranolol, amiodarone, flecainide, tricyclic and selective serotonin reuptake inhibitor antidepressants, phenothiazines, butyrophenones, and opioids. There is racial variation, with 6% of Caucasians and 1% of Asians having reduced activity.[32] The CYP 2C9 enzyme group is important for warfarin metabolism such that individuals with reduced activity of CYP 2C9 are prone to hemorrhagic complications.[33] CYP 2C19 is involved in the oxidation of diazepam and proton pump inhibitors, with reduced activity being more prevalent in Asians (20% versus 3% in Caucasians).[34,35] An important enzyme for the metabolism of midazolam, lidocaine, fentanyl, and alfentanil is CYP 3A4-5, which is responsible for 50% of drug oxidation reactions and has reduced activity in 6% of Caucasians. Metabolism of acetaminophen and the fluorinated volatile anesthetics is predominantly by the CYP 2E1 enzyme.[36]

Plasma Cholinesterase Variants

Plasma cholinesterase (also known as pseudocholinesterase, serum cholinesterase, nonspecific cholinesterase, butyrylcholinesterase, S-type cholinesterase) is most notably responsible for hydrolysis of the depolarizing muscle relaxant succinylcholine to succinyl monocholine and choline. It also accounts for metabolism of the nondepolarizing muscle relaxant mivacurium, and to a lesser extent ester local anesthetics, diamorphine, aspirin, and methylprednisolone. Genetic variation accounts for reduced activity of this enzyme and is most clinically relevant to prolonged succinylcholine paralysis or *scoline apnea*. Investigating scoline apnea involves using inhibitors of plasma cholinesterase such as dibucaine (cinchocaine) and sodium fluoride and quantifying the reduction in activity compared to that for a normal enzyme. Traditionally, four alleles—usual normal (Eu), atypical dibucaine resistant (Ea), silent absent (Es), and fluoride resistant (Ef)—have been identified on chromosome 3, resulting in single amino acid substitutions in each of these variants. Another K-variant has also been described that results in a 30% reduction in enzyme activity.[37,38] Whereas most individuals are homozygous for Eu, up to 4% of the population can be heterozygous and thus demonstrate a prolonged neuromuscular block, which can last between 10 minutes and several hours, in response to succinylcholine.

Glucose-6-Phosphate Dehydrogenase Deficiency

Erythrocytes are obligate glucose users and rely on the pentose phosphate pathway for metabolism. Glucose-6-phosphate dehydrogenase (G6PD) is a rate-limiting enzyme in this pathway, converting glucose-6-phosphate to 6-phosphoglucono-δ-lactone. The reaction usually provides energy for the cell in the form of NADPH, which is needed for the maintenance of reduced glutathione. Reduced glutathione has an important role in combating hydrogen peroxide and other reactive oxygen species produced within the cell during periods of oxidative stress.[39,40] Individuals with G6PD deficiency therefore can have dangerously high levels of hydrogen peroxide (resulting in protein damage and cell death) under periods of oxidative stress. This can occur when oxidizing drugs such as primaquine, chloroquine,

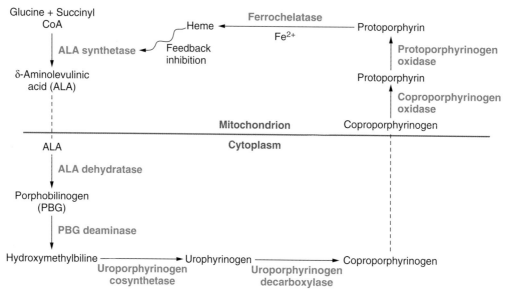

Figure 6-4 Metabolic pathway for heme synthesis. A block in any of the enzymes in the pathway results in accumulation of porphyrin precursors especially following metabolic stress or hemorrhage.

chloramphenicol, some sulphonamides, and vitamin K analogues are administered to susceptible individuals with the ultimate consequence being hemolytic anemia. The highest prevalence of G6PD deficiency appears in falciparum malaria zonal populations, in that this deficiency appears to confer a survival advantage against the parasite. With particular regard to anesthesia, there is some evidence in vitro of G6PD activity being reduced by isoflurane, sevoflurane, diazepam, and midazolam. The specific effect of inhalational general anesthetics in individuals with G6PD deficiency in vivo remains an area for further research.[41]

The Porphyrias

The porphyrias are a group of rare conditions caused by excessive accumulation of porphyrinogens, the precursors of heme (Figure 6-4). In affected individuals these porphyrinogens are excreted in urine and on exposure to light change color, resulting in the classic purple urine. Under normal circumstances, heme tightly controls its own production by feedback inhibition of the first of the seven enzymes in the pathway, aminolevulinic acid (ALA) synthetase. This feedback inhibition can be disrupted in periods of bleeding or metabolic stress (infection, dehydration, fasting) resulting in induced ALA synthetase activity.[42] A block in any of the enzymes in the pathway will result in accumulation of porphyrin precursors. An acute attack results in motor, sensory, and autonomic dysfunction by accumulating porphyrinogen. Of particular importance to anesthesia is the potential for many drugs to induce the activity of ALA synthetase. Drugs such as barbiturates, etomidate, ketamine, benzodiazepines, metoclopramide, mepivacaine, atracurium, vecuronium, diclofenac, and ranitidine all have been implicated in precipitating an acute attack in susceptible individuals.[43] There is some controversy surrounding the effects of propofol. Animal experiments have shown it to induce ALA synthetase activity, and propofol infusions have resulted in raised porphyrin levels in humans with acute porphyria. Nevertheless there are anecdotal reports of its safe use in patients with porphyria.[44,45]

Categorizing drugs as safe or unsafe in porphyria remains difficult. Factors such as stress or infection, which often coincide with the administration of anesthesia, can precipitate an acute crisis. This often results in conflicting anecdotal reports of anesthetic drugs being implicated.

Malignant Hyperthermia

Malignant hyperthermia (MH) is a potentially lethal pharmacogenetic disorder that is attributable to faulty skeletal muscle intracellular calcium (Ca^{2+}) homeostasis. The disorder is genetically heterogeneous but the final common pathophysiologic path is a loss of regulation of Ca^{2+}-release units of myocytes. Fundamental to normal functioning of the Ca^{2+}-release units is a tightly regulated bidirectional interaction between the voltage sensor of the T-tubular sarcolemmal membrane (dihydropyridine receptor, DHPR) and the Ca^{2+} release channel of the sarcoplasmic reticulum (ryanodine receptor isoform 1 [RyR1]) (Figure 6-5). A majority of MH families subjected to genetic investigations have potentially causative variants in *RYR1*, the gene encoding RyR1. In other families, pathologic variants in *RYR1* have been excluded. A small minority of these have variants in *CACNA1S*, the gene encoding the <α-1 subunit of the DHPR. In the remaining 10% to 25% of families, the gene or genes underlying MH remain to be identified. Potential candidate genes encoding proteins known to interact with RyR1 and DHPR number more than 30, but there is currently no evidence that any of these are implicated in MH. Further elucidation of the genetic etiology of MH probably will require genome-wide "next generation" sequencing approaches.

Direct intracellular Ca^{2+} measurements of muscle cells from humans and transgenic mouse models suggest, contrary to previous assumptions, that Ca^{2+} cycling is abnormal in MH-susceptible patients even without exposure to triggering agents. Even though Ca^{2+} sequestration is upregulated, cytoplasmic resting Ca^{2+} concentration is elevated. Evidence is emerging that this might predispose to sarcopenia or even frank myopathy in the long term. The most obvious

Physiologic Activation of RyR1

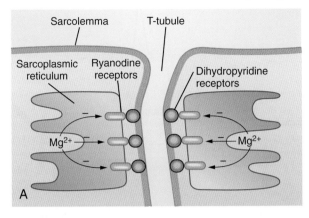

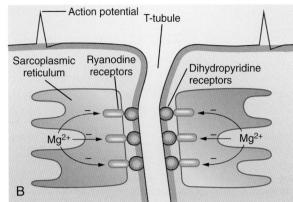

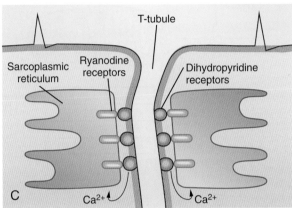

Figure 6-5 Physiologic activation of the ryanodine receptor Ca^{2+} release channel (RyR1). Mg^{2+} exhibits a regulatory role on the RyR1. As an action potential arrives down the T-tubule the dihydropyridine (DHP) receptor acts as a voltage sensor, allowing Ca^{2+} release.

manifestation of MH susceptibility is, however, a pharmacologically triggered massive and persistent increase in cytoplasmic Ca^{2+} concentration resulting in metabolic stimulation and sustained contractile activity with disruption of sarcolemmal integrity (Figure 6-6). The clinical consequences are increased oxygen consumption, carbon dioxide production, tachycardia, hyperthermia, acidosis, rhabdomyolysis, and muscle rigidity. A critical stage appears to be related to mitochondrial failure brought about by mitochondrial Ca^{2+} accumulation secondary to the elevated cytoplasmic Ca^{2+} concentration. Death results from any one, or a combination, of hyperkalemia, disseminated intravascular coagulation (secondary to hyperthermia), profound acidosis, or hyperthermia.

The primary triggers of MH are the potent inhalation anesthetics, including all the currently available agents (isoflurane, sevoflurane, desflurane).[46] They appear to act on RyR1 by overriding the physiologic Mg^{2+} inhibition of the channel (Figure 6-7). The clinical effect can be almost immediate and rapidly progressive or more insidious with signs in some reports delayed for more than 6 hours into anesthesia. Succinylcholine is likely to cause generalized or jaw muscle rigidity and also seems to enhance the onset and severity of a reaction triggered by subsequent exposure to a volatile anesthetic. At worst it is only a weak trigger of the hypermetabolic MH response when administered without a potent inhalation agent. There is no convincing evidence that any other drugs can trigger MH.

Successful treatment of MH depends on early recognition of the evolving reaction. A combination of unexplained tachycardia and unexplained increase in CO_2 production makes the diagnosis likely. An increasing body temperature can be observed almost simultaneously or can be delayed for several minutes. Treatment involves discontinuation and enhancement of elimination of volatile anesthetics, hyperventilation with 100% oxygen, body cooling, and administration of dantrolene. Dantrolene is a hydantoin derivative and was originally classed as a muscle relaxant. It was first reported as a treatment for MH in pigs in 1975 and its efficacy in humans was established several years later.[47,48] The drug is believed to act on the ryanodine receptor within the sarcoplasmic reticulum. By binding to the receptor, it reduces sarcoplasmic reticulum calcium release, thus depressing excitation-contraction coupling in skeletal muscle (see Figure 6-6). General supportive measures are used to treat acidosis, hyperkalemia, myoglobinemia, arrhythmias, and disseminated intravascular coagulation.

Allergic Drug Reactions

Allergic reactions to drugs administered intravenously are acute type I hypersensitivity reactions. This requires an allergen to be exposed to an individual for a second or subsequent time. Epidemiologic data for anesthetic allergic reactions are variable, in that there remains some confusion as to the definitions of allergy and anaphylaxis. Indeed some reactions that are accepted as side effects of certain drugs, for instance, histaminergic reactions due to atracurium and mivacurium, may be underreported.[49] The European Academy of Allergy and Clinical Immunology put forward this definition:

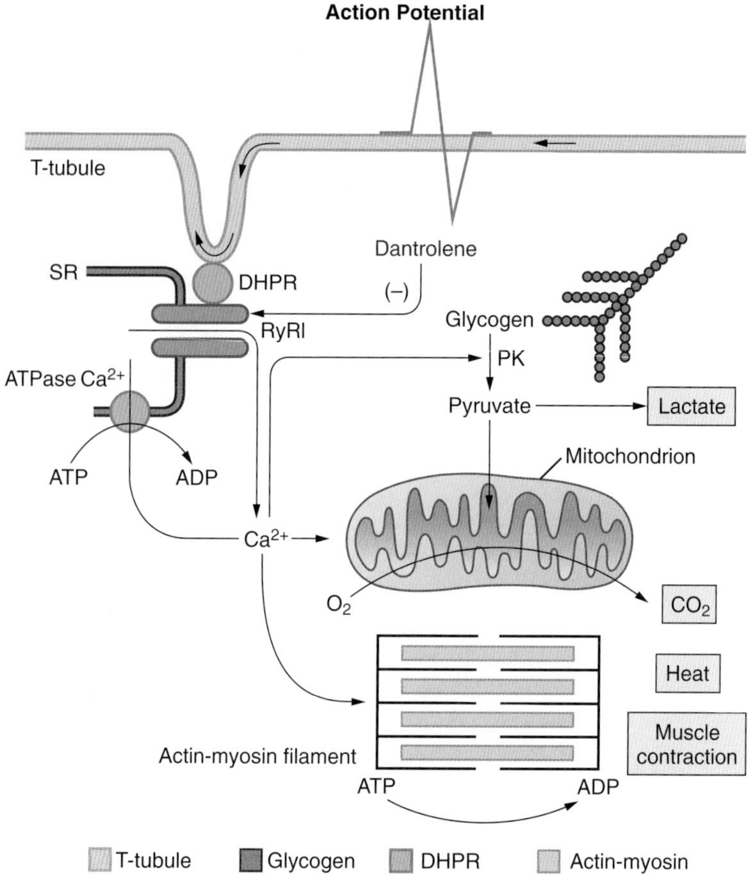

Action Potential

Figure 6-6 Site of dantrolene action preventing a chain of intracellular mechanisms leading to muscle contraction, generation of heat, lactate, and CO_2. Release of Ca^{2+} is central to glycogen metabolism, mitochondrial respiratory function, and contraction of actin-myosin filaments.

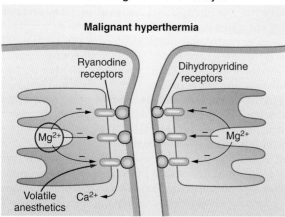

Pharmacologic Activation of RyR1

Malignant hyperthermia

Figure 6-7 Loss of inhibitory effect of Mg^{2+} on ryanodine receptor from inhalational anesthetics. The result is sustained Ca^{2+} release from the sarcoplasmic reticulum. Dantrolene acts by reducing pathologic release of Ca^{2+} from the sarcoplasmic reticulum that leads to muscle contraction, generation of heat, lactate, and CO_2. Release of Ca^{2+} is central to glycogen metabolism, mitochondrial respiratory function, and contraction of actin-myosin filaments.

Allergy is a hypersensitivity reaction initiated by immunologic mechanisms. Allergy can be antibody- or cell-mediated. In the majority of cases the antibody typically responsible for an allergic reaction belongs to the IgE isotype and these individuals may be referred to as suffering from an IgE-mediated allergy. Not all IgE associated "allergic" reactions occur in "atopic" subjects. In non-IgE-mediated allergy the antibody can belong to the IgG isotype, for example, anaphylaxis due to immune complexes containing dextran, and the classical, today rare, serum sickness previously referred to as a type III reaction. Both IgE and IgG antibodies are found in allergic bronchial pulmonary aspergillosis. Allergic contact dermatitis is representative of allergic diseases mediated by lymphocytes.[50]

Anaphylaxis is essentially a severe, life-threatening, generalized or systemic hypersensitivity reaction.[51] The clinical features (hypotension, tachycardia or bradycardia; cutaneous flushing, rash or urticaria; bronchospasm; hypoxia; angioedema and cardiac arrest) usually occur within a few minutes but can be delayed by up to an hour. True allergic anaphylactic reactions involve mast cell degranulation resulting from production of allergen-specific IgE, IgG, or complement activation. Nonallergic anaphylactic (anaphylactoid) reactions can occur through a direct drug action on the mast cell itself, leading to degranulation.

There is little rationale in the use of a test dose in the prevention of allergic drug reactions. True allergic anaphylaxis, of course, can occur after exposure to the smallest dose of antigen. However, direct mast cell degranulation (non-IgE-mediated response) is probably dependent on the mass of drug and its rate of administration. In these circumstances there is unlikely to be any response to a test dose, but the full dose will cause the reaction. It is advisable, therefore, to administer intravenous drugs slowly.

The products of mast cell degranulation responsible for mediating the anaphylactic response include histamine, tryptase, leukotrienes, and prostaglandins. These mediators result in skin flushing or urticaria, vasodilation, increased vascular permeability, bronchoconstriction, and bronchial secretions. Not all of these features occur in every anaphylactic reaction. Some reactions are predominated by vasodilation, whereas others are by bronchoconstriction. This may be due to the presence of two main types of mast cell: mucosal mast cells that are located in the lungs and the gut, and connective tissue mast cells that are ubiquitous.[52] Drugs such as atracurium and morphine characteristically cause cutaneous reactions without the respiratory or systemic vascular responses, suggesting that cutaneous connective tissue mast cells are particularly sensitive to these drugs.

The ability to investigate suspected anaphylactic reactions is not yet precise. Because of its short serum half-life release, histamine is difficult to measure. Its more stable metabolite, methylhistamine, can be detected in the urine. Mast cell degranulation can be demonstrated by serum mast cell tryptase levels measured immediately after the reaction, followed by subsequent measurements at 2 hours and 24 hours. Additional blood tests include specific IgE tests (also known as radioallergosorbent tests), although false-negative findings are possible due to consumption in the initial reaction. Although not diagnostic, complement assays can also be performed and might point to a particular mechanism. Skin-prick testing is commonly performed, but the diagnostic value of a positive result remains in doubt due to a lack of subsequent challenge data. A positive wheal and flare reaction occurring 30 minutes after an allergen is introduced intradermally, usually on the volar aspect of the arm, is indicative of true anaphylaxis.

True to its bizarre nature, anaphylaxis has curious epidemiologic traits. Neuromuscular blocking drugs and latex appear to cause anaphylaxis more commonly in female patients. Individuals with a history of atopy, asthma, or allergy to some foods appear to be at increased risk of latex allergy but not anaphylaxis to neuromuscular blocking drugs or antibiotics.[53] There is an association with smoking status and antibiotic anaphylaxis, possibly due to such patients being repeatedly exposed to antibiotics for respiratory infections. Antibiotics account for approximately 15% of anesthesia-related anaphylactic reactions, with penicillins and cephalosporins (both sharing a β-lactam ring) being responsible for 70% of these.

There continues to be great controversy surrounding the anaphylactic potential of nondepolarizing neuromuscular drugs. A study in France demonstrated that muscle relaxants were implicated in 60% of anesthesia-associated type I hypersensitivity reactions; the largest proportion of these was attributed to succinylcholine followed by rocuronium.[54] In North America and Australia, the incidence of reactions to muscle relaxants other than succinylcholine is low. One explanation for this epidemiologic disparity is the use and interpretation of intradermal testing, which has a high false-positive rate. A growing body of evidence suggests that dilutions of at least 1:1000 improve the specificity of this test.[55,56] Another explanation for these findings is that certain individuals become sensitized to neuromuscular drugs by exposure to environmental factors such as perfumes, toothpastes, or cough medicines, but no strong evidence exists to support this idea.

The difficulty in making an accurate diagnosis makes quantifying the incidence of anaphylaxis challenging, with estimates ranging from 1:10,000 to 1:20,000 anesthetics. Other drug groups commonly implicated are intravenous anesthetic agents and plasma substitutes. With the decline in use of latex gloves, sensitivity to this allergen is becoming less of a problem. Reactions to latex are characterized by their development after 30 to 60 minutes of surgery, whereas drug reactions tend to occur within seconds or a few minutes of drug administration. The use of chlorhexidine as an antiseptic skin wash but also as an antibacterial coating to bladder and central venous catheters has also been associated with severe systemic hypersensitivity reactions.[57] Anaphylactic reactions to local anesthetics are extremely uncommon with the esters more likely than amides to induce a reaction (due to hydrolysis to the allergen para-aminobenzoic acid [PABA]). Similarly it is unlikely that a cutaneous histamine reaction to opioids (particularly morphine, meperidine, and codeine) is attributable to anaphylaxis. A careful history in this instance can prevent a patient from being labeled as allergic, which might deprive the patient of effective perioperative analgesia. It is well known that reactions to nonsteroidal anti-inflammatory drugs (NSAIDs) can occur in susceptible individuals due to the inhibition of the PGE_2 pathway resulting in excessive leukotriene synthesis.[58] Subsequent mediator release is associated with bronchospasm and urticaria, yet the IgE-mediated reaction is reportedly rare. A recently published UK guideline is a useful resource for managing allergy and anaphylaxis.[59]

C—CHRONIC—DIRECT ORGAN DAMAGE: DOSE RELATED AND TIME RELATED

Over time, drugs can exert a cumulative unwanted effect. Examples in anesthesia include bleomycin causing oxygen-induced lung damage or volatile anesthetics causing hepatocellular and renal toxicity.

Bleomycin is a well-established chemotherapeutic agent used to treat metastatic germ cell cancer and, in some regimens, non-Hodgkin lymphoma.[60] The principal dose-related problem associated with the use of bleomycin is progressive pulmonary fibrosis in 10% of patients, occurring more commonly in older adults, at cumulative doses greater than 400 units, and with creatinine clearance less than 35 mL/min.[61] Both iron and oxygen are cofactors for DNA cleavage by bleomycin.[62] Treatment with bleomycin should be terminated if basal lung crepitations or suspicious chest radiograph changes are seen. Patients who have received extensive treatment with bleomycin are at risk for respiratory failure if a general anesthetic using a high inspired oxygen concentration is given within 6 to 12 months. A case series suggested that intraoperative inspired oxygen concentrations of 35% to 42% were responsible for respiratory failure and subsequent death of five patients.[63] This led to the recommended use of low concentrations of oxygen in such cases. In contrast, a 6-year audit of 13 similar patients showed no difference in lung complications between bleomycin-treated patients having surgery with either 24% or 41% inspired oxygen.[64] However, a difference between these two studies was the presence of restricted lung disease and decreased carbon monoxide diffusion capacity secondary to bleomycin treatment in the former group, while the other study did not perform pulmonary function tests on all patients and the majority of those who had were normal. This would suggest that preexisting bleomycin lung damage as shown on lung function tests is a key factor in the risk of hyperoxic lung injury. Several case reports using differing fractions of inspired oxygen in patients with varied cumulative bleomycin exposure have shown mixed results, but it appears prudent to use the lowest concentration and shortest duration of oxygen possible.[65-67]

The volatile anesthetics used in current practice can also lead to direct end-organ damage. All contain fluorine that can be released following metabolism; it is the fluoride ion that can lead to nephropathy. Halothane undergoes the greatest amount of metabolism by hepatic cytochrome P450 (up to 25%) and desflurane the least (0.02%). Fluoride toxicity was first recognized in the 1960s with the introduction of the now obsolete methoxyflurane. A serum fluoride concentration greater than 50 μM over a prolonged time was associated with polyuria, proteinuria, glycosuria, and impaired renal concentrating ability. However, approximately 5% of inhaled sevoflurane undergoes metabolic biotransformation (oxidative defluoridation), readily releasing fluoride concentrations exceeding 50 μM, yet studies have failed to demonstrate subsequent renal damage.[68]

Another by-product of sevoflurane metabolism is compound A (fluoromethyl-2,2-difluoro-1-[trifluoromethyl] vinyl ether), which is produced by its interaction with carbon dioxide absorbents. There is debate surrounding the mechanism leading to renal toxicity, with the renal cysteine conjugating β-lyase pathway (involved in the biotransformation of compound A) playing a significant role. The β-lyase pathway is up to 30-fold less active in humans than in rats; therefore if this is responsible, humans could be less susceptible to compound A renal toxicity than rats. Studies in humans have shown that long (8-hour) sevoflurane exposures and low fresh gas flow rates can result in significant production of compound A.[69] Urinalysis revealed transient changes in biochemical markers of renal injury; however, other studies using prolonged sevoflurane administration at low flow rates suggest no risk of this compound. A useful review of the association of sevoflurane and renal injury is available.[70]

Direct liver damage from halothane (halothane hepatitis) is becoming less of a problem in the developed world due to its decline in use. Its estimated incidence is 1 in 35,000 administrations with risk factors including late middle age, female sex, and obesity. There are two reported types of halothane hepatitis. Type 1 is an asymptomatic, spontaneously resolving rise in serum transaminases within 2 weeks of exposure, likely attributable to hepatic hypoxia secondary to hypoperfusion. A reductive pathway leading to addition of a single electron into the halothane molecule produces a highly reactive metabolite that undergoes debromination to another free radical intermediate (Figure 6-8). These free radicals can then lead to destruction of hepatocytes.

Type 2 hepatitis leads to fulminant hepatic necrosis with a mortality rate between 50% and 75%. There appears to be a correlation between amount of halothane used and severity of liver failure but not the likelihood of occurrence. An immune basis is probably responsible with the metabolites (trifluoroacetyl chloride and trifluoroacetic acid) behaving as haptens, covalently bonding to hepatic proteins and inducing antibody formation (Figure 6-9). Onset can be by the seventh day after administration or relatively delayed compared to direct hepatotoxic drugs such as acetaminophen for up to 28 days.

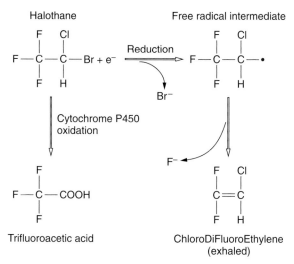

Figure 6-8 Proposed metabolic pathway implicated in halothane hepatitis. A reductive pathway leading to addition of a single electron into the halothane molecule produces a highly reactive metabolite that then undergoes debromination to another free radical intermediate. These free radicals lead to destruction of hepatocytes and trifluoroacetic acid can react with proteins to form neoantigens.

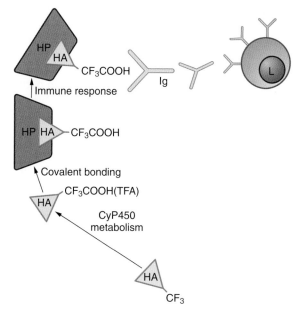

Figure 6-9 Neoantigen (hapten) formation. Halogenated anesthetics (HA) are metabolized by cytochrome P450 enzymes into metabolites such as trifluoroacetic acid (TFA) that form covalent bonds with hepatic proteins (HP). The modified proteins act as neoantigens that trigger an immune response, with immunoglobulin (Ig) production by lymphocytes (L) that then interact with the newly formed neoantigen.

D—DELAYED—TIME RELATED

Certain adverse drug reactions are not apparent until a significant amount of time has elapsed since the initial administration of the drug. Nitrous oxide has been well reported to increase the risk of megaloblastic bone marrow changes and subsequent neurologic complications (subacute combined degeneration of the spinal cord) due to vitamin B_{12} deficiency. Short exposure for a few hours can lead to bone marrow changes and more prolonged exposure of several days can lead to agranulocytosis. The cobalt ion present in vitamin B_{12} is

Nitrous Oxide Effect on Tetrahydrofolate Synthesis

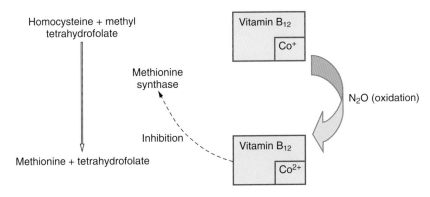

Figure 6-10 Mechanism of nitrous oxide toxicity. The cobalt ion in vitamin B$_{12}$ is oxidized by nitrous oxide, thus preventing it from activating methionine synthase. This enzyme is responsible for the conversion of homocysteine to methionine, and subsequently thymidine and tetrahydrofolate, which are essential for DNA synthesis.

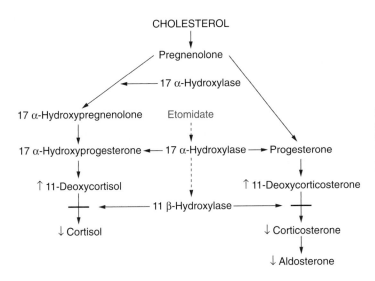

Figure 6-11 Mechanism of immunosuppression by etomidate. Steroid synthetic pathway is shown highlighting enzymes (11β-hydroxylase and 17α-hydroxylase) essential for cortisol and aldosterone synthesis. 11β-Hydroxylase is inhibited by etomidate *arrows* leading to reduced adrenocortical steroid synthesis with possible adverse effects. (Dashed line = inhibitory.)

oxidized by nitrous oxide, thus preventing it from activating methionine synthase. This enzyme is responsible for conversion of homocysteine into methionine, thymidine, and tetrahydrofolate (Figure 6-10). The subsequent accumulation of plasma homocysteine could in theory increase the risk of perioperative myocardial events but no strong evidence appears to support this theory. An attempt to prevent this adverse effect with preoperative vitamin B infusions was not successful.[71]

The use of etomidate as an induction agent in septic patients continues to be a matter of great debate. There is no doubt that a single dose of etomidate suppresses adrenocortical function by inhibiting enzymes (11β-hydroxylase and 17α-hydroxylase) essential for cortisol and aldosterone synthesis (Figure 6-11). The effect can appear as early as 30 minutes after administration or several hours later. These hormones play an important role in the stress response and while there is evidence of increased mortality if etomidate is used in septic patients, the studies are limited by their observational design.

E—END OF USE—WITHDRAWAL

Acute withdrawal of drugs has been well documented to cause harmful effects. Of interest to anesthesiologists is the withdrawal of common addictive drugs such as alcohol, nicotine, and opioids. These effects usually result in detrimental psychiatric, neurologic, and cardiorespiratory consequences. Acute opioid withdrawal in children managed in intensive care has been shown to induce anxiety, agitation, grimacing, insomnia, increased muscle tone, abnormal tremors, and choreoathetoid movements.[72] More recently the withdrawal of cardioprotective agents such as β-blockers and statins has been suggested to increase the risk of perioperative cardiac events. Continuation of preoperative antihypertensive medication is advocated for similar reasons.

Owing to differences in blood-gas partition coefficients, acute withdrawal of inhaled nitrous oxide can in theory lead to diffusion hypoxia. At the end of anesthesia, if an N$_2$O/O$_2$ mixture is replaced by air/O$_2$, the volume of N$_2$O which enters the alveolus from the blood will be greater than the volume of N$_2$ (from the air) entering the pulmonary capillaries. This could create an unwanted dilution of all the alveolar gases, so supplemental oxygen is advised.

F—DRUG FAILURE

There can be a multitude of reasons why any drug can fail to produce its desired effect, but by far the most common reason is inadequate dosing. Due to variation in response within a population, those at the lower end of the dose-response curve might not attain the desired effect of the drug. Another common reason for drug failure involves drug interactions (see Chapter 5).

There are other specific reasons why a drug might fail within an individual depending on the pharmacogenomic profile of the patient. Many drugs rely on active enzyme systems in order to take effect. As discussed earlier, the CYP enzymes are responsible for the metabolism of numerous drugs of relevance to anesthesiologists. For example, CYP 2D6 is responsible for metabolism of the weaker opioids codeine, dihydrocodeine, tramadol, oxycodone, and hydrocodone. The clinical effect of these drugs requires formation of more potent hydroxyl metabolites such as morphine, dihydromorphine, and oxymorphone. The gene encoding CYP 2D6 exhibits significant polymorphism, with 100 variant alleles. This results in a number of clinical phenotypes with approximate frequencies in Caucasians of poor metabolizers (5%-10%), intermediate metabolizers (10%-15%), extensive metabolizers (65%-80%), and ultra-rapid metabolizers (5%-10%).[73] The poor metabolizers are unlikely to attain beneficial effects of these drugs.

Another way drugs can fail involves depletion of critical substrates at the cellular level. Ephedrine, for example, increases release of norepinephrine from synaptic vesicles at the nerve terminal. The released norepinephrine acts postsynaptically (in this case ultimately leading to positive inotropy and chronotropy as well as vasoconstriction). However the synthesis of norepinephrine from the amino acid tyrosine is time-dependent such that if its rate of release and consumption exceeds the rate of synthesis, ephedrine will fail to act (Figure 6-12).[74] This is an example of tachyphylaxis. Other drugs that also depend on intracellular mechanisms subject to depletion include nitroglycerine (nitric oxide release) and hydralazine (guanosine monophosphate release). Another term sometimes used synonymously with tachyphylaxis is *desensitization*. This results from a structural change in receptor conformation or downregulation of receptor numbers. An example of a drug demonstrating this effect is dobutamine, which shows signs of desensitization after 2 hours of continuous infusion and is most significant after 72 hours.[75] Measurable reductions in β2 receptors have been demonstrated after 4 hours.[76] In such examples, by introducing drug-free intervals and replenishment of transmitter stores, restoration of the desired effect of the drug can be possible.

EMERGING DEVELOPMENTS

Much current and future work surrounding adverse drug reactions focuses on prevention, in particular the prevention of drug errors. In practice there are many stages where error can occur, ultimately leading to an adverse drug reaction. A Swiss cheese model depicting human error has been described.[77] In the anesthetic context, patients can present for emergency operation involving a multidisciplinary health care team whereby the anesthesiologist will ultimately administer a drug (Figure 6-13). An adverse drug reaction can occur if all the deficiencies in the system (or holes in the cheese slices) align.

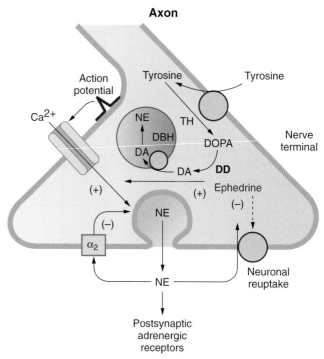

Figure 6-12 Tachyphylaxis with ephedrine. Synthesis of norepinephrine (NE) depends on the hydroxylation of tyrosine by tyrosine hydroxylase (TH) to dihydroxyphenylalanine (DOPA). DOPA is metabolized to dopamine (DA) by DOPA decarboxylase (DD). DA enters vesicles where it is hydroxylated by dopamine β-hydroxylase (DBH) into norepinephrine. Release of norepinephrine is enhanced by ephedrine; if the rate of release exceeds norepinephrine synthesis, then ephedrine can fail to work.

The focus of modern medical practice is in the delivery of safe, effective care. Any adverse event or serious untoward incident is usually subject to an investigation or root cause analysis. The aim of these investigations is not to blame individuals but to understand deficiencies in a patient's care pathway that led to the unwanted incident. This is based on the logic that humans are prone to error and a system should be created to mitigate that error. The hope is that lessons learned from previous mistakes will guide alterations in future management, thus preventing further harm. A perfect flawless pathway is a goal that health care systems continue to strive for.

New developments that might prevent adverse drug reactions include toxigenomics, which embraces the latest technology for compound classification, mechanistic studies, and detection of toxicity markers.[78] Also pharmacogenomics may help us understand more about genetic polymorphisms that underpin individual variance in drug response; however, this rapidly expanding field brings new ethical considerations regarding informed consent for clinical trials, pharmacogenomic profiling, and storage of genetic material.[79] Another developing area is metabonomics.[80] This is a powerful tool for translating disturbances in normal homeostasis of metabolic processes into drug-induced pathology. Using latest advances in mass spectrometry and nuclear magnetic resonance spectroscopy, specific biomarkers can be detected, which is resulting in traditional chemical laboratories being replaced.

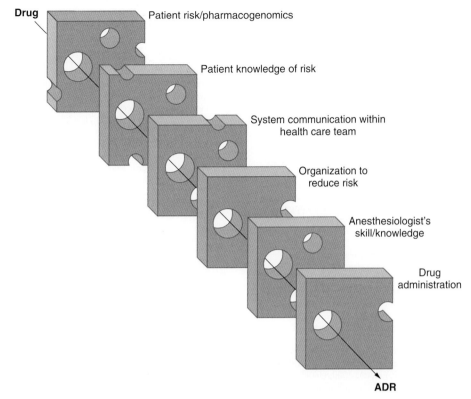

Drug
Patient risk/pharmacogenomics
Patient knowledge of risk
System communication within
health care team
Organization to
reduce risk
Anesthesiologist's
skill/knowledge
Drug
administration
ADR

Figure 6-13 Swiss cheese model of anesthetic drug errors. Error can occur at any point in the medical care pathway, appearing as holes in cheese slices. If a patient has the genetic profile or an unknown risk factor for an adverse drug reaction (ADR), it is up to the health care team to elucidate this potential risk, communicate it to the team, and arrange appropriate measures to mitigate the risk of a hazardous drug being administered. If the anesthesiologist is unaware of which drugs are potentially hazardous or how to administer, then all the holes in the cheese slices align and an ADR occurs.

KEY POINTS

- A large preventable proportion of adverse drug reactions is due to administration error, which can include prescription, formulation, or dosing.
- Drugs exhibit predictable dose-dependent adverse reactions, yet the unpredictable idiosyncratic reactions are often the most life threatening and most challenging to manage.
- Some drugs exhibit their adverse effect over a period of time, occasionally a long time after its initial administration. For example, past use of bleomycin can leave the lungs vulnerable in the presence of high concentrations of inspired oxygen.
- Many drugs have been implicated in precipitating an acute porphyria crisis yet very little conclusive evidence exists as to which drugs should be avoided. Nevertheless it appears prudent to avoid barbiturates in susceptible patients.
- Anaphylaxis remains a relatively unpredictable and potentially fatal complication. The ability to investigate allergic and nonallergic anaphylaxis remains crude.

- Genetic variations within populations can have a major influence on the effect of the drug in an individual and can be a basis for an adverse drug reaction. Well-known genetic variations responsible for adverse drug reactions in anesthesia include pseudocholinesterase deficiency and malignant hyperthermia.
- The volatile anesthetics can lead to direct damage to the kidneys and liver with halothane hepatitis being the most severe complication.
- Withdrawal effect from a drug can be a serious complication, which is of interest to anesthesiologists who usually have direct control over withholding patient medications.
- Some drugs can fail to act either because of pharmacogenetics or because of tachyphylaxis (ephedrine, nitroglycerine).
- Prevention of adverse drug reactions is evolving with the use of root cause analysis and critical incident reporting. Recently the use of modern techniques in pharmacogenomics, toxigenomics, and metabonomics has provided a greater chance of identifying individuals likely to suffer from a reaction.

Key References

Edwards R, Aronson JK. Adverse drug reactions: definitions, diagnosis, and management. *Lancet*. 2000;356:1255-1259. Provides a means of making sense of various existing definitions of adverse drug reaction, adverse drug effect, side effect, and toxic effect. It also proposed a novel classification system, as described in this chapter. (Ref. 8)

Elyassi AR, Rowshan HH. Perioperative management of the glucose-6-phosphate dehydrogenase deficient patient: a review of literature. *Anesthesia Progress*. 2009;56(3):86-91. A review of the background, pathophysiology, and clinical implications of glucose-6-phosphate dehydrogenase deficiency including key recommendations. (Ref. 39)

Harper NJ, Dixon T, Dugué P, et al. Suspected anaphylactic reactions associated with anaesthesia. *Anaesthesia*. 2009;64:199-211. A comprehensive up-to-date guideline on the prevention, detection, and management of suspected anaphylactic reactions in anesthesia. Of particular relevance to anesthesiologists is an appended question and answer section as well as guidance surrounding the use of muscle relaxants, antibiotics, and latex amongst other drugs. (Ref. 59)

Holdcroft A. UK drug analysis prints and anaesthetic adverse drug reactions. *Pharmacoepidemiology Drug Safety*. 2007;16:316-328. A useful insight into the epidemiologic data of adverse drug reactions in nearly all of the commonly used drugs by anesthesiologists. It provides data on incidence, fatalities, and type of reaction. (Ref. 6)

Hopkins PM. Malignant hyperthermia—pharmacology of triggering. *Br J Anaesth*. 2011;107:48-56. A useful review of not only the established known triggers for MH but also some less well known, as well as drugs that might protect against triggering. (Ref. 46)

James MF, Hift RJ. Porphyrias. *Br J Anaesth*. 2009;85:143-153. An in-depth description of porphyria and its implication in anesthesia, including identifying susceptible individuals, identification of porphyrinogenic drugs and anesthetic management of such patients. (Ref. 43)

Lockridge O. Genetic variants of human serum cholinesterase influence metabolism of the muscle relaxant succinylcholine. *Pharmacol Therapeut*. 1990;47:35-60. A useful description of cholinesterase variants and its implications to succinylcholine apnea. (Ref. 37)

Searle R, Hopkins PM. Pharmacogenomic variability and anaesthesia. *Br J Anaesth*. 2009;103(1):14-25. A comprehensive review of pharmacogenetic variability and its influence on the metabolism of drugs important to anesthesiologists such as opioids, inhalational, and intravenous agents. (Ref. 73)

References

1. World Health Organisation. http://www.who.int/mediacentre/factsheets/fs293/en/. Accessed October 2011.
2. Williams V. A classification of antiarrhythmic actions reassessed after a decade of new drugs. *J Clin Pharmacol*. 1984;24:129-147.
3. European Good Clinical Practice Guideline. Page 2. http://www.ich.org/fileadmin/Public_Web_Site/ICH_Products/Guidelines/Efficacy/E6_R1/Step4/E6_R1__Guideline.pdf. Accessed October 2011.
4. Lazarou J, Pomeranz BH, Corey PN. Incidence of adverse drug reactions in hospitalized patients: a meta-analysis of prospective studies. *JAMA*. 1998;279:1200-1205.
5. Samoy LJ, Zed PJ, Wilbur K, et al. Drug-related hospitalizations in a tertiary care internal medicine service of a Canadian hospital: a prospective study. *Pharmacotherapy*. 2006;26(11):1578-1586.
6. Holdcroft A. UK drug analysis prints and anaesthetic adverse drug reactions. *Pharmacoepidemiology and Drug Safety*. 2007;16:316-328.
7. Rawlins MD. Drug interactions and anaesthesia. *Br J Anaesth*. 1978;50:689.
8. Edwards R, Aronson JK. Adverse drug reactions: definitions, diagnosis, and management. *Lancet*. 2000;356:1255-1259.
9. Aspden P, Wolcott JA, Bootman JL, et al. *Preventing medication errors—Committee on Identifying and Preventing Medication Errors. Board on Health Care Services. Institute of Medicine of the National Academies*. Washington, DC: The National Academies Press. http://www.nap.edu/catalog.php?record_id=11623.

10. National Patient Safety Agency UK. Safety in doses: improving the use of medicines in the NHS 2009. http://www.nrls.npsa.nhs.uk/EasySiteWeb/getresource.axd?AssetID=61626&type=full&servicetype=Attachment. Accessed October 2011.
11. Catchpole K, Bell MDD, Johnson S. Safety in anesthesia: a study of 12,606 reported incidents from the UK National Reporting and Learning System. *Anaesthesia*. 2008;63:340-346.
12. Llewellyn RL, Gordon PC, Wheatcroft D, et al. Drug administration errors: a prospective study survey from three South African teaching hospitals. *Anaesth Intens Care*. 2009;37:93-98.
13. Glavin RJ. Drug errors: consequences, mechanisms, and avoidance. *Br J Anaesth*. 2010;105(1):76-82.
14. Jensen LS, Merry AF, Webster CS, et al. Evidence based strategies for preventing drug administration errors during anaesthesia. *Anaesthesia*. 2004;59:493-504.
15. Evley R, Russel J, Mathew D, et al. Confirming the drugs administered during anaesthesia: a feasibility study in the pilot National Health Service sites, UK. *Br J Anaesth*. 2010,105(3):289-296.
16. Williams DJP. Medication errors. *J R Coll Phys Edinburgh*. 2007;37:343-346.
17. Lesar TS, Briceland L, Stein DS. Factors related to errors in medication prescribing. *JAMA*. 1997;277(4):312-317.
18. Beecher HK. Pain in men wounded in battle. *Ann Surg*. 1946;123(1):96-105.
19. McDowell SA, Dundee JW. Neurolept anaesthesia: a comparison with a conventional technique for major surgery. *Can J Anaesth*. 1971;18(5):541-551.
20. Wilkinson GR. Drug metabolism and variability among patients in drug response. *N Engl J Med*. 2005;352:2211-2221.
21. Leino KA, Kuusniemi KS, Palve HK, et al. Spread of spinal block in patients with rheumatoid arthritis. *Acta Anaesthesiol Scand*. 2010;54(1):65-69.
22. Harten JM, Boyne I, Hannah P, et al. Effects of a height and weight adjusted dose of local anaesthetic for spinal anaesthesia for elective caesarean section. *Anaesthesia*. 2005;60(4):348-353.
23. Arzola C, Wieczorec PM. Efficacy of low-dose bupivacaine in spinal anaesthesia for Caesarean delivery: systematic review and meta-analysis. *Br J Anaesth*. 2011;107:308-318.
24. Beaussier M, Paugam C, Deriaz H, et al. Haemodynamic stability during moderate hypotensive anaesthesia for spinal surgery. A comparison between desflurane and isoflurane. *Acta Anaesthesiol Scand*. 2000;44(9):1154-1159.
25. Kanagasundram SA, Lane LJ, Cavaletto BP, et al. Efficacy and safety of nitrous oxide in alleviating pain and anxiety during painful procedures. *Arch Dis Child*. 2001;84:492-495.
26. Finkel R, Cubeddu LX, Clark MA. *Pharmacology*. 4th ed. Philadelphia: Lippincott Williams & Wilkins; 2009.
27. Pandit NK. *Introduction to the pharmaceutical sciences*. 1st ed. Philadelphia: Lippincott Williams & Wilkins; 2007.
28. Bouvet L, Da-Col X, Chassard D, et al. ED_{50} and ED_{95} of intrathecal levobupivacaine with opioids for caesarian delivery. *Br J Anaesth*. 2011;106(2):215-220.
29. Schaller SJ, Fink H, Ulm K, Blobner M. Sugammadex and neostigmine dose-finding study for reversal of shallow residual neuromuscular block. *Anesthesiology*. 2010;113(5):1054-1060.
30. Masui K, Upton RN, Doufas AG, et al. The performance of compartmental and physiologically based recirculatory pharmacokinetic models for propofol: a comparison using bolus, continuous, and target-controlled infusion data. *Anesth Analg*. 2010;111:368-379.
31. Ma MK, Woo MH, McLeod HL. Genetic basis of drug metabolism. *Am J Health Syst Pharm*. 2002;59(21):2061-2069.
32. Kalow W, Otton SV, Kadar D, et al. Ethnic difference in drug metabolism: debrisoquinine 4-hydroxylation in Caucasians and Orientals. *Can J Physiol Pharmacol*. 1980;58:1142-1144.
33. Steward DJ, Haining RL, Henne KR, et al. Genetic association between sensitivity to warfarin and expression of CYP2C9*3. *Pharmacogenetics*. 1997;7:361-367.
34. Wilkinson GR, Guengerich FP, Branch RA, et al. Genetic polymorphism of S-mephenytoin hydroxylation. *Pharmacol Ther*. 1989;43:53-76.
35. Nakamura K, Goto F, Ray WA, et al. Interethnic differences in genetic polymorphism of debrisoquin and mephenytoin hydroxylation between Japanese and Caucasian populations. *Clin Pharmacol Ther*. 1985;38:402-408.
36. Kharasch ED. Adverse drug reactions with halogenated anesthetics. *Clin Pharmacol Ther*. 2008;84(1):158-162.

37. Lockridge O. Genetic variants of human serum cholinesterase influence metabolism of the muscle relaxant succinylcholine. *Pharmacol Ther*. 1990;47:35-60.

38. Soliday FK, Conley YP, Henker R. Pseudocholinesterase deficiency: a comprehensive review of genetic, acquired, and drug influences. *Am Assoc Nurse Anaesth J*. 2010;78(4):313-320.

39. Elyassi AR, Rowshan HH. Perioperative management of the glucose-6-phosphate dehydrogenase deficient patient: a review of literature. *Anesth Progr*. 2009;56(3):86-91.

40. Luzzatto L, Metha A, Vulliany T. Glucose-6-phosphate dehydrogenase deficiency. In: Scriver CR, Beaudet AL, Sly WS, et al, eds. *The Metabolic and Molecular Basis of Inherited Disease*. 8th ed. Columbus, Ohio: McGraw-Hill; 2001:4517-4553.

41. Altikat S, Ciftci M, Buyukokuroglu ME. In vitro effects of some anesthetic drugs on enzymatic activity of human red blood cell glucose-6-phosphate dehydrogenase. *Polish J Pharmacol*. 2002;54:67-71.

42. Thandani H, Deacon A, Peters T. Diagnosis and management of porphyria. *Br Med J*. 2000;320:1647-1651.

43. James MF, Hift RJ. Porphyrias. *Br J Anaesth*. 2000;85:143-153.

44. Bhatia R, Vibha D, Padma Srivastava MV, et al. Use of propofol anesthesia and adjunctive treatment with levetiracetam and gabapentin in managing status epilepticus in a patient of acute intermittent porphyria. *Epilepsia*. 2008;49(5):934-936.

45. Sarantopoulos CD, Bratanow N, Stowe D, et al. Uneventful propofol anesthesia in a patient with coexisting hereditary coproporphyria and hereditary angioneurotic edema. *Anesthesiology*. 2000;92(2):607.

46. Hopkins PM. Malignant hyperthermia—pharmacology of triggering. *Br J Anaesth*. 2011;107:48-56.

47. Harrison GG. Control of the malignant hyperpyrexic syndrome in MHS swine by dantrolene sodium. *Br J Anaesth*. 1975;47(1):62-65.

48. Kolb ME, Horne ML, Martz R. Dantrolene in human malignant hyperthermia. *Anesthesiology*. 1982;56(4):254-262.

49. Axon AD, Hunter JM. Editorial III: Anaphylaxis and anaesthesia—all clear now? *Br J Anaesth*. 2004;93:501-504.

50. The European Academy of Allergy and Clinical Immunology. Allergy definitions glossary. http://eaaci.net/attachments/304_English.pdf. Accessed December 21, 2010.

51. Johansson SGO, Bieber T, Dahl R, et al. Revised nomenclature for allergy for global use: Report of the Nomenclature Review Committee of the World Allergy Organization, October 2003. *J Allergy Clin Immunol*. 2004;113:832-836.

52. Irani AA, Schechtert NM, Craigt SS, et al. Two types of human mast cells that have distinct neutral protease compositions (tryptase/chymotryptic proteinase). *Proc Natl Acad Sci U S A*. 1986;83(12):4464-4468.

53. Mertes PM, Laxenaire MC, Alla F. Groupe d'Etudes des Réactions Anaphylactoïdes Peranesthésiques. Anaphylactic and anaphylactoid reactions occurring during anesthesia in France in 1999–2000. *Anesthesiology*. 2003;99:536-545.

54. Laxenaire MC, Mertes PM. Groupe d'Etudes des Reactions Anaphylactoides Peranesthesiques. Anaphylaxis during anaesthesia. Results of a two-year survey in France. *Br J Anaesth*. 2001;87:549-558.

55. Dhonneur G, Combes X, Chassard D, et al. Skin sensitivity to rocuronium and vecuronium: a randomized controlled prick-testing study in healthy volunteers. *Anesth Analg*. 2004;98(4):986-989.

56. Mertes PM, Moneret-Vautrin DA, Leynadier F, et al. Intradermal neuromuscular blocking agent injections: a randomized multicenter trial in healthy volunteers. *Anesthesiology*. 2007;107(2):245-252.

57. Krautheim AB, Jermann TH, Bircher AJ. Chlorhexidine anaphylaxis: case report and review of the literature. *Contact Dermatitis*. 2004;50(3):113-116.

58. Funk CD. Prostaglandins and leukotrienes: advances in eicosanoid biology. *Science*. 2001;294:1871-1875.

59. Harper NJ, Dixon T, Dugué P, et al. Suspected anaphylactic reactions associated with anaesthesia. *Anaesthesia*. 2009;64:199-211.

60. Blum RH, Carter SK. A clinical review of bleomycin—a new antineoplastic agent. *Cancer*. 1973;31(4):903-914.

61. O'Sullivan JM, Huddart RA, Norman AR, et al. Predicting the risk of bleomycin lung toxicity in patients with germ-cell tumours. *Ann Oncol*. 2003;14(1):91-96.

62. Burger RM, Peisach J, Horwitz SB. Activated bleomycin: a transient complex of drug, iron, and oxygen that degrades DNA. *J Biol Chem*. 1981;256:11636-11644.

63. Goldiner PL, Carlon GC, Cvitkovic E, et al. Factors influencing postoperative morbidity and mortality in patients treated with bleomycin. *Br Med J*. 1978;1:1664-1667.

64. LaMantia KR, Glick JH, Marshall BE. Supplemental oxygen does not cause respiratory failure in bleomycin-treated surgical patients. *Anesthesiology*. 1984;60:65-67.

65. Donat M, Levy DA. Bleomycin associated pulmonary toxicity: is perioperative oxygen restriction necessary? *J Urol*. 1998;160(4):1347-1352.

66. Mathes DD. Bleomycin and hyperoxia exposure in the operating room. *Anaesth Analg*. 1995;81:624-629.

67. Huettemann E, Sakka SG. Anaesthesia and anti-cancer chemotherapeutic drugs. *Curr Opin Anaesthesiol*. 2005;18:307-314.

68. Munday IT, Stoddart PA, Jones RM, et al. Serum fluoride concentration and urine osmolality after enflurane and sevoflurane anesthesia in male volunteers. *Anesth Analg*. 1995;81(2):353-359.

69. Ebert TJ, Frink EJ, Kharasch ED. Absence of biochemical evidence for renal and hepatic dysfunction after 8 hours of 1.25 minimum alveolar concentration sevoflurane anesthesia in volunteers. *Anesthesiology*. 1998;88:601-610.

70. Gentz BA, Malan TP Jr. Renal toxicity with sevoflurane: a storm in a teacup? *Drugs*. 2001;61(15):2155-2162.

71. Rao LK, Francis AM, Wilcox U, et al. Pre-operative vitamin B infusion and prevention of nitrous oxide-induced homocysteine increase. *Anaesthesia*. 2010;65(7):710-715.

72. Anand KJS, Willson DF, Berger J, et al. Tolerance and withdrawal from prolonged opioid use in critically ill children. *Pediatrics*. 2010;12(5):e1208-e1225.

73. Searle R, Hopkins PM. Pharmacogenomic variability and anaesthesia. *Br J Anaesth*. 2009;103(1):14-25.

74. Patil PN, Tye A, LaPidus JB. A pharmacological study of the ephedrine isomers. *J Pharmacol Exp Ther*. 1965;148(2):158-168.

75. Unverferth DV, Blanford M, Kates RE, et al. Tolerance to dobutamine after a 72 hour continuous infusion. *Am J Med*. 1980;69:262-266.

76. Tohmeh JF, Cryer PE. Biphasic adrenergic modulation of β-adrenergic receptors in man: agonist-induced early increment and late decrement of β-adrenergic receptor number. *J Clin Invest*. 1980;65:836-840.

77. Reason J. Human error: models and management. *Br Med J*. 2000;320:768-770.

78. Suter L, Babiss LE, Wheeldon EB. Toxicogenomics in predictive toxicology in drug development. *Chem Biol*. 2004;11(2):161-171.

79. Issa AM. Ethical perspectives on pharmacogenomic profiling in the drug development process. *Nat Rev Drug Disc*. 2002;1:300-308.

80. Vangala S, Tonelli A. Biomarkers, metabonomics, and drug development: can inborn errors of metabolism help in understanding drug toxicity? *Am Assoc Pharmaceut Scientists J*. 2007;9(3):E284-297.

Section II

NERVOUS SYSTEM

Chapter 7

CENTRAL NERVOUS SYSTEM PHYSIOLOGY: NEUROPHYSIOLOGY

Aeyal Raz and Misha Perouansky

The neuron is the fundamental unit of information processing and transfer in the central nervous system (CNS). It is, however, the collective activity of hierarchically organized neuronal circuits and networks that underlies its behavioral and homeostatic functions. These functions are *emerging* properties of a complex system. Therefore the CNS has to be examined on different organizational levels: properties characteristic of a functional unit on one level of organization are absent from lower level elements and cannot predict properties of a higher level unit. How exactly behavior emerges from the activity of individual neurons, circuits, and networks is a question at the cutting edge of research. Neurons, however, carry the primary molecular targets of anesthetic drugs. Conventional thinking attributes most of the desirable effects of general anesthetics to the modulation of membrane ion channels. Drug-induced alterations in the function of individual voltage-, transmitter-, and otherwise gated channels are not exhaustively but relatively well characterized; how these alterations propagate through increasing levels of complexity to finally result in sedation, amnesia, hypnosis, and immobility, less so. General anesthetics also affect second messenger systems either directly or via effects on G protein-coupled receptors. The significance of the latter effects for anesthesia is unclear.

HISTORICAL PERSPECTIVE

The ancient Egyptians tossed it when they prepared for mummification, Aristotle thought it a radiator to cool the heart. More than 2000 years and dozens of Nobel prizes later, the Society for Neuroscience counts more than 35,000 members, many of whom devote their lives to study it: the brain

Except in the last decade of the 19th century, brain science in the 1800s was dominated by physicians such as Broca, Wernicke, Fritsch, and Brodmann, who started the process of a functional localization of the brain but were limited in their ability to resolve the underlying matrix. Pavlov linked psyche to behavior and learning with the development of the conditioned reflex concept, which is still widely used in neuroscience today; he received a Nobel Prize in 1904. Methodologic breakthroughs, the result of decades of hard work, paired with visionary thinking led to fundamental advances that made neuroscience possible by bridging function and structure. The grand debate spanning the 19th and 20th century between scientific giants on whether the brain, like other organs, consisted of discrete cells or was a reticulum-like structure was not settled by the development of the "reazione nera" (known by its eponym Golgi's method). For his revolutionary staining method as well as other discoveries, Golgi shared the 1906 Nobel Prize with Ramon y Cajal—his brilliant opponent in the grand debate. Golgi thought that the fine processes visualized by his staining method maintained continuity between cells, Cajal (using Golgi's impregnation method) was the most eloquent proponent of the opposing view that the cell doctrine (developed by Schleiden and Schwan earlier in the 19th century) also applied to the CNS—the so-called neuron doctrine. The neuron doctrine is accepted today but, as nature is not doctrinaire, some neurons (and parts of the glia) do act syncytially by maintaining specialized intercellular channels, common during embryogenesis, into adulthood. Sherrington postulated communication via the synapse on theoretical grounds in 1897 but only the development of electron microscopy provided incontrovertible proof its existence more than half a century later.

The 20th century witnessed an exponential growth of science as an enterprise that becomes more and more a collaborative endeavor. The names of outstanding individuals give progressively less justice to all those who made important advances possible but are doomed to oblivion. Nevertheless, the names of Nobel Prize laureates are used here to anchor a flash review of concepts particularly relevant to this chapter.[1] Barany studied the physiology and pathology of the vestibular system and received the 1915 Nobel Prize while held in a Russian prisoner of war camp. Action potentials were first recorded by Douglas who shared the Nobel Prize with Sherrington in 1932. Dale and Loewi shared the Prize in 1936 for work on transmitter release. Dale's principle stating that each neuron releases only one type of neurotransmitter was proved false by the end of the 20th century but underlies the familiar classification in widespread use today (e.g., adrenergic, GABAergic). Hodgkin and Huxley shared the Nobel Prize with Eccles in 1963 for discovering the ionic mechanisms involved in excitation and inhibition of the nerve cell membrane. Their biologic model—the giant axon of the Atlantic squid—was so central to this quantum leap in understanding that a contemporary remarked that *Loligo pealei* should have been awarded the prize. Axelrod, Svante von Euler, and Katz shared the prize in 1970 for work on neurotransmitter storage, release, and inactivation in the axon terminal. The Nobel prize to Hubel, Wiesel, and Sperry in 1981 marked a shift in neuroscience toward a comprehensive, system-level understanding of the brain that remains the frontier of neuroscience today. Hubel and Wiesel suggested a hierarchical model for the identification of complex visual themes. Sperry was awarded the prize for his work on lateralized specialization of brain function. Newer models being developed help shed new light on the behavior of the brain.

GLIA

Glial cells (or neuroglia: "nerve glue") are nonneuronal cells that outnumber neurons and are ubiquitous in the CNS. Glia take up, metabolize, respond to, and release neurotransmitters and modulators, control the microenvironment that surrounds neurons, and support communication. Glial cells also play a number of other roles in CNS homeostasis. However, glia are not known to actively transfer and process discrete information.

Two basic types of neuroglial cells can be distinguished: macroglia (oligodendrocytes, astrocytes) and microglia. Oligodendrocytes fulfill in the CNS the role that Schwann cells play in the peripheral nervous system with some adaptations. In order to conserve space, one oligodendrocyte cell body myelinates multiple axons and the myelin itself consists of a single sheet of oligodendrocyte plasma membrane without cytoplasm wrapped tightly around an axonal segment. Each myelinated segment is termed an internode because of the bare segments of axon present at each end of it—the node of Ranvier. The action potential can leap from node to node—a process known as saltatory conduction, allowing rapid conduction even along thin axons.[2]

Astrocytes constitute 20% to 50% of the volume in most brain regions. Two main forms predominate, protoplasmic in the gray and fibrous in the white matter. Astrocytes isolate the brain from the rest of the body by covering the surface of capillaries and ensheathing the nodes of Ranvier, synapses, and dendrites with extensions of their bodies, creating the blood-brain barrier. Astrocytes are connected to each other by gap junctions forming a syncytium that facilitates the diffusion of small molecules across the CNS. They also communicate with neurons via Ca^{2+}-induced transmitter release.[3] Astrocyte precursors (radial glia) guide neuronal migration in early development. Throughout life, astrocytes synthesize a plethora of growth factors and are the major source of extracellular matrix proteins and adhesion molecules.

Microglial cells are immune competent cells, termed the *macrophages of the CNS*. They are the least understood cell type of the CNS even though they account for a substantial fraction of all cells (5%-20% in the mouse brain; human white matter has more microglia than its rodent counterpart).[4,5]

Glial cells are not known to be materially affected by anesthetics in a way that can be linked to acute behavioral changes.

NEURON

The neuron is the fundamental building block of the nervous system. Neurons are diverse in nature, interconnected, adaptive, and therefore, as ensembles, give rise to the stunning complexity of the brain. A *complex* system is endowed with *emerging properties*, that is, properties that appear only in ensembles as opposed to being present fully in the individual element. The human brain contains more than 10^{11} neurons. Their cell bodies are located in gray matter areas of the CNS whereas the white matter consists of fibers connecting neurons from different regions.

Neurons are excitable cells. This property is harnessed to receive, process, integrate, and transmit signals. Their structure is optimized to integrate multiple inputs and deliver what used to be thought of as an all-or-none (binary) signal in the form of an action potential to other, potentially distant, elements. Action potentials, however, should not be interpreted as isolated events where information transfer is concerned. Both their rate modulation and their phase relationship with respect to ongoing oscillations encode information. Neurons in the CNS are connected by approximately 10^{14} synapses, which are specialized structures allowing information transfer and hence networking.

Basic Structure

Neurons display a dazzling variety of shapes. However, the typical neuron contains three basic elements: dendrites (signal reception and processing), soma (signal integration and cellular housekeeping apparatus), and axon (information output). These three elements vary in complexity, shape, and length, but their basic structure and functional properties are similar (Figure 7-1).

The *soma* is the part of a neuron that is most reminiscent of a conventional cell. It contains all the standard cellular components found in other cells, such as nucleus, protein production (ribosomes), and modification machineries and energy generators (mitochondria). The soma also undergoes neuron-specific long-term changes during development, plasticity, degeneration, and aging. In addition, the soma is the hub linking signal input to information output.

The *dendrites* are elongated cytoplasmic processes. Usually a neuron has more than one dendrite. Each dendrite bifurcates multiple times, creating a dendritic arbor in the vicinity of the soma; it can stretch to other cortical layers, but does not spread to distant regions of the brain. The dendritic arbor creates a large, intricately organized membrane surface area to receive input from other neurons. The arbor hosts vast numbers of the postsynaptic component of chemical synapses—transmitter receptors—targeted by incoming axon terminals that form the presynaptic side. A typical pyramidal cell (e.g., in the hippocampus) receives many thousand synapses: excitatory inputs on the dendrites, inhibitory on the soma, and the dendrites. The structure of the dendritic tree and the location of each synapse on it determine the nature of input summation and local integration and hence their relative strength. Spines are small processes of varying shapes found on many dendrites. These processes are specialized sites of synaptic connections, increasing the dendritic membrane but also providing a compartmentalization of subsynaptic structures (Figures 7-2 and 7-3). Spines are highly dynamic and can change their size and composition on a time scale of minutes in response to neuronal activity, thereby creating, changing, or eliminating synaptic points of contact.

The *axon* is a very thin cytoplasmic process that carries the output signal of the neuron (the action potential) to its targets. Typically, a single axon originates from and terminates in specialized structures termed *axon hillock* at the soma and *presynaptic terminal* at its destination. Normally, it bifurcates multiple times on the way and creates an axonal arbor connecting with many other neurons. The axonal lengths range from less than a millimeter (local interneurons) to more than 1 m (spinal α-motoneurons).

Axons are usually much longer and thinner than dendrites; hence they require mechanisms that enable them to reliably and efficiently transfer information over long distances, supporting the presynaptic machinery in the terminal at the target while maintaining their own structural integrity. The myelin envelope and the axonal transport system are two mechanisms to this end.

Myelin is a composite of multiple layers of lipid membranes formed by the oligodendroglia in the CNS (Schwann cells in the peripheral nervous system). Myelin electrically insulates the axon enabling high-speed propagation of action potentials with minimal energy expenditure (varying with the degree of insulation).

Axonal transport is a "housekeeping" mechanism that moves vesicles and proteins from their site of synthesis in the soma along the whole length of the axon, and reverse transport relays signals back to the soma. It is an active, energy-consuming process using the cytoskeleton to meet the metabolic needs of the axon, its collaterals, and the presynaptic terminals since diffusion alone would not suffice.[6]

Excitability

Excitable cells are characterized by the ability to dynamically change the electrical potential across their cell membrane. Typical examples are muscle cells and neurons. Neurons use this property to integrate and disseminate information; their structure and function are optimized to precisely control the membrane potential and can be regulated independently for the different functional compartments of a neuron. Alterations in excitability are an important aspect of anesthetic drug action.

A living cell is defined by its ability to remain segregated from its environment. This fundamental property is made possible by the selective permeability of *the cell membrane* (the lipid bilayer and the proteins embedded into it). The intracellular ions are dominated by K^+, while extracellularly high Na^+ and Cl^- hark back to the ionic composition of sea water (Table 7-1). Because of its hydrophobic interior, the lipid bilayer prevents charged molecules and most ions from crossing the membrane. By contrast, water and other small uncharged molecules (e.g., urea) diffuse freely. Membrane-spanning proteins control the movement of ions and other small molecules across the membrane, rendering this lipid envelope semipermeable. Importantly, the permeability for specific ions is controllable. Membrane transport systems can be divided into two principal categories: catalytic and stoichiometric.[7] The proteins responsible for this property are traditionally grouped into pores and channels (catalytic) on one hand and pumps and transporters (stoichiometric) on the other. Catalytic systems carry out movement only "downhill," that is, toward the equilibrium, while stoichiometric systems can carry out transport "uphill," away from the equilibrium with energy expenditure. Cells also have special mechanisms to transport large molecules across the cytoplasmic membrane. Excitable cells in particular are endowed with a rich assortment of ion channels.

The differential distributions of ions inside and outside the cell create chemical concentration gradients. For example, the concentration of K^+ is high inside and low outside the neuron. This creates a tendency for K^+ ions to diffuse out of the cell through K^+ channels that are typically open at *the resting membrane potential (RMP)*. Because K^+ is positively charged, this creates a redistribution of electrical charge, with the inside of the cell becoming more negative because the membrane is impermeable to large molecules like negatively charged proteins. The excess negative charge inside the cell attracts K^+ ions and, at some point, the tendency to diffuse out of the cell along the chemical concentration gradient will be offset by the electrical attraction from inside the cell, reaching electrochemical equilibrium. The equilibrium is a dynamic state as ions continue to cross the membrane but the

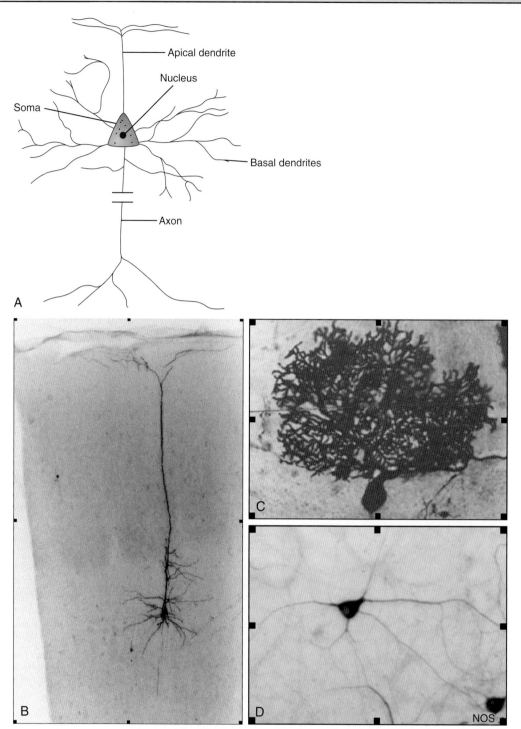

Figure 7-1 A basic plan **(A)** underlies the stunning variety of neuronal shapes found in the mammalian brain. The morphology reflects individual computational needs and architectural constraints. Three examples are shown to illustrate this diversity. **A,** Schematic plan of a pyramidal neuron; notice the apical and basal dendritic arbors providing ample space for synaptic inputs and the long axon projecting to a distant location (symbolized by the interruption). **B,** Photomicrograph of a biocytin-filled cortical pyramidal neuron. Notice the dendritic arbor stretching toward the superficial layers. **C,** Golgi-impregnated Purkinje cell in the cerebellum. **D,** Photomicrograph of striatal interneuron immunostained by antinitric oxide synthase antibodies. *(**B,** Adapted from Cauller LJ, Connors BW. Synaptic physiology of horizontal afferents to layer I in slices of rat SI neocortex.* J Neurosci. *1994;14:751-762;* **C,** *Adapted from Calvet MC, Calvet J, Camacho-Garcia R. The Purkinje cell dendritic tree: a computer-aided study of its development in the cat and in culture.* Brain Res. *1985;331:235-250;* **D,** *Adapted from Schock SC, Jolin-Dahel KS, Schock PC, et al. Striatal interneurons in dissociated cell culture.* Histochem Cell Biol. *2010;134:1-12.)*

net flow of charge at equilibrium is zero. The relation between an ion's concentration gradient and the electrical gradient it creates was described in the 19th century by Nernst in his classic equation:

$$E = \frac{RT}{zF} \ln\left(\frac{[Ion]_{out}}{[Ion]_{in}}\right) \qquad [1]$$

where E is the electric potential across the membrane in mV at equilibrium, R is the ideal gas constant, T is the temperature

in Kelvin, z is the ion's charge, F is Faraday's constant and $[ion]_{out}$ and $[ion]_{in}$ are the concentration of the ion on the two sides of the membrane. All the ions that are differentially distributed between the inside and the outside of a neuron create electrical gradients/potentials across the cell membrane.[8]

Because most of the values in the Nernst equation are constant under biologic conditions, the equation can be simplified assuming intracellular and extracellular K+ concentrations of 140 and 5 mmol/L at 37°C as:

$$E = 60\log\left(\frac{[K^+_{out}]}{[K^+_{in}]}\right) = 60\log\left(\frac{5}{140}\right) = -86.8mV \qquad [2]$$

This means that, at −86.8 mV and the K+ concentrations given above, no net flow of K+ occurs even if the membrane is freely permeable to K+. Similarly, for each ion there is a membrane potential at which its concentration gradient will be balanced by its electrical gradient. These equilibrium potentials become significant determinants of the membrane potential when the membrane becomes permeable to an ion by opening the appropriate channels, for example, for Na+ during an action potential during which the membrane potential rapidly shifts toward the equilibrium potential of Na+. The Nernst potential of some of the common ions that display a major effect on neuronal membrane potential is given in Table 7-1.

The membrane potential of a cell is determined by the gradients of all the intracellular and extracellular ions, scaled according to their permeability through the membrane: the greater the permeability of the cell membrane to a specific ion, the stronger its effect on the membrane voltage. This is described by the Goldman-Hodgkin-Katz (GHK) equation[9]:

$$E = \frac{RT}{F} \ln\left(\frac{\sum_i^N P_{Ci}[Ci]_{out} + \sum_j^M P_{Aj}[Aj]_{in}}{\sum_i^N P_{Ci}[Ci]_{in} + \sum_j^M P_{Aj}[Aj]_{out}}\right) \qquad [3]$$

where P is the permeability, Ci the cations, and Aj the anions; the rest of the variables are the same as in the Nernst equation. In a "resting" neuron, the membrane potential typically is −60 to −70 mV; increasing the membrane permeability to K+, which has an equilibrium potential of −90 mV, will "pull" the membrane potential toward −90 mV, that is, hyperpolarize the cell, whereas increasing the membrane permeability to Na+ (equilibrium potential of +70 mV) will depolarize it. Under resting conditions, the permeability of the cell membrane for K+ dominates and therefore the RMP is largely determined by the equilibrium potential for K+.[8]

Ion channels are pores allowing diffusion of ions across the cell membrane along their electrochemical gradient.

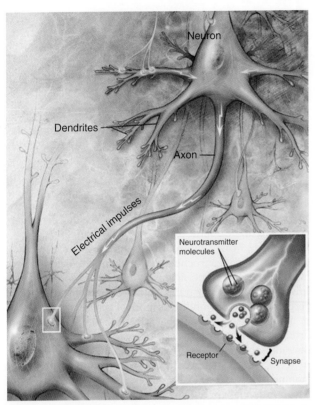

Figure 7-2 Schematic representation of synaptic connections between two neurons. The action potential travels along the axon of neuron A and leads to the release of neurotransmitter containing synaptic vesicles from the presynaptic terminal of A. Neurotransmitter molecules diffuse across the synaptic cleft to activate receptors on the postsynaptic membrane of neuron B. The axon of A contributes to multiple synapses on B and will also innervate many other neurons. The axons of interneurons in particular target specific areas of the postsynaptic neuron (e.g., distal apical dendrites, proximal basal dendrites, or soma). This target specificity has been well characterized in hippocampal interneurons (not shown). The content of one vesicle is thought to lead to a miniature postsynaptic potential that can be either inhibitory or excitatory. (*Adapted from* http://en.wikipedia.org/wiki/File:Chemical_synapse_schema_cropped.jpg#file.)

Table 7-1. Cytoplasmic and Extracellular Ion Concentrations

ION	INTRACELLULAR CONCENTRATION (mM)	EXTRACELLULAR CONCENTRATION (mM)	STEADY STATE POTENTIAL AT 37°C (mV)
Na+	10	145	+70
K+	140	5	−87
Ca2+	10^{-4}	1.5	+125
Mg2+	6.5	2	−15
Cl−	4	110	−86
HCO3−	12	25	−19

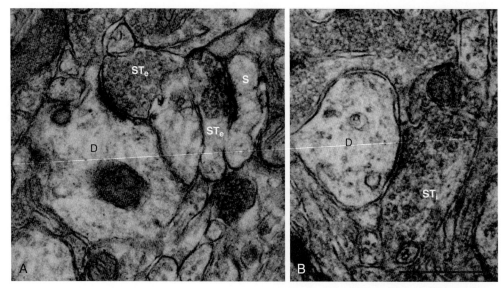

Figure 7-3 Chemical synapses are the mainstay of interneuronal communication. Morphology of excitatory **(A)** and inhibitory **(B)** synapses as seen with the electron microscope. Note that in **A** one excitatory terminal (ST_e) forms a synapse with a dendrite *(D)* and a dendritic spine *(S)*. Note the cloudlike electron-dense material spanning the synaptic cleft. The inhibitory terminal (ST_i) forms a synapse with a dendrite *(D)*. Scale bar = 500 nm. *(Courtesy of S. L. Feig, PhD, University of Wisconsin, Madison, Wisc.)*

Typically, these proteins are composed of a number of subunits, each containing multiple transmembrane domains (Figure 7-4). The three-dimensional folding of the subunits and their arrangement with respect to each other create a hydrophilic pore across the membrane lined by specialized sections of the transmembrane domains, which determine the ion-selectivity of the channel. When open, channels are typically permeable either for cations or anions, but within each group the degree of permeability can vary widely depending on the selectivity of the specific channel.

Changes in the structural conformation of the subunits lead to opening and closing of the channel pore. Opening and closing of a channel are controlled by the electrical potential gradient across the membrane (voltage-gated channels), by the action of a chemical substance on receptors linked to the channel (ligand-gated receptor-channel complexes) (Figure 7-4), by the intrinsic gating properties of the channel itself (e.g., many voltage-gated Ca^{2+} exists within the presynaptic terminal sharing voltage-sensitivity and ion selectivity but nevertheless having different functional properties), and by its sensitivity to modulation. Channel modulators include intracellular and extracellular factors, such as neuromodulators, phosphorylation state, pH, temperature, membrane tension, metabolic products, and preceding activity of the neuron. Table 7-2 is a partial list of ion channels that are abundant in the CNS and are implicated in anesthetic action.

Ion pumps are proteins that deliver ions across the cell membrane against their electrochemical gradient. They are distinguished from transporters by the coupling of transport to an external energy source, in that this process is energy consuming. The energy cost of maintaining the gradient across the membrane is tremendous and may be more than 50% of the total energy expenditure in a spiking neuron. The most common ion pump—the Na,K-ATPase—uses the energy released by hydrolysis of one ATP molecule to pump three Na^+ out in exchange for admitting two K^+ into the cell.

This process, resulting in the net transfer of one positive charge out of the cell for each ATP molecule, generates a hyperpolarizing current.

Transporters carry molecules across the membrane along or against their electrochemical gradient following enzyme kinetics. Transportation against the gradient is achieved by transporting two substrates simultaneously, utilizing the energy from the downhill transport of one substrate to drive the uphill transport of another substrate. This type of transporter is termed *cotransporter* or *symporter;* for example, the potassium-chloride cotransporter (KCC2). KCC2 delivers one K^+ together with one Cl^- across the membrane along their combined electrochemical gradient. Because the internal K^+ concentration is kept high by the activity of the Na,K-ATPase, the transporter carries K^+ and Cl^- out of the cell. In this example, the transporter allows the cell to use energy stored in the K^+ gradient to create a Cl^- gradient across the membrane.

Communication

The nervous system is a network of units communicating on each organizational level, from the individual neuron to the whole brain. An important part of integration and communication is carried by changes in electrical potentials.

CHANGES IN MEMBRANE POTENTIAL

Depolarization is a positive change from the resting potential achieved by increased permeability to an ion with a Nernst potential above the RBP. Ion flux drives the membrane potential closer to the Nernst potential of this ion. The distribution of important ions is shown in Table 7-1. Na^+ and Ca^{2+} are typical "depolarizers" of the membrane potential.

Hyperpolarization and *shunting* are a negative change of the membrane potential from the RMP and an increase of the cell membrane permeability or conductance without a change in the membrane potential, respectively. Increasing

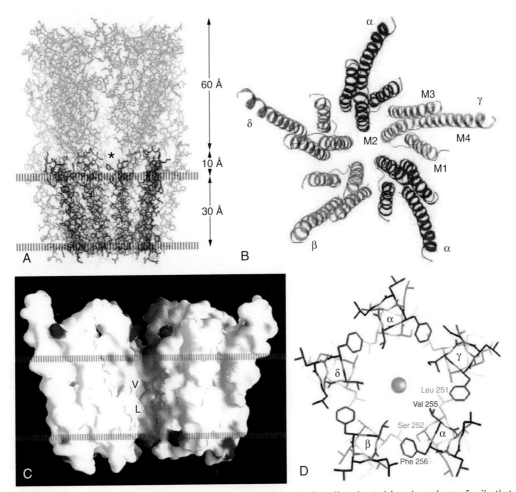

Figure 7-4 The structure of a ligand-gated ion channel. Like other members of the Cys-loop ligand-gated ion channel superfamily that also includes the GABA$_A$, 5-HT$_3$ and glycine receptors, the nicotinic acetylcholine receptor-channel complex consists of five subunits (i.e., it is a pentamer), with each subunit containing multiple transmembrane domains and their intracellular and extracellular connecting loops. **A,** View along the receptor axis showing the pore structure (blue, pore-facing; red, lipid-facing helices) in relation to the membrane surfaces *(broken lines)* and the β-sheet structure *(green)* comprising the ligand-binding domain; the *asterisk* denotes open space at a subunit interface. **B,** View of the pore from the synaptic cleft, with the five subunits shown in different colors (note two α-subunits in red). **C,** Molecular surface of the pore domain with front subunit removed. Red and blue colors indicate areas of high negative and high positive charge, respectively; the hydrophobic gate-containing area is highlighted in yellow; the letters *V* and *L* identify individual amino acids (α-Val 255 and α-Leu 251). **D,** Symmetrical arrangement of side chains forming the gate. The blue spheres in **C** and **D** indicate the size of a sodium ion. *(Adapted from Miyazawa A, Fujiyoshi Y, Unwin N, et al. Nature. 2003;423:949-955.)*

the permeability of ions with a Nernst potential negative to or equal to the RMP will hyperpolarize or shunt the membrane, respectively. K$^+$ and Cl$^-$ conductances underlie both processes. Functionally, both processes are inhibitory because they both impede depolarization.

MEMBRANE TIME CONSTANT AND PASSIVE PROPAGATION

The cell membrane of the neuron can be modeled as an electrical circuit composed of a resistor and a capacitor (RC circuit). The lipid bilayer functions as a capacitor. Ion channels and transporters that allow ion flow across it function as resistors. When ions pass through a channel, the potential across the membrane does not change instantly. Rather, like in the RC circuit, the current needs time to charge the capacitance of the membrane. The inverse process occurs after a channel closes. Rise and fall of the membrane potential follow exponential patterns and lag behind the current. The time course of voltage change is described in the following equation:

$$\Delta V = IR_m\left(1 - e^{\frac{-t}{R_m C_m}}\right) \qquad [4]$$

where V is the potential, I is the current, R$_m$ is the resistance, and C$_m$ is the capacitance of a membrane segment. The term R$_m$C$_m$ is the time constant of the membrane, the dimensionless τ. The larger the value of τ, the faster the change in voltage. τ is an important factor in the ability of a cell to perform temporal summation of different inputs.[10]

Current spreads spatially as charged molecules diffuse along the membrane. This spread allows neurons to perform summation of inputs from neighboring synapses—one type of intraneuronal integration. The electrical potential caused by the current decays along a segment of membrane with a first order exponential (determined by the length constant λ). λ depends on the membrane properties (e.g., conductance) and determines the spread of the potential change.[11]

Table 7-2. Common Ion Channels of the Brain

RECEPTOR (R)/CHANNEL	ION PERMEABILITY AND NORMAL FLOW DIRECTION	TRANSMITTER/GATING MECHANISM	PRINCIPAL ROLES
GABA$_A$R	Cl$^-$ ↓ HCO$^-$ ↑	GABA	Major inhibitory transmitter
Nicotinic Acetylcholine R	Na$^+$,K$^+$ ↓	Acetylcholine	Synaptic transmission in the brain and at the neuromuscular junction
Glutamate R			Major excitatory transmitter
AMPA type GluR	Na$^+$,K$^+$ ↓	Glutamate, provides depolarization for NMDAR	Depolarization
NMDA type GluR	Na$^+$,Ca^{2+} ↓	Glutamate/glycine is coagonist depolarization (to release the Mg^{2+} block) required	Depolarization, synaptic plasticity, excitotoxicity if excessive
Voltage gated Na	Na$^+$ ↓	Membrane depolarization	Action potential initiation/propagation
Voltage gated K$^+$	K$^+$ ↑	Membrane depolarization	Action potential termination and repolarization of the membrane
Voltage gated Ca^{2+}, many subtypes	Ca^{2+} ↓	Membrane depolarization	Burst firing (T-type); dendritic depolarization (H-type) neurotransmitter release (P, N, R types)
Ca^{2+}-activated K$^+$ channels	K$^+$ ↑	Intracellular Ca^{2+} concentration increase	Synaptic plasticity, after hyperpolarization and smooth muscle tone
Hyperpolarization-activated cyclic nucleotide-gated channels (HCN)	K$^+$ ↑ (I$_{funny}$)	Membrane hyperpolarization Intracellular cAMP	Pacemaker/rhythmic oscillation activity Synaptic plasticity
Cyclic nucleotide gated ion channels	Na$^+$,K$^+$,Ca^{2+},Mg^{2+}	Intracellular cGMP and cAMP	Light detection in photoreceptors
Two-pore-domain K$^+$ channel	K$^+$ ↑	Oxygen tension, pH, mechanical stretch, etc.	Resting membrane potential, "leak channels"

Common ion channels of neuronal cell membranes. Transmitter-activated receptor channel complexes are organized by the principal transmitter, voltage-activated channels by principal ion. Down/up pointing arrows indicate inward/outward flow of ions.
AMPA, 2-amino-3-(5-methyl-3-oxo-1,2-oxazol-4-yl) propanoic acid; cAMP, cyclic adenosine monophosphate; cGMP, cyclic guanosine monophosphate; GABA, gamma[use greek symbol]-aminobutyric acid; NMDA, N-methyl-D-aspartate; NMDAR, NMDA receptor.

ACTION POTENTIAL

Frequently referred to as a "spike," describing its rapid time course, the action potential (AP) is driven by the sudden opening of voltage-gated Na$^+$ channels, activated by a local depolarization of the cell membrane beyond the activation "threshold" (typically around −50 mV) when a positive feedback loop results in an extremely fast regenerative process. Within 1 ms, the cell membrane potential is driven beyond 0 mV and toward the Nernst equilibrium for Na$^+$. The AP is rapidly terminated by inactivation of Na$^+$ channels and opening of K$^+$ channels limiting the duration of an AP to a few milliseconds (Figure 7-5).[12]

The threshold of AP generation is the basis of "neuronal calculation." A neuron integrates the barrage of many inputs it constantly receives: positive (depolarizing) and negative (hyperpolarizing) and shunting (increase in conductance without voltage change). Whenever the sum of these signals pushes the membrane potential beyond the threshold, the neuron "fires" an AP. After the AP, the Na$^+$ channels are inactivated and, for a few milliseconds, the cell cannot fire again. This is the refractory period. The threshold is dynamic: the amount of available voltage-gated Na$^+$ channels and the threshold for AP generation change depending on the activity of the cell. For example, hyperpolarization increases the number of available Na$^+$ channels, thereby facilitating AP generation once hyperpolarization terminates. Subthreshold depolarization, by contrast, inactivates Na$^+$ channels and a stronger depolarizing current is necessary to force the cell to fire.

An AP is initiated in a specialized area of the membrane, extending from the axon hillock to the end of the unmyelinated axon initial segment (AIS) (Figure 7-6). Synaptic inputs have been demonstrated at the distal end of the AIS and together with a specialized and diverse set of ion channels support the notion that the AIS is capable of signal integration in addition to being a low-threshold area for AP triggering.[13] From there it invades the axon and rapidly travels along the axon either by a rolling depolarization or by saltatory conduction. In principle, a segment of axon can conduct APs in either direction. The directionality of spread is given by the gating state of Na$^+$ channels on both sides of the depolarized segment. Na$^+$ channels that were just open are now inactivated refractory and cannot open again. Hence the AP will spread into the direction of nonrefractory channels but with exogenous stimulation a "retrograde" spread of an AP can be initiated (see Chapter 17).

SYNAPSE

The synapse is an information relay between two neurons usually located between the axon terminal of one (the presynaptic element) and the dendrite of another (the postsynaptic element) cell. Synapses can be either electrical or chemical and are also found between axon and soma, between two axons, and between two dendrites.

The *electrical synapse* (also called *Gap-junction*) is a channel formed of proteins. Electrical synapses form a minority of all synapses and are enriched in specific areas, such as the thalamus. This channel bridges the membranes of two neurons, creating a syncytium-like continuity of their cytoplasm and membrane. Gap junctions pass current directly. They can transmit action potentials, as well as subthreshold membrane

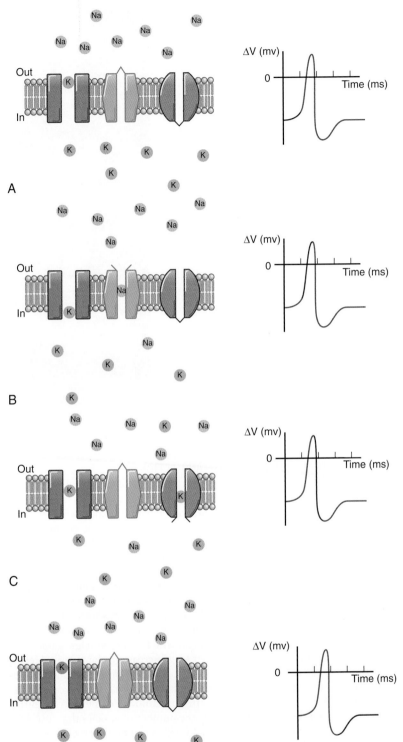

A

B

C

D

Figure 7-5 The action potential (AP, schematic A-D) originates in the axon initial segment (AIS, E). **A,** Membrane at rest; voltage-activated Na⁺ (triangular) and K⁺ (circular) channels are closed. K⁺ leak current *(square)* dominates the membrane potential. **B,** When the membrane potential crosses the threshold for activation, Na⁺ channels open. Because during this phase, Na⁺ permeability dominates, the membrane rapidly depolarizes. **C,** Na⁺ channels slowly become inactivated, and voltage-activated K⁺ channels open. The membrane potential rapidly hyperpolarizes to below baseline. **D,** Na⁺ and K⁺ channels are inactivated. The cell is refractory and an AP cannot be initiated.

potential fluctuations practically without any delay. Gap junctions also undergo plasticity.[14]

The chemical synapse consists of specialized presynaptic and a postsynaptic elements separated by the synaptic cleft. Communication between the two elements is via neurotransmitter. The presynaptic axon terminal stores vesicles containing neurotransmitter. An AP arriving via the axon initiates a cascade of events that leads to the release of neurotransmitter via fusion of vesicles with the plasma membrane of the terminal. This complicated process critically depends on the influx of extracellular Ca^{2+}, the trigger for exocytosis. The neurotransmitter then diffuses through the synaptic cleft, binds to transmitter-specific receptors on the postsynaptic membrane, and sets off a signaling cascade. Release, diffusion, and

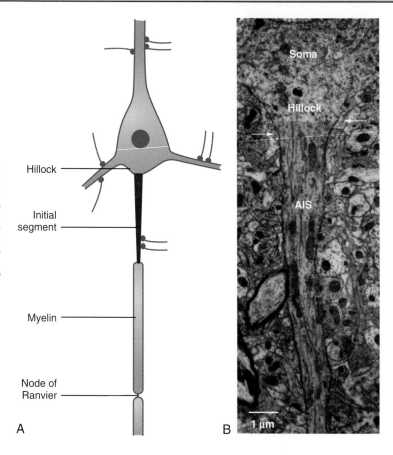

Figure 7-6 A, Schematic of a pyramidal neuron axon showing the location of the axon hillock, the axon initial segment (AIS; red), and the axon proper. Synaptic input onto the AIS is shown in blue. **B,** Electron micrograph of the AIS (in red) of a cortical pyramidal neuron, including the soma and the axon hillock. Blue areas indicate presynaptic terminals onto the AIS. *Arrows* (white) point to the beginning of the AIS. *(Adapted from Peters A, Proskauer CC, Kaiserman-Abramof IR. The small pyramidal neuron of the rat cerebral cortex. The axon hillock and initial segment. J Cell Biol. 1968;39:604-619; Kole MH, Stuart GJ. Signal processing in the axon initial segment. Neuron. 2012;73:235-247.)*

activation of receptors impose a delay typically on the order of 1 ms on signal transfer. If the transmitter binds to receptor-ion channel complexes, it leads to the opening of ion channels (fast synaptic transmission). If it binds to G protein-coupled receptors, a second messenger cascade in the postsynaptic cell is activated (slow synaptic transmission). Transmitter-specific mechanisms ensure that the chemical signal is limited to a brief pulse that barely outlasts the incoming electric signal but exceptions are well known (see later). Chemical synapses are classified according to the transmitter released. Neurotransmitters are typically small organic molecules, some derived from amino acids (γ-aminobutyric acid, L-glutamate, dopamine). Each transmitter substance can activate multiple subtypes of receptors of different classes, providing a tremendous flexibility of signal transmission; for example, GABA, glutamate, and acetylcholine all activate different subtypes of both ionotropic and metabotropic receptor classes. Anatomically defined synapses are typically excitatory or inhibitory in nature but neurotransmitters act also on receptors outside of classic synapses where their action is more modulatory in nature. Some synapses simultaneously release more than one transmitter for example, a fast-acting excitatory or inhibitory transmitter in combination with a slower acting or modulatory one. GABA and substance P are released by the same striatal spiny projection neurons. In addition to falsifying Dale's rule with respect to transmitter-exclusivity, recent research has also uncovered that the long-held belief that the identity of the transmitters expressed by neurons is stable and unchanging is incorrect. Electrical activity can respecify the neurotransmitter phenotype of an individual neuron both during development and in the mature nervous system.[15]

TRANSMITTER RELEASE AND ACTION

Depolarization of the axon terminal of neuron 1 by an AP releases neurotransmitter from the terminal that affects neuron 2. In this case, neuron 1 is presynaptic while neuron 2 is postsynaptic. If neuron 2 is reciprocally connected to neuron 1 and fired first, the order would be reversed. Release of neurotransmitter can be either conventional (quantal) or unconventional.

Conventional (quantal) release indicates that transmitter release occurs in discrete quantities or quanta (singular: quantum) dictated by the storage of transmitter in discrete membrane vesicles of defined capacity within the terminal. An AP depolarizes the terminal, which opens voltage-gated Ca^{2+} channels. The subsequent Ca^{2+} increase in the terminal leads, via a complex cascade, to fusion of transmitter-loaded vesicles with the presynaptic membrane and release of neurotransmitter into the synaptic cleft. The amount of neurotransmitter released is determined by the number of vesicles that fuse with the membrane. Individual vesicles can be observed when APs are blocked, for example, with the selective Na^+ channel blocker tetrodotoxin, spontaneous fusions of individual vesicles with the membrane cause "quantal" postsynaptic events.[16] The released transmitter diffuses across the cleft and binds to receptors on the postsynaptic membrane. The result of receptor activation will depend on the nature of the receptor: an ionotropic receptor will cause excitatory or inhibitory postsynaptic potentials (dependent on the ion it allows to pass), that is, a phasic response. Metabotropic receptors excite or inhibit via G proteins. Some ionotropic channels (e.g., the NMDA type of glutamate receptor) can pass Ca^{2+} in addition to Na^+. Ca^{2+} is a universal second messenger triggering

Table 7-3. Common Neurotransmitter Receptors

NEUROTRANSMITTER	RECEPTOR	TYPE	EFFECT	STRUCTURE
Glutamate	NMDA	Ionotropic	Na^+, K^+, Ca^{2+} permeability	4 subunits: 2GluN1,2GluN2
	AMPA	Ionotropic	Na^+, K^+ permeability	4 subunits: out of GluA1-4, usually
	KA	Ionotropic/metabotropic	Na^+, K^+, Ca^{2+} permeability	2GluA2 and 2 of either GluA1,3
	$mGluR_{1-8}$	Metabotropic	Different types exert different second messenger effects	or 4
Acetylcholine	Nicotinic	Ionotropic	Na^+, K^+, Ca^{2+} permeability	5 subunits: $3\alpha,2\beta$ (neuron) $2\alpha,\beta,\varepsilon,\delta$ (NMJ)
	Muscarinic	Metabotropic	↑ IP_3/DAG	
GABA	$GABA_A$	Ionotropic	Cl^- permeability	5 subunits: 3α:2β:γ
	$GABA_B$	Metabotropic	↓ cAMP	
Glycine	Glycine	Ionotropic	Cl^- permeability	5 subunits: $3\alpha,2\beta$ or $4\alpha,1\beta$
Serotonin (5-hydroxytryptamine)	$5\text{-}HT_1$	Metabotropic	↓ cAMP	
	$5\text{-}HT_2$	Metabotropic	↑ IP_3/DAG	
	$5\text{-}HT_3$	Ionotropic	Na^+, K^+, Ca^{2+} permeability	5 subunits
Norepinephrine	$\alpha_{1,2}$	Metabotropic	↑ IP_3/DAG	
	$\beta_{1,2}$	Metabotropic	↑ cAMP	
Dopamine	$D_{1,5}$	Metabotropic	↑ cAMP	
	$D_{2,3,4}$	Metabotropic	↓ cAMP	
Substance P	NK_1	Metabotropic	↑ IP_3/DAG	
Opioids	μ,δ,κ	Metabotropic	↓ cAMP	

complex physiologic or pathologic cascades ranging, in the case of NMDA receptors, from synaptic plasticity to necrosis (Table 7-3).

Unconventional release and action is frequently associated with slower and longer lasting but spatially localized modulatory effects: a slow background "offset" signal as opposed to the brief quantal information packet. The terms *paracrine* and *neurocrine release of transmitter* fall into this category. The release is typically still AP-dependent and hence it allows rapid communication over long distances to a larger population of cells but it is more selective than neuroendocrine communication via the bloodstream. For obvious reasons, small, gaseous molecules including carbon monoxide and nitric oxide as well as others that are difficult to store such as cannabinoids (and probably other, yet undiscovered, substances) are released in a nonquantal fashion.[17] Some of these mediators make feedback communication from the post- to the presynaptic side of a chemical synapse possible (e.g., endocannabinoids modulate transmitter release from hippocampal GABAergic synapses).[18] Nonquantal release of conventional neurotransmitter such as acetylcholine also occurs under certain circumstances, as during embryonic development.[19]

Under certain conditions, transmitter that diffuses out of the synaptic cleft activates other receptor populations located extrasynaptically. This is best described for GABA. Extrasynaptic $GABA_A$ receptors have distinct gating properties, they are activated by low concentrations of ambient GABA, and they inactivate only very slowly.[20] This mode of transmitter action is called *tonic* as opposed to the classic phasic action outlined earlier. Intermediate forms of transmitter action, such as on receptors located perisynaptically, also exist and give rise to slow phasic synaptic potentials.[21] Extrasynaptic NMDA receptors have also been described.

Termination of transmitter action can be effected in a number of ways: diffusion away from the synapse, active enzymatic degradation and reuptake either into the terminal or into glial cells. The latter processes allow local recycling of the transmitter.

PLASTICITY

Structural and functional refinements of neural circuits, including those underlying learning and memory, are essential processes throughout the entire life of an organism. With few known exceptions, no new neurons are generated after the neonatal period. Therefore, modifications of connections between existing neurons underlie all forms of behavioral modification based on experience. Information is stored by modifying the synaptic strength of connections in a process called *synaptic plasticity*. Synaptic plasticity occurs on a number of time scales and is present from the ganglion of an invertebrate to the neocortex of a mammal. The forms of plasticity usually associated with long-term storage in the mammalian brain are termed long-term potentiation (LTP) (Figure 7-7) and long-term depression (LTD). LTP and LTD have been best described at glutamatergic synapses but occur also at GABAergic synapses. In the most generic terms, rapid repeated depolarization of a presynaptic terminal causes, via release of glutamate, depolarization of the postsynaptic neuron, and Ca^{2+} entry through NMDA receptors with or without spiking of the postsynaptic neuron.[22] Under appropriate conditions, the strength of the synapse connecting these cells will be strengthened or potentiated by an increase in the number of postsynaptic AMPA receptors, which is a postsynaptic expression of LTP (*neurons that fire together wire together*). Some synapses express LTP via an increase in presynaptic transmitter release and a mixed form might also exist.

The fundamental principle of synaptic plasticity was postulated by Hebb in 1949.[23] Repeated activation of the same synapse but with long intervals between stimuli can cause depotentiation or LTD in a previously potentiated or naïve synapse, respectively. The temporal requirements of plasticity are captured in the concept of spike-timing dependent plasticity (STDP): when a synaptic input is followed within a narrow temporal window by the firing of an AP in the postsynaptic cell, LTP can result. Firing outside this window has either no effect or results in LTD. The temporal window varies

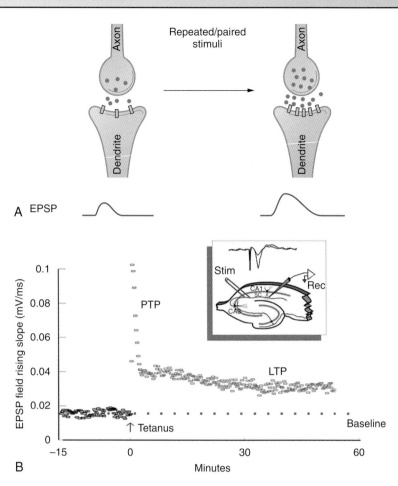

Figure 7-7 Synaptic plasticity illustrated by long-term potentiation *(LTP)*. **A,** LTP can be caused by a variety of mechanisms that can be primarily presynaptic or postsynaptic. The preponderance of mechanisms varies between circuits and the exact mechanisms are still debated. The end result is a use-dependent increase in the postsynaptic response illustrated here as occurring via an increase in both the number of postsynaptic receptors and the amount of transmitter release. Typically, an individual synapse will show only one of these changes. **B,** Time course of experimental LTP induction in the CA1 area of the hippocampus where plasticity has been studied since the 1970s. The inset shows the iconic cross-section of the hippocampus as seen in a transverse slice. Areas of projection neurons are shown in green and the principal excitatory pathways in red. Tetanic stimulation of the Schaffer collaterals (excitatory axon collaterals connecting the hippocampal areas CA3 and CA1) with one electrode (Stim) leads to an increase in field EPSPs recorded by a second electrode (Rec) placed in the termination zone of the Schaffer collaterals in the dendritic arbor of CA1. Stimulation using a different pattern results in long-term depression (LTD) of the same pathway. *(From http:// en.wikipedia.org/wiki/File:LTP_exemplar.jpg.)*

depending on the nature of the connection and the cell types involved.[24,25] Obviously, synchronization between cell populations is necessary for appropriate timing of synaptic inputs and APs for STDP to occur and might be one of the functions of high-frequency brain oscillations.[26] Depotentiation/LTD-like processes are thought to occur during slow wave sleep in order to "reset" the brain for a new day of learning.[27]

TRANSMITTERS AND RECEPTORS

Most major neurotransmitters have both ionotropic and metabotropic receptors, frequently simultaneously activated by transmitter released from the same presynaptic terminal. Ionotropic receptors are ligand-gated ion channels that pass either anions or cations, resulting in either inhibitory or excitatory transmitter binding. Metabotropic receptors add a major flexibility component; the same transmitter can activate inhibitory and excitatory metabotropic receptors, depending on the type of G proteins coupled to it.

L-Glutamate, the major excitatory transmitter in the brain and the spinal cord, follows this pattern. The three major types of ionotropic glutamate receptors (KA, AMPA, and NMDA) are named after their selective agonists (kainic acid, α-amino acid-3-hydroxy-5-methyl-4-isoxazole, and *N*-methyl-D-aspartate). The non-NMDA group (KA and AMPA) is permeable to monovalent cations and underlies fast excitatory postsynaptic potentials (EPSPs).[28]

NMDA receptors are blocked by extracellular Mg^{2+} at the concentration present in the extracellular fluid (see Table 7-1).

Therefore the NMDA channel does not contribute substantially to a regular EPSP. However, as the Mg^{2+}-block is relieved by depolarization, repetitive or particularly strong stimuli can depolarize the postsynaptic membrane sufficiently to open NMDA receptor-associated channels, such as when the postsynaptic cell fires an AP. Open NMDA channels allow Ca^{2+} into the cell. NMDA receptors act therefore as "voltage-sensors" and allow a "conditional" Ca^{2+} signal to occur. For this reason, NMDA receptors play a pivotal role in processes that lead to synaptic plasticity. The Ca^{2+} influx via NMDA receptors is also responsible for glutamate toxicity (excitotoxicity) that occurs when high levels of glutamate are sustained for a long time, such as during status epilepticus. NMDA receptors have slower kinetics than their non-NMDA counterparts and, under appropriate conditions such as when the cell is depolarized or when Mg^{2+} is omitted from the extracellular fluid, slow NMDA EPSPs can be observed. The NMDA receptor is a target of the hallucinogen phencyclidine (PCP) and of the anesthetic drug ketamine.[29]

Metabotropic G protein-coupled glutamate receptors can be excitatory or inhibitory. Glutamate binding to the receptor stimulates the activity of phospholipase C, leading to the formation of inositol 1,4,5-triphosphate (IP_3) and diacylglycerol (DAG), which function as intracellular second messengers. Similar to NMDA receptors, this pathway leads to increase in intracellular Ca^{2+}, but in this case by release of Ca^{2+} from intracellular stores. This release causes a slow depolarization by reducing membrane permeability to K^+. On the other hand, glutamate binding to these receptors on the presynaptic terminal (autoactivation) causes presynaptic inhibition.[29]

GABA is the major inhibitory neurotransmitter in the brain and follows the ionotropic and metabotropic pattern with GABA$_A$ and GABA$_B$ receptor types, respectively. GABA$_A$ receptors are receptor/channel complexes passing anions: mostly Cl$^-$, but also HCO$_3^-$. The receptor has two binding sites for GABA, and the channel opens when both sites are occupied. This channel is the major target for a variety of drugs, including many anesthetics.[30] Interneurons are the main source of GABAergic synaptic transmission. They display a remarkable morphologic and neurochemical diversity that reflects a "computational" role of GABAergic transmission.[31,32] GABA$_B$ receptors are G protein-coupled receptors, the activation of which leads to opening of K$^+$ channels via a second messenger cascade.[33]

Glycine is also a major inhibitory neurotransmitter, primarily in the spinal cord. It is released by local inhibitory interneurons and activates ligand-gated Cl$^-$ channels. Metabotropic glycine receptors have not been described. The structure of the glycine receptor is very similar to that of GABA$_A$ and nicotinic acetylcholine receptors (they are all members of the cys-loop family of pentameric ligand-gated ion channels). However, it requires three glycine molecules to open the channel.[34] Glycine also acts as coagonist of glutamate at NMDA receptors.

Acetylcholine also follows the ionotropic-metabotropic scheme with nicotinic and muscarinic receptors, respectively. Nicotinic receptors are ionotropic and are present at the CNS in addition to their well-known role at the neuromuscular junction and in the autonomic nervous system. Structurally, they are related to GABA$_A$ and glycine receptors.[34] There are several types of muscarinic G protein-coupled receptors. Acetylcholine is released by neurons of brainstem nuclei that send projections to wide areas of the cortex and striatum. It is involved in regulation of wakefulness, attention, learning, and motivation.[35,36]

Neuronology

The brain displays a large variety of neurons of many different shapes and functions.

Principal neurons, also referred to as projection neurons, send their projections to distant locations, either at a different brain structure or, for some cortical neurons, to a different area of cortex. The white matter is composed of their axons crossing from their origin to their targets. Projection neurons can be glutamatergic (e.g., layer five pyramidal neurons, hippocampal pyramidal cells) or GABAergic (e.g., cerebellar Purkinje cells, striatal medium spiny neurons). Pyramidal neurons are the major excitatory neurons in the cortex and hippocampus. They are named so due to the triangular shape of their soma. They have an axon leaving the base of the pyramid, a long dendrite arising from the apex to higher layers of the cortex, and a number of basal dendrites arising from the base and branching in the same layer. The populations of pyramidal and principal neurons overlap to a large degree. Interneurons typically synapse within local circuits. Their axons do not cross via the white matter. Interneurons in the cortex are mostly inhibitory. However, excitatory and modulatory interneurons exist in other brain areas. In some areas of the brain

such as the hippocampus, interneurons display a dazzling variety that is reflected in the picturesque nomenclature (e.g., chandelier cells, ivy cells, neurogliaform cells). Recent work has begun to unravel the functional implications of their highly diverse anatomy (especially the highly selective projections of their axons).

THE BRAIN: STRUCTURE DETERMINES FUNCTION

For obvious reasons, the brain is frequently compared to a computer.[37] While the similarities are obvious on a superficial level, the fundamental differences illuminate why brains, unlike computers, are complex (in addition to being complicated) systems.

- Diversity: individual transistors are homogenous while neurons are diverse.
- Adaptation: transistors lack adaptability while neurons and their connections adapt constantly and on different time scales.
- Connectivity: the interconnectivity of transistors is very low, typically in the single digits per gate, while interneuronal convergence and divergence rates range in the (tens of) thousands.
- Integration: strict separation between memory and computation as well as hardware and software are standard features of computer architecture but are interwoven on multiple levels in the brain.
- Last but not least, in contrast to computers, brains wire themselves up during development and continue to "rewire" during their functional life.

Structure

Brains evolved to allow movement. Once in place, sensors to find food and avoid harm as well as adjusting activity to the dark/light cycle became indispensable for evolutionary success. On top of the basic circuitry necessary to allow the aforementioned functions, additional parallel circuits (neuronal loops) were superimposed during evolution and linked "vertically," generating a hierarchical organization among parallel loops. Older loops are located at the bottom while the more recently added rest on top. The more layers (i.e., the more complex the animal), the more complex and controlled the response to an identical stimulus becomes.

Connectivity is the essential challenge as the number of potential connections between the 10^{11} neurons of the human brain is both unimaginable and inefficient. The solution has to accommodate two competing principles: the degree of local clustering (the density of connections) and the degree of separation (synaptic path length) between distant parts of the brain. High clustering is desirable for coordinated computation—as between neurons in a single visual column. Low synaptic path length is also essential for fast integration of information between physically remote areas, a particular feature of the cortex. Both are expensive with respect to axonal length. The proposed solution is known as "small world networks" (originally proposed outside the field of neuroscience) in which, by replacing a small fraction of local connections with random long-distance connections, the average path length can be dramatically shortened with minimal reduction of clustering.[38] Furthermore, the larger the network, the greater the impact of each random link: a smaller fraction of random connections is required in the human brain than in the mouse brain to achieve the same short synaptic path length despite the difference in size. Nevertheless, cortical white matter volume expands more than gray matter volume with increasing brain size (Figure 7-8).[39]

The *cortex* is a scalable structure that has expanded greatly during mammalian evolution: the neocortical gray matter and the adjacent white matter occupy 10% to 20% of total brain volume in insectivores but 80% in humans. It has been suggested that the smallest functional division of the monkey cerebral cortex (analogous to a single nephron) that can perform the typical "cortical" computational tasks (e.g., a single location in visual space) is about 1 mm^2.[40] Even though the boundaries of a module are difficult to determine, it can be estimated that the total number of cortical modules increases about 10,000-fold from the smallest mammal to the human brain. The human brain, however, is of course not like thousands of mouse brains lumped together.

The cortex can be subdivided into the isocortex, which has a six-layer structure, and the allocortex (heterotypical cortex), which has a variable number of layers. The modular plan of the cortex is identical in all mammals: the isocortex consists of five layers of neurons and a superficial layer of mostly dendrites and axons. Its thickness is only about 1 to 3 mm. The cortex is built-up by multiplication of fundamentally identical "modules" that are variably referred to as *columns*, *barrels*, or *stripes*, and each contains roughly 50,000 to 100,000 neurons. The allocation of space to different functions is a compromise of evolutionary needs, metabolic and wiring costs, and spatial constraints. This is optimized for making predictions and inferences most valuable in the physical niche inhabited by the owner of the brain: echolocation for bats, accurate topography using snout whiskers for many rodents, or pictorial representation of the environment in the primarily visual primates.[31] In the most complex brains, a large proportion of the cortical mantle specializes in processing and generating activity only indirectly related to immediate sensory input or direct motor output; these areas are referred to as *associational areas* and are also hierarchically organized. Importantly, connections between functional brain areas are always bidirectional. With ascending hierarchy, an area becomes ever less directly linked to it sensory modality and ever more interconnected with associational areas of other modalities, as proposed in the convergence-divergence-zone framework (Figure 7-9).[41]

The hippocampal formation includes the hippocampus proper, dentate gyrus, subiculum, and entorhinal cortex, and is the main constituent of the allocortex. In addition to being part of the limbic circuit, it is the brain's ultimate memory machine specialized for, on the one hand, forming quickly updatable cognitive maps of the environment and, on the other hand, forming the flexible expression of declarative, episodic memories.[42] As a corollary, it is also essential for projecting one's experience forward in time and space, thereby "predicting the future." While it is not the long-term storage site for memories, the hippocampal formation remains the "librarian of the brain," facilitating the retrieval of stored memory traces.

The need to organize individual experiences within temporal space is shared by both spatial and episodic memories. Coincidentally, the hippocampal formation expresses one of the most prominent synchronized rhythmic oscillations of the mammalian CNS—the theta (θ)-rhythm that serves as a timing mechanism (see later). The distinct anatomy of the allocortex reflects these specialized computational needs. Contrary to the small-world organization of the neocortex, the whole hippocampus forms a single huge neuronal space, analogous to one oversized cortical module creating a giant random connection space that is necessary for combining arbitrary information (analogous to RAM in computers). The circuitry is dominated by the famous trisynaptic excitatory loop from entorhinal cortex to dentate gyrus granule cells to pyramidal cells of the hippocampal CA3 and on to CA1 pyramidal cells, which then project back to the entorhinal cortex. The distribution of contacts in the dentate gyrus/CA3/CA1 network is reminiscent of a random graph with very low clustering—only about 2% to 5% connection probability—but with equal likelihood of contacting near and remote neurons (unlike the small-world arrangement of the neocortex). The axon of a CA3 neuron in the rat is between 150 and 400 mm long establishing 25,000 to 50,000 synapses within the ipsilateral and about half as many within the contralateral hippocampus. This amounts to a total of 40,000 meters of axon collaterals and 5 to 10 billion synaptic contacts in each hemisphere of the walnut-sized rat brain.[43] The mnemonic functions of the hippocampal formation can be conceptualized and allocated to the components of the trisynaptic circuit as follows: dentate gyrus—pattern separation or disambiguation, that is, differentiation between similar-appearing contexts; CA3—pattern completion, that is, reconstruction of a whole representation based on fragmentary information; CA1—mismatch detection, that is, detection of unpredicted novelty in the environment, a task essential for survival.

Sequential, recurrent, and reentrant excitatory connections have the propensity to create runaway excitation. However, through tight control by intricate multifaceted inhibitory networks, excitation can be harnessed into useful computation.[44,45] Because these powerful excitatory loops are notorious for becoming unbalanced, the medial temporal lobe has become the preferred substrate for in vitro studies of epilepsy, and the target of surgical attempts to cure this disease. In the healthy brain, a complex array of inhibitory loops consisting of diverse, specialized interneurons precisely controls the balance and timing of excitation and inhibition.

The *thalamus* is located in the very center between the two hemispheres, minimizing the length of reciprocal wiring and maximizing communication speed, which is optimal to function as a relay of information transmission to the cortex. It is a collection of nuclei that receives and processes all primary sensory input to the neocortex with the exception of olfaction; however, there are many more nuclei than sensory modalities and a large part of the thalamic circuitry is unrelated to early processing of sensory information. Thalamocortical neurons send their axons predominantly to layer 4 of the neocortex but also to layers 5 and 6. In return, thalamic nuclei are the only target outside the cortex of cortical layer 6 pyramidal cells. Thalamocortical neurons support a complement of membrane channels that can convert them into oscillators—nature's delta-frequency clocks. Unlike the cortex, most GABAergic inhibitory cells are localized in the reticular nucleus, forming a shell surrounding the thalamic space. Reticular thalamic neurons are connected not only by classic chemical synapses but also by dendrodendritic synapses and gap junctions.[46,47]

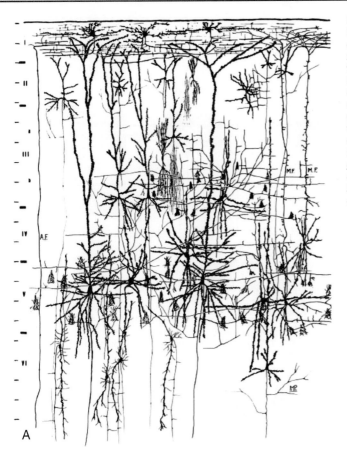

A

Figure 7-8 The neocortex: layers and the demands of connectivity. **A,** Camera lucida drawing based on a Golgi preparation of the motor cortex. Note layered organization with diverse types of neurons dominating in the different horizontal layers. This basic structure is typical for the neocortex. Neurons are tightly packed: a column with a cortical surface area of 1 mm² is populated by thousands of neurons. In order to function, cortical modules must be well connected to their neighbors and to more distal areas. **B,** With increasing cortical size, more space is required for efficient communication pathways. The cortical white and gray matter volumes are related by a power law that spans five to six orders of magnitude in extant mammals demonstrating the "real estate" cost of maintaining high interconnectivity characteristic of advanced brains. (**A,** *Adapted from Marín-Padilla M. Prenatal and early postnatal ontogenesis of the human motor cortex: a Golgi study. I. The sequential development of the cortical layers.* Brain Res. *1970;23:167-183;* **B,** *Adapted from Zhang K, Sejnowski TJ. A universal scaling law between gray matter and white matter of cerebral cortex.* Proc Natl Acad Sci U S A. *2000;97:5621-5626.*)

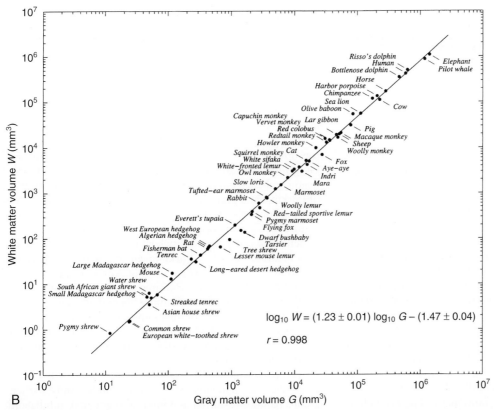

B

$$\log_{10} W = (1.23 \pm 0.01) \log_{10} G - (1.47 \pm 0.04)$$

$$r = 0.998$$

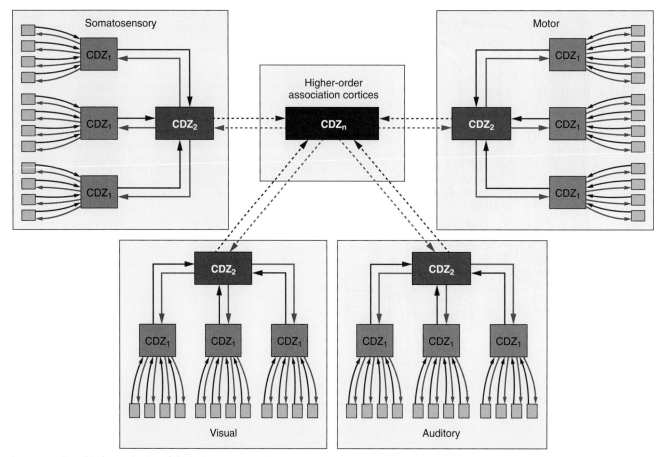

Figure 7-9 Hierarchical organization of the brain. Contrary to the Jamesian view, the model proposed by Damasio's laboratory in the "convergence-divergence zone" (CDZ) framework accentuates the bidirectionality and cross-modality of intracortical communication on each level of information processing. Neuronal ensembles in early sensorimotor cortices of different modalities (represented by the smallest rectangles) send converging forward projections *(red arrows)* to first-order CDZs (CDZ_1s), which, in turn, project back divergently *(blue arrows)* to the early cortical sites. Similar convergent-divergent connectivity patterns interlink CDZ_1s with CDZ_2s and CDZ_2s with CDZ_ns in higher-order association cortices (via several steps not represented here; *dashed arrows*). *(Reprinted with permission from Meyer K, Damasio A. Convergence and divergence in a neural architecture for recognition and memory. Trends Neurosci. 2009;32:376-382.)*

The dense reciprocal connectivity with the cortex paired with the special oscillatory propensity of thalamocortical neurons generates the diverse array of thalamocortical oscillations in different frequency bands. These oscillations show dramatic transitions between waking and sleep states and, in fact, might be the driving force behind them. A pivotal role of these thalamocortical oscillations in the mechanisms underlying consciousness and anesthetic action has been suggested.[48]

The *cerebellum* is, from the point of view of circuitry, the antipode of the neocortex in that its distinctive computational arrangement is in parallel loops favoring autonomic (as opposed to interactive) activity. The cerebellum contains as many cells as the rest of the human brain combined—the granule cells alone are more numerous ($\sim 10^{11}$) than all neurons of the neocortex. The cerebellum continuously monitors the activity of skeletal muscles and communicates with brain areas controlling these muscles. These computations, carried out in the anterior and posterior lobes, are largely subconscious and can therefore take place at speeds unattainable via conscious sensory systems. The phylogenetically older flocculonodular lobe attends to posture and eye movement. The cerebellum exists in all vertebrates. Deep cerebellar nuclei (interposed, fastigial, and dentate) act as relays for incoming and outgoing information controlling ipsilateral limb movements, trunk movements, and motor planning, respectively. There is no

equivalent to the corpus callosum and no intermediate or long-range associational paths within the cerebellum.

The granule cells are the only intrinsic excitatory neurons, the other four neuron types (Purkinje, basket, stellate, and Golgi) involved in computation are all inhibitory and target deep cerebellar nuclei, soma of Purkinje cells, and dendrites of Purkinje and granule cells, respectively. The elaborate dendritic arbor of the Purkinje cell is one of the most recognizable features of CNS histology. In diametric difference to the three-dimensional expansion and rich lateral connectivity of cortical pyramidal cell dendrites, Purkinje cells appear two-dimensional with minimal contacts to their neighbors providing for maximal computational autonomy. Purkinje cells receive a direct excitatory input by way of the climbing fibers that originate in the inferior olivary nucleus of the brainstem. This pathway can be seen as a shortcut. The overall organization of the cerebellum results in two parallel feed-forward inhibitory loops that control the output of deep cerebellar nuclei.[49]

The *basal ganglia* are a group of nuclei located below the cerebral cortex. It includes the striatum (caudate and putamen), globus pallidus (external and internal segments), subthalamic nucleus, and substantia nigra (pars compacta and pars reticulata). These nuclei create a feed-forward loop that receives information from most of the cerebral cortex, and after processing returns its output to the frontal and motor cortex via the thalamus. These nuclei are unique in that the major neurotransmitter they use is GABA, which is used in this system not only locally by interneurons but by the projection neurons as well, creating a variety of inhibitory and disinhibitory responses (inhibition of inhibition that leads to excitation). Other important neurotransmitters in this system are the neuromodulator dopamine that is released in the striatum by substantia nigra neurons and acetylcholine released from local interneurons.[50]

The basal ganglia play a major role in the motor system. This was deduced from the clinical manifestations of basal ganglia disorders: loss of dopaminergic cells in the substantia nigra leads to Parkinson's disease, a disease manifested by difficulty initiating movement, slowness of movement, and tremor during rest. Loss of striatal neurons in Huntington's chorea on the other hand leads to uncontrollable jerking movements. Basal ganglia also play a role in other tasks such as procedural learning, motivation, and response to reward and addiction.[50]

SPINAL CORD

Despite the anatomic separation, the spinal cord and the brain share most of the molecular targets of anesthetic drugs. The spinal cord does, however, have distinct arrangements on the circuit and network levels that can influence its responsiveness to anesthetic drugs. The spinal cord is organized segmentally (31 segments in the human); pairs of spinal nerves exit the cord at each segment. The nerve rootlets forming the sensory (dorsal) and motor (ventral) component combine into a mixed nerve. Each segment of the spinal cord is associated with a pair of dorsal root ganglia located just outside the cord and harboring the cell bodies of sensory neurons.[49]

Behavior is determined by the motor output of the CNS, and the absence of movement is an important component of anesthesia. Motor output, in turn, is the function of three inputs: sensory (reflexive), cognitive (voluntary), and intrinsic (behavioral) state. The relative importance of these inputs varies from species to species and between individuals. All three are affected by anesthesia.

The main determinant of movement in the context of anesthesia is the skeletal muscle system. It is organized hierarchically with the α-motoneurons (their cholinergic axons synapse directly on muscles) on the bottom. The next higher level consists of motor pattern generators (MPGs)—circuits of interneurons that innervate unique sets of motoneuron pools. MPGs are also organized hierarchically. For locomotion, simple MPGs coordinate antagonistic muscle movement across one joint, more complex MPGs coordinate activity of simpler MPGs for all joints of an extremity, and higher order MPGs coordinate activity between limbs. A still higher level consists of motor pattern initiators that "plan" movements. Each of the three types of inputs (sensory, voluntary, intrinsic) can go directly to each hierarchical level.[51]

Interneurons are the critical components of MPGs; in the spinal cord, interneurons have many convergent and divergent connections allowing them to integrate signals from different sources including both supraspinal and primary sensory. The most common fast inhibitory transmitters in the spinal cord are glycine and GABA, while glutamate dominates excitation (with one notable exception being the cholinergic α-motoneuron to Renshaw-cell synapse). Interneurons are also organized in pools that can be partially activated by an input. The activation by two inputs can produce a greater output than the sum of the individual inputs. This can lead to spatial and/or temporal facilitation depending on timing and origin of the stimuli. However, once the whole pool is activated, further increases in stimulation intensity have no effect. On the output side, interneurons connect to several different targets including other interneurons and motoneurons. Those interneurons synapsing on motoneurons are called *last-order interneurons*.[51]

In order for a movement to be considered valid for the purpose of minimum alveolar concentration (MAC) determination of anesthetic potency (see Chapter 3), it has to be "gross and purposeful."[52] This definition, while practical, disregards the "neural content" of a movement. Considering the complexity of circuitry underlying any but the most basic reflexes (which are excluded by the definition of MAC), it is almost surprising that systematically reproducible results are obtained at all. Nevertheless, more in-depth analysis reveals that accurate interpretation of the movement response under anesthesia is more complicated than the deceptively simple all-or-none definition suggests.[53] Moreover, whether explicitly stated or not, an assumption implicit in the definition is that anesthetic suppression of movement involves a "higher agency" and hence that the state of the brain should be predictive of the occurrence of movement in response to noxious stimulation under general anesthesia. However, in the decades after the introduction of the MAC concept into research and clinical practice, it became obvious that, no matter what analytical techniques were applied to extract information from the electroencephalogram (EEG), attempts to predict movement under anesthesia remained unsuccessful.[54] The reason for this conundrum was discovered in the 1990s—anesthetic-induced immobility (with the exception of some injectable agents) is mediated by action in the spinal cord.[55,56] It is noteworthy that experiments early in the 20th century had already indicated that the spinal cord contains circuits, now collectively referred to as *central pattern generators* (CPGs), capable of generating coordinated patterns of muscle activity including actual locomotion. Therefore, the spinal cord even on the segmental level provides a rich substrate for anesthetic action.

Interestingly, the brain, far from mediating anesthetic-induced immobility, appears to counteract it. After the description of this finding in goats, the site mediating this antagonism has been identified (at least in the rat): the mesencephalic locomotor region facilitates ventral spinal locomotor centers—a potential mediator of the "anti-immobilizing" effect of the brain on anesthetic action in the spinal cord.[57]

Function

The traditional Jamesian view of the brain as an organ whose function is primarily determined by responses to sensory input is undergoing a thorough revision. The brain is a foretelling not a reflecting device whose power to predict relies on a variety of synchronous rhythmic activities it constantly generates internally. Simultaneously, the brain is also a highly adapted observational device of the environment, an ability rooted in flexible neuronal firing patterns within rhythmic oscillatory activity of networks organized in hierarchical structures. CPGs of varying complexity have long been recognized as underlying rhythmic activities from peristalsis of the gut,

Table 7-4. Electroencephalogram Wave Categorization by Frequency

RHYTHM	FREQUENCY (HZ)	TYPICAL OCCURRENCE	COMMENTS
Slow	<1	Slow wave sleep	Cortical up-down states, generated by corticothalamocortical loops
δ-delta	0.5-4	Frontal, slow wave sleep, deep sedation	
θ-theta	4-8	Frontal and midline Hippocampal θ difficult to record in humans unless implanted electrodes used	Hippocampal θ linked to mnemonic function; Surface θ appears with altered states of vigilance, also meditation
α-alpha	8-13	Occipital with eyes closed and mental relaxation	Intermittent, waxing-waning pattern during SWS stage II as sleep spindles
β	13-30	Frontal, sensorimotor systems	Preparation and inhibitory control
γ	30-90	Diffuse, generated by local circuitry	Awake, hypervigilant desynchronized EEG; REM sleep; nested into hippocampal θ
Ultra-γ	>100		Hippocampal ripples during non-θ states

Commonly described rhythms observable in mammals. The frequency range varies somewhat between species. The δ-range has been recently further subdivided into various slow rhythms, particularly during sleep. Slower rhythms have higher power density than faster ones. Rhythms faster than slow γ-spectrum cannot be resolved with surface electrodes. Rhythms of different frequencies occur concurrently: θ-γ nesting, sleep spindles during δ. Same frequency does not indicate same mechanism and physiology: continuous α and intermittent sleep spindles share frequency but nothing else.
EEG, electroencephalography; REM, rapid eye movement; SWS, slow wave sleep.

writhing of lampreys to locomotion—from bipedal to centipede walking, respiration, and so on. An exciting breakthrough in the neurosciences of the past 2 decades was the recognition that (complex) rhythmic activity patterns (but without an easily definable generator) also underlie higher cognitive functions. A corollary of this view is that, far from being primarily driven by external inputs, the brain constantly generates a dynamic internal state that is only gradually perturbed by exogenous input. However, these external perturbations are necessary in order to generate behaviorally useful computations that sculpt the familiar "real world" experience.

DEFAULT MODE NETWORK
The advent of magnetic resonance imaging (MRI) in its manifold permutations has opened a new dimension of in vivo human brain structure and activity investigation. Functional MRI (fMRI) looks at changes in blood oxygen level dependent (BOLD) signal to detect changes in ongoing neural activity.[58] fMRI has revealed a task-independent constellation of brain areas that are functionally linked in a distributed network during "intrinsic" brain activity, that is, in the absence of goal-directed behavior. This network is reproducible both within and across subjects and has come to be called the default mode network (DMN).[59] The DMN includes discrete brain regions whose metabolic activity (which is indirectly measured by fMRI) predictably covaries during seemingly "idle" (not directed at specific activity) states of the brain. The exact nature of the processes underlying this signal and their quantitative contribution to it has not been fully clarified because the BOLD signal is a composite measure of changes in cerebral oxygenation, blood volume, and blood flow. Recent research indicates that BOLD signal changes in the cerebral cortex are linked closer to synaptic than to spiking activity.[60] Whatever its underlying content, the existence of the DMN supports the notion of a dynamic intrinsically generated state of the brain.

BRAIN RHYTHMS
The brain constantly generates macroscopic electrical signals that vary with physiologic activities and pathologic states. With the exception of high-resolution implantable electrodes, all electrical brain signals reflect the sum of the activity of large neuronal pools. The surface EEG, in particular, is driven by the activity of layer V cortical pyramidal cells. The

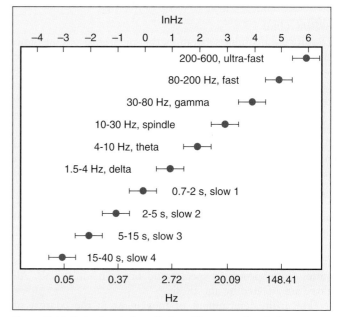

Figure 7-10 Brain electrical oscillations. The mammalian brain generates oscillations in electroencephalographic recordings ranging from ultra-slow to ultra-fast without major gaps to allow neuronal networks of different sizes to cooperate in a coordinated manner. Slower frequencies are thought to allow more complex integrations. Higher frequencies enable more precise and spatially limited representations. The analysis of Pentonen and Buzsaki demonstrates the peak frequencies of discrete oscillation bands forming a geometric progression on a linear scale or a linear progression on a natural logarithmic scale. *(From Penttonen M, Buzsaki G. Natural logarithmic relationship between brain oscillators. Thalamus Relat Syst. 2003;2:145-152.)*

dendritic trees of these neurons extend toward and then parallel to the surface of the cortex. The synaptic inputs to these dendrites cause alternating potential differences that are the predominant basis of the EEG signal rather than action potentials (somewhat similar to the BOLD signal). The activity in the dendritic trees of approximately 50-500,000 pyramidal neurons are reflected in each surface EEG electrode. A summary of commonly observed EEG rhythms is presented in Table 7-4. Oscillations in a mammalian brain do not present a continuum even though their period ranges from seconds to milliseconds. As illustrated in Figure 7-10, discrete oscillation bands form a linear progression on a natural logarithmic scale (a geometric progression on a linear scale) thereby avoiding unwanted harmonic interference that would be a hazard with integer steps between peak frequencies. As a general rule, higher frequency patterns emerge locally whereas slower frequencies involve larger brain areas.[61]

While the functional significance of these rhythms has long been questioned—they were seen as mere epiphenomena with respect to higher cognitive functions—research in the past 20 years has changed this interpretation dramatically. Synchronized activity in different frequency bands is now thought to allow communication and integration of information between physically separate brain areas, an indispensable functionality for all manifestations of the mind, even though it remains elusive to conclusively demonstrate a causal relationship between specific brain processes and synchronous oscillations.[62]

KEY POINTS

- Neuroglial cells are nonneuronal support cells that outnumber neurons in the central nervous system. Oligodendrocytes, astrocytes, and microglia form myelin sheaths, create the blood-brain barrier and attend to immune functions, respectively.
- The generic neuron receives and integrates information in the dendrites and soma and sends out information via its axon.
- The synapse is the physical contact point between neurons that mediates intercellular communication.
- A generic cortical neuron receives thousands of synaptic inputs on its dendrites that form dendritic arbors to provide the necessary surface area. The axon is typically ensheathed in myelin, making rapid communication with hundreds to thousands of other, sometimes remote, neurons possible.
- The typical neuron has a resting membrane potential of −60 to −70 mV (inside relative to outside). The underlying electrochemistry is described in the Nernst and Goldman-Hodgkin-Katz equations. The resting cell membrane is permeable mostly to K^+, hence the resting membrane potential is close to the K^+ equilibrium potential.
- Focal changes in membrane potential, such as depolarization and hyperpolarization from excitatory and inhibitory synaptic inputs, respectively, spread along the membrane, decaying exponentially over time and space.
- Chemical synapses are the mainstay of communication between neurons. Physiologic transmitter release occurs in response to an action potential depolarizing the presynaptic terminal and allowing Ca^{2+} entry through voltage-gated channels to trigger synaptic vesicle fusion and transmitter release.
- Transmitter release occurs in discrete increments (quanta) that reflect the fusion of prepackaged transmitter-containing synaptic vesicles with the membrane of the terminal. Electrical synapses are common in certain brain areas.
- The strength of synaptic connections between neurons undergoes constant, use-dependent modification—both increase and decrease—termed synaptic plasticity.

- L-Glutamate (Glutamate) and γ-aminobutyric acid (GABA) are the major excitatory and inhibitory neurotransmitters, respectively, in the brain.
- The architecture of neuronal circuits and the mode of long-range connectivity differ strikingly between brain areas. The modular "small world" organization of the neocortex, the random synaptic space of the hippocampus, and the strictly parallel organization of the cerebellum are examples.

Key References

Barry PH, Lynch JW. Ligand-gated channels. *IEEE Trans Nanobioscience*. 2005;4:70-80. A review of the biology of ligand-gated ion channels, detailing the biology of the nicotinic/glycine/GABA receptor family. (Ref. 34)

Buzsaki G. Rhythms of the Brain. Oxford: Oxford University Press; 2006. An engaging masterpiece of neuroscience literature from one of the leading contemporary brain scientists (co-laureate of the 2011 Brain Prize). This book provides the coherence only possible with a single author together with a stunning breadth and depth of multidisciplinary knowledge, as well as a wealth of references. (Ref. 62)

Hodgkin AL, Huxley AF. A quantitative description of membrane current and its application to conduction and excitation in nerve. *Bull Math Biol*. 1990;52:25-71. A summary paper of Hodgkin and Huxley's masterpiece (the project includes five papers). In this paper they describe the changes in the Na^+ and K^+ concentration and currents that lead to the action potential. Their new method and insights led to a new era of physiology and neuroscience research. (Ref. 12)

Jasper HH, Sourkes TL. Nobel laureates in neuroscience: 1904-1981. *Annu Rev Neurosci*. 1983;1-42. A somewhat dry gallery of the founders of contemporary neuroscience. (Ref. 1)

Paulsen O, Sejnowski TJ. Natural patterns of activity and long-term synaptic plasticity. *Curr Opin Neurobiol*. 2000;10:172-179. This review describes the mechanisms underlying LTP in the context of Hebbian learning and synaptic plasticity. (Ref. 24)

Rall W. Membrane time constant of motoneurons. *Science*. 1957;126:454. In this brief letter, Wilfrid Rall first described the membrane time constant of neurons. This was the first step in the development of the cable theory in neuroscience and was the basis for the compartmental models of neurons. (Ref. 10)

References

1. Jasper HH, Sourkes TL. Nobel laureates in neuroscience: 1904-1981. *Annu Rev Neurosci*. 1983;6:1-42.
2. Nave KA. Myelination and support of axonal integrity by glia. *Nature*. 2010;468(7321):244-252.
3. Nag S. Morphology and properties of astrocytes. *Methods Mol Biol*. 2011;686:69-100.
4. Ransohoff RM, Cardona AE. The myeloid cells of the central nervous system parenchyma. *Nature*. 2010;468(7321):253-262.
5. Tremblay ME, Stevens B, Sierra A, et al. The role of microglia in the healthy brain. *J Neurosci*. 2011;31(45):16064-16069.
6. Goldstein AYN, Wang X, Schwarz TL. Axonal transport and the delivery of pre-synaptic components. *Curr Opin Neurobiol*. 2008;18(5):495-503.
7. Post RL. Active transport and pumps. In Deamer DW, Kleinzeller A, Fambrough DM, eds. Current Topics In Membranes. Vol 48. San Diego, CA: Academic Press; 1999:397-417.
8. Wright SH. Generation of resting membrane potential. *Adv Physiol Educ*. 2004;28(1-4):139-142.
9. Goldman DE. Potential, impedance, and rectification in membranes. *J Gen Physiol*. 1943;27(1):37-60.
10. Rall W. Membrane time constant of motoneurons. *Science*. 1957; 126:454.
11. Rall W, Burke RE, Holmes WR, et al. Matching dendritic neuron models to experimental data. *Physiol Reviews*. 1992;72(4 Suppl):S159-S186.

12. Hodgkin AL, Huxley AF. A quantitative description of membrane current and its application to conduction and excitation in nerve. 1952. *Bull Math Biol.* 1990;52(1-2):25-71.

13. Kole Maarten HP, Stuart Greg J. Signal processing in the axon initial segment. *Neuron.* 2012;73(2):235-247.

14. Haas JS, Zavala B, Landisman CE. Activity-dependent long-term depression of electrical synapses. *Science.* 2011;334(6054):389-393.

15. Demarque M, Spitzer NC. Neurotransmitter phenotype plasticity: an unexpected mechanism in the toolbox of network activity homeostasis. *Dev Neurobiol.* 2012;72(1):22-32.

16. Stevens CF. Neurotransmitter release at central synapses. *Neuron.* 2003;40(2):381-388.

17. Alger BE, Kim J. Supply and demand for endocannabinoids. *Trends Neurosci.* 2011;34(6):304-315.

18. Kreitzer AC, Regehr WG. Retrograde signaling by endocannabinoids. *CurrOpin Neurobiol.* 2002;12(3):324-330.

19. Young SH, Poo MM. Spontaneous release of transmitter from growth cones of embryonic neurones. *Nature.* 1983;305(5935):634-637.

20. Brickley SG, Mody I. Extrasynaptic GABA(A) receptors: their function in the CNS and implications for disease. *Neuron.* 2012;73(1):23-34.

21. Capogna M, Pearce RA. GABA A, slow: causes and consequences. *Trends Neurosci.* 2011;34(2):101-112.

22. Malenka RC. The long-term potential of LTP. *Nat Rev Neurosci.* 2003;4(11):923-926.

23. Cooper SJ, Donald O. Hebb's synapse and learning rule: a history and commentary. *Neurosci Biobehav Rev.* 2005;28(8):851-874.

24. Paulsen O, Sejnowski TJ. Natural patterns of activity and long-term synaptic plasticity. *Curr Opin Neurobiol.* 2000;10(2):172-179.

25. Caporale N, Dan Y. Spike timing-dependent plasticity: a hebbian learning rule. *Annu Rev Neurosci.* 2008;31:25-46.

26. Wang XJ. Neurophysiological and computational principles of cortical rhythms in cognition. *Physiol Rev.* 2010;90(3):1195-1268.

27. Liu ZW, Faraguna U, Cirelli C, et al. Direct evidence for wake-related increases and sleep-related decreases in synaptic strength in rodent cortex. *J Neurosci.* 2010;30(25):8671-8675.

28. Lerma J. Kainate receptor physiology. *Curr Opin Pharmacol.* 2006;6(1):89-97.

29. Ozawa S, Kamiya H, Tsuzuki K. Glutamate receptors in the mammalian central nervous system. *Prog Neurobiol.* 1998;54(5):581-618.

30. Sieghart W. Structure, pharmacology, and function of GABAA receptor subtypes. *Adv Pharmacol.* 2006;54:231-263.

31. Buzsaki G, Geisler C, Henze DA, et al. Interneuron diversity series: circuit complexity and axon wiring economy of cortical interneurons. *Trends Neurosci.* 2004;27(4):186-193.

32. Mody I, Pearce RA. Diversity of inhibitory neurotransmission through GABA(A) receptors. *Trends Neurosci.* 2004;27(9):569-575.

33. Pinard A, Seddik R, Bettler B. GABAB receptors: physiological functions and mechanisms of diversity. *Adv Pharmacol.* 2010;58:231-255.

34. Barry PH, Lynch JW. Ligand-gated channels. *IEEE Trans Nanobioscience.* 2005;4(1):70-80.

35. Klinkenberg I, Sambeth A, Blokland A. Acetylcholine and attention. *Behav Brain Res.* 2011;221(2):430-442.

36. Platt B, Riedel G. The cholinergic system, EEG and sleep. *Behav Brain Res.* 2011;221(2):499-504.

37. Koch C, Laurent G. Complexity and the nervous system. *Science.* 1999;284(5411):96-98.

38. Watts DJ, Strogatz SH. Collective dynamics of 'small-world' networks. *Nature.* 1998;393(6684):440-442.

39. Zhang K, Sejnowski TJ. A universal scaling law between gray matter and white matter of cerebral cortex. *Proc Natl Acad Sci U S A.* 2000;97(10):5621-5626.

40. Hubel DH, Wiesel TN. Uniformity of monkey striate cortex: a parallel relationship between field size, scatter, and magnification factor. *J Comparative Neurol.* 1974;158(3):295-305.

41. Meyer K, Damasio A. Convergence and divergence in a neural architecture for recognition and memory. *Trends Neurosci.* 2009;32(7):376-382.

42. Perouansky M, Pearce RA. How we recall (or don't): the hippocampal memory machine and anesthetic amnesia. *Can J Anaesth.* 2011;58(2):157-166.

43. Amaral DG, Witter MP. The three-dimensional organization of the hippocampal formation: a review of anatomical data. *Neuroscience.* 1989;31:571-591.

44. Freund TF. Interneuron diversity series: rhythm and mood in perisomatic inhibition. *Trends Neurosci.* 2003;26(9):489-495.

45. Maccaferri G, Lacaille JC. Interneuron diversity series: hippocampal interneuron classifications—making things as simple as possible, not simpler. *Trends Neurosci.* 2003;26(10):564-571.

46. Deschenes M, Madariaga-Domich A, Steriade M. Dendrodendritic synapses in the cat reticularis thalami nucleus: a structural basis for thalamic spindle synchronization. *Brain Res.* 1985;334(1):165-168.

47. Landisman CE, Long MA, Beierlein M, et al. Electrical synapses in the thalamic reticular nucleus. *J Neurosci.* 2002;22(3):1002-1009.

48. Alkire MT, Hudetz AG, Tononi G. Consciousness and anesthesia. *Science.* 2008;322(5903):876-880.

49. Szentagothai J. The modular architectonic principle of neural centers. *Rev Physiol Biochem Pharmacol.* 1983;98:11-61.

50. DeLong M, Wichmann T. Update on models of basal ganglia function and dysfunction. *Parkinsonism Relat Disord.* 2009;15(Suppl 3):S237-S240.

51. Burke RE. The central pattern generator for locomotion in mammals. *Adv Neurol.* 2001;87:11-24.

52. Quasha AL, Eger EI 2nd, Tinker JH. Determination and applications of MAC. *Anesthesiology.* 1980;53:315-334.

53. Antognini JF, Wang XW, Carstens E. Quantitative and qualitative effects of isoflurane on movement occurring after noxious stimulation. *Anesthesiology.* 1999;91(4):1064-1071.

54. Rampil IJ, Laster MJ. No correlation between quantitative electroencephalographic measurements and movement response to noxious stimuli during isoflurane anesthesia in rats. *Anesthesiology.* 1992;77(5):920-925.

55. Antognini JF, Schwartz K. Exaggerated anesthetic requirements in the preferentially anesthetized brain. *Anesthesiology.* 1993;79(6):1244-1249.

56. Rampil IJ, Mason P, Singh H. Anesthetic potency (MAC) is independent of forebrain structures in the rat. *Anesthesiology.* 1993;78(4):707-712.

57. Jinks SL, Bravo M, Satter O, et al. Brainstem regions affecting minimum alveolar concentration and movement pattern during isoflurane anesthesia. *Anesthesiology.* 2010;112(2):316-324.

58. Logothetis NK, Wandell BA. Interpreting the BOLD signal. *Annu Rev Physiol.* 2004;66:735-769.

59. Raichle ME, MacLeod AM, Snyder AZ, et al. A default mode of brain function. *Proc Natl Acad Sci U S A.* 2001;98(2):676-682.

60. Viswanathan A, Freeman RD. Neurometabolic coupling in cerebral cortex reflects synaptic more than spiking activity. *Nat Neurosci.* 2007;10(10):1308-1312.

61. Penttonen M, Buzsaki G. Natural logarithmic relationship between brain oscillators. *Thalamus Rel Systems.* 2003;2:145-152.

Chapter 8

CENTRAL NERVOUS SYSTEM PHYSIOLOGY: CEREBROVASCULAR

Brian P. Lemkuil, John C. Drummond, and Piyush M. Patel

This chapter focuses on central nervous system physiology relevant to anesthesiology and pharmacology. The molecular and cellular substrates of specific drugs affecting the nervous system are covered in Chapter 7 and in the appropriate chapters in this section.

CEREBROVASCULAR ANATOMY

The cerebral arterial vasculature is divided into anterior and posterior circulations that are interconnected through a vascular loop referred to as the *circle of Willis*. This anastomotic loop provides potential for collateral blood flow between the anterior and posterior circulations, as well as between cerebral hemispheres in case of impaired flow in one of the proximal feeding vessels. As one of the most highly perfused organs in the body, the brain is supplied by two paired arteries, the right and left vertebral and the right and left internal carotid arteries. Flow is then distributed throughout the cranium primarily by three paired cerebral arteries arising from the *circle of Willis*, the anterior cerebral, middle cerebral, and posterior cerebral arteries (Figure 8-1). However, a complete *circle of Willis* is present in only 42% to 52% of human adults.[1,2] A variety of incomplete (containing a noncontinuous, hypoplastic, or absent segment) variants that can compromise collateral flow have been identified. In such cases, secondary sources of collateral flow can occur through distal leptomeningeal connections, or by way of retrograde flow though the ophthalmic artery from the external carotid circulation to the internal carotid artery.

Vascular Architecture

ARTERIES AND ARTERIOLES

The cerebral arteries distributing flow from the *circle of Willis* continuously branch into smaller arteries and arterioles that course along the surface of the brain. At their distal end, before entering the brain parenchyma, they are known as leptomeningeal vessels. The leptomeningeal vessels are found within the pia-arachnoid membrane and are surrounded by cerebral spinal fluid (CSF). The highly branched pial arterioles form an extensive collateral network on the surface of the brain before giving rise to relatively unbranched system of penetrating and intraparenchymal arterioles.

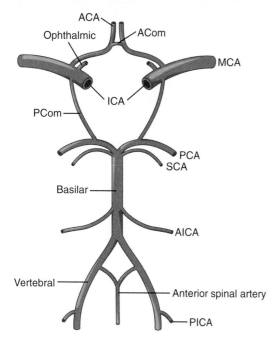

Figure 8-1 *Circle of Willis,* major supply and distributing vessels. Supply vessels include the left and right internal carotid arteries (ICA) and the left and right vertebral arteries. The major distributing vessels include the anterior cerebral arteries (ACA), middle cerebral arteries (MCA), and posterior cerebral arteries (PCA). The anterior and posterior communicating arteries (ACom, PCom) complete this vascular loop and allow for collateral blood flow between vascular territories. The major branches of the vertebrobasilar system are also labeled. *AICA,* Anterior inferior cerebellar artery; *PICA,* posterior inferior cerebellar artery; *SCA,* superior cerebellar artery.

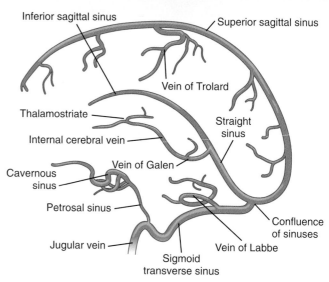

Figure 8-2 Cerebral venous anatomy. The venous drainage of the brain is composed of an interconnected system of superficial and deep veins and sinuses that return blood to the central circulation. Superficial veins, such as the vein of Trolard (most often found in the post-central sulcus), typically empty into the superior sagittal sinus. Labbe is a superficial vein of the temporal convexity with drainage toward the transverse/sigmoid sinus. Many of the deep veins, including the inferior sagittal sinus, internal cerebral vein, and the vein of Galen, are directed toward the confluence of sinuses via the straight sinus. Flow from the confluence is directed through the transverse sinus, sigmoid sinus, and internal jugular vein before reaching the right atrium. The petrosal sinus provides drainage of the cavernous sinus directly into the sigmoid sinus.

VENOUS CIRCULATION

The venous circulation consists of an interconnected system of veins and sinuses. Venous outflow from the cerebral hemispheres occurs via cortical veins within the pia mater on the surface of the brain as well as deep central veins. Cortical and deep veins may empty into the superior sagittal sinus, and the latter may also empty into the inferior sagittal sinus or great vein of Galen. Venous flow is directed toward a confluence of sinuses (torcular herophili) then on toward the central circulation via the transverse sinus, sigmoid sinus, and jugular vein (Figure 8-2). Cerebellar drainage occurs primarily via the inferior cerebellar veins and occipital sinuses. Extensive collateralization between cortical veins as well as the deep veins and sinuses can augment venous drainage when primary routes are compromised.

ANTERIOR CIRCULATION

The anterior circulation arises from the intracranial extension of the internal carotid arteries. The most prominent branches of the anterior circulation are the anterior cerebral, middle cerebral, and posterior communicating (PCom) arteries. The PCom provides communication with the posterior circulation through direct connection with the posterior cerebral artery (PCA). An absent or hypoplastic PCom potentially compromises collateral flow between the anterior and posterior circulations. Likewise, collateral flow between the left and right anterior circulation can be compromised by a hypoplastic or aplastic anterior communicating (ACom) artery.

POSTERIOR CIRCULATION

The posterior circulation arises from paired vertebral arteries. At their rostral end, the vertebral arteries typically join together on the anterior surface of the brainstem to form the basilar artery. The vertebral and basilar arteries have multiple branches that supply the cerebellum, brainstem, and spinal cord (see Figure 8-1). The basilar artery branches distally into the left and right posterior cerebral arteries (PCAs). The branches of the PCA provide blood flow to the brainstem, choroid plexus, and cerebrum (occipital and portions of parietal and temporal lobes) as well as provide a point of connection with the anterior circulation. Like the anterior circulation, there are many anatomic variants that may compromise collateral blood flow and predispose to ischemia in certain clinical scenarios.

REGULATION OF CEREBRAL BLOOD FLOW

The adult brain represents about 2% of total body weight (1350 g), but receives almost 15% of cardiac output. This high flow reflects its significant metabolic demand. At rest, the brain consumes oxygen at an average rate of 3.5 mL/100 g of brain tissue/min, or 50 mL/min overall, which represents nearly 20% of total body oxygen utilization. Normal values for cerebral blood flow (CBF), cerebral metabolic rate (CMR), and other physiologic variables are provided in Table 8-1.

Approximately 60% of cerebral energy consumption is used to support electrophysiologic function in the form of maintenance and restoration of ionic gradients as well as the synthesis, transport, and reuptake of neurotransmitters.[3] This variable and modifiable component of cerebral energy

Table 8-1. Normal Cerebral Physiologic Variables

Cerebral Blood Flow	
Global	45-55 mL/100 g/min
Cortical (mostly gray matter)	75-80 mL/100 g/min
Subcortical (mostly white matter)	20 mL/100 g/min
Cerebral metabolic rate of oxygen (CMRO$_2$)	3-3.5 mL/100 g/min
Cerebral venous Po$_2$	32-44 mm Hg
Cerebral venous So$_2$	55%-70%
Intracranial pressure (supine)	10-15 mm Hg

Adapted with permission from Patel P, Drummond JC. CNS physiology and effects of anesthetic drugs. In: Miller RD, Eriksson LI, Fleisher LA, et al. *Miller's Anesthesia*. Philadelphia: Elsevier; 2009.
CMRO$_2$, Cerebral metabolic rate of oxygen.

Table 8-2. Factors Influencing Cerebral Blood Flow

Chemical/Metabolic/Humoral
Cerebral metabolic rate*
  Anesthetics
  Temperature
  Arousal/seizures
PaCO$_2$
PaO$_2$
Vasoactive drugs
  Anesthetics
  Vasodilators
  Vasopressors
Myogenic
Autoregulation†/mean arterial pressure
Rheologic
Blood viscosity
Neurogenic‡
Extracranial sympathetic and parasympathetic pathways
Intraaxial pathways

Adapted with permission from Patel P, Drummond JC. CNS physiology and effects of anesthetic drugs. In: Miller RD, Eriksson LI, Fleisher LA, et al. *Miller's Anesthesia*. Philadelphia: Elsevier; 2009.
*CMR influence assumes intact flow-metabolism coupling.
†The autoregulation mechanism is fragile, and in many pathologic states CBF is regionally pressure passive.
‡The contribution and clinical significance is poorly defined.

consumption is reflected by electrical activity on electroencephalography (EEG). Maintenance of cellular homeostasis, which includes synthesis and transport of cellular components, accounts for the remainder of oxygen consumption. This second component of neuronal energy consumption related to basic cellular housekeeping function is largely independent of electrophysiologic activity and is sensitive to temperature manipulation.[4,5]

Glucose is the primary substrate of brain metabolism. In the presence of adequate oxygen delivery, glucose is metabolized to pyruvate by oxidative phosphorylation. In the absence of sufficient oxygen delivery, glucose is anaerobically metabolized, resulting in insufficient adenosine triphosphate (ATP) production and energy failure. Therefore, the brain's considerable metabolic demands must be met by adequate delivery of both oxygen and glucose. There are elaborate mechanisms in place for regulating CBF to ensure these demands are met. The various mechanisms, which include chemical, myogenic, and neurogenic factors, are listed in Table 8-2.

Chemical Regulation of Cerebral Blood Flow

A number of factors, by altering the biochemical milieu of the brain, modulate CBF; these include CMR, PaCO$_2$, and PaO$_2$.

CEREBRAL METABOLIC RATE
CMR is directly proportional to neuronal activity.[6] Although the mechanism is not entirely understood, an increase in neuronal activity and CMR is proportionally matched by an increase in CBF.[6-10] This physiologic process, wherein blood flow and metabolism are matched, is referred to as *flow-metabolism coupling*. In summary, coupling of flow and metabolism in the brain is a complex physiologic process that is mediated by a combination of metabolic, glial, neural, and vascular factors. Local by-products of metabolism (K$^+$, H$^+$, lactate, adenosine, and ATP) and increased production of nitric oxide (NO) directly modulate vascular resistance and alter local blood flow.[11,12] Glia are in direct contact with neurons and capillaries, and more recent data highlight the role of glia as a possible conduit for coupling neuronal activity with regional blood flow.[13] Cerebral vessels are densely innervated, and peptidergic neurotransmitters released by nerves also contribute to vascular regulation and flow-metabolism coupling.

In the neurosurgical and critical care environments, CMR is influenced by the functional state of the nervous system, anesthetic agents, and temperature.

FUNCTIONAL STATE
CMR decreases during sleep and increases during sensory stimulation, mental tasks, or arousal of any cause. CMR is markedly increased during epileptic activity and substantially reduced in coma.

ANESTHETIC AGENTS
In general, anesthetics suppress CMR, with the exception of ketamine and N$_2$O. Specifically, the component of CMR related to electrophysiologic function is reduced.[14] With several agents, including barbiturates, isoflurane, sevoflurane, desflurane, propofol, and etomidate, increasing plasma concentrations cause progressive suppression of EEG activity with a concomitant reduction in CMR.[13,15-19] Increasing the plasma level beyond that required to achieve suppression of the EEG results in no further depression of CMR. The component of CMR related to basic cellular homeostatic activities is unaffected by anesthetics (Figure 8-3).

TEMPERATURE
CMR decreases by 6% to 7% per degree Celsius of temperature reduction, and can cause complete suppression of the EEG at about 18° C to 20° C.[3] In contrast to anesthetic agents, temperature reduction beyond that at which EEG suppression first occurs does produce a further decrease in CMR. This occurs because hypothermia decreases the rate of energy utilization associated with both electrophysiologic function and basal maintenance of cellular integrity (Figure 8-4). While these decreases were once assumed to be proportional, more recent data show preferential suppression of the basal component (with mild hypothermia).[4,5] Global CMRO$_2$ at 18° C is less than 10% of normothermic control values, which likely accounts for the brain's tolerance of circulatory arrest for moderate periods at these temperatures.

Hyperthermia leads to substantial increases in CMR and CBF.[20] However, above 42° C a dramatic reduction in

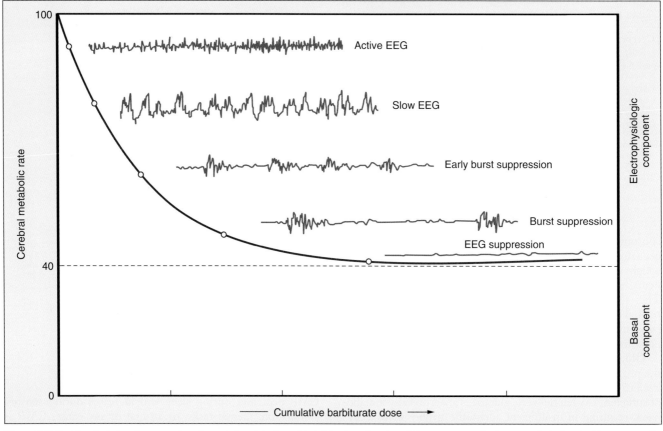

Figure 8-3 Barbiturate induced suppression of cerebral metabolism. Administration of various intravenous anesthetic agents including barbiturates results in a dose-related reduction in cerebral metabolic rate (CMR) and cerebral blood flow. Anesthetic induced-reductions are maximal at the point of electroencephalographic silence. At this point, additional drug administration does not result in a further $CMRO_2$ reduction. The basal component of CMR responsible for maintaining cellular homeostasis is not altered. *BS,* Burst suppression; *$CMRO_2$,* cerebral metabolic rate; *EEG,* electroencephalogram.

$CMRO_2$ occurs, possibly due to neuronal injury and protein denaturation.

$PACO_2$

CBF varies directly with $PaCO_2$ (Figure 8-5). For each change of 1 mm Hg in $PaCO_2$ from normal values, CBF changes 1 to 2 mL/100 g/min.[21] This response is attenuated below a $PaCO_2$ of 25 mm Hg,[21] and is sensitive to the baseline CBF.[22] Hypocapnia causes a greater reduction in CBF when the resting CBF is high (as can occur with volatile anesthetics), an effect that is attenuated with lower resting CBF. Therefore, anesthetic agents have the capacity to alter CO_2 responsiveness of the cerebral circulation by changing basal CBF.

The changes in CBF caused by $PaCO_2$ depend upon pH in the extracellular fluid of the brain.[23] Extracellular pH and CBF changes occur rapidly after $PaCO_2$ adjustments because CO_2 (neutral charge) diffuses freely across the cerebrovascular endothelium. In contrast, acute systemic *metabolic* acidosis has little immediate effect on CBF because the blood-brain barrier (BBB) excludes hydrogen ion (H^+) from the perivascular space.

Although changes to CBF induced by $PaCO_2$ are rapid, they are not sustained. Despite maintenance of increased arterial pH (through hyperventilation), CBF returns toward baseline over 6 to 18 hours because CSF pH gradually normalizes through bicarbonate extrusion[24,25] (Figure 8-6). Therefore, patients with sustained periods of hyperventilation or hypoventilation deserve special consideration. Acute normalization of

$PaCO_2$ results in a significant CSF acidosis (after hypocapnia) or alkalosis (after hypercapnia). The former results in increased CBF with a concomitant intracranial pressure (ICP) increase, depending on the prevailing intracranial compliance. The latter conveys the theoretical risk of ischemia.

PAO_2

The effects of PaO_2 on CBF are minimal within the normal physiologic range (PaO_2 from 60 to over 300 mm Hg). Below a PaO_2 of 60 mm Hg, CBF increases rapidly (see Figure 8-5). The mechanisms mediating cerebral vasodilation during hypoxemia are not fully understood, but are influenced, at least in part, by nitric oxide of neuronal origin, hypoxemia-induced hyperpolarization of vascular smooth muscle, and stimulation of the rostral ventrolateral medulla.[26,27] The response to hypoxemia is synergistic with hypercarbia-induced hyperemia.

Myogenic Regulation (Autoregulation) of Cerebral Blood Flow

Autoregulation refers to the capacity of the cerebral circulation to alter vascular resistance in order to maintain a relatively constant CBF over a range of mean arterial pressure (MAP). Although animal models suggest a lower limit of autoregulation (LLA) near a MAP of 50 mm Hg, available human data suggest a higher threshold (with considerable interindividual variation).[28] In normal nonanesthetized humans, the limits of

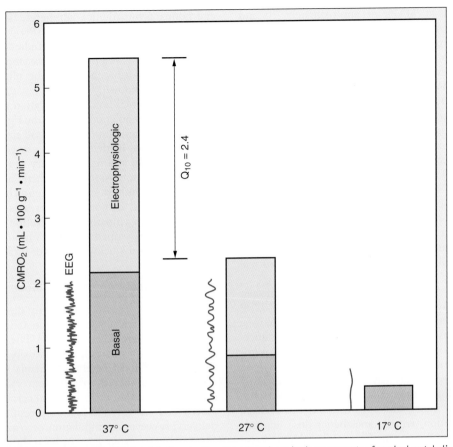

Figure 8-4 Temperature induced suppression of cerebral metabolic rate. Hypothermia reduces both components of cerebral metabolic activity: that associated with neuronal electrophysiologic activity and that associated with the maintenance of cellular homeostasis ("basal"). This is in contrast to anesthetic agents that alter only the electrophysiologic component. The ratio of CMR at 37° C to that at 27° C, the Q10 ratio, is shown in the graph. *CMRO$_2$*, Cerebral metabolic rate for oxygen; *EEG*, electroencephalogram. *(Adapted from Michenfelder JD. Anesthesia and the Brain: Clinical, Functional, Metabolic, and Vascular Correlates. New York: Churchill Livingstone; 1988.)*

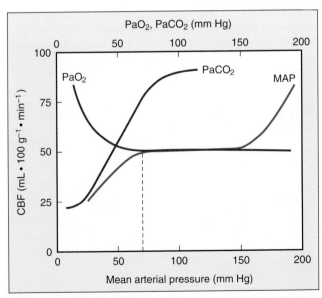

Figure 8-5 Cerebral autoregulation. Changes in cerebral blood flow (CBF) caused by independent alterations in PaCO$_2$, PaO$_2$, and mean arterial pressure.

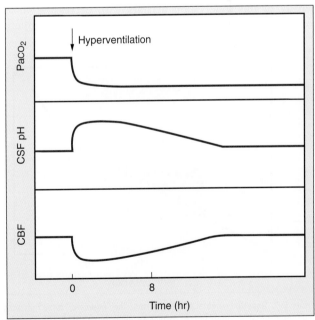

Figure 8-6 Effect of sustained hyperventilation on cerebrospinal fluid pH and cerebral blood flow. Sustained hyperventilation results in almost immediate pH change in cerebrospinal fluid (CSF)/brain extracellular fluid and cerebral blood flow (CBF) as indicated in this nonquantitative graph. These changes are relatively brief, with return toward baseline over a period of 6 to 18 hours.

autoregulation occur at MAPs of approximately 70 and 150 mm Hg[29-33] (see Figure 8-5). These limits are shifted toward the right in patients with poorly controlled, long-standing hypertension.[29] Note that the units used on the x-axis of "autoregulation curves" will influence the correct inflection points of the curve. When the x-axis is "mean arterial pressure," the normal average LLA is near 70 mm Hg. However, cerebral perfusion pressure (CPP) is the ideal independent variable. But, ICP is usually not measured in normal subjects, so CPP (MAP-ICP) is rarely available. Assuming a normal ICP in a supine subject of 10 to 15 mm Hg, a lower limit of autoregulation of 70 mm Hg MAP corresponds to 55 to 60 mm Hg expressed as CPP. Above and below the autoregulatory limits, CBF becomes pressure dependent (pressure-passive) and varies linearly with CPP. The autoregulatory response to a change in arterial pressure occurs over the course of 1 to 2 minutes, such that a rapid change in arterial pressure will transiently alter CBF even within the normal autoregulatory range.[34]

The mechanisms governing autoregulation are unclear. According to the myogenic hypothesis, changes in CPP directly influence alterations in vascular smooth muscle tone independent of extrinsic factors. However, autonomic innervation of cerebral blood vessels might also contribute to autoregulation (discussed later).

Autoregulatory mechanisms may be absent or significantly attenuated in pathologic conditions, such as cerebral ischemia, traumatic brain injury, and subarachnoid hemorrhage (Figure 8-7). In addition, volatile anesthetics dose dependently attenuate autoregulation, an effect attributable to direct vasodilation.

Neurogenic Regulation of Cerebral Blood Flow

The cerebral vasculature is extensively innervated; the density of this innervation declines with decreasing vessel size.[35,36] Innervation includes cholinergic (parasympathetic

and nonparasympathetic), adrenergic (sympathetic and non-sympathetic), serotonergic, and VIPergic systems of extraaxial and intraaxial origin.[37-41] Animal studies have established both extracranial sympathetic and parasympathetic influence on CBF autoregulation; however, the clinical implications in humans are unknown.[37,39,42-48]

In experimental animals, activation of sympathetic fibers shifts the autoregulation curve to the right. Beyond the upper limit of autoregulation, sympathetic activation is considered to be protective in that cerebral vasoconstriction limits the increase in CBF and reduces injury to the BBB. By contrast, in states of hypotension, sympathetic activation might limit CBF further.[49] Indeed, stellate ganglion blockade in the setting of subarachnoid hemorrhage increases CBF considerably.[50] The role of parasympathetic innervation is less clearly defined. In animals, parasympathetic denervation augments CBF when arterial pressure is below the lower limit of autoregualtion.[51]

Viscosity Effects on Cerebral Blood Flow

Blood viscosity variation, primarily determined by hematocrit, results in trivial alterations in CBF in healthy subjects (hematocrit range 33%-45%).[52,53] The benefit of improved CBF resulting from reduced viscosity is more relevant in the setting of focal cerebral ischemia when vasodilation in response to impaired oxygen delivery is probably already maximal.[54,55] In the setting of focal cerebral ischemia, a hematocrit of 30% to 34% probably results in optimal oxygen delivery; however, manipulation of viscosity in patients with acute ischemic stroke has not been shown to reduce cerebral injury.[56,57]

Vasoactive Agents

A number of pharmacologic agents have cerebrovascular effects (Table 8-3). Paramount in the care of patients with intracranial pathology are anesthetic agents (see Chapters 9 and 10) and vasoactive drugs used specifically for hemodynamic manipulation (see Chapters 22 and 23).

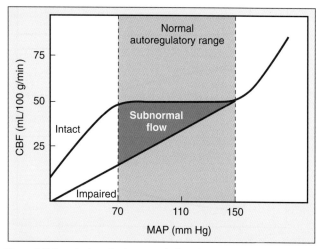

Figure 8-7 Impaired cerebral autoregulation. The *"impaired"* curve indicates a pressure-passive condition in which cerebral blood flow (CBF) varies directly with cerebral perfusion pressure. This *curve* is drawn to indicate subnormal CBF *(green area)* despite mean arterial pressures within the typical autoregulatory range. This has been demonstrated following various central nervous system insults such as traumatic head injury and subarachnoid hemorrhage. The potential even for modest hypotension to cause ischemia is apparent.

Table 8-3. Vasoactive Agents and Their Effects on Cerebral Metabolic Rate and Blood Flow

Systemic vasodilators (e.g., nitroglycerine, nitroprusside, nicardipine)	Increase CBF/CBV*
Catecholamine agonists/antagonists	
α1 agonist	Minimal direct effect on CBF
β agonist (BBB intact)	Minimal direct effect on CBF
β agonist (BBB disrupted)	Increase CMR/CBF
β antagonist	Minimal effect, can reduce CMR/CBF
Dopamine	Poorly defined
Intravenous anesthetics	
Ketamine	Increase CBF
Others	Decrease CMR/CBF
Inhaled anesthetics	Decrease CMR/variable effect on CBF†

BBB, Blood-brain barrier; CBF, cerebral blood flow; CBV, cerebral blood volume; CMR, cerebral metabolic rate.
*Most systemic vasodilators result in cerebral vasodilation and increased CBF/CBV. The notable exception is enalapril, which does not cause cerebral vasodilation.
†See text for discussion.

SYSTEMIC VASODILATORS

The majority of the drugs used to lower systemic blood pressure (including sodium nitroprusside, nitroglycerin, hydralazine, adenosine, and calcium channel blockers) also induce cerebral vasodilation. Agents that vasodilate both the cerebral and systemic circulations can increase CBV, and therefore ICP, by two mechanisms: direct cerebral vascular smooth muscle relaxation and autoregulation-mediated vasodilation. The result is either increased CBF or maintenance of CBF despite inducing systemic hypotension. The hypotensive threshold at which CBF begins to decrease is lower if hypotension is induced with a cerebral vasodilator rather than with hypovolemia or a noncerebral vasodilator.[58] In contrast to direct vasodilators, the angiotensin-converting enzyme inhibitor enalapril has no significant impact on CBF.[59]

CATECHOLAMINE AGONISTS/ANTAGONISTS

Numerous drugs with activity at catecholamine receptors (α1, α2, β, and dopamine) have effects on cerebral physiology that depend on basal blood pressure, the systemic blood pressure change induced, the autoregulatory capacity, and the status of the BBB. A given agent can have direct effects on cerebral vascular smooth muscle and/or indirect effects mediated by cerebral autoregulation. When autoregulation is preserved, increases in systemic pressure increase CBF only if arterial pressure is below or above the limits of autoregulation. When the basal pressure is within the normal autoregulation range, systemic pressure changes do not significantly affect CBF as a result of cerebral vasodilation or vasoconstriction. When autoregulation is defective, CBF varies in direct relation to the systemic pressure.

α1-RECEPTOR AGONISTS

A frequent clinical concern is that the administration of agents with α1-agonist activity (phenylephrine/norepinephrine) will reduce CBF. However, when used in the typical clinical dose ranges, neither intraarterial nor intravenous injection of potent α1-agonists significantly affects CBF.[60-62]

Increases in CBF attributable to norepinephrine can occur when autoregulation is defective or MAP is beyond the limits of autoregulation. Agonists of β-adrenergic receptors (such as norepinephrine and epinephrine) can also increase cerebral metabolism with a coupled increase in CBF.[63] This effect is likely most apparent in the presence of a defective BBB, which allows greater access to the brain parenchyma.[61,64,65]

β-RECEPTOR AGONISTS

In low doses, β-receptor agonists (epinephrine, norepinephrine) have little direct effect on the cerebral vasculature. In large doses, particularly in the presence of a defective BBB, they can cause an increase in CMR accompanied by an increase in CBF.[61,65,66] These effects are likely mediated by the β1 receptor.[67]

β RECEPTOR BLOCKERS

β-Blockers have been reported to either reduce CBF or have no effect on CBF (and/or CMR).[68,69] Catecholamine levels at the time of β-blocker administration and/or the status of the BBB might influence their effects. Adverse effects due to β-blocker administration to patients with intracranial pathology is unlikely, apart from effects related to changes in perfusion pressure.

DOPAMINE

The effects of dopamine on CBF and CMR have not been defined with certainty. The available data suggest slight vasodilation with minimal change in CMR when administered in low doses with normal cerebral vasculature and the absence of cerebral vasoconstriction in high doses (100 μg/kg/min).[70-72]

INTRAVENOUS ANESTHETICS.

In general, the intravenous anesthetic agents (propofol, etomidate, lidocaine, barbiturates, benzodiazepines) produce parallel reductions in CMR and CBF.[73-78] With controlled ventilation and maintenance of normocapnia, it is likely that opioids have relatively little effect on CBF and CMR in the normal, unstimulated nervous system.[79] Many investigations involving ketamine suggest that it increases CBF, particularly within the anterior cingulate cortex, without significantly altering CMR.[79-84] This has the potential to increase ICP; based on this concern, it has been suggested to avoid ketamine for neurosurgical anesthesia. More recent data, however, indicate that ICP can be effectively reduced in patients with increased ICP that is refractory to conventional management.[85] Nonetheless, caution should be exercised with ketamine as the sole anesthetic in patients with impaired intracranial compliance.

Intravenous agent-induced changes in CBF largely reflect coupling between CMR reduction and CBF. In addition, variable direct effects on cerebral vascular smooth muscle make minor contributions to the net CBF/CMR ratio. In general, autoregulation and $PaCO_2$ responsiveness are preserved.

INHALED ANESTHETICS

All volatile anesthetics, in a manner similar to intravenous sedative-hypnotic agents, suppress cerebral metabolism in a dose-related manner.[16,86-90] In contrast, they also directly affect vascular smooth muscle, resulting in cerebral vasodilation.[91] The net effect on CBF is a balance between CBF reduction caused by CMR suppression and augmentation of CBF due to direct cerebral vasodilation. Although the data vary, depending on the agent (isoflurane vs. desflurane vs. sevoflurane), method/location of measuring CBF, and level to which systemic pressure is maintained, they may be best conceptualized in the following way.[78] At low doses (about 0.5 MAC), the CMR reducing effect likely predominates over direct vasodilation, resulting in a net decrease in CBF compared to the awake state. In an intermediate range (roughly 0.5-1.0 MAC), direct cerebral vasodilation offsets the effects of CMR suppression, and CBF is relatively unchanged compared to the awake state. In high does (exceeding 1.0 MAC), the direct vasodilatory effect can predominate and CBF can be increased.

Although the available data suggest that volatile anesthetics will have minimal effect on cerebral hemodynamics when intracranial compliance is normal, they have the potential to induce increases in CBV and ICP in certain clinical scenarios (intracranial hypertension significant enough to produce changes in the level of consciousness). Furthermore, when near maximal reduction of CMR has occurred due to antecedent drug administration, introduction of a volatile agent will have a predominantly vasodilating effect.[92,93]

The cerebrovasculature responsiveness to $PaCO_2$ is well maintained during anesthesia with all volatile anesthetic agents.[21,94-97] By contrast, volatile anesthetics impair autoregulation of CBF in a dose-dependent manner.[98,99] Rising MAP results in increased CBF, while CBF is preserved to a lower MAP during administration of volatile agents.

AGE

Aging, from childhood to late adulthood, is associated with progressive reduction of CBF and $CMRO_2$.[100,101] This might reflect the progressive reduction in gray matter volume that occurs with increasing age. The precise mechanism underlying this reduction is not clear; loss of neurons, loss of spines and synapses, and shrinkage of spines may play a role.[102]

CEREBRAL SPINAL FLUID DYNAMICS

Production

The volume of CSF in human adults is about 150 mL, half of which resides within the cranium and the other half in the spinal CSF space. Approximately 70% is produced by the choroid plexus, and the remainder is largely a product of transependymal diffusion from the brain interstitium. The choroid plexus refers to the ependyma-lined epithelium covering the roof of the third and fourth ventricles as well as the medial walls of the lateral ventricles. The vasculature of the choroid plexus is characterized by relatively large-diameter capillaries with thin fenestrated walls. Although various drugs are capable of altering the rate of CSF formation, total CSF volume is typically turned over three to four times per day.[103]

Circulation

CSF circulates primarily from sites of production in the lateral and third ventricles toward the fourth ventricle (by way of the aqueduct of Sylvius). CSF then exits the fourth ventricle, located between the brainstem and cerebellum, by way of paired lateral openings (foramina of Luschka) and a single midline opening (foramen of Magendie), into the cisterna magna. From the cisterna magna, CSF fluid flows superiorly in the subarachnoid space bathing the cerebral hemispheres or inferiorly toward the spinal subarachnoid space (Figure 8-8). Caudal movement of CSF in the spinal subarachnoid space occurs primarily posterior to the spinal cord whereas the overall direction of flow ventral to the cord is cephalad. Movement for circulation of CSF is provided by hydrostatic pressure created at the sites of production, coordinated ciliary movement on the surface of ependymal cells, and ventricular excursion created by respiratory variation and vascular pulsations. CSF is absorbed primarily through arachnoid villi into the superior sagittal sinus and returned to the central circulation.

Function

The CSF functions both as a supportive and protective cushion for the CNS and as an excretory system for unwanted and potentially harmful substances from the CNS. The buoyancy afforded the brain by the specific gravity difference between the brain and CSF acts to reduce the effective weight of the brain to approximately 4% of its mass.[104] The CSF may also help provide the brain parenchyma a stable biochemical environment essential for proper function. Differences in composition between plasma and CSF (Table 8-4) are maintained by the blood-brain barrier (BBB).

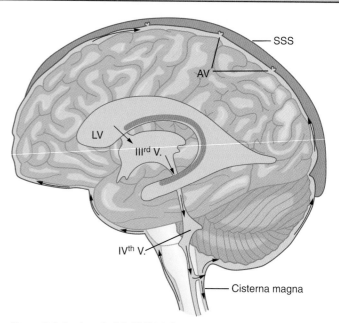

Figure 8-8 Cerebrospinal fluid (CSF) flow. The overall flow of CSF is demonstrated by *black arrows*. At the level of the cisterna magna, CSF can flow upward around the cerebral hemispheres or downward into the spinal subarachnoid space. The overall direction of flow in the spinal subarachnoid space is caudal posteriorly and rostral anteriorly. CSF is primarily absorbed into the superior sagittal sinus (SSS) through small arachnoid protrusions called arachnoid villi (AV). *LV*, Lateral ventricle; *IIIrd V*, third ventricle; *IVth V*, fourth ventricle.

Table 8-4. Normal composition of Cerebrospinal Fluid and Serum

	CSF	SERUM
Osmolarity (mOsm/L)	295	295
Sodium (mEq/L)	138	138
Potassium (mEq/L)	2.8	4.5
Chloride (mEq/L)	119	102
Bicarbonate (mEq/L)	22	24
Phosphorus (mg/dL)	1.6	4.0
Calcium (mEq/L)	2.1	4.8
Magnesium (mEq/L)	2.3	1.7
Iron (g/dL)	1.5	15
Creatinine (mg/dL)	1.2	1.8
Uric acid (mg/dL)	0.25	5.5
CO_2 tension (mm Hg)	47	41
pH	7.33	7.41
O_2 (mm Hg)	43	104
Glucose (mg/dL)	60	90
Lactate:pyruvate ratio	26	17.6
Protein (mg/dL)	35	7000

Adapted from Fishman RA. *Cerebrospinal Fluid in Disease of the Nervous System.* Philadelphia: WB Saunders; 1992.

Blood-Brain Barrier

Most capillary beds contain fenestrations between endothelial cells that are approximately 65 Ångstroms in diameter. In the brain, with the exception of the choroid plexus, pituitary, and area postrema, tight junctions reduce this pore size to approximately 8 Ångstroms. As a result, large molecules and most ions (including pharmacologic agents with these characteristics) are prevented from entering the brain's interstitium or from passing between the plasma and CSF.

PATHOPHYSIOLOGY OF CEREBRAL ISCHEMIA

Critical CBF Thresholds

The brain has a high demand for metabolic substrate (oxygen and glucose) and is quite vulnerable to interruptions in metabolic substrate supply. With declining CBF, and therefore oxygen supply, neuronal function deteriorates in a progressive fashion (Figure 8-9).[105,107] Normal CBF typically provides a substantial reserve in energy substrate delivery; it is not until CBF reaches 20 mL/100 g/min that EEG evidence of ischemia manifests. Further reduction in CBF to 15 mL/100 g/min results in complete suppression of cortical electrical activity as indicated by an isoelectric EEG. When CBF reaches about 6 mL/100 g/min, indications of potentially irreversible membrane failure occur (elevated extracellular K^+, loss of the direct cortical response).[105,108] Between 15 and 6 mL/100 g/min there is a progressive decrease in energy supply that will result in membrane failure and death, although the time course is hours rather than minutes.[107] Regions of brain within this intermediate flow range, termed the ischemic penumbra, reflect tissue with potentially reversible dysfunction that will progress to neuronal death if flow is not restored.[105,109]

Cerebral ischemia can occur with complete global ischemia (e.g., cardiac arrest) or incomplete ischemia from either occlusion of a major cerebral vessel or severe hypotension. With the former, there is cessation of CBF and there is a rapid reduction in cellular ATP.[110] In focal ischemia, the severity of ischemia is greatest within the core of the ischemic lesion with rapid neuronal injury. Surrounding the core is a region (penumbra) in which ischemia is severe enough to abolish electrical activity but in which the neurons are viable for short periods of time (from minutes to 2-3 hours). From a clinician's perspective, the difference is that incomplete ischemia can allow adequate ATP generation to stave off the catastrophic irreversible membrane failure that occurs within minutes during normothermic complete cerebral ischemia (Figure 8-10).[110,111] The duration of viability of the penumbra is dependent upon residual CBF and the extent of collateral circulation. Importantly, autoregulation is abolished in the penumbra and collateral perfusion is critically dependent upon cerebral perfusion pressure. Hypotension can dramatically increase the size of the penumbra, whereas modest increases in perfusion pressure can reduce the extent of injury (see Figure 8-10).

Energy Failure and Excitotoxicity

Central to the pathophysiology of cerebral ischemia is energy failure.[112,113] ATP supply is critical for maintaining normal membrane ion gradients within neurons. Energy failure therefore is rapidly associated with membrane depolarization and influx of Na^+ and Ca^{2+} with subsequent activation of voltage-gated Ca^{2+} channels and increases in intracellular Ca^{2+}. Depolarization also results in release of massive quantities of excitatory neurotransmitter release, particularly glutamate, into the synaptic cleft from presynaptic terminals.[114] Postsynaptic activation of glutamate receptors then further augments Na^+ and Ca^{2+} influx (Figure 8-11). Activation of metabotropic glutamate receptors leads to the release of stored Ca^{2+} from endoplasmic reticulum via IP_3 receptors. Ionic influx is accompanied by water and results in neuronal swelling. Neuronal injury that is initiated by excessive glutamate receptor activation is referred to as excitotoxicity.

Calcium ion (Ca^{2+}), a ubiquitous second messenger, is required for the activation of a number of enzyme systems. The rapid, uncontrolled increase in cytosolic Ca^{2+}

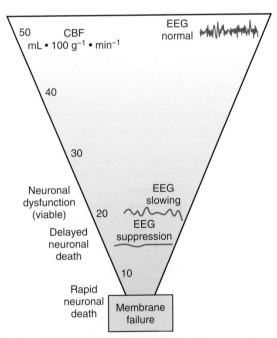

Figure 8-9 Relationships between cerebral blood flow (CBF), electrophysiologic dysfunction, and neuronal viability. As CBF decreases, there is a progressive deterioration in electrophysiologic function, which is perhaps best demonstrated with electroencephalogram (EEG) recordings. Evidence of electrophysiologic dysfunction manifests in the form of EEG slowing at CBF < 20 mL/100 g/min. CBF in the range of 6 to 12 mL/100 g/min provides insufficient metabolic substrate delivery to support electrophysiologic function (EEG suppression), but is adequate to prevent immediate membrane failure and neuronal death. When CBF is reduced below 6 mL/100 g/min, irreversible and rapid membrane failure ensues, resulting in neuronal death.

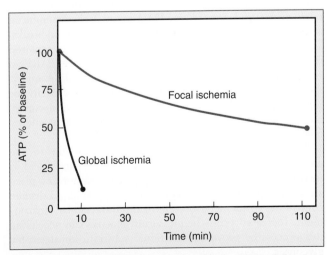

Figure 8-10 Relative rates of ischemic energy failure. Energy failure rates following experimental global (decapitation) and focal ischemia (middle cerebral artery occlusion). In the presence of residual cerebral blood flow, energy failure is substantially delayed. *ATP*, Adenosine triphosphate.

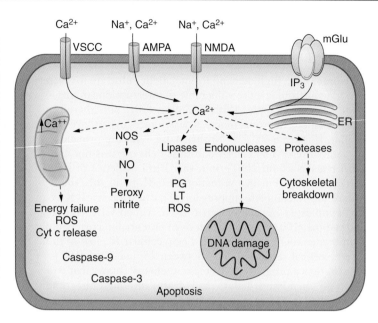

Figure 8-11 Pathophysiology of neuronal energy failure. During ischemia, inadequate neuronal adenosine triphosphate (ATP) supply, required for maintenance of ionic gradients, which leads to presynaptic depolarization and the subsequent excessive unregulated release of excitatory neurotransmitters, especially glutamate. Activation of voltage-gated Ca^{2+} channels and excessive stimulation of ligand-gated ion channels result in rapid Ca^{2+} entry. Stimulation of metabotropic glutamate receptors (mGlu) generates inositol 1,4,5-triphosphate (IP_3), which causes endoplasmic reticulum (ER) release of Ca^{2+}. Activation of the α-amino-3-hydroxy-5-methyl-4-isoaxolepropionic acid (AMPA) receptor-gated subtype of glutamate receptors also permits excessive entry of Na^+. Excessive free Ca^{2+} results in activation of numerous enzymes detrimental to the neuron: protease activation causes cytoskeleton breakdown; lipases damage plasma membrane lipids and release prostaglandins (PG), leukotrienes (LT), and reactive oxygen species (ROS); activation of nitric oxide synthase (NOS) leads to formation of nitric oxide (NO) and the generation of peroxynitrite, a highly reactive free radical; and activated endonucleases cleave DNA. Mitochondrial injury leads to energy failure, ROS, and mitochondrial release of cytochrome c (Cyt c); the latter is one of the means by which neuronal apoptosis is initiated. *LT,* Leukotrienes; *NMDA,* N-methyl-D-aspartate; *PG,* prostaglandins; *VGCC,* voltage-gated Ca^{2+} channels.

concentration initiates a number of cellular processes that contribute to neuronal injury (see Figure 8-11). Activated proteases degrade cytoskeletal proteins[115] and other proteins. Lipases hydrolyze cellular lipids and thus cause damage to cellular membranes. Phospholipase A_2 releases fatty acids such as arachidonic acid[116] that is metabolized into prostaglandins and leukotrienes by cyclo-oxygenase and lipoxygenase with the generation of superoxide free radicals. The latter, in combination with other free radicals generated in response to mitochondrial injury, can lead to lipid peroxidation and membrane injury. Prostaglandins and leukotrienes evoke an inflammatory response and are powerful chemotactic agents. Platelet activation within cerebral microvessels as well as inflammatory cell infiltration into damaged areas aggravates ischemic injury through microvasculature occlusion.

DNA damage is also an important consequence of ischemic neuronal injury[117] (see Figure 8-11). Generation of free radicals from arachidonic acid metabolism, from injured mitochondria and from the production of peroxynitrite (from nitric oxide), leads to oxidative DNA injury. Ischemia induced activation of endonucleases also produces DNA strand breaks. Under normal circumstances, these breaks are repaired through activation of poly-ADP ribose-polymerase (PARP), a DNA repair enzyme. However, with excessive DNA injury, depletion of the PARP substrate NAD limits the capacity for DNA repair.[117] NAD is an important co-enzyme in energy metabolism and its depletion further exacerbates energy failure.

Lactate formation is an additional component to the pathophysiologic process of energy failure. Lactic acid is formed as a result of anaerobic glycolysis that takes place after the failure of oxygen supply. The associated pH decline contributes to the deterioration of the intracellular environment. Increased pre-ischemic serum glucose can accelerate this process by providing additional substrate for anaerobic glycolysis.[118]

Collectively, the simultaneous and unregulated activation of a number of cellular pathways overwhelms reparative and restorative processes and ultimately leads to neuronal death.

Nature of Neuronal Death

Neuronal death that occurs as a result of ischemia can be either necrotic or apoptotic. The excitotoxic injury described above, characteristically leads to necrosis, which is associated with local inflammatory cell infiltration and considerable "collateral damage." Neuronal necrosis mediated by excitotoxic injury is characterized by rapid cellular swelling, condensation and pyknosis of the nucleus, and swelling of the mitochondria and endoplasmic reticulum.

Neuronal apoptosis, a form of programmed cell death or cellular suicide, has also been demonstrated in a variety of cerebral ischemia models. Apoptosis is characterized by chromatin condensation, involution of the cell membrane, swelling of mitochondria and cellular shrinkage. In the later stages of apoptosis, neurons fragment into apoptotic bodies that are then cleared from the brain. The absence of a substantial inflammatory response to apoptotic death limits injury to surrounding neurons that have survived the initial insult.

Neuronal injury in response to ischemia cannot easily be divided into necrosis or apoptosis, but encompasses a spectrum in which some neurons undergo necrosis or apoptosis while others undergo cell death that has features of both necrosis and apoptosis.

Timing of Neuronal Death

Initial concepts of ischemia-induced neuronal death were restricted to the time of ischemia and early reperfusion period. More recent data indicate that post-ischemic neuronal injury is a dynamic process extending for a long period after the initiating ischemic insult.[119-121] Delayed neuronal death, which was first demonstrated in models of global cerebral ischemia, also occurs following focal ischemia. The extent of delayed neuronal death depends upon the severity of the ischemic insult. With severe ischemia, most neurons undergo rapid death. With more moderate insults, neurons that survive the initial insult undergo delayed death, which contributes to the gradual expansion of cerebral infarction after focal ischemia.

Evidence of cerebral inflammation, which theoretically can contribute to further injury, has been demonstrated even 6 to 8 months after the primary ischemic event.

KEY POINTS

- The brain has a high metabolic rate; it receives about 15% of the cardiac output, or about 50 mL/100 g/min.
- About 60% of brain energy consumption supports electrophysiologic functions; the remainder supports cellular homeostasis.
- CBF is tightly coupled to local cerebral metabolism. When cerebral activity in a particular brain region increases, a corresponding increase in blood flow to that region occurs. Conversely, reduced activity/metabolism leads to reduced blood flow.
- CBF is autoregulated, such that flow is normally constant over a range of mean arterial pressure of 70 to 150 mm Hg. CBF is pressure passive below or above the limits of autoregulation.
- Autoregulation can be impaired or absent following insults such as traumatic brain injury or subarachnoid hemorrhage. In such cases, CBF is pressure passive and can be reduced despite normal mean arterial pressure.
- CBF is also under chemical regulation: it varies directly with arterial carbon dioxide tension ($PaCO_2$) in the range of 25 to 70 mm Hg and inversely with PaO_2 below 60 mm Hg.
- Systemic vasodilators (nitroglycerin, nitroprusside, hydralazine, calcium channel blockers) cause cerebral vasodilation and, depending upon the MAP, can increase CBF.
- Vasopressors such as phenylephrine, norepinephrine, ephedrine, and dopamine do not have significant direct cerebrovascular effects.
- Volatile anesthetics suppress CMR and, with the exception of halothane, can produce EEG burst suppression.
- Volatile agents have dose-dependent effects on CBF. At subanesthetic doses, reduced metabolic rate offsets direct cerebral vasodilation and CBF is not significantly altered. Above minimum alveolar concentration, direct cerebral vasodilation increases CBF and volume.
- Barbiturates, etomidate, and propofol decrease CMR and can produce EEG burst suppression. Flow and metabolism coupling is preserved such that CBF decreases. Opioids and benzodiazepines effect minor decreases in CBF and metabolism. Ketamine can significantly increase metabolic rate with a corresponding increase in blood flow.
- Brain stores of metabolic substrate are limited; therefore, the brain is exquisitely sensitive to reductions in blood flow. Severe reductions in CBF (<6 mL/100 g/min) lead to neuronal death within minutes. Ischemic injury is characterized by cell death due to early excitotoxicity and delayed apoptosis.

Key References

Maekawa T, Tommasino C, Shapiro HM, Keifer-Goodman J, Kohlenberger RW. Local cerebral blood flow and glucose utilization during isoflurane anesthesia in the rat. *Anesthesiology.* 1986;65:144-151. This study demonstrated the effect of incremental dose administration of isoflurane on CBF and cerebral glucose uptake in 27 brain segments using quantitative autoradiography in normal rats. Specifically, it demonstrated the dose-related, heterogenous effect of increasing CBF and decreasing $CMRO_2$. (Ref. 91)

Michenfelder JD. *Anesthesia and the Brain: Clinical, Functional, Metabolic, and Vascular Correlates.* New York: Churchill Livingstone; 1989. A classic CNS physiology text that summarizes the functional, metabolic, and vascular sequelae of various physiologic and pharmacologic cerebral manipulations. (Ref. 3)

Michenfelder JD. The interdependency of cerebral functional and metabolic effects following massive doses of thiopental in the dog. *Anesthesiology.* 1974;41:231-236. This early investigation helped confirm the hypothesis that anesthetics act primarily on cerebral function rather than on metabolism. This study demonstrated two separate components of CMR: (1) the part associated with electrophysiologic function and (2) the basal component of CMR that is independent of function and unaffected by anesthetic administration. (Ref. 14)

Patel PM, Drummond JC. Cerebral physiology and the effects of anesthetics and techniques. In: Miller RD, ed. *Miller's Anesthesia.* Vol 1. Philadelphia: Elsevier, Churchill Livingstone; 2005. Provides synthesis of the available literature related to CNS physiology and anesthetic effects as well as a more comprehensive discussion and evaluation of specific studies. (Ref. 78)

Siesjo BK. Pathophysiology and treatment of focal cerebral ischemia. Part I: Pathophysiology. *J Neurosurg.* 1992;77:169-184. A review of the pathophysiology of energy failure, specifically the effects on intracellular and extracellular pH, ion homeostasis, and structural integrity. (Ref. 112)

Siesjo BK. Pathophysiology and treatment of focal cerebral ischemia. Part II: Mechanisms of damage and treatment. *J Neurosurg.* 1992;77:337-354. This review outlines and discusses the cellular and molecular mechanisms responsible for brain injury following neuronal energy failure. (Ref. 113)

References

1. Krabbe-Hartkamp MJ, van der Grond J, de Leeuw FE, et al. Circle of Willis: morphologic variation on three-dimensional time-of-flight MR angiograms. *Radiology.* 1998;207(1):103-111.
2. Alpers BJ, Berry RG, Paddison RM. Anatomical studies of the circle of Willis in normal brain. *AMA Arch Neurol Psychiatry.* 1959;81: 409-418.
3. Michenfelder JD. *Anesthesia and the Brain: Clinical, Functional, Metabolic, and Vascular Correlates.* New York: Churchill Livingstone; 1988.
4. Nemoto EM, Klementavicius R, Melick JA, Yonas H. Suppression of cerebral metabolic rate for oxygen ($CMRO_2$) by mild hypothermia compared with thiopental. *J Neurosurg Anesthesiol.* 1996;8(1): 52-59.
5. Klementavicius R, Nemoto EM, Yonas H. The Q10 ratio for basal cerebral metabolic rate for oxygen in rats. *J Neurosurg.* 1996;85(3): 482-487.
6. Miyauchi Y, Sakabe T, Maekawa T, Ishikawa T, Takeshita H. Responses of EEG, cerebral oxygen consumption and blood flow to peripheral nerve stimulation during thiopentone anaesthesia in the dog. *Can Anaesth Soc J.* 1985;32(5):491-498.
7. Frostig RD, Lieke EE, Ts'o DY, Grinvald A. Cortical functional architecture and local coupling between neuronal activity and the microcirculation revealed by in vivo high-resolution optical imaging of intrinsic signals. *Proc Natl Acad Sci U S A.* 1990;87(16):6082-6086.
8. Lou HC, Edvinsson L, MacKenzie ET. The concept of coupling blood flow to brain function: revision required? *Ann Neurol.* 1987; 22(3):289-297.
9. Hyder F, Behar KL, Martin MA, Blamire AM, Shulman RG. Dynamic magnetic resonance imaging of the rat brain during forepaw stimulation. *J Cereb Blood Flow Metab.* 1994;14(4):649-655.
10. Perlmutter JS, Lich LL, Margenau W, Buchholz S. PET measured evoked cerebral blood flow responses in an awake monkey. *J Cereb Blood Flow Metab.* 1991;11(2):229-235.

11. Ayata C, Ma J, Meng W, Huang P, Moskowitz MA. L-NA-sensitive rCBF augmentation during vibrissal stimulation in type III nitric oxide synthase mutant mice. *J Cereb Blood Flow Metab.* 1996;16(4): 539-541.

12. Cholet N, Seylaz J, Lacombe P, Bonvento G. Local uncoupling of the cerebrovascular and metabolic responses to somatosensory stimulation after neuronal nitric oxide synthase inhibition. *J Cereb Blood Flow Metab.* 1997;17(11):1191-1201.

13. Bonvento G, Lacombe P, Seylaz J. Effects of electrical stimulation of the dorsal raphe nucleus on local cerebral blood flow in the rat. *J Cereb Blood Flow Metab.* 1989;9(3):251-255.

14. Michenfelder JD. The interdependency of cerebral functional and metabolic effects following massive doses of thiopental in the dog. *Anesthesiology.* 1974;41(3):231-236.

15. Newberg LA, Milde JH, Michenfelder JD. The cerebral metabolic effects of isoflurane at and above concentrations that suppress cortical electrical activity. *Anesthesiology.* 1983;59(1):23-28.

16. Scheller MS, Tateishi A, Drummond JC, Zornow MH. The effects of sevoflurane on cerebral blood flow, cerebral metabolic rate for oxygen, intracranial pressure, and the electroencephalogram are similar to those of isoflurane in the rabbit. *Anesthesiology.* 1988;68(4): 548-551.

17. Rampil IJ, Laster M, Dwyer RC, Taheri S, Eger EI II. No EEG evidence of acute tolerance to desflurane in swine. *Anesthesiology.* 1991;74(5):889-892.

18. Bruhn J, Bouillon TW, Shafer SL. Onset of propofol-induced burst suppression may be correctly detected as deepening of anaesthesia by approximate entropy but not by bispectral index. *Br J Anaesth.* 2001;87(3):505-507.

19. Milde LN, Milde JH, Michenfelder JD. Cerebral functional, metabolic, and hemodynamic effects of etomidate in dogs. *Anesthesiology.* 1985;63(4):371-377.

20. Busija DW, Leffler CW, Pourcyrous M. Hyperthermia increases cerebral metabolic rate and blood flow in neonatal pigs. *Am J Physiol.* 1988;255(2 Pt 2):H343-H346.

21. Smith AL, Wollman H. Cerebral blood flow and metabolism: effects of anesthetic drugs and techniques. *Anesthesiology.* 1972; 36(4):378-400.

22. Sato M, Pawlik G, Heiss WD. Comparative studies of regional CNS blood flow autoregulation and responses to CO_2 in the cat. Effects of altering arterial blood pressure and $PaCO_2$ on rCBF of cerebrum, cerebellum, and spinal cord. *Stroke.* 1984;15(1):91-97.

23. Koehler RC, Traystman RJ. Bicarbonate ion modulation of cerebral blood flow during hypoxia and hypercapnia. *Am J Physiol.* 1982; 243(1):H33-H40.

24. Muizelaar JP, van der Poel HG, Li ZC, Kontos HA, Levasseur JE. Pial arteriolar vessel diameter and CO_2 reactivity during prolonged hyperventilation in the rabbit. *J Neurosurg.* 1988;69(6):923-927.

25. Raichle ME, Posner JB, Plum F. Cerebral blood flow during and after hyperventilation. *Arch Neurol.* 1970;23(5):394-403.

26. Hudetz AG, Shen H, Kampine JP. Nitric oxide from neuronal NOS plays critical role in cerebral capillary flow response to hypoxia. *Am J Physiol.* 1998;274(3 Pt 2):H982-H989.

27. Golanov EV, Reis DJ. Contribution of oxygen-sensitive neurons of the rostral ventrolateral medulla to hypoxic cerebral vasodilatation in the rat. *J Physiol.* 1996;495(Pt 1):201-216.

28. Drummond JC. The lower limit of autoregulation: time to revise our thinking? *Anesthesiology.* 1997;86(6):1431-1433.

29. Strandgaard S. Autoregulation of cerebral blood flow in hypertensive patients. The modifying influence of prolonged antihypertensive treatment on the tolerance to acute, drug-induced hypotension. *Circulation.* 1976;53(4):720-727.

30. Waldemar G, Schmidt JF, Andersen AR, Vorstrup S, Ibsen H, Paulson OB. Angiotensin converting enzyme inhibition and cerebral blood flow autoregulation in normotensive and hypertensive man. *J Hypertens.* 1989;7(3):229-235.

31. Larsen FS, Olsen KS, Hansen BA, Paulson OB, Knudsen GM. Transcranial Doppler is valid for determination of the lower limit of cerebral blood flow autoregulation. *Stroke.* 1994;25(10):1985-1988.

32. Olsen KS, Svendsen LB, Larsen FS, Paulson OB. Effect of labetalol on cerebral blood flow, oxygen metabolism and autoregulation in healthy humans. *Br J Anaesth.* 1995;75(1):51-54.

33. Olsen KS, Svendsen LB, Larsen FS. Validation of transcranial near-infrared spectroscopy for evaluation of cerebral blood flow autoregulation. *J Neurosurg Anesthesiol.* 1996;8(4):280-285.

34. Greenfield JC Jr., Rembert JC, Tindall GT. Transient changes in cerebral vascular resistance during the Valsalva maneuver in man. *Stroke.* 1984;15(1):76-79.

35. Branston NM. Neurogenic control of the cerebral circulation. *Cerebrovasc Brain Metab Rev.* 1995;7(4):338-349.

36. Dahl E. The innervation of the cerebral arteries. *J Anat.* 1973;115(Pt 1):53-63.

37. Hara H, Zhang QJ, Kuroyanagi T, Kobayashi S. Parasympathetic cerebrovascular innervation: an anterograde tracing from the sphenopalatine ganglion in the rat. *Neurosurgery.* 1993;32(5):822-827; discussion 827.

38. Iadecola C, Reis DJ. Continuous monitoring of cerebrocortical blood flow during stimulation of the cerebellar fastigial nucleus: a study by laser-Doppler flowmetry. *J Cereb Blood Flow Metab.* 1990;10(5):608-617.

39. Tuor UI. Local distribution of the effects of sympathetic stimulation on cerebral blood flow in the rat. *Brain Res.* 1990;529(1-2):224-231.

40. Underwood MD, Bakalian MJ, Arango V, Smith RW, Mann JJ. Regulation of cortical blood flow by the dorsal raphe nucleus: topographic organization of cerebrovascular regulatory regions. *J Cereb Blood Flow Metab.* 1992;12(4):664-673.

41. Hara H, Jansen I, Ekman R, et al. Acetylcholine and vasoactive intestinal peptide in cerebral blood vessels: effect of extirpation of the sphenopalatine ganglion. *J Cereb Blood Flow Metab.* 1989;9(2): 204-211.

42. Busija DW. Sympathetic nerves reduce cerebral blood flow during hypoxia in awake rabbits. *Am J Physiol.* 1984;247(3 Pt 2):H446-H451.

43. Fitch W, MacKenzie ET, Harper AM. Effects of decreasing arterial blood pressure on cerebral blood flow in the baboon. Influence of the sympathetic nervous system. *Circ Res.* 1975;37(5):550-557.

44. Tuor UI. Acute hypertension and sympathetic stimulation: local heterogeneous changes in cerebral blood flow. *Am J Physiol.* 1992;263(2 Pt 2):H511-H518.

45. Reis DJ, Berger SB, Underwood MD, Khayata M. Electrical stimulation of cerebellar fastigial nucleus reduces ischemic infarction elicited by middle cerebral artery occlusion in rat. *J Cereb Blood Flow Metab.* 1991;11(5):810-818.

46. Koketsu N, Moskowitz MA, Kontos HA, Yokota M, Shimizu T. Chronic parasympathetic sectioning decreases regional cerebral blood flow during hemorrhagic hypotension and increases infarct size after middle cerebral artery occlusion in spontaneously hypertensive rats. *J Cereb Blood Flow Metab.* 1992;12(4):613-620.

47. Shibata M, Einhaus S, Schweitzer JB, Zuckerman S, Leffler CW. Cerebral blood flow decreased by adrenergic stimulation of cerebral vessels in anesthetized newborn pigs with traumatic brain injury. *J Neurosurg.* 1993;79(5):696-704.

48. Johansson BB, Auer LM. Neurogenic modification of the vulnerability of the blood-brain barrier during acute hypertension in conscious rats. *Acta Physiol Scand.* 1983;117(4):507-511.

49. Paulson OB, Strandgaard S, Edvinsson L. Cerebral autoregulation. *Cerebrovasc Brain Metab.* 1990;2(2):161-192.

50. Prabhakar H, Jain V, Rath GP, Bithal PK, Dash HH. Stellate ganglion block as alternative to intrathecal papaverine in relieving vasospasm due to subarachnoid hemorrhage. *Anesth Analg.* 2007;104(5): 1311-1312.

51. Morita Y, Hardebo JE, Bouskela E. Influence of cerebrovascular parasympathetic nerves on resting cerebral blood flow, spontaneous vasomotion, autoregulation, hypercapnic vasodilation and sympathetic vasoconstriction. *J Auton Nerv Syst.* 1994;49(Suppl):S9-14.

52. Harrison MJ. Influence of haematocrit in the cerebral circulation. *Cerebrovasc Brain Metab Rev.* 1989;1(1):55-67.

53. Thomas DJ, Marshall J, Russell RW, et al. Effect of haematocrit on cerebral blood-flow in man. *Lancet.* 1977;2(8045):941-943.

54. Cole DJ, Drummond JC, Shapiro HM, Hertzog RE, Brauer FS. The effect of hypervolemic hemodilution with and without hypertension on cerebral blood flow following middle cerebral artery occlusion in rats anesthetized with isoflurane. *Anesthesiology.* 1989; 71(4):580-585.

55. Korosue K, Ishida K, Matsuoka H, Nagao T, Tamaki N, Matsumoto S. Clinical, hemodynamic, and hemorheological effects of isovolemic hemodilution in acute cerebral infarction. *Neurosurgery.* 1988; 23(2):148-153.

56. Kee DB Jr., Wood JH. Rheology of the cerebral circulation. *Neurosurgery.* 1984;15(1):125-131.

57. Lee SH, Heros RC, Mullan JC, Korosue K. Optimum degree of hemodilution for brain protection in a canine model of focal cerebral ischemia. *J Neurosurg.* 1994;80(3):469-475.

58. Maekawa T, McDowall DG, Okuda Y. Brain-surface oxygen tension and cerebral cortical blood flow during hemorrhagic and drug-induced hypotension in the cat. *Anesthesiology.* 1979;51(4):313-320.

59. Akopov S, Simonian N. Comparison of isradipine and enalapril effects on regional carotid circulation in patients with hypertension with unilateral carotid artery stenosis. *J Cardiovasc Pharmacol.* 1997;30(5):562-570.

60. Olesen J. The effect of intracarotid epinephrine, norepinephrine, and angiotensin on the regional cerebral blood flow in man. *Neurology.* 1972;22(9):978-987.

61. MacKenzie ET, McCulloch J, O'Kean M, Pickard JD, Harper AM. Cerebral circulation and norepinephrine: relevance of the blood-brain barrier. *Am J Physiol.* 1976;231(2):483-488.

62. Rogers AT, Stump DA, Gravlee GP, et al. Response of cerebral blood flow to phenylephrine infusion during hypothermic cardiopulmonary bypass: influence of $PaCO_2$ management. *Anesthesiology.* 1988;69(4):547-551.

63. Nemoto EM, Klementavicius R, Melick JA, Yonas H. Norepinephrine activation of basal cerebral metabolic rate for oxygen ($CMRO_2$) during hypothermia in rats. *Anesth Analg.* 1996;83(6):1262-1267.

64. Berntman L, Dahlgren N, Siesjo BK. Influence of intravenously administered catecholamines on cerebral oxygen consumption and blood flow in the rat. *Acta Physiol Scand.* 1978;104(1):101-108.

65. Artru AA, Nugent M, Michenfelder JD. Anesthetics affect the cerebral metabolic response to circulatory catecholamines. *J Neurochem.* 1981;36(6):1941-1946.

66. Abdul-Rahman A, Dahlgren N, Johansson BB, Siesjo BK. Increase in local cerebral blood flow induced by circulating adrenaline: involvement of blood-brain barrier dysfunction. *Acta Physiol Scand.* 1979;107(3):227-232.

67. Sercombe R, Aubineau P, Edvinsson L, Mamo H, Owman C, Seylaz J. Pharmacological evidence in vitro and in vivo for functional beta 1 receptors in the cerebral circulation. *Pflugers Arch.* 1977;368(3):241-244.

68. Madsen PL, Vorstrup S, Schmidt JF, Paulson OB. Effect of acute and prolonged treatment with propranolol on cerebral blood flow and cerebral oxygen metabolism in healthy volunteers. *Eur J Clin Pharmacol.* 1990;39(3):295-297.

69. Schroeder T, Schierbeck J, Howardy P, Knudsen L, Skafte-Holm P, Gefke K. Effect of labetalol on cerebral blood flow and middle cerebral arterial flow velocity in healthy volunteers. *Neurol Res.* 1991;13(1):10-12.

70. Tuor UI, Edvinsson L, McCulloch J. Catecholamines and the relationship between cerebral blood flow and glucose use. *Am J Physiol.* 1986;251(4 Pt 2):H824-H833.

71. von Essen C, Zervas NT, Brown DR, Koltun WA, Pickren KS. Local cerebral blood flow in the dog during intravenous infusion of dopamine. *Surg Neurol.* 1980;13(3):181-188.

72. Bandres J, Yao L, Nemoto EM, Yonas H, Darby J. Effects of dobutamine and dopamine on whole brain blood flow and metabolism in unanesthetized monkeys. *J Neurosurg Anesthesiol.* 1992;4(4):250-256.

73. Stephan H, Sonntag H, Schenk HD, Kohlhausen S. Effect of Disoprivan (propofol) on the circulation and oxygen consumption of the brain and CO_2 reactivity of brain vessels in the human. *Anaesthesist.* 1987;36(2):60-65.

74. Renou AM, Vernhiet J, Macrez P, et al. Cerebral blood flow and metabolism during etomidate anaesthesia in man. *Br J Anaesth.* 1978;50(10):1047-1051.

75. Lam AM, Mayberg TS. Opioids and cerebral blood flow velocity. *Anesthesiology.* 1993;79(3):616-617.

76. Albrecht RF, Miletich DJ, Rosenberg R, Zahed B. Cerebral blood flow and metabolic changes from induction to onset of anesthesia with halothane or pentobarbital. *Anesthesiology.* 1977;47(3):252-256.

77. Cotev S, Shalit MN. Effects on diazepam on cerebral blood flow and oxygen uptake after head injury. *Anesthesiology.* 1975;43(1):117-122.

78. Patel PM, Drummond JC. Cerebral physiology and the effects of anesthetics and techniques. In: Miller RD, ed. *Miller's Anesthesia.* Vol 1. Philadelphia: Elsevier, Churchill Livingstone; 2005.

79. Hoehner PJ, Whitson JT, Kirsch JR, Traystman RJ. Effect of intracarotid and intraventricular morphine on regional cerebral blood flow and metabolism in pentobarbital-anesthetized dogs. *Anesth Analg.* 1993;76(2):266-273.

80. Vollenweider FX, Leenders KL, Oye I, Hell D, Angst J. Differential psychopathology and patterns of cerebral glucose utilisation produced by (S)- and (R)-ketamine in healthy volunteers using positron emission tomography (PET). *Eur Neuropsychopharmacol.* 1997;7(1):25-38.

81. Strebel S, Kaufmann M, Maitre L, Schaefer HG. Effects of ketamine on cerebral blood flow velocity in humans. Influence of pretreatment with midazolam or esmolol. *Anaesthesia.* 1995;50(3):223-228.

82. Takeshita H, Okuda Y, Sari A. The effects of ketamine on cerebral circulation and metabolism in man. *Anesthesiology.* 1972;36(1):69-75.

83. Hougaard K, Hansen A, Brodersen P. The effect of ketamine on regional cerebral blood flow in man. *Anesthesiology.* 1974;41(6):562-567.

84. Langsjo JW, Maksimow A, Salmi E, et al. S-ketamine anesthesia increases cerebral blood flow in excess of the metabolic needs in humans. *Anesthesiology.* 2005;103(2):258-268.

85. Bar-Joseph G, Guilburd Y, Tamir A, Guilburd JN. Effectiveness of ketamine in decreasing intracranial pressure in children with intracranial hypertension. *J Neurosurg Pediatr.* 2009;4(1):40-46.

86. Newberg LA, Milde JH, Michenfelder JD. The cerebral metabolic effects of isoflurane at and above concentrations that suppress cortical electrical activity. *Anesthesiology.* 1983;59:23-28.

87. Michenfelder JD, Milde JH. Influence of anesthetics on metabolic, functional and pathological responses to regional cerebral ischemia. *Stroke.* 1975;6:405-410.

88. Michenfelder JD, Sundt TM, Fode N, Sharbrough FW. Isoflurane when compared to enflurane and halothane decreases the frequency of cerebral ischemia during carotid endarterectomy. *Anesthesiology.* 1987;67(3):336-340.

89. Todd MM, Drummond JC. A comparison of the cerebrovascular and metabolic effects of halothane and isoflurane in the cat. *Anesthesiology.* 1984;60(4):276-282.

90. Lutz LJ, Milde JH, Milde LN. The cerebral functional, metabolic, and hemodynamic effects of desflurane in dogs. *Anesthesiology.* 1990;73(1):125-131.

91. Maekawa T, Tommasino C, Shapiro HM, Keifer-Goodman J, Kohlenberger RW. Local cerebral blood flow and glucose utilization during isoflurane anesthesia in the rat. *Anesthesiology.* 1986;65:144-151.

92. Drummond JC, Todd MM, Scheller MS, Shapiro HM. A comparison of the direct cerebral vasodilating potencies of halothane and isoflurane in the New Zealand white rabbit. *Anesthesiology.* 1986;65:462-467.

93. Matta BF, Mayberg TS, Lam AM. Direct cerebrovasodilatory effects of halothane, isoflurane and desflurane during propofol-induced isoelectric electroencephalogram in humans. *Anesthesiology.* 1995;83:980-985.

94. Madsen JB, Cold GE, Hansen ES, Bardrum B. The effect of isoflurane on cerebral blood flow and metabolism in humans during craniotomy for small supratentorial cerebral tumors. *Anesthesiology.* 1987;66:332.

95. Ornstein E, Young WL, Ostapkovich N, et al. Comparative effects of desflurane and isoflurane on cerebral blood flow [abstract]. *Anesthesiology.* 1991;75:A209.

96. Drummond JC, Todd MM. The response of the feline cerebral circulation to $PaCO_2$ during anesthesia with isoflurane and halothane and during sedation with nitrous oxide. *Anesthesiology.* 1985;62(3):268-273.

97. Cho S, Fujigaki T, Uchiyama Y, Fukusaki M, Shibata O, Sumikawa K. Effects of sevoflurane with and without nitrous oxide on human cerebral circulation. *Anesthesiology.* 1996;85:755-760.

98. Morita H, Bleyaert AL, Stezoski SW, Nemoto EM. The effect of halothane anesthesia on cerebral blood flow, autoregulation and cerebral metabolism of oxygen and glucose [abstract]. Abstracts of the Annual Meeting of the American Society of Anesthesiologists, 1974;63-64.

99. Strebel S, Kaufmann M, Anselmi L, Schaefer HG. Nitrous oxide is a potent cerebrovasodilator in humans when added to isoflurane. A transcranial Doppler study. *Acta Anaesthesiol Scand.* 1995;39(5):653-658.

100. Marchal G, Rioux P, Petit-Taboue MC, et al. Regional cerebral oxygen consumption, blood flow, and blood volume in healthy human aging. *Arch Neurol*. 1992;49(10):1013-1020.

101. Meyer JS, Terayama Y, Takashima S. Cerebral circulation in the elderly. *Cerebrovasc Brain Metab Rev*. 1993;5(2):122-146.

102. Fjell AM, Walhovd KB. Structural brain changes in aging: courses, causes and cognitive consequences. *Rev Neurosci*. 2010;21(3):187-221.

103. Cutler RW, Spertell RB. Cerebrospinal fluid: a selective review. *Ann Neurol*. 1982;11(1):1-10.

104. Praetorius J. Water and solute secretion by the choroid plexus. *Pflugers Arch*. 2007;454(1):1-18.

105. Astrup J, Symon L, Branston NM, Lassen NA. Cortical evoked potential and extracellular K+ and H+ at critical levels of brain ischemia. *Stroke*. 1977;8(1):51-57.

106. Branston NM, Symon L, Crockard HA, Pasztor E. Relationship between the cortical evoked potential and local cortical blood flow following acute middle cerebral artery occlusion in the baboon. *Exp Neurol*. 1974;45(2):195-208.

107. Jones TH, Morawetz RB, Crowell RM, et al. Thresholds of focal cerebral ischemia in awake monkeys. *J Neurosurg*. 1981;54(6):773-782.

108. Carter LP, Yamagata S, Erspamer R. Time limits of reversible cortical ischemia. *Neurosurgery*. 1983;12(6):620-623.

109. Hossmann KA. Viability thresholds and the penumbra of focal ischemia. *Ann Neurol*. 1994;36(4):557-565.

110. Michenfelder JD, Theye RA. The effects of anesthesia and hypothermia on canine cerebral ATP and lactate during anoxia produced by decapitation. *Anesthesiology*. 1970;33(4):430-439.

111. Michenfelder JD, Sundt TM Jr. Cerebral ATP and lactate levels in the squirrel monkey following occlusion of the middle cerebral artery. *Stroke*. 1971;2(4):319-326.

112. Siesjo BK. Pathophysiology and treatment of focal cerebral ischemia. Part I: Pathophysiology. *J Neurosurg*. 1992;77(2):169-184.

113. Siesjo BK. Pathophysiology and treatment of focal cerebral ischemia. Part II: Mechanisms of damage and treatment. *J Neurosurg*. 1992;77:337-354.

114. Benveniste H, Drejer J, Schousboe A, Diemer NH. Elevation of the extracellular concentrations of glutamate and aspartate in rat hippocampus during transient cerebral ischemia monitored by intracerebral microdialysis. *J Neurochem*. 1984;43(5):1369-1374.

115. Furukawa K, Fu W, Li Y, Witke W, Kwiatkowski DJ, Mattson MP. The actin-severing protein gelsolin modulates calcium channel and NMDA receptor activities and vulnerability to excitotoxicity in hippocampal neurons. *J Neurosci*. 1997;17(21):8178-8186.

116. Chen ST, Hsu CY, Hogan EL, Halushka PV, Linet OI, Yatsu FM. Thromboxane, prostacyclin, and leukotrienes in cerebral ischemia. *Neurology*. 1986;36(4):466-470.

117. Pieper AA, Verma A, Zhang J, Snyder SH. Poly (ADP-ribose) polymerase, nitric oxide and cell death. *Trends Pharmacol Sci*. 1999;20(4):171-181.

118. Chopp M, Welch KM, Tidwell CD, Helpern JA. Global cerebral ischemia and intracellular pH during hyperglycemia and hypoglycemia in cats. *Stroke*. 1988;19(11):1383-1387.

119. Dirnagl U, Iadecola C, Moskowitz MA. Pathobiology of ischaemic stroke: an integrated view. *Trends Neurosci*. 1999;22(9):391-397.

120. Du C, Hu R, Csernansky CA, Hsu CY, Choi DW. Very delayed infarction after mild focal cerebral ischemia: a role for apoptosis? *J Cereb Blood Flow Metab*. 1996;16(2):195-201.

121. Kawaguchi M, Kimbro JR, Drummond JC, Cole DJ, Kelly PJ, Patel PM. Isoflurane delays but does not prevent cerebral infarction in rats subjected to focal ischemia. *Anesthesiology*. 2000;92(5):1335-1342.

Chapter 9

INTRAVENOUS ANESTHETICS

Paul Garcia, Matthew Keith Whalin, and Peter S. Sebel

HISTORY OF INTRAVENOUS ANESTHESIA

The concept of blood delivery of medication can be traced to the middle of the 17th century soon after Harvey described the function of the vascular system. Not only did Sir Christopher Wren study blood transfusions in dogs, but he also experimented with intravenous delivery of injected opium solution into these animals via a feather quill.[1] In the mid-19th century, technologic advancements in needle and syringe manufacturing led to injectable morphine for analgesia but attempts to produce general anesthesia through intravenous drugs came later. Initial attempts with agents such as diethyl ether, chloral hydrate, magnesium sulfate, barbituric acid, and ethyl alcohol were stalled by prolonged side effects and limited techniques for ventilatory support.[2] Local anesthetics were also tested as intravenous agents for general anesthesia in the early 20th century before their primary clinical application in regional anesthesia was established.[3] The major historical developments in intravenous agents for general anesthesia lagged behind those of the inhaled anesthetics until Lundy and Waters began using barbiturates in the 1930s.[4]

General Anesthesia by Intravenous Agents

For the pedagogic purposes of this chapter, *intravenous anesthetic* is defined as a clinically available substance that when administered directly to the patient via the bloodstream can be used to induce or maintain a state of general anesthesia. Many injectable substances, such as antihistamines or antipsychotics (see Chapter 11), have obvious effects on the central nervous system (CNS) and can depress cognitive status and induce sleep. These drugs are potentially useful for several perioperative situations where sedation is required but they are neither appropriate nor safe as primary agents for producing general anesthesia. Similarly, medications like the benzodiazepines can be classified as intravenous anesthetics yet are currently used primarily in the perioperative setting for premedication and sedation, not anesthesia. The intravenous opioids (see Chapter 15) form the backbone of modern surgical analgesia yet are not considered true intravenous anesthetics because awareness and recall can occur despite very high doses that produce deep sedation.[5]

The concept of balanced anesthesia was originally used by Lundy to describe premedication and light sedation as adjuncts to regional anesthesia, but the term was almost

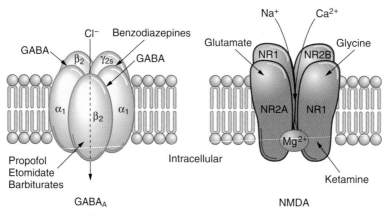

Figure 9-1 Key targets of intravenous anesthetics. GABA$_A$ receptors are critical targets for benzodiazepines, barbiturates, etomidate, and propofol. Although it is possible for the drugs and ligands to interact with this protein in multiple areas, it is generally agreed that the endogenous ligand GABA binds to the receptor in a pocket between the α and β subunits. Many of the intravenous anesthetics have their main influence on the activity of this protein in the transmembrane portion of the β subunit, while the benzodiazepines modulate the protein through interactions with transmembrane amino acids between the α and γ subunits near the intracellular side. NMDA receptors are activated by the agonist glutamate and co-agonist glycine only when voltage changes displace Mg^{2+} from the ion channel pore. Ketamine also acts primarily by a pore-blocking mechanism.

Table 9-1. Comparison of Molecular Targets for Common Intravenous Anesthetic Agents

	GABA$_A$ RECEPTORS	NMDA RECEPTORS	2PK RECEPTORS	GLYCINE RECEPTORS	AMPA RECEPTORS	5-HT RECEPTORS
Thiopental	↑↑			↓	↓↓	↓
Benzodiazepines	↑↑			↑*	↓*	↑*
Etomidate	↑↑		↑	↑		
Propofol	↑↑	↓		↑↑	↓	↓
Ketamine	↑	↓↓	↑			↑
Dexmedetomidine (α2 agonist)	↑*	↓*				
Isoflurane	↑↑	↓	↑↑	↑↑	↓↓	↑↑

*Asterisks indicate a complex relationship between drug and receptor—either evidence for direct allosteric interaction between these drugs and receptors is suspected but has yet to be found, or receptor activity and/or expression is known to be influenced through administration of the drugs. Isoflurane is also shown for comparison. Data summarized from Key References.

universally adopted when nitrous oxide anesthetics supplemented with thiopental and d-tubocurarine grew in popularity in the middle of the 20th century.[6] At present time, it is usually accepted that the state of general anesthesia can best be described as a delicate balance of the following effects: unconsciousness, analgesia, amnesia, suppression of the stress response, and sufficient immobility. The relative importance of each of these separate components varies for each case depending on specific surgical and patient factors; anesthesiologists must tailor combinations of intravenous drugs to match these priorities.

Intravenous Anesthesia Mechanisms and Theory

Modern anesthetic techniques have transformed surgery from a traumatic and barbaric affair to an acceptable, routine, and essential part of modern medicine. Despite technologic advances that have been made in perioperative medicine and surgical techniques, the drugs administered by anesthesiologists to render patients unconscious continue to be used without a clear understanding of how they produce anesthesia. Fortunately, through recent advances in molecular pharmacology and neuroscience, clinicians and investigators understand better than ever before how anesthetic chemicals can alter the function of the nervous system.

The elucidation of general anesthetic mechanisms was not accessible to traditional pharmacology methods; anesthesia is

a clinical state in which multiple behavioral endpoints are caused by a structurally diverse group of drugs. Nevertheless, it appears that certain membrane proteins (Figure 9-1) possess binding sites that interact with many of the currently used anesthetics (Table 9-1).[7,8] In general, the halogenated volatile anesthetic agents (see Chapter 10) exhibit less specificity for molecular targets than the intravenous agents.

At the cellular and network levels, intravenous anesthetics alter signaling between neurons by interacting directly with a small number of ion channels. Under normal conditions, these specialized membrane proteins are activated by chemical signals or changes in the membrane environment. Upon activation, channels modify the electrical excitability of neurons by controlling the flow of ions across the cell membrane via channels that are coupled with specific receptors that sense the initial signal (see Chapter 1).

The majority of intravenous anesthetics exert their primary clinical anesthetic action by enhancing inhibitory signaling via γ-aminobutyric acid type A (GABA$_A$) receptors. Ketamine and dexmedetomidine are notable exceptions. From a neurophysiology perspective, unconsciousness can be considered as a disruption of the precisely timed cortical integration necessary to produce what is considered the conscious state.[7] It is interesting to note that the unconsciousness produced by ketamine is phenotypically different from that produced by the GABA-ergic agents (e.g., propofol, thiopental, or etomidate). Although many talented scientists worked diligently throughout the 20th century to discover a unifying mechanism by which diverse chemicals cause what is loosely defined as the anesthetic state, molecular investigations into the action of individual drugs have revealed that this one true "grail" does not exist. It should rather be interpreted that the anesthetized state (and its separate components) can be arrived at by any disruption of the delicately constructed and precisely timed neuronal networks that underlie the normal awake, un-anesthetized state.

PHARMACOLOGIC TARGETS OF INTRAVENOUS ANESTHETICS IN THE CENTRAL NERVOUS SYSTEM

GABA$_A$ Receptors

GABA is the most abundant inhibitory neurotransmitter in the brain. GABA$_A$ receptors represent the most abundant receptor type for this ubiquitous inhibitory signaling molecule. GABA$_A$ receptors are broadly distributed in the CNS and regulate neuronal excitability.[9] They appear to mediate unconsciousness, arguably the most recognizable phenotype associated with general anesthesia.[10] There is also strong evidence that GABA$_A$ receptors are involved in mediating some of the other classic components of general anesthesia including depression of spinal reflexes and amnesia.[11,12] The contribution of GABA$_A$ receptors in mediating immobility and analgesia is less clear.

GABA$_A$ receptors are ligand-gated ion channels, more specifically members of the "Cys-loop" superfamily that also includes nicotinic acetylcholine (nAChR), glycine, and serotonin type 3 (5-hydroxytryptamine type 3, or 5-HT$_3$) receptors. Each of these receptors is formed as a pentameric combination of transmembrane protein subunits (see Figure 9-1). This superfamily is named for the fixed loops formed in each of the subunits by a disulfide bond between two cysteine residues. No protein crystallization of the GABA$_A$ receptor has been accomplished, but high quality molecular models exist.[13] Binding pockets for neurotransmitters are located at two or more extracellular interfaces: In the case of GABA$_A$ receptors, the endogenous ligand GABA binds between the α and β subunits. Thus far, 19 genes have been identified for GABA$_A$ receptor subunits (α1 – 6, β1 – 3, γ1 – 3, δ, ε, θ, π, ρ1 – 3).[14] Although millions of subunit arrangements are possible, only a subset of receptor configurations is actually expressed in significant amounts in the brain. Preferred subunit combinations distribute among different brain regions and even among different subcellular domains.[15] Each type of GABA$_A$ receptor exhibits subtly distinct biophysical and pharmacologic properties that in turn have diverse influences on synaptic transmission and synaptic integration.

Specific behavioral effects of drugs have been linked to different subunit assemblies present in different brain regions. For example, benzodiazepines are thought to interact with GABA$_A$ receptors between the α and γ subunits[16] (see Figure 9-1) and specific clinical effects have been linked to receptors containing specific α and β subunits. Propofol, etomidate, and barbiturates interact with GABA$_A$ receptors within, or proximal to, β subunits. The β subunits show less specific subcellular localization compared to α subunits, and the distribution of β subunits in mammalian brain does not share the same clear distinctions as α subunits.[17-21] Therefore distinguishing specific differences between the GABA-mediated anesthetic

effects of non-benzodiazepine intravenous anesthetics has been more elusive. However, research involving genetically manipulated mice has suggested that the sedation produced by etomidate can be primarily associated with activity at the β2 subunit while unconsciousness produced by the same drug can be associated with β3 subunits (see GABA$_A$ Insights from Mutagenic Studies).[22,23] Subtle pharmacodynamic differences between intravenous anesthetics (e.g., effects on postoperative nausea and vomiting) might also be mediated by interactions with targets in addition to GABA$_A$ receptors.

Almost all general anesthetics enhance GABA$_A$ receptor-induced chloride currents by enhancing receptor sensitivity to GABA, thereby inhibiting neuronal activation. Most of these drugs, at high concentrations, also directly open the channel as an agonist in the absence of GABA. By virtue of the specific distribution of these receptors in the cerebral cortex and other brain regions, in addition to being involved in producing anesthesia, GABA$_A$ receptors function in thalamic circuits necessary for sensory processing and attention, hippocampal networks involved in memory, and thalamocortical circuits underlying conscious awareness. Computational neuronal modeling studies have been important in revealing the impact of propofol and etomidate on dynamic changes in these networks.[24,25]

GABA$_A$ Insights from Mutagenic Studies

The critical role that the GABA$_A$ receptor plays in the pharmacodynamics of anesthetic drugs has been established through laboratory experimentation using genetic modifications of this protein. In the early 1990s, in vitro studies aimed at determining the interactions of the endogenous ligand GABA with its receptor revealed that specific amino acid substitutions in the GABA$_A$ receptor conferred the sensitivity of the channel to agonist or allosteric modulator activity.[26-28] By 1995, several functional domains of the GABA$_A$ receptor associated with binding of agonists and allosteric modulators were identified (reviewed by Smith and Olsen[29]). Following the discovery of the site of benzodiazepine action, investigators discovered that mutation of a pair of transmembrane amino acids on the α subunit of GABA$_A$ renders the receptors insensitive to inhaled anesthetics.[27,30] That same year, a corresponding area on the β3 subunit was determined to be critical for the action of etomidate.[31] Further studies have determined this location to be essential to the actions of other intravenous agents such as propofol and pentobarbital.[19,32] A different amino acid residue appears to be involved with the specific actions of propofol only (Figure 9-2).[17]

The strategy behind these discoveries was to examine the subtle differences among the amino acid sequences in receptor isoforms known to have different sensitivities to anesthetics. Originally receptor chimeras of unnatural subunit configurations were used, eventually giving way to specifically modified subunits via site-directed mutagenesis. Potential residues and amino acid sequence domains that mediate anesthetic sensitivity can be anticipated by comparing data among different mutated and chimeric receptors. Typically, functional studies are carried out in vitro by virally transfecting this DNA into living cells which results in expression of these receptors on their cell surface. Immortal cells derived from human embryonic kidney cells (HEK cells) and the eggs of the amphibian *Xenopus laevis* (oocytes) have been

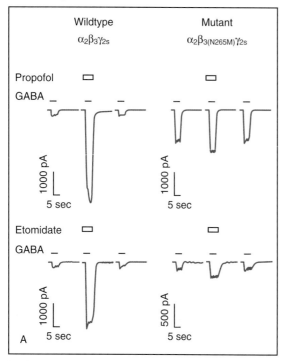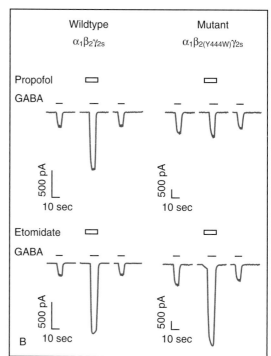

Figure 9-2 Site-directed mutagenesis elucidates specific amino acid residues involved in anesthetic actions at the GABA_A receptor in patch clamp experiments. Treatment with GABA (duration shown with black line) alone or in combination with anesthetics (indicated by white box) triggers depolarization of wild type and mutant receptors. **A,** The substitution of a methionine (M) residue for an asparagine (N) residue in the 265th position on the β3 subunit (β3 N265M mutation) renders that GABA_A receptor immune to enhancement of chloride current via etomidate and propofol administration. **B,** In a similar study of the β2 subunit, substitution of tryptophan (W) for the native tyrosine (Y) blocks propofol enhancement but the receptor remains sensitive to etomidate. (*A, Adapted from Siegwart R, Jurd R, Rudolph U. Molecular determinants for the action of general anesthetics at recombinant alpha(2)beta(3)gamma(2) gamma-aminobutyric acid(A) receptors. J Neurochem. 2002;80:140-148; B, Adapted from Richardson JE, Garcia PS, O'Toole KK, et al. A conserved tyrosine in the beta2 subunit M4 segment is a determinant of gamma-aminobutyric acid type A receptor sensitivity to propofol. Anesthesiology. 2007;107:412-418.*)

invaluable as conduits for this type of research; establishing electrical access in these cells using conventional patch-clamp technique is relatively straightforward and measurements of their chloride-currents in response to opening of the GABA_A channel is robust (see Figure 9-2).

By now a great body of literature exists in which anesthetic sensitivity has been mapped to specific point mutations on GABA_A receptors.[8] Some of these point mutations, so-called silent mutations, do not affect the natural function of the receptor but only its modulation by specific anesthetics. The introduction of mutations such as these into genetically modified mice can be used to determine the importance of this receptor to the production of certain qualities of an anesthetic in vivo.[33] In vivo experimentation on animals possessing these "knock-in" point mutations has advantages over traditional gene knockout studies. Specifically, if the receptor is unaltered except with respect to its response to exogenous anesthesia, there exists less potential for compensatory changes that could influence the results of in vivo experiments. Mouse geneticists have successfully bred mice with attenuated sensitivity to benzodiazepines as well as etomidate and propofol.[18,34-36]

By creating a point mutation that confers anesthetic selectivity in a single specific subunit, the phenotypic effects attributable to that drug and that subunit can be dissected (Figure 9-3). For example, the substitution of a methionine (M) residue for an asparagine (N) residue in the 265th position on the β3 subunit (β3 N265M mutation) results in a phenotypically normal animal that is essentially immune to the hypnotic effects of propofol and etomidate while maintaining its sensitivity to inhaled anesthetics.[18] Similarly, by substituting an arginine (R) for the histidine (H) residue in the 101st position on the α1 subunit (α1 H101R mutation) essentially renders that GABA_A receptor unresponsive to benzodiazepines.[34] By making analogous substitutions in the other α subunits, scientists have been able to map particular behavioral effects from benzodiazepines to specific subunits. For example, the α1 subunit appears to mediate the sedative, amnestic, and anticonvulsant actions of some benzodiazepines, while benzodiazepine muscle relaxation and anxiolysis are mainly mediated via α2 and α3 subunits.[34,35,37,38]

These amino acid substitutions (in vitro and in vivo) alter the molecular environment in the anesthetic binding cavity by reducing the number of favorable interactions between the receptor and the anesthetic molecule, thus reducing the efficacy of that anesthetic drug on enhancing GABA-ergic transmission. Although this work has greatly increased insight into anesthetic mechanisms, a complete description of the biophysical interactions between specific residues and specific anesthetics remains as incomplete as understanding of the spike-coded pattern of neuronal network activity responsible for the transitions between consciousness and unconsciousness.

N-Methyl-D-Aspartate Receptors

Whereas augmentation of endogenous inhibitory chemical signaling is important to mechanisms of anesthesia, mitigation

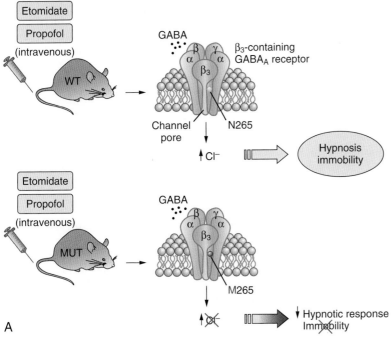

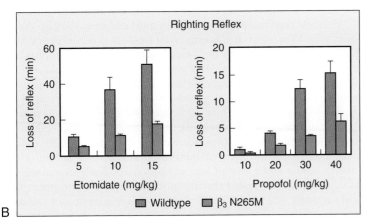

Figure 9-3 Genetic manipulation of GABA$_A$ receptors in mice facilitates the study of behavioral effects of different anesthetic drugs. **A,** In this schematic diagram, intravenous anesthetics (e.g., propofol and etomidate) are administered to a mouse with normal or wild type (WT) GABA$_A$ receptors and, as expected, general anesthesia ensues. When these same drugs are administered to an animal with a specific knock-in mutation at the 265th position on the β3 subunit, the effects of these drugs are mitigated. **B,** Quantitative data comparing the effect of propofol and etomidate on wild type and β3 N265M knock-in mutants in the loss of righting reflex test, an animal correlate of unconsciousness. *(Adapted from Jurd R, Arras M, Lambert S, et al. General anesthetic actions in vivo strongly attenuated by a point mutation in the GABA(A) receptor beta3 subunit. FASEB J. 2003;17:250-252.)*

of excitatory signaling also depresses neuronal activity. Of the many excitatory chemical signals in the CNS, blockade of the N-methyl-D-aspartate (NMDA)-type glutamate receptors appears to be most relevant to mechanisms of anesthesia. There are two broad categories of excitatory synaptic receptors that use the amino acid L-glutamate as their chemical messenger: NMDA receptors and non-NMDA receptors.[39] The latter group can be subdivided into AMPA (α-amino-3-hydroxy-5-methyl-4-isoxazole propionic acid) receptors and kainate receptors. Both AMPA and kainate receptors mediate fast excitatory postsynaptic currents (EPSCs) and show relatively little anesthetic sensitivity.[40] NMDA receptors, by contrast, mediate EPSCs of relatively prolonged duration. NMDA receptors are found presynaptically, postsynaptically, and extrasynaptically[41]; they are important targets for xenon, nitrous oxide and the dissociative anesthetic ketamine.[42]

NMDA receptors are tetramers consisting of four subunits arranged circumferentially around a central ion channel pore (see Figure 9-1).[39] All NMDA receptors contain an obligatory NR1 subunit and at least one of four types of NR2 subunits (A–D). Other subunits (NR3) and numerous splice variants

exist that translate to considerable variability in the kinetic and pharmacologic profile of each receptor isoform.[43] In contrast to non-NMDA glutamate receptors, which are selective for sodium ions (Na$^+$), the pore of NMDA receptors permit entry of both monovalent and divalent cations (Na$^+$ and Ca^{2+}) into the cell upon activation. The Ca^{2+} flux is important for activating Ca^{2+}-dependent processes in the postsynaptic cell such as long-term potentiation (LTP), a form of synaptic plasticity thought to play an important role in memory.[44]

NMDA receptors are unique among ligand-gated ion channels in that their probability of opening depends not only on presynaptic release of neurotransmitter but also on the voltage across the membrane containing the receptor. Until membrane depolarization occurs, Mg^{2+} blocks the channel pore whether or not agonist is present. High-frequency excitatory input causes membrane depolarization, so NMDA receptors play a significant role in CNS functions that require activity-dependent changes in cellular physiology such as learning and processing of sensory information.[45] In the nociceptive circuitry of the spinal cord, repeated peripheral nerve stimulation results in an increase in response to subsequent stimuli through activation of NMDA receptors. This "wind up" phenomenon is associated with hyperalgesia, and both knockout and knockdown of NR1 blocks inflammatory pain in animals.[46,47] This, combined with their ability to modify opioid tolerance, makes NMDA receptor antagonists promising treatments for chronic pain.[48]

NMDA antagonists are classified by their mechanism of action. Volatile anesthetics may exert some of their effects as competitive antagonists by displacing the coagonist glycine from NMDA receptors.[49] The intravenous NMDA antagonists in current clinical use are primarily channel blockers that bind to the pore only in its open confirmation. They are considered uncompetitive antagonists and, because their binding requires prior activation by agonist, they are termed *use-dependent*.[39] Blockers such as ketamine, which remain bound after channel closure, cause prolonged disruption of the associative aspects of neuronal communication. High concentrations of ketamine cause sedation and loss of consciousness with a significant incidence of dysphoric effects. This may reflect a lack of selectivity among various NMDA isoforms or activity at other receptors (see Table 9-1). Noncompetitive antagonists, which bind to allosteric sites with some NMDA receptor subunit specificity, may have more specific clinical effects and a better side-effect profile.[39]

Other Molecular Targets

Other receptors, such as glycine receptors, voltage-gated Na^+ channels, and two-pore domain potassium channels deserve attention in that they probably contribute to certain components of the balanced anesthetic state with intravenous anesthetics. Glycine receptors colocalize with $GABA_A$ receptors near the cell body. Propofol, etomidate, and thiopental all have some positive modulation of the glycine receptors, but ketamine does not. Glycine receptors have an inhibitory role, particularly in the lower brainstem and spinal cord. They are likely major contributors to anesthetic immobility, especially that produced by the volatiles: An investigation of spinal neurons estimated that propofol's effects on immobility were mediated almost entirely via GABA receptors, whereas the immobility caused by sevoflurane was predominantly mediated by glycine receptors.[50] Propofol inhibits some subtypes of voltage-gated Na^+ channels, which could contribute to its antiepileptic activity.[51] In high doses, ketamine can also block Na^+ channel activity.[52]

Two-pore domain K^+ (2PK) channels modulate neuronal excitability through control of the transmembrane potential. There are 15 different 2PK isoforms, and functional channels are formed from homomeric or heteromeric dimers. Genetic deletion of several members of this channel family (TREK1, TREK2, TASK1, TASK3, and TRESK) in animal models reduces the immobilizing effect of intravenous and volatile general anesthetics, which suggests a contribution to their anesthetic mechanisms.

Hyperpolarization-activated cation channels (HCN channels) are important in mediating coordinated neuronal firing between the thalamus and cortex. With the exception of propofol, the anesthetic sensitivity of this channel is relatively unexplored despite its important role in setting the frequency of thalamocortical rhythms critical for high-order cognitive processing.[53] These channels are also important for controlling burst firing in the hippocampus, thalamus, and

locus coeruleus. Amnesia and hypnosis are produced upon disruption of signaling in these brain areas via intravenous anesthetics. Some anesthetics like dexmedetomidine exert their sedating effects by activating α2 receptors in the locus coeruleus.[54]

INDIVIDUAL AGENTS

Barbiturates

In 1864, some 20 years after Morton and Long discovered inhaled anesthesia, von Baeyer synthesized barbituric acid, which eventually led to the development of intravenous anesthesia. Barbituric acid is pharmacologically inert, but substitutions at the C5 position impart hypnotic activity. The clinical use of barbiturates as hypnotics began in 1904 with 5,5-diethylbarbituric acid, but their adaptation to anesthesia was pioneered in the late 1920s by Bumm in Germany and Lundy in the United States.[4,55] Lundy's investigations included pentobarbital, also known as nembutal (sodium [N] 5-ethyl-5-[1-methylbutyl]) substituted barbituric acid). Thionembutal, the sulfur substitution of this compound better known as sodium thiopental, became the dominant intravenous induction agent of the next 60 years.

Thiopental was popularized by Lundy but might have been first used in a patient several months earlier in 1934 by Waters in Wisconsin. It was employed in short procedures and early use was limited by the lack of reliable equipment to maintain intravenous access. Over time it evolved from a sole agent to a means of inducing anesthesia without breathing the pungent vapors of that era (e.g., ether).

Both pentobarbital and thiopental are supplied as racemic mixtures (see Chapter 2), with the S(−) isomer exhibiting roughly double the potency of the R(+) form. Methylation of the ring nitrogen of methohexital creates a second chiral center and a total of four stereoisomers. Early animal work at Eli Lilly revealed that the potent β isomers had more excitatory side effects so methohexital is marketed as a racemate of the α isomers.[56] The α-dextrorotatory form is roughly three times more potent than the α-levorotatory (S_bR_b) isomer and recent stereochemical synthesis suggested that the latter is responsible for the residual excitatory effects of commercial methohexital (Figure 9-4, *B*).[57]

Methohexital found use in electroconvulsive therapy and pentobarbital was used as a pediatric premedication, but thiopental was the mainstay for the intravenous induction of anesthesia before the introduction of propofol. American production of thiopental ceased in 2010 and plans to import the drug from Europe stalled over the political controversy associated with thiopental's use for lethal injection in the U.S. penal system. Like etomidate, thiopental enhances $GABA_A$ receptor function in a stereoselective manner.[58] This is also true for other barbiturate sedatives/hypnotics such as hexobarbital and pentobarbital. Thiopental directly gates $GABA_A$ receptors at high concentrations (like propofol and etomidate). Thiopental discriminates between synaptic and extrasynaptic $GABA_A$ receptors in the hippocampus, suggesting a possible role for the δ subunit in barbiturate enhancement of this channel.[59] The β subunit has also been implicated as a molecular site of action of barbiturates at $GABA_A$ receptors.

In addition to $GABA_A$ receptors, barbiturates modulate a variety of ligand-gated ion channels in vitro. They block the

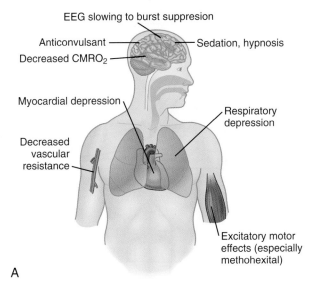

A

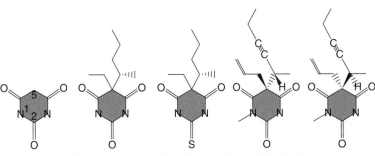

B Barbituric acid S(–)-Pentobarbital S(–)-Thiopental Methohexital racemate

Figure 9-4 A, Selected effects of barbiturates. **B,** Structures of clinically important barbiturates. Pentobarbital and thiopental are supplied as racemic mixtures but only their more potent isomers are shown. Methohexital has two chiral centers and both of the isomers in the commercial formulation are shown.

action of the excitatory neurotransmitter glutamate at AMPA and kainate receptor subtypes, but not at NMDA receptors. They also inhibit neuronal nicotinic acetylcholine receptors. The relevance of these receptors to the clinical action of barbiturates remains unclear. Several clinical effects appear to be modulated by allosteric augmentation at $GABA_A$ receptors. Transgenic mice carrying a point mutation (N265M) of the $GABA_A$ β3 subunit are resistant to the immobilizing effects of pentobarbital.[19] However, this mutation had no effect on the pentobarbital-induced respiratory depression and intermediate blunting of hypnotic and cardiovascular effects. Future studies are needed to determine whether these effects are mediated by some other $GABA_A$ receptor subtype, ionotropic glutamate receptors, or other receptors.

Barbiturates produce dose-dependent CNS depression with characteristic effects on electroencephalography (EEG), progressing from a low-frequency, high-amplitude pattern to isoelectric periods of increasing duration. The cerebral metabolic rate for oxygen ($CMRO_2$) is decreased to a widely quoted maximal extent of 55%, and both cerebral blood flow and intracranial pressure (ICP) are decreased as a result of flow-metabolism coupling. These factors led to widespread use of barbiturates for neuroprotection, although large trials and metaanalyses have failed to show substantial clinical benefit in humans. Thiopental and pentobarbital have anticonvulsant effects in the setting of prolonged high-dose administration, whereas prolonged use of methohexital leads to epileptiform discharges.

Barbiturates cause venodilation with consequent decreases in preload and cardiac output. This effect is particularly pronounced in hypovolemic patients.[60] There is in vitro evidence for direct myocardial depression at doses much higher than those used for anesthesia. Other selected effects of barbiturates are summarized in Figure 9-4.

Barbiturate sodium salts require a pH greater than 10 to remain in aqueous solution and precipitate readily when mixed with nonbasic solutions such as normal saline. They also precipitate when combined in high concentrations with certain weak bases such as the neuromuscular blockers, forming a "conjugate salt" (e.g., sodium thiopental and rocuronium bromide precipitate to form sodium bromide). In the plasma, barbiturates are readily protonated and become quite lipophilic, which leads to profound anesthesia 30 to 60 seconds after bolus injection. Kinetic modeling of bolus administration reveals a rapid peak in effect site (CNS) concentration (Figure 9-5, *A*). The subsequent decline in concentration results primarily from redistribution to other tissues rather than metabolism and elimination (see Chapter 2). Repeated bolus dosing or continuous infusions lead to very prolonged recovery times as depicted by plots of the context-sensitive half-time (see Figure 9-5, *C*).[61] When given in very high doses, thiopental can even exhibit "zero order kinetics," wherein metabolic capacity is saturated, grossly prolonging the duration of action.

Thiopental is highly protein bound (75%-90%) in the plasma, primarily to albumin. Decreased albumin levels such

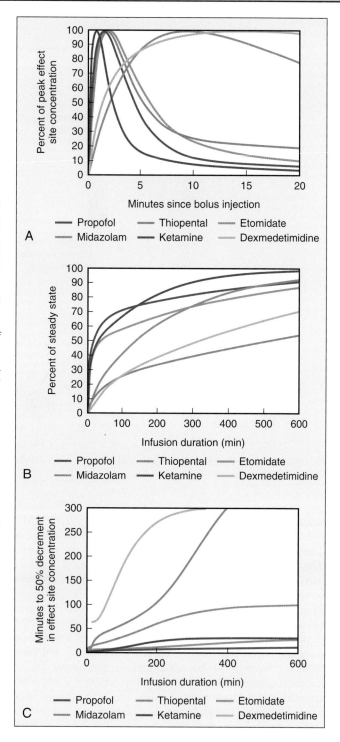

Figure 9-5 A, Bolus front and back-end kinetics comparing the time courses of effect site concentrations after bolus injection based on the pharmacokinetics and rate of plasma-effect site equilibrium. The curves have been normalized to the peak effect site concentration, permitting comparison of the relative rate of rise (and fall) independent of dose. **B,** Infusion front-end kinetics expressed as a percentage of eventual steady-state effect site concentration. After 10 hours, no intravenous anesthetic has reached steady-state concentration. **C,** Infusion back-end kinetics (i.e., the context sensitive half-times) of intravenous anesthetics based on the pharmacokinetics and rate of plasma-effect site equilibrium. *(Simulations courtesy of Dr. Shinju Obara, Fukushima University, Japan, performed with PKPDtools, www.pkpdtools.com. Note that dexmedetomidine is not approved for bolus dosing but the curve was derived from the data of Dyck et al,[154] using PKPDtools with an assumed time to peak effect of 15 minutes. Pharmacokinetics of the intravenous anesthetics derived from studies of propofol, thiopental, etomidate, midazolam, ketamine, and dexmedetomidine in Schnider TW, Minto CF, Gambus PL, et al. The influence of method of administration and covariates on the pharmacokinetics of propofol in adult volunteers. Anesthesiology. 1998;88:1170-1182; Stanski DR, Maitre PO. Population pharmacokinetics and pharmacodynamics of thiopental: the effect of age revisited. Anesthesiology. 1990;72(3):412-422; Arden JR, Holley FO, Stanski DR. Increased sensitivity to etomidate in the elderly: initial distribution versus altered brain response. Anesthesiology. 1986;65:19-27; Greenblatt DJ, Ehrenberg BL, Gunderman J, et al. Pharmacokinetic and electroencephalographic study of intravenous diazepam, midazolam, and placebo. Clin Pharmacol Ther. 1989;45:356-365; Buhrer M, Maitre PO, Hung O, Stanski DR. Electroencephalographic effects of benzodiazepines. I. Choosing an electroencephalographic parameter to measure the effect of midazolam on the central nervous system. Clin Pharmacol Ther. 1990;48:544-554; and Domino EF, Domino SE, Smith RE, et al. Ketamine kinetics in unmedicated and diazepam-premedicated subjects. Clin Pharmacol Ther. 1984;36:645-653.)*

as those seen in chronic renal or hepatic disease can markedly increase free drug levels and may warrant decreased dosing.[62] Thiopental undergoes some desulfurization to form its parent drug pentobarbital. This "metabolite" is likely relevant only to prolonged high-dose administration of thiopental. Both drugs are deactivated by poorly characterized pathways in the liver to form inactive carboxylic acid and alcohol derivatives. Thiopental causes some cytochrome P450 induction but this is generally of no clinical consequence when used as an induction agent. An active porphyric crisis could be exacerbated by this mechanism, but triggering an event in a patient

with latent porphyria is reported to be unusual.[63] Even so, it is prudent to avoid even potential triggers in patients with porphyria.

Benzodiazepines

Benzodiazepines were introduced into clinical use in the 1960s and rapidly gained popularity as anxiolytics with a wider safety margin than barbiturates.[64] Diazepam, lorazepam, and midazolam are three of the most important class members in the practice of anesthesia. Diazepam and lorazepam are

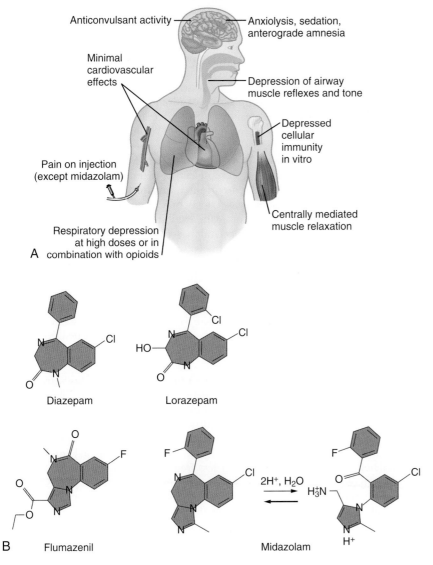

Figure 9-6 **A,** Selected effects of benzodiazepines. **B,** Structures of clinically important benzodiazepines, including both the hydrophilic prodrug (right) and lipophilic (left) conformations of midazolam. Flumazenil is generally considered a benzodiazepine antagonist but has demonstrated some partial agonist effects (see text).

lipophilic and are traditionally formulated in propylene glycol because they are not soluble in water. These formulations are associated with pain on injection and long-term infusions in the intensive care unit (ICU) can lead to glycol toxicity. The imidazole ring of midazolam allows the preparation of acidic aqueous solutions, which cause minimal pain on injection.[65] Once at physiologic pH, midazolam assumes a more lipophilic ring conformation and can gain rapid access to the CNS (Figure 9-6, *B*).

Benzodiazepines act on a subset of $GABA_A$ receptors containing γ subunits to potentiate chloride conductance upon GABA binding. This modulatory mode of action is postulated to create a "ceiling effect" that limits CNS depression, although when combined with other drugs, benzodiazepines can lead to dangerous respiratory depression.[66] Even when respiratory drive is preserved, midazolam increases the likelihood of airway obstruction, and caution is advised in patients with obstructive sleep apnea or advanced age.[67,68] The binding pocket appears to be at the interface of the α and γ2 subunits in receptors containing α1, α2, α3, or α5 subunits. Recent elegant studies of mutant $GABA_A$ subunits in transgenic mice

have raised the possibility of dissecting the effects of the benzodiazepines at a molecular level (see $GABA_A$ insights from Mutagenic Studies earlier).

Benzodiazepines have anxiolytic, sedative, hypnotic, amnestic, and anticonvulsant properties in the CNS. Although they have no intrinsic analgesic effects, they are currently being investigated as adjunct medications to prevent hyperalgesia.[69] The α subunit of the $GABA_A$ receptor appears to differentially mediate the CNS effects of benzodiazepines. For example, α2-containing receptors play an important role in anxiolysis, anti-hyperalgesia, and centrally mediated muscle relaxation, while α1-containing subunits are important mediators of the sedative, amnestic, and anticonvulsive effects of benzodiazepines.[33] Although benzodiazepines can be used for the induction of anesthesia, the high doses required delay emergence unless the surgery is of prolonged duration. Combining midazolam with another induction agent can offer improved hemodynamic stability without affecting emergence. Other selected effects of benzodiazepines are depicted in Figure 9-6.

Oral midazolam in children has an onset of action within 10 minutes and peaks in 20 to 30 minutes; its effects begin to dissipate 45 minutes after administration. These kinetics require some planning to get the child to the operating room within the window of efficacy. As shown in Figure 9-5, *A*, intravenous midazolam does not reach peak effect site concentration until nearly 10 minutes after administration. When titrating midazolam, one must therefore be patient to avoid "stacking" the doses and oversedating the patient. The onset of intravenous diazepam is more than twice as rapid as that of midazolam, but its use is limited by an extremely long duration of action. Not only is the elimination half-life 10 times longer than that of midazolam, but about half of the parent drug is metabolized to the active compound desmethyldiazepam, which has an even longer elimination half-life. Both midazolam and diazepam are metabolized by CYP3A family members in the liver and are subject to interactions with erythromycin and antifungal medications. Diazepam is also metabolized by CYP1A2 and CYP2C19.

Premedication is currently the main role of benzodiazepines in anesthesia; a majority of U.S. practitioners surveyed in the 1990s used intravenous midazolam for adults (>70%) and oral midazolam for children (80%).[70] For patients requiring long-term mechanical ventilation, combinations of an opioid and benzodiazepine have been the traditional method of sedation. Although midazolam is often considered a short-acting benzodiazepine, prolonged infusions in critically ill patients leads to markedly delayed awakening in part due to accumulation of its active metabolite 1-hydroxymidazolam (see Figure 9-5, *B* and *C*). For this reason, recent Society for Critical Care Medicine (SCCM) sedation guidelines recommend limiting midazolam use to 2 to 3 days.[71] For longer periods of sedation, the benzodiazepine of choice is lorazepam, but some formulations of lorazepam are formulated in a glycol-based vehicle and prolonged infusions lead to glycol toxicity. An emerging body of literature links benzodiazepine use to delirium in critically ill patients.[72,73] Because delirium increases time on mechanical ventilation, length of stay, and morbidity and mortality, there has been a movement toward other sedatives in the ICU. Benzodiazepines also have some immunomodulatory effects on monocytes and T cells in vitro, but the clinical significance of these effects is not clear.[74,75]

An important and unique feature of the benzodiazepines compared to the other GABA-ergic sedative hypnotics is that a competitive antagonist for the reversal of benzodiazepine effects is available. As an intravenous rescue agent, flumazenil can rapidly reverse the CNS depression associated with benzodiazepine intoxication. Routine administration of flumazenil to patients presenting to the emergency room with the suspicion of overdose can lead to seizures via precipitating acute withdrawal in chronic benzodiazepine users.[76] But, there is some evidence that flumazenil has anticonvulsant properties suggesting that this drug may have mixed or partial agonist effects on the GABA_A receptor, even in the absence of benzodiazepine administration.[77] In support of this phenomenon is the potential for high doses of flumazenil to potentiate the hypnosis of other positive GABA modulators such as propofol.[78] Its use to augment recovery from general anesthesia is being explored with mixed results (see Emerging Developments). While flumazenil can be life saving in cases of benzodiazepine overdose, its short acting kinetic profile creates the possibility of resedation after the effects of flumazenil dissipate.

Etomidate

Etomidate is a rapidly acting intravenous agent that was introduced into clinical practice in the 1970s. Compared with other induction agents, it has minimal effects on the cardiovascular system.[79] Because of its association with nausea and prolonged suppression of adrenocortical synthesis of steroids, its main clinical use is for inductions in which hemodynamic stability is essential.[80] The R(+) isomer has much greater hypnotic effects (Figure 9-7), and it is formulated as a single enantiomer. Like propofol, etomidate interacts with GABA_A receptors in a stereoselective manner.[81] Its enhancement of GABA-mediated current is smaller on receptors containing the β1 subunit.[82] Of all of the clinically used intravenous anesthetics, etomidate exhibits the greatest selectivity for GABA_A receptors and has the fewest relevant interactions with other ion channels (see Table 9-1).

Following intravenous injection, etomidate is tightly bound to plasma proteins such as albumin. The uncharged drug is highly lipophilic so etomidate rapidly penetrates the blood-brain barrier; peak brain levels are achieved within 2 minutes of injection (see Figure 9-5, *A*). Etomidate is metabolized in the liver by ester hydrolysis to a pharmacologically inactive metabolite.

The effects of etomidate on the CNS are similar to those of propofol and the barbiturates. Induction doses are associated with a high incidence of myoclonus, possibly via a loss of cortical inhibition during the transition from consciousness to unconsciousness. Although this myoclonic activity could be mistaken for generalized tonic-clonic seizures, etomidate has anticonvulsant activity in several experimental models. Epileptic attacks occur less frequently during etomidate anesthesia but it is likely that propofol and thiopental possess greater anticonvulsant effects; etomidate is therefore a viable option for electroconvulsive therapy.

Etomidate causes less depression of ventilation compared to the barbiturates (see Figure 9-7).[83,84] Despite its favorable hemodynamic profile it should be noted that patients with high sympathetic tone such as those suffering from shock, intoxication or drug withdrawal can have a precipitous drop in blood pressure even when etomidate is used to induce anesthesia.

In 1983, investigators reported increased mortality in ICU patients sedated for days with etomidate.[85] The increased mortality was attributed to suppression of cortisol synthesis since etomidate is a potent inhibitor of the synthetic enzyme 11β-hydroxylase in the adrenal cortex. The original retrospective study has been criticized for failing to control for the severity of illness and for the potential role played by concurrent administration of adjuncts to ICU sedation (e.g., opioids) in those patients. Randomized controlled trials in elective cardiac surgery and critically ill patients verified the adrenal suppression but did not show differences in clinical outcome.[80,86] Nevertheless, a recent meta-analysis reported a weak association between etomidate use and mortality in critically ill patients, and new etomidate analogs with rapid metabolism are currently under development to avoid endocrine disturbance (see Emerging Developments).[87]

Propofol

The most important factor in increasing use of total intravenous anesthesia (TIVA) since the late 1980s has been the

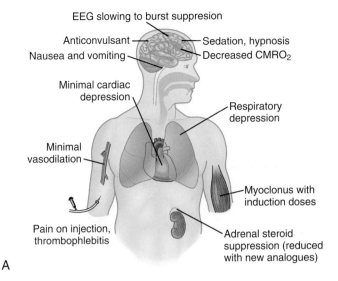

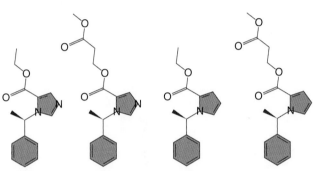

B   Etomidate   MOC-etomidate   Carboetomidate   MOC-carboetomidate

Figure 9-7 **A,** Selected effects of etomidate. **B,** Structures of etomidate and its analogs.

availability of the alkylated phenol propofol (Figure 9-8). Propofol (2,6, diisopropylphenol) potentiates GABA responses in neurons and directly activates GABA$_A$ receptor function.[88] Other receptors respond to propofol in the therapeutic concentration range but the majority of its clinical effects are likely mediated through GABA receptors. The specific interaction between propofol and GABA$_A$ receptors is not fully characterized, but likely involves residues in the transmembrane domains on β subunits.[17] Site-directed mutagenesis studies with recombinant GABA$_A$ receptors have contributed to precise knowledge regarding the molecular interactions between this drug and GABA$_A$ receptors. Initially, only the property of direct activation of the GABA$_A$ receptor by propofol was thought to depend on the β subunit while the modulatory effects were considered to involve other subunits.[89] There is now evidence that α, β, and γ subunits all contribute to GABA$_A$ sensitivity to propofol.[90]

The necessity to formulate propofol in a lipid emulsion (because of its extremely poor water solubility) has some very important clinical implications. The original preparation of propofol used a polyethoxylated castor oil (Cremophor EL) in its formulation, but this mixture was abandoned out of concern for allergic reactions to the excipient.[91] The most commonly available propofol formulations today involve a mixture of soy bean oil, glycerol, and purified egg phospholipid to solubilize the drug.[92] Despite initial concerns that the egg-derived lecithin might precipitate anaphylaxis in egg allergic individuals, it appears that propofol can be safely used

in egg allergic patients.[93] Most egg allergies are related to egg albumin (in egg whites) as opposed to lecithin (primarily in the egg yolk), and a small study revealed no hypersensitivity to propofol in egg allergic patients undergoing skin prick testing.[94]

Perhaps most important among concerns over the lipid formulation of propofol involves the promotion of rapid microbial growth. This issue received much attention after a high-impact epidemiologic investigation described unusual outbreaks of postoperative infections at seven hospitals.[95] In 2007, the Food and Drug Administration (FDA) mandated that all propofol emulsions in the United States contain an antimicrobial agent (EDTA or sodium metabisulfite).[96,97] The FDA also recommended that, to minimize the potential for bacterial contamination, both the vial and prefilled syringe formulations must be used on only one patient, administration must commence immediately after the vial or syringe has been opened, and administration from a single vial or syringe must be completed within 6 hours of opening.[98] Failing to follow these practices and usual aseptic technique for intravenous administration of medication can lead to transmission of viral particles between patients and bacterial sepsis.[99-102]

Although pain on injection was a contributing factor to changing the initial formulation of propofol, the change to the current isotonic, emulsified, soybean-based formulation has not eliminated pain on injection of propofol. Pain on intravenous injection of any medication has multiple etiologies and can be influenced by the temperature of the drug,

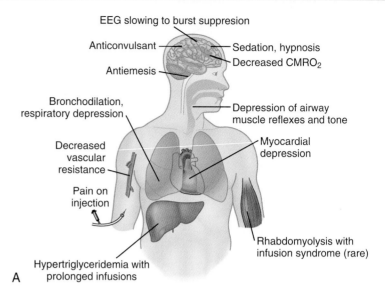

Figure 9-8 A, Selected effects of propofol. **B,** Structures of propofol and the water-soluble prodrug fospropofol.

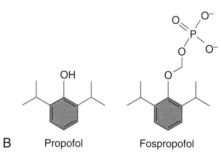

B   Propofol   Fospropofol

the site of administration, the size of the vein, the speed of injection, and the rate of infusion of the carrier fluid. Some common hyperosmolar formulations of diazepam and etomidate also cause pain on injection and this pain is often reduced with formulations that are closer to blood in osmolarity.[103,104] However, the modern formulation of propofol is not hyperosmolar and has a pH in the physiologic range. It is thought that the pain on injection of propofol is related to its free aqueous concentration, because the pain on injection appears to be less when the propofol concentration is reduced in its current formulation.[105] Coadministration of lidocaine (either as a pretreatment or mixed with propofol) can reduce the incidence of pain on injection, although other strategies have been suggested.[106]

The rapid effects of propofol on the brain make it a frequent choice for sedation in monitored anesthesia care (MAC) settings and for induction and maintenance of general anesthesia. Its rapid metabolic clearance is useful in pediatric procedures like magnetic resonance imaging (MRI), in the critical care arena for sedation during mechanical ventilation, and in neuroanesthesia to temporarily reduce cerebral metabolic rate (i.e., burst suppression or isoelectric EEG). Propofol also possesses unique antiemetic qualities that are beneficial for ambulatory procedures.

Propofol is metabolized via conjugation into inactive metabolites, however its clearance (total body clearance estimated at 25 mL/kg/min) exceeds that of hepatic blood flow and continues even during the anhepatic phase of liver transplantation; this argues for some extrahepatic metabolism of

the drug.[107] Like most of the intravenous anesthetics, the offset of the hypnotic effect after bolus administration occurs mainly through redistribution of propofol from the brain to less well-perfused sites. Plasma concentrations for inducing unconsciousness are 2 to 2.5 µg/mL and for maintenance of anesthesia are 2 to 6 µg/mL. The elimination half-life of propofol is prolonged because of the slow mobilization from adipose tissue. Regardless, obesity should not be considered a contraindication to its use for induction or maintenance. Obesity does not drastically prolong recovery and dose adjustments based on lean body weight have been suggested.[108] However, there is some controversy about this as other groups have demonstrated total body weight as the best predictor of propofol pharmacokinetics.[109]

Moderate hepatic or renal impairment has little effect on the duration of clinical effect. The dose requirement for propofol is reduced in the elderly because of reduced metabolic clearance of drugs and reduced relative volume of the central compartment. Dosing is increased in pediatric populations because relative central compartment volume is larger and clearance and metabolism are increased.

Propofol has a number of advantages over other intravenous agents for induction and maintenance of anesthesia. It depresses airway reflexes, reduces nausea, does not induce adrenocortical suppression, and has a short context-sensitive half-time even after prolonged infusion (see Figure 9-5, *C*).[110,111] Simulations of bolus kinetics indicate that it is second only to ketamine in speed of onset and offset (see Figure 9-5, *A*).

The primary disadvantage of propofol is its depressive effect on the cardiovascular system. Patients who are hypovolemic, debilitated, or reliant on high sympathetic tone to maintain blood pressure require careful titration of propofol to avoid severe hypotension. Animal models of hemorrhagic shock suggest that the induction dose should be reduced to between 10% and 20% of usual doses if given before fluid resuscitation and decreased 50% if given after resuscitation.[112] Use of propofol in patients with cardiac tamponade or critical aortic stenosis can result in hemodynamic collapse. Mixtures of low-dose ketamine infusions (10-20 µg/kg/min) with propofol infusions (100-200 µg/kg/min) have been used to mitigate the cardiovascular effects of both drugs, especially in pediatric anesthesia.[113] However, there is no improvement in respiratory complications compared with using propofol alone.[114]

Early clinical trials in the late 1980s and early 1990s consistently reported faster time to eye-opening and other recovery criteria for propofol-based anesthetics compared with "traditional" regimens of thiopental and volatile agents such as enflurane or isoflurane. More recent studies comparing propofol-based techniques to newer inhaled agents with lower blood and tissue solubility (desflurane and sevoflurane) have either failed to show benefit or have shown only minimal benefits in speed of recovery.[115] Propofol-based TIVA probably confers advantages over volatile agents in anesthetic maintenance for patients at high risk for postoperative nausea and vomiting.[111] It is beneficial not only for patients at high risk for malignant hyperthermia or postoperative nausea and vomiting but it also led to improved operating conditions for endoscopic sinus surgery and decreased pain and opioid consumption in gynecologic procedures.[116,117]

Anesthetic depth is an important consideration when comparing propofol-based TIVA techniques with volatile anesthesia. The concentration of expired anesthetic gases measured by modern anesthesia monitors correlates with the concentration of inhaled agent in the CNS.[118] Because propofol blood concentrations are not easily measured in the operating room, many practitioners choosing TIVA with propofol as their maintenance anesthetic attempt to control for individual variability in drug clearance through the use of an EEG-based depth of anesthesia monitor becasue it has been proven to decrease anesthetic use and facilitate postoperative recovery.[119] Favorable pharmacokinetic properties and effects on cerebral blood flow (CBF) and cerebral metabolic requirement for oxygen (CMRO$_2$) have made propofol popular for neuroanesthesia. In animal studies, reduction of CBF occurs even when mean arterial blood pressure is held constant, and propofol can reduce ICP even when cerebral perfusion pressure is fixed.[120] Cerebral autoregulation also appears to be preserved in the setting of propofol anesthesia.[121] In comparison, the volatile agents tend to increase ICP and at high doses compromise cerebral autoregulation. Although propofol and thiopental have similar effects on brain physiology, propofol might suppress apoptosis in models of ischemia in vitro (see Chapter 8).[122-124]

The latest Society for Critical Care Medicine sedation guidelines recommended the use of propofol when rapid or frequent interruptions of sedation are required, such as serial neurologic evaluations.[71] Awakening times were similar after 24-, 48-, 72-, and 96-hour constant rate infusions of propofol. Prolonged, high-dose infusions can lead to hypertriglyceridemia or a constellation of metabolic acidosis, rhabdomyolysis,

renal failure, and hemodynamic instability, known as propofol infusion syndrome. These complications are not common but patients should be monitored closely for propofol infusions greater than 48 hours. Although moderate-dose infusions (>40 µg/kg/min) can increase triglyceride levels in critically ill patients after just 3 days, low-dose propofol infusions (<33 µg/kg/min) showed no detectable increase in triglycerides after 2 weeks of constant infusion.[125]

It is difficult to imagine the practice of anesthesia without propofol. It is also essential outside of the operating room in settings such as the ICU, pediatric imaging procedures, and endoscopy suites. Propofol has numerous advantages (see Figure 9-8), but its depression of respiration makes it potentially dangerous in unskilled hands. Propofol appears to have greater relaxation effects on the pharyngeal musculature than thiopental and should be administered only by persons trained in the rescue of patients who experience deeper-than-intended sedation, including general anesthesia, (and who are not involved in the conduct of the procedure).[110]

Currently, no widely accepted method is available to anesthesia providers in the United States that allows estimates of blood concentrations of intravenous drugs being infused for maintenance of anesthesia during TIVA. This presents a disadvantage of intravenous anesthetics in comparison to inhaled anesthetics which are typically used in conjunction with monitors equipped with gas sampling for measurements of expired concentrations. Using computer-based models of drug pharmacokinetics, mathematical modeling of a drug's disposition can provide a convenient way to estimate these blood concentrations of intravenous agents.[126] Target-controlled infusion devices (e.g., Diprifusor) have been used successfully in maintaining anesthesia for both inpatient and outpatient surgery.[127] Despite obvious advantages of these devices in predicting blood concentrations some controversy exists in regard to which pharmacokinetic model should be used.[128,129] Another impediment to widespread use of these devices has been the unfamiliarity of providers in targeting an actual blood concentration range, as it is more common to think in terms of infusion rates rather than blood concentrations for infusions of other medications in the hospital.[130] There has been some attempts to improve the adoption of these devices by targeting depth of anesthesia using a processed EEG device rather than targeting a desired blood concentration (see Emerging Developments).[131]

Ketamine

Ketamine, an arylcyclohexylamine related to phencyclidine, was developed in the 1960s and approved for use in the United States in 1970. Early test subjects described a sense of disconnection from their environment, leading to the term "dissociative anesthesia."[132] Its combination of hypnosis and analgesia showed great promise as a complete anesthetic with minimal effects on cardiovascular function, respiratory drive, and airway reflexes. Concern over psychologic side effects such as hallucinations and emergence delirium limited its clinical use as a primary anesthetic agent, but there is an increasing body of evidence supporting the use of subanesthetic doses for treatment of acute and chronic pain (see Emerging Developments).

Ketamine was originally produced as a racemic mixture and most commercial preparations continue to be a racemic

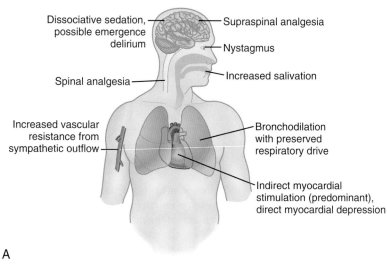

Figure 9-9 **A,** Selected effects of ketamine. **B,** Structures of S(+) ketamine and its parent drug phencyclidine. Ketamine is usually supplied as a racemic mixture but the more active S(+) isomer is available in some countries.

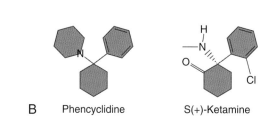

mix of the R and S enantiomers (see Chapter 2). S(+) ketamine, a single enantiomer formulation that is available in some areas of Europe and South America, is more potent in most clinical and experimental settings (Figure 9-9).

Despite more than 40 years of clinical use, the key site or sites of ketamine action have not been fully elucidated. The diverse effects of ketamine are likely mediated by a variety of receptors and signaling pathways. Landmark studies in the 1980s identified ketamine as an NMDA receptor antagonist in the spinal cord and brain.[133,134] Ketamine binds uncompetitively within the ion channel pore in a use-dependent fashion, but there is some evidence for allosteric binding as well.[39,135] Experimental data support a role for NMDA receptors in mediating analgesia, but their role in ketamine anesthesia is unclear.[46,47] Ketamine also inhibits nicotinic acetylcholine receptors at clinically relevant concentrations, which could contribute to analgesia but does not appear to influence its sedative properties.[136] Ketamine has some local anesthetic properties on Na⁺ channels and binds μ- and κ-opioid receptors.[137] Although blunted responses to ketamine have been noted in μ-opioid receptor knockout mice, the limited effect of naloxone on ketamine actions in humans suggests a limited role for these receptors. Finally, knockout of the HCN1 receptor in mice abolishes the hypnotic effect of ketamine and propofol but not of etomidate.[138] Further research is needed to confirm the significance of this pathway in humans.

In the brain, ketamine has a unique profile combining depressed consciousness with increased sympathetic tone. This sympathetic activation leads to increases in cardiac output in patients with normal catecholamine stores, which can make ketamine a useful induction agent in patients with hypovolemia. In patients with shock and depleted catecholamine reserves, the inability to mount a sympathetic surge unmasks a direct myocardial depressant effect of ketamine.[139] Respiratory effects of ketamine include bronchodilation,

preservation of respiratory drive, and maintenance of respiratory muscle tone.[140,141] It produces direct relaxation of airway smooth muscle ex vivo but may also cause bronchodilation indirectly through the modulation of vagal tone.[142,143] Ketamine has a number of other effects detailed in Figure 9-9.

Compared to other intravenous anesthetics, ketamine has relatively low plasma protein binding. This, in conjunction with its lipid solubility, allows rapid accumulation in the CNS. Intravenous bolus administration leads to peak effect site concentration within a minute (see Figure 9-5, *A*). Peak effects for other routes of administration are 10 to 15 minutes for intramuscular injection and 15 to 30 minutes following oral administration. Hepatic cytochrome P450 enzymes (especially CYP3A4) metabolize ketamine to norketamine by N-methylation in a perfusion-limited manner. Extensive first-pass metabolism leads to less than 20% bioavailability of orally administered ketamine. Norketamine is roughly one-third as potent as ketamine; its contribution to clinical effects appears relatively more significant in settings of long infusions or chronic use.

Although ketamine continues to play a major role in perioperative care in developing nations, concerns over side effects have limited its use in modern operating rooms to special situations. Low doses are frequently used to augment regional anesthesia during caesarean sections when the regional block is inadequate. It can be used for inductions in patients with asthma or hypovolemia; in a randomized controlled trial of acutely ill patients requiring rapid sequence intubation it was as effective as etomidate.[80] Ketamine is sometimes used in critical care in cases of status asthmaticus as an adjunctive bronchodilator, and as an analgesic for dressing changes in the burn ICU.

The role of ketamine in patients with neurologic injury is controversial. Its blockade of NMDA receptors could attenuate excitotoxicity, but animal studies have demonstrated neurotoxic effects on the developing brain.[144] The tradeoffs are presently unclear but recent German guidelines have outlined a role for ketamine in brain injured patients whose PaCO₂ is being controlled with mechanical ventilation.[145] The sympathomimetic properties of ketamine allow sedation with preserved or augmented blood pressure to improve cerebral perfusion. In general, however, ketamine has traditionally been avoided in neuroanesthesia (see Chapter 8).

The analgesic properties of ketamine and preservation of respiratory drive are useful for procedures in which it is critical to maintain spontaneous ventilation and preserve airway reflexes. These cases include patients with large anterior mediastinal masses who may suffer airway collapse if they become apneic or those patients whose airways must be secured while awake. Ketamine increases salivation and airway secretions that can impair visualization during fiberoptic intubation, but dexmedetomidine has emerged as an alternative with antisialagogue effects.[146]

Dexmedetomidine

Evidence of analgesic effects of the α-adrenergic agonist clonidine emerged in animal studies in the 1970s and led to the development of agents with greater α₂ specificity. Medetomidine was developed in the 1980s and found to have an α2/α1 selectivity ratio of 1620, almost eight times higher than clonidine's ratio. The α-adrenergic effects were mediated exclusively by the d-enantiomer now known as dexmedetomidine (Figure 9-10).[147] Even at high doses it does not produce general anesthesia but it is a valuable sedative in a number of settings.

Dexmedetomidine has effects both on the spinal cord and in the locus coeruleus. A number of elegant studies in transgenic mice suggest that the α2A subtype receptor mediates the majority of the analgesic and sedative effects on the CNS.[148] Dexmedetomidine leads to hyperpolarization via K⁺ influx with a subsequent decrease in neuronal firing as well as reduced norepinephrine release mediated by inhibitory presynaptic autoreceptors. It also decreases cAMP concentration by inhibiting adenylyl cyclase. Many of its effects stem from this decreased sympathetic outflow, but in some cases direct effects on peripheral α2B and α2A receptors predominate and blood pressure increases.[149] This hypertensive response is sometimes seen during loading doses and is the reason that dexmedetomidine should not be administered as a bolus.

The sedation produced by dexmedetomidine is different in that patients tend to be easily arousable. This feature, in combination with its minimal effects on respiratory drive, allows continuation of infusions during weaning from mechanical ventilation and after extubation without the need for dose titration.[150] It has some analgesic qualities and augments the effects of opioids by both spinal and supraspinal mechanisms.[54,151] In contrast to other agents, dexmedetomidine has limited amnestic effect and so should be avoided as a sole agent in patients with neuromuscular blockade. Dexmedetomidine also reduces shivering in an additive fashion with meperidine, raising the possibility that effects of both are mediated by α2 receptors.[152]

The sympatholytic effects of dexmedetomidine lead to decreased heart rate and blood pressure, which can be helpful, harmful, or of no clinical consequence. In many scenarios these effects are minimal and well tolerated. In patients

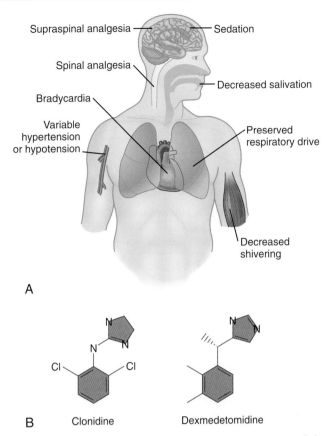

Figure 9-10 **A,** Selected effects of dexmedetomidine. **B,** Structures of the α₂ agonists clonidine and dexmedetomidine.

with cardiac disease there is a potential benefit of decreased myocardial demand in response to painful stimuli. A recent meta-analysis found decreased mortality in vascular surgery patients, but with increased bradycardia and hypotension.[153] Bradycardia can be dangerous in the setting of heart block and dexmedetomidine should be used with caution in this setting. Significant hypotension is more likely in patients with high sympathetic tone such as diabetics, the elderly, and those with hypovolemia. Selected other effects are shown in Figure 9-10.

Dexmedetomidine is metabolized in the liver primarily by glucuronidation with a small portion undergoing hydroxylation by CYP2A6. The distribution half-life is 6 to 8 minutes and its lipophilicity leads to a high volume of distribution. The context-sensitive half-times range from 25 to 120 minutes for a 1-hour infusion to 87 to 250 minutes for infusions greater than 6 hours (Figure 9-11).[154-156]

Dexmedetomidine sedation is increasingly used in the ICU and is associated with less delirium than benzodiazepine sedation.[157,158] Dexmedetomidine may reduce delirium in part because its sedation closely mimics physiologic sleep in adults and children.[159,160] The ability to extubate patients without weaning dexmedetomidine can facilitate earlier extubation in those patients who become agitated when sedation is held. In the United States, dexmedetomidine is approved for infusions up to 24 hours, but much longer infusions have been reported in the literature. There are concerns for withdrawal phenomena for prolonged infusions but no clear withdrawal syndrome has been reported.

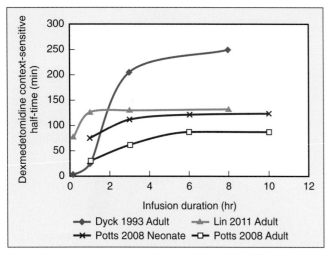

Figure 9-11 Context-sensitive half-times of dexmedetomidine reported in adults and neonates based on various pharmacokinetic models. *(Modified from Dyck JB, Maze M, Haack C, et al. Computer-controlled infusion of intravenous dexmedetomidine hydrochloride in adult human volunteers. Anesthesiology. 1993;78:821-828; Potts AL, Warman GR, Anderson BJ. Dexmedetomidine disposition in children: a population analysis. Paediatr Anaesth. 2008;18:722-730; and Lin L, Guo X, Zhang MZ, et al. Pharmacokinetics of dexmedetomidine in Chinese post-surgical intensive care unit patients. Acta Anaesthesiol Scand. 2011;55:359-367.)*

Controversy over the use of propofol by non-anesthesiologists has prompted a number of studies of dexmedetomidine as an alternative in sedation practice.[161] A small clinical trial suggested it was comparable to propofol but had longer recovery times; conventional doses up to 1 µg/kg/hr often require supplementation with other drugs. One group reported success of dexmedetomidine as a sole agent in over 97% of pediatric MRI scans by escalating the loading dose to 3 µg/kg and the infusion to 2 µg/kg/hr.[162]

The clinical applications of dexmedetomidine continue to expand. Although initially approved by regulatory agencies only for ICU sedation, dexmedetomidine was recently approved for monitored anesthesia care (MAC) sedation in the United States. The antisialagogue effect of dexmedetomidine represents an advantage over ketamine for awake fiberoptic intubations.[146] It has also been administered intranasally for premedication of children.[163] The specific and distinctive mechanism of action of dexmedetomidine provides an important alternative amid ongoing uncertainty about short- and long-term cognitive effects of more established anesthetics in both young and old patients.[73]

EMERGING DEVELOPMENTS

Ongoing efforts to improve the safety of intravenous anesthetics include both new systems to titrate existing drugs and new compounds with the potential for improved safety profiles.

High-Tech Delivery Systems

The development of a computer-aided device that dynamically adjusts anesthetic administration based on measured physiologic parameters has been explored for both inhaled[164] and intravenously administered drugs.[164,165] Commonly referred to as closed-loop anesthesia delivery systems (CLADS), these devices are typically associated with feedback controls based on predicting depth of hypnosis via EEG analysis or other brain monitor (e.g., auditory evoked potentials).[166] Recently, a Canadian group has developed an automated system that titrates dose based on three separate parameters: pain, muscle relaxation, and depth of hypnosis (measured via EEG analysis).[167] Several studies have shown some benefit to CLADS over manual infusion rates and open-loop target controlled infusions, but there is some controversy regarding their economic efficiency and the choice of physiologic parameters to which dosage is titrated.[131,166,168,169] Controversy surrounding the supervision of these automated devices for use in endoscopic and other office-based procedures will also necessitate discussions regarding the safety of traditional anesthesia drugs in the hands of nonanesthesiologists.

Novel Sedatives

The rapid growth in outpatient and office-based procedures has stimulated the development of several new drugs. One example is fospropofol, a water-soluble prodrug of propofol. Circulating phosphatases metabolize the drug into propofol, formaldehyde, and a phosphate group (Figure 9-12, *A*).[170] It was envisioned during the drug development process that the slower onset of drug effect associated with the metabolism of the propofol prodrug would allow safe bolus administration in the setting of procedural sedation. However, the FDA product labeling ultimately recommended that fospropofol should only be administered by persons trained in general anesthesia as unanticipated transitions to general anesthesia remain a possibility. The formaldehyde levels measured after routine fospropofol administration are indistinguishable from baseline levels.[171] After administration of the drug, formaldehyde is rapidly metabolized to formate. Although high formate levels can lead to metabolic acidosis, there has been no reported formate toxicity from fospropofol. Other supposed advantages from this alternative formulation of propofol are decreased risk of bacteremia, decreased risk of hyperlipidemia, and decreased pain on injection, although pruritus and perineal paresthesias are reported side effects of its administration.[172]

Other intravenous anesthetics have been designed to mimic the rapid, end-organ independent metabolism of drugs such as remifentanil. The benzodiazepine CNS-7056, also known as remimazolam, undergoes ester hydrolysis to form a carboxylic acid metabolite which is 300 times less potent (see Figure 9-12, *B*).[173] It may offer sedation with less postprocedure cognitive effects than midazolam and is now being investigated in humans.

A similar strategy has been applied to modify etomidate and reduce its adrenal suppression effects. Investigators have developed an ultrarapid metabolizing etomidate named methoxycarbonyletomidate (MOC-etomidate), which is broken down via nonspecific esterases (see Figure 9-12, *C*).[174] The in vitro half-life of MOC-etomidate is approximately one-tenth that of its parent compound etomidate. The rapid metabolism of MOC-etomidate into a carboxylic acid metabolite, which has low affinity for 11β-hydroxylase, results in less adrenocortical suppression than its parent compound.[175] This compound, as well as carboetomidate (see Figure 9-7), a pyrrole analog of etomidate specifically designed not to

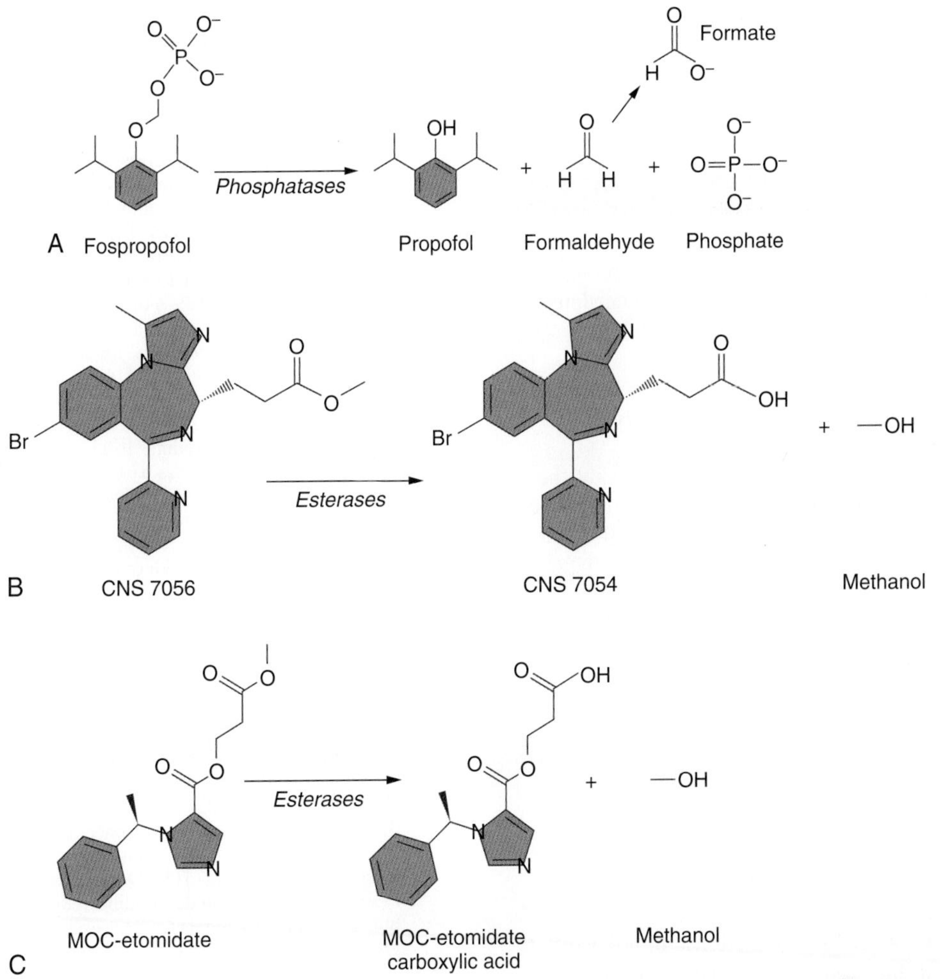

Figure 9-12 Metabolism of next generation intravenous anesthetics. Fospropofol **(A)** is a prodrug, which is activated by phosphatases.[172] The benzodiazepine remimazolam/CNS-7056 **(B)** and the etomidate analog MOC-etomidate **(C)** are rapidly metabolized by esterases to carboxylic acid derivatives with very low activity.[173,174]

bind 11β-hydroxylase with high affinity, both maintain the beneficial qualities of etomidate including rapid induction of general anesthesia with significant hemodynamic stability in animal models.[176] MOC-carboetomidate combines rapid esterase metabolism with the minimal adrenal effects of carboetomidate.[177]

Novel Applications of Existing Sedatives

There is ongoing investigation of NMDA antagonists in chronic pain. Although the opioid-sparing effects of low-dose intraoperative ketamine infusions are well-established, there is renewed interest in its use in patients with chronic pain.[178] In opioid-tolerant patients undergoing back surgery, intraoperative ketamine reduced pain scores and opioid consumption not only in the acute postoperative period, but also 6 weeks after the operation.[48] Post-hoc analysis suggested that the greatest benefit was in those patients whose preoperative opioid consumption exceeded the equivalent of 0.55 mg/hour of intravenous morphine. In the long-term management of chronic pain, small studies have found that multiday ketamine infusions may provide weeks of benefit for patients with complex regional pain syndrome type 1 and neuropathic spinal cord pain.[179,180] Nevertheless, a trial in fibromyalgia

patients showed no benefit and reversible hepatotoxicity has occurred in three patients receiving multiday infusions.[181,182] Preclinical data suggests that NR2B-selective NMDA antagonists may offer a better therapeutic index and the search continues for a viable oral drug for chronic pain.[183]

Reversal of General Anesthesia

Anesthesiologists have several intravenous "antidotes" for certain features of the anesthetized state at their disposal (e.g., neostigmine for neuromuscular blocking agents or naloxone for opioids). Since the arrival of flumazenil, reversal of general anesthesia or sedation has been investigated to facilitate and expedite recovery from benzodiazepine-based procedural sedation or general anesthesia.[184,185] Early studies showed little effect on recovery from enflurane or propofol anesthesia, but concurrent opioid administration may have contaminated the results.[186,187] More recent studies have shown improvements in the quality of recovery, including reduced shivering and expedited recovery endpoints in un-premedicated patients receiving volatile anesthesia.[188,189] Interestingly, flumazenil may also find a role in reducing postoperative narcotic usage.[190] Although the GABA_A receptor may play a prominent role in emergence and recovery, the partial agonist properties of this drug may make it difficult to study as a pure reversal agent of general anesthesia. Studies investigating the role of dopamine and nicotine in anesthesia recovery are also promising.[191,192]

KEY POINTS

- Intravenous anesthetics are used both to induce and maintain general anesthesia in the operating room, for sedation and anxiolysis preoperatively, for procedures outside the operating room, and in the ICU.
- Potentiation of the effect of the inhibitory neurotransmitter GABA at $GABA_A$ receptors is the most important mechanism of action for barbiturates, benzodiazepines, etomidate, and propofol.
- Ongoing molecular studies are dissecting not only the specific binding pockets for intravenous anesthetics but also the receptor subunit combinations that differentially mediate effects such as sedation, anxiolysis, and amnesia.
- Etomidate plays an important role in the induction of anesthesia in patients with significant cardiovascular comorbidities such as congestive heart failure or hemorrhagic shock.
- Propofol-based TIVA has advantages over anesthetic maintenance with volatile anesthetics in some patient populations.
- Ketamine blocks glutamate signaling at NMDA-type glutamate receptors, but its clinical effects are broader and more profound than those of more specific NMDA receptor antagonists.
- Subanesthetic doses of ketamine are useful adjuvants for chronic pain patients and its combination of low cost, analgesia, and preserved respiratory drive make it an important anesthetic, especially in developing nations.
- Dexmedetomidine is a highly specific α_2 adrenergic receptor agonist that produces sedation with preserved respiratory drive. Dexmedetomidine has seen an increasing role in perioperative and ICU sedation.
- The combination of intravenous anesthetics can be tailored for each patient and procedure to optimize the key aspects of the anesthetic and minimize toxicity.

Key References

Anis NA, Berry SC, Burton NR, Lodge D. The dissociative anaesthetics, ketamine and phencyclidine, selectively reduce excitation of central mammalian neurones by N-methyl-aspartate. *Br J Pharmacol.* 1983;79(2):565-575. Representative of several seminal publications by Lodge demonstrating blockade of NMDA action in isolated spinal cord cells as well as after intravenous administration in intact animals. (Ref. 133)

Belelli D, Lambert JJ, Peters JA, Wafford K, Whiting PJ. The interaction of the general anesthetic etomidate with the gamma-aminobutyric acid type A receptor is influenced by a single amino acid. *Proc Natl Acad Sci U S A.* 1997;94(20):11031-11036. A pioneering demonstration of manipulating the sensitivity of $GABA_A$ receptors to intravenous anesthetics by specific amino-acid substitutions. (Ref. 31)

Cummings GC, Dixon J, Kay NH, et al. Dose requirements of ICI 35,868 (propofol, 'Diprivan') in a new formulation for induction of anaesthesia. *Anaesthesia.* 1984;39(12):1168-1171. First demon-

stration of propofol's clinical usage in humans with its new soy-based emulsion. (Ref. 92)

Glen JB. Animal studies of the anaesthetic activity of ICI 35 868. *Br J Anaesth.* 1980;52(8):731-742. Glen's original characterization of the phenolic compound now known as propofol. Glen would later go on to prepare propofol in the soy-based emulsion suitable for human anesthesia after concerns of adverse reactions to its original carrier solution (Cremaphor EL) surfaced. (Ref. 91)

Loftus RW, Yeager MP, Clark JA, et al. Intraoperative ketamine reduces perioperative opiate consumption in opiate-dependent patients with chronic back pain undergoing back surgery. *Anesthesiology.* 2010;113(3):639-646. In a population of opioid-tolerant patients, sub-anesthetic ketamine infusion decreased pain and opioid consumption not only immediately postoperatively but also 6 weeks after surgery. (Ref. 48)

Lundy JS. The barbiturates as anesthetics, hypnotics and antispasmodics. *Anesthesia & Analgesia.* 1929;8(1-6):360-364. After verifying that barbiturates reduce local anesthetic toxicity in dogs, Lundy outlined their use as part of a balanced anesthetic in over 1000 patients. The lessons gleaned from his progression from oral premedication to sole anesthetic laid the foundation for his later work with thiopental. (Ref. 55)

Pandharipande PP, Pun BT, Herr DL, et al. Effect of sedation with dexmedetomidine vs lorazepam on acute brain dysfunction in mechanically ventilated patients: the MENDS randomized controlled trial. *JAMA.* 2007;298(22):2644-2653. First of the large clinical trials showing a reduction in delirium with dexmedetomidine compared to benzodiazepine sedation. (Ref. 157)

Unwin N. Refined structure of the nicotinic acetylcholine receptor at 4A resolution. *J Mol Biol.* 2005;346(4):967-989. Our current best understanding of the structure of the $GABA_A$ receptor is based on homology to this high resolution structure. (Ref. 13)

Vickery RG, Sheridan BC, Segal IS, Maze M. Anesthetic and hemodynamic effects of the stereoisomers of medetomidine, an alpha 2-adrenergic agonist, in halothane-anesthetized dogs. *Anesth Analg.* 1988;67(7):611-615. Demonstrated not only that the racemic compound medetomidine reduces MAC for halothane but also that its effects were exclusively mediated by the D-enantiomer now marketed as dexmedetomidine. (Ref. 47)

References

1. Bergman NA. Early intravenous anesthesia: an eyewitness account. *Anesthesiology.* 1990;72(1):185-186.
2. Adams RC. Intravenous anesthesia. *Anesthesiology.* 1947;8(5):489-496.
3. Hatcher RA, Eggleston C. A contribution to the pharmacology of Novocain. *J Pharmacol Exp Ther.* 1916;8(Jul):385-405.
4. Dundee JW, McIlroy PD. The history of barbiturates. *Anaesthesia.* 1982;37(7):726-734.
5. Hilgenberg JC. Intraoperative awareness during high-dose fentanyl—oxygen anesthesia. *Anesthesiology.* 1981;54(4):341-343.
6. Lundy J. Balanced anesthesia. *Minn Med.* 1926;(9):399.
7. Alkire MT, Hudetz AG, Tononi G. Consciousness and anesthesia. *Science.* 2008;322(5903):876-880.
8. Franks NP. General anaesthesia: from molecular targets to neuronal pathways of sleep and arousal. *Nat Rev Neurosci.* 2008;9(5):370-386.
9. Sieghart W, Sperk G. Subunit composition, distribution and function of GABA(A) receptor subtypes. *Curr Top Med Chem.* 2002;2(8):795-816.
10. Antkowiak B, Kirschfeld K. [Neural mechanisms of anesthesia.] *Anasthesiol Intensivmed Notfallmed Schmerzther.* 2000;35(12):731-743.
11. Collins JG, Kendig JJ, Mason P. Anesthetic actions within the spinal cord: contributions to the state of general anesthesia. *Trends Neurosci.* 1995;18(12):549-553.
12. McGaugh JL, Izquierdo I. The contribution of pharmacology to research on the mechanisms of memory formation. *Trends Pharmacol Sci.* 2000;21(6):208-210.
13. Unwin N. Refined structure of the nicotinic acetylcholine receptor at 4A resolution. *J Mol Biol.* 2005;346(4):967-989.

14. Simon J, Wakimoto H, Fujita N, Lalande M, Barnard EA. Analysis of the set of GABA(A) receptor genes in the human genome. *J Biol Chem.* 2004;279(40):41422-41435.

15. Mody I, Pearce RA. Diversity of inhibitory neurotransmission through GABA(A) receptors. *Trends Neurosci.* 2004;27(9):569-575.

16. Sieghart W, Schuster A. Affinity of various ligands for benzodiazepine receptors in rat cerebellum and hippocampus. *Biochem Pharmacol.* 1984;33(24):4033-4038.

17. Richardson JE, Garcia PS, O'Toole KK, Derry JM, Bell SV, Jenkins A. A conserved tyrosine in the beta2 subunit M4 segment is a determinant of gamma-aminobutyric acid type A receptor sensitivity to propofol. *Anesthesiology.* 2007;107(3):412-418.

18. Jurd R, Arras M, Lambert S, et al. General anesthetic actions in vivo strongly attenuated by a point mutation in the GABA(A) receptor beta3 subunit. *FASEB J.* 2003;17(2):250-252.

19. Zeller A, Arras M, Jurd R, Rudolph U. Identification of a molecular target mediating the general anesthetic actions of pentobarbital. *Mol Pharmacol.* 2007;71(3):852-859.

20. Laurie DJ, Seeburg PH, Wisden W. The distribution of 13 GABAA receptor subunit mRNAs in the rat brain. II. Olfactory bulb and cerebellum. *J Neurosci.* 1992;12(3):1063-1076.

21. Wisden W, Laurie DJ, Monyer H, Seeburg PH. The distribution of 13 GABAA receptor subunit mRNAs in the rat brain. I. Telencephalon, diencephalon, mesencephalon. *J Neurosci.* 1992;12(3):1040-1062.

22. Reynolds DS, Rosahl TW, Cirone J, et al. Sedation and anesthesia mediated by distinct GABA(A) receptor isoforms. *J Neurosci.* 2003;23(24):8608-8617.

23. O'Meara GF, Newman RJ, Fradley RL, Dawson GR, Reynolds DS. The GABA-A beta3 subunit mediates anaesthesia induced by etomidate. *Neuroreport.* 2004;15(10):1653-1656.

24. Ching S, Cimenser A, Purdon PL, Brown EN, Kopell NJ. Thalamocortical model for a propofol-induced alpha-rhythm associated with loss of consciousness. *Proc Natl Acad Sci U S A.* 2010;107(52):22665-22670.

25. Talavera JA, Esser SK, Amzica F, Hill S, Antognini JF. Modeling the GABAergic action of etomidate on the thalamocortical system. *Anesth Analg.* 2009;108(1):160-167.

26. Sigel E, Baur R, Kellenberger S, Malherbe P. Point mutations affecting antagonist affinity and agonist dependent gating of GABAA receptor channels. *EMBO J.* 1992;11(6):2017-2023.

27. Kleingoor C, Wieland HA, Korpi ER, Seeburg PH, Kettenmann H. Current potentiation by diazepam but not GABA sensitivity is determined by a single histidine residue. *Neuroreport.* 1993;4(2):187-190.

28. Amin J, Weiss DS. GABAA receptor needs two homologous domains of the beta-subunit for activation by GABA but not by pentobarbital. *Nature.* 1993;366(6455):565-569.

29. Smith GB, Olsen RW. Functional domains of GABAA receptors. *Trends Pharmacol Sci.* 1995;16(5):162-168.

30. Mihic SJ, Ye Q, Wick MJ, et al. Sites of alcohol and volatile anaesthetic action on GABA(A) and glycine receptors. *Nature.* 1997;389(6649):385-389.

31. Belelli D, Lambert JJ, Peters JA, Wafford K, Whiting PJ. The interaction of the general anesthetic etomidate with the gamma-aminobutyric acid type A receptor is influenced by a single amino acid. *Proc Natl Acad Sci U S A.* 1997;94(20):11031-11036.

32. Siegwart R, Jurd R, Rudolph U. Molecular determinants for the action of general anesthetics at recombinant alpha(2)beta(3)gamma(2)gamma-aminobutyric acid(A) receptors. *J Neurochem.* 2002;80(1):140-148.

33. Rudolph U, Mohler H. Analysis of GABAA receptor function and dissection of the pharmacology of benzodiazepines and general anesthetics through mouse genetics. *Annu Rev Pharmacol Toxicol.* 2004;44:475-498.

34. Rudolph U, Crestani F, Benke D, et al. Benzodiazepine actions mediated by specific gamma-aminobutyric acid(A) receptor subtypes. *Nature.* 1999;401(6755):796-800.

35. Low K, Crestani F, Keist R, et al. Molecular and neuronal substrate for the selective attenuation of anxiety. *Science.* 2000;290(5489):131-134.

36. Crestani F, Keist R, Fritschy JM, et al. Trace fear conditioning involves hippocampal alpha5 GABA(A) receptors. *Proc Natl Acad Sci U S A.* 2002;99(13):8980-8985.

37. McKernan RM, Rosahl TW, Reynolds DS, et al. Sedative but not anxiolytic properties of benzodiazepines are mediated by the GABA(A) receptor alpha1 subtype. *Nat Neurosci.* 2000;3(6):587-592.

38. Morris HV, Dawson GR, Reynolds DS, Atack JR, Stephens DN. Both alpha2 and alpha3 GABAA receptor subtypes mediate the anxiolytic properties of benzodiazepine site ligands in the conditioned emotional response paradigm. *Eur J Neurosci.* 2006;23(9):2495-2504.

39. Traynelis SF, Wollmuth LP, McBain CJ, et al. Glutamate receptor ion channels: structure, regulation, and function. *Pharmacol Rev.* 2010;62(3):405-496.

40. Harris RA, Mihic SJ, Dildy-Mayfield JE, Machu TK. Actions of anesthetics on ligand-gated ion channels: role of receptor subunit composition. *FASEB J.* 1995;9(14):1454-1462.

41. Duguid IC, Smart TG. Presynaptic NMDA Receptors. In: Van Dongen AM, ed. *Biology of the NMDA Receptor.* Boca Raton, FL: CRC Press; 2009 [chapter 14].

42. Grasshoff C, Drexler B, Rudolph U, Antkowiak B. Anaesthetic drugs: linking molecular actions to clinical effects. *Curr Pharm Des.* 2006;12(28):3665-3679.

43. Paoletti P, Neyton J. NMDA receptor subunits: function and pharmacology. *Curr Opin Pharmacol.* 2007;7(1):39-47.

44. Nicoll RA, Malenka RC. Expression mechanisms underlying NMDA receptor-dependent long-term potentiation. *Ann N Y Acad Sci.* 1999;868:515-525.

45. Daw NW, Stein PS, Fox K. The role of NMDA receptors in information processing. *Annu Rev Neurosci.* 1993;16:207-222.

46. South SM, Kohno T, Kaspar BK, et al. A conditional deletion of the NR1 subunit of the NMDA receptor in adult spinal cord dorsal horn reduces NMDA currents and injury-induced pain. *J Neurosci.* 2003;23(12):5031-5040.

47. Garraway SM, Xu Q, Inturrisi CE. siRNA-mediated knockdown of the NR1 subunit gene of the NMDA receptor attenuates formalin-induced pain behaviors in adult rats. *J Pain.* 2009;10(4):380-390.

48. Loftus RW, Yeager MP, Clark JA, et al. Intraoperative ketamine reduces perioperative opiate consumption in opiate-dependent patients with chronic back pain undergoing back surgery. *Anesthesiology.* 2010;113(3):639-646.

49. Dickinson R, Peterson BK, Banks P, et al. Competitive inhibition at the glycine site of the N-methyl-D-aspartate receptor by the anesthetics xenon and isoflurane: evidence from molecular modeling and electrophysiology. *Anesthesiology.* 2007;107(5):756-767.

50. Grasshoff C, Antkowiak B. Propofol and sevoflurane depress spinal neurons in vitro via different molecular targets. *Anesthesiology.* 2004;101(5):1167-1176.

51. Ratnakumari L, Hemmings HC Jr. Effects of propofol on sodium channel-dependent sodium influx and glutamate release in rat cerebrocortical synaptosomes. *Anesthesiology.* 1997;86(2):428-439.

52. Frenkel C, Urban BW. Molecular actions of racemic ketamine on human CNS sodium channels. *Br J Anaesth.* 1992;69(3):292-297.

53. Ying SW, Abbas SY, Harrison NL, Goldstein PA. Propofol block of I(h) contributes to the suppression of neuronal excitability and rhythmic burst firing in thalamocortical neurons. *Eur J Neurosci.* 2006;23(2):465-480.

54. Guo TZ, Jiang JY, Buttermann AE, Maze M. Dexmedetomidine injection into the locus ceruleus produces antinociception. *Anesthesiology.* 1996;84(4):873-881.

55. Lundy JS. The barbiturates as anesthetics, hypnotics and antispasmodics. *Anesth Analg.* 1929;8(1-6):360-364.

56. Gibson WR, Doran WJ, Wood WC, Swanson EE. Pharmacology of stereoisomers of 1-methyl-5-(1-methyl-2-pentynyl)-5-allyl-barbituric acid. *J Pharmacol Exp Ther.* 1959;125(1):23-27.

57. Brunner H, Ittner K-P, Lunz D, Schmatloch S, Schmidt T, Zabel M. Highly enriched mixtures of methohexital stereoisomers by palladium-catalyzed allylation and their anaesthetic activity. *Eur J Organic Chem* 2003;2003:855-862.

58. Tomlin SL, Jenkins A, Lieb WR, Franks NP. Preparation of barbiturate optical isomers and their effects on GABA(A) receptors. *Anesthesiology.* 1999;90(6):1714-1722.

59. Bieda MC, Su H, Maciver MB. Anesthetics discriminate between tonic and phasic gamma-aminobutyric acid receptors on hippocampal CA1 neurons. *Anesth Analg.* 2009;108(2):484-490.

60. Bennetts FE. Thiopentone anaesthesia at Pearl Harbor. *Br J Anaesth.* 1995;75(3):366-368.

61. Hughes MA, Glass PS, Jacobs JR. Context-sensitive half-time in multicompartment pharmacokinetic models for intravenous anesthetic drugs. *Anesthesiology.* 1992;76(3):334-341.

62. Russo H, Bressolle F. Pharmacodynamics and pharmacokinetics of thiopental. *Clin Pharmacokinet.* 1998;35(2):95-134.

63. Mustajoki P, Heinonen J. General anesthesia in "inducible" porphyrias. *Anesthesiology.* 1980;53(1):15-20.

64. Martin IL. The benzodiazepines and their receptors: 25 years of progress. *Neuropharmacology.* 1987;26(7B):957-970.

65. Gerecke M. Chemical structure and properties of midazolam compared with other benzodiazepines. *Br J Clin Pharmacol.* 1983;16 Suppl 1:11S-16S.

66. Bailey PL, Pace NL, Ashburn MA, Moll JW, East KA, Stanley TH. Frequent hypoxemia and apnea after sedation with midazolam and fentanyl. *Anesthesiology.* 1990;73(5):826-830.

67. Gueye PN, Lofaso F, Borron SW, et al. Mechanism of respiratory insufficiency in pure or mixed drug-induced coma involving benzodiazepines. *J Toxicol Clin Toxicol.* 2002;40(1):35-47.

68. Sun GC, Hsu MC, Chia YY, Chen PY, Shaw FZ. Effects of age and gender on intravenous midazolam premedication: a randomized double-blind study. *Br J Anaesth.* 2008;101(5):632-639.

69. Shih A, Miletic V, Miletic G, Smith LJ. Midazolam administration reverses thermal hyperalgesia and prevents gamma-aminobutyric acid transporter loss in a rodent model of neuropathic pain. *Anesth Analg.* 2008;106(4):1296-1302.

70. Kain ZN, Mayes LC, Bell C, Weisman S, Hofstadter MB, Rimar S. Premedication in the United States: a status report. *Anesth Analg.* 1997;84(2):427-432.

71. Jacobi J, Fraser GL, Coursin DB, et al. Clinical practice guidelines for the sustained use of sedatives and analgesics in the critically ill adult. *Crit Care Med.* 2002;30(1):119-141.

72. Pisani MA, Murphy TE, Araujo KL, Slattum P, Van Ness PH, Inouye SK. Benzodiazepine and opioid use and the duration of intensive care unit delirium in an older population. *Crit Care Med.* 2009;37(1):177-183.

73. Hughes CG, Pandharipande PP. Review articles: the effects of perioperative and intensive care unit sedation on brain organ dysfunction. *Anesth Analg.* 2011;112(5):1212-1217.

74. Taupin V, Jayais P, Descamps-Latscha B, et al. Benzodiazepine anesthesia in humans modulates the interleukin-1 beta, tumor necrosis factor-alpha and interleukin-6 responses of blood monocytes. *J Neuroimmunol.* 1991;35(1-3):13-19.

75. Wei M, Li L, Meng R, et al. Suppressive effect of diazepam on IFN-gamma production by human T cells. *Int Immunopharmacol.* 2010;10(3):267-271.

76. Spivey WH. Flumazenil and seizures: analysis of 43 cases. *Clin Ther.* 1992;14(2):292-305.

77. Scollo-Lavizzari G. The clinical anti-convulsant effects of flumazenil, a benzodiazepine antagonist. *Eur J Anaesthesiol Suppl.* 1988;2:129-138.

78. Adachi YU, Watanabe K, Higuchi H, Satoh T. Flumazenil reduces the hypnotic dose of propofol in male patients under spinal anesthesia. *J Anesth.* 2002;16(1):9-12.

79. Ray DC, McKeown DW. Effect of induction agent on vasopressor and steroid use, and outcome in patients with septic shock. *Crit Care.* 2007;11(3):R56.

80. Jabre P, Combes X, Lapostolle F, et al. Etomidate versus ketamine for rapid sequence intubation in acutely ill patients: a multicentre randomised controlled trial. *Lancet.* 2009;374(9686):293-300.

81. Tomlin SL, Jenkins A, Lieb WR, Franks NP. Stereoselective effects of etomidate optical isomers on gamma-aminobutyric acid type A receptors and animals. *Anesthesiology.* 1998;88(3):708-717.

82. Hill-Venning C, Belelli D, Peters JA, Lambert JJ. Subunit-dependent interaction of the general anaesthetic etomidate with the gamma-aminobutyric acid type A receptor. *Br J Pharmacol.* 1997;120(3):749-756.

83. McCollum JS, Dundee JW. Comparison of induction characteristics of four intravenous anaesthetic agents. *Anaesthesia.* 1986;41(10):995-1000.

84. Choi SD, Spaulding BC, Gross JB, Apfelbaum JL. Comparison of the ventilatory effects of etomidate and methohexital. *Anesthesiology.* 1985;62(4):442-447.

85. Ledingham IM, Watt I. Influence of sedation on mortality in critically ill multiple trauma patients. *Lancet.* 1983;1(8336):1270.

86. Morel J, Salard M, Castelain C, et al. Haemodynamic consequences of etomidate administration in elective cardiac surgery: a randomized double-blinded study. *Br J Anaesth.* 2011;107(4):503-509.

87. Albert SG, Ariyan S, Rather A. The effect of etomidate on adrenal function in critical illness: a systematic review. *Intensive Care Med.* 2011;37(6):901-910.

88. Orser BA, McAdam LC, Roder S, MacDonald JF. General anaesthetics and their effects on GABA(A) receptor desensitization. *Toxicol Lett.* 1998;100-101:217-224.

89. Sanna E, Mascia MP, Klein RL, Whiting PJ, Biggio G, Harris RA. Actions of the general anesthetic propofol on recombinant human GABAA receptors: influence of receptor subunits. *J Pharmacol Exp Ther.* 1995;274(1):353-360.

90. Jones MV, Harrison NL, Pritchett DB, Hales TG. Modulation of the GABAA receptor by propofol is independent of the gamma subunit. *J Pharmacol Exp Ther.* 1995;274(2):962-968.

91. Glen JB. Animal studies of the anaesthetic activity of ICI 35 868. *Br J Anaesth.* 1980;52(8):731-742.

92. Cummings GC, Dixon J, Kay NH, et al. Dose requirements of ICI 35,868 (propofol, 'Diprivan') in a new formulation for induction of anaesthesia. *Anaesthesia.* 1984;39(12):1168-1171.

93. Dewachter P, Mouton-Faivre C, Castells MC, Hepner DL. Anesthesia in the patient with multiple drug allergies: are all allergies the same? *Curr Opin Anaesthesiol.* 2011;24(3):320-325.

94. Murphy A, Campbell DE, Baines D, Mehr S. Allergic reactions to propofol in egg-allergic children. *Anesth Analg.* 2011;113(1):140-144.

95. Bennett SN, McNeil MM, Bland LA, et al. Postoperative infections traced to contamination of an intravenous anesthetic, propofol. *N Engl J Med.* 1995;333(3):147-154.

96. Jansson JR, Fukada T, Ozaki M, Kimura S. Propofol EDTA and reduced incidence of infection. *Anaesth Intensive Care.* 2006;34(3):362-368.

97. Thompson KA, Goodale DB. The recent development of propofol (DIPRIVAN). *Intensive Care Med.* 2000;26 Suppl 4:S400-S404.

98. FDA. Information for Healthcare Professionals: propofol (marketed as Diprivan and as generic products). 2007; http://www.fda.gov/Drugs/DrugSafety/PostmarketDrugSafetyInformationforPatientsandProviders/ucm125817.htm. Accessed December 16, 2011.

99. Germain JM, Carbonne A, Thiers V, et al. Patient-to-patient transmission of hepatitis C virus through the use of multidose vials during general anesthesia. *Infect Control Hosp Epidemiol.* 2005;26(9):789-792.

100. Fischer GE, Schaefer MK, Labus BJ, et al. Hepatitis C virus infections from unsafe injection practices at an endoscopy clinic in Las Vegas, Nevada, 2007-2008. *Clin Infect Dis.* 2010;51(3):267-273.

101. Henry B, Plante-Jenkins C, Ostrowska K. An outbreak of Serratia marcescens associated with the anesthetic agent propofol. *Am J Infect Control.* 2001;29(5):312-315.

102. Muller AE, Huisman I, Roos PJ, et al. Outbreak of severe sepsis due to contaminated propofol: lessons to learn. *J Hosp Infect.* 2010;76(3):225-230.

103. Klement W, Arndt JO. Pain on I.V. injection of some anaesthetic agents is evoked by the unphysiological osmolality or pH of their formulations. *Br J Anaesth.* 1991;66(2):189-195.

104. Bretschneider H. Osmolalities of commercially supplied drugs often used in anesthesia. *Anesth Analg.* 1987;66(4):361-362.

105. Klement W, Arndt JO. Pain on injection of propofol: effects of concentration and diluent. *Br J Anaesth.* 1991;67(3):281-284.

106. Tan CH, Onsiong MK. Pain on injection of propofol. *Anaesthesia.* 1998;53(5):468-476.

107. Veroli P, O'Kelly B, Bertrand F, Trouvin JH, Farinotti R, Ecoffey C. Extrahepatic metabolism of propofol in man during the anhepatic phase of orthotopic liver transplantation. *Br J Anaesth.* 1992;68(2):183-186.

108. Ingrande J, Brodsky JB, Lemmens HJ. Lean body weight scalar for the anesthetic induction dose of propofol in morbidly obese subjects. *Anesth Analg.* 2011;113(1):57-62.

109. Cortinez LI, Anderson BJ, Penna A, et al. Influence of obesity on propofol pharmacokinetics: derivation of a pharmacokinetic model. *Br J Anaesth.* 2010;105(4):448-456.

110. McKeating K, Bali IM, Dundee JW. The effects of thiopentone and propofol on upper airway integrity. *Anaesthesia.* 1988;43(8):638-640.

111. Apfel CC, Korttila K, Abdalla M, et al. A factorial trial of six interventions for the prevention of postoperative nausea and vomiting. *N Engl J Med.* 2004;350(24):2441-2451.

112. Shafer SL. Shock values. *Anesthesiology*. 2004;101(3):567-568.

113. Weatherall A, Venclovas R. Experience with a propofol-ketamine mixture for sedation during pediatric orthopedic surgery. *Paediatr Anaesth*. 2010;20(11):1009-1016.

114. Hui TW, Short TG, Hong W, Suen T, Gin T, Plummer J. Additive interactions between propofol and ketamine when used for anesthesia induction in female patients. *Anesthesiology*. 1995;82(3):641-648.

115. Gupta A, Stierer T, Zuckerman R, Sakima N, Parker SD, Fleisher LA. Comparison of recovery profile after ambulatory anesthesia with propofol, isoflurane, sevoflurane and desflurane: a systematic review. *Anesth Analg*. 2004;98(3):632-641.

116. Eberhart LH, Folz BJ, Wulf H, Geldner G. Intravenous anesthesia provides optimal surgical conditions during microscopic and endoscopic sinus surgery. *Laryngoscope*. 2003;113(8):1369-1373.

117. Cheng SS, Yeh J, Flood P. Anesthesia matters: patients anesthetized with propofol have less postoperative pain than those anesthetized with isoflurane. *Anesth Analg*. 2008;106(1):264-269.

118. Katoh T, Suguro Y, Nakajima R, Kazama T, Ikeda K. Blood concentrations of sevoflurane and isoflurane on recovery from anaesthesia. *Br J Anaesth*. 1992;69(3):259-262.

119. Punjasawadwong Y, Boonjeungmonkol N, Phongchiewboon A. Bispectral index for improving anaesthetic delivery and postoperative recovery. *Cochrane Database Syst Rev*. 2007(4):CD003843.

120. Artru AA, Shapira Y, Bowdle TA. Electroencephalogram, cerebral metabolic, and vascular responses to propofol anesthesia in dogs. *J Neurosurg Anesthesiol*. 1992;4(2):99-109.

121. Fox J, Gelb AW, Enns J, Murkin JM, Farrar JK, Manninen PH. The responsiveness of cerebral blood flow to changes in arterial carbon dioxide is maintained during propofol-nitrous oxide anesthesia in humans. *Anesthesiology*. 1992;77(3):453-456.

122. Hans P, Bonhomme V. Why we still use intravenous drugs as the basic regimen for neurosurgical anaesthesia. *Curr Opin Anaesthesiol*. 2006;19(5):498-503.

123. Sagara Y, Hendler S, Khoh-Reiter S, et al. Propofol hemisuccinate protects neuronal cells from oxidative injury. *J Neurochem*. 1999;73(6):2524-2530.

124. Iijima T, Mishima T, Akagawa K, Iwao Y. Neuroprotective effect of propofol on necrosis and apoptosis following oxygen-glucose deprivation–relationship between mitochondrial membrane potential and mode of death. *Brain Res*. 2006;1099(1):25-32.

125. Carrasco G, Cabre L, Sobrepere G, et al. Synergistic sedation with propofol and midazolam in intensive care patients after coronary artery bypass grafting. *Crit Care Med*. 1998;26(5):844-851.

126. Roberts FL, Dixon J, Lewis GT, Tackley RM, Prys-Roberts C. Induction and maintenance of propofol anaesthesia. A manual infusion scheme. *Anaesthesia*. 1988;43(Suppl):14-17.

127. Coates D. 'Diprifusor' for general and day-case surgery. *Anaesthesia*. 1998;53 Suppl 1:46-48.

128. Servin FS. TCI compared with manually controlled infusion of propofol: a multicentre study. *Anaesthesia*. 1998;53 Suppl 1:82-86.

129. Enlund M. TCI: Target controlled infusion, or totally confused infusion? Call for an optimised population based pharmacokinetic model for propofol. *Ups J Med Sci*. 2008;113(2):161-170.

130. Egan TD. Target-controlled drug delivery: progress toward an intravenous "vaporizer" and automated anesthetic administration. *Anesthesiology*. 2003;99(5):1214-1219.

131. Absalom AR, Kenny GN. Closed-loop control of propofol anaesthesia using bispectral index: performance assessment in patients receiving computer-controlled propofol and manually controlled remifentanil infusions for minor surgery. *Br J Anaesth*. 2003;90(6):737-741.

132. Domino EF. Taming the ketamine tiger. 1965. *Anesthesiology*. 2010;113(3):678-684.

133. Anis NA, Berry SC, Burton NR, Lodge D. The dissociative anaesthetics, ketamine and phencyclidine, selectively reduce excitation of central mammalian neurones by N-methyl-aspartate. *Br J Pharmacol*. 1983;79(2):565-575.

134. Thomson AM, West DC, Lodge D. An N-methylaspartate receptor-mediated synapse in rat cerebral cortex: a site of action of ketamine? *Nature*. 1985;313(6002):479-481.

135. Orser BA, Pennefather PS, MacDonald JF. Multiple mechanisms of ketamine blockade of N-methyl-D-aspartate receptors. *Anesthesiology*. 1997;86(4):903-917.

136. Udesky JO, Spence NZ, Achiel R, Lee C, Flood P. The role of nicotinic inhibition in ketamine-induced behavior. *Anesth Analg*. 2005;101(2):407-411.

137. Hirota K, Okawa H, Appadu BL, Grandy DK, Devi LA, Lambert DG. Stereoselective interaction of ketamine with recombinant mu, kappa, and delta opioid receptors expressed in Chinese hamster ovary cells. *Anesthesiology*. 1999;90(1):174-182.

138. Chen X, Shu S, Bayliss DA. HCN1 channel subunits are a molecular substrate for hypnotic actions of ketamine. *J Neurosci*. 2009;29(3):600-609.

139. Gelissen HP, Epema AH, Henning RH, Krijnen HJ, Hennis PJ, den Hertog A. Inotropic effects of propofol, thiopental, midazolam, etomidate, and ketamine on isolated human atrial muscle. *Anesthesiology*. 1996;84(2):397-403.

140. Hemmingsen C, Nielsen PK, Odorico J. Ketamine in the treatment of bronchospasm during mechanical ventilation. *Am J Emerg Med*. 1994;12(4):417-420.

141. Drummond GB. Comparison of sedation with midazolam and ketamine: effects on airway muscle activity. *Br J Anaesth*. 1996;76(5):663-667.

142. Gateau O, Bourgain JL, Gaudy JH, Benveniste J. Effects of ketamine on isolated human bronchial preparations. *Br J Anaesth*. 1989;63(6):692-695.

143. Brown RH, Wagner EM. Mechanisms of bronchoprotection by anesthetic induction agents: propofol versus ketamine. *Anesthesiology*. 1999;90(3):822-828.

144. Paule MG, Li M, Allen RR, et al. Ketamine anesthesia during the first week of life can cause long-lasting cognitive deficits in rhesus monkeys. *Neurotoxicol Teratol*. 2011;33(2):220-230.

145. Martin J, Heymann A, Basell K, et al. Evidence and consensus-based German guidelines for the management of analgesia, sedation and delirium in intensive care–short version. *Ger Med Sci*. 2010;8:Doc02.

146. Abdelmalak B, Makary L, Hoban J, Doyle DJ. Dexmedetomidine as sole sedative for awake intubation in management of the critical airway. *J Clin Anesth*. 2007;19(5):370-373.

147. Vickery RG, Sheridan BC, Segal IS, Maze M. Anesthetic and hemodynamic effects of the stereoisomers of medetomidine, an alpha 2-adrenergic agonist, in halothane-anesthetized dogs. *Anesth Analg*. 1988;67(7):611-615.

148. Fairbanks CA, Stone LS, Wilcox GL. Pharmacological profiles of alpha 2 adrenergic receptor agonists identified using genetically altered mice and isobolographic analysis. *Pharmacol Ther*. 2009;123(2):224-238.

149. Seyrek M, Halici Z, Yildiz O, Ulusoy HB. Interaction between dexmedetomidine and alpha-adrenergic receptors: emphasis on vascular actions. *J Cardiothorac Vasc Anesth*. 2011;25(5):856-862.

150. Herr DL, Sum-Ping ST, England M. ICU sedation after coronary artery bypass graft surgery: dexmedetomidine-based versus propofol-based sedation regimens. *J Cardiothorac Vasc Anesth*. 2003;17(5):576-584.

151. Sullivan AF, Kalso EA, McQuay HJ, Dickenson AH. The antinociceptive actions of dexmedetomidine on dorsal horn neuronal responses in the anaesthetized rat. *Eur J Pharmacol*. 1992;215(1):127-133.

152. Doufas AG, Lin CM, Suleman MI, et al. Dexmedetomidine and meperidine additively reduce the shivering threshold in humans. *Stroke*. 2003;34(5):1218-1223.

153. Wijeysundera DN, Bender JS, Beattie WS. Alpha-2 adrenergic agonists for the prevention of cardiac complications among patients undergoing surgery. *Cochrane Database Syst Rev*. 2009(4):CD004126.

154. Dyck JB, Maze M, Haack C, Azarnoff DL, Vuorilehto L, Shafer SL. Computer-controlled infusion of intravenous dexmedetomidine hydrochloride in adult human volunteers. *Anesthesiology*. 1993;78(5):821-828.

155. Potts AL, Warman GR, Anderson BJ. Dexmedetomidine disposition in children: a population analysis. *Paediatr Anaesth*. 2008;18(8):722-730.

156. Lin L, Guo X, Zhang MZ, Qu CJ, Sun Y, Bai J. Pharmacokinetics of dexmedetomidine in Chinese post-surgical intensive care unit patients. *Acta Anaesthesiol Scand*. 2011;55(3):359-367.

157. Pandharipande PP, Pun BT, Herr DL, et al. Effect of sedation with dexmedetomidine vs lorazepam on acute brain dysfunction in mechanically ventilated patients: the MENDS randomized controlled trial. *JAMA*. 2007;298(22):2644-2653.

158. Riker RR, Shehabi Y, Bokesch PM, et al. Dexmedetomidine vs midazolam for sedation of critically ill patients: a randomized trial. *JAMA*. 2009;301(5):489-499.

159. Huupponen E, Maksimow A, Lapinlampi P, et al. Electroencephalogram spindle activity during dexmedetomidine sedation and physiological sleep. *Acta Anaesthesiol Scand.* 2008;52(2):289-294.

160. Mason KP, O'Mahony E, Zurakowski D, Libenson MH. Effects of dexmedetomidine sedation on the EEG in children. *Paediatr Anaesth.* 2009;19(12):1175-1183.

161. Mason KP. Sedation trends in the 21st century: the transition to dexmedetomidine for radiological imaging studies. *Paediatr Anaesth.* 2010;20(3):265-272.

162. Mason KP, Zurakowski D, Zgleszewski SE, et al. High dose dexmedetomidine as the sole sedative for pediatric MRI. *Paediatr Anaesth.* 2008;18(5):403-411.

163. Yuen VM, Hui TW, Irwin MG, Yuen MK. A comparison of intranasal dexmedetomidine and oral midazolam for premedication in pediatric anesthesia: a double-blinded randomized controlled trial. *Anesth Analg.* 2008;106(6):1715-1721.

164. Locher S, Stadler KS, Boehlen T, et al. A new closed-loop control system for isoflurane using bispectral index outperforms manual control. *Anesthesiology.* 2004;101(3):591-602.

165. Struys MM, Mortier EP, De Smet T. Closed loops in anaesthesia. *Best Pract Res Clin Anaesthesiol.* 2006;20(1):211-220.

166. Mi WD, Sakai T, Kudo T, Kudo M, Matsuki A. Performance of bispectral index and auditory evoked potential monitors in detecting loss of consciousness during anaesthetic induction with propofol with and without fentanyl. *Eur J Anaesthesiol.* 2004;21(10):807-811.

167. Hemmerling TM, Charabati S, Zaouter C, Minardi C, Mathieu PA. A randomized controlled trial demonstrates that a novel closed-loop propofol system performs better hypnosis control than manual administration. *Can J Anaesth.* 2010;57(8):725-735.

168. Liu N, Chazot T, Hamada S, et al. Closed-loop coadministration of propofol and remifentanil guided by bispectral index: a randomized multicenter study. *Anesth Analg.* 2011;112(3):546-557.

169. Suttner S, Boldt J, Schmidt C, Piper S, Kumle B. Cost analysis of target-controlled infusion-based anesthesia compared with standard anesthesia regimens. *Anesth Analg.* 1999;88(1):77-82.

170. Gan TJ. Pharmacokinetic and pharmacodynamic characteristics of medications used for moderate sedation. *Clin Pharmacokinet.* 2006;45(9):855-869.

171. Fechner J, Schwilden H, Schuttler J. Pharmacokinetics and pharmacodynamics of GPI 15715 or fospropofol (Aquavan injection)—a water-soluble propofol prodrug. *Handb Exp Pharmacol.* 2008;182:253-266.

172. Pergolizzi Jr JV, Gan TJ, Plavin S, Labhsetwar S, Taylor R. Perspectives on the role of fospropofol in the monitored anesthesia care setting. *Anesthesiol Res Pract.* 2011;2011:458920.

173. Kilpatrick GJ, McIntyre MS, Cox RF, et al. CNS 7056: a novel ultra-short-acting Benzodiazepine. *Anesthesiology.* 2007;107(1):60-66.

174. Cotten JF, Husain SS, Forman SA, et al. Methoxycarbonyl-etomidate: a novel rapidly metabolized and ultra-short-acting etomidate analogue that does not produce prolonged adrenocortical suppression. *Anesthesiology.* 2009;111(2):240-249.

175. Ge RL, Pejo E, Haburcak M, Husain SS, Forman SA, Raines DE. Pharmacological studies of methoxycarbonyl etomidate's carboxylic acid metabolite. *Anesth Analg.* 2011.

176. Cotten JF, Forman SA, Laha JK, et al. Carboetomidate: a pyrrole analog of etomidate designed not to suppress adrenocortical function. *Anesthesiology.* 2010;112(3):637-644.

177. Pejo E, Cotten JF, Kelly EW, et al. In vivo and in vitro pharmacological studies of methoxycarbonyl-carboetomidate. *Anesth Analg.* 2011.

178. Laskowski K, Stirling A, McKay WP, Lim HJ. A systematic review of intravenous ketamine for postoperative analgesia. *Can J Anaesth.* 2011;58(10):911-923.

179. Sigtermans MJ, van Hilten JJ, Bauer MC, et al. Ketamine produces effective and long-term pain relief in patients with Complex Regional Pain Syndrome Type 1. *Pain.* 2009;145(3):304-311.

180. Amr YM. Multi-day low dose ketamine infusion as adjuvant to oral gabapentin in spinal cord injury related chronic pain: a prospective, randomized, double blind trial. *Pain Physician.* 2010;13(3):245-249.

181. Noppers I, Niesters M, Swartjes M, et al. Absence of long-term analgesic effect from a short-term S-ketamine infusion on fibromyalgia pain: a randomized, prospective, double blind, active placebo-controlled trial. *Eur J Pain.* 2011;15(9):942-949.

182. Noppers IM, Niesters M, Aarts LP, et al. Drug-induced liver injury following a repeated course of ketamine treatment for chronic pain in CRPS type 1 patients: a report of 3 cases. *Pain.* 2011;152(9):2173-2178.

183. Swartjes M, Morariu A, Niesters M, Aarts L, Dahan A. Nonselective and NR2B-selective N-methyl-D-aspartic acid receptor antagonists produce antinociception and long-term relief of allodynia in acute and neuropathic pain. *Anesthesiology.* 2011;115(1):165-174.

184. Ricou B, Forster A, Bruckner A, Chastonay P, Gemperle M. Clinical evaluation of a specific benzodiazepine antagonist (RO 15-1788). Studies in elderly patients after regional anaesthesia under benzodiazepine sedation. *Br J Anaesth.* 1986;58(9):1005-1011.

185. Nilsson A, Persson MP, Hartvig P. Effects of flumazenil on post-operative recovery after total intravenous anesthesia with midazolam and alfentanil. *Eur J Anaesthesiol Suppl.* 1988;2:251-256.

186. Schwieger IM, Szlam F, Hug Jr CC. Absence of agonistic or antagonistic effect of flumazenil (Ro 15-1788) in dogs anesthetized with enflurane, isoflurane, or fentanyl-enflurane. *Anesthesiology.* 1989;70(3):477-480.

187. Fan SZ, Liu CC, Yu HY, Chao CC, Lin SM. Lack of effect of flumazenil on the reversal of propofol anaesthesia. *Acta Anaesthesiol Scand.* 1995;39(3):299-301.

188. Weinbroum AA, Geller E. Flumazenil improves cognitive and neuromotor emergence and attenuates shivering after halothane-, enflurane- and isoflurane-based anesthesia. *Can J Anaesth.* 2001;48(10):963-972.

189. Karakosta A, Andreotti B, Chapsa C, Pouliou A, Anastasiou E. Flumazenil expedites recovery from sevoflurane/remifentanil anaesthesia when administered to healthy unpremedicated patients. *Eur J Anaesthesiol.* 2010;27(11):955-959.

190. Holtman JR, Jr., Sloan JW, Jing X, Wala EP. Modification of morphine analgesia and tolerance by flumazenil in male and female rats. *Eur J Pharmacol.* 2003;470(3):149-156.

191. Solt K, Cotten JF, Cimenser A, Wong KF, Chemali JJ, Brown EN. Methylphenidate actively induces emergence from general anesthesia. *Anesthesiology.* 2011;115(4):791-803.

192. Alkire MT, McReynolds JR, Hahn EL, Trivedi AN. Thalamic microinjection of nicotine reverses sevoflurane-induced loss of righting reflex in the rat. *Anesthesiology.* 2007;107(2):264-272.

Chapter 10

PHARMACOLOGY OF INHALED ANESTHETICS

Andrew E. Hudson, Karl F. Herold, and Hugh C. Hemmings, Jr.

This chapter focuses on the pharmacology of the inhaled anesthetics, including their mechanisms of action and clinical effects (pharmacodynamics). Related pharmacokinetic principles are covered in Chapter 3.

HISTORICAL PERSPECTIVE

Discovery of Inhaled Anesthetics

The German physician and botanist Valerius Cordus (1515-1544) described a method for preparing ether by combining sulfuric acid with alcohol, which he called *oleum dulci vitrioli* or "sweet oil of vitriol." Paracelsus (1493-1541), the father of toxicology, recognized the analgesic properties of ether:

"...in diseases which are treated by allaying the pain, it cures all of the disorders, relieves all of the pains, reduces the fever, and prevents the disagreeable complications of all sicknesses..."[1]

Paracelsus was unknowingly close to the discovery of the anesthetic effects of ether. Two centuries later in the 18th century, despite flammability issues and the lack of appropriate delivery systems, Friedrich Hoffman of Halle recommended the introduction of ether into medicine.

In 1772, nitrous oxide (N_2O) was discovered by the English philosopher and chemist Joseph Priestley (1733-1804). He and other scientists such as Joseph Black (1728-1799) and Antoine Lavoiser (1743-1794) identified many other atmospheric gases including oxygen, hydrogen, and carbon dioxide, pioneering the field of "pneumatic medicine" and elucidating the basic properties of gases. Thomas Beddoes (1760-1808) established in 1799 the Pneumatic Institution for Relieving Diseases by Medical Airs in England. Together with young assistant Humphrey Davy (1778-1829), who ultimately became more successful than he, Beddoes experimented with nitrous oxide. Davy performed numerous experiments on himself and discovered both the mood-enhancing effects, leading to the name *laughing gas*, and the analgesic effect of nitrous oxide. Despite these pain-relieving effects and its potential use for surgical procedures, nitrous oxide did not meet expectations as a cure for diseases, and the Pneumatic Institution soon closed.

Decades later Gardner Quincy Colton (1814-1898), a self-proclaimed professor of chemistry, went on tour with his (lucrative) "scientific exhibits" and public demonstrations of nitrous oxide. In 1844, dentist Horace Wells (1815-1848) attended one of Colton's demonstrations of the effects of "laughing gas" and observed its analgesic effects in a fallen volunteer. The next morning, a fellow dentist removed one of Wells' molars with only little pain while Colton administered nitrous oxide.[2] Wells saw potential in nitrous oxide and scheduled a demonstration at Harvard Medical School in 1845 with help of his assistant William T. G. Morton (1819-1868). During the demonstration the patient cried out and moaned, probably due to failure of continuous delivery of the gas, an incident that discredited nitrous oxide as an anesthetic. Wells later committed suicide.

Morton, who was present at that demonstration, was searching for another suitable substance to relieve pain during tooth extractions. He met Charles T. Jackson (1805-1880), a Harvard professor in chemistry who introduced him to ether. Morton's experiments on himself and on his pet animals were promising, and in September 1846 he performed a painless tooth extraction. This caught the attention of Harvard surgeon Henry J. Bigelow (1818-1890), who helped schedule a successful public demonstration at Massachusetts General Hospital on October 16, 1846, which is considered by many the beginning of the era of anesthesia. Morton did not reveal the identity of the substance he called *Letheon*, which was ether he masked with additional fragrances and colors. Most likely he saw a potential for profit, and unsuccessfully attempted to patent Letheon. Under pressure from the hospital, Morton revealed the identity of the main ingredient ether, and after further procedures with ether followed, Bigelow published the results of ether as a suitable agent for use in surgical procedures.[3] The term *anesthesia* is derived from Greek *an-* "without" and *aisthētikos* "perception" or "sensation."

Controversy regarding who first discovered anesthesia arose with contenders including Wells, Jackson, and especially Crawford W. Long (1815-1878), a physician in rural Georgia who had used ether anesthesia since 1842, but did not publish his work until after Bigelow's report.[4] Morton with his perseverance is generally credited with the discovery of anesthesia, although there are regional sentiments favoring Wells or Long. The use of both ether and nitrous oxide was quickly adopted by many institutions, revolutionizing surgery and defining the field of anesthesia.

The science of anesthesia began with the introduction and development of chloroform as an anesthetic by John Snow (1813-1858) in England.[5] He conducted experiments on the physical and pharmacologic properties of chloroform and other inhaled anesthetics, developed methods for their administration by introducing the chloroform inhaler, studied their side effects and complications, and developed specific clinical applications. His work established the scientific basis of anesthesia by determining the relationships between anesthetic solubility, vapor pressure, and potency. He also described five stages of etherization in response to increasing doses, presaging Guedel's description, and the first dose-response relationship for an anesthetic. These are among the seminal foundation studies of inhalational anesthesia.[6]

Development of Modern Inhaled Anesthetics

The development of the modern potent inhaled anesthetics was facilitated by developments in fluoride chemistry that accelerated with the atomic weapons program in the mid-20th century. This allowed the synthesis and testing of many fluorinated alkane and ether compounds that were safer and less combustible than ether or cyclopropane. Robbins demonstrated the potential of fluorinated hydrocarbons as nonflammable inhaled anesthetics with greater therapeutic ratios than ether or chloroform.[7] This work led to the synthesis and testing of the polyhalogenated alkane halothane, which showed outstanding anesthetic properties in animals and humans.[8] This was followed by the pioneering work of Ross Terrell (1925-2010) and colleagues who synthesized and evaluated over 700 fluorinated compounds that included the essential agents of the last 40 years of modern inhalational anesthesia, the fluorinated methyl ethyl ethers: enflurane, isoflurane, sevoflurane, and desflurane (Figure 10-1).[9]

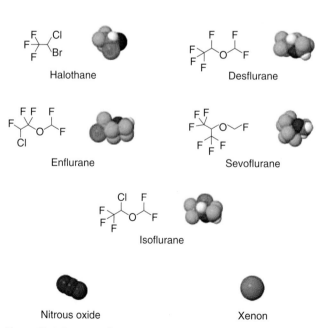

Figure 10-1 Structure of representative inhaled anesthetics shown as two-dimensional and space-filling models. Note the similarities among the modern methyl ethyl ethers, in particular desflurane and isoflurane which differ by a single substitution.

STRUCTURE-ACTIVITY RELATIONSHIPS

Meyer-Overton Correlation

At the beginning of the 20th century, German pharmacologists Meyer and Overton independently noted that the potency of volatile anesthetics for sedating tadpoles was inversely correlated with their solubility in olive oil (Figure 10-2, *A*). Subsequent investigations confirmed that for a majority of anesthetic agents potency is proportional to lipid solubility as measured by the oil-gas partition coefficient. Remarkably, this correlation holds across multiple animal phyla from invertebrates to humans and spans over five orders of magnitude in potency. Another way of stating this correlation is that the product of the oil-gas partition coefficient and anesthetic potency defined as minimum alveolar concentration (MAC; see Chapter 3) is constant between anesthetics. This implies that at MAC the concentration of inhaled anesthetic molecules in the hydrophobic phase is approximately 50 mM. This observation formed the basis for a unitary hypothesis that argued that the mechanism of action of inhaled anesthetics derived from their effects on bulk lipid membrane properties. A modern form fruste of the lipid hypothesis suggests that anesthetics interact with lipids in the vicinity of membrane proteins to indirectly alter their functional properties.[10]

Despite its central position in mechanistic theories of anesthesia, the Meyer-Overton correlation had limitations. While Meyer and Overton both used olive oil as their reference solvent, similar correlations have been obtained using other hydrophobic solvents that are more hydrophobic than olive oil, such as benzene, which do not produce as strong a correlation as olive oil. The amphipathic (having both hydrophobic and hydrophilic qualities) solvents methanol, octanol, and lecithin produce even better correlations than olive oil, correctly predicting that enflurane is less potent than isoflurane. However, lipid solubility alone does not predict anesthetic potency, in that a number of chemically similar compounds with lipid solubilities comparable to known anesthetics lack anesthetizing capacity themselves. These so-called nonimmobilizers have been useful experimentally as a negative test in evaluating potential anesthetic targets.[11] Although the Meyer-Overton correlation does constrain the possible mechanisms of action of anesthetics (the site at which anesthetics bind must be hydrophobic, and likely amphipathic), in practice this is not a particularly restrictive constraint on possible anesthetic binding sites because lipid membrane bilayers, membrane proteins, and most water-soluble proteins have amphipathic domains.

Stereoselectivity

Isoflurane, enflurane, halothane, and desflurane all have a chiral carbon atom, and thus exist as racemic mixtures of enantiomeric pairs that are mirror images of each other, but with identical physical and chemical properties other than their ability to polarize light in opposite directions (see Chapter 1). While they are synthesized as racemic mixtures, separation of the enantiomers of isoflurane and halothane by gas chromatography allowed testing of the anesthetic properties of the individual enantiomers, which have identical lipid solubilities. Rats are about 1.5-fold more sensitive to the

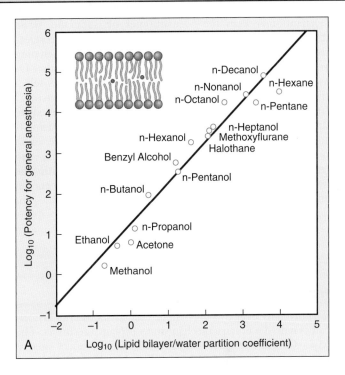

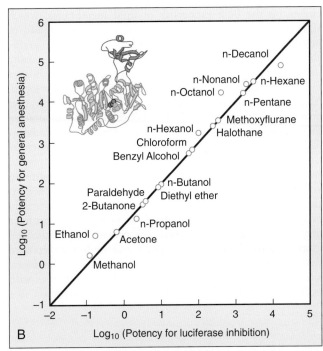

Figure 10-2 General anesthetics act by binding directly to proteins. **A,** The Meyer-Overton correlation (c. 1900) suggested that lipids were the principal target for anesthetics based on the correlation between anesthetic potency and lipid-water partition coefficients. **B,** General anesthetic potencies correlate equally well with their potency for inhibition of the soluble enzyme firefly luciferase. The crystal structure of luciferase is shown in the inset. (*Reprinted with permission from Macmillan Publishers Ltd. Nature copyright 2007. Franks NP. Molecular targets underlying general anaesthesia. Br J Pharmacol. 2006;147[Suppl 1]:S72-81.*)

(+)enantiomer than the (-)enantiomer of isoflurane, while its lipid perturbing effects are equivalent (nonstereoselective).[12,13] A number of putative targets (see later), including γ-aminobutyric acid (GABA)$_A$ receptors and N-methyl-D-aspartate (NMDA) receptors, have demonstrated stereoselectivity in vitro, although not to the degree seen in vivo.[14,15] Interestingly, L-type Ca^{2+} channels (which partially mediate the cardiodepressive effects of volatile agents) do not demonstrate stereoselectivity in vitro, suggesting that the more potent enantiomer should have an increased therapeutic ratio (reduced cardiovascular depression) compared with the racemic mixture.[16] Importantly, stereoselective effects on anesthetic potency indicate that lipid solubility alone does not determine anesthetic potency.

MECHANISMS OF ACTION

From Lipid to Protein-Based Mechanisms

The diversity of agents that can be used as anesthetics historically favored a unitary mechanism to explain anesthesia. The Myer-Overton correlation suggested that the effect sites of anesthetics were lipophilic or amphipathic. As a result, initial concepts of general anesthetic mechanisms of action favored effects on the bulk properties of lipid membranes, which allowed for the vast chemical diversity of agents found to produce an anesthetic state (see earlier). However, no verifiable hypothesis of a lipid-based mechanism, which usually invoked effects on lipid membrane properties (e.g., bilayer fluidity, thickness, curvature, permeability) was developed. Moreover, comparable effects on membrane biophysical properties could be achieved by small changes in temperature that do not cause anesthesia. Subsequently, the nonimmobilizers were found to violate the basic Meyer-Overton correlation between potency and lipophilicity.[11] The improved correlation between anesthetic potency and solubility in amphipathic rather than purely hydrophobic solvents is consistent with a protein-based mechanism, or perhaps a lipid bilayer with phospholipoproteins. The proof of concept for a protein as an anesthetic target was provided by Ueda and extended unambiguously by Franks and Lieb who reported that the bioluminescent function of the protein luciferase was inhibited by a large range of anesthetic molecules with potencies predicted by the Meyer-Overton correlation (see

Figure 10-2, B).[17,18] This concept was strengthened by the demonstration of stereoselective anesthetic effects, which implies a specific chiral binding site.[19]

Diversity of Molecular Targets

Anesthesia is a composite pharmacologic endpoint that is commonly defined as reversible amnesia, loss of consciousness, and immobility. It is not surprising then that these diverse effects result from multiple mechanisms, and that the relative potency and efficacy of various general anesthetics in producing these effects vary between specific anesthetics (Figure 10-3). The prevailing view is that inhaled anesthetics have multiple, agent-specific molecular effects on a number of targets critical to neuronal communication and excitability, as summarized in Table 10-1.[20,21] These multiple actions work in concert or individually to produce the pleiotropic effects characteristic of inhaled anesthetics.[22]

Criteria for identifying targets of inhaled anesthetics are shown in Table 10-2. Volatile anesthetics at clinically relevant concentrations positively modulate inhibitory GABA$_A$ receptors and inhibitory glycine receptors, inhibit excitatory NMDA-type glutamate receptors and neuronal nicotinic acetylcholine receptors, activate certain two-pore domain (K_{2P}) and leak K^+ channels, and inhibit multiple voltage-gated Na^+ channel subtypes. The gaseous inhaled anesthetics (cyclopropane, nitrous oxide, xenon) at clinically relevant concentrations do not affect GABA$_A$ receptors but block NMDA receptors and activate K_{2P} channels.[23,24]

Putative anesthetic targets are not distributed evenly throughout the nervous system. For example, multiple subtypes of GABA$_A$ receptors exist, each with its own expression profiles at the regional, cellular, and subcellular levels. Specific receptor isoforms appear to mediate various anesthetic endpoints, as shown for certain intravenous anesthetics (see Chapter 9).

Multiple Behavioral Endpoints

Anesthesia is a drug-induced comatose state with multiple behavioral components including the essential triad of unconsciousness, amnesia, and immobility, and in some cases also analgesia and autonomic stability.[25] These effects are dose-related: amnesia at low doses is followed by sedation, unconsciousness, and eventually immobility (Figure 10-4, A).

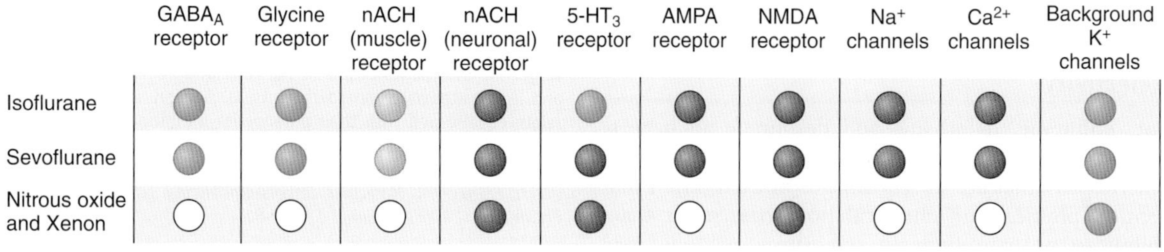

Figure 10-3 Ligand-gated and voltage-gated ion channels are thought to be among the most relevant targets for general anesthetics. The activities of representative inhaled anesthetics on these targets in vitro are summarized above. A dark green or pink spot indicates significant potentiation or inhibition, respectively, by the anesthetic at clinically relevant concentrations; a light pink spot indicates some inhibition, and an empty spot indicates no effect at clinically relevant concentrations. This summary represents a synthesis of major effects, but important differences exist between various receptor and channel isoforms (not indicated here). *nACh*, Nicotinic acetylcholine. *(Modified from Rudolph U, Antkowiak B. Molecular and neuronal substrates for general anaesthetics. Nat Rev Neurosci. 2004;5:709-720.)*

Table 10-1. Overview of Putative Sites of Inhaled Anesthetic Action

LEVEL	SITE	EFFECT	TARGET(S)
Proteins	Amphipathic binding sites	Conformational flexibility, ligand binding	Ion channels, receptors, signaling proteins
Action potential	Nervous system	Small reduction in amplitude	Na$^+$ channels
	Cardiovascular system	Reduced amplitude, duration	Ca^{2+} channels, K$^+$ channels
Synaptic transmission			
Inhibitory	Presynaptic terminal	Enhanced transmitter release	
	Postsynaptic receptors	Enhanced transmitter effects	Glycine, GABA$_A$ receptors
Excitatory	Presynaptic terminal	Reduced transmitter release	Na$^+$ channels, K$_{2P}$ channels
	Postsynaptic receptors	Reduced transmitter effects	NMDA receptors, nicotinic acetylcholine receptors
Neuronal networks	Neuronal circuit	Altered long-term potentiation/depression	Synaptic plasticity
	Neuronal integration	Altered rhythmicity, coherence	HCN channels, K$_{2P}$ channels, extrasynaptic GABA$_A$ receptors etc.
Central nervous system	Neocortex, hippocampus, amygdala	Sedation, amnesia	θ-rhythms, γ-rhythms, synchrony
	Diencephalon (thalamus), brainstem (reticular formation)	Unconsciousness	γ-band transfer entropy? Thalamic deafferentation?
	Spinal cord	Immobility	Nocifensive reflex
Cardiovascular system	Heart		
	Myocardium	Negative inotropy	Excitation-contraction coupling
	Conduction system	Dysrhythmias	Cardiac action potential
	Vasculature	Vasodilation	Direct and indirect vasoregulation
Pulmonary system	Vasculature	Vasodilation, reduced	Direct and indirect vasoregulation
	Bronchioles	Bronchodilation	Direct and indirect bronchiolar smooth muscle tone

(Modified from Perouansky M, Pearce RA, Hemmings Jr HC. Inhaled anesthetic agents: mechanisms of action. In: Miller RD, ed. *Miller's Anesthesia*. 7th ed. Philadelphia: Churchill Livingstone Elsevier; 2010:515-538.)

Table 10-2. Criteria for Identifying Targets of Anesthetic Action

The anesthetic reversibly and directly alters the target function at clinically relevant concentrations (sensitivity).

The target is expressed in appropriate anatomical locations to mediate the specific behavioral effects of the anesthetic (plausibility).

The stereoselective effects of the anesthetic or nonimmobilizer in vivo parallel effects on the target in vitro.

Pharmacologic or genetic disruption of the sensitivity of the target abolishes the effect of the anesthetic on the relevant endpoint.

Current evidence favors the hypothesis that the multiple behavioral endpoints of anesthesia result from multiple distinct molecular and anatomic effect sites (see Figure 10-4, *B*). Unconsciousness is likely due to enhanced inhibition at multiple sites in cerebral cortex, thalamus, and brainstem involved in arousal. While the neuronal correlates of consciousness remain unknown, it has been proposed that anything that sufficiently perturbs activity in thalamocortical loops, and hence long-range cortical connectivity, could disorder consciousness.[26] Moreover, individual lesions to brainstem arousal areas and intralaminar thalamus result in transient coma, suggesting that severe pharmacologic inhibition of these areas is also likely to induce a state of unarousable unresponsiveness.[27] Amnesia is likely due to altered neurotransmission in frontal cortex, hippocampus, and amygdala critical to memory acquisition and storage. Immobility is due to effects on spinal cord networks, likely through suppression of central pattern generators critical to coordinated movement.[28,29] Analgesia is likely due to disruption of spinothalamic tract transmission

and possible effects on peripheral nociception. A shortcoming of the volatile anesthetics is their poor control of the autonomic nervous system response to painful stimuli. In the modern era, inhalation anesthesia is routinely supplemented with opioids to achieve optimal anesthetic conditions.[30]

Molecular and Cellular Sites of Action

Because of the ability to precisely define and monitor immobilization, this anesthetic endpoint has been investigated more completely than amnesia and unconsciousness. Inhaled anesthetics produce immobilization at increasing doses primarily via effects on the spinal cord. A series of elegant experiments in vivo showed that the potency of volatile anesthetics for immobilization was determined by effects on the spinal cord.[28,29] Volatile anesthetic immobility does not appear to be mediated by GABA$_A$ receptor effects. The GABA$_A$ receptor antagonist bicuculline does not antagonize the immobility induced by isoflurane.[31] This is in contrast to the intravenous anesthetics propofol and etomidate, whose immobilizing effects are mediated primarily by GABA$_A$ receptors, as evident in their effective antagonism by bicuculline (see Chapter 9). In contrast mice harboring mutations that reduce sensitivity of GABA$_A$ receptor α$_1$ or β$_3$ subunits to volatile anesthetics exhibit only slight resistance to the immobilizing and hypnotic effects of volatile anesthetics, whereas analogous mutations that greatly reduce the effects of propofol or etomidate on the β$_3$ GABA$_A$ receptor subunit essentially abolish their hypnotic effects.[32,33] This indicates that other targets likely play a more important role in these volatile anesthetic actions.

The amnestic effect of volatile anesthetics, like that of the intravenous anesthetics, probably involves potentiation of

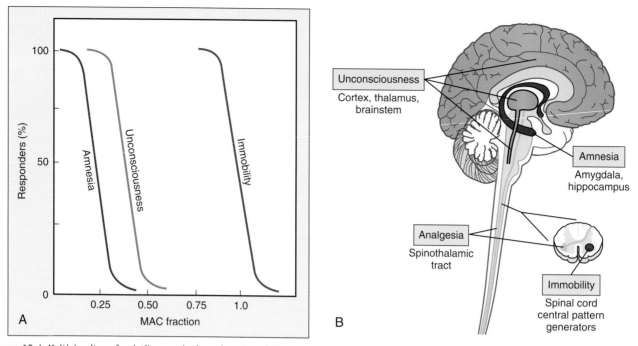

Figure 10-4 Multiple sites of volatile anesthetic action. **A,** Volatile anesthetics lead to multiple dose-dependent behavioral endpoints. Cardiovascular responses occur at even greater doses (not shown). **B,** Amnesia, the most sensitive anesthetic endpoint, probably involves the hippocampus, amygdala, mediotemporal lobe, and possibly other cortical structures involved in learning and memory. Unconsciousness likely involves the cerebral cortex, thalamus, and brainstem reticular formation essential to consciousness and arousal. Immobility occurs by anesthetic action on the spinal cord central pattern generators. Anesthetic effects on the spinal cord blunts ascending impulses arising from noxious stimulation, leading to analgesia, and might indirectly contribute to anesthetic-induced unconsciousness.

specific GABA$_A$ receptor subtypes (Figure 10-5). For example, amnesia during anesthesia has been attributed to enhanced activation of α_5 subunit containing GABA$_A$ receptors, which are known to regulate hippocampal dependent synaptic plasticity and short-term memory.[34] Long-term potentiation (LTP), a cellular model of hippocampal memory, is suppressed by isoflurane, an effect that is reversed by the GABA$_A$ receptor antagonist bicuculline.[35] The finding that both β_3 and α_4 subunit knockout mice are resistant to the amnestic effects of isoflurane indicates a role for GABA$_A$ receptors containing these subunits in the amnestic action of volatile anesthetics.[36,37]

Glycine receptors, members of the ligand-gated ion channel superfamily that are closely related to GABA$_A$ receptors both structurally and functionally, are likewise potentiated by volatile anesthetics (see Figure 10-5). Their high level of expression in the spinal cord makes them putative targets for the immobilizing effects of anesthetics. Pharmacologic evidence shows partial antagonism of the immobilizing effect of isoflurane by the glycine receptor antagonist strychnine, consistent with a contribution to this anesthetic endpoint.[38]

Neuronal nicotinic acetylcholine receptors (nAChRs) are, like GABA$_A$ and glycine receptors, pentameric cys-loop ligand-gated ion channels, but in contrast they are cation selective excitatory channels and are inhibited rather than potentiated by volatile anesthetics. Administration of mecamylamine (an antagonist of nAChRs) does not affect MAC for several inhaled anesthetics, suggesting that nAChRs do not contribute to inhaled anesthetic immobility.[39,40] However they might contribute to the amnestic and hyperalgesic effects of very low dose volatile anesthetics, consistent with their

roles in learning and memory in that both isoflurane and nonimmobilizers, both of which produce amnesia, block nAChRs.[41,42]

Voltage-gated Na$^+$ channels are integral to all facets of central nervous system (CNS) function, and thus are well positioned to mediate multiple aspects of general anesthesia. Clinical concentrations of volatile anesthetics inhibit Na$^+$ channels in isolated rat nerve terminals and neurons. Although not as sensitive to volatile anesthetics as cys-loop ligand-gated ion channels, Na$^+$ channels are inhibited in vitro in a clinical concentration range.[21,43] Moreover, reductions in neurotransmitter release by volatile anesthetics involve inhibition of presynaptic action potentials as a result of Na$^+$ channel blockade.[44,45] The presynaptic effects of isoflurane are selective for inhibition of release of the excitatory transmitter glutamate over the inhibitor transmitter GABA, consistent with their neurodepressive actions.[46] Intrathecal administration of the specific Na$^+$ channel blocker tetrodotoxin reduces MAC in rats, while the activator veratridine increases MAC, supporting a role for Na$^+$ channel block in immobility produced by isoflurane.[47,48]

There is also some evidence for K$^+$ channels as targets for inhaled anesthetics. The MAC of chloroform, desflurane, halothane, and sevoflurane is variably increased in a knockout of the TREK-1 two-pore domain (K$_{2P}$) K$^+$ channel.[49] This variable effect on MAC is not paralleled by the effect of these anesthetics to increase channel opening in vitro, which argues against a causal connection between TREK-1 and anesthetic mechanism.[49,50] Nitrous oxide, xenon, and cylopropane also activate TREK-1. The MAC of halothane is increased significantly by knockout of the TASK-3 channel, but the MAC of

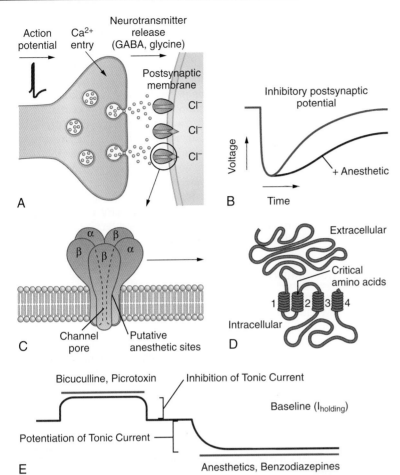

Figure 10-5 Effects of volatile anesthetics on inhibitory synaptic transmission. **A,** On binding of released GABA (γ-aminobutyric acid) or glycine (blue dots) to the pentameric GABA$_A$ or glycine receptor complexes, chloride flows into the postsynaptic neuron, leading to hyperpolarization. **B,** Volatile anesthetics prolong channel opening and increase postsynaptic inhibition. **C,** A pentameric GABA$_A$ receptor complex in the lipid bilayer membrane showing the likely binding sites in the transmembrane domains and the chloride conducting ion channel pore. **D,** Membrane topology of a single receptor subunit showing the extracellular domain that forms the ligand binding site, and the four transmembrane domains, including the critical amino acid residues in transmembrane domain 2 (TM2) that potentially contribute to the anesthetic binding site. **E,** Synaptic GABA$_A$ receptors have a low potency and a high efficacy, whereas extrasynaptic GABA$_A$ receptors have a high potency and a low efficacy for GABA, and contribute to tonic inhibitory currents in response to low ambient extrasynaptic GABA. Extrasynaptic GABA$_A$ receptors usually contain the δ subunit, have increased sensitivity to anesthetics, and might be important targets for general anesthetics. The role of the tonic current is demonstrated schematically in the depolarization in response to the GABA$_A$ receptor inhibitors bicuculline and picrotoxin, and the hyperpolarization in response to anesthetics and benzodiazepines.

isoflurane is not.[51] Increased pH opens TASK K$^+$ channels, but decreases in PaCO$_2$ (with associated increases in pH) do not decrease MAC.[52,53] Reduced pH blocks TASK channels, but increases in PaCO$_2$ that decrease pH also decrease MAC.[54] Finally, intravenous and intrathecal infusions of the KCNK type K$^+$ channel activator riluzole decrease isoflurane MAC equipotently in rats, which suggests that, while activation of K$^+$ channels might affect anesthetic requirement, the effect is primarily on higher centers rather than the spinal cord.[55] The issue is complicated by the nonspecificity of riluzole, which blocks slowly inactivating Na$^+$ channels (important for maintaining repetitive firing, and thus likely MAC) even more potently than KCNK channels.[56]

Blockade of receptors for glutamate, the principal excitatory neurotransmitter in the CNS, provides a plausible mechanism for depression of excitatory synaptic transmission and thereby CNS depression by inhaled anesthetics. NMDA-type and AMPA-type receptors are critical for all forms of synaptic function and plasticity, and are critical to learning, memory, and nociception among other roles. Blockade of NMDA receptors, as well as HCN1 channels, appears important to the anesthetic mechanisms of ketamine (see Chapter 9), and might contribute to inhaled anesthetic effects as well. Isoflurane and xenon inhibit NMDA and AMPA receptors in vitro due to competitive blockade of the glycine co-agonist site.[57,58] In addition to K$_{2P}$ channels and nAChRs, NMDA receptors are among the most sensitive targets in vitro to nitrous oxide and xenon, and are therefore important to their anesthetic actions, although this conclusion awaits confirmation in vivo.[59] Thus

nitrous oxide, xenon, and cyclopropane have a distinct pharmacologic profile with little or no effect on GABA$_A$ receptors, but strong inhibition of NMDA and activation of the two-pore-domain K$^+$ channel TREK-1.[60]

Compared to the intravenous anesthetics (see Chapter 9), inhaled anesthetics are generally more promiscuous in their molecular targets, lacking the receptor-specific, and sometimes receptor subtype-specific, effects of certain intravenous anesthetics. This complicates their pharmacologic characterization, but might also provide considerable redundancy contributing to their marked efficacy across phyla and within species. Such redundancy might also explain the relatively minor effects on anesthetic potency in vivo of mutations that reduce sensitivity of specific molecular targets to inhaled anesthetics in vitro.

Drug Class Effects

Inhaled anesthetics are characterized by their diverse chemical classes, including the volatile ethers and alkanes, and the gases nitrous oxide and xenon. The molecular effects of inhaled anesthetics are also diverse, in that their low potency leads to pleiotropic interactions with multiple molecular targets. This includes a large number of systemic (nonanesthetic) effects. It is instructive to consider the effects of the volatile ethers and alkanes, which exert predominantly GABA-ergic effects (Figure 10-6), separately from the gases (Figure 10-7), which exert predominantly NMDA blocking effects (see Figure 10-3).

Effect Sites of Volatile Anesthetics

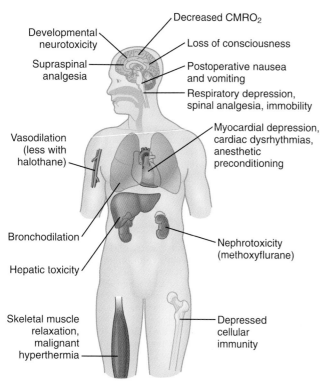

Figure 10-6 Major sites of action of the volatile anesthetics are shown schematically.

Effect Sites of Nitrous Oxide and Xenon

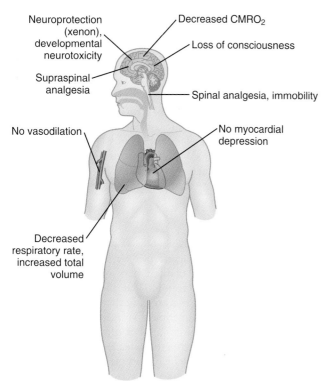

Figure 10-7 Major sites of action of the gaseous anesthetics nitrous oxide and xenon are shown schematically.

Bronchodilation

Volatile anesthetics relax airway smooth muscle through block of voltage-gated Ca^{2+} channels, depletion of Ca^{2+} stores in the sarcoplasmic reticulum, and possibly through potentiation of GABAergic mechanisms.[61] Since the airways normally have low tone this effect is evident almost exclusively in the setting of bronchospasm. Baseline pulmonary resistance and dynamic pulmonary compliance are unchanged by 1 or 2 MAC halothane, enflurane, isoflurane, or sevoflurane. However, in subjects challenged with intravenous histamine, volatile anesthetics attenuate the increase in pulmonary resistance.[62] In contrast to other volatile anesthetics, this effect is not observed with desflurane.[63]

Neuromuscular Effects

In contrast to intravenous anesthetics, which either have excitatory myoclonic effects or produce weak myorelaxation (propofol), volatile anesthetics produce dose-dependent skeletal muscle relaxation and potentiate both depolarizing and nondepolarizing neuromuscular blockers. The mechanisms of skeletal muscle relaxation include decreasing the depolarizing current at the neuromuscular junction in response to acetylcholine due to direct inhibition of nicotinic acetylcholine receptors and enhancement of spinal cord glycine receptors.[38,64-66] Potentiation of nondepolarizing neuromuscular blockers is likely due to potentiation of antagonist affinity at the nicotinic acetylcholine receptor.[67] Elimination of residual volatile anesthetic facilitates recovery from neuromuscular blockade.

Analgesia and Neuroprotection

Inhibition of NMDA receptors by nitrous oxide, xenon, and cyclopropane probably underlies their unique analgesic properties, and their propensity to produce excitement and euphoria, and therefore abuse as psychotomimetics. In addition, NMDA receptor blockers including xenon and nitrous oxide are both neuroprotective and neurotoxic in animal models (see Emerging Developments).[59]

The promiscuous pharmacologic actions of inhaled anesthetics result in numerous undesirable effects that are summarized herein by system.

Respiratory Depression

All halogenated ethers cause dose-dependent respiratory depression. Even subanesthetic concentrations blunt both the hypoxic and hypercarbic ventilatory responses.[68] The acute hypoxic response can remain suppressed for several hours after anesthesia.[69] These effects are multifactorial. The peripheral drive from hypoxia detected by the carotid bodies is blunted. There is a general depression of the central respiratory centers and arousal centers, and motor neurons and respiratory muscles are suppressed, leading both to reduced respiratory drive and upper airway muscular tone and patency.[70]

Hypoxia is sensed by glomus type I cells of the carotid bodies by reduced opening of K^+ channels, although the specific type is difficult to determine and might be species dependent.[71] Volatile anesthetic suppression of peripheral hypoxic respiratory drive might be mediated by reactive oxygen species, altering the redox state of K^+ channels that detect hypoxia. Halothane, with a relatively large degree of peripheral metabolism and associated production of reactive oxygen species, dramatically suppresses the carotid body response to hypoxia. Desflurane, with minimal metabolism, minimally suppresses the carotid body reflex.[72] Isoflurane, with an intermediate degree of metabolism, moderately inhibits the carotid bodies. Pretreatment with a mixture of antioxidants prevents suppression of the respiratory response by subanesthetic doses of halothane and isoflurane.[71,73,74]

Cardiovascular Depression

Volatile anesthetics universally produce concentration-dependent myocardial depression, especially halothane. This is due primarily to altered Ca^{2+} entry and sarcoplasmic reticulum function.[75,76] The most significant cardiodepressant effect of halothane is direct myocardial depression. The negative inotropy is compounded by decreases in systemic vascular resistance (SVR) by enflurane, isoflurane, desflurane, and sevoflurane. In contrast, nitrous oxide and especially xenon have minimal direct cardiovascular effects (Table 10-3). In contrast to the volatile agents, xenon does not affect the major cation currents in isolated cardiomyocytes, which probably explains the minimal cardiovascular depression. Reduced SVR is most prominent with isoflurane, leading to suggestions that it could promote a steal phenomenon in patients with coronary artery disease. However there is no convincing clinical evidence that isoflurane is riskier than other inhaled anesthetics in patients with coronary artery disease as long as perfusion pressure is maintained.[77] Rapid increases in inhaled concentrations of isoflurane and especially desflurane can lead to increases in heart rate and blood pressure secondary to sympathetic activation due to an irritant effect.[78] Sevoflurane has minimal effects on heart rate.

Table 10-3. Cardiovascular Effects of Various Inhalational Anesthetics Compared

	CARDIAC OUTPUT	SYSTEM VASCULAR RESISTANCE	MEAN ARTERIAL PRESSURE	HEART RATE
Halothane	↓	↔	↓	↓↓
Enflurane	↓↓	↓	↓↓	↑
Isoflurane	↓	↓	↓↓	↑
Desflurane	↔	↓	↓	↑
Sevoflurane	↔	↓	↓	↔
Nitrous oxide	↓	↑	↔	↑
Xenon	↔	↔	↔	↓

Reprinted with permission from Hemmings Jr HC, Hopkins PM, eds. *Foundations of Anesthesia: Basic Sciences for Clinical Practice.* 2nd ed. London: Mosby Elsevier; 2006:316.

Arrows indicate an increase, decrease, or no change in the parameter. The number of arrows signifies the approximate magnitude of the effect.

Cardiac Dysrhythmias

Isoflurane, desflurane, and sevoflurane all prolong the electrocardiographic QT interval, potentially increasing the risk of torsades de pointe polymorphic ventricular tachycardia. There is some controversy as to whether halothane presents a similar risk.[79] Prolongation of the QT interval is likely due to inhibition of the delayed rectifier K^+ current through hERG channels that normally contribute to cardiomyocyte repolarization (see Chapter 24).[80]

Halothane and cyclopropane are notorious for myocardial sensitization to catecholamine-induced arrhythmias. This has been proposed to result from disruption of muscarinic regulation of myocardial adenylyl cyclase.[81,82] These arrhythmias are suppressed by calcium channel blockers and β-adrenergic blockers.[83] The ether anesthetics, xenon, and nitrous oxide have minimal proarrhythmic effects.

Neurophysiologic Effects

Volatile anesthetics decrease cerebral metabolic rate of oxygen consumption ($CMRO_2$; see Chapter 8). Because of flow-metabolism coupling this should result in a decrease in cerebral blood flow (CBF) and intracranial pressure (ICP). However, these effects are offset by the direct vasodilation effect of volatile anesthetics on the cerebral vasculature particularly at higher doses. Nitrous oxide increases cerebral blood flow with a mild increase in $CMRO_2$. Coadministration of propofol, barbiturates, or opioids counteracts these vasodilatory effects.

Volatile anesthetics lead to characteristic changes in the electroencephalogram (EEG; see Chapter 7). During quiet wakefulness, α and β activity predominate. As anesthetic concentration increases, the EEG shifts to larger amplitude, lower frequency activity in the θ and δ range. As concentration increases further, the EEG shows burst suppression, alternating periods of isoelectric activity and bursts of activity. By the time concentration reaches 1.5 to 2 MAC, the EEG becomes isoelectric. These characteristic shifts in the EEG power spectrum have been exploited to create multiple measures of depth of anesthesia, including the bispectral index (BIS), spectral entropy, and spectral edge. Unfortunately, none has proven to be a compelling monitor for awareness, in that the BAG-RECALL trial failed to demonstrate superiority for awareness prevention when following BIS compared to a protocol to maintain a minimum end-tidal volatile anesthetic concentration.[84] Ketamine and nitrous oxide do not reduce bispectral index or suppress midlatency auditory evoked potentials, while xenon does. Thus anesthetic depth monitors are inaccurate when ketamine and nitrous oxide are used.

Sevoflurane, isoflurane, and enflurane are notable for producing epileptiform EEG activity at high concentrations.[85,86] This effect is particularly pronounced with hyperventilation, and has been detected during pediatric inhalational induction with sevoflurane. This activity is of unclear clinical significance, but raises concerns of possible neurotoxicity.

Mutagenic and Immunomodulatory Effects

Postoperative immunocompromise in surgical patients is primarily related to the neuroendocrine stress response to surgery through activation of the autonomic nervous system and the hypothalamic-pituitary-adrenal axis.[87,88] Monocytes, macrophages, and T cells all have β_2-adrenoreceptors and glucocorticoid receptors through which the perioperative surge in catecholamines, adrenocorticotropic hormone, and cortisol can directly suppress function. This immunomodulatory effect has the potential for significant impact on postoperative outcome, particularly for cancer surgery, because pain and surgery increase tumor metastasis in cancer surgery when comparing groups that received systemic or epidural analgesia in addition to general anesthesia during surgery.[89] This argues that the immune effects of anesthesia are significantly smaller than the effects of surgery, but volatile anesthetics also have immunomodulatory effects.[90]

Data concerning the immunomodulatory effects of volatile anesthetics are somewhat contradictory. Volatile anesthetics generally inhibit inflammatory cytokines, either directly or through stimulation of helper T-cell cytokines such as interleukin (IL)-4 and IL-10 that normally function to limit the inflammatory response. Studies have shown decreased lymphocyte proliferation, inhibition of neutrophil function, and suppression of alveolar monocyte responses to cytokines.[91-96] Additionally, volatile anesthetics reversibly inhibit voltage-gated Ca^{2+} channels, decrease intracellular Ca^{2+} concentration, and reduce expression of inducible nitric oxide synthase (iNOS) in lymphocytes, while iNOS expression is increased in alveolar macrophages exposed to isoflurane.[97,98]

Volatile anesthetics inhibit human neutrophil bacterial killing in vitro by reducing production of reactive oxygen species (ROS).[94,99,100] The resulting decrease in ROS suppresses the initial inflammatory response by directly limiting neutrophil mediated local tissue injury, which itself is responsible for upregulation of endothelial adhesion molecules that recruit more immune cells and launch the systemic immune response. While inhibition of neutrophil ROS production could compromise the immune response, neutrophil ROS release is also a significant contributor to the initial tissue injury that is responsible for reperfusion injury.

Hepatotoxicity

Anesthetic-induced hepatitis was first recognized in the 19th century with chloroform but not ether. Hepatotoxicity has been traced to biotransformation of volatile agents by cytochrome P450 enzymes, producing trifluoroacetylated protein antigens (see Chapter 6).[101] Halothane-induced hepatitis is most common and is classified into two types. Type I occurs commonly (estimates range from 5% to 30% of patients) and results in asymptomatic elevation of serum transaminases 1 to 2 weeks after exposure. No prior exposure is required, and the mechanism of injury is unclear. Leading explanations include a direct toxic effect of halothane itself or an indirect effect as halothane metabolism produces free radicals that interact with cellular components leading to an autocatalytic peroxidative chain reaction.

Type II halothane hepatitis is much less common (1 in 35,000 halothane anesthetics). An immune-mediated response directed against hepatocytes leads to fulminant hepatitis with high mortality. In most cases there is prior exposure to halothane. Delayed onset jaundice or postoperative fever is also common. The presentation can be delayed up to 1 month following anesthesia. Cytochrome P450 2E1 (CYP 2E1) oxidation of halothane produces trifluoroacetyl chloride, which is highly reactive and covalently binds to hepatic proteins, producing trifluoroacetylated protein neoantigens that initiate the immune response responsible for the hepatitis.[102] The trifluoroacetylated sites act as haptens to establish an antibody reaction, and serum from patients with type II halothane hepatitis contains antibodies that react with acyl halides bound to liver proteins. Patients also develop autoantibodies against CYP 2E1, but the same autoantibodies have been found in unaffected pediatric anesthesiologists who were routinely exposed to halothane during inhalational inductions, suggesting that these CYP 2E1 antibodies do not have a pathogenic role.[103]

Nephrotoxicity

There are two potential pathways by which volatile anesthetics contribute to nephrotoxicity, either by metabolism leading to inorganic fluoride production or via degradation products, as described earlier for sevoflurane. Fluoride production has a well-documented history of inducing nephrotoxicity, while the other degradation product pathways lack reported clinical significance in humans.

Methoxyflurane was withdrawn after reports of severe nephrotoxicity due to production of inorganic fluoride. A high output renal failure unresponsive to vasopressin develops in association with serum fluoride concentrations in excess of $50\ \mu M$. Sevoflurane is the modern anesthetic with the highest associated serum fluoride concentrations, with some reports of serum levels exceeding $50\ \mu M$ after as little as 2 MAC hours of exposure, although nephrotoxicity from sevoflurane exposure has not been reported and controlled studies have failed to detect an impact of sevoflurane anesthesia on renal function.[104-106] This is likely secondary to the metabolism of methoxyflurane by cytochrome P450 enzymes 2E1, 2A6, and 3A4 within the kidney, producing fluoride locally within the nephrons themselves. In contrast there is less renal metabolism of sevoflurane.[107] Sevoflurane metabolism leads to formation of compound A, a nephrotoxic vinyl halide (see Chapters 3 and 6). However, the dose-dependent nephrotoxicity of compound A has only been demonstrated in rats, and multiple human studies have not shown evidence of renal impairment.[108]

Malignant Hyperthermia

Malignant hyperthermia is an uncommon inherited genetic disorder of skeletal muscle that can produce a potentially lethal hypermetabolic state after certain triggers (see Chapter 6), which include all the volatile anesthetics, but not nitrous oxide or xenon. A trigger leads to excessive release of Ca^{2+} from intracellular stores, which leads to muscle rigidity and rhabdomyolysis. The associated hypermetabolism increases body temperature, CO_2 production, and O_2 consumption. Untreated, malignant hyperthermia has an estimated mortality of 80%. Mortality is reduced to near 10% by early dantrolene treatment to terminate the hypermetabolic reaction by blocking intracellular Ca^{2+} release and supportive care to manage the sequelae of rhabdomyolysis. A molecular lesion underlying malignant hyperthermia was first traced to a single point mutation in the ryanodine receptor RyR1 in pigs, but it is now known that a variety of mutations can lead to this pharmacogenetic reaction (discussed further in Chapter 6).[109]

Postoperative Nausea and Vomiting

All inhaled anesthetics are emetogenic, including the volatile anesthetics, nitrous oxide and xenon; there are no significant differences between the modern volatile ether inhaled agents in their propensity for inducing postoperative nausea and vomiting (PONV). General anesthesia increases the risk of PONV significantly relative to regional anesthesia techniques (see Chapter 29). The incidence of PONV following general inhalational anesthesia involving the use of two triggering agents (opioids and volatile anesthetics) is 25% to 30%. Substituting propofol, which is not emetogenic (but rather is antiemetic), for the volatile anesthetic reduces the relative risk of PONV by 19%, and using nitrogen as a carrier gas rather than nitrous oxide reduces the relative risk by 12%.[110,111]

Metabolic Effects

Nitrous oxide can produce megaloblastic bone marrow changes and neurologic complications due to vitamin B_{12} deficiency (see Chapter 6). The cobalt ion in vitamin B_{12} is oxidized, which inhibits the activity of methionine synthase, which is responsible for conversion of homocysteine to methionine, thymidine, and tetrahydrofolate. Accumulation of plasma homocysteine could in theory increase the risk of perioperative myocardial events, but its clinical significance is currently unknown.[112]

UNIQUE FEATURES OF INDIVIDUAL AGENTS

Agents with Prominent GABA$_A$ Receptor Activity

HALOTHANE, ENFLURANE, METHOXYFLURANE

Halothane, enflurane, and methoxyflurane are no longer used in clinical practice in North America, although halothane is still widely used in the developing world due to its low cost. The following information is included for historical interest. Halothane, a halogenated alkane, is not very pungent and hence is compatible with inhalational induction. Use of halothane is associated with a lower risk of nausea and vomiting than the flourinated methyl ethyl ether agents. Its principle limitations include sensitizing myocardium to catecholamine-induced arrhythmias and occasional, but severe, hepatic necrosis. In pediatric patients, halothane notably causes bradyarrhythmias.

Enflurane, a halogenated methyl ethyl ether, is relatively pungent and high concentrations are associated with seizure-like EEG activity. Enflurane metabolism can release fluoride, which rarely can inhibit renal concentrating ability. Methoxyflurane is a halogenated methyl ethyl ether that provides more analgesia than other volatile agents. However, methoxyflurane produces significant levels of inorganic fluoride due to its high degree metabolism, and it is associated with high-output renal failure.

ISOFLURANE

Isoflurane is an isomer of enflurane, introduced to clinical practice almost simultaneously, with a more favorable side-effect profile. Isoflurane is highly pungent. It is also chemically quite stable.

SEVOFLURANE

Sevoflurane is a fluorinated methyl isopropyl ether. It is sweet smelling and minimally pungent, and hence well-suited to inhalational inductions. Because of its complete fluorination, sevoflurane has a very low blood solubility (among commonly used volatile anesthetics only desflurane has a lower solubility). It is approximately half as potent as isoflurane. Metabolism of sevoflurane leads to release of inorganic fluoride, similar to enflurane and methoxyflurane. Sevoflurane can form carbon monoxide when exposed to certain dehydrated CO_2 absorbants in an exothermic reaction that can ignite a fire (see Chapter 3). Sevoflurane appears to induce the least cerebral vasodilation of the modern agents, which likely makes sevoflurane the volatile agent of choice for neurosurgical patients with elevated ICP.[113]

DESFLURANE

Desflurane is a fluorinated methyl ethyl ether that is identical to isoflurane save for the substitution of a fluorine atom for the α-ethyl chlorine in isoflurane. The complete fluorination greatly reduces blood solubility and potency, and increases vapor pressure relative to isoflurane, to near atmospheric pressure (672 mm Hg at 20°C). The low boiling point of desflurane requires a specialized pressurized vaporizer (see Chapter 3). Desflurane is the most pungent of the inhaled anesthetics, potentially causing coughing, sialorrhea, breath holding, and laryngospasm. Rapid increases in desflurane concentration cause increased sympathetic activity, with associated tachycardia and hypertension.[78] Desflurane undergoes almost no metabolism, minimizing the risk of hepatitis and nephrotoxicity. Desflurane is, however, degraded to carbon monoxide by certain dehydrated CO_2 absorbants (see Chapter 3).

ETHER AND CHLOROFORM

Diethyl ether (ether) is notable for its high aqueous solubility compared to other anesthetic ethers. Ether is sweet smelling and mildly pungent; while it can be used for inhalational induction, an ether induction is very slow and risks laryngospasm. Ether is still used as an anesthetic in some developing countries because of its low cost and high therapeutic index with minimal cardiac and respiratory depression. Its explosive flammability has eliminated its use in most developed nations. Ether is not a cardiac depressant and maintains the baroreceptor reflex, making it relatively safe in patients with septic shock. Ether has a high incidence of PONV.

Chloroform (trichloromethane) is a sweet smelling volatile anesthetics that can be used for inhalational induction. While initially developed as an alternative to ether, chloroform was abandoned due to its association with hepatotoxicity and fatal cardiac arrhythmias.

Agents with Prominent NMDA Receptor Activity

NITROUS OXIDE

Nitrous oxide is a sweet-smelling gas with low solubility, low anesthetic potency (MAC of 104 vol%) and good analgesic properties. Although nitrous oxide is not flammable, it is a powerful oxidizing agent that supports combustion. Nitrous oxide is usually used as an anesthetic adjuvant because its low potency prevents it from being used as a sole agent. It does not produce skeletal muscle relaxation. Nitrous oxide should be avoided in pregnant patients due to its teratogenic effects. Because of the high delivered concentrations and solubility of nitrous oxide, it has a tendency to rapidly accumulate in closed spaces (see Chapter 3). It is associated with stable hemodynamics in that it does not produce cardiac depression.

XENON

Xenon is an odorless and nonpungent noble gas with low solubility, leading to rapid induction and emergence, and was first demonstrated to produce human anesthesia in 1951.[114] It is nontoxic and lacks teratogenicity, produces excellent analgesia, and is associated with stable hemodynamics in that it does not produce cardiac depression.

Xenon is relatively expensive to obtain and has low potency (MAC ~ 71 vol%), and hence is not in common use. Systems designed to minimize waste either by recycling xenon or using closed breathing circuits might eventually make its widespread use practical.

CYCLOPROPANE

The cycloalkane cyclopropane is a sweet-smelling and nonpungent gas, and hence suitable for inhalational induction. Because of the large amount of potential energy attributed to the strain in the carbon-carbon bonds of cylcopropane, it is prone to explosive decomposition when stored in large quantities or when mixed with an oxygen-enriched atmosphere; hence it is no longer in clinical use. Cyclopropane is associated with a high risk for PONV.[115]

Environmental Considerations

All of the inhaled anesthetics except xenon are greenhouse gases that have potential global warming effects based on their infrared absorption and atmospheric lifetimes. The impact of the volatile anesthetics is relatively small compared to that of nitrous oxide, which is usually used at higher concentrations and flow rates, and is also destructive to the ozone layer.[116,117]

DRUG INTERACTIONS

Given their multiple mechanisms and pleiotropic effects, it is not surprising that inhaled anesthetics are subject to a number of drug interactions.

Reduction in MAC by Anesthetic Adjuvants

Sedative and hypnotic drugs decrease the MAC of volatile anesthetics (see Chapter 5). GABAergic agents (propofol, benzodiazepines, and barbiturates), opioids, NMDA antagonists (ketamine, nitrous oxide, xenon), and α_2 agonists (dexmedetomidine, clonidine) all reduce the MAC of volatile anesthetics (Table 10-4).[118-121] This fact is exploited in balanced anesthesia to minimize the hemodynamic side effects associated with high-dose volatile agents. The β blocker esmolol appears to potentiate the MAC-reducing effect of opioids.[122]

MAC Additivity

When using more than one agent, MAC equivalents of the agents combine additively with no synergism between inhaled

Table 10-4. Factors That Alter the Value of Minimal Alveolar Concentration

FACTORS THAT DECREASE MAC	FACTORS THAT INCREASE MAC
Drugs	**Drugs**
α_2 Agonists	Alcohol (chronic)
Barbiturates	**Other Factors**
Benzodiazepines	Young age
Opioid analgesia	Hyperthermia
Other anesthetics	
Other Factors	
Increasing age	
Hypothermia	
Hypoxia	
Hypotension	
Pregnancy	

Reprinted with permission from Hemmings Jr HC, Hopkins PM, eds. *Foundations of Anesthesia: Basic Sciences for Clinical Practice.* 2nd ed. London: Mosby Elsevier; 2006:316.

anesthetics. For example, the combination of 0.5 MAC desflurane and 0.5 MAC sevoflurane sums to 1 MAC equivalent and thus inhibits movement in response to incision in 50% of subjects. In practice, modern anesthetic vaporizers have a lockout to prohibit delivery of multiple volatile agents at the same time to reduce the risk of overdose. Hence the most common application of MAC additivity is the delivery of a volatile anesthetic with nitrous oxide.

Synergy with Opioid-Induced Respiratory Depression

The combination of volatile anesthetic and opioid causes synergistic respiratory depression. For example, the combination of alfentanil and sevoflurane leads to more depression of minute ventilation and heart rate than does the summed effect of each drug administered separately.[123]

FACTORS INFLUENCING MAC

Despite the surprisingly narrow population range in sensitivity to inhaled anesthetics, certain subject-dependent factors consistently influence individual susceptibility to inhaled anesthetics. MAC is increased by anxiety, thyrotoxicosis, and stimulants (e.g., amphetamines). MAC is decreased by hypothyroidism, hypothermia, hypotension, and pregnancy (see Table 10-4), as well as pharmacogenetic factors.

Age

A major physiologic determinant of the MAC for an anesthetic gas is age.[25] In humans, MAC increases in the first few months of life, peaks, and then declines approximately exponentially with age, with a drop of 6% to 7% per decade of life (Figure 10-8). When quoting MAC for an anesthetic, the standard age of 40 years is the usual default unless otherwise specified.

Temperature

The MAC for potent inhaled anesthetics decreases with decreasing body temperature by 4% to 5% per 1°C decrease,

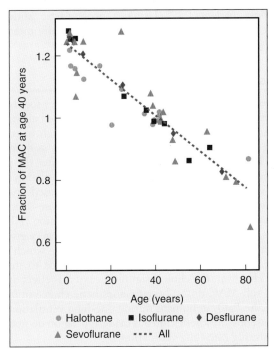

Figure 10-8 Variation of anesthetic potency with age for volatile anesthetics. There is a progressive increase in anesthetic potency with age older than 1 year, with MAC decreasing by 6.7% with each increasing decade of life. *(Modified from Eger EI. Age, minimum alveolar anesthetic concentration, and minimum alveolar anesthetic concentration-awake.* Anesth Analg. *2001;93:947-953.)*

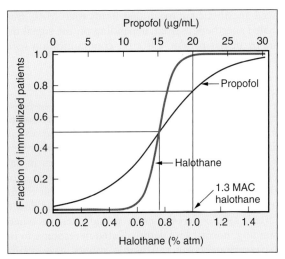

Figure 10-9 Potency population responses of halothane compared to propofol. The curves are drawn so the minimum alveolar concentration for halothane (MAC; lower scale) corresponds to the plasma EC_{50} for surgical incision for propofol (upper scale). The vertical lines indicate the 1.0 MAC and 1.3 MAC (resulting in 99% immobilization) for halothane. At 1.3 times the EC_{50} for propofol, only 75% of subjects are immobilized by propofol (upper horizontal line). *(Modified with permission from Dilger JP. From individual to population: the minimum alveolar concentration curve.* Curr Opin Anaesthesiol. *2006;19:390-396.)*

with complete elimination of the requirement for anesthesia at 20°C in laboratory mammals. However, this effect is not observed for nitrous oxide.[25]

Pharmacogenetic Effects on Potency

Fortuitously for anesthesiologists, the population range in anesthetic potency around the median is narrow, with a standard deviation of ~10% of its median value (MAC). This is much narrower than the distribution of effects for most other drugs (Figure 10-9). Additionally, the MAC is roughly the same order of magnitude across multiple species that are widely separated phylogenetically, including *Caenorhabditis elegans* (nematode), *Drosophila* (insect), and vertebrates. This argues that susceptibility to general anesthesia evolved in a very early, likely unicellular, common ancestor and its persistence must contribute to reproductive fitness or is an epiphenomenon of a beneficial trait, although at present it is unclear how.[124]

Given that metabolic factors affect MAC, it should not be surprising that genetic differences can contribute to anesthetic sensitivity. There is a statistically significant difference in MAC between Jews of three different ethnicities (European, Caucasian, and Asian) with the Caucasian population having a 24% higher MAC than the European population.[125] Additional evidence for specific mutations affecting anesthetic requirements originates with the observation that red-haired patients seem to have greater analgesic requirements. Interestingly, 75% of individuals with red hair and pale skin carry at least two inactivating variants of the melanocortin-1 receptor (MC1R).[126] MC1R mediates kappa opioid receptor-induced analgesia, which appears to be more effective in women than men.[126-128] This probably explains the

observation that redheads are both more sensitive to thermal pain and relatively resistant to subcutaneous lidocaine.[129] A functional consequence of these differences in pain sensation is that redheaded women are more difficult to sedate. Redheaded subjects are less sedated by a plasma-concentration targeted midazolam infusion than non-redheads.[130] The concentration of desflurane required to suppress movement to a noxious electrical stimulus is significantly higher in redheaded as opposed to dark-haired women; 9 of the 10 redheaded women in the study were either MC1R homozygous or compound heterozygous mutants.[131]

COMMON CLINICAL INDICATIONS AND CONSIDERATIONS

Choices of anesthetic agent for induction and maintenance of anesthesia depend on multiple patient and procedure dependent factors. Type and length of surgery, expected disposition, patient comorbidities, and economic factors all figure into the decision making process for agent selection.

Induction and Maintenance of Anesthesia

Induction of anesthesia with an inhaled anesthetic requires a nonpungent, nonirritating agent, such as halothane, sevoflurane, or nitrous oxide. Since the MAC of nitrous oxide exceeds 1 atm, sevoflurane is frequently used to reliably induce general anesthesia by inhalation due to its lower solubility and thus more rapid equilibration compared to halothane.

Neuroanesthesia and Neuromonitoring

Neuromonitoring can be substantially affected by the potent inhaled anesthetics. Somatosensory evoked potential magnitude is diminished and latency prolonged, such that a balanced anesthetic approach that limits total MAC fraction of inhaled anesthetic is used, depending on the signal quality for the particular patient. Effective communication with the clinical neurophysiology team is important.

Cardiac Anesthesia

Anesthetic preconditioning (see Emerging Developments: Anesthetic Preconditioning), which limits the extent of postanesthetic exposure ischemic infarction, represents a potential advantage of using volatile anesthetics in cardiac surgery patients who are predisposed to ischemia. Volatile anesthetics can induce coronary vasodilation. This prompted a theoretical fear of coronary steal, whereby blood flow distal to a fixed, atherosclerotic lesion would decrease when the surrounding, normal vasculature dilated in response to isoflurane, triggering ischemia. Multiple studies have confirmed that this concern is unfounded with isoflurane.[132-134] Interestingly, data from a recent randomized controlled clinical trial suggest patients given a sevoflurane anesthetic for surgery requiring cardiopulmonary bypass may have better cognitive performance in the immediate postoperative period than patients given propofol.[135]

Pediatric Anesthesia

Most pediatric cases are initiated with an inhalational induction using sevoflurane, particularly in day surgery cases where the patient arrives without intravenous access. Maintenance of anesthesia can be provided using the agent of choice, adjusting for the higher MAC in children.

Obstetric Anesthesia

Three main concerns dominate the choice of agent for the pregnant patient:
1. Throughout pregnancy efforts should be maintained to ensure adequate uterine blood flow, so blood pressure should be maintained in a normal range.
2. In the first trimester, teratogenic agents such as nitrous oxide should be avoided.
3. During delivery, maintenance of uterine tone is essential to achieve adequate postpartum hemostasis. The volatile agents all decrease smooth muscle tone, although this effect might be less with desflurane.[136,137] Hence it has been recommended that volatile agent concentration be minimized, ideally to less than 0.5 MAC with sevoflurane or to less than 1 MAC with desflurane, to ensure adequate uterine muscle tone.[137]

Ambulatory Anesthesia

Ambulatory cases represent an increasing fraction of all anesthetic procedures performed. In order to maximize throughput in busy surgery centers, it is essential to provide a cost-effective anesthetic that minimizes side effects and allows a rapid recovery. Use of the minimally soluble agents desflurane, sevoflurane, and nitrous oxide improves recovery time and drug cost compared to propofol infusion.[138-141] While the intermediate and late recovery profiles of desflurane, sevoflurane, and propofol are similar for the majority of patients, desflurane might have the best intermediate recovery profile

for obese patients.[142-144] Using a prophylactic antiemetic regimen to minimize PONV when using a volatile anesthetic-based technique can avoid discharge delays.[145,146]

Thoracic Anesthesia

The volatile anesthetics offer several advantages for thoracic surgery, including bronchodilation and decreased airway irritability, as well as the ability to maintain a high fraction of inspired oxygen when compared to anesthetics using nitrous oxide. Rapid clearance of volatile anesthetics after the procedure minimizes the need for postoperative ventilation (especially when combined with local anesthetic-based analgesic techniques). Volatile anesthetics cause a dose-dependent attenuation of hypoxic pulmonary vasoconstriction (HPV).[147] This is of particular significance for thoracic surgery given the frequent use of one-lung ventilation, during which HPV diminishes the shunt fraction and hence tends to improve PaO_2. However, the clinical significance of this effect appears low at sub-MAC doses, because anesthetic choice minimally affects the PaO_2 in humans during one-lung ventilation.[148-150] The gaseous anesthetics nitrous oxide and xenon do not affect HPV during one-lung ventilation.

EMERGING DEVELOPMENTS

It has been generally assumed that anesthetics have minimal or no persistent effects after elimination. However, general anesthetics act on multiple receptors and second messenger systems in the central nervous system with increasing evidence for more durable changes in gene and protein expression, posttranslational modification, and epigenetic effects.[20] It is therefore not surprising that the assumption that volatile anesthetics have no lasting effects has been called into question. This is particularly true at the extremes of the human life cycle. Data are accumulating that neonatal exposure to anesthetics is neurotoxic in animals, although evidence remains scant in humans. In older adults, there is concern that anesthesia contributes to postoperative cognitive dysfunction (POCD) and possibly to the progression of neurodegenerative diseases, although again there is a lack of direct evidence in humans.

Developmental Neurotoxicity

Animal data in multiple species indicate that inhaled anesthetics have profound and long-lasting effects when administered during key developmental periods. In the perinatal period, mammals undergo a brain "growth spurt," characterized by a burst of neurogenesis and synaptogenesis. The neural network is then pruned to produce an adult functional architecture through synaptic pruning and programmed cell death, or apoptosis, with ultimate removal of 50% to 70% of neonatal neurons.[151,152] In immature rodents and monkeys at critical developmental periods, exposure to either NMDA antagonist and/or GABAergic agents can lead to increased apoptosis. What remains unclear is the functional consequences of this apoptosis. Does this represent acceleration of a physiologic process, or is this excessive cell death above what would normally occur over time? If so, does this have consequences for cognitive function later in life? In rodents and monkeys, anesthetic exposure can lead to long-term cognitive deficits, but translating these findings to humans is difficult due to differences in neurodevelopment and difficulty in comparing duration of exposure.

NMDA receptor blockade by ketamine in the developing rodent brain causes excessive apoptosis.[153,154] A compelling study of more commonly used drugs exposed postnatal day 7 (P7) rat pups to a cocktail of isoflurane, midazolam, and nitrous oxide at levels sufficient to maintain a surgical plane of anesthesia for 6 hours. The rat pups developed excessive and widespread neuronal apoptosis immediately following exposure. This had persistent behavioral consequences with impairment of hippocampal long-term potentiation and of spatial reference memory as juveniles that lasted into adulthood. While isoflurane exposure in isolation led to significant apoptosis, the addition of other agents to the cocktail substantially increased the degree of apoptosis, suggesting that drug combinations might be more detrimental.[155]

The increased neuronal death with additional agents from other drug classes suggests that the significant event might be the pharmacologically induced coma itself rather than the particular agent employed to achieve the anesthetic state. Thus equipotent exposure of neonatal mice to desflurane, isoflurane, and sevoflurane produced similar increases in apoptotic cell death.[156] While data for some drugs are conflicting, most anesthetic agents produce increased apoptosis after exposure.[157] Disruption of neurotrophic factor secretion in the developing nervous system by anesthetic suppression of spontaneous activity might underlie anesthetic neurotoxicity.[158] At sensitive ages (P0-14 rats), the chloride gradient is reversed compared to adults due to developmental changes in expression of the KCC2 chloride transporter. Hence, in the immature brain, the increase in chloride permeability associated with $GABA_A$ receptor activation leads to depolarization of neurons, with resultant excitation and possibly excitotoxicity. A significant number of P7 rats have seizures with sevoflurane anesthesia and postanesthetic apoptosis could be mitigated by bumetanide, a N^+-K^+-$2Cl^-$ cotransporter 1 inhibitor, suggesting that apoptosis after anesthesia involves excitotoxicity rather than withdrawal of trophic factors.[159] The idea that perturbation of neonatal neuronal chloride gradients can rescue neurons from apoptosis is provocative, suggesting that pharmacologic prophylaxis for long-term cognitive deficits after neonatal anesthesia might be possible.

Despite robust laboratory evidence of increased apoptosis after anesthesia in neonatal animal models, the clinical significance of these observations remains controversial. Exposure of rhesus monkey fetuses and newborns to 24 hours of ketamine produced neurodegeneration both at day 122 of gestation and at postnatal day 5 (P5), but not at P35, while a smaller exposure of 3 hours at P5 demonstrated no neurodegeneration.[160] Cognitive deficits have been demonstrated in rhesus monkeys after exposure to 24 hours of ketamine anesthesia at P5-6, but it remains unclear what the minimum required exposure is for a significant effect on neurodevelopment.[161] Significant apoptotic and necrotic cell death occurred in neonatal monkeys exposed to ketamine for 9 hours or isoflurane for 5 hours.[160,162] Anesthetic exposure must occur during the critical period of neurogenesis and synaptogenesis to have significant apoptotic sequelae and it is unclear when this period is in humans. The rat peak critical period for anesthesia exposure approximates the 20th week of gestation in humans,

while the rhesus critical period approximates the 26th week of gestation in humans.[163] Translation to humans suggests that anesthetic neurotoxicity is likely most significant for the premature human fetus rather than term neonates or infants.

Available clinical data on cognitive deficits after exposure to anesthesia are necessarily retrospective. In one series, children exposed to multiple anesthetics before the age of 4 years had a doubled incidence of learning disability diagnoses later in life.[164] Another retrospective cohort study found that children who underwent hernia repair before 3 years of age were more than twice as likely as controls to have a developmental or behavioral disorder diagnosis.[165] Because of the retrospective nature of these studies, the relative contributions of surgery, anesthesia, and other comorbid conditions remain undefined. Other studies have not supported an association between early anesthetic exposure and long-term cognitive deficits. Several prospective studies are ongoing to attempt to address this problem. These include the GAS study to compare cognitive function at 5 years in infants undergoing hernia repair using general anesthesia or spinal anesthesia, and the PANDA study prospectively assessing cognitive function in children younger than 3 years exposed to general anesthesia compared to sibling controls.[166]

Anesthesia and Neurodegenerative Disease

The existence and prevalence of POCD in older adults were established in the International Study of Post-Operative Cognitive Dysfunction.[167] While short-term cognitive dysfunction was associated with multiple comorbid medical conditions, the predominant risk factor for prolonged cognitive decline was advanced age. Research to determine what role, if any, anesthesia plays in POCD is ongoing, with suggestive laboratory models finding parallels between neurodegenerative disorders and effects of anesthesia.

POCD could reflect altered drug responses, loss of functional reserve, or the cumulative effects of chronic disease over time. With aging, neurogenesis and synaptogenesis slow, the total number of neurons decreases, and potentially toxic by-products accumulate. These processes gradually deplete physiologic reserves, potentially increasing the vulnerability of the brain to insults, including exposure to perioperative stressors. Current hypotheses of POCD posit roles for direct toxic effects via alterations in Ca^{2+} homeostasis, systemic inflammatory effects secondary to surgical insult leading to neuroinflammation, age-sensitive suppression of neuronal stem cell function, and/or acceleration of ongoing endogenous neurodegenerative processes such as production of aggregated amyloid beta (Aβ) peptide oligomers and tau hyperphosphorylation, thereby unmasking the patient's preexisting pathophysiology.[168-173]

Alzheimer disease is a neurodegenerative process resulting in diffuse atrophy of the cerebral cortex, characteristic plaques composed of Aβ, and accumulation of neurofibrillary tangles made up of hyperphosphorylated tau protein.[174] Research has focused on the toxic effects that result from selective proteolysis of the amyloid precursor protein (APP) into Aβ peptide oligomers.[175] Aβ formation and apoptosis are increased in rodent brains exposed to isoflurane, isoflurane with nitrous oxide, sevoflurane, and desflurane with hypoxia.[173,176-179] However, not all data implicate a postanesthetic Aβ mechanism for POCD. In a transgenic mouse model of Alzheimer disease, increased production of amyloid plaque had no associated cognitive deficits after daily exposure to halothane or isoflurane, while wild-type mice developed cognitive impairment after repeated isoflurane exposure.[180] Aβ might not be the only neurodegenerative component increased by anesthetic exposure, in that multiple anesthetic agents appear to promote hyperphosphorylation of the protein tau, either associated with hypothermia or normothermia.[181,182] Interpreting these data is further complicated in that the choice of anesthetic exposure duration, and total dose all matter, with several studies suggesting a potential neuroprotective preconditioning effect with lower exposures.[183-185]

Neuroinflammation and Cognitive Dysfunction

Systemic inflammation resulting from a surgical insult could lead to neuroinflammation and reduced neurogenesis, and possibly be involved in POCD. Adult rats undergoing splenectomy with neuroleptanesthesia had impaired cognitive function on postoperative days 1 and 3 compared to rats anesthetized without surgery (which were indistinguishable from nonanesthetized controls). Increased IL-1β mRNA and protein expression in hippocampus suggests that systemically triggered neuroinflammation contributes to cognitive impairment.[169] In a similar model, memory dysfunction after surgery was mitigated both by nonspecific immunosuppression with minocycline and by pretreatment with an IL-1 receptor antagonist, and was less prominent in IL-1 receptor knockout mice.[186] This IL-1 response appears to be mediated by tumor necrosis factor alpha (TNF-α) as peripheral TNF-α blockade attenuates both the neuroinflammatory response mediated by IL-1 and its associated postoperative cognitive decline, suggesting that pretreatment with an anti-TNF antibody might prevent POCD. This neuroinflammatory response appears to be more prominent in older mice, consistent with POCD in humans.[187,188] However, anesthesia might also contribute to the neuroinflammatory response, as increased levels of TNF-α, IL-6, and IL-1β have been observed following isoflurane anesthesia. This increase was more marked in transgenic Alzheimer disease model mice, suggesting that neuroinflammation might contribute to the increase in neurodegenerative markers after anesthesia.[189]

Despite animal data linking Alzheimer disease pathophysiology to anesthesia exposure, data linking Alzheimer disease and anesthetic exposure in humans are contradictory. There was no significant difference in mean cumulative duration of general anesthesia between controls and Alzheimer patients and no association between number of surgical operations and risk of Alzheimer disease, or between exposures to anesthesia in a 1 to 5 year window preceding onset of Alzheimer disease.[172,190] However, an association between cumulative anesthesia exposure prior to age 50 years and earlier onset of Alzheimer disease suggests that the time horizon for accumulating effects might be quite long.[172]

A recent retrospective cohort study calls into question the severity of POCD as a clinical problem. Long-term cognitive decline could be independently attributed to illness or surgery and neither illness nor surgery appeared to speed progression to dementia, though patients who had initial dementia declined more rapidly over the course of the study than those who did not.[191] Multicenter prospective clinical trials to determine the contributions of anesthesia, surgery, and illness to

cognitive dysfunction will be essential to resolve the possible association between anesthesia and POCD and progression of neurodegenerative disease.

Anesthetic Preconditioning

Volatile anesthetic exposure prior to induction of myocardial ischemia decreases severity of the ensuing ischemia-reperfusion injury, a property known as *anesthetic preconditioning*. Isoflurane concentrations as low as 0.25 MAC confer protection, although higher concentrations might have greater efficacy.[192] Preconditioning appears to involve production of reactive oxygen species (ROS) during the anesthetic exposure, as bracketing the anesthetic exposure with ROS scavengers attenuates the anesthetic preconditioning effect.[193] A similar phenomenon known as *ischemic preconditioning* has been observed whereby brief episodes of ischemia minimize the ischemia-reperfusion injury sustained from a subsequent, more profound episode of ischemia. While exposure to isoflurane and to brief episodes of ischemia upregulate several common cell defense signaling pathways and genes, ischemic and anesthetic preconditioning appear to have distinct phenotypes.[194] The magnitude of the anesthetic preconditioning effect diminishes with age in animal models.[195]

Exposure to anesthetic agents after the ischemic event also diminishes ischemia-reperfusion injury, an effect known as *anesthetic post-conditioning*. It appears that anesthetic preconditioning and postconditioning have similar effects and are not additive.[196]

In addition to cardiac protection, anesthetic preconditioning by volatile anesthetics has been demonstrated in other organs as well including brain, kidney, and lung.[197]

Immunomodulation and Cancer

Volatile anesthetics suppress the activity of natural killer (NK) cells.[198] Significant suppression of NK cell function in the perioperative period has been associated with an increase in cancer patient mortality.[198-201] This argues that volatile anesthetics might increase the risk of retained tumor metastasis due to reduced immune surveillance by NK cells, but on balance the effect is significantly smaller than the immune suppression triggered by the stress response to surgery without general anesthesia.[89] There is currently insufficient evidence to wholly avoid volatile anesthetics for cancer patients. Yet anesthesiologists should remain aware of their possible contributions to postoperative immune function, particularly in patients who are immunosuppressed at baseline.

KEY POINTS

- Inhaled anesthetics as single agents provide all of the essential features of general anesthesia, including amnesia, unconsciousness, and immobility. Each of these components results from agent-specific actions on distinct neuronal pathways in the central nervous system.
- The characteristic immobilizing effect of volatile anesthetics involves a site in the spinal cord. Amnesia and unconsciousness involve poorly understood supraspinal mechanisms.

- The principal effects of inhaled anesthetics on the nervous system involve alterations in synaptic transmission, the mechanism for chemical transmission between neurons.
- The precise mechanisms by which inhaled anesthetics produce each of their principal actions have not been fully elucidated despite a number of promising candidate molecular targets. The physicochemical nature of the typical anesthetic binding site is hydrophobic and amphipathic.
- In contrast to intravenous anesthetics, inhaled anesthetics can act at a number of membrane bound ion channels and receptors at clinically relevant effect site concentrations. The volatile anesthetics have potentiating effects on inhibitory $GABA_A$ and glycine receptors and K^+ channels, and inhibitory effects on excitatory Na^+ and Ca^{2+} channels. The gaseous anesthetics nitrous oxide and xenon have predominant NMDA-type glutamate receptor blocking effects.
- Inhaled anesthetics have a diverse range of clinically significant effects on multiple organ systems, both beneficial and potentially adverse. Potentially beneficial effects include organ protection, while adverse effects include respiratory and cardiovascular depression.
- Specific inhaled anesthetics have agent-specific pharmacologic, pharmacokinetic, and side-effect profiles that determine their optimal clinical applications based on patient and procedure specific applications.
- Anesthetic-induced neurotoxicity occurs in animal models at critical periods in early brain development; its clinical significance is not yet clear.

Key References

Antognini JF, Schwartz K. Exaggerated anesthetic requirements in the preferentially anesthetized brain. *Anesthesiology*. 1993;79:1244-1249; Rampil IJ, Mason P, Singh H. Anesthetic potency (MAC) is independent of forebrain structures in the rat. *Anesthesiology* 1993;78:707-712. First demonstrations of a spinal site of action for the immobilizing action volatile anesthetics in two distinct animal models. (Refs. 28 and 29)

Bigelow HJ. Insensibility during surgical operations produced by inhalation. *Boston Med Surg J*. 1846;35:309-317, 379-382. October 16, 1846 marked the first successful public operation on a patient under ether anaesthesia at Massachusetts General Hospital. The account of Dr. Henry J. Bigelow, printed in *The Boston Medical and Surgical Journal* on November 18, is the first medical publication on this groundbreaking achievement. (Ref. 3)

Franks NP, Lieb WR. Do general anaesthetics act by competitive binding to specific receptors? *Nature*. 1984;310:599-601. A landmark demonstration that a large range of anesthetic molecules can act on a single protein binding site in a lipid-free preparation, thus providing proof of concept that the Meyer-Overton correlation is not incompatible with a protein site of action for anesthetics. (Ref. 18)

Jevtovic-Todorovic V, Hartman RE, Izumi Y, et al. Early exposure to common anesthetic agents causes widespread neurodegeneration in the developing rat brain and persistent learning deficits. *J Neurosci*. 2003;23:1066-1082. Landmark study that demonstrates persistent cognitive deficits after exposure to anesthetic agents during a critical period of rat brain development. (Ref. 155)

References

1. Ph. Aureoli. Theophrasti Paracelsi Op., vol. II, p. 197, Geneva, 1658. [Interpretation by C.D. Leake, "Valerius Cordus and the Discovery of Ether", Isis, Vol. 7, No. 1 (1925), pp. 14-24, The University of Chicago Press.]
2. Erwing HW. The discoverer of anaesthesia: Dr. Horace Wells of Hartford. *Yale J Bio Med*. 1933;5:426.
3. Bigelow HJ. Insensibility during surgical operations produced by inhalation. *Boston Med Surg J*. 1846;35:309-317, 379-382.
4. Long CW. An account of the first use of sulphuric ether by inhalation as an anaesthetic in surgical operation. *South Med Surg J*. 1849;5:705-713.
5. Snow J. *On Chloroform and Other Anaesthetics: Their Action and Administration*. London: Churchill; 1858.
6. Hemmings Jr HC. General anaesthetic agents. In: Webster NR, Galley HF, eds. *Landmark Papers in Anaesthesia*. Oxford: Oxford University Press; 2012 (in press).
7. Robbins BH. Preliminary studies of the anesthetic activity of fluorinated hydrocarbons. *J Pharmacol Exp Ther*. 1946;86:197-204.
8. O'Brien HD. The introduction of halothane into clinical practice: the Oxford experience. *Anaesth Intensive Care*. 2006;34(Suppl 1):27-32.
9. Terrell RC. The invention and development of enflurane, isoflurane, sevoflurane, and desflurane. *Anesthesiology*. 2008;108:531-533.
10. Cantor R. The lateral pressure profile in membranes: a physical mechanism of general anesthesia. *Biochemistry*. 1997;36:2339–2344.
11. Perouansky M. Non-immobilizing inhalational anesthetic-like compounds. *Handb Exp Pharmacol*. 2008;(182):209-223.
12. Lysko GS, Robinson JL, Casto R, Ferrone RA. The stereospecific effects of isoflurane isomers in vivo. *Eur J Pharmacol*. 1994;263:25-29.
13. Eger EI 2nd, Koblin DD, Laster MJ, et al. Minimum alveolar anesthetic concentration values for the enantiomers of isoflurane differ minimally. *Anesth Analg*. 1997;85:188–192.
14. Quinlan JJ, Firestone S, Firestone LL. Isoflurane's enhancement of chloride flux through rat brain gamma-aminobutyric acid type A receptors is stereoselective. *Anesthesiology*. 1995;83:611-615.
15. Keshavaprasad B, Liu C, Au JD, Kindler CH, Cotten JF, Yost CS. Species-specific differences in response to anesthetics and other modulators by the K2P channel TRESK. *Anesth Analg*. 2005;101:1042-1049.
16. Moody EJ, Harris B, Hoehner P, Skolnick P. Inhibition of [^{3}H] isradipine binding to L-type calcium channels by the optical isomers of isoflurane. Lack of stereospecificity. *Anesthesiology*. 1994;81:124-128.
17. Ueda I. Effects of diethyl ether and halothane on firefly luciferin bioluminescence. *Anesthesiology*. 1965;26:603-606.
18. Franks NP, Lieb WR. Do general anaesthetics act by competitive binding to specific receptors? *Nature*. 1984;310:599-601.
19. Dickinson R, Franks NP, Lieb WR. Can the stereoselective effects of the anesthetic isoflurane be accounted for by lipid solubility? *Biophys J*. 1994;66:2019-2023.
20. Hemmings Jr HC, Akabas MH, Goldstein PA, Trudell JR, Orser BA, Harrison NL. Emerging molecular mechanisms of general anesthetic action. *Trends Pharmacol Sci*. 2005;26:503-510.
21. Eger EI 2nd, Raines DE, Shafer SL, Hemmings Jr HC, Sonner JM. Is a new paradigm needed to explain how inhaled anesthetics produce immobility? *Anesth Analg*. 2008;107:832-848.
22. Sonner JM, Antognini JF, Dutton RC, et al. Inhaled anesthetics and immobility: mechanisms, mysteries, and minimum alveolar anesthetic concentration. *Anesth Analg*. 2003;97:718-740.
23. Mennerick S, Jevtovic-Todorovic V, Todorovic SM, Shen W, Olney JW, Zorumski CF. Effect of nitrous oxide on excitatory and inhibitory synaptic transmission in hippocampal cultures. *J Neurosci*. 1998;18:9716-9726.
24. Franks NP, Dickinson R, de Sousa SL, Hall AC, Lieb WR. How does xenon produce anaesthesia? *Nature*. 1998;396:324.
25. Eger EI. Age, minimum alveolar anesthetic concentration, and minimum alveolar anesthetic concentration-awake. *Anesth Analg*. 2001;93:947-953.
26. Sanders RD, Tononi G, Laureys S, Sleigh JW. Unresponsiveness ≠ unconsciousness. *Anesthesiology*. 2012;116:946-959.

27. Posner J, Saper C, Schiff N, Plum F. *Plum and Posner's Diagnosis of Stupor and Coma*. 4th ed. New York, NY: Oxford University Press; 2007.
28. Antognini JF, Schwartz K. Exaggerated anesthetic requirements in the preferentially anesthetized brain. *Anesthesiology*. 1993;79:1244-1249.
29. Rampil IJ, Mason P, Singh H. Anesthetic potency (MAC) is independent of forebrain structures in the rat. *Anesthesiology*. 1993;78:707-712.
30. Zbinden AM, Petersen-Felix S, Thomson DA. Anesthetic depth defined using multiple noxious stimuli during isoflurane/oxygen anesthesia. II. Hemodynamic responses. *Anesthesiology*. 1994;80:261-267.
31. Sonner JM, Zhang Y, Stabernack C, Abaigar W, Xing Y, Laster MJ. GABA(A) receptor blockade antagonizes the immobilizing action of propofol but not ketamine or isoflurane in a dose-related manner. *Anesth Analg*. 2003;96:706-712.
32. Sonner JM, Werner DF, Elsen FP, et al. Effect of isoflurane and other potent inhaled anesthetics on minimum alveolar concentration, learning, and the righting reflex in mince engineered to express alpha 1 gamma-aminobutyric acid type A receptors unresponsive to isoflurane. *Anesthesiology*. 2007;106:107-113.
33. Jurd R, Arras M, Lambert S, et al. General anesthetic actions in vivo strongly attenuated by a point mutation in the GABA(A) receptor beta3 subunit. *FASEB J*. 2003;17:250-252.
34. Martin LJ, Zurek AA, MacDonald JF, Roder JC, Jackson MF, Orser BA. Alpha5GABA_A receptor activity sets the threshold for long-term potentiation and constrains hippocampus-dependent memory. *J Neurosci*. 2010;30:5269–5282.
35. Simon W, Hapfelmeier G, Kochs E, Zieglgänsberger W, Rammes G. Isoflurane blocks synaptic plasticity in the mouse hippocampus. *Anesthesiology*. 2001;94:1058-1065
36. Rau V, Oh I, Liao M, et al. Gamma-aminobutyric acid type A receptor β3 subunit forebrain-specific knockout mice are resistant to the amnestic effect of isoflurane. *Anesth Analg*. 2011;113:500-504.
37. Rau V, Iyer SV, Oh I, et al. Gamma-aminobutyric acid type A receptor alpha 4 subunit knockout mice are resistant to the amnestic effect of isoflurane. *Anesth Analg*. 2009;109:1816-1822.
38. Zhang Y, Laster MJ, Hara K, et al. Glycine receptors mediate part of the immobility produced by inhaled anesthetics. *Anesth Analg*. 2003;96:97-101.
39. Flood P, Sonner JM, Gong D, Coates KM. Heteromeric nicotinic inhibition by isoflurane does not mediate MAC or loss of righting reflex. *Anesthesiology*. 2002;97:902-905.
40. Eger EI II, Zhang Y, Laster MJ, Flood P, Kendig JJ, Sonner JM. Acetylcholine receptors do not mediate the immobilization produced by inhaled anesthetics. *Anesth Analg*. 2002;94:1500–1504.
41. Flood P, Sonner JM, Gong D, Coates KM. Isoflurane hyperalgesia is modulated by nicotinic inhibition. *Anesthesiology*. 2002;97:192-198.
42. Matsuura T, Kamiya Y, Itoh H, Higashi T, Yamada Y, Andoh T. Inhibitory effects of isoflurane and nonimmobilizing halogenated compounds on neuronal nicotinic acetylcholine receptors. *Anesthesiology*. 2002;97:1541-1549.
43. Hemmings Jr HC. Sodium channels and the synaptic mechanisms of inhaled anaesthetics. *Br J Anaesth*. 2009;103:61-69.
44. Wu XS, Sun JY, Evers AS, Crowder M, Wu LG. Isoflurane inhibits transmitter release and the presynaptic action potential. *Anesthesiology*. 2004;100:663-670.
45. OuYang W, Hemmings Jr HC. Depression by isoflurane of the action potential and underlying voltage-gated ion currents in isolated rat neurohypophysial nerve terminals. *J Pharmacol Exp Ther*. 2005;312:801-808.
46. Westphalen RI, Hemmings Jr HC. Selective depression by general anesthetics of glutamate vs. GABA release from isolated nerve terminals. *J Pharmacol Exp Ther*. 2003;304:1188-1196.
47. Zhang Y, Guzinski M, Eger EI 2nd, et al. Bidirectional modulation of isoflurane potency by intrathecal tetrodotoxin and veratridine in rats. *Br J Pharmacol*. 2010;159:872-878.
48. Zhang Y, Sharma M, Eger EI 2nd, Laster MJ, Hemmings Jr HC, Harris RA. Intrathecal veratridine administration increases minimum alveolar concentration in rats. *Anesth Analg*. 2008;107:875-878.
49. Heurteaux C, Guy N, Laigle C, et al. TREK-1, a K(+) channel involved in neuroprotection and general anesthesia. *EMBO J*. 2004;23:2684-2695.
50. Patel AJ, Honore E, Lesage F, Fink M, Romey G, Lazdunski M. Inhalational anesthetics activate two-pore-domain background K⁺ channels. *Nat Neurosci*. 1999;2:422-426.
51. Linden AM, Sandu C, Aller MI, et al. TASK-3 knockout mice exhibit exaggerated nocturnal activity, impairments in cognitive functions, and reduced sensitivity to inhalation anesthetics. *J Pharmacol Exp Ther*. 2007;323:924-934.
52. Leonoudakis D, Gray AT, Winegar BD, et al. An open rectifier potassium channel with two pore domains in tandem cloned from rat cerebellum. *J Neurosci*. 1998;18:868-877.
53. Eisele JH, Eger EI, II, Muallem M. Narcotic properties of carbon dioxide in the dog. *Anesthesiology*. 1967;28:856-865.
54. Brosnan RJ, Eger EI, II, Laster MJ, Sonner JM. Anesthetic properties of carbon dioxide in the rat. *Anesth Analg*. 2007;105:103-106.
55. Xing Y, Zhang Y, Stabernack CR, Eger EI II, Gray AT. The use of the potassium channel activator riluzole to test whether potassium channels mediate the capacity of isoflurane to produce immobility. *Anesth Analg*. 2003;97:1020-1024.
56. Urbani A, Belluzzi O. Riluzole inhibits the persistent sodium current in mammalian CNS neurons. *Eur J Neurosci*. 2000;12:3567-3574.
57. De Sousa SL, Dickinson R, Lieb WR, Franks NP. Contrasting synaptic actions of the inhalational general anesthetics isoflurane and xenon. *Anesthesiology*. 2000;92(4):1055-1066.
58. Dickinson R, Peterson BK, Banks P, et al. Competitive inhibition at the glycine site of the N-methyl-D-aspartate receptor by the anesthetics xenon and isoflurane: evidence from molecular modeling and electrophysiology. *Anesthesiology*. 2007;107:756-767.
59. Jevtović-Todorović V, Todorović SM, Mennerick S, et al. Nitrous oxide (laughing gas) is an NMDA antagonist, neuroprotectant and neurotoxin. *Nat Med*. 1998;4:460-463.
60. Gruss M, Bushell TJ, Bright DP, Lieb WR, Mathie A, Franks NP. Two-pore-domain K⁺ channels are a novel target for the anesthetic gases xenon, nitrous oxide, and cyclopropane. *Mol Pharmacol*. 2004;65:443-452.
61. Pabelick CM, Ay B, Prakash YS, Sieck GC. Effects of volatile anesthetics on store-operated Ca(2+) influx in airway smooth muscle. *Anesthesiology*. 2004;101:373-380.
62. Katoh T, Ikeda K. A comparison of sevoflurane with halothane, enflurane, and isoflurane on bronchoconstriction caused by histamine. *Can J Anaesth*. 1994;41:1214-1219.
63. Goff MJ, Arain SR, Ficke DJ, Uhrich TD, Ebert TJ. Absence of bronchodilation during desflurane anesthesia: a comparison to sevoflurane and thiopental. *Anesthesiology*. 2000;93:404-408.
64. Waud BE, Waud DR. The effects of diethyl ether, enflurane, and isoflurane at the neuromuscular junction. *Anesthesiology*. 1975;42:275-280.
65. Scheller M, Bufler J, Schneck H, Kochs E, Franke C. Isoflurane and sevoflurane interact with the nicotinic acetylcholine receptor channels in micromolar concentrations. *Anesthesiology*. 1997;86:118-127.
66. Zhang Y, Laster MJ, Hara K, et al. Glycine receptors mediate part of the immobility produced by inhaled anesthetics. *Anesth Analg*. 2003;96:97-101.
67. Paul M, Fokt RM, Kindler CH, Dipp NC, Yost CS. Characterization of the interactions between volatile anesthetics and neuromuscular blockers at the muscle nicotinic acetylcholine receptor. *Anesth Analg*. 2002;95:362-367.
68. van den Elsen M, Sarton E, Teppema L, Berkenbosch A, Dahan A. Influence of 0.1 minimum alveolar concentration of sevoflurane, desflurane and isoflurane on dynamic ventilatory response to hypercapnia in humans. *Br J Anaesth*. 1998;80:174-182.
69. Dahan A, Teppema LJ. Influence of anaesthesia and analgesia on the control of breathing. *Br J Anaesth*. 2003;91:40-49.
70. Eikermann M, Malhotra A, Fassbender P, et al. Differential effects of isoflurane and propofol on upper airway dilator muscle activity and breathing. *Anesthesiology*. 2008;108:897-906.
71. López-Barneo J, Ortega-Sáenz P, Pardal R, Pascual A, Piruat JI. Carotid body oxygen sensing. *Eur Respir J*. 2008;32:1386-1398.
72. Dahan A, Sarton E, van den Elsen M, van Kleef J, Teppema L, Berkenbosch A. Ventilatory response to hypoxia in humans. Influences of subanesthetic desflurane. *Anesthesiology*. 1996;85:60-68.
73. Teppema LJ, Nieuwenhuijs D, Sarton E, et al. Antioxidants prevent depression of the acute hypoxic ventilatory response by subanaesthetic halothane in men. *J Physiol*. 2002;544:931-938.

74. Teppema LJ, Romberg RR, Dahan A. Antioxidants reverse reduction of the human hypoxic ventilatory response by subanesthetic isoflurane. *Anesthesiology.* 2005;102:747-753.

75. Wheeler DM, Katz A, Rice RT, Hansford RG. Volatile anesthetic effects on sarcoplasmic reticulum Ca content and sarcolemmal Ca flux in isolated rat cardiac cell suspensions. *Anesthesiology.* 1994;80:372-382.

76. Connelly TJ, Coronado R. Activation of the Ca2+ release channel of cardiac sarcoplasmic reticulum by volatile anesthetics. *Anesthesiology.* 1994;81:459-469.

77. Agnew NM, Pennefather SH, Russell GN. Isoflurane and coronary heart disease. *Anaesthesia.* 2002;57:338-347.

78. Ebert TJ, Perez F, Uhrich TD, Deshur MA. Desflurane-mediated sympathetic activation occurs in humans despite preventing hypotension and baroreceptor unloading. *Anesthesiology.* 1998;88:1227-1232.

79. Booker PD, Whyte SD, Ladusans EJ. Long QT syndrome and anaesthesia. *Br J Anaesth.* 2003;90:349-366.

80. Yamada M, Hatakeyama N, Malykhina AP, Yamazaki M, Momose Y, Akbarali HI. The effects of sevoflurane and propofol on QT interval and heterologously expressed human ether-a-go-go related gene currents in Xenopus oocytes. *Anesth Analg.* 2006;102:98-103.

81. Bovill JG. Inhalation anaesthesia: from diethyl ether to xenon. *Handb Exp Pharmacol.* 2008;182:121-142

82. Böhm M, Schmidt U, Gierschik P, Schwinger RH, Böhm S, Erdmann E. Sensitization of adenylate cyclase by halothane in human myocardium and S49 lymphoma wild-type and cyc- cells: evidence for inactivation of the inhibitory G protein Gi alpha. *Mol Pharmacol.* 1994;45:380-389.

83. Hashimoto K. Arrhythmia models for drug research: classification of antiarrhythmic drugs. *J Pharmacol Sci.* 2007;103:333-346.

84. Avidan MS, Jacobsohn E, Glick D, et al; BAG-RECALL Research Group. Prevention of intraoperative awareness in a high-risk surgical population. *N Engl J Med.* 2011;365:591-600.

85. Constant I, Seeman R, Murat I. Sevoflurane and epileptiform EEG changes. *Paediatr Anaesth.* 2005;15:266-274.

86. Harrison JL. Postoperative seizures after isoflurane anesthesia. *Anesth Analg.* 1986; 65:1235-1236.

87. Chrousos GP. The hypothalamic-pituitary-adrenal axis and immune-mediated inflammation. *N Engl J Med.* 1995;332:1351-1362.

88. Kennedy BC, Hall GM. Neuroendocrine and inflammatory aspects of surgery: do they affect outcome? *Acta Anaesthesiol Belg.* 1999;50:205-209.

89. Page GG, Blakely WP, Ben-Eliyahu S. Evidence that postoperative pain is a mediator of the tumor-promoting effects of surgery in rats. *Pain.* 2001;90:191-199.

90. Kurosawa S, Kato M. Anesthetics, immune cells, and immune responses. *J Anesth.* 2008;22:263-277.

91. Salo M, Eskola J, Nikoskelainen J. T and B lymphocyte function in anaesthetists. *Acta Anaesthesiol Scand.* 1984;28:292-295.

92. Ferrero E, Ferrero ME, Marni A, et al. In vitro effects of halothane on lymphocytes. *Eur J Anaesthesiol.* 1986;3:321-330.

93. Hamra JG, Yaksh TL. Halothane inhibits T cell proliferation and interleukin-2 receptor expression in rats. *Immunopharmacol Immunotoxicol.* 1996;18:323-336.

94. Welch WD. Halothane reversibly inhibits human neutrophil bacterial killing. *Anesthesiology.* 1981;55:650-654.

95. Tait AR, Davidson BA, Johnson KJ, Remick DG, Knight PR. Halothane inhibits the intraalveolar recruitment of neutrophils, lymphocytes, and macrophages in response to influenza virus infection in mice. *Anesth Analg.* 1993;76:1106-1113.

96. Kotani N, Hashimoto H, Sessler DI, et al. Intraoperative modulation of alveolar macrophage function during isoflurane and propofol anesthesia. *Anesthesiology.* 1998;89:1125-1132.

97. Schneemilch CE, Schilling T, Bank U. Effects of general anaesthesia on inflammation. *Best Pract Res Clin Anaesthesiol.* 2004;18:493-507.

98. Tschaikowsky K, Ritter J, Schröppel K, Kühn M. Volatile anesthetics differentially affect immunostimulated expression of inducible nitric oxide synthase: role of intracellular calcium. *Anesthesiology.* 2000;92:1093-1102.

99. Nakagawara M, Takeshige K, Takamatsu J, Takahashi S, Yoshitake J, Minakami S. Inhibition of superoxide production and Ca2+ mobilization in human neutrophils by halothane, enflurane, and isoflurane. *Anesthesiology.* 1986;64:4-12.

100. Fröhlich D, Rothe G, Schwall B, et al. Effects of volatile anaesthetics on human neutrophil oxidative response to the bacterial peptide FMLP. *Br J Anaesth.* 1997;78:718-723.

101. Van Pelt FN, Kenna JG. Formation of trifluoroacetylated protein antigens in cultured rat hepatocytes exposed to halothane in vitro. *Biochem Pharmacol.* 1994;48:461-471.

102. Njoku D, Laster MJ, Gong DH, Eger EI 2nd, Reed GF, Martin JL. Biotransformation of halothane, enflurane, isoflurane, and desflurane to trifluoroacetylated liver proteins: association between protein acylation and hepatic injury. *Anesth Analg.* 1997;84:173-178.

103. Njoku DB, Greenberg RS, Bourdi M, et al. Autoantibodies associated with volatile anesthetic hepatitis found in the sera of a large cohort of pediatric anesthesiologists. *Anesth Analg.* 2002;94:243-249.

104. Kharasch ED, Frink Jr EJ, Artru A, Michalowski P, Rooke GA, Nogami W. Long-duration low-flow sevoflurane and isoflurane effects on postoperative renal and hepatic function. *Anesth Analg.* 2001;93:1511-1520.

105. Kharasch ED, Frink Jr EJ, Zager R, Bowdle TA, Artru A, Nogami WM. Assessment of low-flow sevoflurane and isoflurane effects on renal function using sensitive markers of tubular toxicity. *Anesthesiology.* 1997;86:1238-1253.

106. Obata R, Bito H, Ohmura M, et al. The effects of prolonged low-flow sevoflurane anesthesia on renal and hepatic function. *Anesth Analg.* 2000;91:120-128.

107. Kharasch ED, Hankins DC, Thummel KE. Human kidney methoxyflurane and sevoflurane metabolism. Intrarenal fluoride production as a possible mechanism of methoxyflurane nephrotoxicity. *Anesthesiology.* 1995;82:689-699.

108. Story DA, Poustie S, Liu G, McNicol PL. Changes in plasma creatinine concentration after cardiac anesthesia with isoflurane, propofol, or sevoflurane: a randomized clinical trial. *Anesthesiology.* 2001;95:842-848.

109. Fujii J, Otsu K, Zorzato F, et al. Identification of a mutation in porcine ryanodine receptor associated with malignant hyperthermia. *Science.* 1991;253:448-451.

110. Apfel CC, Stoecklein K, Lipfert P. PONV: a problem of inhalational anaesthesia? *Best Pract Res Clin Anaesthesiol.* 2005;19:485-500.

111. Apfel CC, Korttila K, Abdalla M, et al. A factorial trial of six interventions for the prevention of postoperative nausea and vomiting. *N Engl J Med.* 2004;350:2441-2451.

112. Sanders RD, Weimann J, Maze M. Biologic effects of nitrous oxide: a mechanistic and toxicologic review. *Anesthesiology.* 2008;109:707-722.

113. Holmstrom A, Akeson J. Sevoflurane induces less cerebral vasodilation than isoflurane at the same A-line autoregressive index level. *Acta Anaesthesiol Scand.* 2005;49:16-22.

114. Cullen S, Gross E. The anesthetic properties of xenon in animals and human beings, with additional observations on krypton. *Science.* 1951;113:580-582.

115. Kenny GN. Risk factors for postoperative nausea and vomiting. *Anaesthesia.* 1994;49(Suppl):6-10.

116. Langbein T, Sonntag H, Trapp D, et al. Volatile anaesthetics and the atmosphere: atmospheric lifetimes and atmospheric effects of halothane, enflurane, isoflurane, desflurane and sevoflurane. *Br J Anaesth.* 1999;82:66-73.

117. Ryan SM, Nielsen CJ. Global warming potential of inhaled anesthetics: application to clinical use. *Anesth Analg.* 2010;111:92-98.

118. Inagaki Y, Sumikawa K, Yoshiya I. Anesthetic interaction between midazolam and halothane in humans. *Anesth Analg.* 1993;76:613-617.

119. Glass PS, Gan TJ, Howell S, Ginsberg B. Drug interactions: volatile anesthetics and opioids. *J Clin Anesth.* 1997;9:18S-22S.

120. Daniell LC. The noncompetitive N-methyl-D-aspartate antagonists, MK-801, phencyclidine and ketamine, increase the potency of general anesthetics. *Pharmacol Biochem Behav.* 1990;36:111-115.

121. Aho M, Lehtinen A-M, Erkola O, Kallio A, Korttila K. The effect of intravenously administered dexmedetomidine on perioperative hemodynamics and isoflurane requirements in patients undergoing abdominal hysterectomy. *Anesthesiology.* 1991;74:997-1002.

122. Johansen JW, Schneider G, Windsor AM, Sebel PS. Esmolol potentiates reduction of minimum alveolar isoflurane concentration by alfentanil. *Anesth Analg.* 1998;87:671-676.

123. Dahan A, Nieuwenhuijs D, Olofsen E, Sarton E, Romberg R, Teppema L. Response surface modeling of alfentanil-sevoflurane interaction on cardiorespiratory control and bispectral index. *Anesthesiology.* 2001;94:982-991.

124. Sonner JM. A hypothesis on the origin and evolution of the response to inhaled anesthetics. *Anesth Analg.* 2008;107:849-854.

125. Ezri T, Sessler D, Weisenberg M, et al. Association of ethnicity with the minimum alveolar concentration of sevoflurane. *Anesthesiology.* 2007;107:9-14.

126. Mogil JS, Ritchie J, Smith SB, et al. Melanocortin-1 receptor gene variants affect pain and mu-opioid analgesia in mice and humans. *J Med Genet.* 2005;42:583-587.

127. Mogil JS, Wilson SG, Chesler EJ, et al. The melanocortin-1 receptor gene mediates female-specific mechanisms of analgesia in mice and humans. *Proc Natl Acad Sci U S A.* 2003;100:4867-4872.

128. Gear RW, Miaskowski C, Gordon NC, Paul SM, Heller PH, Levine JD. Kappa-opioids produce significantly greater analgesia in women than in men. *Nat Med.* 1996;2:1248-1250.

129. Liem EB, Joiner TV, Tsueda K, Sessler DI. Increased sensitivity to thermal pain and reduced subcutaneous lidocaine efficacy in redheads. *Anesthesiology.* 2005;102:509-514.

130. Chua MV, Tsueda K, Doufas AG. Midazolam causes less sedation in volunteers with red hair. *Can J Anaesth.* 2004;51:25-30.

131. Liem EB, Lin CM, Suleman MI, et al. Anesthetic requirement is increased in redheads. *Anesthesiology.* 2004;101:279-283.

132. Sologoff S, Keats AS. Randomized trial of primary anesthetic agents on outcome of coronary artery by pass operations. *Anesthesiology.* 1989;70:179-188.

133. Forrest JB, Cahalan MK, Rehder K, et al. Multicenter study of general anesthesia: II: results. *Anesthesiology.* 1990;72:262-268.

134. Leung JM, Goehner P, O'Kelly BF, et al. Isoflurane anesthesia and myocardial ischemia: comparative risk versus sufentanil anesthesia in patients undergoing coronary artery bypass graft surgery. *Anesthesiology.* 1991;74:838-847.

135. Schoen J, Husemann L, Tiemeyer C, et al. Cognitive function after sevoflurane- vs propofol-based anaesthesia for on-pump cardiac surgery: a randomized controlled trial. *Br J Anaesth.* 2011;106:840-850.

136. Munson ES, Embro WJ. Enflurane, isoflurane, and halothane and isolated human uterine muscle. *Anesthesiology.* 1977;46:11-14.

137. Yildiz K, Dogru K, Dalgic H, et al. Inhibitory effects of desflurane and sevoflurane on oxytocin-induced contractions of isolated pregnant human myometrium. *Acta Anaesthesiol Scand.* 2005;49:1355-1359.

138. Dolk A, Cannerfelt R, Anderson RE, Jakobsson J. Inhalation anaesthesia is cost-effective for ambulatory surgery: a clinical comparison with propofol during elective knee arthroscopy. *Eur J Anaesthesiol.* 2002;19:88.

139. Watson KR, Shah MV. Clinical comparison of "single agent" anaesthesia with sevoflurane versus target controlled infusion of propofol. *Br J Anaesth.* 2000;85:541.

140. Elliott RA, Payne K, Moore JK. Clinical and economic choices in anaesthesia for day surgery: a prospective randomized controlled trial. *Anaesthesia.* 2003;58:412.

141. Visser K, Hassink EA, Bonsel GJ, et al. Randomized controlled trial of total intravenous anesthesia with propofol vs inhalation anesthesia with isoflurane-nitrous oxide: postoperative nausea and vomiting and economic analysis. *Anesthesiology.* 2001;95:616.

142. Rapp SE, Conahan TJ, Pavlin DJ, et al. Comparison of desflurane with propofol in outpatients undergoing peripheral orthopedic surgery. *Anesth Analg.* 1992;75:572.

143. Van Hemelrijck J, Smith I, White PF. Use of desflurane for outpatient anesthesia: a comparison with propofol and nitrous oxide. *Anesthesiology.* 1991;75:197.

144. Juvin P, Vadam C, Malek L, et al. Postoperative recovery after desflurane, propofol, or isoflurane anesthesia among morbidly obese patients: a prospective, randomized study. *Anesth Analg.* 2000;91:714.

145. Tang J, Chen L, White PF, et al. Recovery profile, costs, and patient satisfaction with propofol and sevoflurane for fast-track office-based anesthesia. *Anesthesiology.* 1999;91:253.

146. Tang J, White PF, Wender RH, et al. Fast-track office-based anesthesia: a comparison of propofol vs desflurane with antiemetic prophylaxis in spontaneously breathing patients. *Anesth Analg.* 2001; 92:95.

147. Marshall C, Lindgren L, Marshall BE. Effects of halothane, enflurane, and isoflurane on hypoxic pulmonary vasoconstriction in rat lungs in vitro. *Anesthesiology.* 1984;60:304–308.

148. Rogers SN, Benumof JL. Halothane and isoflurane do not decrease PaO$_2$ during one-lung ventilation in intravenously anesthetized patients. *Anesth Analg.* 1985;64:946.

149. Kazuo A, Mashimo T, Yoshiya I. Arterial oxygenation and shunt fraction during one-lung ventilation: a comparison of isoflurane and sevoflurane. *Anesth Analg.* 1998;86:1266–1270.

150. Benumof JL, Augustine SD, Gibbons JA. Halothane and isoflurane only slightly impair arterial oxygenation during one lung ventilation in patients undergoing thoracotomy. *Anesthesiology.* 1987;67:910.

151. Oppenheim RW. Cell death during development of the nervous system. *Annu Rev Neurosci.* 1991;14:453-501.

152. Rakic S, Zecevic N. Programmed cell death in the developing human telencephalon. *Eur J Neurosci.* 2000;12:2721-2734.

153. Ikonomidou C, Bosch F, Miksa M, et al. Blockade of NMDA receptors and apoptotic neurodegeneration in the developing brain. *Science.* 1999;283:70-74.

154. Scallet AC, Schmued LC, Slikker Jr W, et al. Developmental neurotoxicity of ketamine: morphometric confirmation, exposure parameters, and multiple fluorescent labeling of apoptotic neurons. *Toxicol Sci.* 2004;81:364-370.

155. Jevtovic-Todorovic V, Hartman RE, Izumi Y, et al. Early exposure to common anesthetic agents causes widespread neurodegeneration in the developing rat brain and persistent learning deficits. *J Neurosci.* 2003;23:1066-1082

156. Istaphanous GK, Howard J, Nan X, et al. Comparison of the neuroapoptotic properties of equipotent anesthetic concentrations of desflurane, isoflurane, or sevoflurane in neonatal mice. *Anesthesiology.* 2011;114:578-587.

157. Young C, Jevtovic-Todorovic V, Qin YQ, et al. Potential of ketamine and midazolam, individually or in combination, to induce apoptotic neurodegeneration in the infant mouse brain. *Br J Pharmacol.* 2005;146:189-197.

158. Olney JW, Young C, Wozniak DF, Ikonomidou C, Jevtovic-Todorovic V. Anesthesia-induced developmental neuroapoptosis. Does it happen in humans? *Anesthesiology.* 2004;101:273-275.

159. Edwards DA, Shah HP, Cao W, Gravenstein N, Seubert CN, Martynyuk AE. Bumetanide alleviates epileptogenic and neurotoxic effects of sevoflurane in neonatal rat brain. *Anesthesiology.* 2010; 112:567-575.

160. Slikker Jr W, Zou X, Hotchkiss CE, et al. Ketamine-induced neuronal cell death in the perinatal rhesus monkey. *Toxicol Sci.* 2007;98:145-158.

161. Paule MG, Li M, Allen RR, et al. Ketamine anesthesia during the first week of life can cause long-lasting cognitive deficits in rhesus monkeys. *Neurotoxicol Teratol.* 2011;33:220-230.

162. Brambrink AM, Evers AS, Avidan MS, et al. Isoflurane-induced neuroapoptosis in the neonatal rhesus macaque brain. *Anesthesiology.* 2010;112:834-841.

163. Clancy B, Finlay BL, Darlington RB, Anand KJ. Extrapolating brain development from experimental species to humans. *Neurotoxicology.* 2007;28:931-937.

164. Wilder RT, Flick RP, Sprung J, et al. Early exposure to anesthesia and learning disabilities in a population-based birth cohort. *Anesthesiology.* 2009;110:796-804.

165. DiMaggio C, Sun LS, Kakavouli A, Byrne MW, Li G. A retrospective cohort study of the association of anesthesia and hernia repair surgery with behavioral and developmental disorders in young children. *J Neurosurg Anesthesiol.* 2009;21:286-291.

166. Sun L. Early childhood general anaesthesia exposure and neurocognitive development. *Br J Anaesth.* 2010;105(Suppl 1):i61-68.

167. Moller JT, Cluitmans P, Rasmussen LS, et al. Long-term postoperative cognitive dysfunction in the elderly ISPOCD1 study. ISPOCD investigators. International Study of Post-Operative Cognitive Dysfunction. *Lancet.* 1998;351:857-861.

168. Wei H, Xie Z. Anesthesia, calcium homeostasis and Alzheimer's disease. *Curr Alzheimer Res.* 2009;6:30-35.

169. Wan Y, Xu J, Ma D, Zeng Y, Cibelli M, Maze M. Postoperative impairment of cognitive function in rats: a possible role for

cytokine-mediated inflammation in the hippocampus. *Anesthesiology.* 2007;106:436-443.

170. Stratmann G, Sall JW, May LD, et al. Isoflurane differentially affects neurogenesis and long-term neurocognitive function in 60-day-old and 7-day-old rats. *Anesthesiology.* 2009;110:834-848.

171. Sall JW, Stratmann G, Leong J, et al. Isoflurane inhibits growth but does not cause cell death in hippocampal neural precursor cells grown in culture. *Anesthesiology.* 2009;110:826-833.

172. Bohnen NI, Warner MA, Kokmen E, Beard CM, Kurland LT. Alzheimer's disease and cumulative exposure to anesthesia: a case-control study. *J Am Geriatr Soc.* 1994a;42:198-201.

173. Xie Z, Culley DJ, Dong Y, et al. The common inhalation anesthetic isoflurane induces caspase activation and increases amyloid beta-protein level in vivo. *Ann Neurol.* 2008;64:618-627.

174. Alonso A, Zaidi T, Novak M, Grundke-Iqbal I, Iqbal K. Hyperphosphorylation induces self-assembly of tau into tangles of paired helical filaments/straight filaments. *Proc Natl Acad Sci U S A.* 2001;98:6923-6928.

175. Tanzi RE, Bertram L. Twenty years of the Alzheimer's disease amyloid hypothesis: a genetic perspective. *Cell.* 2005;120:545-555.

176. Wei H, Liang G, Yang H, et al. The common inhalational anesthetic isoflurane induces apoptosis via activation of inositol 1,4,5-trisphosphate receptors. *Anesthesiology.* 2008;108:251-260.

177. Zhen Y, Dong Y, Wu X, et al. Nitrous oxide plus isoflurane induces apoptosis and increases beta-amyloid protein levels. *Anesthesiology.* 2009;111:741-752.

178. Dong Y, Zhang G, Zhang B, et al. The common inhalational anesthetic sevoflurane induces apoptosis and increases beta-amyloid protein levels. *Arch Neurol.* 2009;66:620-631.

179. Zhang B, Dong Y, Zhang G, et al. The inhalation anesthetic desflurane induces caspase activation and increases amyloid beta-protein levels under hypoxic conditions. *J Biol Chem.* 2008;283:11866-11875.

180. Bianchi SL, Tran T, Liu C, et al. Brain and behavior changes in 12-month-old Tg2576 and nontransgenic mice exposed to anesthetics. *Neurobiol Aging.* 2008;29:1002-1010.

181. Planel E, Richter KE, Nolan CE, et al. Anesthesia leads to tau hyperphosphorylation through inhibition of phosphatase activity by hypothermia. *J Neurosci.* 2007;27:3090-3097.

182. Whittington RA, Virág L, Marcouiller F, et al. Propofol directly increases tau phosphorylation. *PLoS One.* 2011;6:e16648.

183. Li L, Peng L, Zuo Z. Isoflurane preconditioning increases B-cell lymphoma-2 expression and reduces cytochrome c release from the mitochondria in the ischemic penumbra of rat brain. *Eur J Pharmacol.* 2008;586:106-113.

184. Codaccioni JL, Velly LJ, Moubarik C, Bruder NJ, Pisano PS, Guillet BA. Sevoflurane preconditioning against focal cerebral ischemia: inhibition of apoptosis in the face of transient improvement of neurological outcome. *Anesthesiology.* 2009;110:1271-1278.

185. Wei H, Liang G, Yang H. Isoflurane preconditioning inhibited isoflurane-induced neurotoxicity. *Neurosci Lett.* 2007;425:59-62.

186. Cibelli M, Fidalgo AR, Terrando N, et al. Role of interleukin-1beta in postoperative cognitive dysfunction. *Ann Neurol.* 2010;68:360-368.

187. Terrando N, Monaco C, Ma D, Foxwell BM, Feldmann M, Maze M. Tumor necrosis factor-alpha triggers a cytokine cascade yielding postoperative cognitive decline. *Proc Natl Acad Sci U S A.* 2010;107:20518-20522.

188. Rosczyk HA, Sparkman NL, Johnson RW. Neuroinflammation and cognitive function in aged mice following minor surgery. *Exp Gerontol.* 2008;43:840-846.

189. Wu X, Lu Y, Dong Y, et al. The inhalation anesthetic isoflurane increases levels of proinflammatory TNF-α, IL-6, and IL-1β. *Neurobiol Aging.* 2012;33:1364-1378.

190. Gasparini M, Vanacore N, Schiaffini C, et al. A case-control study on Alzheimer's disease and exposure to anesthesia. *Neurol Sci.* 2002;23:11-14.

191. Avidan MS, Searleman AC, Storandt M, et al. Long-term cognitive decline in older subjects was not attributable to noncardiac surgery or major illness. *Anesthesiology.* 2009;111:964-970.

192. Kehl F, Krolikowski JG, Mraovic B, Pagel PS, Warltier DC, Kersten JR. Is isoflurane-induced preconditioning dose related? *Anesthesiology.* 2002;96:675-680.

193. Novalija E , Varadarajan SG, Camara AKS, et al. Anesthetic preconditioning: triggering role of reactive oxygen and nitrogen species in isolated hearts. *Am J Physiol Heart Circ Physiol.* 2002;283:H44-H52.

194. Sergeev P, da Silva R, Lucchinetti E, et al. Trigger-dependent gene expression profiles in cardiac preconditioning: evidence for distinct genetic programs in ischemic and anesthetic preconditioning. *Anesthesiology.* 2004;100:474-488.

195. Sniecinski R, Liu H. Reduced efficacy of volatile anesthetic preconditioning with advanced age in isolated rat myocardium. *Anesthesiology.* 2004;100:589-597.

196. Deyhimy DI, Fleming NW, Brodkin IG, Liu H. Anesthetic preconditioning combined with postconditioning offers no additional benefit over preconditioning or postconditioning alone. *Anesth Analg.* 2007;105:316-324.

197. Minguet G, Joris J, Lamy M. Preconditioning and protection against ischaemia-reperfusion in non-cardiac organs: a place for volatile anaesthetics? *Eur J Anaesthesiol.* 2007;24:733-745.

198. Woods GM, Griffiths DM. Reversible inhibition of natural killer cell activity by volatile anaesthetic agents in vitro. *Br J Anaesth.* 1986;58:535-539.

199. Markovic SN, Murasko DM. Anesthesia inhibits interferon-induced natural killer cell cytotoxicity via induction of CD8+ suppressor cells. *Cell Immunol.* 1993;151:474-480.

200. Tartter PI, Steinberg B, Barron DM, Martinelli G. The prognostic significance of natural killer cytotoxicity in patients with colorectal cancer. *Arch Surg.* 1987;122:1264-1268.

201. Schantz SP, Brown BW, Lira E, Taylor DL, Beddingfield N. Evidence for the role of natural immunity in the control of metastatic spread of head and neck cancer. *Cancer Immunol Immunother.* 1987;25:141-148.

Chapter 11

DRUGS FOR NEUROPSYCHIATRIC DISORDERS

Kane O. Pryor and Kingsley P. Storer

HISTORICAL PERSPECTIVE

In 2008, more than 250 million prescriptions for antidepressants and benzodiazepines were dispensed in the United States. This was approximately three times as many prescriptions as for calcium channel blockers, twice as many as for beta blockers, and 90 million more than for angiotensin converting enzyme (ACE) inhibitors.[1] Antidepressants are the most frequently used drugs in adults aged 20 to 59 years and are taken by 11% of persons aged 12 and older.[2,3] Psychopharmacology also includes a heterogeneous and expanding collection of antipsychotics, mood stabilizer agents, and psychostimulants. Considered together, drugs used to treat mental health are encountered by anesthesiologists as a matter of routine daily practice. They have diverse effects on neuronal systems, and many are associated with significant unwanted actions on central and peripheral signaling across broad transmitter classes. Many alter hepatic cytochrome P450 isoenzyme activity and thus can have significant drug interactions by affecting the metabolism of other agents. The potential impact of psychopharmacologic drugs on perioperative physiology is enormous: In addition to altering the central nervous system (CNS) response to sedative and hypnotic agents, they can alter autonomic responsiveness, cardiac conduction, bleeding, seizure potential, the endocrine response to stress, and multiple other physiologic variables that fall under the purview of the anesthesiologist.

Constituting a smaller group in terms of aggregate population usage are the neurologic drugs. Of the many drugs in this class, only a subset have particular relevance to the practice of anesthesia. Of import with regard to the neuromuscular blockers are the anticholinesterases used in the treatment of myasthenia gravis. The anticonvulsant drugs, a number of which are also mood stabilizers, as well as the anti-Parkinsonian drugs have a number of potential adverse physiologic effects. Finally, drugs of abuse, with wide-ranging effects on the CNS, have important implications for the safe delivery of anesthesia in abusing patients.

Because the clinical foci of psychiatry and neurology are so distinct from that of anesthesiology, and because many psychopharmacologic agents have emerged only very recently, anesthesiologists might have less awareness of the actions and adverse effects associated with these drugs. This chapter presents a focused introduction to most of the drugs encountered in perioperative patients. An exhaustive description can be found in dedicated reference texts.[4]

ANTIDEPRESSANT DRUGS

Tricyclic Antidepressants

HISTORY
The iminodibenzyl derivatives were initially investigated in humans in the 1950s for their sedative and antihistaminic properties. The sedative properties of the archetypal drug imipramine proved to be of little benefit in the treatment of agitated patients, but serendipitously it was noted to relieve the symptoms of depression.[5] Subsequently, several other tricyclic compounds were developed, and the class remained the first-line treatment for depression until the rapid expansion in use of selective serotonin reuptake inhibitors (SSRIs) in the 1990s. Early advances in the neuropsychopharmacology of depression—including the importance of the serotonin and noradrenergic pathways—owed much to the study of this class of compounds.

BASIC PHARMACOLOGY
Structure-activity
The tricyclic antidepressants are named because of their central three-ring complex with a single side-chain. The class is then further divided into two subgroups on the basis of the side chain: the *tertiary amines* have two methyl groups at the end of the side chain, whereas the *secondary amines* possess a single methyl group (Figure 11-1). Although all compounds block both the serotonin transporter and the norepinephrine transporter, the relative potency for each is largely determined by the nature of the side chains. The tertiary amines have dominant effects on serotonin reuptake, whereas the secondary amines have greater potency norepinephrine reuptake.[6] Amoxapine is a structurally unique tricyclic antidepressant derived from the antipsychotic loxapine; it is characterized by potent inhibition of norepinephrine reuptake and dopamine receptor block by the metabolite 7-hydroxy-amoxapine.[7] Maprotiline is unique in possessing a four-ring central structure, and is referred to as a tetracyclic or heterocyclic. It possesses the secondary amine side chain, and predictably has dominant effects on norepinephrine transport.

Mechanism
The antidepressant effects of the tricyclic drugs are mediated by effects on two monoaminergic systems—serotonin and norepinephrine—although it is not clear to what extent this implicates specific abnormalities of serotonin and norepinephrine pharmacology in the biochemical pathogenesis of depression (Figure 11-2). Although modulation of reuptake occurs rapidly, clinical benefit is not seen until several weeks of treatment, suggesting that downstream changes in gene expression are critically involved. The decreased uptake initially causes feedback inhibition via presynaptic 5-HT$_{1A}$ autoreceptors, but this is followed by desensitization and a return to normal firing rate after 2 weeks.[8] Postsynaptic 5-HT$_{1A}$ receptors become sensitized, while antagonism of postsynaptic 5-HT$_2$ receptors further increases the effects of serotonin.[9] In contrast, presynaptic α2 receptors do not desensitize, and the firing rate of noradrenergic neurons remains inhibited

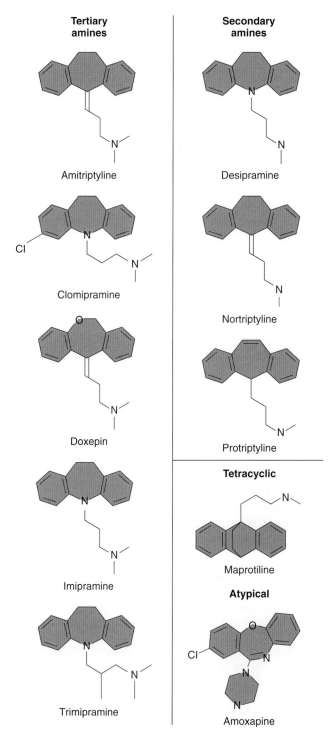

Figure 11-1 Chemical structure of the tricyclic and tetra cyclic antidepressants.

throughout treatment.[10] The noradrenergic mechanism likely includes complex modulatory effects on the expression of postsynaptic α1, α2, and β adrenergic receptors, and on their second messenger systems. Tricyclic antidepressants also have variable antagonist activity at 5-HT$_6$, 5-HT$_7$, *N*-methyl-D-aspartate (NMDA)-type glutamate, H$_1$ and H$_2$ histaminergic, and muscarinic acetylcholine receptors. They also have variable agonist activity at σ$_1$ opioid receptors.[11]

Metabolism

Metabolism is almost exclusively hepatic and dominantly involves either hydroxylation of the ring structure or demethylation of the side chain. The tertiary amines are demethylated to active secondary amines (e.g., imipramine to desipramine), which incurs an increase in noradrenergic activity. Many of the hydroxy metabolites are also active. The principal cytochrome P450 (CYP) isoenzymes are 2D6, 1A2, 3A4, and 2C19. Variability in metabolism and plasma levels can be dramatic, due to both exogenous modulation of the CYP system and to genetic polymorphisms occurring in up to 20% of Asian and 10% of Caucasian patients.[12]

CLINICAL PHARMACOLOGY

Pharmacokinetics

The tricyclic antidepressants are rapidly absorbed from the small intestine and mostly attain peak plasma levels in 2 to 8 hours. They are highly protein bound (>90%) and lipophilic, with large volumes of distribution up to 60 L/kg. Bioavailability is variable, with on average about 50% to hepatic first-pass metabolism. Plasma half-life is longer than 24 hours for most drugs (the exception being amoxapine), allowing for once-a-day dosing. However, variation is significant, and determined largely by genetic variability. The daily dose is thus not a reliable determinant of steady-state plasma levels. Further, a relationship between plasma concentration and therapeutic response, while demonstrated for some drugs, has not been established across the entire class.[13] Thus monitoring of plasma levels, though often suggested, remains controversial because of the lack of validated interpretation studies. Dosing is often started low and increased gradually based on therapeutic response, with monitoring of plasma levels reserved for patients suspected to be at the extremes of rapid and slow metabolizers.

Pharmacodynamics

THERAPEUTIC EFFECTS. Tricyclic antidepressants have demonstrated efficacy in the treatment of major depression.[14] Response rates for patients completing treatment with imipramine, the most studied drug, exceed 65%. They are also effective for maintenance therapy, with up to 80% of patients successfully maintained for 3 years.[15] Relative to other classes of antidepressants, the tricyclics might be especially efficacious in patients with severe or endogenous depression, or in those who are hospitalized, although this is not clearly established. They have no particular advantage over other agents in the treatment of anxious, atypical, psychotic, bipolar, or late-life depression. Because of its high serotonergic activity, clomipramine is effective and is used for the treatment of obsessive-compulsive disorder.[16] The tricyclics are also used in panic disorder. Desipramine is effective in the treatment of attention deficit/hyperactivity disorder,[17] but is contraindicated in children because of reports of sudden cardiac death. Tricyclics are also widely used in the treatment of chronic and neuropathic pain syndromes (see Chapter 16), and are more effective than the SSRIs in this regard. A recent Cochrane review showed a number-needed-to-treat of 3.6 and a relative risk of 2.1 for at least moderate relief of neuropathic pain with tricyclic antidepressants.[18] The effects appear independent of those on depression, and generally occur at lower doses, consistent with a distinct underlying mechanism, with antinociceptive actions mediated by effects on descending serotonin and norepinephrine spinal pathways.[19]

Adverse Effects

The most common side effects associated with tricyclic antidepressants result from their antimuscarinic and antihistaminic actions. Amitriptyline and clomipramine have the greatest antimuscarinic potency, and desipramine the lowest. Dry mouth, urinary hesitancy, decreased gastric motility, and blurred vision are relatively common. Ocular crisis can be precipitated in patients with narrow-angle glaucoma. H_1-histaminic blockade results in sedation. Confusion and delirium are dose-dependent, and result from the combination of anticholinergic and antimuscarinic activity. Patients with preexisting dementia or psychotic depression are especially at risk, and the incidence is highest with amitriptyline. There is also a dose-dependent risk of seizure. The incidence is poorly defined, although it is less than 1% across the drug class if plasma level monitoring is appropriately used.[20] Use of these drugs in patients with elevated seizure risk is not advisable. The overall incidence of CNS toxicity is approximately 6%.[21] Tricyclic antidepressants cause orthostatic hypotension, especially in patients receiving antihypertensive therapy, and also cause a persistent increase in heart rate. They inhibit Na^+/K^+-ATPase and act like class Ia (quinidine-like) antiarrhythmics by stabilizing excitable membranes and delaying His bundle conduction, and so they must be used cautiously in patients with prolonged QTc interval. In overdose, sudden death can occur from cardiac arrhythmia at doses of only 10 times the therapeutic dose.[22] Largely because of this arrhythmia risk, the mortality associated with tricyclic overdose is 17 times that associated with SSRI overdose—a significant factor in the rapid acceptance of SSRIs as first-line therapy for treatment of depression.[23]

Drug Interactions

The complex effect of tricyclic antidepressants on presynaptic and postsynaptic noradrenergic signaling can alter the response of patients to sympathomimetic drugs used in the perioperative period. During initial treatment, patients can have an exaggerated response to indirect-acting sympathomimetics such as ephedrine due to increased presynaptic availability of norepinephrine. In contrast, adrenergic desensitization and catecholamine depletion can result in a relatively refractory response to sympathomimetics in patients treated long term; such patients might respond best to the potent direct-acting sympathomimetic norepinephrine.[24] Rebound hypertension following discontinuation of antihypertensives has been reported and likely results from changes in norepinephrine uptake.[25] Tricyclic antidepressants can increase arrhythmogenicity in the presence of volatile anesthetics, although these observations are dominantly with halothane, and have not been seen with newer volatile anesthetics.[26,27] The anticholinergic effects of tricyclic antidepressants are expected to be additive to those of other drugs used in the perioperative period, and special caution should be used in administering centrally acting anticholinergics in those patients taking tricyclics who are at increased risk of delirium and dementia. Barbiturates are potent inducers of CYP3A4 and when chronically administered can increase metabolism of tricyclic antidepressants, but significant effects

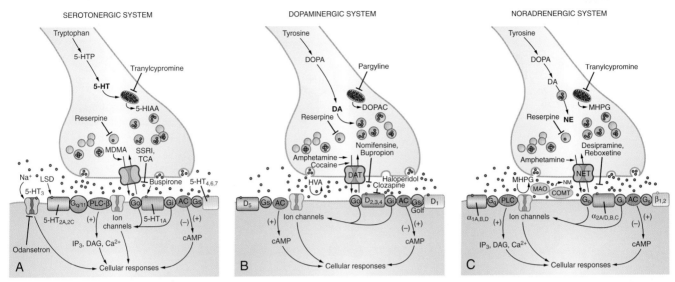

Figure 11-2 The serotonergic, dopaminergic, and noradrenergic systems in psychopharmacology. **A,** In the serotonergic system, L-tryptophan is converted to 5-hydroxytryptophan (5-HTP), and then to serotonin (5-HT). Presynaptic regulation occurs through somatodendritic 5-HT$_{1A}$ and 5-HT$_{1B,1D}$ autoreceptors (not shown). Binding to G protein-coupled receptors (G$_o$, G$_i$, etc.) that are coupled to adenylyl cyclase (AC) and phospholipase C-β (PLC-β) results in a cascade of second messenger and cellular effects. Reuptake occurs via the 5-HT transporter (5-HTT), after which 5-HT is either repackaged into vesicles or metabolized to 5-hydroxyindolacetic acid (5-HIAA) by mitochondrial monoamine oxidase (MAO). The SSRIs and TCAs block reuptake at the 5-HTT. Tranylcypromine inhibits mitochondrial MAO. Reserpine, an antipsychotic, causes depletion of storage vesicles. Buspirone is a presynaptic and postsynaptic partial 5-HT$_{1A}$ agonist. Lysergic acid diethylamide (LSD) likely interacts with numerous 5-HT receptors, while MDMA ("ecstasy") alters 5-HTT function. **B,** In the dopaminergic system, L-tyrosine is converted to L-dihydroxyphenylalanine (L-DOPA), and then to dopamine (DA). Presynaptic regulation occurs through somatodendritic and nerve terminal D$_2$ receptors (not shown). Reuptake is via the dopamine transporter (DAT), after which DA is either sequestered into vesicles, or metabolized to dihydroxyphenylalanine (DOPAC) by mitochondrial MAO. DA can also be degraded to homovanillic acid (HVA) through synaptic MAO and catechol-O-methyltransferase (COMT). Reserpine causes depletion of storage vesicles. Pargyline inhibits MAO selectively in DA neurons. Haloperidol is a D$_2$ antagonist, and clozapine is an nonspecific D$_2$/D$_4$ antagonist. Bupropion interacts with the DA system, but its exact action is unclear. Cocaine and amphetamine alter DAT function. **C,** In the noradrenergic system, L-tyrosine is metabolized through L-DOPA and DA to norepinephrine (NE). Presynaptic regulation occurs through somatodendritic and nerve terminal α2 adrenoreceptors (not shown). Reuptake occurs via the NE transporter (NET), after which NE is either sequestered into vesicles or metabolized to 3-methoxy-4-hydroxyphenylglycol (MHPG) by mitochondrial MAO and aldehyde reductase. Metabolism also occurs synaptically, to MHPG via MAO or to normetanephrine (NM) via COMT. Reserpine causes depletion of NE in storage vesicles. Tranylcypromine inhibits mitochondrial MAO. The selective NE reuptake inhibitor and antidepressant reboxetine and TCA desipramine interfere with the reuptake of NE. Amphetamine facilitates NE release by altering NET function. *DAG,* Diacylglycerol; *IP3,* inositol-1,4,5-triphosphate. *(Modified from Schatzberg AF, Nemeroff CB. The American Psychiatric Publishing Textbook of Psychopharmacology. 4th ed. Arlington: Va: American Psychiatric Publishing; 2009.)*

are unlikely after a single anesthetic administration. Tricyclics are not known to have any effects on CYP isoenzyme induction or inhibition that are of significance to common anesthetic management.

Selective Serotonin Reuptake Inhibitors

HISTORY

The SSRIs were developed in the early 1970s. A series of compounds derived from 3-phenoxy-3-phenylpropylamine—which is structurally similar to diphenhydramine—were tested for selective inhibition of serotonin (5-HT) reuptake. The most potent and selective of the compounds was identified and named fluoxetine, and was eventually approval by the US Food and Drug Administration (FDA) for the treatment of major depression in 1987 (Prozac). This was followed by sertraline (Zoloft) in 1991, paroxetine (Paxil) and fluvoxamine (Luvox) in 1993, citalopram (Celexa) in 1998, and escitalopram (Lexapro) in 2002.[28] A highly favorable safety profile compared to the tricyclic antidepressants rapidly propelled fluoxetine and later SSRIs to become the dominant antidepressant agents, although in recent years their success relative to their clinical efficacy has been questioned.[29]

BASIC PHARMACOLOGY

Structure-Activity

There is considerable diversity in the chemical structure-activity relations among the SSRIs (Figure 11-3). Fluoxetine exists as a racemate, with both the (S)- and (R)-enantiomers pharmacologically active. Citalopram was initially introduced as a racemate, with the more potent (S)-enantiomer (escitalopram) subsequently isolated. All SSRIs possess relatively high affinity for serotonin uptake sites, low affinity for norepinephrine uptake sites, and very low affinity for neurotransmitter receptors, although there is considerable variability. Fluoxetine is the least selective of the class, with citalopram and escitalopram the most selective.[30] Sertraline is unique as a more potent inhibitor of dopamine uptake than any of the SSRIs or tricyclic antidepressants. Activity at H$_1$-histaminergic, α1-adrenergic, and muscarinic receptors is minimal and unlikely to be of clinical significance, which is responsible for the absence of many of the side effects associated with tricyclic antidepressants.

Mechanism

The mechanisms for the therapeutic effects of the SSRIs are not clearly established, but are believed to derive from

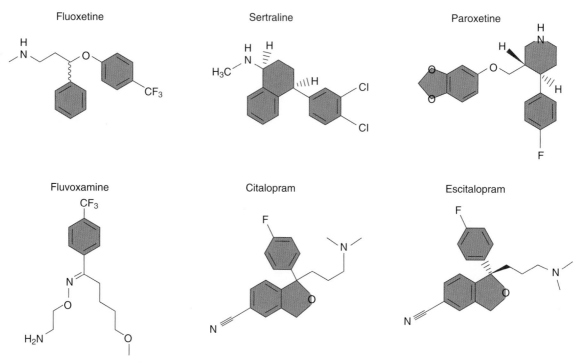

Fluoxetine

Sertraline

Paroxetine

Fluvoxamine

Citalopram

Escitalopram

Figure 11-3 Chemical structure of selective serotonin reuptake inhibitors.

blockade of 5-HT reuptake into serotonergic neurons, prolonging the duration of exposure to 5-HT at postsynaptic binding sites (see Figure 11-2).[31] In contrast to direct 5-HT receptor agonists, SSRI action is dependent on presynaptic 5-HT release, and they are ineffective if release of 5-HT is compromised. Because therapeutic effects are not fully realized within 2 to 8 weeks, it is unlikely that reuptake inhibition, which occurs far sooner, is mechanistically sufficient. Several downstream effects have been mechanistically postulated. Initially, inhibitory autoreceptors in the soma (5-HT$_{1A}$) and terminals (5-HT$_{1B}$) are stimulated, and neuronal firing rates decrease. Normalization of firing rates occurs with downregulation of these autoreceptors and decreased production of 5-HT$_{1B}$ mRNA, and coincides temporally with the onset of therapeutic efficacy.[32] In the same temporal window there is increased production of neuroprotective proteins, including brain-derived neurotrophic factor (Figure 11-4).[33]

Metabolism
SSRIs are oxidatively metabolized in the liver. Several CYP isoenzymes are involved, including 2D6, 2C9, 2C19, 1A2, and 3A4, with significant differences between the drugs in relevant importance. While all SSRIs except fluvoxamine have pharmacologically active major metabolites, only that of fluoxetine (norfluoxetine) is likely of therapeutic significance.

CLINICAL PHARMACOLOGY
Pharmacokinetics[34]
The SSRIs are well absorbed from the small intestine and most attain peak plasma levels in 2 to 8 hours. Protein binding is high (>80%), except with escitalopram, with volumes of distribution mostly in the range of 10 to 20 L/kg, somewhat less than seen with the tricyclic antidepressants. Plasma half-life is mostly around 20 to 30 hours, with fluoxetine somewhat

longer (24-72 hours) and fluvoxamine shorter (15 hours). Norfluoxetine, the active metabolite of fluoxetine, has a half-life of 1 to 3 days. Once-a-day dosing is commonly used for all drugs except fluvoxamine, for which twice-daily dosing is preferred. There are known age and gender effects on plasma concentrations: sertraline concentrations are approximately 40% lower in young males than in older males or females, while fluvoxamine concentrations are 40% to 50% lower in males across all ages. Because no clear relationship between therapeutic efficacy and steady-state plasma concentrations has been established and because the therapeutic index is wide, plasma level monitoring is not used.[35]

Pharmacodynamics
THERAPEUTIC EFFECTS. SSRIs are efficacious in the initial treatment of major depression. There is little evidence to support that SSRIs as a class are more efficacious than other classes of antidepressants, including the tricyclic antidepressants, although one 2009 metaanalysis suggests that sertraline and escitalopram could have therapeutic advantages over other drugs, including other SSRIs.[36] Although frequently prescribed for less severe depression, recent metaanalyses—some including trial data submitted to the FDA—question whether SSRIs have any significant therapeutic benefit.[29,37,38] The onset of clinical improvement takes 2 to 3 weeks and might not be maximal for up to 8 weeks, suggesting that downstream effects, rather than 5-HT reuptake inhibition per se, are responsible. SSRIs are also prescribed and are probably efficacious in several other psychiatric disorders believed to involve abnormalities of 5-HT systems. Metaanalysis has demonstrated SSRIs to be effective in the initial treatment of obsessive-compulsive disorder, although it is unclear how serotonergic selectivity confers therapeutic benefit.[39] SSRIs are also used for the prevention of panic

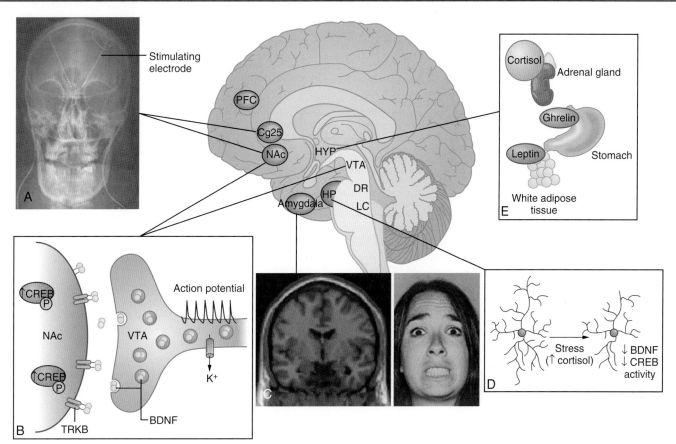

Figure 11-4 The neural circuitry of depression beyond monoamines. Several brain regions are implicated in the pathophysiology of depression. **A,** Deep brain stimulation of the subgenual cingulate cortex (Cg25) or the nucleus accumbens (NAc) has an antidepressant effect on individuals with treatment-resistant depression thought to be mediated through inhibition of these regions either by depolarization blockade or by stimulation of passing axonal fibers. **B,** Increased activity-dependent release of brain-derived neurotrophic factor (BDNF) within the mesolimbic dopamine circuit (dopamine-producing ventral tegmental area [VTA] to dopamine-sensitive NAc) mediates susceptibility to social stress, occurring in part through activation of the transcription factor CREB (cyclic-AMP-response-element-binding protein) by phosphorylation (P). **C,** Neuroimaging studies implicate the amygdala (red pixels show activated areas) as an important limbic node for processing emotionally salient stimuli, such as fearful faces. **D,** Stress decreases the concentrations of neurotrophins (such as BDNF), the extent of neurogenesis, and the complexity of neuronal processes in the hippocampus (HP). These effects are mediated in part through increased cortisol concentrations and decreased CREB activity. **E,** Peripherally released metabolic hormones in addition to cortisol, such as ghrelin and leptin, produce mood-related changes through their effects on the hypothalamus (HYP) and several limbic regions. *DR,* Dorsal raphe; *LC,* locus coeruleus; *PFC,* prefrontal cortex. *(Reproduced from Krishnan V, Nestler EJ. The molecular neurobiology of depression. Nature. 2008;455:894-902.)*

attacks in panic disorder, and, because of postulated involvement of 5-HT in feeding behaviors, have been used in bulimia nervosa, anorexia nervosa, and obesity.[40] They reduce symptoms of premenstrual dysphoric disorder and posttraumatic stress disorder, and are effective in the treatment of premature ejaculation.[41-43]

ADVERSE EFFECTS. The SSRIs have a highly favorable side-effect profile when compared with other classes of antidepressants. The most common side effects include sexual dysfunction, weight changes, dizziness, and insomnia. Although the effects of SSRIs on suicidality in adults are unclear, they increase suicidality in patients younger than 24 and carry an FDA black box warning for use in this age group.[44] SSRIs have effects on cardiac Na^+, K^+, and Ca^{2+} channels, and can theoretically cause QTc prolongation, but there is no observable increase in the risk of dysrhythmia.[45] SSRIs decrease platelet 5-HT content and inhibit platelet aggregation, and can increase bleeding, especially when combined with other anticoagulants.[46,47] One retrospective study of orthopedic patients demonstrated a significantly increased risk of transfusion in patients taking serotonergic

antidepressants, but not with those taking nonserotonergic agents.[48] However, there is insufficient consensus to support perioperative changes in SSRI therapy on the basis of bleeding risk. SSRIs have effects on bone metabolism, and are associated with increased risk of fracture.[49] Overdose with a single SSRI is very rarely fatal, and is usually associated with minimal sequelae. Citalopram is the most likely to cause QTc prolongation, but even with extremely high doses, arrhythmias are exceedingly rare.[50]

Serotonin syndrome is a potentially fatal adverse reaction to serotonergic drugs resulting in mental status changes, autonomic hyperactivity, and neuromuscular hyperactivity. Initially this can be very difficult to distinguish from malignant hyperthermia.[51] Although theoretically possible, induction of serotonin syndrome by a single SSRI is rare, and they are usually only implicated in combination with other drugs. Several drugs used in the perioperative period—notably cocaine, ondansetron, and fentanyl—have the potential to directly or indirectly augment serotonergic activity, and this should be considered when assessing patients exhibiting hypermetabolic activity.

Drug Interactions

Significant drug interactions are less likely with SSRIs than with earlier classes of antidepressants. Perhaps the most likely source of interaction results from SSRI-induced inhibition of specific CYP isoenzymes, notably 2D6 and 2C19. However, this effect is of little relevance to the vast majority of drugs handled by anesthesiologists. Anesthesiologists should be aware of the potential for SSRIs to potentiate the QTc-prolongation and antiplatelet effect of other drugs used in the perioperative period, and the serotonergic effect of methylene blue.

Monoamine Oxidase Inhibitors

The antidepressant actions of monoamine oxidase inhibitors (MAOIs) were identified in the 1950s. One member of this class—iproniazid—historically represents one of the earliest attempts to treat depression pharmacologically. MAOIs continue to have clinical utility in the treatment of resistant depression, and can be particularly effective in treating atypical depression. However, because of their severe and dangerous food and drug interactions, the classic MAOIs remain a treatment of last resort, and are encountered relatively rarely. However, it is critical for anesthesiologists to recognize and be aware of these drugs, in that the potential for adverse interactions with agents used in the perioperative period exceeds that of any other psychopharmacologic class.

BASIC PHARMACOLOGY

Monoamine oxidase (MAO) exists as two isoenzymes, MAO-A and MAO-B. MAO-A preferentially deaminates serotonin, epinephrine, norepinephrine, and melatonin, whereas MAO-B preferentially deaminates phenylethylamine, phenylethanolamine, tyramine, and benzylamine. Dopamine and tryptamine are deaminated by both isoenzymes. In the CNS, MAO-A is concentrated in dopaminergic and noradrenergic neurons, whereas MAO-B is concentrated in serotonergic neurons.[52] Both are also found in glial cells. Outside the CNS, MAO-A is found in the gastrointestinal tract, liver, and placenta, and MAO-B in platelets. The reason for the apparent discrepancy between the dominant substrates and localization is unknown.

MAOIs act by inhibiting MAO, thereby increasing the availability of monoaminergic transmitters (see Figure 11-2). All MAOIs currently available in the United States bind irreversibly, inhibiting enzyme activity for up to 2 weeks. Changes in $\alpha1$-, $\alpha2$-, 5-HT$_1$, and 5-HT$_2$ receptors emerge after several weeks. Phenelzine is a hydrazine derivative and nonselective, while tranylcypromine is nonselective and chemically related to amphetamine. Selegiline is selective for MAO-B at lower doses, but becomes nonselective at higher doses; metabolites of selegiline include L-amphetamine and L-methamphetamine. In 2006, selegiline became available as a transdermal patch. This system avoids inhibition of intestinal and hepatic MAO-A, thereby reducing food-drug interactions and obviating the need for dietary restriction.

CLINICAL PHARMACOLOGY

MAOIs are used to treat a variety of psychiatric conditions, but have received greatest acceptance for atypical depression, which is characterized by early age of onset, dysthymia, alcohol abuse, and sociopathy. They are more effective than the tricyclic antidepressants in treating this disorder.[53] MAOIs are also therapeutic in typical major depression, panic disorder, bulimia nervosa, atypical facial pain, and treatment-resistant depression.[54] The transdermal patch form of selegiline is approved for use in major depression, although its efficacy relative to other drugs is not well studied.[55]

Adverse effects, dietary interactions, and drug interactions

Common adverse effects of MAOIs include dizziness, headache, dry mouth, nausea, weight gain, peripheral edema, urinary hesitancy, and myoclonic movements. Orthostatic hypotension is common in older patients, and can necessitate mineralocorticoid treatment. MAOIs can augment the response to insulin and other hypoglycemic agents increasing the risk of hypoglycemia. Phenelzine has anticholinergic action.

Dietary interactions

Orally ingested MAOIs inhibit the catabolism of dietary amines. The consumption of foods containing tyramine can lead to severe hypertensive crisis within an hour of eating. Decreased first-pass breakdown of tyramine leads to elevated systemic levels. Tyramine is transported via vesicular monoamine transporter (VMAT) into synaptic vessels, where it displaces norepinephrine, and the release of norepinephrine precipitates the hypertensive crisis.[56] Patients using oral MAOIs must adhere to dietary restrictions to avoid precipitation of a crisis. Key foods that must be avoided include cheese, sausage meats, red wine, overripe fruits, fermented products, and some yeasts. Transdermal selegiline does not require dietary restrictions.

Drug interactions

Irreversible inhibition of MAO by MAOIs leads to several potentially dangerous drug interactions when therapy is combined with sympathomimetic agents. In the outpatient setting, significant caution is required when crossing over to or from other psychopharmacologic agents that alter monoaminergic activity, such as SSRIs, tricyclic antidepressants, or stimulants. Several over-the-counter medications contain indirect-acting sympathomimetics and are able to precipitate a hypertensive crisis. In the perioperative setting, several drugs have the potential for dangerous interactions. The most notable of these is meperidine, which can precipitate a type I excitatory response with hypertension, clonus, agitation, and hyperthermia, or a type II depressive response with hypotension, hypoventilation, and coma.[57] This effect is believed to result from meperidine's serotonin reuptake inhibition properties. Members of the phenylpiperidine opioids, which include tramadol, fentanyl, alfentanil, sufentanil, and remifentanil, are also serotonin reuptake inhibitors and have been associated with perioperative serotonergic toxicity, as has methadone. Morphine does not appear to precipitate serotonergic crisis and is perhaps the drug of choice when opioids must be used in patients taking MAOIs. Indirect sympathomimetics, such as ephedrine, can precipitate an exaggerated pressor response due to increased release of norepinephrine and so should be avoided. Direct-acting drugs such as phenylephrine are preferable, although the response can be exaggerated due to receptor hypersensitivity.[58] Ketamine should similarly be avoided, although its safe use has been described.[59]

Atypical Antidepressants

Several drugs currently used in the treatment of depression and related disorders have structures and mechanisms that cannot be placed in any of the broad classes described and are commonly referred to as atypica, second-generation antidepressants. The most important of these are summarized in Table 11-1. Like the tricyclic antidepressants and SSRIs, the therapeutic mechanism of these agents is poorly understood. All drugs share effects on signaling or transmitter availability in at least one monoaminergic (serotonergic, noradrenergic, or dopaminergic) pathway.

ANXIOLYTIC DRUGS

Benzodiazepines

HISTORY

The first benzodiazepine, chlordiazepoxide (Librium) was introduced in 1960. This was followed in 1963 by diazepam (Valium), the archetypal compound from which many derivatives were synthesized. The benzodiazepines were rapidly embraced as treatments for anxiety because they were considerably safer than the barbiturate alternatives and were extensively prescribed until the 1980s. In the past 25 years, benzodiazepine use has declined, partly because of awareness and concerns regarding addiction, withdrawal, and recreational abuse, and also because of the evolution of the SSRIs as a safe and effective first-line therapy for anxiety and panic disorder. Nonetheless, alprazolam (Xanax), a triazolo-benzodiazepine introduced in 1981 for the treatment of panic disorder, remains the single most prescribed psychiatric medication, with 44.4 million prescriptions in 2009.[60]

BASIC PHARMACOLOGY
Structure-activity

The core structure of the benzodiazepines is the fusion of benzene and diazepine ring systems. All therapeutically active drugs are substituted 1,4-benzodiazepines, with many containing a 5-phenyl-1 H-benzo[e][1,4]diazepin-2(3H)-one substructure (Figure 11-5).

Mechanism

Benzodiazepines act by binding at the interface of the α and γ subunits of the GABA$_A$ receptor. This binding site is distinct from that of endogenous agonist GABA (which binds between the α and β subunits), and also from other GABAergic drugs,

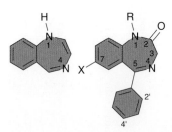

Figure 11-5 Benzodiazepine structure. The 1,4-benzodiazepine ring system is shown on the left. The right shows the most common skeleton, which contains a 5-phenyl-1 H-benzo[e][1,4]diazepin-2(3H)-one substructure.

such as barbiturates (Figure 11-6). Benzodiazepines allosterically modulate the receptor such that it has greater affinity for GABA. This increases the opening time of the associated chloride channel, which leads to hyperpolarization or stabilization of the resting membrane potential near the chloride equilibrium potential. Because binding requires a specific histidine residue in the α subunit, benzodiazepines act only at receptors containing α1, α2, α3, or α5 subunits, and have no action on receptors containing α4 or α6 subunits. Benzodiazepines are heterogeneous in their affinities for various GABA$_A$ receptor subtypes, which underlies the differences in their pharmacologic effects. For example, anxiolysis is associated with greater relative affinity for the α2 subunit.[61]

Metabolism

Most benzodiazepines are highly protein bound and undergo microsomal oxidation in the liver via CYP enzymes, especially CYP 3A4. Their metabolism is therefore altered by the presence of drugs that either inhibit or induce CYP activity, as well as by age and disease. Several benzodiazepines have active metabolites, including a number with half-lives considerably longer than the parent compound; the half-life of the partial agonist N-desmethyldiazepam, the principal metabolite of diazepam, can exceed 100 hours. Three benzodiazepines—oxazepam, lorazepam, and temazepam—are metabolized by glucuronidation and have no significantly active metabolites; these are therefore preferred in older adults and in patients with hepatic disease.

CLINICAL PHARMACOLOGY
Pharmacokinetics

Benzodiazepines vary substantially in their absorption and rate of elimination (Table 11-2). Although differences in affinities for specific GABA$_A$ receptor subtypes lead to greater or lesser propensity to alter a particular cognitive function, heterogeneity in pharmacokinetic properties largely determines the clinical application of individual drugs. Duration of action is principally a function of α phase (distribution-redistribution) dynamics rather than rate of elimination in most applications.

Pharmacodynamics
THERAPEUTIC EFFECTS. Benzodiazepines have a wide spectrum of uses in psychopharmacology due to their sedative, hypnotic, amnesic, anxiolytic, anticonvulsant, and muscle relaxant properties. They are efficacious in the short-term treatment of panic disorder, but have largely been replaced by SSRIs as the first-line pharmacotherapy and are generally not regarded as appropriate for long-term therapy.[62] Similarly, they are effective in the initial management of generalized anxiety disorder, but do not modify the course when used long term.[63] Benzodiazepines remain a common therapy for short-term treatment of insomnia, although their use has declined with greater awareness of dependence and cognitive side effects in older adults. The time to onset and duration of sleep are prolonged, but there is a characteristic reduction in rapid eye movement (REM) sleep, increase in non-REM sleep, and reduction in delta electroencephalographic activity.[64] They are also used as second-line treatment in the nonacute management of seizure disorders and as first-line treatment in alcohol withdrawal syndrome. Benzodiazepines are also used for their muscle relaxant properties. Despite clear evidence

Table 11-1. Atypical Antidepressants

	BUPROPION	TRAZODONE	MIRTAZAPINE	VENLAFAXINE	DULOXETINE
Structure					
Common trade name	Wellbutrin	Oleptro	Remeron	Effexor	Cymbalta
Class	Dopamine and norepinephrine reuptake inhibitor	Serotonin antagonist and reuptake inhibitor (SARI)	Noradrenergic and specific serotonergic antidepressant	Serotonin-norepinephrine reuptake inhibitor (SNRI)	Serotonin-norepinephrine reuptake inhibitor (SNRI)
Metabolism	CYP2B6 to hydroxybupropion (active)	CYP3A4 to m-chlorophenylpiperazine (active)	CYP1A2, 2C9, 2D6, 3A4	CYP2D6 to O-desmethylvenlafaxine (active) and others	CYP1A2, 2D6
Half-life	21 hours	7-10 hours	20-40 hours	5 hours	12 hours
Approved therapeutic indications	Major depression Seasonal depression Smoking cessation	Major depression	Major depression	Major depression Generalized anxiety Social anxiety Panic disorder	Major depression Generalized anxiety Diabetic neuropathy Fibromyalgia Musculoskeletal pain
Adverse effects	Common: nausea, dry mouth Dose-related increase in seizures May cause increased blood pressure and tachycardia.	Common: sedation, headache, dizziness May cause orthostatic hypotension, priapism, and QT prolongation. Arrhythmias have been reported. May impair platelet aggregation and increase bleeding risk.	Common: sedation, weight gain, hypercholesterolemia May cause decreased gastric motility, urinary retention, hyponatremia, and akathisia. Agranulocytosis is rare.	Common: nausea, dry mouth, dizziness, sexual dysfunction May cause increased blood pressure, tachycardia, and hypercholesterolemia. May impair platelet aggregation and increase bleeding risk.	Common: nausea, sexual dysfunction May impair platelet aggregation and increase bleeding risk. May increase serum glucose in diabetic patients. May cause hepatotoxicity in at-risk patients.
Drug interactions	May reduce the effectiveness of codeine and tramadol due to CYP2D6 inhibition. Caution should be used when combining with other drugs that lower the seizure threshold.	May potentiate action of antiplatelet drugs, drugs that prolong QTc, antihypertensives, and sedatives, including anesthetic drugs, and drugs that can trigger serotonin syndrome. Should not be combined with MAOIs.	May potentiate action of sedatives, including anesthetic drugs, anticholinergic drugs, drugs that lower the seizure threshold, and drugs that can trigger serotonin syndrome. May potentiate the effect of warfarin. Should not be combined with MAOIs.	May potentiate action of antiplatelet drugs, drugs that lower seizure threshold, and drugs that can trigger serotonin syndrome. Should not be combined with MAOIs. No known significant anesthetic interactions.	Ciprofloxacin may significantly increase serum concentration and toxicity. May potentiate action of antiplatelet drugs, drugs that lower seizure threshold, and drugs that can trigger serotonin syndrome. Should not be combined with MAOIs. No known significant anesthetic interactions

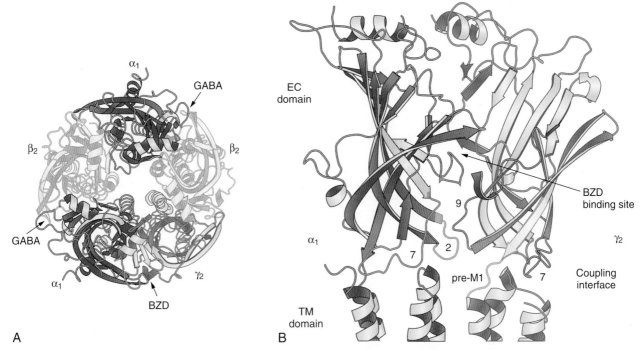

Figure 11-6 GABA$_A$ receptor structure and benzodiazepine binding site. **A,** Homology model of the $\alpha_1\beta_2\gamma_2$ GABA$_A$ receptor as seen from the extracellular membrane surface. The α_1, β_2, and γ_2 subunits are highlighted in red, yellow, and blue, respectively. *Arrows* indicate that GABA binds at the β_2/α_1 interfaces whereas benzodiazepines (BZDs) bind at the α_1/γ_2 interface of the receptor. **B,** Side view of the α_1 and γ_2 extracellular domains, with the location of the BZD binding site is indicated by an *arrow*. Relevant loops at the coupling interface are highlighted as follows: γ_2Loop 9, purple; γ_2 pre-M1, yellow; γ_2 Loop 7, red; α_1 Loop2, green; α_1 Loop 7, blue. *(Reproduced from Hanson SM, Morlock EV, Satyshur KA, Czajkowski C. Structural requirements for eszopiclone and zolpidem binding to the gamma-aminobutyric acid type-A (GABA$_A$) receptor are different. J Med Chem. 2008;51:7243-7252.)*

Table 11-2. Benzodiazepine Pharmacokinetics

CLASS	DRUG	COMMON TRADE NAME	ONSET (min)	DURATION (hr)	Vd (L/kg)	PROTEIN BINDING	t½ (hr)
Desmethyldiazepam	Diazepam	Valium	30	2-3	0.8-1.0	98%	20-50
	Chlordiazepoxide	Librium	60-120	≤24	3.3	90%-98%	6.6-25
Desalkylfurazepam	Flurazepam	Dalmane	15-20	7-8	3.4	97%	74-90
	Clonazepam	Klonopin	20-60	≤12	1.5-4.4	85%	19-50
Triazolobenzodiazepine	Triazolam	Halcion	15-20	6-7	0.8-1.8	89%	1.5-5.5
	Alprazolam	Xanax	60	3.5-7	0.9-1.2	80%	11.2
Thienodiazepine	Nitrazepam	Mogadon	20-50	6-10	2.4	87%	30
	Flunitrazepam	Rohypnol	15-30	7-8	4.6	78%	22
Oxazolobenzodiazepine	Oxazepam	Serax	45-90	6-12	1.0-1.3	86%-99%	2.8-5.7
	Lorazepam	Ativan	5-20	6-8	1.3	85%	12.9
	Temazepam	Restoril	20-40	6-8	1.4	96%	9.5-12.4

that long-term benzodiazepine use is rarely helpful and can be harmful, long-term use remains common.

ADVERSE EFFECTS. Benzodiazepines can cause prolonged sedation, impaired cognition and psychomotor performance, and unwanted amnesia. In older patients, they can precipitate delirium states and increase the risk of accidents and falls. Drugs with long-acting metabolites pose the greatest risk. However, the most significant risks associated with benzodiazepine use occur due to dependence and withdrawal effects. Abrupt withdrawal can precipitate delirium, anxiety, panic, seizures, insomnia, and muscle spasm.[65]

Drug Interactions
Although widely believed, it is not clear that patients on chronic benzodiazepine therapy have significant cross-tolerance to nonbenzodiazepine GABAergic anesthetic

agents, or that the risk of intraoperative recall is elevated with long-term use.[66] Acutely, benzodiazepines augment the CNS depressant effects of sedative-hypnotic anesthetic drugs and opioids, such that dosage reduction is appropriate. Although many benzodiazepines are metabolized by CYP3A4, they are generally not strong inducers or inhibitors, and effects on the metabolism of other drugs used in the perioperative period are generally not significant.[66a]

ANTIPSYCHOTIC DRUGS

First-Generation (Typical) Antipsychotics

The introduction of chlorpromazine (Thorazine) in 1952 arguably represents the most significant single development in psychopharmacology. Before that, treatment for psychosis was largely supportive and ineffective, with only electroconvulsive therapy and psychosurgery standing as controversial therapeutic options. The ability to treat psychosis effectively with drugs heralded massive deinstitutionalization as patients were discharged from psychiatric long-term care facilities and integrated into the community.

PHARMACOLOGY

The first-generation, or *typical*, antipsychotics (FGAs) include drugs from several classes: phenothiazines, butyrophenones, thioxanthenes, dihydroindolones, dibenzepines, diphenylbutylpiperidines, benzamides, and iminodibenzyls (Table 11-3). The butyrophenone class includes haloperidol (Haldol) and droperidol, two of the only psychopharmacologic agents commonly administered by anesthesiologists, although the latter is usually used for its antiemetic rather than its antipsychotic actions (see Chapter 28).

The principal mechanism for treatment of schizophrenia and other psychoses is blockade of D_2 dopamine receptors in the mesolimbic dopamine system. Dopamine receptors are G protein-coupled receptors that exist in multiple subtypes (Table 11-4). They can be grouped as D_1-like (activate adenylyl cyclase) or D_2-like (inhibit adenylyl cyclase) based on their signaling mechanisms. However, FGAs are not selective and have variable effects on D_1, D_3, and D_4 receptors, M_1 muscarinic cholinergic receptors, H_1 histamine receptors, α1- and α2-adrenergic receptors, and both 5-HT_1 and 5-HT_2 serotonergic receptors. The effects on these other receptors appear to have little influence on the therapeutic efficacy, but are of considerable importance to the side effect profile of individual drugs. Most FGAs are highly protein bound and lipophilic, and have large volumes of distribution (10-40 L/kg) with very significant variation in steady-state plasma concentrations. Oral preparations undergo extensive hepatic first-pass metabolism through hydroxylation, demethylation, and glucuronidation via CYP enzymes, and metabolites are dominantly eliminated in urine and bile. Elimination half-lives vary from 18 to 40 hours, allowing for once-a-day dosing. In the United States, depot preparations of haloperidol and fluphenazine are available as the decanoate ester suspended in sesame oil. After intramuscular injection, the esterified drug is slowly excreted from the oil and hydrolyzed, permitting dosing at intervals of 2 to 4 weeks.

SIDE EFFECTS

Extrapyramidal Side Effects

FGAs are associated with a spectrum of potentially severe side effects involving multiple organ systems. The most characteristic are a cluster of movement disorders termed extrapyramidal symptoms (EPS) with an overall incidence of over 50%.[67] The precise mechanism of EPS is unclear, but is in part related to D_2 receptor effects in the nigrostriatal pathway.[68] *Dystonia* is the earliest of the acute-onset EPS and is characterized by involuntary and frequently painful sustained muscle contractions, most often involving head and neck muscles. Although dystonic torticollis appears to have no significant effect on anesthetic airway management, sudden death due to laryngeal dystonia has been described.[69,70] Dystonic reactions are most likely following treatment with high-affinity D_2 receptor antagonists, which include haloperidol and droperidol. Acute dystonic reactions are usually responsive to the anticholinergic benztropine (2 mg every 30 minutes until symptom abatement) or the antihistamine diphenhydramine (25-50 mg). *Akathisia* is an unpleasant sensation of motor restlessness with an irresistible urge to move, leading patients to continuously perform patterns of complex motor activity. Symptomatically, akathisia resembles restless legs (Wittmaack-Ekbom) syndrome. Propranolol (20-120 mg/day) is the most consistently effective treatment, although antihistamines, anticholinergics, benzodiazepines, and serotonin antagonists are also used.[71] *Neuroleptic-induced pseudoparkinsonism* mimics classical Parkinson's disease, and must further be distinguished from depression or the negative symptoms of schizophrenia. Symptoms usually develop after several weeks of treatment, and acute events are rare. Approaches to treatment resemble those for akathisia, with the addition of dopaminergic agents such as amantadine. *Tardive dyskinesia* is a late development following chronic use of FGAs and is characterized by persistent and often stereotyped choreoathetoid movements that can involve any part of the body, but most commonly involve conspicuous oral and facial dyskinesias. Tetrabenazine is considered first-line treatment, but is associated with significant side effects; other agents include amantadine, benzodiazepines, β-blockers, vitamin E, and botulinum toxin for focal dystonias.[72] The overall effectiveness of treatment is poor, and the development of symptoms can be irreversible. Patients who develop tardive dyskinesia on FGAs can be changed to clozapine or another second-generation antipsychotic (see later), in that these agents decrease the incidence and severity of symptoms. In contrast to their efficacy in other forms of EPS, anticholinergics worsen tardive dyskinesia and should be avoided. Furthermore, anesthesiologists must be aware that the D_2-receptor antagonist metoclopramide, used perioperatively for its antiemetic and gastroprokinetic properties, can also trigger or exacerbate tardive dyskinesia and is contraindicated in patients receiving FGAs.[73]

Neuroleptic Malignant Syndrome

Neuroleptic malignant syndrome (NMS) is a life-threatening emergency that closely resembles malignant hyperthermia (MH). It is characterized by hyperthermia, muscle rigidity, severe hypermetabolic dysautonomia, and mental status changes. It can be triggered by a single dose of any antipsychotic, but is most commonly associated with the high potency FGAs, including haloperidol and droperidol. Rhabdomyolysis with elevated creatine kinase and renal failure are common secondary features. Overall mortality has been reported as in excess of 50%, but is probably closer to 10% to 20%.[74]

As with MH, first-line management is dantrolene (0.5-2.5 mg/kg every 6-12 hours), aggressive hydration, and supportive management. The dopamine agonist bromocriptine is also used. Although NMS is sometimes described as a neurogenic form of MH, the genetic and mechanistic relationship between the two is unclear.[75] Evidence relating MH-susceptibility on muscle contraction testing with a history of NMS is inconsistent, but is sufficient to manage such patients with full MH precautions.[76]

Other Side Effects

Several of the FGAs—notably thioridazine, haloperidol, droperidol, and pimozide—are associated with QTc prolongation and sudden cardiac death due to *torsades de pointes*, likely via

Table 11-3. First-Generation Antipsychotic Drugs

CLASS	STRUCTURE	POTENCY	DRUGS
Phenothiazines Aliphatic		Low/medium	Chlorproethazine, chlorpromazine, cyamemazine, levomepromazine, promazine, triflupromazine
Piperidine		Low/medium	Mesoridazine, pericyazine, piperacetazine, pipotiazine, peopericiazine, sulforidazine, thioridazine
Piperazine		Medium/high	Acetophenazine, butaperazine, dixyrazine, fluphenazine, perazine, perphenazine, propchlorperazine, thiopropazate, thioproperazine, trifluoperazine
Butyrophenones		High	Benperidol, bromperidol, droperidol, fluanisone, haloperidol, melperone, moperone, pipamperone, timiperone, trifluperidol
Thioxanthenes		Low/medium	Chlorprothixene, clopenthixol, flupenthixol, thiothixene, zuclopenthixol
Dihydroindolones		Low/medium	Molindone, oxypertine
Dibenzepines		Low/medium	Clotiapene, loxapine
Diphenylbutylpiperidines		High	Fluspirilene, penfluridol, pimozide

Continued

Table 11-3. First-Generation Antipsychotic Drugs—cont'd

CLASS	STRUCTURE	POTENCY	DRUGS
Benzamides		Low	Nemonapride, sulpiride, sultopride, tiapride
Iminodibenzyl		Medium	Clocapramine, mosapramine

Modified from Nasrallah HA, Tandon R. Classic antipsychotic medications. In: *American Psychiatric Publishing Textbook of Psychopharmacology*. 4th ed. Washington, DC: American Psychiatric Publishing; 2009:534.

Table 11-4. Dopamine Receptor Subtypes

DOPAMINE RECEPTOR SUBTYPE	D_1	D_{2S}	D_{2L}	D_3	D_4	D_5
Gene symbol	*DRD1*	*DRD2*	*DRD2*	*DRD3*	*DRD4*	*DRD5*
Molecular weight	49,300	47,347	50,619	44,225	41,487	52,951
Amino acids	446	414	443	400	387	477
Family classification	D_1	D_2	D_2	D_2	D_2	D_1
Adenylyl cyclase action	Stimulate	Inhibit	Inhibit	Inhibit	Inhibit	Stimulate
G protein coupling	$G\alpha_s$, $G\alpha_{olf}$	$G\alpha_i$, $G\alpha_o$	$G\alpha_i$, $G\alpha_o$	$G\alpha_i$, $G\alpha_o$	$G\alpha_i$, $G\alpha_o$	$G\alpha_s$, $G\alpha_q$
Principal brain expression sites	Striatum, NA, SN, olfactory bulb, amygdala	Striatum, NA, olfactory tubercle	Striatum, NA, olfactory tubercle	NA, olfactory tubercle, islands of Calleja	Frontal cortex, amygdala, hippocampus	PFC, PMC, entorhinal cortex, SN, hypothalamus, hippocampus, dentate gyrus
Clinical selective agonists	Fenoldopam	Bromocriptine, pergolide, cabergoline, ropinirole	Bromocriptine, pergolide, cabergoline, ropinirole	Pramipexole, rotigotine	None	None
Clinical selective antagonists	None	Haloperidol, spiperone, raclopride, sulpiride, risperidone	Haloperidol, spiperone, raclopride, sulpiride, risperidone	Nafadotride	None	None

NA, Nucleus accumbens; *SN*, substantia nigra; *PFC*, prefrontal cortex; *PMS*, premotor cortex. Modified from Beaulieu JM, Gainetdinov RR. The physiology, signaling, and pharmacology of dopamine receptors. *Pharmacol Rev.* 2011;63:182-217.

blocking the rapidly activating component of the delayed rectifier K^+ current.[77] In December 2001, the FDA issued a black box warning for droperidol, and a safety alert was issued for haloperidol in September 2007. The warning for droperidol refers to doses greater than 2.5 mg, which is greater than the common antiemetic dose of 0.625 to 1.25 mg.[78] Nonetheless, its use in anesthesia has virtually disappeared in the United States. The risk with haloperidol is greatest with intravenous administration, which, although off-label, is commonly used in the treatment of delirium in the intensive care setting. The QTc should be assessed in all patients before the administration of droperidol or intravenous haloperidol, and the electrocardiogram monitored following administration.

The M_1 anticholinergic activity of FGAs contributes to cognitive impairment, such as sedation, decreased memory function, and delirium, as well as to gastrointestinal effects such as nausea, vomiting, ileus, dry mouth, and urinary retention. Weight gain, dyslipidemia, hypertension, and the induction of diabetes mellitus secondary to H_1 histaminic, M_1 cholinergic, and $5\text{-}HT_{2C}$ serotonergic blockade are most pronounced with the second-generation antipsychotics, but can occur with the FGAs. Antagonism of tuberoinfundibular dopaminergic tracts causes hyperprolactinemia, with several secondary endocrine effects. The α1-adrenergic blockade can cause orthostatic hypertension and dizziness, especially early in the treatment course.

Second-Generation (Atypical) Antipsychotics

The description of an antipsychotic medication as *atypical* is pharmacologically imprecise, but is historically based only on a lower incidence of EPS. The group is, in fact, pharmacologically heterogeneous. When clozapine was introduced in 1961, there was little interest in conducting human trials because primate studies had demonstrated minimal EPS effects, and the prevailing theory was that EPS was a necessary (albeit unwanted) feature of antipsychotic efficacy. It was introduced in Europe in the early 1970s, but withdrawn in 1975 following reports of fatal agranulocytosis. However, a large trial demonstrated that it was effective in otherwise treatment-resistant schizophrenia, and clozapine received cautionary approval from the FDA in 1990.[79] The search for agents with a similarly low incidence of EPS but lower risk of agranulocytosis led to several other second-generation antipsychotic (SGA) drugs during the 1990s and 2000s. The newer SGAs—largely under patent protection and considerably more expensive—have replaced FGAs as the dominant pharmacotherapy for schizophrenia and other psychotic disorders. However, recent non–industry-sponsored trials suggest that, with the exception of clozapine, SGAs might have no better therapeutic efficacy than FGAs and offer no consistent advantage in long-term quality of life indicators.[80,81]

INDIVIDUAL AGENTS
Clozapine (Clozaril)
Clozapine is a dibenzodiazepine that is structurally related to loxapine. The mechanism of its low incidence of EPS and unique efficacy in treatment-refractory patients remains unclear. It is a weak antagonist at D_1, D_2, D_3, and D_5 dopamine receptors, but a strong antagonist at D_4 receptors. Positron emission tomography (PET) ligand studies demonstrate that clozapine is therapeutically effective when it occupies 20% to 67% of D_2 receptors, in contrast to FGAs, which only become therapeutic at 80% D_2 occupancy.[82] This reduced affinity for D_2 receptors might underlie the lower incidence of EPS and further suggests that the therapeutic efficacy is related to activity other than D_2 receptor antagonism. Clozapine also has high affinity for adrenergic, cholinergic, and $5\text{-}HT_{2C}$ and $5\text{-}HT_{2A}$ serotonergic receptors. Like most SGAs, it has a pK_i $(5\text{-}HT_{2A})$:pK_i (D_2) ratio higher than is observed with FGAs, an observation central to the *serotonin–dopamine hypothesis* of SGA action. This hypothesis suggests that interactions between the serotonin and dopamine systems play an important role in the mechanism of action of SGAs because relatively potent blockade of $5\text{-}HT_{2A}$ receptors coupled with weaker antagonism of dopamine D_2 receptors has been found as the only pharmacologic feature shared by most atypical antipsychotic drugs.[83-85] Clozapine is highly protein bound and is extensively metabolized in the liver via CYP 1A2; monitoring of plasma levels and adjustments in dosage must be considered when agents that induce or inhibit CYP activity are added or removed.

Clozapine carries five FDA black box warnings. Agranulocytosis is most likely in the first 3 months of treatment. The incidence in the absence of monitoring is as high as 1% to 2%; however, strict adherence to monitoring reduces the incidence to less than 0.5%.[86] Treatment should not be initiated if the white blood cell count is less than 3500 cells/μL or the absolute neutrophil count is less than 2000 cells/μL, and cell counts should be monitored. A number of cardiovascular side effects are reported, and a boxed warning exists for myocarditis. Myocarditis and cardiomyopathy are most common in the first 2 months of therapy and might involve an immunoglobulin E-mediated hypersensitivity reaction.[87] Boxed warnings also exist for orthostatic hypotension, seizures, and an increased risk of death in older patients receiving clozapine for dementia-related psychosis. Hyperglycemia and other diabetogenic effects, including ketoacidosis, are also seen. Because of the severity and incidence of these and other

adverse effects, although clozapine is clearly the most effective antipsychotic in the treatment of schizophrenia, its use is usually restricted to patients who have failed therapy with at least two other pharmacologic agents.

Olanzapine (Zyprexa)
Olanzapine is a thienobenzodiazepine structurally similar to clozapine that received FDA approval in 1997 and in 2004 was approved for the long-term treatment of bipolar disorder. Olanzapine is also available in a combined preparation with fluoxetine. Like other SGAs, selectivity for D_2 dopamine receptors is significantly less than for FGAs, although it does have relatively greater selectivity for D_2 than does clozapine. Antagonist affinity for the $5\text{-}HT_{2A}$ receptor is greater than for dopamine receptors, while affinity for the $5\text{-}HT_{2C}$ receptor is similar to that for D_2. There is also antagonism of α1-adrenergic, H_1-histaminergic, and M_{1-5} muscarinic receptors. Olanzapine also has weak activity at $GABA_A$ receptors; although interaction with GABAergic anesthetics is not defined, olanzapine is considered to potentiate the effects of benzodiazepines, and fatalities due to cardiorespiratory depression have been reported when intramuscular olanzapine has been combined with benzodiazepines.[88] Olanzapine is highly protein bound and predominantly metabolized by CYP 1A2.

Olanzapine is associated with weight gain, diabetogenesis, and dyslipidemia, with an incidence and magnitude greater than other SGAs or FGAs.[89,90] Boxed warnings exist for increased risk of death in older patients receiving olanzapine for dementia-related psychosis, and for excessive sedation and delirium following intramuscular injection. The incidence of EPS is less than that of the FGAs, but greater than that with clozapine. Although a small number of cases of olanzapine-induced leukopenia and agranulocytosis have been reported, scheduled monitoring is not required. Similarly, while cardiac conduction abnormalities have been reported, myocarditis and cardiomyopathy are not features, and the overall cardiac risk is significantly less than that associated with clozapine.

Quetiapine (Seroquel)
Quetiapine is a dibenzothiazepine approved by the FDA for the treatment of schizophrenia in 1997 and for the treatment of bipolar disorder in 2004. At 12 hours after the last dose, PET ligand studies demonstrate that quetiapine occupies only 30% of D_2 receptors, which is significantly less than that considered necessary for therapeutic efficacy.[91] However, occupancy is higher when measured at shorter intervals; this has led to the theory that transient occupancy of D_2 receptors provides clinical potency, but also permits dynamics of dopamine release in nigrostriatal and tuberoinfundibular pathways, accounting for the low incidence of EPS and hyperprolactinemia.[92] Quetiapine has high affinity for $5\text{-}HT_{2A}$ receptors, but relatively weak affinity for $5\text{-}HT_{2C}$ or $5\text{-}HT_1$ receptors. It has very strong affinity for H_1-histamine receptors, which likely accounts for it being the most sedating of the SGAs and also for α1-adrenergic receptors, accounting for postural hypotension. Protein binding is 83%, and it is metabolized by CYP 3A4. Its active metabolite, norquetiapine, has similar or even greater potency than the parent compound at many receptors. The most characteristic side effect of quetiapine is sedation. It is associated with weight gain,

diabetogenesis, and dyslipidemia, although the effect is not as great as that seen with clozapine or olanzapine. It can also cause orthostatic hypotension, but unlike clozapine it does not carry a boxed warning for this effect. Boxed warnings exist for an increased risk of death in older patients receiving quetiapine for dementia-related psychosis, and also for suicidality in children, adolescents, and young adults. The incidence of EPS and hyperprolactinemia is especially low compared to other FGAs and SGAs.[93] Dysrhythmias have been reported, but earlier concerns that quetiapine causes prolongation of QTc are probably unfounded.[77]

Aripiprazole (Abilify)

Aripiprazole is a dihydroquinolinone antipsychotic that is chemically and pharmacologically distinct from other FGA or SGA drugs. It received FDA approval for the treatment of schizophrenia in 2002, for acute manic and mixed episodes associated with bipolar disorder in 2004, as an adjunctive therapy for major depression in 2007, and for irritability in autistic children in 2009. In contrast to other antipsychotics, which are D_2 and 5-HT_{1A} receptor antagonists, aripiprazole is a *partial agonist* at these receptors and at 5-HT_{2C} receptors.[94,95] It is a strong antagonist at 5-HT_{2A}, 5-HT_7, and D_3 receptors, and has moderate effects at D_4, H_1 histamine, and α1-adrenergic receptors. It has virtually no affinity for muscarinic cholinergic receptors. Protein binding is at least 99%, and it is metabolized by CYP 2D6 and CYP 3A4. Its active metabolite, dehydro-aripiprazole, has similar affinity for D_2 receptors. Because of its partial agonist activity on nigrostriatal and tuberoinfundibular pathways, aripiprazole causes minimal EPS or hyperprolactinemia despite D_2 receptor occupancy of 70% to 95%. It also appears to be largely free of the adverse weight gain, diabetogenesis, and dyslipidemia associated with other SGAs. Aripiprazole does not cause prolongation of the QTc.[96] It is generally well tolerated. As with all the SGAs, aripiprazole carries a boxed warning for increased risk of death in older patients receiving antipsychotics for dementia-related psychosis and for suicidality in children, adolescents, and young adults.

Risperidone (Risperdal)

Risperidone is a benzisoxazole derivative approved by the FDA for treatment of schizophrenia in 1994, for short-term treatment of the mixed and manic states of bipolar disorder in 2003, and for treatment of irritability in children with autism in 2006. In 2007 it was approved as a treatment for schizophrenia and bipolar disorder in children. Its pharmacology is characterized by binding affinity for 5-HT_{2A} receptors that is 20 times that for D_2 dopamine receptors. D_2 receptor affinity is approximately 50 times, and 5-HT_{2A} receptor affinity approximately 20 times, that of clozapine. Risperidone also has strong affinity for α1/α2-adrenergic and H_1 histamine receptors. Affinity for D_1 receptors is low, and it has no affinity at muscarinic receptors. Protein binding is 90%, and it is metabolized by CYP 2D6. D_2 receptor occupancy at therapeutic doses is 63% to 89%, which would be expected to be associated with a significant incidence of EPS.[97] The addition of strong serotonergic antagonism, with a 5-HT_2 receptor occupancy of 95%, is thought to confer protection against D_2 antagonist effects on the nigrostriatal pathway, and the incidence of EPS is low. Nonetheless, unlike other SGAs with relatively lower affinities for D_2 receptors that permit

dynamic responses to surges in dopamine, risperidone is tightly bound and does cause significant hyperprolactinemia.[98] It can also cause orthostatic hypotension during early treatment. Risperidone does not cause prolongation of the QTc and is less arrhythmogenic than other antipsychotics. It carries a boxed warning for increased risk of death in older patients receiving antipsychotics for dementia-related psychosis.

Lithium

HISTORY

Lithium was first used medicinally in the late 19th century as a treatment for gout and other disorders, and was used as a substitute for table salt in the first half of the 20th century until several deaths from toxicity were reported. Just as cocaine was initially added to Coca-Cola for medicinal purposes, lithium was part of the original recipe for the beverage 7 Up. It was first identified as a treatment for mania in 1949, but at least partly because of concerns about toxicity, did not receive FDA approval for the treatment of acute mania until 1970, and for prophylaxis for bipolar disorder in 1974.

BASIC PHARMACOLOGY

Structure-Activity

Lithium is the third element of the periodic table and exists as a monovalent cation. It shares some properties with sodium and potassium, and substitution or competition with other cations can contribute to its effects.[99]

Mechanism

The therapeutic mechanism of lithium remains fundamentally unknown, although several proposals have been developed. Lithium depletes free intracellular inositol through noncompetitive inhibition of inositol monophosphate. This depletion can lead to changes in G protein-coupled second messenger systems and protein kinase C actions linked to inositol phosphate signaling, which are important in adrenergic, serotonergic, and cholinergic signaling.[100,101] Lithium also inhibits glycogen synthase kinase-3 (GSK-3), mimicking the Wnt protein signaling pathway to stimulate protein kinase C activity.[102,103] Effects on glutamate and gene expression have also been proposed. Lithium has effects on serotonin and norepinephrine signaling, and is an antagonist at 5-HT_{1A} and 5-HT_{1B} autoreceptors, increasing serotonin availability.[104,105] Lithium also causes a resetting of hypothalamic circadian oscillators, which are dysfunctional in bipolar disorder and depression.

Metabolism

As a monovalent cation, lithium undergoes no metabolism.

CLINICAL PHARMACOLOGY

Pharmacokinetics[106]

Lithium is rapidly and completely absorbed from the gastrointestinal tract and attains peak plasma concentration in 1 to 2 hours with rapid release preparations and 4 to 12 hours in extended release preparations. It is not protein bound and is evenly distributed in the total body water. The initial volume of distribution is 0.3 to 0.4 L/kg and in steady-state is 0.7 to

1 L/kg. Bioavailability is nearly 100% for the rapid release preparations, and 60% to 90% with the extended release preparations. It is excreted unchanged in the urine with an elimination half-time of 18 to 24 hours, or longer in older adults and those with renal impairment. Time to steady-state is 5 to 7 days. Filtered Li⁺ (80%) is reabsorbed in the proximal convoluted tubule, which is competitive with Na⁺ reabsorption. As a consequence, changes in renal functional dynamics such as diuretic therapy, sodium intake, and hydration status can alter plasma concentration, so monitoring of serum Li⁺ concentrations is required. The target concentration is 0.8 to 1.2 mM. Although there is no clear recommendation for therapeutic monitoring in surgical patients, there are numerous pharmacologic and physiologic events in the perioperative period that can affect Li⁺ plasma concentrations.

Pharmacodynamics

THERAPEUTIC EFFECTS. Lithium remains a first-line therapy for the treatment of acute mania, with a response rate in excess of 70%, and is at least as effective as other first-line agents.[107-109] It is also first-line treatment for bipolar depression and significantly reduces suicide attempts and successful suicide.[110,111] It is effective as prophylaxis and maintenance therapy in bipolar disorder, which is usually a lifelong disease characterized by recurrent acute mood episodes.[112] Lithium can also be effective as adjunctive therapy in treatment-resistant unipolar depression.[113] Although less well tolerated in older adults, lithium appears to have neuroprotective effects, and in animal models it is protective against Alzheimer's disease. Early data suggest that it might modify the course of Alzheimer's in humans.[114,115]

ADVERSE EFFECTS. Lithium is associated with a number of significant adverse effects and has a narrow therapeutic index. The most common side effects at therapeutic concentrations are weight gain and disturbed cognition and coordination. Lithium impairs renal concentrating ability, and a significant number of patients experience diabetes insipidus with polyuria and polydipsia, which is usually responsive to amiloride.[116] Renal tubular damage and even acute renal failure are reported. Neurotoxic reactions such as encephalopathy, delirium, memory changes, and movement disorders are possible and can be irreversible. Hypothyroidism is common and is more prevalent in females. Abnormal thyroid function occurs in excess of 35% of patients on long-term lithium therapy.[117] Clinically significant cardiac conduction abnormalities are unusual in patients without preexisting cardiac disease, but sinus node dysfunction, atrioventricular block, and T wave flattening can occur.[118] Caution and monitoring is essential in patients with elevated cardiac risk. Tremor may occur in up to 65% of patients.[119]

Drug Interactions

A number of drugs used in the perioperative period can alter plasma lithium concentrations. Thiazide diuretics increase concentrations by a compensatory increase in proximal tubule reabsorption, while loop diuretics such as furosemide generally have minimal effect, as do the potassium-sparing diuretics. Osmotic diuretics lower lithium concentrations and so are useful in the treatment of toxicity. Angiotensin converting enzyme (ACE) inhibitors increase lithium levels, as do angiotensin II receptor blockers, many nonsteroidal antiinflammatory agents, and several antibiotics.[120,121] Caution should be observed in using neuroleptic medications such as droperidol and haloperidol, in that the risk of extrapyramidal side effects and neuroleptic malignant syndrome is increased. Lithium prolongs the action of both depolarizing and nondepolarizing neuromuscular blocking drugs.[122,123]

Anticonvulsant Mood Stabilizers

Several heterogeneous compounds used initially as anticonvulsants possess or have been investigated for therapeutic benefit in bipolar disorder. The anticonvulsant properties of valproate were serendipitously established in 1963 when its incidental mood-enhancing effects stimulated interest in its use as a mood stabilizer. It received FDA approval for the treatment of mania in 1995. Lamotrigine was approved for maintenance therapy of bipolar disorder in 2003, and carbamazepine for the treatment of mania and mixed episodes in 2004. Valproate and carbamazepine are considered alternative first-line agents to lithium for the treatment of mania, although they are frequently used in combination therapy.[124,125] Valproate might be superior to lithium in the treatment of patients with mixed states.[126] Several other anticonvulsant drugs, including gabapentin, pregabalin, and topiramate have been investigated but do not have clearly established efficacy.

INDIVIDUAL AGENTS (Figure 11-7)
Valproate (Depakote)
Valproate is an eight-carbon, branched-chain carboxylic acid that suppresses seizures without affecting focal activity. The therapeutic mechanism for suppression of mania is unclear. Valproate facilitates GABAergic transmission through increased expression of mRNA for glutamate decarboxylase (the GABA synthetic enzyme), reduces protein kinase C activity in manic patients, and inhibits inositol cycling and GSK-3, although via different pathways than lithium.[100,127-129] It is 80% to 90% protein bound and attains peak plasma concentration in approximately 4 hours. It is hepatically metabolized via glucuronide conjugation and mitochondrial β oxidation. Elimination half life is 9 to 16 hours.

Valproate carries FDA black box warnings for hepatic failure, acute pancreatitis, and use in pregnancy. Hepatotoxicity is greatest in children under 2 years of age, but fatalities have been reported in adults. Fatal acute pancreatitis has been reported in both adults and children, including in those who have been on stable, long-term therapy. Hyperammonemia with encephalopathy is reported. Of special significance to surgical patients, valproate can cause thrombocytopenia, inhibition of platelet aggregation, and increased bleeding, but modification of therapy during the perioperative period is not

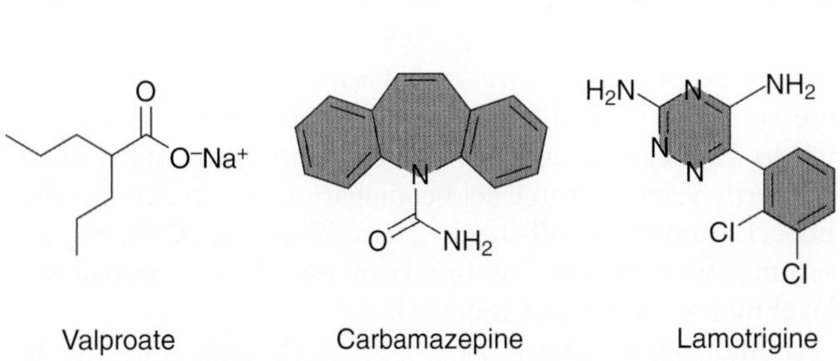

Figure 11-7 Anticonvulsant mood stabilizers.

recommended.[130] No drug interactions specific to anesthetic care are known.

Carbamazepine (Tegretol)

Carbamazepine is an iminostilbene derivative with a dibenzazepine nucleus, and thus has a tricyclic structure similar to imipramine. Like lithium and valproate, carbamazepine increases limbic GABA$_B$ receptors and has effects on inositol cycling. It has unique effects at peripheral-type benzodiazepine receptors, increases stimulatory G protein alpha subunits (G$_s\alpha$), and decreases inhibitory G protein subunits (G$_i\alpha$). It appears to lack the effects on GSK-3 and protein kinase C possessed by lithium and valproate. It has anticholinergic, antidiuretic, and muscle relaxant properties. Carbamazepine is 75% to 90% protein bound, with a volume of distribution of 0.6 to 2 L/kg in adults. It is hepatically metabolized via CYP 3A4 to an active epoxide metabolite, and is a strong CYP inducer. Elimination half life is highly variable and is initially 25 to 65 hours, but reduces to 12 to 17 hours after several weeks of therapy due to autoinduction. Plasma level monitoring is not required.

Carbamazepine carries two FDA black box warnings for blood dyscrasias and dermatologic reactions. A spectrum of hematologic abnormalities, including agranulocytosis, aplastic anemia, neutropenia, leukopenia, and thrombocytopenia have been reported, and monitoring standards similar to those for clozapine are recommended.[131] Severe dermatologic reactions include fatal toxic epidermal necrolysis and Stevens-Johnson syndrome. The risk of dermatologic reactions is strongly linked to the HLA-B*1502 allele, which is prevalent in Asian populations. Patients of Asian descent should be screened for HLA-B*1502 and carbamazepine avoided if the test is positive.[132] An SIADH-like syndrome is occasionally observed in older patients. Cardiac conduction abnormalities, including atrioventricular nodal block, have also been reported. Carbamazepine has strong induction effects on CYP 1A2, 2B6, 2C8, 2C9, 2C19, 3A4, and P-glycoprotein, and thus has the potential for significant drug interactions. The metabolism of midazolam, alfentanil, fentanyl, methadone, tramadol, and most nondepolarizing muscle relaxants is increased, but the effect of reduced plasma concentration is countered by generalized enhancement of the CNS depressant effects of anesthetic drugs.[133]

Lamotrigine (Lamictal)

Lamotrigine is a phenyltriazine that is structurally unrelated to the other anticonvulsant mood stabilizers. It reduces folate activity via inhibition of dihydrofolate reductase. It suppresses paroxysmal bursts from Na$^+$ channels, and inhibits glutamate release in response to ischemia and to the Na$^+$ channel activator veratrine.[134] It has no demonstrated effects on reuptake of dopamine, norepinephrine, or serotonin, and has minimal affinity for α1, α2, β, D$_1$, D$_2$, GABA, H$_1$, M$_1$, M$_2$, or κ and σ opioid receptors. It is a weak inhibitor of 5-HT$_3$.[135] Lamotrigine is 55% protein bound, with a volume of distribution of 0.9 to 1.3 L/kg. It undergoes hepatic and renal metabolism, primarily via glucuronic acid conjugation to inactive metabolites. Elimination half-life is 25 to 33 hours. A therapeutic serum concentration has not been established, and plasma level monitoring is not required.

Lamotrigine carries an FDA black box warning for dermatologic reactions, including potentially fatal Stevens-Johnson syndrome and toxic epidermal necrolysis. Other significant concerns include an increased risk of aseptic meningitis and the development of blood dyscrasias, including neutropenia, leukopenia, thrombocytopenia, and pancytopenia.[136,137] Most of the common adverse effects are relatively mild. No characteristic cardiac conduction defect is described, although rare events of arrhythmias in patients taking lamotrigine have been reported. When used as monotherapy, induction and inhibition of CYP isoenzymes does not occur, and changes in the metabolism of other drugs is not of significance. In general, lamotrigine augments the CNS depressant effects of drugs used in the perioperative period, but no interaction with any specific anesthetic drug is known.

PSYCHOSTIMULANTS

Amphetamine, first synthesized in 1887, was available without prescription as a decongestant inhalant under the trade name Benzedrine from the 1930s to 1960s. Its utility as a stimulant was recognized during World War II, when it was used to combat fatigue in soldiers. Methylphenidate, identified as a stimulant in the 1950s, was used to treat children with the conditions that would subsequently be named attention deficit disorder (ADD) or attention deficit/hyperactivity disorder (ADHD), marketed under the name Ritalin. Diagnosis and treatment of ADD/ADHD has exploded over the past 20 years and has expanded to include a greater number of adult patients. Modafinil was approved for use in the United States in 1998 and has significantly improved the pharmacologic treatment of narcolepsy and other disorders of wakefulness.[138] The psychostimulant drugs are briefly summarized in Table 11-5.

Long-term use of amphetamine and methylphenidate leads to catecholamine depletion, which can blunt the sympathetic response to hemodynamic stress. Significant perioperative events, including cardiac arrest during induction of anesthesia, have been rarely reported.[139] However, there is no basis to recommend discontinuation of therapy before surgery.[140] Direct-acting sympathomimetics such as phenylephrine are preferred, and pretreatment with atropine can be used in selected pediatric patients.

DRUGS USED IN THE TREATMENT OF PARKINSON'S DISEASE

Levodopa

HISTORY

The discovery in the 1950s that the loss of dopaminergic neurons in the substantia nigra leads to Parkinson's disease (PD) was swiftly followed by the introduction of the dopamine precursor levodopa for the treatment of motor symptoms.[141-143] Levodopa has remained the gold standard treatment for the last 50 years, but is associated with the development of long-term motor complications.[144] Appreciation of these problems has led to the preferential use of dopamine agonists and MAO-B inhibitors as initial therapy in patients with milder motor symptoms and without cognitive impairment.

Table 11-5. Psychostimulants

	AMPHETAMINE	METHYLPHENIDATE	MODAFINIL
Structure			
Common trade names	Adderall (amphetamine, dextroamphetamine mixed salts) Dexedrine (dextroamphetamine) Desoxyn (methamphetamine)	Ritalin Metadate Concerta Focalin (dexmethylphenidate)	Provigil Nuvigil (armodafinil)
Class and mechanism	Noncatecholamine sympathomimetic amine. Enhances dopaminergic, serotonergic, and noradrenergic release in neural network specific regions via complex transporter effects	Norepinephrine and dopamine (dominant) reuptake inhibitor. Blocks the dopamine transprter (DAT). Has regionally specific effects similar to amphetamine	Mechanism is unclear. Does not appear to involve dopamine or noradrenergic pathways. May involve glutamatergic and GABAergic effects.
Metabolism	CYP2D6 with no significantly active metabolites	Hepatic via carboxylesterase CES1A1 to inactive metabolites	CYP3A4
Half-life	10-15 hours	1-4 hours	15 hours
Approved therapeutic indications	ADHD Narcolepsy Obesity (methamphetamine)	ADHD Narcolepsy	Narcolepsy Shift work sleep disorder Obstructive sleep apnea/ hypopnea syndrome (OSAHS)
Adverse effects	Common: insomnia, headache, anxiety, weight loss, tachycardia, hypertension May cause cardiac arrhythmia, seizure, and hyperpyrexia in susceptible patients. High potential for abuse Abrupt discontinuation may precipitate withdrawal.	Common: insomnia, headache, anxiety, weight loss, tachycardia, hypertension May cause cardiac arrhythmia, seizure, and hyperpyrexia in susceptible patients. High potential for abuse Discontinuation symptoms generally less pronounced than for amphetamine	Common: headache, nausea Generally less arrhythmogenic than amphetamine and methylphenidate, but events are described. May cause severe rashes, including Stevens-Johnson syndrome.
Drug interactions	May reduce the sedative effect of drugs used in anesthesia, and potentiate the analgesic effect of opiates. May unpredictably alter the response of the sympathomimetic drugs. May potentiate the action of arrhythmogenic drugs and drugs that lower the seizure threshold.	May reduce the sedative effect of drugs used in anesthesia, and potentiate the analgesic effect of opiates. May unpredictably alter the response of the sympathomimetic drugs. May potentiate the action of arrhythmogenic drugs and drugs that lower the seizure threshold.	May unpredictably alter the response to sympathomimetic drugs. No known significant anesthetic interactions.

BASIC PHARMACOLOGY

Structure-Activity

Levodopa is the levorotatory isomer of 3,4-dihydroxyphenyl-alanine. The dextrorotatory isomer has no biologic activity. Levodopa is an intermediate in the biosynthesis of dopamine. It is formed endogenously in humans by the action of tyrosine hydroxylase on the amino acid L-tyrosine.[145]

Mechanism

Unlike exogenous dopamine that cannot cross the blood-brain barrier, levodopa is actively transported into the CNS and is rapidly converted to dopamine by the enzyme aromatic L-amino acid decarboxylase (AAAD). The converted dopamine is available throughout the CNS and binds to presynaptic and postsynaptic dopamine receptors. In the corpus striatum, increased levels of dopamine normalize the levels of this neurotransmitter caused by dopaminergic neuronal loss.

Metabolism

Only a fraction of levodopa reaches the CNS, while the majority is converted to dopamine peripherally by AAAD.[146]

For this reason, levodopa is always coadministered with an AAAD inhibitor (carbidopa or benserazide). These agents increase cerebral bioavailability and reduce adverse effects associated with peripheral excesses of dopamine, including nausea and hypotension.

Decarboxylation of levodopa by endogenous catechol-O-methyltransferase (COMT) reduces bioavailability and shortens half-life. This leads to phasic stimulation of dopamine receptors in the basal ganglia, which can contribute to the development of motor fluctuations and dyskinesias.[147] To ameliorate this, COMT inhibitors (entacapone or tolcapone) are often given concurrently. Tolcapone is rarely associated with severe liver injury and frequent monitoring of liver function is now recommended on initiation of therapy.[148]

Clinical Pharmacology

Pharmacokinetics

The absorption of levodopa approaches 100% in the presence of an AAAD inhibitor. The duration of action of the immediate-release formulation is 2 to 4 hours and of the sustained-release formulation is 3 to 6 hours.[145] It is not appreciably bound to plasma proteins.[146] Elimination of levodopa and metabolites is primarily renal.

Because of the short half-life and the absence of a parenteral formulation, levodopa should be continued perioperatively including shortly before induction of anesthesia.[149] Interruption of administration can lead to exacerbation of motor symptoms and interfere with ventilation. During longer procedures, consideration should be given to administration of levodopa via a gastric tube.

Pharmacodynamics
THERAPEUTIC EFFECTS. Levodopa is effective in treatment of bradykinesias, gait disturbances and tremor at all stages of PD. It does not have any appreciable effect on nondopaminergic aspects of the disease such as dementia or autonomic dysfunction.

ADVERSE EFFECTS. Adverse effects not already mentioned include somnolence, psychosis, cardiac irritability, and orthostatic hypotension. Neuroleptic malignant syndrome has been reported on sudden discontinuation and responds to reinstatement of levodopa.[150] Earlier concerns that levodopa hastens progress of PD have not been borne out by recent clinical studies.

Dopamine Agonists

HISTORY
Motor complications arising from PD treatment with levodopa led to the search for other agents. The ergot derivative and dopamine agonist, bromocriptine, was first used for the treatment of PD in the mid 1970s. Since that time a number of other ergot (cabergoline, lisuride) and non-ergot derivatives (pramipexole and ropinirole) have been approved for PD therapy. The association of the oral ergot derivatives with pulmonary, valvular, and retroperitoneal fibrosis has severely curtailed their use for the management of PD.[151,152] One of the oldest known non-ergot derivatives, apomorphine, has only recently been approved for PD management but the technical challenges of delivery due to high first pass metabolism have prevented wider use.

BASIC PHARMACOLOGY
Structure-Activity
Agents from this class have chemically distinct structures. Pramipexole is a synthetic aminothiazole while ropinirole is an indole derivate. Apomorphine is a derivative of the quinolone alkaloid aporphine. The name refers to its historical derivation as a morphine decomposition product but there are no structural elements of morphine present in apomorphine. Apomorphine has two stereoisomers with only the R-enantiomer having dopaminergic activity. All three of these agents are chemically unrelated to the ergoline dopamine agonists.

Mechanism
The dopamine agonists activate presynaptic and postsynaptic dopamine receptors directly. The enteral nonergot derivatives preferentially bind D_2 and D_3 receptors. The affinity for D_3 receptors is up to ten times higher than for D_2 receptors. Apomorphine has affinities for the D_1, D_2, D_3, and D_4 receptors similar to those of dopamine.[153] Enteral ergot derivatives not only bind D_1 and D_2 but also some serotonin and adrenergic receptors.

Metabolism
Ropinirole is inactivated in the liver by CYP 1A2 with none of the major metabolites having pharmacologic activity. Pramipexole has negligible metabolism and more than 90% is excreted unchanged in the urine. Apomorphine undergoes extensive first pass inactivation in the liver and is largely metabolized by systemic oxidation.

CLINICAL PHARMACOLOGY
Pharmacokinetics
The two most commonly used enteral agents, pramipexole and ropinirole, have distinct pharmacokinetic profiles. Bioavailability for pramipexole is greater than 90% while ropinirole is around 50%. These agents remain in the body longer than levodopa with the immediate release formulations of pramipexole and ropinirole, having elimination half-lives of 8 hours and 6 hours, respectively.[154,156] Pramipexole is largely renally cleared while ropinirole is predominantly cleared by the liver.

Because apomorphine has extensive first pass metabolism, it is not effective as an oral agent. Instead it is most commonly administered subcutaneously or intranasally. The drug has a clinical effect within 20 minutes of subcutaneous administration and has an elimination half-life of 30 to 60 minutes.

Pharmacodynamics
THERAPEUTIC EFFECTS. The oral dopamine agonists in clinical use are effective in the treatment of the major motor symptoms of PD, in particular bradykinesias and tremor. They are used as sole agents in PD patients with mild-moderate motor symptoms and as an adjunct to levodopa in more severe disease. Ropinirole and pramipexole are also approved for the treatment of restless legs syndrome.

Apomorphine can be used as a touching type therapy to improve mobility in patients experiencing "off" periods. It is as effective as levodopa in the management of motor symptoms but technical difficulties associated with long-term subcutaneous delivery have limited its clinical utility. Apomorphine can be used as an alternative to gastric administration of levodopa during longer anesthetics.[149]

ADVERSE EFFECTS. As a class the dopamine agonists are generally well tolerated and have a similar side effect profile to levodopa. The prevalence of dyskinesias and motor fluctuations are reduced, which is postulated to result from longer elimination half-lives of the enteral agents. Unlike levodopa, the enteral agents can cause headaches and psychiatric symptoms including confusion, compulsive gambling, and hypersexuality.[153] Apomorphine is associated with nausea and vomiting, necessitating the concurrent administration of domperidone.[149]

There are no significant interactions between the dopamine agonists and anesthetic agents. Because of the longer half-life of the enteral agents, concerns regarding interruption of administration are not as pertinent as for levodopa.

MAO-B Inhibitors

MAO-B inhibitors act by reducing synaptic and glial metabolism of dopamine, leading to enhanced activity and reuptake.

They are effective as monotherapy in early PD and are used as adjuncts to either dopamine agonists or levodopa in more severe disease.

Selegiline and rasagiline are approved for PD treatment. Unlike selegiline, rasagiline has no amphetamine metabolites, which may account for the lower incidence of cognitive side effects.[157] Details of the pharmacology of these agents have been presented earlier in this chapter.

DRUGS USED IN THE TREATMENT OF MYASTHENIA GRAVIS

Myasthenia gravis (MG) is an antibody-mediated disorder of neuromuscular transmission. Modern therapy is based on increasing the availability of acetylcholine (ACh) at the neuromuscular junction with anticholinesterases and modulating the immune response. Agents that moderate autoimmune injury include corticosteroids, cyclosporine, azathioprine, tacrolimus, and rituximab. A discussion of these agents is outside the scope of this chapter and the reader is referred to recent reviews for further information.[158,159]

Anticholinesterases

HISTORY
In 1934, the anticholinesterase physostigmine was demonstrated to markedly improve muscle strength in a patient with myasthenia. This finding strongly implicated the neuromuscular junction in the etiology of MG. Physostigmine was the mainstay of treatment for 3 decades before the introduction of the longer acting oral agent pyridostigmine. Substantial improvements in the life expectancy of patients with MG during the middle of last century owed much to the introduction of the anticholinesterases and improved therapies for respiratory failure.

Pyridostigmine remains the most frequently used anticholinesterase for MG treatment, with neostigmine only rarely used due to a shorter duration of action and higher rate of gastrointestinal side effects. The short acting edrophonium is used as an aid in the diagnosis of MG and cholinesterase inhibitor overdose.

BASIC PHARMACOLOGY
Structure-Activity
Pyridostigmine, neostigmine, and edrophonium all contain a quaternary ammonium group, limiting lipid solubility and preventing passage through the blood-brain barrier. Physostigmine lacks the quaternary ammonium group enabling it to pass freely into the CNS.[160] The longer acting agents, pyridostigmine, neostigmine, and physostigmine, contain a carbamate group that forms a reversible covalent bond with acetylcholinesterase. Edrophonium, lacking a carbamate group, forms short-lived electrostatic and hydrogen bonds with acetylcholinesterase, accounting for its shorter activity.

Mechanism
Binding of acetylcholinesterase inhibits the breakdown of ACh, increasing the amount of neurotransmitter available to stimulate the reduced number of ACh receptors in the synaptic cleft of the neuromuscular junction.

Metabolism
The carbamate containing anticholinesterases undergo hydrolysis by cholinesterases and are also metabolized by microsomal enzymes in the liver. While physostigmine is extensively metabolized, the majority of neostigmine and pyridostigmine is excreted unchanged by the kidneys.

CLINICAL PHARMACOLOGY
Pharmacokinetics
Agents containing a quaternary ammonium group are poorly absorbed and have oral bioavailabilities of only 2% for neostigmine and between 7% and 25% for pyridostigmine.[161] The duration of action is between 3 to 6 hours and elimination half-life varies from 2 to 4 hours. Slow release formulations can help patients who become symptomatic during the night but due to variable absorption are not used for awake patients. Around 90% of pyridostigmine is renally cleared unchanged and dose reductions are recommended for MG patients with reduced renal function and in older adults.[162]

Edrophonium acts within 2 minutes of administration. It has an elimination half-life of 30 to 110 minutes but a duration of action much shorter due to transient binding to acetylcholinesterase.[163] It is predominantly renally cleared.

Pharmacodynamics
THERAPEUTIC EFFECTS. Pyridostigmine is the most commonly used initial treatment for MG. It is particularly effective at reversing muscle weakness and fatigability early in the course of the disease. Over time tolerance can develop, necessitating higher doses. Beyond single doses of 120 to 180 mg, little clinical benefit is seen and the rate of adverse effects increases significantly. Babies of myasthenic mothers can have muscle weakness lasting for up to 4 weeks that responds to pyridostigmine but occasionally requires mechanical ventilation.

ADVERSE EFFECTS. Pyridostigmine is well tolerated in most patients but at standard doses the muscarinic side effects of nausea and abdominal cramps are frequent. For some, intractable diarrhea prevents continued usage. Uncommonly bradycardia can lead to orthostatic hypotension and require dose reduction.

An increase in airway secretions can worsen reactive airway disease and can be confused with respiratory muscle involvement with MG.[158] The development of respiratory failure requiring intubation during a myasthenic crisis often leads to discontinuation of the cholinesterase inhibitors due to excessive airway secretions. Increased nicotinic activity can lead to muscle cramps and fasciculation that rarely leads to dose adjustment. Excessive administration of an anticholinesterase can lead to increased muscle weakness and muscarinic side effects ("cholinergic crisis"). Increased weakness in response to edrophonium can be used to help differentiate this from a myasthenic crisis.

Drug Interactions
The decision to continue anticholinesterase treatment perioperatively should be individualized.[158] These agents interfere with neuromuscular blockers, if used, during general anesthesia. The cholinesterase inhibitors also act on plasma cholinesterase and can slow the metabolism of ester-type local anesthetics and succinylcholine.

Table 11-6. Pharmacokinetics of the Antiepileptic Drugs

	STRUCTURE	ELIMINATION	BIOAVAILABILITY	HALF-LIFE	PROTEIN BINDING
Phenytoin	Related to barbiturates	Hepatic	Oral and IV: 70%-100%	Highly variable avg. 20-30 hr	90%
Oxcarbazepine	Carbamazepine derivative	Renal	>95%	1-2.5 hr active metabolite (MHD): 9 hr	40%
Topiramate	Aminosulfonic derivative of monosaccharide	Renal	>90%	19-23 hr	9%-17%
Gabapentin	Cyclic analog of GABA	Renal	55%-65%	6-8 hr	<5%
Pregabalin	Cyclic analog of GABA	Renal	>90%	5-7 hr	<5%
Levetiracetam	Pyrollidine derivative	Renal	>95%	7 hr	10%
Ezogabine	Carbamic acid ethyl ester	Renal	60%	8 hr	60%-80%

Table 11-7. Mechanism of Action of the Antiepileptic Drugs

	INCREASED GABA LEVELS	GABA$_A$ RECEPTOR AFFINITY	SODIUM CHANNEL BLOCKADE	CALCIUM CHANNEL BLOCKADE	GLUTAMATE INHIBITION	POTASSIUM CHANNEL ACTIVATION
Phenytoin			+			
Oxcarbazepine			+	+ (N, P-type)		
Topiramate	+	+	+	+ (L-type)	+	
Gabapentin				+ (N, P/Q–type)		
Pregabalin				+ (N, P/Q–type)		
Levetiracetam		+		+ (N-type)		
Ezogabine	+	+				+Kv7.2-7.5

Adapted from Lasoń W, Dudra-Jastrzębska M, Rejdak K, Czuczwar SJ. Basic mechanisms of antiepileptic drugs and their pharmacokinetic/pharmacodynamics interactions: an update. *Pharmacol Rep.* 2011;63:271-292.

ANTIEPILEPTIC DRUGS

The chronic neurologic disorder of epilepsy, which affects more than 50 million people worldwide, is characterized by seizures and hypersynchronous firing of neuronal networks. The antiepileptic drugs (AEDs) constitute a chemically diverse class. Some of these agents (carbamazepine, valproate, and lamotrigine) are also approved for use as mood stabilizers and details of their pharmacology are reviewed earlier in this chapter.

History

In the latter half of the 19th century, bromides were introduced as the first AEDs. While effective, they had numerous toxicities and were supplanted by phenobarbital on its introduction after World War I. The low cost of phenobarbital has helped it remain a popular first-line antiepileptic in developing countries to this day. It was in 1938 that the antiseizure properties of phenytoin were discovered. With a similar efficacy to phenobarbital but without excessive sedation, it continues to be widely used.[164] Through the 1990s, the discovery of new AEDs was infrequent but saw the introduction of the benzodiazepines, valproate, and carbamazepine to the armamentarium. Since then, a continuing stream of drugs has been released, including lamotrigine, topiramate, gabapentin, pregabalin, levetiracetam, and the carbamazepine-derivative oxcarbazepine.[165] Ezogabine (retigabine) is the most recently added AED drug with FDA approval in 2011 for treatment of partial-onset seizures.[166,167] With a novel action as a neuronal K$^+$ channel opener and with early indications of efficacy in drug resistant epilepsy, it holds promise for wide use.

BASIC PHARMACOLOGY
Structure-Activity

All of the AEDs are synthetic compounds. Individual structural details are listed in Table 11-6. Phenytoin is related to the barbiturates but contains a five-member carbon ring instead of the four-carbon basic structure.[168] Gabapentin and pregabalin are both cyclic analogs of GABA, although pregabalin is around three times more potent.[169] Oxcarbazepine is a keto-analog of carbamazepine.

Mechanism

Agents in this class act through a variety of mechanisms. Molecular targets of action include voltage-gated Na$^+$, K$^+$, and Ca^{2+} channels, GABA$_A$ receptors, glutamate receptors, some enzymes, and synaptic proteins. Table 11-7 summarizes the targets of each member of the AEDs. They all act by tilting the balance in favor of inhibition, thereby preventing abnormal neuronal excitation and suppressing the spread of ongoing pathologic activity. The AEDs also affect neuroplastic processes and have genetic and epigenetic effects with longer term changes on the evolution of the disease.[164]

Metabolism

Phenytoin is extensively metabolized in the liver to an inactive metabolite by CYP 2C9. This process is capacity-limited and at higher doses demonstrates zero-order kinetics. Around 20% of topiramate is also metabolized by CYP 3A4 but most is renally cleared unchanged.[170] Oxcarbazepine is rapidly metabolized by reduction to a pharmacologically active metabolite, which is subsequently glucuronidated and renally excreted. Ezogabine is metabolized in the liver by glucuronidation and acetylation by enzymes independent of the CYP system. It has an active metabolite with some antiepileptic activity but lower potency than the parent drug.[166] The agents levetiracetam, gabapentin, and pregabalin are not appreciably metabolized and are excreted unchanged in the urine.[170]

CLINICAL PHARMACOLOGY
Pharmacokinetics
Pharmacokinetic parameters of the AEDs are summarized in Table 11-7.

At therapeutic doses, the metabolism of phenytoin is nonlinear (first-order kinetics) but becomes linear at toxic doses. Plasma level monitoring is required due to its unpredictable pharmacokinetics and narrow therapeutic index.

Pharmacodynamics
THERAPEUTIC EFFECTS. There are no placebo-controlled trials of the AEDs as monotherapy for seizure control but there is widespread consensus that these drugs are effective.[170] The addition of newer AEDs as second-line agents in epilepsy refractory to standard monotherapy is supported by clinical data, but is associated with a higher rate of adverse effects. With optimal pharmacotherapy, around 50% of patients will have total seizure control and a further 25% will have significant improvement. AEDs are often used prophylactically in patients with brain tumors, severe traumatic head injuries and intracerebral hemorrhages.[171,172] Definitive data demonstrating efficacy for brain tumors and hemorrhages are lacking and there is a paucity of information on the use of the newer AEDs for prophylaxis.

ADVERSE EFFECTS. Unlike older AEDs, some of which carry FDA black box warnings (see earlier), the newer AEDs are generally well tolerated. Adverse effects that are common to most agents in the group include dizziness, somnolence, headaches, and memory impairment.

Phenytoin is more frequently associated with adverse effects than other members of this class. Specific problems include gingival hyperplasia, nystagmus, Stevens-Johnson syndrome, and osteomalacia.[173] Phenytoin is also linked with an increased risk of congenital birth defects. Rapid intravenous administration of phenytoin can lead to hypotension and arrhythmias, hence the recommendation to limit delivery rate to 50 mg/min in adults. Gabapentin and pregabalin are associated with an increased risk of depression and suicide. Sudden withdrawal of these agents can precipitate seizures, even in patients who have not seized previously. Rarely, hepatotoxicity is linked to gabapentin use. Oxcarbazepine causes syndrome of inappropriate antidiuretic hormone (SIADH) in around 3% of patients.[174] It has been associated with photosensitivity and, given its similarity to carbamazepine, is considered to be a potential teratogen.

Drug Interactions
Phenytoin and oxcarbazepine induce CYP enzymes, increasing the metabolism of commonly used anesthetic agents including midazolam, fentanyl, alfentanil, and aminosteroidal muscle relaxants. All drugs in this class enhance the CNS depressant effects of agents used in the perioperative period.[175]

DRUGS OF ABUSE

The abuse of legal and illicit substances remains an intractable problem in modern society. The number of Americans abusing or dependent on ethanol is over 17 million and an estimated 19 million are current users of illicit drugs. Anesthesiologists often see acutely intoxicated patients during anesthesia for trauma. In the elective setting, many patients are chronic drug abusers and if acutely intoxicated or withdrawing should have their procedures postponed.

The social history is often unreliable in detecting substance abuse. A history of alcohol abuse in younger patients should raise concerns over concurrent use of illicit substances. For nonurgent procedures in which suspicion is high, urine drug screening is useful. Routine drug screens do not test for designer drugs unless regional prevalence makes this cost effective. It is important to understand how these substances adversely interact with anesthetic agents and to recognize withdrawal syndromes.

Drugs of abuse are used for their pleasurable effects, which are due to activation of the mesolimbic dopaminergic reward system, either directly or indirectly.

Ethanol

Ethanol is an organic compound (C_2H_5OH) that has been consumed since prehistoric times. It is produced for human consumption by fermentation. It remains unclear how ethanol produces its neurologic effects. Historically, it was thought that ethanol acted by perturbing the neuronal lipid membrane. More recent evidence suggests that there are multiple sites of action including $GABA_A$ and glycine receptor potentiation and NMDA glutamate receptor inhibition.[176,177] Ethanol is rapidly absorbed into the bloodstream and metabolized by alcohol dehydrogenase in the liver to acetaldehyde. This unstable intermediate is metabolized to acetic acid by aldehyde dehydrogenase. Ethanol is also oxidized by CYP 2E1 in the liver. This pathway is minor except under conditions of chronic consumption, in which CYP 2E1 is dramatically upregulated.[178]

Acutely intoxicated patients have decreased anesthetic requirements while chronic abusers can have higher requirements, partly due to CYP induction. Perioperative concerns for the alcoholic patient include cardiomyopathy, alcoholic hepatitis, cirrhosis, and varices. Postoperatively, generalized grand mal withdrawal seizures can occur around 24 to 36 hours after abstinence. Within 72 hours of cessation, delirium tremens occur in around 5% to 10% of alcoholics and is characterized by confusion, hallucinations, agitation, and autonomic hyperactivity. Treatment and prophylaxis are with the benzodiazepines. The older chronic alcoholic is also at an increased risk for postoperative cognitive dysfunction.

Cocaine

Since the time of the Incas, cocaine has been used as a stimulant. Originally consumed by chewing the leaves of the South American plant *Erythroxylon coca*, it was popularized in Europe and North America by its use in Coca-Cola and Vin Mariani. Modern pharmaceutical techniques allowed purification of the active ingredient in the 1880s and cocaine hydrochloride was marketed as a panacea for a wide range of illnesses. Identification of the anesthetic properties of the drug saw its widespread use for local and regional anesthesia. Early experimenters including Freud and Halsted often self-administered to study the drug but succumbed to its addictive potential. With increasing evidence of problems associated with abuse, cocaine fell out of favor for medicinal use and was banned from distribution in 1914. It remains the second most commonly abused illicit substance, with around 2.7% of adults in the United States reporting recent use.[179]

Cocaine produces intense euphoria and feelings of increased energy. The drug acts by blocking the reuptake of the neurotransmitters dopamine, serotonin, and norepinephrine into nerve terminals, thereby increasing the synaptic concentrations of these neurotransmitters. Effects on dopaminergic neurons are thought to be responsible for the high addictive potential of this drug.[180]

Cocaine is usually consumed orally or by snorting. The alkalinized form ("crack cocaine") can be injected, smoked, or snorted and has even greater addictive potential due to very rapid absorption with high peak plasma levels. The elimination half-life is 0.5 to 1.5 hours and metabolism is by liver and plasma cholinesterases.

The sympathetic effects of cocaine can precipitate vasoconstriction or vasospasm in arteries supplying the brain and heart, leading to strokes and myocardial infarction or ischemia. Higher doses lead to ventricular arrhythmias and death. Users who smoke crack cocaine can induce asthma or develop pulmonary hemorrhages. Several serious complications are associated with anesthesia in the setting of acute cocaine use. Patients can become severely hypertensive, particularly during laryngoscopy.[181] Direct acting vasodilators including nitroglycerin and hydralazine or calcium channel blockers are appropriate for treatment and prophylaxis although they worsen preexisting tachycardia. Caution should be exercised in the use of beta blockers, in that unopposed α-receptor action can worsen hypertension and lead to myocardial ischemia. The induction agents, ketamine and etomidate, can exacerbate the underlying hemodynamic abnormalities. Halothane should be avoided in that it sensitizes the myocardium to catecholamines, with a potential for arrhythmias.[182]

Chronic cocaine users can develop intraoperative hypotension that is unresponsive to ephedrine that will usually respond to direct acting vasoconstrictors such as phenylephrine.

Physical and psychologic dependence to the drug develops, and abrupt cessation perioperatively is associated with a non–life-threatening withdrawal syndrome characterized by depression and fatigue.

Amphetamines

Amphetamine derivatives from the plant *Ephedra sinica* have been used for medicinal purposes for millennia. Modern pharmaceutical processes allowed the synthesis of amphetamine in 1887. Other members of the class, methamphetamine and 3,4-methylenedioxymethamphetamine (MDMA) were first synthesized in the early 20th century. Methamphetamine was used widely by the German military during World War II as a stimulant to prevent fatigue. Over the past 2 decades, methamphetamine ("crystal meth") abuse has become a vast social problem, particularly in the American Midwest. MDMA (ecstasy) was first used as an appetite suppressant before finding use in psychotherapy circles during the 1970s. The euphoric and energizing effects of the drug led to use in the club and bar scene. Although scheduled in the United States in 1984, usage spread to the mainstream

and around the world, with ecstasy being amongst the top four most widely consumed illicit substances.

The basic amphetamine structure is comprised of a phenethylamine backbone with a methyl group attached to the alpha carbon. Substitutions generate the related compounds, methamphetamine and MDMA. Methamphetamine abusers commonly administer the drug intravenously, by smoking or snorting. Less commonly it is taken orally. MDMA is usually taken orally, but can be snorted or delivered rectally. Metabolism of the amphetamines is by CYP 2D6 in the liver. The elimination half-life is 6 to 10 hours for MDMA and 10 to 15 hours for methamphetamine.[183,184] The effects of amphetamines are mediated by enhanced neuronal release of dopamine, serotonin, and norepinephrine in specific regions of the brain.

Abuse of methamphetamine is associated with cognitive impairment, psychosis, Parkinson's disease, extensive dental disease, and hypertension. Amphetamine and methamphetamine have high addictive potential, particularly when administered intravenously or by smoking. Idiosyncratic effects of MDMA include severe hyperthermia that can lead to rhabdomyolysis and disseminated intravascular coagulation. On occasion, patients present with seizures or obtundation due to severe hyponatremia. Ecstasy is commonly adulterated with other agents, leading to a wide range of other adverse effects.[182]

In the setting of acute intoxication, amphetamines increase volatile anesthetic requirements and reduce the duration of thiopental. These agents have unpredictable effects on the response to sympathomimetic drugs. Hypertensive effects akin to those seen with cocaine can be observed and are managed similarly. Severe hyperthermia is treated by supportive measures. It is unclear if dantrolene is useful in this setting. Postoperatively, discontinuance of amphetamine and methamphetamine can lead to a withdrawal syndrome similar to that seen with cocaine.

KEY POINTS

- Psychopharmacologic drugs are among the most frequently prescribed agents. The pharmacology and clinical significance of these drugs in the perioperative setting are often underappreciated.
- The underlying mechanisms for most of the drugs remains elusive, although theories for many converge in effects centered in serotonergic, noradrenergic, and dopaminergic pathways; other receptor groups important to anesthetic pharmacology, including GABA, acetylcholine, and glutamate receptors, are also frequently implicated.
- A number of psychopharmacologic agents are potent inducers or inhibitors of specific cytochrome P450 isoenzymes and thus have the potential to alter the metabolism of many drugs used in the perioperative period.
- Many antipsychotic and mood stabilizer drugs have a narrow therapeutic index with multiple warnings in the product labeling. Pharmacologic and physiologic changes in the perioperative period have the potential to alter plasma concentrations and therapeutic/toxic effects.

- Several psychopharmacologic agents are associated with effects on cardiac conduction, seizure threshold, CNS depression, autonomic and serotonergic responsivity, the neuroendocrine response to stress, bleeding tendency, and other parameters relevant to anesthetic care. Interaction between some drugs, such as meperidine with monoamine oxidase inhibitors, can be severe or fatal.
- Neuroleptic malignant syndrome (NMS), which can be triggered by many antipsychotics, very closely resembles malignant hyperthermia (MH) and is treated similarly. Patients with a history of NMS should be regarded as MH-susceptible.
- Most psychopharmacologic drugs, including the commonly prescribed antidepressants and anxiolytics, cause changes in receptor expression and function, and are associated with withdrawal syndromes if discontinued abruptly. Psychopharmacologic agents should almost always be continued during the perioperative period.
- Levodopa for Parkinson's disease should be continued perioperatively and consideration given to enteral administration for longer procedures.
- The decision to continue anticholinesterase therapy for myasthenia gravis should be individualized. These agents interact with neuromuscular blockers and inhibit the metabolism of ester-type local anesthetics and succinylcholine.
- Substance abuse is common in patients undergoing anesthesia. Acute intoxication can lead to adverse interactions with anesthetic agents and vasoactive drugs.

Key References

Birkmayer W, Hornykiewicz O. [The L-3,4-dioxyphenylalanine (DOPA)-effect in Parkinson-akinesia.] *Wien Klin Wochenschr.* 1961;73:787-788. This landmark work led to the establishment of L-DOPA as the principal treatment of Parkinson's disease. (Ref. 143)
Fournier JC, DeRubeis RJ, Hollon SD, et al. Antidepressant drug effects and depression severity: a patient-level meta-analysis. *JAMA.* 2010;303:47-53. Confirming a 2008 study using previously unpublished data from the FDA that suggested antidepressants might be ineffective in patients with mild to moderate baseline symptoms, this large and controversial meta-analysis casts doubt on the utility of widespread antidepressant use and suggests that only patients with severe baseline symptoms will benefit. (Ref. 29)
Kane J, Honigfeld G, Singer J, Meltzer H. Clozapine for the treatment-resistant schizophrenic. A double-blind comparison with chlorpromazine. *Arch Gen Psychiatry.* 1988;45:789-796. This large muticenter trial demonstrated the efficacy of clozapine in otherwise treatment-resistant schizophrenia, setting a path for FDA approval despite the risk of agranulocytosis associated with the drug. (Ref. 79)
Lieberman JA, Stroup TS, McEvoy JP, et al. Effectiveness of antipsychotic drugs in patients with chronic schizophrenia. *N Engl J Med.* 2005;353:1209-1223. This study broke ground in evaluating the effectiveness of the second-generation antipsychotics in comparison to the first generation agents. Efficacies were similar, but the clinical course was dominated by a 74% rate of discontinuation. (Ref. 81)
Meltzer HY. Clinical studies on the mechanism of action of clozapine: the dopamine-serotonin hypothesis of schizophrenia. *Psychopharmacology (Berl).* 1989;99(Suppl):S18-S27. This landmark paper put forward the hypothesis that antagonism of D_2 and $5\text{-}HT_2$ receptors and enhancement of DA and 5-HT release are critical elements in the action of clozapine to minimize both positive and negative symptoms of schizophrenia, and offers insights into the underlying pathologic mechanisms. (Ref. 83)
Melvin MA, Johnson BH, Quasha AL, Eger 3rd EI. Induction of anesthesia with midazolam decreases halothane MAC in humans. *Anesthesiology.* 1982;57:238-241. This study established an interaction between the benzodiazepines and volatile anesthetics at a time when the mechanisms for neither were well elucidated, and formed a foundation for predicting how nonanesthetic sedatives would affect anesthetic management. (Ref. 66a)
Wong DT, Horng JS, Bymaster FP, et al. A selective inhibitor of serotonin uptake: Lilly 110140, 3-(p-trifluoromethylphenoxy)-N-methyl-3-phenylpropylamine. *Life Sci.* 1974;15:471-479. Principally of historical import, this paper represents the initial description of an SSRI, describing the drug that would come to be named fluoxetine and be marketed under the name Prozac. (Ref. 28)

References

1. National Prescription Audit PLUS. Plymouth Meeting, CT, IMS Health, 2009.
2. Pratt LA, Brody DJ, Gu Q. *Antidepressant use in persons aged 12 and over: United States, 2005-2008, NCHS data brief, no 76.* Hyattsville, MD: National Center for Health Statistics; 2011.
3. Gu Q, Dillon C, Burt V. *Prescription drug use continues to increase: U.S. prescription drug data for 2007-2008., NCHC data brief, no 42.* Hyattsville, MD: National Center for Health Statistics; 2010.
4. Schatzberg AF, Nemeroff CB. *The American Psychiatric Publishing Textbook of Psychopharmacology.* 4th ed. Arlington, Va: American Psychiatric Publishing; 2009.
5. Kuhn R. The treatment of depressive states with G 22355 (imipramine hydrochloride). *Am J Psychiatry.* 1958;115:459-464.
6. Tatsumi M, Groshan K, Blakely RD, Richelson E. Pharmacological profile of antidepressants and related compounds at human monoamine transporters. *Eur J Pharmacol.* 1997;340:249-258.
7. Coupet J, Rauh CE, Szues-Myers VA, Yunger LM. 2-Chloro-11-(1-piperazinyl)dibenz[b, f] [1, 4]oxazepine (amoxapine), an antidepressant with antipsychotic properties—a possible role for 7-hydroxyamoxapine. *Biochem Pharmacol.* 1979;28:2514-2515.
8. Tremblay P, Blier P. Catecholaminergic strategies for the treatment of major depression. *Curr Drug Targets.* 2006;7:149-158.
9. Marek GJ, Carpenter LL, McDougle CJ, Price LH. Synergistic action of 5-HT2A antagonists and selective serotonin reuptake inhibitors in neuropsychiatric disorders. *Neuropsychopharmacology.* 2003;28:402-412.
10. Szabo ST, Blier P. Effect of the selective noradrenergic reuptake inhibitor reboxetine on the firing activity of noradrenaline and serotonin neurons. *Eur J Neurosci.* 2001;13:2077-2087.
11. Narita N, Hashimoto K, Tomitaka S, Minabe Y. Interactions of selective serotonin reuptake inhibitors with subtypes of sigma receptors in rat brain. *Eur J Pharmacol.* 1996;307:117-119.
12. Madsen H, Nielsen KK, Brosen K. Imipramine metabolism in relation to the sparteine and mephenytoin oxidation polymorphisms—a population study. *Br J Clin Pharmacol.* 1995;39:433-439.
13. Tricyclic antidepressants—blood level measurements and clinical outcome: an APA Task Force report. Task Force on the Use of Laboratory Tests in Psychiatry. *Am J Psychiatry.* 1985;142:155-162.
14. Rush AJ. Depression in primary care: detection, diagnosis and treatment. Agency for Health Care Policy and Research. *Am Fam Physician.* 1993;47:1776-1788.
15. Frank E, Kupfer DJ, Perel JM, et al. Three-year outcomes for maintenance therapies in recurrent depression. *Arch Gen Psychiatry.* 1990;47:1093-1099.
16. Greist JH, Jefferson JW, Kobak KA, Katzelnick DJ, Serlin RC. Efficacy and tolerability of serotonin transport inhibitors in obsessive-compulsive disorder. A meta-analysis. *Arch Gen Psychiatry.* 1995;52:53-60.
17. Wilens TE, Biederman J, Prince J, et al. Six-week, double-blind, placebo-controlled study of desipramine for adult attention deficit hyperactivity disorder. *Am J Psychiatry.* 1996;153:1147-1153.

18. Saarto T, Wiffen PJ. Antidepressants for neuropathic pain. *Cochrane Database Syst Rev.* 2007: CD005454.
19. Yoshimura M, Furue H. Mechanisms for the anti-nociceptive actions of the descending noradrenergic and serotonergic systems in the spinal cord. *J Pharmacol Sci.* 2006;101:107-117.
20. Preskorn SH, Fast GA. Tricyclic antidepressant-induced seizures and plasma drug concentration. *J Clin Psychiatry.* 1992;53:160-162.
21. Preskorn SH, Jerkovich GS. Central nervous system toxicity of tricyclic antidepressants: phenomenology, course, risk factors, and role of therapeutic drug monitoring. *J Clin Psychopharmacol.* 1990;10:88-95.
22. Woolf AD, Erdman AR, Nelson LS, et al. Tricyclic antidepressant poisoning: an evidence-based consensus guideline for out-of-hospital management. *Clin Toxicol (Phila).* 2007;45:203-233.
23. Bronstein AC, Spyker DA, Cantilena Jr LR, Green J, Rumack BH, Heard SE. 2006 Annual Report of the American Association of Poison Control Centers' National Poison Data System (NPDS). *Clin Toxicol (Phila).* 2007;45:815-917.
24. Sprung J, Schoenwald PK, Levy P, Krajewski LP. Treating intraoperative hypotension in a patient on long-term tricyclic antidepressants: a case of aborted aortic surgery. *Anesthesiology.* 1997;86:990-992.
25. Stiff JL, Harris DB. Clonidine withdrawal complicated by amitriptyline therapy. *Anesthesiology.* 1983;59:73-74.
26. Edwards RP, Miller RD, Roizen MF, et al. Cardiac responses to imipramine and pancuronium during anesthesia with halothane or enflurane. *Anesthesiology.* 1979;50:421-425.
27. Spiss CK, Smith CM, Maze M. Halothane-epinephrine arrhythmias and adrenergic responsiveness after chronic imipramine administration in dogs. *Anesth Analg.* 1984;63:825-828.
28. Wong DT, Horng JS, Bymaster FP, Hauser KL, Molloy BB. A selective inhibitor of serotonin uptake: Lilly 110140, 3-(p-trifluoromethylphenoxy)-N-methyl-3-phenylpropylamine. *Life Sci.* 1974;15:471-479.
29. Fournier JC, DeRubeis RJ, Hollon SD, et al. Antidepressant drug effects and depression severity: a patient-level meta-analysis. *JAMA.* 2010;303:47-53.
30. Hiemke C, Hartter S. Pharmacokinetics of selective serotonin reuptake inhibitors. *Pharmacol Ther.* 2000;85:11-28.
31. Blier P. Pharmacology of rapid-onset antidepressant treatment strategies. *J Clin Psychiatry.* 2001;62(Suppl 15):12-17.
32. Anthony JP, Sexton TJ, Neumaier JF. Antidepressant-induced regulation of 5-HT(1b) mRNA in rat dorsal raphe nucleus reverses rapidly after drug discontinuation. *J Neurosci Res.* 2000;61:82-87.
33. Krishnan V, Nestler EJ. The molecular neurobiology of depression. *Nature.* 2008;455:894-902.
34. Preskorn SH. Clinically relevant pharmacology of selective serotonin reuptake inhibitors. An overview with emphasis on pharmacokinetics and effects on oxidative drug metabolism. *Clin Pharmacokinet.* 1997;32(Suppl 1):1-21.
35. Rasmussen BB, Brosen K. Is therapeutic drug monitoring a case for optimizing clinical outcome and avoiding interactions of the selective serotonin reuptake inhibitors? *Ther Drug Monit.* 2000;22:143-154.
36. Cipriani A, Furukawa TA, Salanti G, et al. Comparative efficacy and acceptability of 12 new-generation antidepressants: a multiple-treatments meta-analysis. *Lancet.* 2009;373:746-758.
37. Ioannidis JP. Effectiveness of antidepressants: an evidence myth constructed from a thousand randomized trials? *Philos Ethics Humanit Med.* 2008;3:14.
38. Kirsch I, Deacon BJ, Huedo-Medina TB, Scoboria A, Moore TJ, Johnson BT. Initial severity and antidepressant benefits: a meta-analysis of data submitted to the Food and Drug Administration. *PLoS Med.* 2008;5:e45.
39. Soomro GM, Altman D, Rajagopal S, Oakley-Browne M. Selective serotonin re-uptake inhibitors (SSRIs) versus placebo for obsessive compulsive disorder (OCD). *Cochrane Database Syst Rev.* 2008: CD001765.
40. Michelson D, Allgulander C, Dantendorfer K, et al. Efficacy of usual antidepressant dosing regimens of fluoxetine in panic disorder: randomised, placebo-controlled trial. *Br J Psychiatry.* 2001;179:514-518.
41. Brown J, O'Brien PM, Marjoribanks J, Wyatt K. Selective serotonin reuptake inhibitors for premenstrual syndrome. *Cochrane Database Syst Rev.* 2009: CD001396.
42. Stein DJ, Ipser JC, Seedat S. Pharmacotherapy for post traumatic stress disorder (PTSD). *Cochrane Database Syst Rev.* 2006: CD002795.
43. Giuliano F, Hellstrom WJ. The pharmacological treatment of premature ejaculation. *BJU Int.* 2008;102:668-675.
44. Olfson M, Marcus SC, Shaffer D. Antidepressant drug therapy and suicide in severely depressed children and adults: a case-control study. *Arch Gen Psychiatry.* 2006;63:865-872.
45. Alvarez PA, Pahissa J. QT alterations in psychopharmacology: proven candidates and suspects. *Curr Drug Saf.* 2010;5:97-104.
46. Li N, Wallen NH, Ladjevardi M, Hjemdahl P. Effects of serotonin on platelet activation in whole blood. *Blood Coagul Fibrinolysis.* 1997;8:517-523.
47. Schalekamp T, Klungel OH, Souverein PC, de Boer A. Increased bleeding risk with concurrent use of selective serotonin reuptake inhibitors and coumarins. *Arch Intern Med.* 2008;168:180-185.
48. Movig KL, Janssen MW, de Waal Malefijt J, Kabel PJ, Leufkens HG, Egberts AC. Relationship of serotonergic antidepressants and need for blood transfusion in orthopedic surgical patients. *Arch Intern Med.* 2003;163:2354-2358.
49. Richards JB, Papaioannou A, Adachi JD, et al. Effect of selective serotonin reuptake inhibitors on the risk of fracture. *Arch Intern Med.* 2007;167:188-194.
50. Kelly CA, Dhaun N, Laing WJ, Strachan FE, Good AM, Bateman DN. Comparative toxicity of citalopram and the newer antidepressants after overdose. *J Toxicol Clin Toxicol.* 2004;42:67-71.
51. Boyer EW, Shannon M. The serotonin syndrome. *N Engl J Med.* 2005;352:1112-1120.
52. Cesura AM, Pletscher A. The new generation of monoamine oxidase inhibitors. *Prog Drug Res.* 1992;38:171-297.
53. Quitkin FM, McGrath PJ, Stewart JW, et al. Atypical depression, panic attacks, and response to imipramine and phenelzine. A replication. *Arch Gen Psychiatry.* 1990;47:935-941.
54. McGrath PJ, Stewart JW, Fava M, et al. Tranylcypromine versus venlafaxine plus mirtazapine following three failed antidepressant medication trials for depression: a STAR*D report. *Am J Psychiatry.* 2006;163:1531-1541; quiz 1666.
55. Frampton JE, Plosker GL. Selegiline transdermal system: in the treatment of major depressive disorder. *Drugs.* 2007;67:257-267.
56. Jacob G, Gamboa A, Diedrich A, Shibao C, Robertson D, Biaggioni I. Tyramine-induced vasodilation mediated by dopamine contamination: a paradox resolved. *Hypertension.* 2005;46:355-359.
57. Gillman PK. Monoamine oxidase inhibitors, opioid analgesics and serotonin toxicity. *Br J Anaesth.* 2005;95:434-441.
58. Wells DG, Bjorksten AR. Monoamine oxidase inhibitors revisited. *Can J Anaesth.* 1989;36:64-74.
59. Doyle DJ. Ketamine induction and monoamine oxidase inhibitors. *J Clin Anesth.* 1990;2:324-325.
60. IMS National Prescription Audit. Norwalk, Conn, IMS Health, 2010.
61. Mohler H, Fritschy JM, Rudolph U. A new benzodiazepine pharmacology. *J Pharmacol Exp Ther.* 2002;300:2-8.
62. Batelaan NM, Van Balkom AJ, Stein DJ. Evidence-based pharmacotherapy of panic disorder: an update. *Int J Neuropsychopharmacol.* 2011:1-13.
63. Martin JL, Sainz-Pardo M, Furukawa TA, Martin-Sanchez E, Seoane T, Galan C. Benzodiazepines in generalized anxiety disorder: heterogeneity of outcomes based on a systematic review and meta-analysis of clinical trials. *J Psychopharmacol.* 2007;21:774-782.
64. Tobler I, Kopp C, Deboer T, Rudolph U. Diazepam-induced changes in sleep: role of the alpha 1 GABA(A) receptor subtype. *Proc Natl Acad Sci U S A.* 2001;98:6464-6469.
65. Chouinard G. Issues in the clinical use of benzodiazepines: potency, withdrawal, and rebound. *J Clin Psychiatry.* 2004;65(Suppl 5):7-12.
66. Mashour GA, Orser BA, Avidan MS. Intraoperative awareness: from neurobiology to clinical practice. *Anesthesiology.* 2011;114:1218-1233.
67. McCreadie RG. The Nithsdale schizophrenia surveys. An overview. *Soc Psychiatry Psychiatr Epidemiol.* 1992;27:40-45.
68. Kapur S, Zipursky R, Jones C, Remington G, Houle S. Relationship between dopamine D(2) occupancy, clinical response, and side effects: a double-blind PET study of first-episode schizophrenia. *Am J Psychiatry.* 2000;157:514-520.
69. Mac TB, Girard F, McKenty S, et al. A difficult airway is not more prevalent in patients suffering from spasmodic torticollis: a case series. *Can J Anaesth.* 2004;51:250-253.

70. Christodoulou C, Kalaitzi C. Antipsychotic drug-induced acute laryngeal dystonia: two case reports and a mini review. *J Psychopharmacol.* 2005;19:307-311.

71. Miller CH, Fleischhacker WW. Managing antipsychotic-induced acute and chronic akathisia. *Drug Saf.* 2000;22:73-81.

72. Aia PG, Revuelta GJ, Cloud LJ, Factor SA. Tardive dyskinesia. *Curr Treat Options Neurol.* 2011;13:231-241.

73. Rao AS, Camilleri M. Review article: metoclopramide and tardive dyskinesia. *Aliment Pharmacol Ther.* 2010;31:11-19.

74. Shalev A, Hermesh H, Munitz H. Mortality from neuroleptic malignant syndrome. *J Clin Psychiatry.* 1989;50:18-25.

75. Gurrera RJ. Is neuroleptic malignant syndrome a neurogenic form of malignant hyperthermia? *Clin Neuropharmacol.* 2002;25:183-193.

76. Caroff SN, Rosenberg H, Fletcher JE, Heiman-Patterson TD, Mann SC. Malignant hyperthermia susceptibility in neuroleptic malignant syndrome. *Anesthesiology.* 1987;67:20-25.

77. Glassman AH, Bigger Jr JT. Antipsychotic drugs: prolonged QTc interval, torsade de pointes, and sudden death. *Am J Psychiatry.* 2001;158:1774-1782.

78. Ludwin DB, Shafer SL. Con: The black box warning on droperidol should not be removed (but should be clarified!). *Anesth Analg.* 2008;106:1418-1420.

79. Kane J, Honigfeld G, Singer J, Meltzer H. Clozapine for the treatment-resistant schizophrenic. A double-blind comparison with chlorpromazine. *Arch Gen Psychiatry.* 1988;45:789-796.

80. Jones PB, Barnes TR, Davies L, et al. Randomized controlled trial of the effect on Quality of Life of second- vs first-generation antipsychotic drugs in schizophrenia: Cost Utility of the Latest Antipsychotic Drugs in Schizophrenia Study (CUtLASS 1). *Arch Gen Psychiatry.* 2006;63:1079-1087.

81. Lieberman JA, Stroup TS, McEvoy JP, et al. Effectiveness of antipsychotic drugs in patients with chronic schizophrenia. *N Engl J Med.* 2005;353:1209-1223.

82. Farde L, Nordstrom AL, Wiesel FA, Pauli S, Halldin C, Sedvall G. Positron emission tomographic analysis of central D1 and D2 dopamine receptor occupancy in patients treated with classical neuroleptics and clozapine. Relation to extrapyramidal side effects. *Arch Gen Psychiatry.* 1992;49:538-544.

83. Meltzer HY. Clinical studies on the mechanism of action of clozapine: the dopamine-serotonin hypothesis of schizophrenia. *Psychopharmacology (Berl).* 1989;99(Suppl):S18-S27.

84. Meltzer HY, Matsubara S, Lee JC. Classification of typical and atypical antipsychotic drugs on the basis of dopamine D-1, D-2 and serotonin2 pKi values. *J Pharmacol Exp Ther.* 1989;251:238-246.

85. Kuroki T, Nagao N, Nakahara T. Neuropharmacology of second-generation antipsychotic drugs: a validity of the serotonin-dopamine hypothesis. *Prog Brain Res.* 2008;172:199-212.

86. Honigfeld G. Effects of the clozapine national registry system on incidence of deaths related to agranulocytosis. *Psychiatr Serv.* 1996;47:52-56.

87. Kilian JG, Kerr K, Lawrence C, Celermajer DS. Myocarditis and cardiomyopathy associated with clozapine. *Lancet.* 1999;354:1841-1845.

88. Marder SR, Sorsaburu S, Dunayevich E, et al. Case reports of postmarketing adverse event experiences with olanzapine intramuscular treatment in patients with agitation. *J Clin Psychiatry.* 2010;71:433-441.

89. Komossa K, Rummel-Kluge C, Hunger H, et al. Olanzapine versus other atypical antipsychotics for schizophrenia. *Cochrane Database Syst Rev.* 2010: CD006654.

90. Newcomer JW. Second-generation (atypical) antipsychotics and metabolic effects: a comprehensive literature review. *CNS Drugs.* 2005;19(Suppl 1):1-93.

91. Kapur S, Zipursky R, Jones C, Shammi CS, Remington G, Seeman P. A positron emission tomography study of quetiapine in schizophrenia: a preliminary finding of an antipsychotic effect with only transiently high dopamine D2 receptor occupancy. *Arch Gen Psychiatry.* 2000;57:553-559.

92. Nemeroff CB, Kinkead B, Goldstein J. Quetiapine: preclinical studies, pharmacokinetics, drug interactions, and dosing. *J Clin Psychiatry.* 2002;63(Suppl 13):5-11.

93. Larmo I, de Nayer A, Windhager E, et al. Efficacy and tolerability of quetiapine in patients with schizophrenia who switched from haloperidol, olanzapine or risperidone. *Hum Psychopharmacol.* 2005;20:573-581.

94. Burris KD, Molski TF, Xu C, et al. Aripiprazole, a novel antipsychotic, is a high-affinity partial agonist at human dopamine D2 receptors. *J Pharmacol Exp Ther.* 2002;302:381-389.

95. Jordan S, Koprivica V, Chen R, Tottori K, Kikuchi T, Altar CA. The antipsychotic aripiprazole is a potent, partial agonist at the human 5-HT1A receptor. *Eur J Pharmacol.* 2002;441:137-140.

96. Stip E, Tourjman V. Aripiprazole in schizophrenia and schizoaffective disorder: a review. *Clin Ther.* 2010;32(Suppl 1):S3-S20.

97. Kapur S, Zipursky RB, Remington G. Clinical and theoretical implications of 5-HT2 and D2 receptor occupancy of clozapine, risperidone, and olanzapine in schizophrenia. *Am J Psychiatry.* 1999;156:286-293.

98. Seeman P. Atypical antipsychotics: mechanism of action. *Can J Psychiatry.* 2002;47:27-38.

99. Ward ME, Musa MN, Bailey L. Clinical pharmacokinetics of lithium. *J Clin Pharmacol.* 1994;34:280-285.

100. Hahn CG, Umapathy, Wang HY, Koneru R, Levinson DF, Friedman E. Lithium and valproic acid treatments reduce PKC activation and receptor-G protein coupling in platelets of bipolar manic patients. *J Psychiatr Res.* 2005;39:355-363.

101. Einat H, Kofman O, Itkin O, Lewitan RJ, Belmaker RH. Augmentation of lithium's behavioral effect by inositol uptake inhibitors. *J Neural Transm.* 1998;105:31-38.

102. Li X, Friedman AB, Zhu W, et al. Lithium regulates glycogen synthase kinase-3beta in human peripheral blood mononuclear cells: implication in the treatment of bipolar disorder. *Biol Psychiatry.* 2007;61:216-222.

103. Williams RS, Harwood AJ. Lithium therapy and signal transduction. *Trends Pharmacol Sci.* 2000;21:61-64.

104. Price LH, Charney DS, Delgado PL, Heninger GR. Lithium and serotonin function: implications for the serotonin hypothesis of depression. *Psychopharmacology (Berl).* 1990;100:3-12.

105. Haddjeri N, Szabo ST, de Montigny C, Blier P. Increased tonic activation of rat forebrain 5-HT(1A) receptors by lithium addition to antidepressant treatments. *Neuropsychopharmacology.* 2000;22:346-356.

106. Grandjean EM, Aubry JM. Lithium: updated human knowledge using an evidence-based approach. Part II: Clinical pharmacology and therapeutic monitoring. *CNS Drugs.* 2009;23:331-349.

107. Bowden CL, Grunze H, Mullen J, et al. A randomized, double-blind, placebo-controlled efficacy and safety study of quetiapine or lithium as monotherapy for mania in bipolar disorder. *J Clin Psychiatry.* 2005;66:111-121.

108. Smith LA, Cornelius V, Warnock A, Tacchi MJ, Taylor D. Pharmacological interventions for acute bipolar mania: a systematic review of randomized placebo-controlled trials. *Bipolar Disord.* 2007;9:551-560.

109. Perlis RH, Welge JA, Vornik LA, Hirschfeld RM, Keck Jr PE. Atypical antipsychotics in the treatment of mania: a meta-analysis of randomized, placebo-controlled trials. *J Clin Psychiatry.* 2006;67:509-516.

110. Geddes JR, Burgess S, Hawton K, Jamison K, Goodwin GM. Long-term lithium therapy for bipolar disorder: systematic review and meta-analysis of randomized controlled trials. *Am J Psychiatry.* 2004;161:217-222.

111. Tondo L, Baldessarini RJ. Reduced suicide risk during lithium maintenance treatment. *J Clin Psychiatry.* 2000;61(Suppl 9):97-104.

112. Tondo L, Baldessarini RJ, Floris G. Long-term clinical effectiveness of lithium maintenance treatment in types I and II bipolar disorders. *Br J Psychiatry Suppl.* 2001;41:S184-S190.

113. Nierenberg AA, Fava M, Trivedi MH, et al. A comparison of lithium and T(3) augmentation following two failed medication treatments for depression: a STAR*D report. *Am J Psychiatry.* 2006;163:1519-1530; quiz 1665.

114. Chuang DM. Neuroprotective and neurotrophic actions of the mood stabilizer lithium: can it be used to treat neurodegenerative diseases? *Crit Rev Neurobiol.* 2004;16:83-90.

115. Forlenza OV, Diniz BS, Radanovic M, Santos FS, Talib LL, Gattaz WF. Disease-modifying properties of long-term lithium treatment for amnestic mild cognitive impairment: randomised controlled trial. *Br J Psychiatry.* 2011;198:351-356.

116. Bendz H, Aurell M. Drug-induced diabetes insipidus: incidence, prevention and management. *Drug Saf.* 1999;21:449-456.

117. Fagiolini A, Kupfer DJ, Scott J, et al. Hypothyroidism in patients with bipolar I disorder treated primarily with lithium. *Epidemiol Psychiatr Soc.* 2006;15:123-127.

118. Oudit GY, Korley V, Backx PH, Dorian P. Lithium-induced sinus node disease at therapeutic concentrations: linking lithium-induced blockade of sodium channels to impaired pacemaker activity. *Can J Cardiol*. 2007;23:229-232.

119. Gelenberg AJ, Jefferson JW. Lithium tremor. *J Clin Psychiatry*. 1995;56:283-287.

120. Wilting I, Movig KL, Moolenaar M, et al. Drug-drug interactions as a determinant of elevated lithium serum levels in daily clinical practice. *Bipolar Disord*. 2005;7:274-280.

121. Finley PR, Warner MD, Peabody CA. Clinical relevance of drug interactions with lithium. *Clin Pharmacokinet*. 1995;29:172-191.

122. Hill GE, Wong KC, Hodges MR. Lithium carbonate and neuromuscular blocking agents. *Anesthesiology*. 1977;46:122-126.

123. Saarnivaara L, Ertama P. [Interactions between lithium/rubidium and six muscle relaxants. A study on the rat phrenic nerve-hemidiaphragm preparation]. *Anaesthesist*. 1992;41:760-764.

124. Yatham LN, Kennedy SH, Schaffer A, et al. Canadian Network for Mood and Anxiety Treatments (CANMAT) and International Society for Bipolar Disorders (ISBD) collaborative update of CANMAT guidelines for the management of patients with bipolar disorder: update 2009. *Bipolar Disord*. 2009;11:225-255.

125. Macritchie K, Geddes JR, Scott J, Haslam D, de Lima M, Goodwin G. Valproate for acute mood episodes in bipolar disorder. *Cochrane Database Syst Rev*. 2003: CD004052.

126. Swann AC, Bowden CL, Morris D, et al. Depression during mania. Treatment response to lithium or divalproex. *Arch Gen Psychiatry*. 1997;54:37-42.

127. Tremolizzo L, Carboni G, Ruzicka WB, et al. An epigenetic mouse model for molecular and behavioral neuropathologies related to schizophrenia vulnerability. *Proc Natl Acad Sci U S A*. 2002;99:17095-17100.

128. Shaltiel G, Shamir A, Shapiro J, et al. Valproate decreases inositol biosynthesis. *Biol Psychiatry*. 2004;56:868-874.

129. Harwood AJ, Agam G. Search for a common mechanism of mood stabilizers. *Biochem Pharmacol*. 2003;66:179-189.

130. DeVane CL. Pharmacokinetics, drug interactions, and tolerability of valproate. *Psychopharmacol Bull*. 2003;37(Suppl 2):25-42.

131. Sobotka JL, Alexander B, Cook BL. A review of carbamazepine's hematologic reactions and monitoring recommendations. *DICP*. 1990;24:1214-1219.

132. Locharernkul C, Shotelersuk V, Hirankarn N. Pharmacogenetic screening of carbamazepine-induced severe cutaneous allergic reactions. *J Clin Neurosci*. 2011;18(10):1289-1294.

133. Backman JT, Olkkola KT, Ojala M, Laaksovirta H, Neuvonen PJ. Concentrations and effects of oral midazolam are greatly reduced in patients treated with carbamazepine or phenytoin. *Epilepsia*. 1996;37:253-257.

134. Prica C, Hascoet M, Bourin M. Antidepressant-like effect of lamotrigine is reversed by veratrine: a possible role of sodium channels in bipolar depression. *Behav Brain Res*. 2008;191:49-54.

135. Ketter TA, Manji HK, Post RM. Potential mechanisms of action of lamotrigine in the treatment of bipolar disorders. *J Clin Psychopharmacol*. 2003;23:484-495.

136. Seo HJ, Chiesa A, Lee SJ, et al. Safety and tolerability of lamotrigine: results from 12 placebo-controlled clinical trials and clinical implications. *Clin Neuropharmacol*. 2011;34:39-47.

137. Bowden CL, Asnis GM, Ginsberg LD, Bentley B, Leadbetter R, White R. Safety and tolerability of lamotrigine for bipolar disorder. *Drug Saf*. 2004;27:173-184.

138. Kumar R. Approved and investigational uses of modafinil: an evidence-based review. *Drugs*. 2008;68:1803-1839.

139. Perruchoud C, Chollet-Rivier M. Cardiac arrest during induction of anaesthesia in a child on long-term amphetamine therapy. *Br J Anaesth*. 2008;100:421-422.

140. Fischer SP, Schmiesing CA, Guta CG, Brock-Utne JG. General anesthesia and chronic amphetamine use: should the drug be stopped preoperatively? *Anesth Analg*. 2006;103:203-206.

141. Carlsson A, Lindqvist M, Magnusson T. 3,4-Dihydroxyphenylalanine and 5-hydroxytryptophan as reserpine antagonists. *Nature*. 1957;180:1200.

142. Carlsson A, Lindqvist M, Magnusson T, Waldeck B. On the presence of 3-hydroxytyramine in brain. *Science*. 1958;127:471.

143. Birkmayer W, Hornykiewicz O. [The L-3,4-dioxyphenylalanine (DOPA)-effect in Parkinson-akinesia.] *Wien Klin Wochenschr*. 1961;73:787-788.

144. Kostic V, Przedborski S, Flaster E, Sternic N. Early development of levodopa-induced dyskinesias and response fluctuations in young-onset Parkinson's disease. *Neurology*. 1991;41:202-205.

145. Khor SP, Hsu A. The pharmacokinetics and pharmacodynamics of levodopa in the treatment of Parkinson's disease. *Curr Clin Pharmacol*. 2007;2:234-243.

146. Hardie RJ, Malcolm SL, Lees AJ, Stern GM, Allen JG. The pharmacokinetics of intravenous and oral levodopa in patients with Parkinson's disease who exhibit on-off fluctuations. *Br J Clin Pharmacol*. 1986;22:429-436.

147. Gottwald MD, Aminoff MJ. Therapies for dopaminergic-induced dyskinesias in Parkinson disease. *Ann Neurol*. 2011;69:919-927.

148. Olanow CW, Watkins PB. Tolcapone: an efficacy and safety review (2007). *Clin Neuropharmacol*. 2007;30:287-294.

149. Kalenka A, Schwarz A. Anaesthesia and Parkinson's disease: how to manage with new therapies? *Curr Opin Anaesthesiol*. 2009;22:419-424.

150. Ikebe S, Harada T, Hashimoto T, et al. Prevention and treatment of malignant syndrome in Parkinson's disease: a consensus statement of the malignant syndrome research group. *Parkinsonism Relat Disord*. 2003;9(Suppl 1):S47-S49.

151. Tintner R, Manian P, Gauthier P, Jankovic J. Pleuropulmonary fibrosis after long-term treatment with the dopamine agonist pergolide for Parkinson Disease. *Arch Neurol*. 2005;62:1290-1295.

152. Bhattacharyya S, Schapira AH, Mikhailidis DP, Davar J. Drug-induced fibrotic valvular heart disease. *Lancet*. 2009;374:577-585.

153. Smith Y, Wichmann T, Factor SA, Delong MR. Parkinson's disease therapeutics: new developments and challenges since the introduction of levodopa. *Neuropsychopharmacology*. 2012;37(1):213-246.

154. Antonini A, Calandrella D. Pharmacokinetic evaluation of pramipexole. *Expert Opin Drug Metab Toxicol*. 2011;7:1307-1314.

155. Wright CE, Sisson TL, Ichhpurani AK, Peters GR. Steady-state pharmacokinetic properties of pramipexole in healthy volunteers. *J Clin Pharmacol*. 1997;37:520-525.

156. Shill HA, Stacy M. Update on ropinirole in the treatment of Parkinson's disease. *Neuropsychiatr Dis Treat*. 2009;5:33-36.

157. Schapira AH. Progress in neuroprotection in Parkinson's disease. *Eur J Neurol*. 2008;15(Suppl 1):5-13.

158. Kumar V, Kaminski HJ. Treatment of myasthenia gravis. *Curr Neurol Neurosci Rep*. 2011;11:89-96.

159. Sanders DB, Evoli A. Immunosuppressive therapies in myasthenia gravis. *Autoimmunity*. 2010;43:428-435.

160. Komloova M, Musilek K, Dolezal M, Gunn-Moore F, Kuca K. Structure-activity relationship of quaternary acetylcholinesterase inhibitors—outlook for early myasthenia gravis treatment. *Curr Med Chem*. 2010;17:1810-1824.

161. Aquilonius SM, Hartvig P. Clinical pharmacokinetics of cholinesterase inhibitors. *Clin Pharmacokinet*. 1986;11:236-249.

162. Stone JG, Matteo RS, Ornstein E, et al. Aging alters the pharmacokinetics of pyridostigmine. *Anesth Analg*. 1995;81:773-776.

163. Matteo RS, Young WL, Ornstein E, Schwartz AF, Silverberg PA, Diaz J. Pharmacokinetics and pharmacodynamics of edrophonium in elderly surgical patients. *Anesth Analg*. 1990;71:334-339.

164. Stern JM. Overview of evaluation and treatment guidelines for epilepsy. *Curr Treat Options Neurol*. 2009;11:273-284.

165. Kwan P, Schachter SC, Brodie MJ. Drug-resistant epilepsy. *N Engl J Med*. 2011;365:919-926.

166. Stafstrom CE, Grippon S, Kirkpatrick P. Ezogabine (retigabine). *Nat Rev Drug Discov*. 2011;10:729-730.

167. Deeks ED. Retigabine (ezogabine): in partial-onset seizures in adults with epilepsy. *CNS Drugs*. 2011;25:887-900.

168. Camerman A, Camerman N. Diphenylhydantoin and diazepam: molecular structure similarities and steric basis of anticonvulsant activity. *Science*. 1970;168:1457-1458.

169. Belliotti TR, Capiris T, Ekhato IV, et al. Structure-activity relationships of pregabalin and analogues that target the alpha(2)-delta protein. *J Med Chem*. 2005;48:2294-2307.

170. Lason W, Dudra-Jastrzebska M, Rejdak K, Czuczwar SJ. Basic mechanisms of antiepileptic drugs and their pharmacokinetic/pharmacodynamic interactions: an update. *Pharmacol Rep*. 2011;63:271-292.

171. Sperling MR, Ko J. Seizures and brain tumors. *Semin Oncol*. 2006;33:333-341.

172. Formisano R, Barba C, Buzzi MG, et al. The impact of prophylactic treatment on post-traumatic epilepsy after severe traumatic brain injury. *Brain Inj*. 2007;21:499-504.

173. Mockenhaupt M, Messenheimer J, Tennis P, Schlingmann J. Risk of Stevens-Johnson syndrome and toxic epidermal necrolysis in new users of antiepileptics. *Neurology*. 2005;64:1134-1138.

174. Mavragani CP, Vlachoyiannopoulos PG. Is polydipsia sometimes the cause of oxcarbazepine-induced hyponatremia? *Eur J Intern Med*. 2005;16:296-297.

175. Kofke WA. Anesthetic management of the patient with epilepsy or prior seizures. *Curr Opin Anaesthesiol*. 2010;23:391-399.

176. Aguayo LG, Peoples RW, Yeh HH, Yevenes GE. GABA(A) receptors as molecular sites of ethanol action. Direct or indirect actions? *Curr Top Med Chem*. 2002;2:869-885.

177. Howard RJ, Murail S, Ondricek KE, et al. Structural basis for alcohol modulation of a pentameric ligand-gated ion channel. *Proc Natl Acad Sci U S A*. 2011;108:12149-12154.

178. Cederbaum AI. Role of CYP2E1 in ethanol-induced oxidant stress, fatty liver and hepatotoxicity. *Dig Dis*. 2010;28:802-811.

179. Muhuri PK, Gfroerer JC. Mortality associated with illegal drug use among adults in the United States. *Am J Drug Alcohol Abuse*. 2011;37:155-164.

180. Navarro G, Moreno E, Aymerich M, et al. Direct involvement of sigma-1 receptors in the dopamine D1 receptor-mediated effects of cocaine. *Proc Natl Acad Sci U S A*. 2010;107:18676-18681.

181. Hernandez M, Birnbach DJ, Van Zundert AA. Anesthetic management of the illicit-substance-using patient. *Curr Opin Anaesthesiol*. 2005;18:315-324.

182. Steadman JL, Birnbach DJ. Patients on party drugs undergoing anesthesia. *Curr Opin Anaesthesiol*. 2003;16:147-152.

183. Hysek CM, Brugger R, Simmler LD, et al. Effects of the alpha2-adrenergic agonist clonidine on the pharmacodynamics and pharmacokinetics of 3,4 methylenedioxymethamphetamine in healthy volunteers. *J Pharmacol Exp Ther*. 2012;340(2):286-294.

184. Volkow ND, Fowler JS, Wang GJ, et al. Distribution and pharmacokinetics of methamphetamine in the human body: clinical implications. *PLoS One*. 2010;5:e15269.

Chapter 12

AUTONOMIC NERVOUS SYSTEM PHYSIOLOGY

Joel O. Johnson

HISTORICAL CONSIDERATIONS

A specialized taxonomy of the autonomic nervous system (ANS) has been developing since the time of Galen (AD 130-200). In the early 1900s, Langley first referred to the ANS.[1] He used the term *sympathetic nervous system* (SNS) as described by Willis in 1665, and introduced the second division as the *parasympathetic nervous system* (PNS) in 1921.[2] Although Langely initially described only the visceral motor system (efferent fibers), the existence of visceral reflex arcs necessitated the inclusion of the sensory (afferent) portions of the ANS.[3] Early anesthesia textbooks dealt with the practice of anesthesia, elucidating basic considerations, pharmacology and techniques, but did not contain explicit information dealing with the ANS. The evolution of the comprehensive anesthesia textbook has led to extensive chapters on the ANS.[2,4]

The ANS maintains cardiovascular, thermal, and gastrointestinal homeostasis. A firm understanding of the basic anatomy and physiology of the ANS forms an important foundation for the practice of anesthesiology. ANS structure, function, and reflexes are critical to the support of the circulation under anesthesia. This chapter reviews anatomy and physiology of the ANS relevant to anesthesia.

ANATOMY AND PHYSIOLOGY

ANS anatomy is comprised of central control and feedback areas, sensory receptors, peripheral effectors, and reflex conduction pathways. In addition, complex interactions occur between the ANS and the endocrine system (Chapter 30).[4] The renin-angiotensin system, antidiuretic hormone, glucocorticoid and mineralocorticoid responses, and insulin interact via an increasing number of receptor subtypes to maintain physiologic homeostasis (Figure 12-1).

There are no distinct centers of autonomic function in the cerebral cortex. However, input from various sensory systems can impact higher cortical centers, be processed, and result in efferent autonomic activity. Tachycardia and peripheral vasoconstriction heralding a "fight-or-flight" response or a vasovagal response (fainting) are well-known examples of this higher cortical sensory processing.[5] External stimuli representing a threat or danger are detected by the senses of hearing, touch, smell, or sight. These signals are sent to the

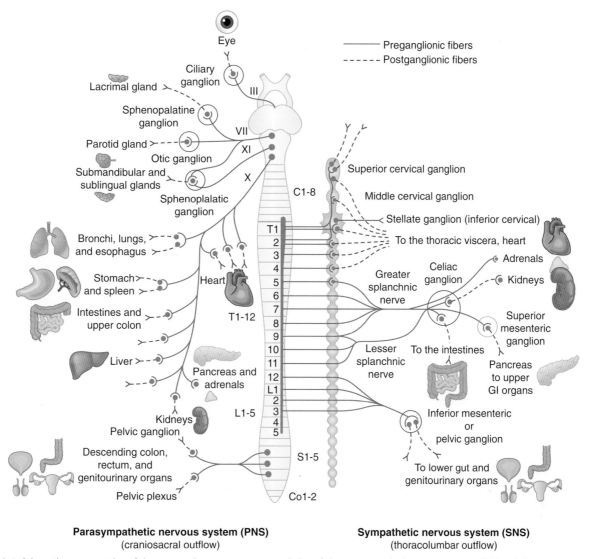

Figure 12-1 Schematic representation of the autonomic nervous system consisting of the parasympathetic nervous system *(left)* and the sympathetic nervous system *(right)*.

brainstem, where reflex responses are processed in the hypothalamus and the limbic forebrain. Higher cortical centers provide descending input to the paraventricular nucleus of the hypothalamus, which has projections to sympathetic and parasympathetic nuclei. Chronic stress alters these structures and their function leading to both sensitization and habituation of the stress response.[6,7]

The hypothalamus is the midbrain center that processes sympathetic and parasympathetic functions, temperature regulation, fluid regulation, neurohumoral control, and stress responses. Hunger, sleep, and sexual function are also regulated by the hypothalamus, dependent upon both cortical input and complex feedback control. The anterior hypothalamus controls temperature, while the posterior hypothalamus is involved in water regulation. The hypothalamic-pituitary axis is a part of the ANS that ultimately regulates long-term blood pressure control and stress responses.[7]

The output centers of the ANS reside in the medulla oblongata and the pons of the brainstem. Immediate control of blood pressure, heart rate, cardiac output, and ventilation is organized and integrated in specific nuclei. Tonic impulses

from nuclei like the nucleus tractus solitarius maintain blood pressure and respond to afferent signals from the sensory side of the ANS. These afferent impulses from the vagus (X) and glossopharyngeal (XI) nerves result in vasodilation and bradycardia (see section on ANS reflexes).

The ANS is anatomically and functionally divided into two complementary systems, the SNS and the PNS (see Figure 12-1). The peripheral SNS is controlled by the thoracolumbar segment of the spinal cord, while PNS control arises from the brainstem nuclei and sacral segments (see Figure 12-1). Activation of the SNS produces diffuse physiologic responses, while the PNS exerts local control of innervated organs.[8]

Both systems have efferent pathways through peripheral ganglia; the SNS ganglia are located close to the thoracolumbar spine, and the PNS ganglia are situated near or inside the innervated organs (see Figure 12-1; Figure 12-2). Ganglia serve as synaptic relay stations, and in the SNS coordinate an efferent mass action response through signal amplification. Thus one preganglionic SNS fiber can activate 20 to 30 postganglionic sympathetic neurons and their fibers. In contrast, PNS preganglionic fibers terminate in ganglia located in

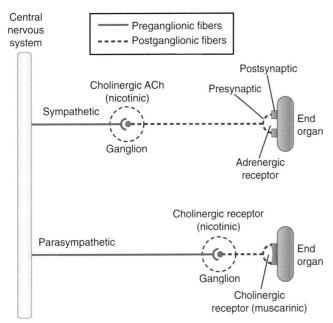

Figure 12-2 Differences between the location of the ganglia in the sympathetic and parasympathetic branches of the autonomic nervous system. The 22 paired sympathetic ganglia are located close to the vertebral column in the sympathetic chain. The unmyelinated postganglionic fibers innervate their respective organs. The exception is the adrenal gland, where the sympathetic preganglionic nerve fibers travel directly to the adrenal medulla. The parasympathetic preganglionic fibers travel directly to the organ of innervation, to synapse with postganglionic neuronal cell bodies.

Table 12-1. Autonomic Nervous System Receptor Types and Subtypes

RECEPTOR	EFFECTOR	RESPONSE TO STIMULATION
Sympathetic Nervous System		
α_1	Smooth muscle (vascular, iris radial, ureter, trigone, bladder sphincters)	Constriction
α_2	Presynaptic SNS nerve endings	Inhibition of NE release
	Brain	Neurotransmission
β_1	Heart	Increase rate, contractility, conduction
	Adipose tissue	Lipolysis
β_2	Blood vessels	Dilation
	Bronchioles	Dilation
	Kidney	Renin secretion
	Liver	Gluconeogenesis, glycogenolysis
	Endocrine pancreas	Insulin secretion
	Uterus	Relaxation
D_1	Blood vessels	Dilation
D_2	Presynaptic SNS nerve endings	Inhibition of NE release
Parasympathetic Nervous System		
M_1	Skeletal prejunctional nerve endings	Facilitate ACh release
M_2	Lung–presynaptic PNS nerve endings	Inhibits ACh release
	Visceral organs	Increase
M_3	Lung smooth muscle, postsynaptic	Bronchoconstriction
N_1	PNS and SNS ganglion	Ganglionic blockade
N_2	Skeletal muscle	Muscle contraction

ACh, Acetylcholine; *D,* dopamine; *M,* muscarinic; *N,* nicotinic; *NE,* norepinephrine; *PNS,* parasympathetic nervous system; *SNS,* sympathetic nervous system.

proximity to the innervated organs and affects only one to three postganglionic neurons.[2] The close proximity of PNS ganglia to their effector organs is the anatomic basis of the more focused and specific responses elicited by PNS activation.

Most organ systems are affected by both the SNS and the PNS. Different organ systems have their resting tone dominated by the SNS or the PNS, and this ratio can change depending on pathophysiologic states and can change over the lifetime of an individual. For instance, newborns are dominated by parasympathetic responses, hence bradycardia can be seen in 20% of unpremedicated infants during stressful situations such as anesthetic induction and airway manipulation, while it is uncommon in adults.[9] Vasoreactivity of the major blood vessels, arteries and arterioles is primarily responsive to the SNS, while PNS cardiovascular effects reside mainly at the level of the heart. Examples of the differential effects of the ANS in various organs and organ systems are summarized in Table 12-1.

In general, the SNS modulates the activity of vascular smooth muscle, cardiac muscle, and various glands (especially the adrenal gland); this modulation is critical for the fight-or-flight response. In contrast, the PNS modulates "rest-and-digest" functions such as salivation, lacrimation, urination, digestion, defecation, and sexual arousal.

Sympathetic Nervous System

The SNS is formed from preganglionic fibers in the thoracolumbar segments (T1-L3) of the spinal cord arising from the intermediolateral gray column (see Figure 12-1). These myelinated fibers enter the paravertebral ganglia and travel a

variable distance up or down the sympathetic chain to synapse with the neuronal cell bodies of postganglionic sympathetic neurons. The unmyelinated postganglionic fibers then innervate their respective organs. An exception to this rule is the adrenal gland, where the preganglionic fibers do not synapse in the thoracic ganglia, but course through the sympathetic chain into the adrenal medulla. The chromaffin cells in the adrenal medulla are derived from neuronal tissue and essentially function as the postganglionic cells.

The stellate ganglion consists of postganglionic neurons that provide sympathetic innervation to the head and neck. Preganglionic fibers from the first four or five thoracic segments form this ganglion as well as the superior cervical and middle cervical ganglia. Blockade of this structure with local anesthetic blocks the sympathetic fibers coursing to the ipsilateral head and neck, resulting in Horner syndrome, characterized by ptosis, miosis, enophthalmos, and anhydrosis on the affected side.[10] This syndrome would be seen as a direct effect of a stellate ganglion block and possibly be experienced as a side effect of a brachial plexus block due to its close proximity to the stellate ganglion.[10] Similarly, blockade of the lumbar plexus produces a sympathectomy in the lower extremities, and peripheral nerve block often produces a sympathectomy in the affected limb because the postganglionic sympathetic nerve fibers travel along the somatic nerves.

Parasympathetic Nervous System

Preganglionic fibers in the PNS arise from the midbrain, medulla oblongata, and sacral segments of the spinal cord. Cranial nerves II, VII, IX, and X carry preganglionic parasympathetic fibers directly to ganglia located near or directly in innervated organs. The sacral segments S2-S4 provide innervation to the rectum and genitourinary tissues (see Figure 12-1).

The vagus nerve (X) is the major carrier of parasympathetic neuronal traffic. These preganglionic fibers affect the heart, lungs, and abdominal organs with the exception of the distal portion of the colon. A combination of the distal location of the ganglion and the smaller 2- to 3-fold amplification factor between preganglionic and postganglionic fibers causes parasympathetic effects to be specific to each organ.

CELLULAR PHYSIOLOGY

Preganglionic Neurons

Synaptic transmission through ANS ganglia is similar in both the SNS and the PNS. Preganglionic neurons in both the SNS and PNS are cholinergic. Acetylcholine (ACh) is stored in synaptic vesicles and released by a Ca^{2+} dependent process upon nerve terminal depolarization (Figure 12-3). ACh then interacts with postsynaptic receptors to depolarize the postsynaptic membrane. The principal ganglionic receptors are excitatory nicotinic ACh receptors, related to the ACh receptors at the neuromuscular junction (see Chapter 18). Thus many neuromuscular blocking agents have cardiovascular side effects mediated by their actions at the level of ANS ganglia. Recent advances in the pharmacology of these drugs have been directed at decreasing these ganglionic actions (see Chapter 19).

There are two distinct nicotinic receptor types, designated neuronal and muscle nicotinic ACh receptors (Figure 12-4).[11] Neuronal ACh receptors expressed in the autonomic ganglia are composed of α3β4 subunits, and are blocked by older neuromuscular blockers (e.g., gallamine), leading to ganglionic blockade. The neuromuscular junction has muscle nicotinic ACh receptors (composed of αβδε subunits in adults) that are blocked selectively by the newer neuromuscular blocking agents, resulting in few side effects. Volatile anesthetics and ketamine are potent inhibitors both at α4β2 in the central nervous system and ganglionic α3β4 receptors.[11] The development of neuromuscular blocking agents has been focused on reduction of muscarinic side effects and elimination of ganglionic blockade. Structure-activity relationships indicate that the presence of quaternary ammonium moieties facilitates binding at the ACh site, while interionic distances may play a role in diminishing ganglionic as well as muscarinic cross-reactivity.[12]

Both nicotinic and muscarinic agonists and blockers interact at the level of the ganglia, the effects of which summate to either excite or inhibit the postganglionic neuron, and subsequently inhibit the effector organ. Thus the ganglionic synapse serves complex integrative and processing functions during normal physiology and while under the influence of anesthetic agents.

Postganglionic Neurons

SYMPATHETIC NERVOUS SYSTEM

Epinephrine, norepinephrine, and dopamine are the classic neurotransmitters of sympathetic synaptic transmission released from postganglionic neurons (Figure 12-5); they interact with adrenergic receptors to effect sympathetic physiologic responses. As shown in Figure 12-6, these neurotransmitters and their receptors can be characterized at different levels. Building on the original observation by Ahlquist,

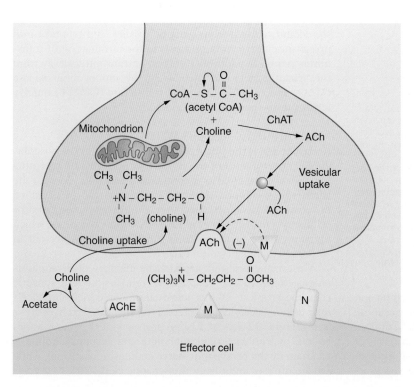

Figure 12-3 The cholinergic synapse. Acetylcholine (ACh) is produced in the presynaptic terminal by the combination of acetyl CoA and choline through the action of choline acetyltransferase (ChAT). This neurotransmitter is stored in vesicles located in the presynaptic terminal and released upon nerve stimulation. ACh can bind to either nicotinic (N) or muscarinic (M) postsynaptic receptors to elicit an effector response (after summation in the postsynaptic membrane). In addition ACh interacts with presynaptic muscarinic receptors to provide negative feedback on ACh release. ACh is broken down in the synapse by acetylcholine esterase (AChE), and choline is taken up into the presynaptic terminal to be reused.

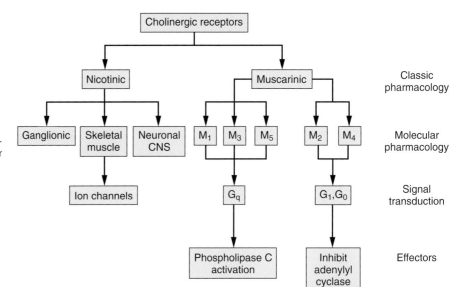

Figure 12-4 Classification of cholinergic receptors. Receptor classification is pharmacologic or based on second messenger signal transduction.

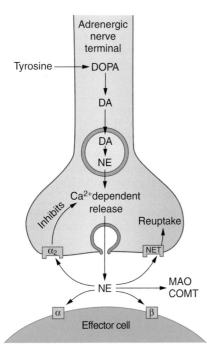

Figure 12-5 The adrenergic presynaptic terminal. Tyrosine (Tyr) is converted to dihydroxyphenylalanine (DOPA) by tyrosine hydroxylase. DOPA decarboxylase produces dopamine (DA) in the cytoplasm, which is taken up into synaptic vesicles. Inside the synaptic vesicles, DA is converted to norepinephrine (NE) by dopamine β-hydroxylase. When NE is released from the presynaptic site by calcium (Ca²⁺)-dependent exocytosis, and the released neurotransmitter interacts with the effector cell adrenergic receptors and receptors located on the presynaptic membrane. Presynaptic α₂ receptors inhibit further NE release. Presynaptic β-receptors enhance NE reuptake, the major factor in removal of NE from the synaptic cleft. NE synthesis is controlled by a negative feedback loop at the level of tyrosine hydroxylase (not shown). Small amounts of NE escape into extraneuronal tissues where it is inactivated by monoamine oxidase (MAO) and catechol-O-methyltransferase (COMT).

adrenergic "receptors" are of two different types (alpha and beta), classified in terms of the overall physiologic response they elicit (the "classic pharmacology" approach).[13] Modern pharmacology further categorizes these receptors in terms of their molecular biology (e.g., DNA sequence and protein structure). From a mechanistic perspective, these receptors

can also be classified in terms of how their signals are transduced (i.e., which G-protein subtype is involved) and how the response is effected (i.e., what ion channels or enzymes are involved).

For example, norepinephrine released from sympathetic postganglionic neurons stimulates both α- and β-adrenergic receptors, eliciting classic adrenergic responses. Alpha-2 (α₂) receptors located presynaptically, provide a negative feedback loop to modulate further release of neurotransmitter (Figure 12-5). The postsynaptic receptors regulate effector cells through second messenger signaling. The various and widespread physiologic actions of adrenergic and dopaminergic receptors are summarized in Table 12-1.

Synthesis of the adrenergic neurotransmitters takes place in the presynaptic varicosities of postganglionic sympathetic neurons. The steps in the enzymatic synthesis of norepinephrine are depicted in Figure 12-5. The neurotransmitters are stored and released from synaptic vesicles, and reuptake into presynaptic nerve endings assists in the termination of transmitter action. In addition, diffusion of transmitters away from the synaptic cleft and metabolism by monoamine oxidase (MAO) and catechol-O-methyl transferase (COMT) quickly terminate the action of norepinephrine.

PARASYMPATHETIC NERVOUS SYSTEM

Acetylcholine is the primary neurotransmitter at the postganglionic effector sites of the PNS. The postsynaptic receptors for ACh are classified as nicotinic or muscarinic. As with the adrenergic receptors, cholinergic receptors can be classified in terms of classic pharmacology, molecular biology and/or cellular mechanisms (Figure 12-4). Nicotinic receptors, which function at the neuromuscular junction, are also present in autonomic ganglia (see earlier).

Muscarinic receptors mediate the majority of PNS physiologic effects (Table 12-2). After release into the synaptic cleft, the action of ACh is quickly terminated by the extracellular enzyme acetylcholinesterase (AChE) through hydrolysis (see Figure 12-3). AChE is postsynaptically membrane-bound; hydrolysis produces choline and acetate. Choline is taken up by the presynaptic nerve endings to be reused, while acetate diffuses away from the synaptic cleft.

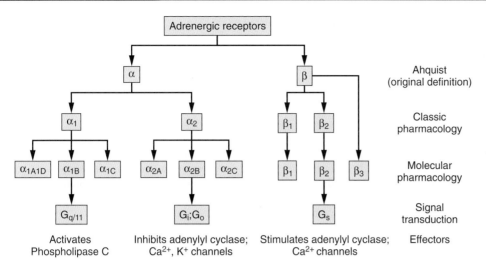

Figure 12-6 Classification of adrenergic receptors. Receptor classification is pharmacologic or based on second messenger signal transduction.

Table 12-2. Homeostatic Balance Between the Parasympathetic and Sympathetic Nervous Systems by Organ System

ORGAN SYSTEM	EFFECTOR	SNS STIMULATION	PNS STIMULATION
Cardiovascular	Sinoatrial node	Increase heart rate	Decrease heart rate
	Atrioventricular node	Increase conduction velocity	Decrease conduction velocity
	His-Purkinje fiber	Increase automaticity, conduction	None or minimal
	Myocardial tissue	Increase contractility	None or minimal
	Coronary arterioles	Constriction (α_2), Dilation (β_2)	Dilation and constriction
Gastrointestinal	Salivary glands	Little increase in secretion	Stimulates secretion
	Gall bladder	Relaxation	Contraction
	Smooth muscle	Inhibits	Stimulates
	Sphincters	Constricts	Relaxes
Ophthalmologic	Iris	Mydriasis	Miosis
	Ciliary muscle	Relaxation (for far vision)	Contraction (for near vision)
Pulmonary	Bronchial smooth muscle	Relaxation	Contraction
Genitourinary	Bladder walls	Relaxes smooth muscle	Smooth muscle contraction
	Bladder sphincter	Contraction	Relaxation
	Ductus deferens, seminal vesicle, prostatic and uterine musculature	Contraction of smooth muscle	Vasodilation and erection
Thermal regulation	Blood vessels	Constriction	Dilation
	Sweat glands	Diaphoresis (postganglionic sympathetic fibers are cholinergic)	Little effect

PNS, Parasympathetic nervous system; SNS, sympathetic nervous system.

There are five distinct subclasses of muscarinic receptors, three of which have pharmacologic significance in the PNS, designated M_1, M_2, and M_3.[14] M_1 receptors exist in autonomic ganglia and the CNS, and are present in the airway. M_1, M_2, and M_3 receptors have effects on the airway smooth muscle with the majority of receptors being M_2 and M_3. M_2 receptors are located presynaptically and function as part of a negative feedback loop to limit release of ACh. M_3 receptors are located postsynaptically and mediate bronchoconstriction.

ENTERIC NERVOUS SYSTEM

The gastrointestinal tract is innervated by sympathetic and parasympathetic efferents arising from preganglionic and postganglionic sites. These neural inputs, along with visceral afferents, interact with intrinsic neural elements (often referred to as the enteric nervous system) to control gut function. The SNS contributes nerve fibers from cell bodies located within the prevertebral sympathetic ganglia, and from celiac, inferior mesenteric, and pelvic ganglia. Vagal (parasympathetic) innervation consists of both sensory and motor fibers. The vagal efferents end on smooth muscle within the walls of the gut, interacting with the intrinsic myenteric ganglion to control motility (see Chapter 27). Efferent outflow from the sympathetic and the parasympathetic systems modulate blood flow, secretory activity, and motility.[15,16] Vagal afferent traffic responds to normal gut function, while sympathetic afferents respond to painful stimuli such as distention and injury.

Anesthetic effects on the enteric nervous system can be divided into direct pharmacologic effects on the intestinal smooth muscle, and effects due to spinal or epidural anesthesia. Muscarinic cholinergic receptors in the gut can be modulated by acetylcholinesterase inhibitors and anticholinergics used for reversal of neuromuscular blockade.[17] Postoperative ileus can be decreased by the use of thoracic epidural anesthesia.[18] Autonomic dysfunction causing gut dysmotility occurs because the SNS exerts more influence in the postoperative period than the parasympathetic system. This inhibitory sympathetic reflex can be interrupted by division of the splanchnic nerves, destruction of afferent sensory nerves, or chemical sympathectomy via thoracic epidural anesthesia. The result is a shortened time to resolution of postoperative ileus.[18]

Second Messengers in the Autonomic Nervous System

Interaction of neurotransmitters with their postsynaptic receptors results in signal transduction, which translates receptor binding into an effector cell response. In the adrenergic system, transduction is mediated by G proteins, which then regulate adenylyl cyclase and phospholipase C to generate second messengers and/or directly modulate various ion channels (see Chapter 1). In contrast, nicotinic ACh receptor binding leads to opening of its intrinsic ion channel, which leads to changes in the cell electrical potential. Muscarinic ACh receptors are G protein-coupled receptors similar to adrenergic receptors. Second messenger responses to muscarinic receptor stimulation depend on the effector site and the muscarinic receptor subtypes expressed (see Table 12-2).

ADRENAL MEDULLA
The paired adrenal medullae are specialized portions of the SNS. Chromaffin cells are homologous to the sympathetic ganglion neurons and are similarly derived from the neural crest. The adrenal medulla can be thought of as a functional sympathetic ganglion in direct communication with the systemic circulation. Stimulation of the SNS results in the release of epinephrine and norepinephrine from the medulla into the bloodstream, eliciting a diffuse (nontargeted) sympathetic response from various effector organs expressing adrenergic receptors. In this way, the adrenal gland represents the general effector of the SNS, an amplification essential to the stress response.[19]

AUTONOMIC NERVOUS SYSTEM REFLEXES

The ANS maintains homeostasis using the SNS and PNS as counteracting regulators (see Table 12-2). The relative tone of each of the two subsystems varies with age, sex, organ system, and environmental effects such as stress.[20] The challenge facing anesthesiologists is to maintain homeostasis while the ANS is modulated by medications, coexisting disease, surgical stimulation, and anesthetic drugs. Understanding of the pathways of ANS reflexes, and the anesthetic/surgical circumstances under which they are accentuated or attenuated, provides a conceptual framework for maintaining homeostasis during anesthesia and critical care.

Central Nervous System Reflexes

CUSHING'S TRIAD
Cushing's triad is the physiologic association of increased intracranial pressure, bradycardia, and hypertension.[21] Intracranial hypertension leads to sympathetically mediated increases in blood pressure; the apparent disparity in reduced heart rate is probably due to medullary ischemia. Activation of parasympathetic medullary centers via the baroreceptor reflex (see later) slows the heart but does not overcome sympathetically mediated hypertension. The result is homeostatically increased blood flow to the brain.

AUTONOMIC HYPERREFLEXIA
Alternatively termed *autonomic dysreflexia*, this condition results from chronic disruption of efferent impulses down the spinal cord, as in spinal cord trauma or tumor impingement.[22] Autonomic hyperreflexia is uncommon if the level of disruption is below T5. Inciting stimuli such as bladder distention, bowel distention, or surgical stimulation can produce an exaggerated sympathetic response. This occurs because there is a loss of normal inhibitory impulses from areas above the level of the lesion. A portion of the exaggeration in the response is due to adrenergic receptor supersensitivity secondary to denervation. Management of the quadriplegic or high paraplegic patient consists of either spinal or general anesthesia combined with careful manipulation of blood pressure due to the alterations in the ANS.[23]

THERMOGENESIS REFLEX
Autonomic control of thermoregulation in mammals consists of reflex pathways from sensory cells originating in diverse tissues including the skin, core organs, and the central nervous system. These signals are processed by the hypothalamus, which maintains body temperature within a narrow range of a few tenths of a degree around 37°C. Daily circadian rhythms result in a sinusoidal variation of about 1. The output of the hypothalamus controls effector responses including peripheral vasculature action (vasodilation or vasoconstriction), sweating, and shivering.[24]

The preoptic area (POA) in the anterior hypothalamus receives thermal afferent signals from peripheral receptors as well as sensors located in the core (spinal cord, some organs). Efferent traffic goes to the principal thermoregulatory effectors: (1) cutaneous blood vessels, which vasoconstrict to reduce heat loss and vasodilate to facilitate heat loss; (2) brown fat and skeletal muscle for thermogenesis and shivering; and (3) sweat glands to provide for evaporative heat loss.[25]

Sweating is controlled by cholinergic fibers that can be blocked by muscarinic antagonists like atropine, or by peripheral nerve block.[26] Shivering can be blocked by the use of neuromuscular blockers, and can be diminished in old age and neuromuscular diseases. Shivering does not occur in newborns and is limited in infants. Nonshivering thermogenesis occurring in newborns and infants is modulated by norepinephrine from adrenergic nerve terminals. Vasoconstriction is controlled by the ANS at the level of the arteriovenous shunts, and is the result of sympathetic nerve traffic and not circulating catecholamines.

All general anesthetics impair thermogenesis reflexes. Sweating threshold is slightly increased and vasoconstriction and shivering thresholds are decreased markedly. These effects of anesthetics can lead to hypothermia during surgery if heat loss through radiation, conduction, convection, and evaporation is not minimized.[27]

Cardiac Reflexes

BARORECEPTOR REFLEX
Stretch receptors in the walls of the carotid artery and aorta sense an increase in pressure (either endovascular or external, such as carotid massage). Afferent impulses are carried via the nerve of Hering and the vagus nerve to the medulla. In the medulla the excitatory baroreceptor inputs interact at the nucleus of the solitary tract to disinhibit inhibitory

interneurons, which then send increased signals to the rostral ventrolateral medulla and onward to the intermediolateral nucleus.[28] A decrease in heart rate, blood pressure, myocardial contractility, and total peripheral vascular resistance is mediated by efferent vagal activity (see Chapter 21). This effect is seen during anesthesia when phenylephrine, an α_1 receptor agonist, is administered intravenously, causing a rise in blood pressure and a fall in heart rate. Halothane attenuates this reflex.[29]

CHEMORECEPTOR REFLEX
Central chemoreceptors are sensitive to increases in arterial CO_2 and decreases in arterial pH. Hypercarbia elicits a rapid and vigorous increase in minute ventilation (see Chapter 25). Volatile anesthetics, opioids, and nitrous oxide attenuate this response in a dose-dependent fashion. Even subanesthetic concentrations of volatile anesthetics have an effect on the ventilation response, thus patients given halogenated agents in the operating room can continue to have an impaired response to hypercarbia in the postanesthesia care unit.[30] Peripheral chemoreceptors are present in the carotid body; volatile anesthetics also produce dose-dependent attenuation of the ventilatory response to hypoxia mediated by these receptors.[31] Hypoxia elicits afferent impulses from the carotid and aortic bodies through Hering's nerve and the vagus to the nucleus tractus solitarius, increasing respiratory rate, tidal volume, and thus minute ventilation. Sympathetic activation causing increased heart rate and cardiac output can also occur.[32]

BAINBRIDGE REFLEX
An increase in central venous pressure (CVP) activates stretch receptors in the atria. Afferent impulses through the vagus nerve impact cardiovascular centers in the brain, which then inhibit tonic parasympathetic output, resulting in tachycardia.[33] The Bainbridge reflex can be seen during childbirth when autotransfusion increases CVP.[34]

BEZOLD-JARISCH REFLEX
This cardiac reflex is characterized by hypotension, bradycardia, and dilation of the coronary arteries (see Chapter 21). The Bezold-Jarisch reflex occurs in response to noxious stimuli detected in the ventricle; historically this was studied using *Veratrum* alkaloids applied intravenously. Chemoreceptors located in the ventricles respond to myocardial ischemia, resulting in an increase in blood flow to the myocardium and a decrease in the work of the heart. This appears to be a cardioprotective reflex. The pathway for this cardioprotective reflex begins with receptors in the ventricles of the heart, which detect mechanical and chemical stimuli. Afferent unmyelinated C-fibers travel through the vagus to enhance the baroreceptor reflex mechanisms, inhibit sympathetic output and inhibit vasomotor tone leading to peripheral vasodilation. The significance of this reflex in the presence of anesthetics continues to be debated, particularly in relation to regional anesthesia. As a cardioinhibitory reflex, the Bezold-Jarish reflex might be functioning in parallel with the baroreceptor reflex but is probably not a predominant cause of physiologic change in humans.[35]

VALSALVA MANEUVER
Forced expiration against a closed glottis leads to multiple ANS-mediated responses. Increased intrathoracic pressure leads to a decrease in venous return, causing an abrupt decrease in cardiac filling and blood pressure. The baroreceptor response leads to an increase in heart rate and inotropy through sympathetic stimulation. Upon glottic opening, the increase in venous return leads to an increase in blood pressure (contractility is still increased). This is detected by the baroreceptors, causing a parasympathetically mediated decrease in heart rate.[36]

OCULOCARDIAC REFLEX (TRIGEMINAL NERVE MEDIATED REFLEXES)
The trigeminal nerve (V) is associated with several autonomic reflexes; the best known is the oculocardiac reflex. Pressure on the globe or pulling on the extraocular musculature elicits afferent signals in the short and long ciliary nerves. These signals converge upon the Gasserian ganglion, causing a parasympathetic response, notably severe bradycardia. Release of the stretch results in a return of normal heart rate. This muscarinic receptor-mediated response can be blocked with glycopyrrolate or atropine, or by retrobulbar nerve block. In addition to the oculocardiac reflex, parasympathetic activation has been reported during intranasal stimulation and is an important part of the diving reflex.[37,38]

EMERGING DEVELOPMENTS

Effects of Anesthetics on Autonomic Nervous System
General anesthetics tend to suppress the ANS, as they do the central nervous system. Many specific drugs used in anesthesia directly or indirectly interact with systems, organs, and receptors of the ANS, which then modify the function of the ANS. For instance, administration of the α_2 agonist clonidine decreases the dose of halothane required to produce general anesthesia.[39] This was followed by further investigation into the use of dexmedetomidine as an agonist of α_2 receptors in the central nervous system as an anesthetic adjunct.[40]

Anesthetics depress the ANS, in part by attenuating homeostatic reflexes and by decreasing the normal variability in measurements seen due to the balance between the sympathetic and parasympathetic systems. Heart rate variability, pulse-to pulse interval and pulse plethysmography amplitude have been used to characterize the state of the ANS.[41,42] Administration of a potent opioid such as fentanyl decreases normal beat-to beat variability, depresses sympathetic tone and promotes vagal activation.[43] Potent inhaled anesthetics such as desflurane depress the ANS as measured by heart rate variability.[44] Xenon, an anesthetic that has less hemodynamic depression than potent inhaled agents, causes increased parasympathetic and decreased sympathetic activity compared with total intravenous anesthesia (TIVA) with propofol.[45] Thus, while inhaled anesthetics have variable effects on the ANS, depression of the SNS appears to dominate.

General anesthesia and regional anesthesia also affect the ANS differently. The balance of sympathetic with parasympathetic tone in the upper body (unaffected by a lumbar epidural block) and the lower body, or the change in the balance between the intraoperative and postoperative state can have consequences in critical cardiac patients.[46] Continued ANS dysfunction in the intensive care unit complicates the perioperative course in the surgical patient.[47]

Autonomic Failure

Aging, diabetes mellitus, and dysautonomia can result in failure or dysfunction of the ANS that affects perioperative management.

Aging. The cardiovascular effects of aging are characterized by hypertension and orthostatic hypotension, two conditions regulated by the ANS.[48] In addition, loss of temperature control can lead to heat stroke or hypothermia. All of these conditions lead to an inability of the older patients to adequately adapt to environmental stress. While the amount of circulating epinephrine and the number of β-adrenergic receptors are not reduced in older adults, the amount of norepinephrine is increased. This leads to a cyclic decline in responsiveness of adrenergic receptors as circulating plasma norepinephrine increases and receptors downregulate, requiring more stimulation.[48] Because older adults have decreased levels of plasma renin and aldosterone and increased levels of atrial natriuretic factor, they are prone to salt-wasting and hypovolemia.[49] The resultant labile blood pressure, particularly with orthostatic changes, makes pharmacologic management challenging. For instance, β-adrenergic agonists have a markedly decreased effect on heart rate, cardiac output, and vasodilation as a result of reduced affinity of the β-adrenergic receptor and a decline in the efficacy of second messenger coupling.[48]

Temperature regulation in older patients is also altered as a consequence of changes in the ANS, and as a result of reduced ability to respond physiologically with shivering and vasoconstriction. Older patients have reduced muscle mass so they are unable to generate heat effectively. They also have reduced subcutaneous fat (even though total fat as measured as a proportion of body weight is increased), leading to a decrease in thermal insulation.[50] Thermoregulatory control of skin blood flow in the elderly is also altered as a result of changes in the ANS. Reflex vasoconstriction and vasodilation are impaired due to diminished sympathetic output and reduced vascular responsiveness.[51] As a consequence, older adults can experience more stress directly related to hypothermia and hyperthermia.

DIABETES MELLITUS

Autonomic neuropathy is common among diabetic patients. Between 20% and 40% of insulin-dependent diabetics have significant peripheral neuropathy, characterized by labile blood pressure, thermoregulatory deficits, and gastroparesis (possibly vagal nerve dysfunction).[52] This constellation of problems can require modification of the typical anesthetic plan, including pretreatment to mitigate the consequences of aspiration of stomach contents, cardiovascular support, and proactive efforts to prevent hypothermia. Perhaps in part because of autonomic dysfunction, diabetic patients experience more stress and are at increased risk for peri-operative complications.

AUTONOMIC DYSAUTONOMIA

Dysautonomia can occur as a result of a genetic defect (e.g., familial dysautonomia, Shy-Drager syndrome), viral infection (Gullain-Barré syndrome), malignancy (Lambert-Eaton syndrome), or unknown reasons. Orthostatic hypotension and a decreased beat-to-beat variability in heart rate are common signs. This can lead to rapid changes in blood pressure and an exaggerated response to sympathomimetic drugs under anesthesia due to an alteration in adrenergic receptor number or function.[53]

KEY POINTS

- The ANS maintains cardiovascular, metabolic, thermal, and gastrointestinal homeostasis.
- Central control of the ANS is primarily mediated in the hypothalamus and medulla oblongata.
- Emerging from the spinal cord, the SNS acts primarily by the effector neurotransmitter norepinephrine to increase critical organ blood flow (i.e., muscles, heart, brain) in response to external challenges. The distribution of sympathetic ganglia close to the central nervous system facilitates a rapid amplification of this generalized fight-or-flight response.
- Emerging from select cranial and sacral nerves, the PNS acts primarily by the effector neurotransmitter acetylcholine (and muscarinic cholinergic receptors) to modulate activities that occur when the body is at rest (e.g., salivation, urination, defecation, sexual function). The distribution of parasympathetic ganglia close to effector organs facilitates the more focused rest-and-digest functions of the parasympathetic system.
- The adrenal medulla is functionally a sympathetic ganglion in direct communication with the systemic circulation that contributes to the amplification of the fight-or-flight response by delivering epinephrine and norepinephrine throughout the body.
- ANS reflexes (e.g., baroreceptor reflex, oculocardiac reflex) have important implications for anesthetic management.
- Anesthetics generally depress the ANS, in part by attenuating homeostatic reflexes.
- Autonomic dysfunction associated with aging, diabetes, and other disease states can have important implications on anesthetic management, especially as it relates to the support of the circulation during anesthesia.

Key References

Ahlquist RP. A study of adrenotropic receptors. *Am J Physiol.* 1948;153:586-600. This famous description led to an improved taxonomy of adrenoreceptors that continues to be utilized today. (Ref. 13)

Bloor BC, Flacke WE. Reduction in halothane anesthetic requirement by clonidine, an α-adrenergic agonist. *Anesth Analg.* 1982;61:741-745. The understanding that the autonomic response to surgery could be modified by α₂ agonists working in the spinal cord and in the brain further contributed to the concept of "balanced anesthesia." Developments in this area would lead to dexmedetomidine as a sedative and supplement to anesthesia, and α₂ agonists in chronic and acute pain. (Ref. 39)

Matsukawa T, Sessler DI, Sessler AM, et al. Heat flow and distribution during induction of general anesthesia. *Anesthesiology.* 1995;82:662-673. The importance of thermoregulation and the effects of anesthetic agents on the autonomic responses governing control of temperature are reviewed. (Ref. 27)

Mustafa HI, Fessel JP, Barwise J, et al. Dysautonomia: perioperative implications. *Anesthesiology.* 2012;116:205-215. Reviews the pathophysiology and perioperative management of dysautonomia. (Ref. 53)

Tassonyi E, Chapantier E, Muller D, et al. The role of nicotinic acetylcholine receptors in the mechanisms of anesthesia. *Brain Res Bull*. 2002;57:133-150. The function of nicotinic receptors in the brain, and their effects on the autonomic nervous system through their ganglionic action receive a critical review in this paper. (Ref. 11)

References

1. Langley J. Observations on the physiological action of extracts of the supra-renal bodies. *J Physiol*. 1901;27:237-256.
2. Carpenter MB, Sutin J. The autonomic nervous system. In: *Human Neuroanatomy*. 8th ed. Baltimore: Williams & Wilkins; 1983:209-210.
3. Johnson JO, Grecu L, Lawson NW. Autonomic nervous system. In: Barash PG, Cullen BF, Stoelting RK, et al, eds. *Clinical Anesthesia*. 6th ed. Philadelphia: Wolters Kluwer; 2009:326-368.
4. Glick DB. The autonomic nervous system. In: Miller RD, Eriksson LI, Fleisher LA, et al, eds. *Miller's Anesthesia*. 7th ed. Philadelphia: Elsevier; 2011:261-304.
5. Hainsworth R. Pathophysiology of syncope. *Clin Auton Res*. 2004; 14(Suppl1):18-24.
6. Goldstein, DS. Adrenal responses to stress. *Cell Mol Neurobiol*. 2010;30:1433-1440.
7. Ulrich-Lai YM, Herman JP. Neural regulation of endocrine and autonomic stress responses. *Nature Reviews/Neurosci*.. 2009;10:397-409.
8. Guyton AC, Hall JE. The autonomic nervous system and the adrenal medulla. In: Guyton AC, Hall JE, eds. *Textbook of Medical Physiology*, 11th ed. Philadelphia: Elsevier & Saunders; 2006:748-760.
9. Shaw CA, Kelleher AA, Gill CP, Murdoch LJ, Stables RH, Black AE. Comparison of the incidence of complications at induction and emergence in infants receiving oral atropine vs no premedication. *Br J Anaesth*. 2000;84:174-178.
10. Winnie AP, Ramamurthy S, Durrani Z, et al. Pharmacologic reversal of Horner's syndrome following stellate ganglion block. *Anesthesiology*. 1974;41:615-617.
11. Tassonyi E, Chapantier E, Muller D, et al. The role of nicotinic acetylcholine receptors in the mechanisms of anesthesia. *Brain Res Bul*. 2002;57:133-150.
12. Bowman WC. Neuromuscular block. *Br J Pharmacol*. 2009;147: S277-S286.
13. Ahlquist RP. A study of adrenotropic receptors. *Am J Physiol*. 1948;153:586-600.
14. Eglen RM. Muscarinic receptor subtypes in neuronal and non-neuronal cholinergic function. *Auton Autacoid Pharmacol*. 2006;26: 219-233.
15. Xue J, Askwith C, Javed NH, Cooke HJ. Autonomic nervous system and secretion across the intestinal mucosal surface. *Aut Neurosci*. 2007;133:55-63.
16. Phillips RJ, Powley TL. Innervation of the gastrointestinal tract: patterns of aging. *Aut Neurosci*. 2007;136:1-19.
17. Caldwell JE. Clinical limitations of acetylcholinesterase antagonists. *J Crit Care*. 2009;24:21-28.
18. Miedema BW, Johnson JO. Methods for decreasing postoperative gut dysmotility. *Lancet Oncol*. 2003;4:365-372.
19. Ledowski T, Bein B, Hanss R, et al. Neuroendocrine response and heart rate variability: a comparison of total intravenous versus balanced anesthesia. *Anesth Analg*. 2005;1700-1705.
20. Buckworth J, Dishman RK, Cureton KJ. Autonomic responses of women with parental hypertension. Effects of physical activity and fitness. *Hypertension*. 1994;24:576-584.
21. Agrawal A, Timothy J, Cincu R, Agarwal T, Waghmare LB. Brady-cardia in neurosurgery. *Clin Neurol Neurosurg*. 2008;110:321-327.
22. Amzallag M. Autonomic hyperreflexia. *Int Anesthesiol Clin*. 1993; 31:87-102.
23. Hambly PR, Martin B. Anaesthesia for chronic spinal cord lesions. *Anaesthesia*. 1998;53:273-289.
24. Sessler DI. Thermoregulatory defense mechanisms. *Crit Care Med*. 2009;37(7):S203-S210.
25. Morrison SF, Nakamura K. Central neural pathways for thermoregulation. *Front Biosci*. 2011;16:74-104.
26. Hemmingway A, Price WM. The autonomic nervous system and regulation of body temperature. *Anesthesiology*. 1968;29:693-701.
27. Matsukawa T, Sessler DI, Sessler AM, et al. Heat flow and distribution during induction of general anesthesia. *Anesthesiology*. 1995;82: 662-673.
28. Pilowsky PM, Goodchild AK. Baroreceptor reflex pathways and neurotransmitters. 10 years on. *J Hyperten*. 2002;20:1675-1688.
29. Ebert TJ, Kotrly KJ, Vucins EJ, Pattison CZ, Kampine JP. Halothane anesthesia attenuates cardiopulmonary baroreflex control of peripheral resistance in humans. *Anesthesiology*. 1985;63:668-674.
30. Dahon A, Sarton E, van den Elsen M, et al. Ventilatory response to hypoxia in humans. Influences of subanesthetic desflurane. *Anesthesiology*. 1996;85:60-68.
31. van den Elsen, MJ, Dahan A, Berkenbosch A, DeGoede J, van Kleef JW, Olievier IC. Does subanesthetic isoflurane affect the ventilator response to acute isocapnic hypoxia in healthy volunteers? *Anesthesiology*. 1994;81:860-867.
32. Nurse CA. Neurotransmitter and neuromodulatory mechanisms at peripheral arterial chemoreceptors. *Exp Physiol*. 2010;95:657-667.
33. Hakümäki MO. Seventy years of the Bainbridge reflex. *Acta Physiol Scand*. 1987;130:177-185.
34. Crystal GJ, Salem MR. The Bainbridge and the "reverse" Bainbridge reflexes: history, physiology, and clinical relevance. *Anesth Analg Sept*. 2011;29 (epub ahead of print).
35. Campagna JA, Carter C. Clinical relevance of the Bezold-Jarisch reflex. *Anesthesiology*. 2003;98:1250-1260.
36. Liang F, Liu H. Simulation of hemodynamic responses to the Valsalva maneuver: an integrative computational model of the cardiovascular system and the autonomic nervous system. *J Physiol Sci*. 2006;56:45-65.
37. Bailey PL. Sinus arrest induced by trivial nasal stimulation during alfentanil-nitrous oxide anesthesia. *Br J Anaesth*. 1990;65:718-720.
38. Paton JFR, Boscan P, Pickering AE, Nalivaiko E. The yin and yang of cardiac autonomic control: vago sympathetic interactions revisited. *Brain Res Rev*. 2005;49:555-565.
39. Bloor BC, Flacke WE. Reduction in halothane anesthetic requirement by clonidine an α-adrenergic agonist. *Anesth Analg*. 1982;61: 741-745.
40. Doze VA, Chen BX, Maze M. Dexmedetomidine produces a hypnotic-anesthetic action in rats via activation of central α2 adrenoreceptors. *Anesthesiology*. 1989;71:75-79.
41. Martín Concho MF, Carasco-Jiménez MS, Lima JR, Luis L, Crisóstomo V, Usón-Gargallo J. The measurement of neurovegatative activity during anesthesia and surgery in swine: an evaluation of different techniques. *Anesth Analg*. 2006;102:133-140.
42. Paloheimo MPJ, Sahanne S, Uutela KH. Autonomic nervous system state: the effect of general anaesthesia and bilateral tonsillectomy after unilateral infiltration of lidocaine. *Br J Anaes*. 2010;104:587-595.
43. Vettorello M, Colombo R, De Grandis CE, et al. Effect of fentanyl on heart rate variability during spontaneous and paced breathing in healthy volunteers. *Acta Anaesthesiol Scand*. 2008;52:1064-1070.
44. Paisansathan C, Hoffman WE, Lee M, et al. Autonomic activity during desflurane anesthesia in patients with brain tumors. *J Clin Monit Comput*. 2007;21:265-269.
45. Hanss R, Bein B, Turowski P, et al. The influence of xewnon on regulation of the autonomic nervous system in patents at high risk of periperative cardiac complications. *Br J Anaesth*. 2006;96:427-436.
46. Fleisher LA, Frank SM, Shir Y, et al. Cardiac sympathovagal balance and peripheral sympathetic vasoconstriction: epidural versus general anesthesia. *Anesth Analg*. 1994;79:165-171.
47. Mazzeo AT, La Monaca E, Di Leo R, Vita G, Santamaria LB. Heart rate variability: a diagnostic and prognostic tool in anesthesia and intensive care. *Acta Anaesthesiol Scand*. 2011;55:797-811.
48. Corcoran TB, Hillyard S. Cardiopulmonary aspects of anaesthesia for the elderly. *Best Pract Res Clin Anaesthesiol*. 2011;25:329-354.
49. Charloux A, Brandenberger G, Piquard F, Geny B. Dysregulation of pulsatility in aging IV. Pulsatile signaling and cardiovascular aging: functions and regulation of natriuretic peptide signaling. *Ageing Res Rev*. 2008;7:151-163.
50. Chester JG, Rudolf JL. Vital signs in older patients: age-related changes. *J Am Med Dir Assoc*. 2011;12:337-343.
51. Holowatz LA, Kenney WL. Peripheral mechanisms of thermoregulatory control of skin blood flow in aged humans. *J Appl Physiol*. 2010;109:1538-1544.
52. Kadoi Y. Perioperative considerations in diabetic patients. *Curr Diabetes Rev*. 2010;6:236-246.
53. Mustafa HI, Fessel JP, Barwise J, et al. Dysautonomia: perioperative implications. *Anesthesiology*. 2012;116:205-215.

Chapter 13

AUTONOMIC NERVOUS SYSTEM PHARMACOLOGY

Thomas J. Ebert

The autonomic nervous system (ANS) maintains homeostasis by integrating signals from peripheral and central sensors to modulate organ perfusion and function. Autonomic "tone" maintains cardiac muscle, visceral organs, and vascular smooth muscle in a state of intermediate function. From this state, rapid increases or decreases in autonomic outflow can adjust blood flow and organ activity in response to the environment. The rapidity of the ANS response is impressive considering that neurotransmitters must be released from terminals, cross a synaptic cleft to an effector site, bind to a receptor, and initiate an intracellular event. For example, in just a few seconds, ANS activation can double heart rate (HR) and arterial blood pressure (BP). In a nearly similar time frame it can cause sweating, nausea, loss of bladder control, and fainting. The sympathetic nervous system (SNS) has been called the "fight-or-flight" response system and is activated under stress. In contrast, the parasympathetic nervous system is responsible for "rest and digest." The anatomy and physiology of the ANS are discussed in Chapter 12.

In the perioperative and intensive care settings, multiple factors disrupt the typically tight ANS control of organ and vascular homeostasis. Thus pharmacologic activation or inhibition of the ANS is commonplace in these settings. For example, both general and regional anesthesia have powerful influences on normal ANS function. When an inhaled anesthetic acts to directly relax vascular smooth muscle and lower BP, the ANS reacts to counteract hypotension via baroreflex adjustments of ANS activity. However, a second effect of volatile anesthetics is to impair baroreflex function. The net effect of these influences requires treatment of unwanted hypotension with sympathomimetic or vagolytic drugs. Laryngoscopy and tracheal intubation or surgical incision powerfully activate the SNS; adrenergic receptor blocking drugs are used to dampen these responses.

HISTORICAL PERSPECTIVE

The sympathomimetic properties of the Ma-huang plant were appreciated in China as early as 3000 BC. Ma-huang was used as a diaphoretic, circulatory stimulant, antipyretic, and sedative for cough.[1] Ephedrine, the main alkaloid of Ma-huang, was isolated in 1886.[2] Over the next 25 years, adrenal extracts were described and analyzed, and the term *sympathomimetic* was coined. Adrenergic receptors were identified and subdivided into two primary types (α and β) according to their responses to epinephrine and norepinephrine.[3] The β-receptors were further divided into β1-, β2-, and β3-receptors based on their actions at receptors and sensitivities to inhibitors.[4-6] The α-receptors were similarly subdivided into α1- and α2-receptors, but have been further subdivided into $\alpha1_a$-, $\alpha1_b$-, $\alpha1_d$-, $\alpha2_a$-, $\alpha2_b$-, and $\alpha2_c$-receptors based on their pharmacology and associated second messenger systems.[7,8]

The history of parasympatholytic drugs dates back to ancient times when Mandragora, the mandrake plant, was used for wounds and sleeplessness. Henbane, which contains atropine, was used in ancient Egyptian times as a mydriatic. In the Middle Ages, henbane extract was used to enhance the inebriating qualities of beer and by "witches" to produce flushed skin and vivid hallucinations.

Muscarine, the first parasympathomimetic drug, derives from the fungus *Amanita muscaria* and was described in 1869. It was found to bind receptors that would be called *muscarinic* and had the same effect on the heart as did stimulation of the vagus nerve. Originally discovered by Loewi, the "heart inhibiting" substance that decreased HR and contractility was acetylcholine.[9] Muscarinic receptors are activated by acetylcholine and are thus called *cholinergic*.

STRUCTURE AND MECHANISM OF ADRENERGIC RECEPTORS

The basic catecholamine structure is an aromatic phenylethylamine with two hydroxyl groups. The name *catecholamine* derives from the molecule 3,4-dihydroxylphenyl, known as *catechol*. Epinephrine and norepinephrine have a chiral center at the hydroxyl group on the β-carbon, where the L-isomer is active, while dopamine has no chiral center (Figure 13-1). Intravenous formulations of epinephrine and norepinephrine consist of the L-isomer; a racemic formulation of epinephrine is available for inhalation.

Epinephrine and norepinephrine are predominantly charged molecules at physiologic pH due to their amine moiety and are unable to cross lipid cellular membranes on their own (although they can cross via transporters). Their actions are mediated following signal transduction by transmembrane receptors that initiate intracellular signaling events. Adrenergic receptors are coupled to guanine nucleotide binding proteins (G proteins) that couple the receptor to an effector system (see Chapter 1). Adrenergic G protein-coupled receptors (GPCRs) are classified according to their actions on adenylyl cyclase and their sensitivity to pertussis toxin. The structure of the β-adrenergic receptor is consistent with most GPCRs, with seven transmembrane segments.[10] The signaling cascade of β1- and β2-adrenergic receptors begins with ligand binding to the amino terminus of the receptor on the extracellular surface, then proceeds to the intracellular carboxyl terminal loop of the receptor coupling to G_s-proteins, which stimulate adenylyl cyclase to convert adenosine triphosphate (ATP) to the second messenger cyclic adenosine monophosphate (AMP). The resulting phosphorylation by cyclic AMP-dependent protein kinase produces cellular responses.[11,12] The atomic resolution structure of the β2-receptor bond to G_s has recently been determined and shows the involvement of the amino- and carboxy-terminal

alpha helices of G_s as the main interaction between the two proteins. The activated receptor demonstrates outward movement of the sixth transmembrane segment and the presence of a second intracellular loop between the β2-adrenergic receptor-G_s complex. The receptor is stabilized extracellularly by fusion of the amino-terminus to T4 lysozyme, and intracellularly by numerous interactions with G_s. The Gβ and Gγ subunits of G_s do not directly interact with the β2-adrenergic receptor.[13]

The α2-receptors are coupled to G_i-proteins to inhibit adenylyl cyclase. The α1-receptors are coupled to G_q-proteins activating phospholipase C that hydrolyzes phosphatidylinositol diphosphates (PIP_2) to the second messengers inositol trisphosphate (IP_3) and diacylglycerol (DAG). IP_3 activates Ca^{2+} release from intracellular stores via IP_3 receptors, while DAG activates lipid mediated signaling pathways including members of the protein kinase C family.[14]

Dopamine receptors also are GPCRs and are classified as D1-type (D1 and D5) and D2-type (D2, D3, and D4) receptors.[15] These receptors are located throughout the central nervous system (CNS), on SNS postganglionic nerve terminals, on afferent and efferent arterioles of the nephron, and in the adrenal glands. D1-like receptors stimulate adenylyl cyclase via G_s, and D2-like receptors inhibit adenylyl cyclase via G_i. D1-receptors are postsynaptic and stimulation mimics β2 effects, leading to regional vascular dilation. D2-like receptors occur at presynaptic and postsynaptic sites. Presynaptic D2-like receptor activation inhibits norepinephrine release from sympathetic terminals, an effect similar to the presynaptic effects of acetylcholine and α2-agonists. Postsynaptic sites mimic α1 and α2 vasoconstriction on blood vessels, but this action is relatively weak.

The α1-adrenoceptors are activated by the selective α1-receptor agonists phenylephrine and methoxamine, and inhibition by low concentrations of the antagonist prazosin. The α1-receptors are widely distributed, and when stimulated mediate primarily arterial and venous vascular constriction (Table 13-1). The α2-adrenoceptors are activated by the selective α2-receptor agonists clonidine and dexmedetomidine and are blocked by the antagonist yohimbine; they exist as three subtypes: $\alpha2_a$, $\alpha2_b$, and $\alpha2_c$.[16] The α2-receptors are located presynaptically on sympathetic neurons where they inhibit the release of norepinephrine. Postsynaptic α2-receptors are located on blood vessels and in tissues including liver, pancreas, platelets, kidney, adipose tissue, and the eye (Figure 13-2). Within the CNS, receptors in the locus ceruleus likely account for the sedative properties of α2-agonists, and in the medullary dorsal horn area for the reduction in sympathetic outflow.[17] The α2-receptors are also in the vagus nerve, intermediolateral cell column, and the substantia gelatinosa. The dorsal horn of the spinal cord contains $\alpha2_a$-adrenoceptors co-localized with opioid receptors that modulate afferent pain signals.

Both β1- and β2-adrenergic receptors are characterized by their stimulation by epinephrine and norepinephrine and are heavily expressed in myocardial tissue including atria, ventricular papillary muscle, sinoatrial and atrioventricular nodes, left and right bundles, and Purkinje fibers. They have inotropic (increased contractility), chronotropic (increased HR), and dromotropic (increased conduction velocity) effects (Figure 13-3). Activation of β1-receptors increases renin and aqueous humor production. The β2-receptors are the major

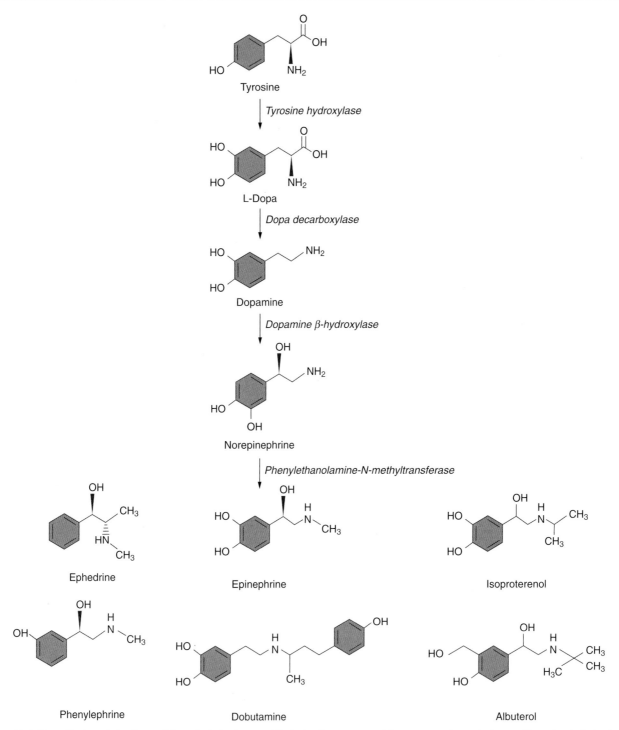

Figure 13-1 Biosynthesis and structures of the catecholamines, and their structures compared to common adrenergic drugs. Stereochemical structure is indicated as shown; Isoproterenol, dobutamine and albuterol are racemates.

β-receptors in arterioles and the only β-receptors in the vena cava, aorta, and pulmonary artery.[18] Activation of β2-receptors leads to uterine relaxation and relaxation of vascular smooth muscle including splanchnic, muscular, and renal vasculature, resulting in a reduction in diastolic pressure and systemic vascular resistance. β2-receptor activation also reduces plasma K$^+$ concentration by promoting uptake into skeletal muscle and reducing aldosterone secretion leading to renal losses of K$^+$ (see Figure 13-3). The β3-receptors are expressed in

visceral adipocytes, gallbladder, and colon. Their activation mediates lipolytic and thermogenesis in brown and white adipose tissue.[19]

ENDOGENOUS CATECHOLAMINES

The biosynthesis of the naturally occurring catecholamines (epinephrine, norepinephrine, and dopamine) begins with the conversion of tyrosine to 3,4-dihydroxyphenylalanine (DOPA) (see Figure 13-1). The rate-limiting step in catecholamine synthesis is conversion of tyrosine to DOPA by the enzyme tyrosine hydroxylase.

Epinephrine

Epinephrine, also known as adrenaline, is an endogenous monoamine with broad clinical applications. Epinephrine is present in chromaffin cells in the adrenal medulla, where it is synthesized, stored, and released upon sympathetic stimulation. On average, 80% of the secreted catecholamine in the adrenal medulla is epinephrine and 20% is norepinephrine. The normal resting rate of secretion by the adrenal medulla

is about 0.2 µg/kg/min of epinephrine and about 0.05 µg/kg/min of norepinephrine. These rates are sufficient to support arterial BP fully if the SNS is denervated. The effects of secreted epinephrine and norepinephrine on organ function lasts 5 to 10 times longer than the effect from a burst of sympathetic stimulation to an organ or vascular bed, in part due to their slow removal from the bloodstream. Because epinephrine has a large β-receptor effect, cardiac function (i.e., HR and contractility) increases far more than for norepinephrine (Table 13-2). The β-receptor effect also constricts precapillary blood vessels and large veins. Epinephrine has a weaker effect on blood vessels in skeletal muscle than norepinephrine due to the greater affinity of epinephrine for β2- than α1-receptors. Epinephrine, due to its greater β-effects, can increase metabolic rate twice normal, and can increase glycogenolysis in liver and muscle, thereby raising blood glucose levels.

Infusions of epinephrine have dose-dependent actions at α- and β-receptors. Low doses (2-10 µg/min) predominantly stimulate β1- and β2-receptors (see Table 13-2). β1-receptor stimulation results in increased HR, cardiac output, contractility, and conduction. Activation of β2-adrenoceptors causes relaxation of bronchial smooth muscle, increased liver glycogenolysis, and vasodilatation in many regional vascular tissues. Blood vessel dilation leads to decreased diastolic BP from redistribution of blood flow to low-resistance circulations. At higher doses of epinephrine (>10 µg/min), α-receptors are activated, leading to vasoconstriction of the skin, mucosa, and renal vascular beds, which promotes blood flow redistribution away from these circulations. Further stimulation of α-receptors decreases skeletal muscle and splanchnic blood flow and inhibits insulin secretion.

Table 13-1. Relative Adrenergic Drug Effects on Peripheral Resistance and Capacitance Vessels*

	Vasoconstriction	
	α1 ARTERIAL	α1 VENOUS
Norepinephrine	+++++	+++++
Phenylephrine	++++	+++++
Epinephrine	0/++++†	0/++++†
Dopamine	0/++++‡	+++
Methoxamine, metaraminol	+++++	++++
Ephedrine	++	+++
Dobutamine	+/0	?
Isoproterenol	0	0

*Drugs are listed in descending order of potency within each vascular region.
†Dose-dependent; β effects of epinephrine predominate at low doses.
‡Dose-dependent; dopamine and β effects predominate at low doses.

Predominant Physiologic Effects of α1 and Dopamine (D) Receptor Activation

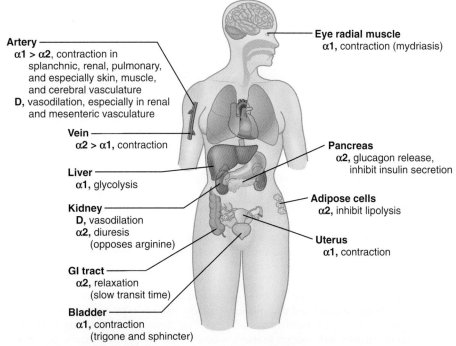

Artery
α1 > α2, contraction in splanchnic, renal, pulmonary, and especially skin, muscle, and cerebral vasculature
D, vasodilation, especially in renal and mesenteric vasculature

Vein
α2 > α1, contraction

Liver
α1, glycolysis

Kidney
D, vasodilation
α2, diuresis (opposes arginine)

GI tract
α2, relaxation (slow transit time)

Bladder
α1, contraction (trigone and sphincter)

Eye radial muscle
α1, contraction (mydriasis)

Pancreas
α2, glucagon release, inhibit insulin secretion

Adipose cells
α2, inhibit lipolysis

Uterus
α1, contraction

Figure 13-2 Predominant physiologic effects of α1-adrenergic and dopamine (D) receptors.

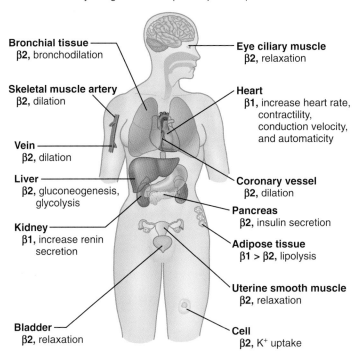

Predominant Physiologic Effects of β1 and β2 Receptor Activation

Bronchial tissue
β2, bronchodilation

Eye ciliary muscle
β2, relaxation

Skeletal muscle artery
β2, dilation

Heart
β1, increase heart rate, contractility, conduction velocity, and automaticity

Vein
β2, dilation

Liver
β2, gluconeogenesis, glycolysis

Coronary vessel
β2, dilation

Pancreas
β2, insulin secretion

Kidney
β1, increase renin secretion

Adipose tissue
β1 > β2, lipolysis

Uterine smooth muscle
β2, relaxation

Bladder
β2, relaxation

Cell
β2, K⁺ uptake

Figure 13-3 Predominant physiologic effects of β₁- and β₂-adrenergic receptor activation.

Epinephrine has broad clinical effects and thus its use has diminished as more selective synthetic adrenergic agonists have become available. However, epinephrine is still commonly added to local anesthetics to prolong their duration of action. Epinephrine is also indicated in anaphylactic shock, localized bleeding, bronchospasm, and stridor related to laryngotracheal edema. Subcutaneous doses of 0.2 to 0.5 mg can be used in early anaphylaxis to stabilize mast cells and reduce degranulation. Epinephrine also stimulates cellular K^+ uptake via β2-receptors and for short periods can be used to treat life-threatening hyperkalemia.

Norepinephrine

Norepinephrine is the principal endogenous mediator of SNS activity secreted from postganglionic terminals to act on adrenergic effector organs. Intravenous administration (4-12 μg/min) results in dose-dependent hemodynamic effects on α1- and β-adrenoceptors (see Table 13-2). Compared with the effects of epinephrine, norepinephrine has a greater effect at α1-receptors and no effect on β2-receptors, thereby creating greater arterial and venous vascular constriction than epinephrine (see Table 13-1). In lower doses, β1 actions predominate, and BP increases due to augmented cardiac output. Larger doses of norepinephrine stimulate the α1-receptors and result in arterial and venous smooth muscle contraction in hepatic, skeletal muscle, splanchnic, and renal vascular systems. At these larger doses, HR and cardiac output can decrease via baroreflex mechanisms.

Intravenous administration of norepinephrine is most often used therapeutically for treatment of profound vasodilation, as in septic shock unresponsive to fluid administration. It will increase BP, left ventricular stroke work index, cardiac output, and urine output. When given to patients already exhibiting marked vasoconstriction, further increases in vascular resistance can lead to compromised limb and organ blood flow, resulting in ischemia. Norepinephrine can produce arrhythmias, but it is less arrhythmogenic than epinephrine. Its effect on pulmonary α1-receptors combined with its increase in venous return can result in pulmonary hypertension and right heart failure. To minimize this effect during open heart surgery, it can be given directly into the left atrium along with a selective pulmonary vasodilator such as prostaglandin E_1.

Dopamine

Dopamine is an endogenous catecholamine that is also involved in central and peripheral neural transmission. Dopamine is synthesized from tyrosine and is the immediate precursor to norepinephrine (see Figure 13-1). Parenteral administration of dopamine does not cross into the CNS; therapy of Parkinson's disease requires use of the precursor L-DOPA that can cross the blood-brain barrier. Dopamine is commonly used for hemodynamic support and maintenance of adequate perfusion during shock. For these hemodynamic effects it must be given via continuous infusion because of rapid metabolism. At low infusion rates (1-3 μg/kg/min), vasodilation of coronary, renal, and mesenteric vasculature occurs and renal blood flow, glomerular filtration, and Na^+ excretion increase due to D1-like receptor agonism (see Figure 13-2). Although this "renal dose" of dopamine was purported to improve kidney function in patients at risk for acute renal failure, metaanalysis has failed to show improvement in renal dysfunction or mortality.[20] At doses of 3 to 10 μg/kg/min, β1-receptor stimulation leads to positive inotropic and chronotropic effects, and at higher doses (>10 μg/kg), α1-receptor activation

Table 13-2. Relative Potency of Common, Naturally Occurring, and Synthetic Adrenergic Agonists

SYMPATHOMIMETICS	α1	α2	Receptors β1	β2	D1	D2	DOSE DEPENDENCE*
Phenylephrine	+++++	?	±	0	0		++
Norepinephrine	+++++	+++++	+++	0	0		+++
Epinephrine	++++	+++	++++	++	0		++++
Ephedrine	++	?	++++	++	0		++
Dopamine	+ to +++++	?	++++	++	+++	?	+++++
Dobutamine†	0 to +	?	++++	++	0		++
Isoproterenol	0	0	+++++	+++++	0		0
Dexmedetomidine	+	+++++	0	0	0		
Clonidine	++	+++++	0	0	0		
Fenoldopam	0	0	0	0	+++++		

†Dobutamine is a racemic mixture; (−)dobutamine is a potent α1-agonist, and (+)dobutamine is a potent α1-antagonist, reducing its net vasoconstrictor effect.
*(α, β, or D).

causes peripheral vasoconstriction and can reduce renal blood flow.

Metabolism of Catecholamines

The catecholamines are metabolized by catechol-*O*-methyltransferase (COMT) and monoamine oxidase (MAO). COMT is an intracellular enzyme located in postsynaptic neurons. MAO is concentrated in the mitochondria of nerve terminals, resulting in a constant turnover of norepinephrine even in the resting nerve terminal. Metabolites can be detected in urine as metanephrines or vanillylmandelic acid. Urine collections and analysis can be useful to follow progress in treatment of pheochromocytoma. There are two primary termination routes for norepinephrine released from nerve terminals: simple diffusion (and metabolism in plasma, kidney, or liver) and reuptake into noradrenergic nerve terminals (which can be blocked by cocaine and most tricyclic antidepressants). Synthetic sympathomimetic drugs that mimic endogenous catecholamines can have longer durations of action due to resistance to metabolism by MAO or COMT.

Synthetic Catecholamine-Like Drugs

Synthetic catecholamines, which are also included as sympathomimetic drugs, are a mainstay of critical care and perioperative medicine for support of the circulation. Depending on their selectivity and potency for different subtypes of α-, β-, and dopamine-receptors, their route of administration, their lipid solubility, and their metabolism, sympathomimetic drugs can be used to achieve a variety of clinical effects. Certain drugs also have indirect sympathomimetic action; these include ephedrine, tyramine, and the amphetamines. They cause release of norepinephrine from its storage vesicles in the sympathetic nerve endings, thereby increasing synaptic concentration and postsynaptic effects.

D1-Receptor Agonists

Fenoldopam is a synthetic, selective D1-agonist without significant D2-, α-adrenergic, or β2-adrenergic effects (see Table 13-2 and Figure 13-2).[21] It is 10-fold more potent than dopamine. The principal use of fenoldopam is to manage hypertension in doses of 0.1 to 0.8 μg/kg/min, with upward titration in 0.1-μg/kg/min steps as needed. A low-dose

infusion of fenoldopam (~0.1-0.2 μg/kg/min) produces renal vasodilation and increases renal blood flow, glomerular filtration rate, and Na+ excretion without changes in systemic BP. A renal protective effect has been observed in aortic and cardiac surgery involving cardiopulmonary bypass.[22,23] When compared with dopamine in acute early renal dysfunction, fenoldopam is more effective at reversing renal hypoperfusion.[24] A metaanalysis indicated that fenoldopam reduces both the need for renal replacement therapy and in-hospital death in cardiovascular surgery.[25]

α1-Receptor Agonists

Agonists of α1-adrenoceptors exert vasoconstrictor actions on arteries and veins, leading to BP increase and redistribution of blood flow (see Figure 13-2).[26] In healthy individuals, cardiac output is maintained because of increased preload. HR typically slows via the baroreflex response to increased BP. Myocardial blood flow and oxygen delivery can be improved due to the longer diastolic filling time from the lower HR, and from improved diastolic coronary blood flow because of the increased aortic BP. In patients with impaired ventricular function, increases in afterload can impair myocardial function. Topical use of α1-agonists can be used for vasoconstriction (e.g., on nasal mucosa).

PHENYLEPHRINE

The effects of phenylephrine were described in the 1930s, and it was first used to maintain BP during spinal anesthesia.[27] It is a nearly pure α1 selective agonist, only affecting β-receptors at very high doses (see Table 13-2). It has similar potency to norepinephrine for α1-receptors but has a longer duration of action. Phenylephrine produces greater venoconstriction than arterial vasoconstriction and therefore increases venous return and stroke volume. Cardiac output typically does not change due to baroreflex slowing of HR. Phenylephrine can be useful as a bolus or continuous infusion for treatment of hypotension, and can be used to reverse unwanted right-to-left shunt in tetralogy of Fallot. Newer evidence suggests that phenylephrine is not detrimental to fetal oxygen delivery in pregnant patients who are hypotensive after neuraxial blockade. However, although not harmful, it still might be inferior to ephedrine in maintaining placental blood flow during cesarean delivery.[28,29] A 0.25%, 0.5%, or 1% phenylephrine solution can be used topically as a nasal decongestant; 2.5% or

10% phenylephrine solutions are used to produce mydriasis when administered into the eye. Both these routes can raise BP. Rarely, more serious side effects such as pulmonary edema and adverse cardiac events result. Thus α1-adrenergic antagonists, such as phentolamine or tolazoline, or direct vasodilating drugs, such as hydralazine or nicardipine, should be available. β-blockers are contraindicated to treat a hypertensive crisis from phenylephrine (such as an accidental overdose). β-blockers in this situation can reduce myocardial contractility and produce acute pulmonary edema in the face of high afterload.[30]

METHOXAMINE

First described in 1948 and used to maintain BP during spinal anesthesia, methoxamine has a longer duration of action, more arterial vasoconstriction, and less venoconstriction compared with phenylephrine.[31] It is not typically used to support BP acutely since it can increase afterload and has a long half-life. Doses of 1 to 5 mg every 15 minutes are typical. Untoward hypertension can occur following its use to treat regional anesthetic-induced hypotension because sympathetic tone returns as the spinal anesthetic recovers before the action of methoxamine dissipates.

MIDODRINE

Midodrine is an orally absorbed α1-agonist with a half-life of about 3 hours and duration of action of 4 to 6 hours. It is used to treat dialysis-related hypotension or autonomic failure resulting in postural hypotension, but hypertension is a possible effect while supine.

α2-Receptor Agonists

Agonists of α2-receptors such as clonidine were originally used as antihypertensive agents because of their central effect to decrease sympathetic outflow from the CNS and to reduce presynaptic norepinephrine release. The α2$_a$-receptor mediates sedation and hypnosis, sympatholysis, neuroprotection, diuresis and inhibition of insulin and growth hormone secretion.[32-34] Rapid intravenous administration of α2-agonists such as dexmedetomidine can transiently increase BP through vasoconstriction at postsynaptic α2$_b$-receptors on arteries and veins. This receptor subtype might also account for their antishivering effect. Postsynaptic α2-receptors exist in a number of other tissues and organs including liver, pancreas, platelets, kidney, fat, and eye (see Figure 13-2).

Within the CNS, a large density of α2-receptors is located in the medullary dorsal motor complex and in the locus ceruleus. The locus ceruleus is an important modulator of wakefulness and the major site of the sedative/hypnotic actions of the α2-agonists. Among the many desirable properties of α2-agonists that promote their use in the perioperative period are anxiolysis, sedation, reductions in minimal alveolar concentration (MAC) of volatile anesthetics, reduced chest wall rigidity from opioids, reduction in intraoperative BP variability from intubation, extubation and surgical stress response, and reductions in postanesthetic shivering.[35] A metaanalysis found that α2-receptor agonists reduce perioperative cardiac mortality and ischemia, a benefit likely attributable to reduced sympathetic outflow and reduced shivering.[36] Side effects include sedation, dry mouth, and bradycardia via reduced sympathetic "tone," and a slight

Table 13-3. Classification of α-Receptors and the Relative α1/α2 Selectivity

| | Order of Selectivity | |
	AGONISTS	ANTAGONISTS
α1	Methoxamine	Prazosin
	Phenylephrine	Phenoxybenzamine
	Norepinephrine	Phentolamine
	Epinephrine	Tolazoline
	Dopamine	Yohimbine
	Clonidine (220:1)	
α2	Dexmedetomidine (1620:1)	

vagomimetic effect. It is likely that some of the effects from α2-receptor agonists are from actions at nonadrenergic imidazoline receptors.

CLONIDINE

Clonidine, first synthesized in the 1960s, has an onset time after oral administration of 30 to 60 minutes, with a half-life of 6 to 24 hours. The α2:α1-receptor affinity is ~220:1 (Table 13-3). It is available in 100-, 250-, and 300-μg tablets for oral administration, a transdermal patch releasing 150 to 200 μg over 24 hours, and an injectable solution of 150 μg/mL. Oral dosing is typically every 8 hours. Clonidine should not be withheld prior to surgery because acute withdrawal can result in rebound hypertension.[37] Neuraxial administration can be used to lessen the requirement for opioids when treating acute and chronic pain. Epidural clonidine is indicated for treatment of severe cancer pain (0.5 μg/kg/hr). When given in this manner, bradycardia and sedation can occur but respiratory drive is maintained. Clonidine also is beneficial in the treatment of opioid withdrawal in an intensive care unit (ICU) setting.[38]

DEXMEDETOMIDINE

Dexmedetomidine is highly selective for α2-adrenoceptors (see Table 13-3), with an α2:α1-receptor affinity of 1620:1. Intravenous administration in the ICU setting is useful for continuous sedation and analgesia while sparing respiratory drive. Sedation is described as "arousable sedation" much like natural sleep, consistent with effects on central sleep mechanisms. Patients receiving dexmedetomidine for postsurgical pain have slower early postoperative HRs and require 50% less morphine in the PACU.[39] In a prospective randomized study, dexmedetomidine initiated at the end of coronary artery bypass surgery and continued into the ICU resulted in reduced use of analgesics, β-blockers, diuretics, antiemetics, and epinephrine, and achieved adequate sedation compared to propofol sedation.[40] In the ICU setting following cardiac surgery, the combination of opioid/dexmedetomidine sedation resulted in less delirium compared to opioid/benzodiazepine sedation.[41,42] Recommended dosage is a 1 μg/kg load given over 10 to 20 minutes followed with a 0.2 to 0.7 μg/kg/hr infusion. Hypotension and bradycardia are common side effects and bradyarrhythmias and sinus arrest are rare but potential serious adverse events. Newer applications for dexmedetomidine include pediatric sedation for hospital procedures, treatment of emergence agitation, and sedation in the ICU setting. Additionally, the FDA approved the use of dexmedetomidine for MAC sedation in 2010.[43]

β1-Receptor Agonists

ISOPROTERENOL

Isoproterenol, the isopropyl derivative of norepinephrine, was the first synthetic β-receptor agonist in clinical use. It is given parenterally due to its short duration of action (less than 1 hour).[44] It has almost purely β-receptor activity, with minimal α-receptor affinity. It is nonselective for β1- and β2-receptors (see Table 13-2). Isoproterenol produces positive chronotropic and inotropic cardiac effects via β1-adrenoceptor stimulation, and bronchodilation and vasodilatation in vascular smooth muscle through β2-activation. Large doses cause tachycardia and decrease diastolic BP, which reduces coronary blood flow and thus can compromise myocardium at risk or worsen dysrhythmias. Dobutamine is a common substitute for isoproterenol due to lesser effects on HR and myocardial oxygen demand. The emergence of phosphodiesterase inhibitors to improve myocardial performance has also reduced the need for isoproterenol as an inotropic agent.[45] The β2 response from isoproterenol can be used for bronchodilation, although other β2 drugs are more typically used. Isoproterenol has been used to manage heart failure secondary to bradycardia, cor pulmonale, pulmonary hypertension, as a chemical "pacer" in third-degree heart block, and in torsades de pointes ventricular tachycardia.

DOBUTAMINE

Dobutamine is a synthetic catecholamine obtained by substitution of a bulky aromatic group on the side chain of dopamine. Dobutamine is a racemic mixture of the (+) and (−) isomers. The (−) isomer acts on α1-adrenergic receptors and increases vascular resistance, and the (+) isomer is a potent β1-adrenergic receptor agonist and a potent α1-adrenergic receptor antagonist that blocks the effects of (−) dobutamine (see Table 13-2). Compared to dopamine, dobutamine has less notable venoconstriction and is less likely to increase HR and more likely to decrease pulmonary vascular resistance. The most prominent effects with increasing infusion rates of dobutamine (2-20 μg/kg/min IV) are a progressive increase in cardiac output, decrease in left ventricular filling pressure, minimal increase in HR until higher doses, and decreases or no change in systematic vascular resistance. However, when given to β-blocked patients, systemic vascular resistance can increase, leading to increases in BP from the unmasked α1-effect. Dobutamine has minimal β2-effects. Thus it often improves cardiac output without major adverse effects on the myocardial oxygen supply/demand ratio because afterload is maintained, thereby improving coronary blood flow.[46] It enhances automaticity of the sinus and atrioventricular nodes and facilitates intraventricular conduction. It does not affect dopamine receptors. Dobutamine is prepared in 5% dextrose in water because it is inactivated in alkaline solutions. Tachyphylaxis can occur with infusions longer than 72 hours. Dobutamine is often used for nonexercise cardiac stress testing and for the treatment of acute heart failure, especially in patients being weaned from cardiopulmonary bypass.

Selective β2-Receptor Agonists

Selective β2-receptor agonists are indicated in the treatment of acute asthma and chronic obstructive pulmonary disease (COPD). These agents work by reducing bronchial airway resistance via smooth muscle relaxation. By changing the catechol ring (3,4-dihydroxylphenyl) to a resorcinol ring (3,5-dihydroxylphenyl), there is improved bioavailability due to reduced action of COMT. Further substitutions on the amino group increase β-receptor activity, reduce α-receptor activity, and increase the duration of action by decreasing metabolism by MAO.

Metaproterenol (orciprenaline), albuterol, salmeterol, and isoetharine (isoetaine) are inhaled, thereby reducing their systemic side effects. These reach therapeutic concentrations in the bronchi with minimal activation of cardiac and peripheral β2-receptors. In addition to bronchodilation, therapeutic effects include suppression of release of leukotrienes and histamine from mast cells and decreased microvascular permeability. However, at higher concentrations all currently used β2-selective agonists also stimulate β1-receptors, which increases the risk for arrhythmias (predominantly atrial fibrillation). Other potential adverse effects, particularly when given orally or parenterally, are skeletal muscle tremor, tachycardia, mismatching of pulmonary ventilation and perfusion, and pulmonary edema. Long-term use can lead to tolerance, bronchial hyperreactivity, and hyperglycemia in diabetic patients.

TERBUTALINE AND RITODRINE

Terbutaline can be administered orally, subcutaneously, or by inhalation. It is rapidly effective by the latter two routes and its effects persist for 36 hours, in part due to its structure with a resorcinol ring preventing COMT action. A subcutaneous dose of 0.25 mg can be useful to treat status asthmaticus. Terbutaline is used primarily long term for obstructive pulmonary disease, and acutely for status asthmaticus, bronchospasm, and acute anaphylactic shock, where it does not have the cardiac stimulating effects of epinephrine.

Terbutaline and ritodrine are also tocolytic drugs used to manage premature labor contractions through relaxation of the myometrium via their β2 effect. Ritodrine is usually started intravenously and is continued orally if tocolysis is achieved. It is metabolized in the liver to inactive conjugates, and about half the drug is excreted unchanged in the urine. Albuterol is similar to terbutaline, although it cannot be given subcutaneously. Continuous use of β-agonists has been associated with hypokalemia as well as tachyphylaxis. The mechanism of hypokalemia involves insulin mediated increase in uptake of extracellular K^+ or increased Na^+/K^+ ATPase activity.[47] Angina, cardiac arrhythmias, hyperglycemia, hypokalemia, and pulmonary edema with normal pulmonary capillary wedge pressures have been attributed to terbutaline and ritodrine therapy.[48]

INDIRECT-ACTING SYMPATHOMIMETICS

Some of the synthetic catecholamine-like drugs have an indirect sympathomimetic action. These drugs include ephedrine, tyramine, and the amphetamines. Because their effects are to cause release of norepinephrine from synaptic vesicles in sympathetic nerve endings, care must be taken when they are administered to patients taking tricyclic antidepressants (TCA) or monoamine oxidase inhibitors (MAOIs).[49] The TCAs inhibit catecholamine reuptake and the MAOIs inhibit catecholamine breakdown. MAOIs in combination with serotonin reuptake inhibitors can also lead to neuromuscular and autonomic hyperactivity and altered mental status (serotonin syndrome).[50]

Ephedrine

Ephedrine is one of the most commonly used noncatecholamine sympathomimetic drugs in the perioperative period. Ephedrine is a natural product of the ephedra plant (*Ephedra sinica*), and is a mixed-acting, noncatecholamine sympathomimetic with both direct and indirect stimulating effects on α- and β-adrenergic receptors. It acts indirectly by competing with norepinephrine for local reuptake into synaptic vesicles, resulting in elevated concentrations of norepinephrine at receptor sites. Intravenous effects resemble those of epinephrine, albeit with a less potent but longer lasting effect. It causes increases in HR, cardiac output, and BP that last 10 to 15 minutes. Tachyphylaxis due to catecholamine depletion can occur with repeat doses.

Ephedrine relaxes bronchial smooth muscle, increases trigone and sphincter muscle tone in the urinary bladder, and has a stimulatory effect on the CNS that increases MAC (minimum alveolar concentration). Uterine and placental artery blood flow are not adversely affected when ephedrine is used to sustain BP during spinal anesthesia for cesarean section, and umbilical artery vascular resistance remains unchanged. This is due to an often unappreciated, pronounced effect of ephedrine to cause venoconstriction, thereby improving preload, cardiac output, and uterine blood flow.

Amphetamine and Other Central Nervous System Stimulants

Amphetamine and methamphetamine are powerful stimulants of the CNS, in addition to having peripheral α and β actions common to indirect acting sympathomimetics. They cause release and inhibit reuptake of stimulatory neurotransmitters in the cortex, motor nuclei, and reticular activating system. Acute effects include wakefulness, alertness, mood elevation, decreased sense of fatigue, and increased initiative, self-confidence, euphoria, and elation. Peripheral indirect activity leads to acute increases in BP with reflex bradycardia; large doses can cause arrhythmias. Chronic use leads to a decrease in BP because the metabolites are false neurotransmitters. Even though therapeutic use has declined, their respective methylenedioxy derivatives (MDA and MDMA) remain popular illicit recreational drugs. Treatment of acute intoxication consists of acidification of urine to enhance elimination, administration of sedatives, and control of cardiovascular side effects. Dantrolene is indicated to prevent hyperthermia.

Methylphenidate (Ritalin, Methylin) is structurally related to amphetamine, but has milder CNS-stimulating activity and less effect on motor function. It is used to treat narcolepsy and attention deficit/hyperactivity disorder. Side effects of insomnia, anorexia, weight loss, suppression of growth, and abdominal pain have been described in children. Overdose causes symptoms similar to those of overdose with amphetamine, including restlessness, agitation, irritability progressing to confusion, aggressive behavior, delirium, and paranoid delusions.

False Transmitters and Monoamine Oxidase Inhibition

MAOIs are powerful drugs used to treat depression and Parkinson's disease. They include phenelzine, iproclozide, isocarboxazid, tranylcypromine, selegiline, rasagiline, and moclobemide. MAO catalyzes the oxidation of monoamines such as norepinephrine, serotonin (MAO-A), phenylethylamine (MAO-B), and dopamine (MAO-A,B). Dietary amines (e.g., tyramine derived from fermentation processes in cheese, wine, and beer) can cause a hypertensive reaction in patients taking MAOIs. In the presence of MAOIs, tyramine displaces norepinephrine from synaptic vesicles leading to profound hypertension. When an indirect acting sympathomimetic drug such as ephedrine is administered, an exaggerated BP increase can occur, especially in the first weeks of therapy with an MAOI. With long-term use, there is downregulation of adrenergic receptors, and tricyclic antidepressants and selective serotonin reuptake inhibitors are usually continued through the perioperative period given their rapid excretion and long latency period for effectiveness.[51] MAOIs require discontinuation before surgery to allow restoration of enzyme activity. Irreversible MAOIs should be discontinued two weeks before surgery or switched to a reversible MAOI (moclobemide), which needs to be stopped only 24 hours before surgery.[52] Because dopamine is a substrate for MAO, it should be administered at much lower doses in patients taking an MAOI or TCA. Use of meperidine with an MAOI can lead to hypertension, convulsions, and coma. Because of their risk for lethal dietary and drug interactions, MAOIs are generally used only when patients are unresponsive to first-line antidepressants.

Ergot Alkaloids

Poisoning caused by the fungus *Claviceps purpurea* on wheat or rye in the Middle Ages was associated with mental disturbances and severe, painful peripheral vasoconstriction frequently leading to gangrene of the extremities. Often termed *St. Anthony's fire*, this effect is from ergot alkaloids that stimulate contraction of a variety of smooth muscles, both directly and indirectly via adrenergic and serotonergic receptors. Contraction of vascular smooth muscle leads to coronary, cerebral, and peripheral vasoconstriction. In clinical practice, the ergot alkaloids are taken orally and are slowly absorbed from the gut with bioavailability of approximately 10%; they are hepatically metabolized and eliminated primarily in the bile. The oral dose of ergotamine to treat an acute migraine is 2 mg, followed by a 1-mg dose every half hour to a maximum of 6 mg. The intramuscular dose is 0.5 mg, repeated every half hour to a maximum of 3 mg. Intramuscular administration of ergonovine is used to enhance postpartum uterine contractions. The usual dose of 0.2 mg can be continued up to a week postpartum as an oral preparation. Ergot alkaloids are contraindicated in patients with sickle cell disease, peripheral and coronary artery disease, thyrotoxicosis, and porphyria.

Other Sympathomimetic Drugs

Pseudoephedrine and phenylpropanolamine are commonly used as oral preparations to treat nasal congestion via vasoconstriction. These sympathomimetic drugs are similar to ephedrine in releasing norepinephrine and epinephrine, but have fewer CNS effects. Several drugs are used primarily as vasoconstrictors via α1-receptor agonism for local application to the nasal mucous membranes or to the conjunctiva, including propylhexedrine, tetrahydrozoline, oxymetazoline, naphazoline, and xylometazoline. Their systemic absorption is minimal when compared with topical phenylephrine solutions. Cocaine is another sympathomimetic still used clinically for its analgesic and vasoconstrictive properties. Intranasal cocaine with a topical local anesthetic has been shown to provide adequate pain control during repair of nasal fractures.[53] However, given the potential for abuse and toxicity, the aforementioned topical drugs have largely replaced the use of cocaine-containing topical solutions for vasoconstriction.

Vasopressin

Vasopressin, commonly known as arginine vasopressin (AVP), is an endogenous hormone that regulates urine volume and plasma osmolality. Although not a sympathomimetic, it, too, is used as a potent vasoconstrictor that preserves splanchnic perfusion.[54,55] It acts on V2-receptors on the collecting ducts to promote water reabsorption and concentration of urine. Higher concentrations of AVP, which result from a baroreflex response to hypotension, act on $V1_a$-receptors located on vascular smooth muscle to promote vasoconstriction via a phosphoinositol pathway. Vasopressin is available in an aqueous solution of 20 units/mL. A dose of 40 units is recommended as an alternative to a first or second dose of epinephrine during resuscitation from cardiac arrest, and can be useful in smaller doses to treat refractory intraoperative hypotension in patients on angiotensin converting enzyme inhibitors or angiotensin II receptor blockers. Doses of 1 to 8 units are typical. Vasopressin also has been cited as a useful pharmacologic aid in hemorrhagic shock due to its augmentation of the neuroendocrine stress response and can reverse severe hypotension, restore cardiovascular function, and decrease catecholamine requirements.[56-59] Furthermore, it has demonstrated these effects in hypotension that had been resistant to fluids and exogenous catecholamines.[59]

ADRENERGIC BLOCKING DRUGS

Sympatholytic drugs oppose the effects transmitted by postganglionic fibers of the SNS. Most drugs of this class act postsynaptically to compete reversibly with agonists for α- and β-adrenergic receptors. Adrenergic activity can be disrupted at several points in the stimulatory process, as follows:

1. Blockade of α-receptors, resulting primarily in dilation of vascular tissue; examples are phenoxybenzamine and phentolamine.
2. Blockade of β-receptors, the major pharmacologic target being the heart and vascular smooth muscle. Propranolol blocks β1- and β2-receptors; atenolol and metoprolol block mainly β1-receptors.
3. Blockade of sympathetic activity by drugs that block transmission of nerve impulses through autonomic ganglia at nicotinic receptors; hexamethonium blocks both sympathetic and parasympathetic transmission through the ganglia.

4. Inhibition of synthesis and storage of norepinephrine in sympathetic nerve endings; examples are reserpine and α-methyldopa.
5. Blockade of release of norepinephrine from sympathetic endings; an example is guanethidine.

α-Antagonists

The "α-blockers" play an important role in regulating the activity of the SNS both peripherally and centrally. Blockade of α2-adrenergic receptors with selective antagonists such as yohimbine can potentiate release of norepinephrine to activate both α1- and α2-receptors. Antagonists of α1-adrenergic receptors such as prazosin also stimulate release of norepinephrine, but the α1-receptor effect is blocked.

PHENOXYBENZAMINE

Phenoxybenzamine is an irreversible, noncompetitive blocker of α-adrenergic receptors (see Table 13-3). It forms a covalent link with the α-receptor such that recovery of receptor function requires synthesis of new receptor molecules with a half-life of 18 to 24 hours. The consequent reduction in peripheral vascular tone leads to orthostatic hypotension and is accompanied by baroreflex-mediated sympathetic activation resulting in increases in HR and cardiac output. Phenoxybenzamine also improves cardiac output by other mechanisms. It blocks presynaptic inhibitory α2-receptors in the heart and decreases elimination of myocardial norepinephrine by inhibition of reuptake. Overdoses are treated with norepinephrine when unopposed β1-receptor effects are present. Epinephrine is not recommended for this purpose in that its β2 effects lead to further hypotension. Oral doses of phenoxybenzamine are used to manage pheochromocytoma or urinary retention caused by neurogenic bladder or benign prostatic hypertrophy. For adults, initial dosing is 10 to 20 mg bid for pheochromocytoma and 10 to 20 mg per day for relief of obstruction in neurogenic bladder.

PHENTOLAMINE AND TOLAZOLINE

Phentolamine and tolazoline are competitive, nonselective α-receptor antagonists (see Table 13-3). Although these drugs have cardiovascular effects similar to those of phenoxybenzamine, α-blockade is short-lived and the effects are reversible with α-receptor agonists. Phentolamine and tolazoline can be used to treat hypertensive crisis due to ingestion of tyramine-containing substances in patients taking MAOIs, or due to clonidine withdrawal. Phentolamine can be given as a 5- to 15-mg intravenous bolus and has an onset in 12 minutes and duration of 10 to 30 minutes. Tolazoline has a plasma half-life of 313 hours and is excreted mainly unchanged by the kidney. The recommended dose for treatment of neonatal persistent pulmonary hypertension is a 0.5 to 2 mg/kg loading dose administered over 10 minutes followed by 0.5 to 2 mg/kg per hour. Their use to treat pulmonary hypertension has fallen out of favor with the advent of newer agents (see Chapter 23). Phentolamine can be infiltrated into tissues to reduce the vasoconstriction from accidental extravasation of norepinephrine.

PRAZOSIN

Prazosin is the prototype of a family of α-adrenergic drugs that contain a piperazinyl quinazole nucleus. Prazosin has a very high affinity for most subtypes of α1-receptors (see Table 13-3). Its α1$_B$-receptor antagonism results in dilation of arteries and veins with a decrease in peripheral vascular resistance and venous return and cardiac filling. The unexpectedly blunted reflex HR response to the hypotensive effect of prazosin might be due to a CNS effect to suppress sympathetic outflow. Prazosin is given orally (15 mg); the starting dose to treat hypertension is usually 0.5 mg at bedtime. The effects of a single dose last about 10 hours.

DOXAZOSIN, TERAZOSIN, TAMSULOSIN

Doxazosin has hemodynamic effects similar to prazosin, but its duration is about three times longer. Terazosin is less potent than prazosin but has higher bioavailability so its effects last longer. Selectivity of α1$_A$-subtype over α1$_B$-subtype receptors for relaxation of bladder neck, prostate capsule, and prostatic urethra make doxazosin and tamsulosin useful for treating benign prostatic hypertrophy with little effect on BP.

β-Antagonists

The β-adrenergic receptor blockers have a range of lipid solubilities that influence their absorption and distribution (Table 13-4). The prototype drug propranolol, developed in the early 1960s, has high lipid solubility and attains high brain concentrations. The lipid-insoluble β-blockers such as atenolol are less well absorbed orally, have fewer CNS side effects, and are excreted primarily via the kidneys (with prolonged excretion in renal failure). β2-blockade can cause bronchospasm and peripheral vasoconstriction; this can be problematic in patients with chronic obstructive pulmonary disease and peripheral vascular disease.

Modifications of the molecular structure of β-blockers can lead to a range of desired pharmacodynamic effects, including enhanced selectivity for β1-receptors, partial agonist activity at β2-receptors (known as intrinsic sympathomimetic activity, ISA), α1-receptor antagonism, and/or quinidine-like membrane stabilizing activity. ISA from drugs such as pindolol leads to less reduction of HR, cardiac output, and peripheral blood flow and reduced risk of bronchoconstriction. Most β-adrenergic antagonists do not block α-adrenergic receptors. Two exceptions are labetalol and carvedilol, which have both

nonselective β-receptor antagonist and α-receptor antagonist activity. Blockade of stimulatory presynaptic β2-receptors reduces release of norepinephrine and contributes to the hypotensive effect of β-receptor antagonists.

The β-receptor antagonists have a number of predictable side effects. They can lead to profound bradycardia, asystole and heart failure. They inhibit gluconeogenesis; in diabetics receiving β-blockers, the common signs of hypoglycemia such as tremors and tachycardia can be masked. Hypoglycemia-induced perspiration, mediated by cholinergic mechanisms, can remain the only warning sign in these patients. Blockade of peripheral β2-receptors can precipitate Raynaud's vascular spasm in susceptible patients. The use of β-blockers to attenuate adrenergic crisis can worsen hypertension (from β2-receptor blockade) if α-receptor blockade is not adequate due to unopposed α effects. Combination of β-blockers with non-dihydropyridine calcium channel blockers can significantly reduce cardiac conduction, and when also combined with H$_2$-receptor blockers, severe negative inotropism can result.

Even though myocardial depression from volatile or intravenous anesthetics is additive with that of pure β-blockers, perioperative use of β-blockers reduces morbidity and mortality in patients with documented coronary artery disease and in patients at high risk for coronary artery disease.[60-65] However, there has been some controversy regarding β-blockade with metoprolol in particular. The POISE trial showed that while those starting metoprolol in the perioperative period experienced fewer myocardial infarctions, this group also had more deaths and nonfatal cerebrovascular accidents. A metaanalysis has shown significant heterogeneity across studies, suggesting that the benefits and risks of initiating a perioperative β-blockade should be carefully weighed for each patient.[65] Clinically, both partial and pure antagonists are used in the treatment of hypertension and tachyarrhythmias, and both decrease mortality after myocardial infarction. Sudden withdrawal of β-receptor blockers can lead to rebound adrenergic effects, including tachycardia, hypertension, arrhythmias, myocardial ischemia, and infarction. The enhanced adrenergic state occurs 2 to 6 days after withdrawal.[66] This has led to the current recommendation to continue β-blockers in the perioperative period to avoid withdrawal.[51]

Table 13-4. β-Adrenergic Blocking Drugs

DRUG	RECEPTOR SELECTIVITY	ISA	PLASMA HALF-LIFE (HR)	ORAL AVAILABILITY (%)	LIPID SOLUBILITY	ELIMINATION	ORAL DOSE	IV DOSE
Propranolol	β1β2	0	3-4	36	+++	Hepatic	40-320 mg	0.5-1 mg to max 3 mg
Metoprolol	β1	0	3-4	38	+	Hepatic	100-400 mg	5 mg q 2 min to 15 mg total
Atenolol	β1	0	6-9	57	0	Renal	50-100 mg	2.5 mg over 2.5 min q 5 min to 10 mg or 0.15 mg·kg^{-1} over 20 min
Esmolol	β1	0	9 min	–	?	RBC esterase	NA	50-100 mg bolus, 0.05-0.3 mg·kg^{-1}·min^{-1} infusion
Timolol	β1β2	0	4-5	50	+	Hepatic > renal	15-45 mg; 60 mg max	Ophthalmic prep for glaucoma, 0.25-0.5 mg·mL^{-1}
Carvedilol	α1β1β2		2-8			Hepatic	12.5-50 mg	NA
Labetalol	α1β1β2		~6			Hepatic	400-1200 mg	5-20 mg IV q 5-10 min to max 300 mg; start infusion at 2 mg·min^{-1}

ISA, Intrinsic sympathomimetic activity; *NA,* not applicable; *RBC,* red blood cells.

ESMOLOL

Esmolol is a selective β1-adrenoceptor antagonist with a rapid onset of 90 seconds. Due to rapid hydrolysis by red blood cell esterase, it has a short duration of action with a half-life of only 9 to 10 minutes (see Table 13-4). Esmolol is not metabolized by plasma cholinesterase. The brevity of esmolol makes it useful as a bolus of 10 to 100 mg to reduce cardiac effects from transient β-adrenergic stimulation in the perioperative period and as an infusion in critically ill patients where it can be withdrawn quickly if adverse cardiac effects (congestive heart failure, bradycardia, hypotension) occur. As an infusion, a loading dose of 500 μg/kg followed by a 50 to 300 μg/kg/min infusion results in steady-state concentrations in 5 minutes.[67,68] β1-selectivity allows esmolol to be used safely in patients with bronchospastic and vascular disease.

LABETALOL

Labetalol is a mixture of four stereoisomers that block α1-, β1-, and β2-receptors, and is therefore considered a mixed antagonist (see Table 13-4). It is considered a peripheral vasodilator that does not cause reflex tachycardia.[69] It has an α:β antagonistic potency ratio of 1:7 when given intravenously and a ratio of 1:3 after oral administration. It is lipid soluble and has substantial first pass hepatic metabolism. The peak hypotensive effect from intravenous labetalol occurs within 5 to 15 minutes and the duration of action is 4 to 6 hours. It can be used to treat hypertension in pregnancy. Despite bradycardia from labetalol, the decreased afterload helps maintain cardiac output. It may be given in 5- to 10-mg bolus doses at 5-minute intervals to control a hypertensive crisis. Uterine blood flow is not affected, due in part to preserved cardiac output.

METOPROLOL AND ATENOLOL

Metoprolol is cardioselective with a ratio of 30:1 in affinity for β1- and β2-receptors (see Table 13-4). It is lipid soluble and has a high first pass hepatic metabolism resulting in the need for high oral doses (100-200 mg/day) compared to intravenous doses of 2.5 to 5 mg, titrated to effect. It is roughly half as potent as propranolol, and maximum β1-blockade effect is achieved at 0.2 mg/kg. Atenolol is also β1 selective, is lipophilic, and has an elimination half-life of 6 hours. Even so, the effect of an oral dose of 25 to 100 mg lasts 24 hours. In a recent study, perioperative blockade with atenolol resulted in a reduced short- and long-term mortality in high-risk patients having noncardiac surgery compared with metoprolol.[70] The differences might be explained by the longer metabolic half-life of atenolol and a higher chance of missing a dose and/or experiencing a "withdrawal" sympathetic response from a missed dose of metoprolol.

INHIBITION OF SYNTHESIS, STORAGE, AND RELEASE OF NOREPINEPHRINE

α-Methyldopa is one of a group of antihypertensive drugs called *false neurotransmitters* that replace norepinephrine in the synaptic vesicles located in postganglionic nerve endings of the SNS. It is metabolized to α-methyldopamine and then to α-methylnorepinephrine, which are less potent at adrenergic receptors than dopamine and norepinephrine, thus accounting for some of their antihypertensive effects. Central effects of the metabolites result from action on α2-receptors to decrease sympathetic outflow and to reduce anesthetic requirements by 20% to 40%. *Reserpine* prevents uptake of norepinephrine into vesicles, thereby inhibiting storage of dopamine and norepinephrine. *Guanethidine* acts by reducing norepinephrine release from sympathetic terminals and by depleting norepinephrine storage. It does not have sedating effects since it does not cross the blood-brain barrier. Side effects from the false transmitters include orthostatic hypotension, drowsiness, diarrhea, bradycardia, hepatitis, and autoimmune hemolytic anemia. Thus their use as antihypertensive drugs has fallen out of favor.

PARASYMPATHETIC PHARMACOLOGY

Cholinergic Receptors

The neurotransmitter acetylcholine (ACh) acts at distinct receptor types: nicotinic and muscarinic. The naturally occurring substances, muscarine and nicotine, were originally used to define and name the two receptor families. They have distinctly different tissue locations (see Chapter 12). Muscarinic receptors are G protein-coupled receptors with a typical seven-transmembrane configuration. There are five subtypes, M1-M5. The odd numbered subtypes are defined by *Pertussis* toxin insensitivity, coupling to G_q/G_{11} protein and stimulating phospholipase C to alter one or more ion channels. This effect generally leads to depolarization or increased excitability.[71,72] The even numbered subtypes M2 and M4 are *Pertussis* toxin sensitive, are coupled to the G_i/G_0 protein, and inhibit adenylyl cyclase to initiate a presynaptic inhibitory effect. Muscarinic subtypes M1 and M4 are found primarily in brain, M3 and M4 are found in lung, gastrointestinal tract, and glandular tissue, and M2-receptors are located in cardiac tissue. Muscarinic receptor activation by ACh at the postsynaptic junction in heart and smooth muscle leads to bradycardia, salivation, bronchoconstriction, miosis, and increased gastrointestinal motility and secretion (Table 13-5). In

Table 13-5. Antimuscarinic Drugs

DRUG	IV	IM	CNS[†]	GI TONE	GASTRIC ACID	AIRWAY SECRETIONS*	HEART RATE
Atropine	15-30 min	2-4 hr	++	--	-	--	+++[††]
Scopolamine	30-60 min	4-6 hr	+++[†]	-	-	----	–0[††]
Glycopyrrolate	2-4 hr	6-8 hr	0	---	---	---	+0

CNS, Central nervous system; *IV*, intravenous; *IM*, intramuscular; *GI*, gastrointestinal.
*Secretions may be reduced by inspissation.
[†]CNS effect often manifest as sedation before stimulation.
[††]May decelerate initially.

addition, "adrenergic" muscarinic receptors are located on presynaptic sympathetic terminals in the cardiovascular and coronary systems, and their activation reduces norepinephrine release. In brain, release of ACh is subject to substantial ongoing autoinhibition as a result of coactivation of presynaptic muscarinic receptors on cholinergic terminals.

Nicotinic receptors activate postganglionic junctions of both the sympathetic and parasympathetic nervous systems (see Chapter 12). Nicotinic receptors are also located at the neuromuscular junction (see Chapter 18). Nicotinic cholinergic receptors are heteropentameric ligand-gated ion channels that allow depolarizing inward flow of monovalent cations.[73] The nicotinic receptor agonists consist primarily of the depolarizing neuromuscular-blocking drugs (e.g., succinylcholine [suxamethonium], hexamethonium) and can simultaneously stimulate autonomic ganglia. The neuromuscular blocking drugs are considered in Chapter 19.

Muscarinic Receptor Agonists

Muscarinic agonists are divided into two general groups:
1. The choline esters (acetylcholine [ACh], methacholine, carbachol, bethanechol) and alkaloids (pilocarpine, muscarine, arecoline) that act directly on muscarinic receptors
2. Acetylcholinesterase inhibitors or anticholinesterases (physostigmine, neostigmine, pyridostigmine, edrophonium, echothiophate) that act indirectly by inhibiting ACh hydrolysis

The anticholinesterase drugs are frequently employed to reverse the action of nondepolarizing neuromuscular blocking drugs (see Chapter 19), to improve neuromuscular function in myasthenia gravis, and for colonic pseudo-obstruction. Newer drugs have been designed to improve cognitive function in Alzheimer's disease.

Due to rapid hydrolysis, direct-acting agonists such as ACh have few clinical applications, with the exception of topical application to produce miosis. Longer activity of the direct acting agonists can be achieved by methylation of the choline moiety as noted with the synthetic drug methacholine. This modification prevents significant nicotinic receptor effects and slows acetylcholinesterase metabolism (Table 13-6). Carbachol and bethanechol are long-acting synthetic parasympathetic agonists; the carbamic-linked ester moiety significantly reduces metabolism. Carbachol has significant nicotinic activity at autonomic ganglia. Bethanechol is similar to methacholine and is highly specific for muscarinic receptors. It is used orally or parenterally, has only minimal cardiac negative chronotropic and inotropic effects, and is useful therapy for postoperative urinary retention and neurogenic bladder from spinal cord injury.

Pilocarpine is a tertiary amine alkaloid with actions similar to methacholine (see Table 13-6). Clinical use includes treatment for xerostomia and glaucoma, where it is employed as a topical drug to produce miosis and reduce intraocular pressure. Pilocarpine has minimal nicotinic effects unless given systemically, in which case hypertension and tachycardia can result.

Echothiophate, a long-acting irreversible anticholinesterase, is instilled into the eye to reduce resistance to aqueous humor outflow and lower intraocular pressure. Echothiophate is absorbed into the circulation and, therefore, can prolong the duration of succinylcholine because of a reduction in cholinesterase levels. The action of ester-based local anesthetics can also be lengthened in patients receiving echothiophate through slower metabolism of the local anesthetic. Enzyme activity might not return to normal for 4 to 6 weeks after discontinuation of long-term therapy.

Muscarinic Receptor Antagonists

Anticholinergic drugs (atropine, scopolamine, glycopyrrolate) competitively inhibit the action of ACh by reversibly binding at muscarinic receptors. Nicotinic ACh receptors are not affected by doses usually employed. The naturally occurring anticholinergic drugs atropine and scopolamine are tertiary amines derived from the belladonna plant. Low doses of atropine and scopolamine (up to 2 µg/kg) have effects within the CNS to augment vagal outflow, which can result in bradycardia.[74]

At usual clinical doses (0.5-1 mg), atropine acts at peripheral muscarinic receptors to block the action of ACh, thereby increasing HR, producing mydriasis (pupil dilation) and cycloplegia (paralysis of accommodation), and inhibiting salivary, bronchial, pancreatic, and gastrointestinal secretions (see Table 13-5). It reduces gastric secretion of acid, mucin and proteolytic enzymes, slows gastric emptying, reduces lower esophageal tone and slows gastric motility. Atropine reduces the activity of sweat glands and thus evaporative heat loss, even in small doses. It relaxes bronchial smooth muscle, reduces airway resistance, inhibits mucociliary clearance in the airways, and thickens bronchial secretions.[75] Atropine and scopolamine are tertiary amines that cross the blood-brain barrier and the placenta. There is no harmful effect on the fetus. Their central effects might account for their antiemetic properties and control of nausea triggered by the vestibular apparatus.[76] Scopolamine skin patches are used to control motion sickness and postoperative nausea and vomiting (see Chapter 29). Atropine can block presynaptic muscarinic receptors on adrenergic terminals leading to a sympathomimetic effect. These drugs should be used with caution in patients with cardiac tachyarrhythmias or severe coronary artery disease, and are contraindicated in narrow angle glaucoma because they can increase intraocular pressure. They are considered safe when given parenterally to patients with the more common open angle glaucoma.

Scopolamine in the usual clinical doses of 0.3 to 0.6 mg displays stronger antisialagogue and ocular activity, but is less likely than glycopyrrolate or atropine to increase HR (see Table 13-5).[77] Scopolamine crosses the blood-brain barrier more effectively than atropine and is commonly associated with amnesia, drowsiness, fatigue, and non-REM sleep. One limitation imposed by the central actions of higher doses of scopolamine (and atropine) is an infrequent side effect termed the *central anticholinergic syndrome*. The origin of the syndrome is due to blockade of the abundant muscarinic ACh receptors in the CNS, which leads to agitation, disorientation, delirium, hallucinations, and restlessness. It can manifest as somnolence and should be considered in the differential diagnosis of delayed awakening from anesthesia. Physostigmine is a tertiary amine anticholinesterase that crosses into the CNS and can be administered in intravenous doses of 15 to 60 mg/kg for the treatment of central anticholinergic syndrome.

Glycopyrrolate is a synthetic quaternary amine that does not cross into the CNS and does not produce the CNS side

Table 13-6. Comparative Muscarinic Actions of Systemic Direct Cholinomimetic Agents

	ACETYLCHOLINE	METHACHOLINE	CARBAMYLCHOLINE	BETHANECHOL	PILOCARPINE
Esterase hydrolysis	+++	+	0	0	0
Eye (topical)					
Iris	++	++	+++	+++	+++
Ciliary	++	++	+++	+++	++
Heart					
Rate	−−−	−−	−	−	?
Contractility	−	−	−	−	
Conduction	−−	−−	−	−	
Smooth muscle					
Vascular	−−−	−−	−	+	−
Bronchial	++	++	+++	+++	++
GI motility	++	++	+++	+++	++
GI sphincters	−−−	−	−−	−−	++
Biliary	++	++	+++	+++	++
Bladder					
Detrusor	++	+	+++	+++	++
Sphincter	−−	−	−−	−−	++
Exocrine glands					
Respiratory	+++	++	+++	++	+++
Salivary	++	+++	++	++	+++
Pharyngeal	++	++	++	++	+++
Lacrimal	++	+++	++	++	+++
Sweat	++	++	++	++	+++
GI acid, secretions	++	+	+++	++	+++
Nicotinic actions	+++	+	+++	−	+++

GI, Gastrointestinal; +, stimulation; −, inhibition.

effects noted with atropine and scopolamine (see Table 13-5). It is more potent and longer acting at peripheral muscarinic receptors than atropine. It is used clinically as an antisialagogue to treat bradycardia and to inhibit cardiac muscarinic receptor side effects when anticholinesterase agents are employed to reverse the effects of muscle relaxants. The antisialagogue dose of 0.004 mg/kg can last up to 8 hours. Similar to atropine, low doses can cause initial bradycardia.

Inhalation of anticholinergics is the most effective route of administration when bronchodilation without systemic side effects is desired. Ipratropium, a derivative of methylatropine, is an inhaled anticholinergic that inhibits muscarinic receptor subtypes with a peak effect of 30 to 60 minutes and a duration of action of 3 to 6 hours.[78] Low doses of ipratropium decrease airway size via preferential blockade of neuronal M2-muscarinic receptors. However, following large ipratropium doses, bronchodilation results from blockade of M3-muscarinic receptors on airway smooth muscle. Ipratropium, unlike atropine, does not affect mucociliary clearance of respiratory secretions. In chronic obstructive pulmonary disease, ipratropium is beneficial in improving pulmonary function, and tachyphylaxis with long-term use has not been demonstrated.[79] In acute asthma exacerbations, ipratropium can provide additional benefit when used with inhaled β2-agonists.

KEY POINTS

- The naturally occurring catecholamines epinephrine, norepinephrine, and dopamine are derived from the amino acid L-tyrosine. Their sites of action are on adrenergic and dopaminergic receptors.
- Adrenergic receptors have been subdivided based on their effector responses. β1-receptors are localized in cardiac tissue and mediate increases in HR, contractility, and conduction velocity whereas β2-receptors are found on arterioles, vena cava, pulmonary artery, aorta, and uterine smooth muscle; both types mediate smooth muscle relaxation. The α1-receptors mediate arterial and venous smooth muscle contraction. The α2-receptors also mediate vascular constriction but have additional actions in the CNS to reduce sympathetic outflow and pain perception and to produce sedation.
- Dopamine is an endogenous catecholamine involved in neural transmission. Parenteral administration can be used for hemodynamic support and, depending on the infusion rate, activates D1-receptors to dilate renal and coronary vessels and β1-receptors to cause chronotropic and inotropic effects, or, at high doses, activates α1-receptors to mediate vasoconstriction. Fenoldopam is a synthetic selective D1-agonist used to treat hypertension or to improve renal function via selective vasodilation.
- Dexmedetomidine is a highly selective α2-agonist used for sedation. It produces an "arousable" sedation much like natural sleep and is associated with less delirium compared to benzodiazepine sedation.
- Dobutamine is a racemic synthetic catecholamine. The (−) isomer acts on α1-receptors to increase vascular resistance and the (+) isomer acts on β1-receptors to increase contractility while antagonizing the increase in

vascular resistance. It increases cardiac output, decreases pulmonary vascular resistance and is unlikely to increase HR.
- Selective β2-agonists are indicated for the treatment of acute asthma and chronic obstructive pulmonary disease by reducing smooth muscle tone and bronchial airway resistance. They are most commonly given via inhalation, with longer duration of action due to structural changes that reduce metabolism.
- Ephedrine is a noncatecholamine sympathomimetic drug with both direct and indirect actions on α- and β-adrenergic receptors.
- Vasopressin is an endogenous hormone that acts on V1- and V2-receptors to promote water reabsorption and to preserve coronary, cerebral, and pulmonary blood flow while constricting splanchnic vessels during severe hypotension and shock.
- β-adrenergic receptor blockers have a number of predictable effects to slow HR and inhibit gluconeogenesis. Their effects to reduce myocardial oxygen demand and myocardial infarction can be overshadowed in select circumstances by their association with a higher risk of stroke and death.
- Muscarinic receptor antagonists inhibit the action of acetylcholine at muscarinic receptors to increase HR and pupil dilation, and reduce production of secretions.

Key References

Brienza N, Malcangi V, Dalfino L, et al. A comparison between fenoldopam and low-dose dopamine in early renal dysfunction of critically ill patients. *Crit Care Med*. 2006;34:707-714. In a prospective, multicenter RCT of critically ill patients in the ICU with early renal dysfunction, fenoldopam improved renal function compared with renal dose dopamine. (Ref. 24)

Flynn RA, Glynn DA, Kennedy MP. Anticholinergic treatment in airways diseases. *Adv Ther*. 2009;26:908-919. An excellent review of the history, pharmacokinetics and effectiveness of anticholinergic treatment for both chronic obstructive pulmonary disease and asthma. (Ref. 78)

Friedrich JO, Adhikari N, Herridge MS, Beyene J. Metaanalysis: low-dose dopamine increases urine output but does not prevent renal dysfunction or death. *Ann Intern Med*. 2005;142:510-524. A meta-analysis of 61 trials to evaluate the renal effects of low-dose dopamine. Compared with placebo, dopamine did not significantly alter mortality, the need for renal replacement therapy, or creatinine clearance. (Ref. 20)

Landoni G, Biondi-Zoccai GG, Marino G, et al. Fenoldopam reduces the need for renal replacement therapy and in-hospital death in cardiovascular surgery: a meta-analysis. *J Cardiothorac Vasc Anesth*. 2008;22:27-33. In a meta-analysis of 13 RCT in patients undergoing cardiovascular surgery, the use of fenoldopam reduced the requirement for renal replacement therapy and reduced overall mortality compared to conventional therapy. (Ref. 25)

POISE Study Group, Devereaux PJ, Yang H, et al. Effects of extended-release metoprolol succinate in patients undergoing non-cardiac surgery (POISE trial): a randomised controlled trial. *Lancet*. 2008;371:1839-1847. In a large (>8300 patients) prospective RCT, patients at risk for atherosclerotic disease undergoing non-cardiac surgery received either extended-release metoprolol or placebo beginning 2 to 4 days before surgery and continued to 30 days postsurgery. The β-blockade group had fewer myocardial infarctions but more strokes and a higher death rate. (Ref. 65)

Raab H, Lindner KH, Wenzel V. Preventing cardiac arrest during hemorrhagic shock with vasopressin. *Crit Care Med*. 2008;

36(Suppl):S474-S480. One-third of traumatic injury deaths are due to uncontrolled hemorrhagic shock. Vasopressin amplifies the neuroendocrine stress response to hemorrhage via activation of receptors in vascular beds other than coronary, cerebral, and pulmonary. The authors review the theory and actions of vasopressin in this setting. (Ref. 56)

Riker RR, Shehabi Y, Bokesch PM, et al. SEDCOM (Safety and Efficacy of Dexmedetomidine Compared With Midazolam) Study Group. Dexmedetomidine vs midazolam for sedation of critically ill patients: a randomized trial. *JAMA.* 2009;301:489-499. A prospective, double-blind RCT comparing the safety and efficacy of dexmedetomidine to midazolam for sedation in critically ill patients on mechanical ventilation. Dexmedetomidine achieved equivalent time in the targeted sedation range compared to midazolam and resulted in less delirium, tachycardia, and hypertension. There was more bradycardia in the dexmedetomidine treatment group. (Ref. 41)

Wallace AW, Au S, Cason BA. Perioperative beta-blockade: atenolol is associated with reduced mortality when compared to metoprolol. *Anesthesiology.* 2011;114:824-836. In a large retrospective analysis of 30-day and 1-year mortality following major inpatient surgery, perioperative β-blockade using atenolol was associated with reduced short- and long-term postoperative mortality compared with metoprolol. (Ref. 70)

References

1. Chen KK, Schmidt GF. The action of ephedrine, the active principle of the Chinese drug ma huang. *J Pharmacol Exp Ther.* 1924;24:339.
2. Nagai T. Ephedrin. *Pharm Zeit.* 1887;32:700.
3. Ahlquist RP. A study of the adrenotropic receptors. *Am J Physiol.* 1948;153:586-600.
4. Wikberg JE. Adrenergic receptors: classification, ligand binding and molecular properties. *Acta Med Scand Suppl.* 1982;665:19-36.
5. Minneman KP, Molinoff PB. Classification and quantitation of beta-adrenergic receptor subtypes. *Biochem Pharmacol.* 1980;29:1317-1323.
6. Lands AM, Arnold A, McAuliff JP, Luduena FP, Brown TG Jr. Differentiation of receptor systems activated by sympathomimetic amines. *Nature.* 1967;214:597-598.
7. Docherty JR. Subtypes of functional alpha1- and alpha2-adrenoceptors. *Eur J Pharmacol.* 1998;361:1-15.
8. Hieble JP, Bylund DB, Clarke DE, et al. International Union of Pharmacology. X. Recommendation for nomenclature of alpha 1-adrenoceptors: consensus update. *Pharmacol Rev.* 1995;47:267-270.
9. Zimmer HG. Otto Loewi and the chemical transmission of vagus stimulation in the heart. *Clin Cardiol.* 2006;3:135-136.
10. Dixon RA, Kobilka BK, Strader DJ, et al. Cloning of the gene and cDNA for mammalian beta-adrenergic receptor and homology with rhodopsin. *Nature.* 1986;321:75-79.
11. Royster RL. Intraoperative administration of inotropes in cardiac surgery patients. *J Cardiothor Anesth.* 1990;4:17S-28S.
12. Berkowitz DE, Schwinn DA. Basic pharmacology of alpha and beta adrenoceptors. In: Bowdle TA, Horita A, Kharasch ED, eds. The Pharmacologic Basis of Anesthesiology. New York: Churchill Livingstone; 1994:581-605.
13. Rasmussen SG, DeVree BT, Zou Y, et al. Crystal structure of the β(2) adrenergic receptor-Gs protein complex. *Nature.* 2011;477(7366):549-555. doi:10.1038/nature10361.
14. Hawrylyshyn KA, Michelotti GA, Coge F, Guenin SP, Schwinn DA. Update on human alpha1-adrenoceptor subtype signaling and genomic organization. *Trends Pharmacol Sci.* 2004;25:449-455.
15. Undieh AS. Pharmacology of signaling induced by dopamine D(1)-like receptor activation. *Pharmacol Ther.* 2010;128:37-60.
16. Bylund DB. Heterogeneity of alpha-2 adrenergic receptors. *Pharmacol Biochem Behav.* 1985;22:835-843.
17. Khan ZP, Ferguson CN, Jones RM. Alpha-2 and imidazoline receptor agonists. Their pharmacology and therapeutic role. *Anaesthesia.* 1999;54:146-165.
18. Kaumann AJ, Lemoine H. Beta 2-adrenoceptor-mediated positive inotropic effect of adrenaline in human ventricular myocardium. Quantitative discrepancies with binding and adenylate cyclase stimulation. *Naunyn Schmiedebergs Arch Pharmacol.* 1987;335:403-411.
19. Lipworth BJ. Clinical pharmacology of beta 3-adrenoceptors. *Br J Clin Pharmacol.* 1996;42:291-300.
20. Friedrich JO, Adhikari N, Herridge MS, Beyene J. Metaanalysis: low-dose dopamine increases urine output but does not prevent renal dysfunction or death. *Ann Intern Med.* 2005;142:510-524.
21. Goldberg LI. Dopamine receptors and hypertension. Physiologic and pharmacologic implications. *Am J Med.* 1984;77:37-44.
22. Halpenny M, Lakshmi S, O'Donnell A, O'Callaghan-Enright S, Shorten GD. Fenoldopam: renal and splanchnic effects in patients undergoing coronary artery bypass grafting. *Anaesthesia.* 2001;56:953-960.
23. Gilbert TB, Hasnain JU, Flinn WR, Lilly MP, Benjamin ME. Fenoldopam infusion associated with preserving renal function after aortic cross-clamping for aneurysm repair. *J Cardiovasc Pharmacol Ther.* 2001;6:31-36.
24. Brienza N, Malcangi V, Dalfino L, et al. A comparison between fenoldopam and low-dose dopamine in early renal dysfunction of critically ill patients. *Crit Care Med.* 2006;34:707-714.
25. Landoni G, Biondi-Zoccai GG, Marino G, et al. Fenoldopam reduces the need for renal replacement therapy and in-hospital death in cardiovascular surgery: a meta-analysis. *J Cardiothorac Vasc Anesth.* 2008;22:27-33.
26. Thiele RH, Nemergut EC, Lynch C 3rd. The physiologic implications of isolated alpha1 adrenergic stimulation. *Anesth Analg.* 2011;113:284-296.
27. Lorhan PH, Oliverio RM. A study of the use of neosynephrine hydrochloride in spinal anesthesia in place of ephedrine for the sustaining of blood pressure. *Curr Res Anesth Analg.* 1938;17:44.
28. Erkinaro T, Kavasmaa T, Pakkila M, et al. Ephedrine and phenylephrine for the treatment of maternal hypotension in a chronic sheep model of increased placental vascular resistance. *Br J Anaesth.* 2006;96:231-237.
29. Erkinaro T, Makikallio K, Kavasmaa T, Alahuhta S, Rasanen J. Effects of ephedrine and phenylephrine on uterine and placental circulations and fetal outcome following fetal hypoxaemia and epidural-induced hypotension in a sheep model. *Br J Anaesth.* 2004;93:825-832.
30. Groudine SB, Hollinger I, Jones J, DeBouno BA. New York State guidelines on the topical use of phenylephrine in the operating room: the Phenylephrine Advisory Committee. *Anesthesiology.* 2000;92:859-864.
31. King BD, Dripps RD. Use of methoxamine for maintenance of the circulation during spinal anesthesia. *Surg Gynec Obstet.* 1950;90:659.
32. Lakhlani PP, MacMillan LB, Guo TZ, et al. Substitution of a mutant alpha2a-adrenergic receptor via "hit and run" gene targeting reveals the role of this subtype in sedative, analgesic, and anesthetic-sparing responses in vivo. *Proc Natl Acad Sci U S A.* 1997;94:9950-9955.
33. Hunter JC, Fontana DJ, Hedley LR, et al. Assessment of the role of alpha2-adrenoceptor subtypes in the antinociceptive, sedative and hypothermic action of dexmedetomidine in transgenic mice. *Br J Pharmacol.* 1997;122:1339-1344.
34. Ma D, Hossain M, Rajakumaraswamy N, et al. Dexmedetomidine produces its neuroprotective effect via the alpha 2A-adrenoceptor subtype. *Eur J Pharmacol.* 2004;502:87-97.
35. Ebert T, Maze M. Dexmedetomidine: another arrow for the clinician's quiver. *Anesthesiology.* 2004;101:568-570.
36. Wijeysundera DN, Naik JS, Beattie WS. Alpha-2 adrenergic agonists to prevent perioperative cardiovascular complications: a meta-analysis. *Am J Med.* 2003;114:742-752.
37. Stevens JE. Rebound hypertension during anaesthesia. *Anaesthesia.* 1980;35:490-491.
38. Aantaa R, Jalonen J. Perioperative use of alpha2-adrenoceptor agonists and the cardiac patient. *Eur J Anaesthesiol.* 2006;23:361-372.
39. Arain SR, Ruehlow RM, Uhrich TD, Ebert TJ. Efficacy of dexmedetomidine versus morphine for post-operative analgesia following major inpatient surgery. *Anesth Analg.* 2004;98:153-158.
40. Herr DL, Sum-Ping ST, England M. ICU sedation after coronary artery bypass graft surgery: dexmedetomidine-based versus propofol-based sedation regimens. *J Cardiothorac Vasc Anesth.* 2003;17:576-584.
41. Riker RR, Shehabi Y, Bokesch PM, et al. SEDCOM (Safety and Efficacy of Dexmedetomidine Compared With Midazolam) Study Group: Dexmedetomidine vs midazolam for sedation of critically ill patients: a randomized trial. *JAMA.* 2009;301:489-499.
42. Pandharipande PP, Pun BT, Herr DL, et al. Effect of sedation with dexmedetomidine vs lorazepam on acute brain dysfunction in

mechanically ventilated patients: the MENDS randomized controlled trial. *JAMA.* 2007;298:2644-2653.

43. Candiotti KA, Bergese SD, Bokesch PM, Feldman MA, Wisemandle W, Bekker AY. Monitored anesthesia care with dexmedetomidine. *Anesth Analg.* 2010;110:47-56.

44. Drugs.com/ppa/isoproterenol.html. Retrieved July 18, 2012.

45. Butterworth JF 4th, Royster RL, Prielipp RC, Lawless ST, Wallenhaupt SL. Amrinone in cardiac surgical patients with left-ventricular dysfunction. A prospective, randomized placebo-controlled trial. *Chest.* 1993;104:1660-1667.

46. Fowler MB, Alderman EL, Oesterle SN, et al. Dobutamine and dopamine after cardiac surgery: greater augmentation of myocardial blood flow with dobutamine. *Circulation.* 1984;70:I103-I111.

47. Braden GL, Germain MJ, Mulhern JG, Hafer JG Jr, Bria WF. Hemodynamic, cardiac, and electrolyte effects of low-dose aerosolized terbutaline in asthmatic patients. *Chest.* 1998;114:380-387.

48. The Canadian Preterm Labor Investigators Group. Treatment of preterm labor with the beta-adrenergic agonist ritodrine. *N Engl J Med.* 1992;327:308-312.

49. Biaggioni I, Robertson D. Chapter 9. Adrenoceptor agonists and sympathomimetic drugs. In: Katzung BG, Masters SB, Trevor AJ, eds. *Basic and Clinical Pharmacology.* 11th ed. New York: McGraw-Hill; 2011.

50. Gillman PK. Monoamine oxidase inhibitors, opioid analgesics and serotonin toxicity. *Br J Anaesth.* 2005;95:434-441.

51. Barash PG, Cullen BF, Stoelting RK, Cahalan MK, Stock MC. *Clinical Anesthesia.* 6th ed. Philadelphia: Lippincott Williams and Wilkins; 2009:358.

52. Huyse FJ, Touw DJ, Strack van Schijndel R, deLange JJ, Slaets JP. Psychotropic drugs and the perioperative period: a proposal guide for elective surgery. *Psychosomatics.* 2006;47:8-22.

53. Chadha NK, Repanos C, Carswell AJ. Local anesthesia for manipulation of nasal fractures: systematic review. *J Laryngol Otol.* 2009; 123:830-836.

54. Mitra JK, Roy J, Sengupta S. Vasopressin: its current role in anesthetic practice. *Ind J Crit Care Med.* 2011;15:71-77.

55. Dunser MW, Mayr AJ, Ulmet H, et al. Arginine vasopressin in advanced vasodilatory shock: a prospective, randomized, controlled study. *Circulation.* 2003;107:2313-2319.

56. Raab H, Lindner KH, Wenzel V. Preventing cardiac arrest during hemorrhagic shock with vasopressin. *Crit Care Med.* 2008;36(Suppl): S474-S480.

57. Stadlbauer KH, Wenzel V, Krismer AC, Voelckel WG, Lindner KH. Vasopressin during uncontrolled hemorrhagic shock: less bleeding below the diaphragm, more perfusion above. *Anesth Analg.* 2005; 101:830-832.

58. Tsuneyoshi I, Onomoto M, Yonetani A, Kanmura Y. Low-dose vasopressin infusion in patients with severe vasodilatory hypotension after prolonged hemorrhage during general anesthesia. *J Anesth.* 2005; 19:170-173.

59. Sharma RM, Setlur R. Vasopressin in hemorrhagic shock. *Anesth Analg.* 2005;101:833-834.

60. Kertai MD, Bax JJ, Klein J, Poldermans D. Is there any reason to withhold beta blockers from high-risk patients with coronary artery disease during surgery? *Anesthesiology.* 2004;100:4-7.

61. Silverman NA, Wright R, Levitsky S. Efficacy of low-dose propranolol in preventing postoperative supraventricular tachyarrhythmias: a prospective, randomized study. *Ann Surg.* 1982;196:194-197.

62. Giles JW, Sear JW, Foex P: Effect of chronic beta-blockade on perioperative outcome in patients undergoing non-cardiac surgery: an analysis of observational and case control studies. *Anaesthesia.* 2004; 59:574-583.

63. Poldermans D, Boersma E, Bax JJ, et al. The effect of bisoprolol on perioperative mortality and myocardial infarction in high-risk patients undergoing vascular surgery. Dutch Echocardiographic Cardiac Risk Evaluation Applying Stress Echocardiography Study Group. *N Engl J Med.* 1999;341:1789-1794.

64. Mangano DT, Layug EL, Wallace A, Tateo I. Effect of atenolol on mortality and cardiovascular morbidity after noncardiac surgery. *N Engl J Med* 1996;335:1713-1720.

65. POISE Study Group, Devereaux PJ, Yang H, et al. Effects of extended-release metoprolol succinate in patients undergoing noncardiac surgery (POISE trial): a randomised controlled trial. *Lancet.* 2008;371:1839-1847.

66. Egstrup K. Transient myocardial ischemia after abrupt withdrawal of antianginal therapy in chronic stable angina. *Am J Cardiol.* 1988; 61:1219-1222.

67. Gorczynski RJ. Basic pharmacology of esmolol. *Am J Cardiol.* 1985; 56:3F-13F.

68. Sum CY, Yacobi A, Kartzinel R, Stampfli H, Davis CS, Lai CM. Kinetics of esmolol, an ultra-short-acting beta blocker, and of its major metabolite. *Clin Pharmacol Ther.* 1983;34:427-434.

69. MacCarthy EP, Bloomfield SS. Labetalol: a review of its pharmacology, pharmacokinetics, clinical uses and adverse effects. *Pharmacotherapy.* 1983;3:193-219.

70. Wallace AW, Au S, Cason BA. Perioperative beta-blockade: atenolol is associated with reduced mortality when compared to metoprolol. *Anesthesiology.* 2011;114:824-836.

71. Brown DA. Muscarinic acetylcholine receptors (mAChRs) in the nervous system: some functions and mechanisms. *J Mol Neurosci.* 2010;41:340-346.

72. Caulfield MP. Muscarinic receptors–characterization, coupling and function. *Pharmacol Ther.* 1993;58:319-379.

73. Barash PG, Cullen BF, Stoelting RK, Cahalan MK, Stock MC. *Clinical Anesthesia.* 6th ed. Philadelphia: Lippincott Williams and Wilkins; 2009:502.

74. Raczkowska M, Ebert TJ, Eckberg DL. Muscarinic cholinergic receptors modulate vagal cardiac responses in man. *J Autonomic Nerv Syst.* 1983;7:271-278.

75. Ali-Melkkila T, Kanto J, Iisalo E. Pharmacokinetics and related pharmacodynamics of anticholinergic drugs. *Acta Anaesthesiol Scand.* 1993;37:633-642.

76. Apfel CC, Zhang K, George E, et al. Transdermal scopolamine for the prevention of postoperative nausea and vomiting: a systematic review and meta-analysis. *Clin Ther.* 2010;32:1987-2002.

77. Renner UD, Oertel R, Kirch W. Pharmacokinetics and pharmacodynamics in clinical use of scopolamine. *Ther Drug Monit.* 2005;27: 655-665.

78. Flynn RA, Glynn DA, Kennedy MP. Anticholinergic treatment in airways diseases. *Adv Ther.* 2009;26:908-919.

79. Gross NJ. Anticholinergic agents in asthma and COPD. *Eur J Pharmacol.* 2006;533:36-39.

Chapter 14

NOCICEPTIVE PHYSIOLOGY

Einar Ottestad and Martin S. Angst

SYSTEMS PHYSIOLOGY

Perioperative Pain

Aggressive management of perioperative pain is a high clinical priority in the current practice of anesthesia. Inadequately treated pain is not only associated with personal suffering but also with increased morbidity and mortality, protracted recovery, and delayed discharge from the hospital.[1] For example, poor perioperative pain control correlates with an increased risk for developing chronic postsurgical pain.[2] Despite relevant progress in our mechanistic understanding of pain and significant clinical efforts directed toward its improved management, a third of patients undergoing surgery continue to suffer from moderate to severe pain. It is unclear whether we can address this shortcoming with current therapies.[3] Consequently, identification of novel therapeutic targets and development of drugs aimed at such targets are current priorities in analgesic research.

This chapter covers the fundamental neuroanatomy, molecular biology, and physiologic function of the nociceptive system as they pertain to the processing of acute pain and the practice of anesthesia. The major objective is to provide a framework that facilitates understanding of current and novel analgesic drug targets and *acute pain* management strategies. Given the focus of this book on the practice of anesthesia rather than the management of *chronic pain*, functional alterations of the nociceptive system in the context of chronic pain will not specifically be reviewed. However, acute pain associated with surgery and tissue trauma can become chronic and maladaptive in that it no longer serves a protective function. During the past decade it has become clear that a significant number of patients develop persistent pain as a direct result of surgery.[2,4] While the mechanisms underlying persistent postsurgical pain (PPP) remain poorly understood, several risk factors have been identified, including the type of surgery, younger age, female sex, preexisting chronic pain conditions, psychologic vulnerability, and the severity of postoperative pain.[2,5,6] Some of these risk factors might reflect a general predisposition to amplified nociceptive responses. Genetic variants predisposing to chronic pain have been identified.[7-9] A shift in balance between pro-nociceptive and anti-nociceptive processes discussed later in the context of acute pain seems to underlie the propensity to develop PPP. Mechanisms might include the exaggerated amplification of nociceptive input (central sensitization) and deficient activation of endogenous inhibitory pathways. Perioperative regimens counteracting central sensitization such as administration of α2-adrenergic agonists, gabapentin, and N-methyl-D-aspartate (NMDA)-type glutamate receptor antagonists have all been associated with a lower incidence of PPP.[10-12]

Nociceptive System

The nociceptive system is a sensory component of the peripheral and central nervous systems that is devoted to signaling potentially harmful stimuli. The system controls the involuntary defensive and adaptive responses to injurious stimuli and mediates perception of pain. Nociception typically starts by activation of peripheral nociceptors that respond to potentially harmful thermal, mechanical, or chemical stimuli. Physical or chemical input is transduced into transmembrane potential changes that can trigger action potentials (see Chapter 7). Primary sensory afferents consisting of nonmyelinated slow-conducting C-fibers and thinly myelinated faster conducting Aδ fibers propagate action potentials to the dorsal horn of the spinal cord where they synapse with spinal neurons. The neuronal architecture of the dorsal horn is complex and largely consists of interneurons that either amplify or inhibit transmission of incoming signals. Nociceptive input is relayed to supraspinal sites by projection neurons ascending in the spinothalamic and spinomedullary tracts, but is also transmitted to spinal sites serving autonomic and motor functions. Integration of nociceptive information in supraspinal brain regions results in complex somatic, emotional, autonomic, and endocrine responses. Finally, descending fibers emerge from supraspinal sites including the cerebral cortex, hypothalamus and brainstem. These project to the spinal cord where they facilitate or inhibit transmission of nociceptive signals.

CELLULAR AND MOLECULAR PHYSIOLOGY

Nociceptors

Nociceptors are a specific set of primary afferent nerve fibers that conduct noxious signals from peripheral somatic and visceral tissue to the spinal cord. They are pseudo-unipolar in architecture with distal and proximal projections arising from their cell bodies located in dorsal root and other sensory (e.g., trigeminal) ganglia. Peripheral nerve endings show significant arborization and cover receptive fields from a few square millimeters to a few square centimeters contingent on body location and fiber type. Membrane receptors and ion channels located on unmyelinated nerve endings transduce nociceptive input into transmembrane potential changes, which trigger the propagation of action potentials if the potential change is of sufficient magnitude (Figure 14-1).

Action potentials are conducted to the dorsal horn of the spinal cord by two distinct populations of nociceptors with fast and slow conduction velocities: small myelinated Aδ-fibers (5-25 m/s) or unmyelinated C fibers (<2 m/s). According to their conduction velocity and their differential neuronal processing in the central nervous system (CNS), Aδ fibers transmit "fast" pain that is well localized and causes a rapid withdrawal of the affected body part, while C-fibers transmit

"slow onset" pain that is diffuse in character, intensifies over time, and often elicits a guarding response.

An important characteristic of nociceptors is their ability to become sensitized in injured tissue. Nociceptor sensitization is the neurophysiologic correlate of primary hyperalgesia. Hyperalgesia corresponds to the increased pain sensitivity that is typically present in injured and inflamed tissue. The term *primary* indicates that hyperalgesia is due to local events at the site of injury rather than central processes that can also amplify nociceptive input (secondary hyperalgesia; see later).

While nociceptors serve prominent afferent functions, they also exert efferent functions. In other words, nociceptors are in "peripheral dialogue" with neighboring resident cells as well as migrating cells that invade tissue upon injury. A phenomenon that has received significant attention and directly relates to the efferent function of nociceptors is known as neurogenic inflammation. Nociceptors synthesizing the neuropeptides substance P and calcitonin gene-related peptide (CGRP) release these peptides peripherally in response to tissue injury. Substance P causes plasma extravasation and CGRP induces vasodilation via activation of their respective receptors on capillaries and terminal arterioles. Just as importantly, these neuropetides bind to neighboring cells triggering release of inflammatory and nociceptive mediators, thereby contributing to inflammation and pain. The release of neuropetides is mediated by N- and L-type voltage-gated Ca^{2+} channels and inhibition of these channels decreases inflammation and pain.[13] In a clinical context, neurogenic inflammation has been implicated as a relevant pathogenic mechanism underlying acute and chronic pain conditions.[14] It is also a prominent feature of migraine headache.

Nociceptor Activation

Nociceptors are activated by endogenous ligands as well as exogenous physical or chemical input including heat, cold, and mechanical or chemical stimuli. Examples of endogenous ligands are bradykinin 2, prostaglandin E2, and 5-hydroxytryptamine, which are released from resident and migrating immune cells in response to tissue injury and inflammation. Examples of exogenous physicochemical input are the pungent capsaicin, an ingredient of red pepper, and exogenous heat, both of which activate the transient receptor potential vanilloid 1 (TRPV1) receptor.[15]

The "naked" terminals of nociceptors contain a mosaic of different receptors that can induce depolarization through conductance changes of voltage-gated ion channels. Stimulus transduction is the result of complex excitatory and inhibitory molecular interactions occurring within the mosaic of these receptors, illustrated schematically for the TRPV1 receptor in Figure 14-1.[16] However, the complexity of signal transduction is not limited to the nociceptor but also comprises interactions between nociceptors and neighboring cells including resident cells (e.g., keratinocytes and mast cells) and migrating immune cells (e.g., neutrophils and lymphocytes).

NOCICEPTIVE SIGNAL TRANSDUCTION
Cell surface proteins studied in detail for the transduction of nociceptive signals fall into three classes: ion channels, metabotropic G-protein coupled receptors, and receptors for neurotrophins or cytokines.[13] Knowledge regarding the role of these ion channels and receptors in nociception is rapidly

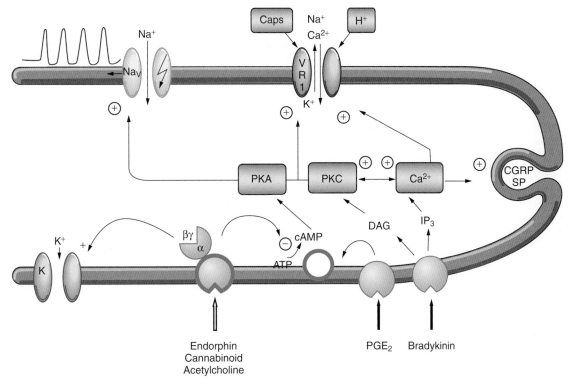

Figure 14-1 Nociceptive signal transduction. Nociceptive signal transduction involves interactions between excitatory and inhibitory molecular mechanisms at the peripheral nerve terminal. Some relevant interactions are illustrated for the transient receptor potential vanilloid 1 receptor (VR1), which plays a critical role in the transduction of noxious heat and directly responds to ligands such as capsaicin and hydrogen ion. Bradykinin and prostaglandin E2 lead to phosphorylation by protein kinase C (PKC) and protein kinase A (PKA) via second messenger systems including inositol trisphosphate (IP$_3$) and diacylglycerol (DAG) and cyclic adenosine monophosphate (cAMP). This leads to increased permeability of VR1 and voltage-gated channels such as the Na$^+$ channel Na$_V$1.8 (NAV). Voltage-gated channels play an important role for the transduction of sensor potentials into spike sequences in the conductile part of the nerve. Increased intracellular Ca^{2+}, which acts as a second messenger, is critical in the secretion of neuropeptides from the peripheral terminal. Calcitonin gene-related peptide (CGRP) and substance P (SP) are sentinel mediators triggering peripheral neurogenic inflammatory events. Endogenous inhibitory ligands including endorphins, endocannabinoids, and acetylcholine modulate the transduction process through activation of their respective G protein-coupled receptors. Cannabinoid and opioid receptors oppose depolarization by activation of K$^+$ channels via the β-subunit of the G-protein, while inhibition of adenylyl cyclase (AC) via the α-subunit reduces production of cAMP from adenosine triphosphate (ATP). cAMP is required for activating PKA. *(Modified from Handwerker HO. Nociceptors: neurogenic inflammation. Handb Clin Neurol. 2006;81:23-33.)*

evolving yet quite incomplete. Complicating our understanding regarding the respective role of various ion channels and receptors in nociception are the multiple interdependent mechanisms that are simultaneously at play and vary according to tissue type (e.g., skin versus viscera) and change contingent on the specific biologic context (e.g., type and time course of injury). Additionally, processing of specific noxious input can be redundant and involve different receptor and second messenger systems.

The complexity, heterogeneity, redundancy, and plasticity underlying the transduction and signaling of nociceptive information make identification of novel analgesic drug targets a challenging task. Most promising might be targets that convene input from various nociceptive events across a wide range of tissue injuries. Examples that might fulfill such requirements are ion channels such as TRPV1, P2X$_3$, Na$_V$1.8, and TRPA1. However, such targets are rare and can vary according to tissue-type. Examples include a particular role of ASIC channels in muscle pain, P2X$_3$ channels in visceral pain, and chloride channels in meningeal pain.[13]

Ion channels
Table 14-1 lists the ionotropic receptors directly transducing nociceptive signals. Relevant examples of inotropic receptors and ion channels involved in signal transduction and propagation including members of the TRP-family, isoforms of the voltage-gated Na$^+$ channel, and K$^+$ channels are discussed in more detail.

The discovery of the TRPV1 receptor, a member of the TRP-family, provided important insight into the transduction of nociceptive heat.[15] TRPV1 is also activated by other noxious modalities including protons, fatty acids, arachidonic acid derivatives, and vanilloids. It is a Ca^{2+} permeable nonselective cation channel with a binding site for capsaicin, the spicy ingredient of red pepper. All TRP channels consist of six-transmembrane segments that assemble tetramerically to form cation-permeable pores in the cell membrane. Other members of the TRP family sense a wide array of noxious and nonnoxious stimuli. Most notable are the TRPM8 and the TRPA1 receptors. The TRPM8 receptor is critical for transduction of noxious cold stimuli, while the TRPA1 receptor transduces input from endogenous and exogenous inflammatory proalgesic agents including bradykinin, mustard oil, and formalin.[17,18]

Voltage-gated Na$^+$ channels (Na$_v$) play an essential role in the initiation and propagation of action potentials. They are large, multimeric complexes that consist of an α-subunit and one or more auxiliary β-subunits (see Chapter 17). The α-subunit contains the ion-conducting aqueous pore that is the essential element of Na$^+$ channel function. The β-subunits

Table 14-1. Ionotropic Nociceptive Transducers*

ABBREVIATION	NAME	STIMULUS TRANSDUCTION	ACTIVATION	SENSITIZATION
ASIC 1-4	Acid sensing ion channels, subtypes 1-4	Chemical	Protons	Ischemia-induced pain, muscle hypersensitivity
TRPV1	Transient receptor potential vanilloid 1 receptor (URI)	Thermal Chemical	Heat, protons, vanilloids, fatty acids, arachidonic acid derivatives	Heat hyperalgesia
TRPV4	Transient receptor potential vanilloid 4 receptor	Mechanical	Osmotic challenge	Visceral and cutaneous hypersensitivity in inflammation and nerve injury
TRPA1	Transient receptor potential subfamily A1 receptor	Chemical Mechanical	Mustard oil, cinimaldehyde, acrolein, formalin	Chemically induced hyperalgesia Mechanical hyperalgesia
TRPM8	Transient receptor potential subfamily M8 receptor	Thermal	Cold	Cold hyperalgesia
P2X3	P2X purinoceptor 3	Mechanical (indirect)	Adenosine triphosphate	Visceral and somatic pain in inflammation and nerve injury
P2X1-6	P2X purinoceptor 1-6	Chemical	Adenosine triphosphate	Pain and hypersensitivity associated with injury in various tissues
TREK 1	TWIK-related potassium channel 1	Mechanical Thermal Chemical	Stretching Heat Protons, arachidonic acid	Inflammatory hyperalgesia
TRAAK	TWIK-activated arachidonic acid potassium channel	Mechanical Thermal Chemical	Stretching Heat Protons, arachidonic acid	No data
5-HT3	5-Hydroxytryptamine receptor	Chemical	Serotonin	Most prominent role in visceral pain
nACh (multiple subunits)	Nicotinic acetylcholine receptor	Chemical	Acetylcholine	May be pro-nociceptive at peripheral terminals, anti-nociceptive at central terminals
Glutamate (GluR1-5 and NR1-2)	Ampakine (GluR1-4), kainate (GluR5), and NMDA (NR1-2) receptors	Chemical	Glutamate and subtype specific agonists	Evidence for peripheral role in pain, but most compelling evidence for role at central terminals
GABA (multiple subunits)	γ-aminobutyric acid receptor	Chemical	GABA and subunit specific agonists	May be inhibitory or excitatory

*Metabotropic receptors exist in large numbers on nociceptive neurons and are not included in this table.
Modified from Gold and Gebhart, Nature Medicine 2010.

modify kinetics and voltage dependence and are involved in channel localization and interaction with cell adhesion molecules, extracellular matrix, and the intracellular cytoskeleton.[19] Nine isoforms of the α-subunit ($Na_v1.1$ through $Na_v1.9$), each with its specific physiologic and pharmacologic function, have been identified. Several Na^+ channels play a role in inflammatory and neuropathic pain.[20] Their expression is altered by tissue injury and such alterations likely contribute to pain and hyperalgesia associated with such injury. Two isoforms, $Na_v1.8$ and $Na_v1.9$, are selectively expressed in the peripheral nervous system and specifically on nociceptive neurons. Both channels have been implicated in processing inflammatory and potentially, neuropathic pain. $Na_v1.7$ is expressed on small diameter sympathetic and nociceptive neurons and is critical for the processing of inflammatory pain. The importance of $Na_v1.7$ in nociception is highlighted by the fact that mutations of SCN9A, the gene encoding $Na_v1.7$, result in loss- or gain-of-function channelopathies that underlie rare pain disorders. Examples are the congenital insensitivity to pain and erythermalgia, a condition with recurrent episodes of severe pain and inflammation.[21,22] Finally, $Na_v1.3$ re-expression on peripheral axons after nerve damage or in dorsal horn neurons after spinal cord injury

is associated with increased neuronal excitability and likely contributes to the genesis of neuropathic pain.[23] Sodium channel isoforms ($Na_v1.3$, $Na_v1.7$, $Na_v1.8$, and $Na_v1.9$) are attractive analgesic drug targets given their essential roles in nociception.

The inhibitory role of K^+ channels in nociceptive signal transduction is well established. Many G-protein coupled receptor ligands including opioids and endocannabinoids exert their anti-nociceptive effects by activating K^+ channels via their respective second messenger systems. Of particular recent interest are two-pore domain (K_2P) K^+ channels (TREK-1, TRAAK) that are directly activated by noxious mechanical, thermal, and chemical stimuli.[24,25] These channels are potential analgesic targets for specific agonists. However, given that ion channels are widely distributed throughout the body and serve multiple physiologic functions, potential off-target effects (e.g., CNS or cardiac toxicity) could limit the utility of pharmacologic agents targeting these channels.

Metabotropic G-protein coupled receptors
Many excitatory and inhibitory G-protein coupled receptors modulate nociceptor excitability by activating or inhibiting

ion channels via their respective second messenger systems. Examples of excitatory receptors include the receptors for CGRP, bradykinin (B1 and B2), protease (PAR 1-4), or prostaglandin (EP1, EP3C, and EP4). The relative abundance of various G-protein coupled receptors on nociceptors might account for why specific receptor antagonists mostly fail as analgesics.[13] Exceptions are CGRP antagonists that are effective for treatment of migraine.[26] Several inhibitory receptors are useful drug targets such as opioid receptors (μ, δ, κ) and serotonin receptors (5HT1B and D). While opioids exert broad analgesic effects, the efficacy of serotonergic antagonists is limited to migraine.

Receptors for neurotrophins

Nociceptors express two classes of neurotrophic factors that are infrequently coexpressed in a specific nociceptor. Neurotrophic factors belong either to the nerve growth factor family (NGF, brain-derived neurotrophic factor [BDNF], and neurotrophin 3 and 4) or the glial cell line-derived family (glial cell derived neurotrophic factors, neurturin, artemin, and persephin). Neurotrophic factors provide a critical link between inflammation and nociception. Each trophic factor affects neurotransmitter expression, as well as ion channel and transducer composition in nociceptors. Consequently, an inflammation-induced surge of neurotrophic factors can profoundly affect nociceptor excitability and result in hyperalgesia.[27] NGF is the most widely studied factor in the context of pain, and pharmacologic approaches sequestering NGF or targeting its high affinity receptor TrkA are actively being pursued. NGF plays a critical role in early and longer term generation of acute and chronic pain conditions.[28] NGF is released from a host of inflammatory and resident cells upon tissue injury. NGF directly binds to nociceptive afferents but also triggers the release of nociceptive mediators from inflammatory cells. Both actions result in nociceptor sensitization and hyperalgesia (e.g., via upregulation of TRPV1, ASID, and Na_V channels). Within hours to days, transcriptional changes are triggered by the retrograde transport of the NGF-TrkA complex. This further contributes to peripheral nociceptor sensitization by upregulating peptides (e.g., CGRP) and ion channels (e.g., $Na_V1.8$) but also induces central sensitization via synthesis of BDNF. Current pharmacologic approaches, either sequestering NGF or antagonizing TrkA receptors, target chronic pain in patients suffering from osteoarthritis, diabetic neuropathy, cancer, or back pain. While proven effective in some of these conditions, safety concerns remain given the wide range of physiologic functions of NGF.[28,29]

Nociceptor classification

Nociceptors are a heterogeneous group of afferents and no single anatomic, biochemical, physiologic, or functional criterion can reliably identify a nociceptor. The degree of heterogeneity among nociceptors might contribute to the difficulties in identifying novel analgesic drug targets.[13] A recent example is the failed attempt to develop neurokinin-1 (substance P) receptor antagonists for the treatment of pain.[30]

The mosaic of receptors on peripheral nerve endings is not homogenous among nociceptors and differences provide a molecular basis for dividing nociceptors into subpopulations. However, such classification remains imperfect because expression profiles overlap and coexpression of receptors and humoral content is variable. Bearing this limitation in mind, nociceptors are commonly divided into peptidergic and nonpeptidergic fibers. Peptidergic fibers are the largest group of nociceptors and contain one or both of the neuropeptides substance P and CGRP. Peptidergic fibers also express TrkA, the high affinity receptor for NFG. TrkA and NGF are critical for the normal development of these nociceptors. In fact, a genetic defect causing loss of TrkA receptor function underlies congenital insensitivity to pain with anhidrosis, a rare autosomal recessive disease.[31] Clinical manifestations include self-mutilating behavior, unexplained fever, mental retardation, and autonomic abnormalities. Nonpeptidergic fibers encode a receptor tyrosine kinase that binds glial cell line–derived neurotrophic factors and often coexpress the purinergic $P2X_3$ receptor.

Nociceptors have also been characterized based on their response properties, but such characterization is incomplete and not uniform across species.[16] Some nociceptors respond to multiple noxious modalities, while others are modality-specific or remain silent until activated by tissue injury or inflammation. Some examples of well characterized nociceptors are "polymodal" mechano-heat sensitive C-fibers that are also responsive to chemical input, mechanoinsensitive C-fibers that can respond to chemical and heat stimulation in regular skin but only become responsive to mechanical stimulation in inflamed skin, and two different types of high-threshold mechanosensitive Aδ fibers that inconsistently respond to noxious heat. Mechanoinsensitive C-fibers constitute up to 20% of nociceptors in human skin and might play a particularly important role in the development and maintenance of tissue hyperalgesia.

DORSAL HORN

Nociceptors terminate in the dorsal horn of the spinal cord where they synapse with interneurons and projection neurons. Incoming signals are processed through a complex neuronal network built by primary afferents, inhibitory and excitatory interneurons, projection neurons, and descending neurons that originate in the brainstem. Projection neurons carry the major neuronal output to various supraspinal structures including nuclei of the brainstem and thalamus. However, neuronal output from the dorsal horn is also conveyed to intermediate and ventral portions of the dorsal horn to elicit nociceptive autonomic and motor responses. Despite recent advances, knowledge regarding the synaptic circuitry and function of dorsal horn neuronal structures is limited. This is partially explained by the tremendous morphologic and neurochemical diversity of primary afferents and dorsal horn neurons.

STRUCTURAL COMPONENTS

Primary afferents originating in skin and deeper tissue terminate in specific regions of the dorsal horn. Interrelated characteristics of primary afferents including their response properties (sensory modality and activation threshold), conduction velocity, and neurochemical phenotype determine their distribution pattern in the gray matter of the dorsal horn.[32] Regions of the gray matter are defined by 10 cytoarchitecturally distinct layers (Figure 14-2). The majority of nociceptive fibers terminate in superficial laminae I and II. Peptidergic nociceptive fibers originating in skin and deeper tissue and nonpeptidergic nociceptive fibers mainly

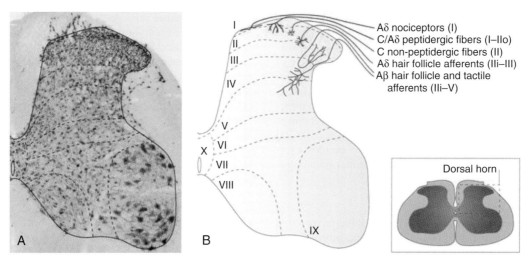

Figure 14-2 Laminar organization of the spinal dorsal horn. The gray matter of the dorsal horn has been subdivided into 10 layers based on variations in size and neuron packing density. **A,** Neurons in a transverse section of the rat spinal cord have been immunostained. Dashed lines indicate the laminar boundaries. **B,** Primary afferents arborize in an orderly manner. The central terminations of the major primary afferents are shown (except proprioceptors). Aβ tactile and hair follicle afferents mainly end in laminae III-V. Aδ hair follicle afferents arborize on the border of laminae II and III. Aδ nociceptors predominantly terminate in lamina I and give some branches to laminae V and X. Peptidergic primary afferents consisting of C and Aδ nociceptors end in lamina I and the outer portion of lamina II, while nonpeptidergic C nociceptors form a band in the central part of lamina II. *(Modified from Todd AJ. Neuronal circuitry for pain processing in the dorsal horn. Nat Rev Neurosci. 2010;11:823-836.)*

originating in skin distribute differently within the dorsal horn, indicating that they serve different functions.

Primary afferents synapse with interneurons and projection neurons in various ways. Characteristic structures of the dorsal horn are multifaceted arrangements known as synaptic glomeruli.[33] These are built by a central axon (mainly nonpeptidergic nociceptors) linked to dendrites and axons of other neuronal structures, thereby allowing for complex modulation of sensory information. However, primary afferents (peptidergic and Aδ nociceptors) also form simpler arrangements including axoaxonic and axodendritic synapses.

The majority of laminae I and II neurons are interneurons that arborize locally but can project across several segments within the spinal cord.[34] Interneurons are much more numerous than projection neurons and are either excitatory or inhibitory. The major neurotransmitter of excitatory interneurons is glutamate, while γ-aminobutyric acid (GABA) and glycine are the main transmitters of inhibitory interneurons. Laminae II interneurons have been studied in great detail. Based on morphologic criteria, these interneurons can be classified as islet, central, vertical, and radial cells (Figure 14-3). Although a relationship between morphology and neurochemical function exists, this relationship is not strict. Islet cells are inhibitory and invariably release GABA. Radial and most vertical cells are excitatory and release glutamate, while central cells are either excitatory or inhibitory. Islet cells, radial cells, and most vertical cells likely represent genuine functional classes. However, central cells and about 30% of all interneurons that do not fit morphologic criteria require further functional characterization and a more refined classification.

Projection neurons are present in high density in lamina I, are virtually absent in lamina II, and are scattered throughout the remaining laminae. Projection neurons belong to two classes. Nociceptive-specific neurons exclusively transmit noxious signals, while wide-dynamic-range (WDR) neurons code for nonnoxious and noxious signals contingent on signal

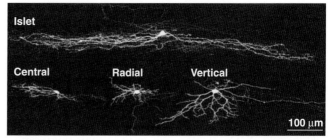

Figure 14-3 Classification of lamina II interneurons. Conofocal images of four lamina II interneurons labeled with the cell indicator neurobiotin are shown. Somatodendritic morphologic criteria allow characterizing these neurons as islet, central, radial, or vertical cells. Islet cells are inhibitory and are characterized by elongated dendritic trees, mainly spreading along the rostrocaudal axis. Central cells are similar in configuration but have much shorter dendritic trees and are either inhibitory or excitatory. Radial cells have compact dendritic trees that spread in multiple directions. Vertical cells have dendritic trees that fan out ventrally in conical shape. Radial and most vertical cells are excitatory. *(Modified from Todd AJ. Neuronal circuitry for pain processing in the dorsal horn. Nat Rev Neurosci. 2010;11:823-836.)*

strength. WDR neurons receive simultaneous input from somatic and visceral structures allowing for viscera-somatic signal convergence, which underlies the perception of referred pain (e.g., myocardial ischemia causing shoulder pain). Many neurons cross the midline and ascend to various supraspinal structures including nuclei in the brainstem and thalamus (Figure 14-4). Neurons also show significant collateralization by simultaneously projecting to different supraspinal sites.

Neurons of the dorsal horn build complex synaptic networks and it is likely that most receive input from primary afferents as well as inhibitory and excitatory interneurons. Interneurons are the primary target of primary afferents. However, there are direct synaptic connections between primary afferents and projection neurons. For example, peptidergic nociceptors widely connect to lamina I and III projection neurons that express the neurokinin 1 receptor (NK1R). Conversely, excitatory interneurons are the primary source of

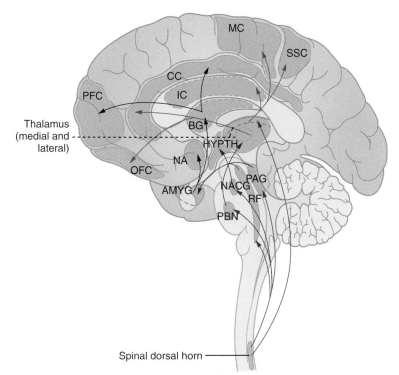

Figure 14-4 Major components of the nociceptive system. An overview of the major anatomic components that process nociceptive information from the periphery to cortical structures. Myelinated and nonmyelinated primary afferent fibers provide nociceptive input to the spinal cord. Major nociceptive projections target the brainstem (spinomedullary tract) and the thalamus (spinothalamic tract). Projections from the brainstem reach the medial thalamus, hypothalamus and amygdala; these structures play a predominant role in regulating autonomic, neuroendocrine, and emotional states. The lateral thalamus projects to the somatosensory cortex, which decodes sensory-discriminative aspects of pain. The amygdala pairs noxious input with affective content. Its critical integrative function is underlined by connections to various cortical and subcortical structures modulating emotional and behavioral processes. *CN*, Caudate nucleus; *GP*, globus pallidus; *MDN*, medial dorsal nucleus; *NA*, nucleus accumbens; *NACG*, noradrenergic cell group; *NSM*, nucleus submedius; *PAG*, periaqueductal gray; *PBN*, parabrachial nucleus; *PUT*, putamen; *RF*, reticular formation; *SI*, primary sensory cortex; *SII*, secondary somatosensory; *SN*, substantia nigra; *VLN*, ventral lateral nucleus; *VMN*, ventral, medial nucleus; *VPN*, ventral posterior nuclei.

nociceptive input to giant lamina I projection neurons that lack neurokinin 1 receptor. There is evidence that different interneurons are innervated by specific classes of afferent fibers. For example, islet cells and most central cells mainly receive input from C-fibers, whereas vertical and radial cells receive input from C and Aδ afferents. Similarly, neurochemically or electrophysiologically distinct C-fibers preferentially connect to different interneurons. For example, C-fibers expressing TRPA1 and TRPV1 receptors build synapses with vertical and radial cells but do not innervate islet and central cells.[35] The complexity of a neuronal circuit involving projection neurons is illustrated in Figure 14-5.

NEUROCHEMISTRY

The neurochemistry of dorsal horn circuits is quite complicated and currently only understood in broad terms. For example, while many dorsal horn receptors and ligands have been identified, precise knowledge regarding their expression in particular neuronal structures is often incomplete. Some details have recently emerged suggesting that receptor expression is quite distinct. For example, somatostatin receptor type 2A is exclusively found on inhibitory interneurons. Conversely, the μ-opioid receptor is found on excitatory interneurons and primary afferents, while neuropeptide Y receptor type 1 is found on excitatory neurons and projection neurons.[32] More detailed knowledge regarding the distribution and colocalization of ligands and their respective receptors on neuronal structures will need to be integrated with morphologic knowledge of distinct neurocircuits to fully understand the functional relevance of individual ligands and receptors.

Virtually all primary afferents exert their excitatory effects on postsynaptic structures by the release of glutamate. Glutamate binds to ionotropic glutamatergic receptors including AMPA (α-amino-3-hydroxy-5-methyl-4-isoxazolepropionic acid), NMDA, and kainate receptors. AMPA receptors are

ubiquitous at glutamatergic synapses of the dorsal horn, while NMDA receptors show more restricted expression. Little is known about the synaptic distribution of kainate receptors. Finally, several metabotropic glutamate receptors are also present in the dorsal horn.

Activation of AMPA and kainate receptors causes rapid depolarization of postsynaptic structures and fast transmission of excitatory signals. Activation of NMDA receptors is strictly voltage-gated (e.g., through AMPA-induced membrane depolarization), requires high-strength synaptic input, and occurs in more delayed fashion (Figure 14-6).[36] NMDA-receptor activation can result in long-term potentiation (LTP), the long-lasting use-dependent enhancement of synaptic signal transmission (see later). The basic arrangement of a nociceptive synapse in the dorsal horn is illustrated in Figure 14-7.

Primary afferent fibers express multiple receptors and release different ligands at their central terminal.[33] AMPA and NMDA receptors likely act as autoregulators of glutamate release. GABA and glycine receptors exert inhibitory influences. All three opioid receptor classes are present (μ, δ, κ) and oppose excitatory neurotransmitter release. Other receptors expressed by primary afferents include α-adrenergic and purinergic (P2X₃) receptors. Neurotransmitters released from peptidergic afferents include CGRP and substance P. Substance P propagates nociceptive signals via neurokinin 1 (NRK1) receptors expressed by many spinal neurons. Other neuropeptides include endomorphin 2 and galanin, which are both inhibitory.

As discussed previously, GABA and glycine are the major neurotransmitters of inhibitory interneurons, while glutamate is the major neurotransmitter of excitatory neurons. However, interneurons synthesize additional neurotransmitters and express receptors that are specific to their inhibitory or excitatory function. Excitatory interneurons synthesize somatostatin, neurotensin, substance P, and neurokinin (A and B), while

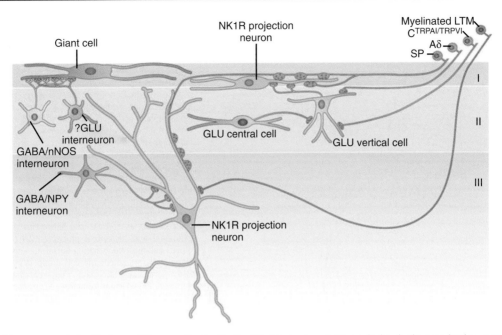

Figure 14-5 Dorsal horn neuronal circuit. Some of the synaptic circuits identified in laminae I-III are depicted. Three projection neurons are shown: the neurokinin 1 receptor (NK1R) expressing neurons found in laminae I and III and giant cells lacking the NK1R in lamina I. Both NK1R projection neurons receive dense input from substance P containing primary afferents, while NK1R projection neurons in lamina III also receive input from low-threshold mechanosensitive (LTM) afferents. Different inhibitory interneurons control neuronal traffic. Interneurons expressing γ-amino butyric acid (GABA) and neuropeptide Y (NPY) are in contact with NK1R projection neurons, while interneurons expressing GABA and nitric oxide synthase (NOS) innervate giant cells. Giant cells also receive excitatory input from glutamatergic (GLU) interneurons. Similarly, glutamatergic interneurons are interconnected (central and vertical cells) and control traffic between primary afferents and NK1R projection neurons in lamina I. Specific primary afferents synapsing with vertical cells include Aδ fibers and C-fibers expressing the transient receptor potential vanilloid 1 (TRPV1) and subfamily A1 (TRPA1) receptors. *(Modified from Todd AJ. Neuronal circuitry for pain processing in the dorsal horn. Nat Rev Neurosci. 2010;11:823-836.)*

inhibitory interneurons produce neuropeptide Y and galanin. Both interneuron classes generate enkephalin. Excitatory interneurons specifically express NRK1, μ-opioid, and neuropeptide Y type 1 receptors. Conversely, inhibitory interneurons express somatostatin 2A and neurokinin 3 receptors. The differential expression of neurotransmitter and their corresponding receptor systems by inhibitory and excitatory interneurons points to a multivariate "dialogue" between these interneurons.

Two receptor systems that are widely distributed in the dorsal horn are the monoaminergic and the GABAergic/glycinergic systems. The monoaminergic system includes adrenergic, dopaminergic, and serotonergic receptor subtypes. Little is known about their precise location on spinal neurons. All monoaminergic ligands are released by descending projection neurons originating in the brainstem. Accordingly, they are reviewed in the section discussing descending control mechanisms. GABA and glycine receptors are expressed by the vast majority of dorsal horn neurons.

SPINAL MECHANISMS OF HYPERALGESIA AND ALLODYNIA

Tissue and nerve injuries are associated with the development of spontaneous pain, hyperalgesia, and allodynia. Hyperalgesia describes the occurrence of amplified pain in response to stimuli that are normally noxious. It can be visualized as a left shift of the stimulus intensity versus pain response relationship (Figure 14-8). Allodynia describes the occurrence

of pain in response to stimuli that are normally nonnoxious (e.g., light touch). Several spinal mechanisms including long-term potentiation (LTP), loss of inhibitory control, gain in excitatory function, and alterations in the properties of low-threshold mechanoreceptive Aβ fibers could underlie these phenomena.[32,37,38]

For example, LTP has been observed in NRK1 expressing projection neurons in lamina 1. LTP is triggered by high-strength synaptic input and can be described as the long-term enhancement of synaptic signal transmission (synaptic plasticity). While various mechanisms underlie LTP, a common theme is the increased excitability of postsynaptic structures. This results in amplified nociceptive signal transmission as well as spontaneous burst firing. Functional changes or increased expression of membrane receptors are important mechanisms underlying LTP.

Loss of inhibitory function could explain the occurrence of spontaneous pain, hyperalgesia, and allodynia. For example, miscoding of tactile input as pain (allodynia) could result from loss of inhibition of excitatory interneurons conveying low-threshold mechanoreceptive input to lamina I projection neurons. Reports documenting reduced GABAergic and glycinergic output from lamina II neurons support the view that loss of inhibitory control could be a relevant mechanism.

A third mechanism is the gain in excitatory function due to intrinsic changes of dorsal horn neurons. For example, inhibition of voltage-gated K⁺ channels by phosphorylation in response to noxious input increases the excitability of lamina II excitatory interneurons, which in turn could enhance activation of lamina I projection neurons.

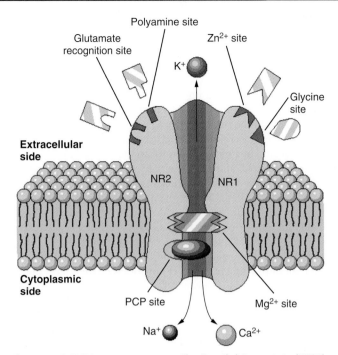

Figure 14-6 NMDA receptor structure. The *N*-methyl-D-aspartate (NMDA)-type glutamate receptor is a hetero-tetramer formed by two obligatory NR1 subunits and two variable NR2 subunits (NR2A-D). The four subunits form a cationic channel that is highly permeable to Ca²⁺ as well as Na⁺ and K⁺. At a resting state the channel is blocked by Mg²⁺. Voltage-gate activation is required for the release of Mg²⁺ from the channel, which is followed by influx of Ca²⁺ upon stimulation by endogenous ligands, further membrane depolarization, and engagement of second messenger systems. The channel has several subunit-specific binding sites for endogenous and exogenous ligands. These include recognition sites for the endogenous agonists glutamate and aspartate, exogenous antagonist including phencyclidine (PCP) and ketamine, the voltage-independent blocker Zn²⁺, and co-agonist modulators enhancing NMDA responses including glycine and polyamines. Glycine and polyamines do not effect channel opening. However, glycine acts as a coagonist and is required for NMDA-receptor activation. *(Modified and adapted from Scatton B. The NMDA receptor complex. Fundam Clin Pharmacol. 1993;7:389-400.)*

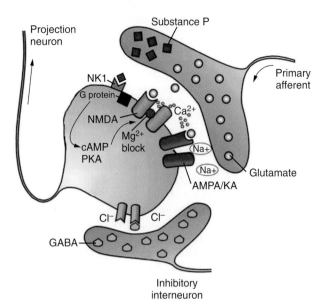

Figure 14-7 Dorsal horn synapse. Arrangement of a dorsal horn synapse between a primary afferent and a projection neuron are shown. The central terminal of the primary afferent contains glutamate and substance P. Release of glutamate results in activation of AMPA (α-amino-3-hydroxy-5-methyl-4-isoxazolepropionic acid) and kainate (KA) receptors and depolarization of the postsynaptic membrane via fast Na⁺-influx. Release of substance P acts synergistically via metabotropic neurokinin 1 receptors (NK1) that upon activation, up-regulate second messenger systems including cyclic adenosine monophosphate (cAMP) and protein kinase A (PKA). Sustained synaptic input can depolarize the postsynaptic membrane sufficiently to activate the voltage-gated NMDA (*N*-methyl-D-aspartate) receptor. Activation of NMDA receptors is associated with long-term enhancement of synaptic transmission (long-term potentiation (LTP), which might underlie hyperalgesic states. The synapse is also under control of other neuronal structures including inhibitory interneurons. Release of GABA (γ-amino butyric acid) enhances influx of Cl⁻, which hyperpolarizes presynaptic or postsynaptic membranes and inhibits activity. *(Modified from Mense, Gerwin. Muscle Pain: Understanding the Mechanisms. Berlin/Heidelberg: Springer-Verlag; 2010.)*

Finally, abnormal function of low-threshold mechanoreceptive Aβ afferents could contribute to tactile allodynia, in that these fibers gain access to nociceptive pathways. Sprouting of Aβ fibers from terminals in the deeper dorsal horn to superficial laminae I and II has been observed after nerve injury.[39] Aβ-fibers can also undergo a phenotypic switch in response to injury and start synthesizing substance P, which could activate the NRK1 receptors of nociceptive lamina I projection neurons.[40]

SUPRASPINAL STRUCTURES

Various nuclei in the brainstem and thalamus receive nociceptive input from the spinal cord and trigeminal nucleus. These structures are important for autonomic regulation and descending modulation of nociceptive information, and act as relays transmitting information to the amygdala and cortical areas. The lateral thalamus mediates sensory-discriminative components of pain, while the medial thalamus modulates affective and behavioral aspects of pain. The amygdala plays a sentinel role for pairing nociceptive input with affective content. Multiple interconnected cortical areas process

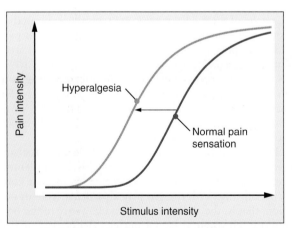

Figure 14-8 Hyperalgesia. Sensitization of peripheral nociceptors results in hyperalgesia which is characterized by a left-shift of the nociceptive stimulus *versus* pain response relationship. This is reflected clinically by an increased sensitivity to painful stimuli.

incoming nociceptive traffic and differentially contribute to the sensory, affective, and cognitive components of pain.[41] The sensory component refers to the ability to discriminate stimuli according to their intensity, location, and temporal relationship. The affective component relates to negative hedonic aspects of pain. The cognitive component represents the evaluation of pain in terms of past experiences, environmental context, and overall significance. An overview of the major components of the nociceptive system and their projections is provided in Figure 14-4.

Brainstem

Neurons in lamina I, V, and VII of the dorsal horn and the trigeminal nucleus build the distinct spinomedullary tract (SMT) that runs in parallel to the spinothalamic tract (STT), thus enabling differential modulation of the two neuronal projections.[42] The SMT terminates at four major brainstem sites including the reticular formation (RF), the noradrenergic cell group (NACG) including the locus coeruleus, the parabrachial nucleus (PBN), and the periaqueductal gray (PAG).[43] Contrasting with the contralateral projections of the STT, neurons of the SMT can terminate bilaterally. This is compatible with their predominant homeostatic role in nociceptive processing including the modulation of autonomic and neuroendocrine responses. Projections of the reticular formation to the dorsal horn and lateral thalamus, the noradrenergic cell group to the dorsal horn and hypothalamus, and the parabrachial nucleus to the hypothalamus, medial thalamus, and amygdala build the neuroanatomic network underlying these functions.

Thalamus

The thalamus is the key relay linking ascending nociceptive input from neurons of the STT to several cortical areas with distinct functions. The sentinel role of the thalamus in nociception is highlighted by clinical studies indicating that lesions of the thalamus can be associated with pain or pain relief. Several thalamic nuclei play a role in the processing of nociceptive signals. While nuclei within the lateral portion of the thalamus mediate sensory and discriminative components of pain, nuclei of the medial portion are typically associated with the processing of affective and motivational aspects of pain.[43] The ventral posterior nuclei (VPN, lateral thalamus) are the major sites receiving somatosensory input. About 10% of VPN neurons process nociceptive information originating from nociceptive and wide dynamic range neurons of the dorsal horn (lamina I and laminae IV-V). The VPN project to the somatosensory cortex (SI and SII), which encodes sensory-discriminative aspects of pain.

The ventral medial nucleus (VMN, lateral thalamus) receives input from nociceptive neurons residing in lamina 1 of the dorsal horn and mainly projects to the insular cortex. Functionally, the VMN might play a particular role in interception, that is, the ability to sense and be aware of the body's condition. The ventral lateral nucleus (VLN; lateral thalamus) also receives input from the STT, projects to the motor cortex, and likely contributes to sensorimotor signal integration. The medial dorsal nucleus (MDN; medial thalamus) receives input from nociceptive neurons located in lamina 1 and projects to the anterior cingulate cortex, a key structure regulating affective and behavioral aspects of pain. Finally, the nucleus submedius (NSM, medial thalamus) receives similar input from lamina 1 but projects to the ventral lateral orbital cortex, a structure regulating descending anti-nociceptive control via the periaqueductal gray.

Basal Ganglia

The basal ganglia are interconnected nuclei located in the white matter of both hemispheres. They include the caudate nucleus, the putamen, the nucleus accumbens, the globus pallidus, the substantia nigra, and the subthalamic nucleus. While the basal ganglia are important for motor function, they might also be relevant for the processing of pain.[44] Afferent input and efferent output to several brain structures are reciprocal and include connections to the cingulate cortex, the prefrontal cortex, and the amygdala. This reciprocal network suggests that the basal ganglia can modulate affective components of pain. The basal ganglia also encode the intensity of noxious input but seem of little importance for localizing pain. Opioids, dopamine, and GABA can alter nociceptive signaling in the substantia nigra, the putamen, and the globus pallidus. Similarly, agonists binding to opioid, dopamine 1, and cholinergic receptors exert anti-nociceptive effects in the nucleus accumbens. However, the overall significance of the basal ganglia for contributing to components of clinical pain is not known.

Amygdala

The amygdala is part of the limbic system and plays a sentinel role for pairing sensory input with emotional significance. In the domain of pain, the amygdala matches nociceptive signals with affective content and serves as the neuronal interface for the reciprocal relationship between pain and an affective state or an affective disorder.[45] The amygdala receives nociceptive information from the spinal cord, brainstem, thalamus, and several cortical regions (insular, anterior cingulate, and association areas). The lateral nucleus of the amygdala serves as the initial site of sensory convergence and connects with the basolateral nucleus, which is critical for associative learning and affective states. Signals carrying affective content are then transmitted to the central nucleus. Nociceptive signals merge in the laterocapsular portion of the central nucleus, which has been labeled the "nociceptive amygdala" because of its high content of nociceptive neurons. Major efferent projections originate from the central nucleus and build widespread connections with the forebrain, thalamus, hypothalamus, and brainstem areas (e.g., periaqueductal gray), thereby regulating autonomic, neuroendocrine, and somatosensory functions related to emotional behavior.

Negative and positive emotions modify neuronal activity in the amygdala, which could therefore exert a dual pain inhibiting and pain enhancing function dependent on the particular affective state.[44] The biochemistry underlying the nociceptive processing in the amygdala is incompletely understood. However, opioid, glutamate, and neuropeptide receptors seem to play an important role. Agonists binding to the μ-opioid receptor, and antagonists binding to ionotropic glutamate receptors, subtypes of metabotropic glutamate receptors (mGluR1, mGluR5), and the CGRP 1 receptor can inhibit nociceptive signaling.[46,47]

Cortical Structures

Interconnected and functionally distinct cortical areas process nociceptive signals in parallel and in series, and build the necessary network underlying the complex experience of pain

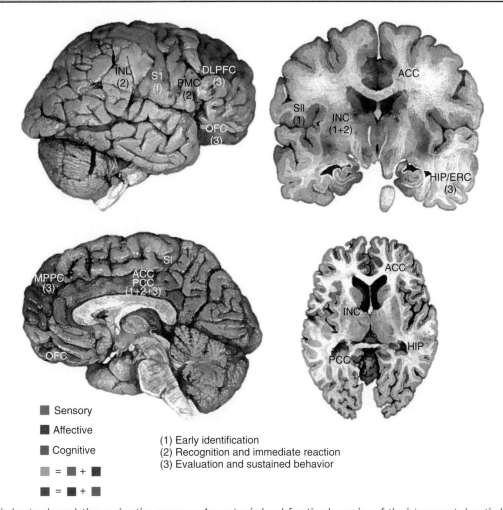

Sensory
Affective
Cognitive
■ = ■ + ■
■ = ■ + ■

(1) Early identification
(2) Recognition and immediate reaction
(3) Evaluation and sustained behavior

Figure 14-9 Cortical network regulating nociceptive processes. An anatomical and functional overview of the interconnected cortical areas of the pain processing network is shown. Areas are coded numerically and by color to indicate their temporal and functional role. For more details see text. *ACC*, Anterior cingulate cortex; *DLPFC*, dorsolateral prefrontal cortex; *ERC*, entorhinal cortex; *HIP*, hippocampus; *INC*, insular cortex; *IPL*, inferior parietal lobule; *MPFC*, medio prefrontal cortex; *OFC*; orbitofrontal cortex; *PCC*, posterior cingulate cortex; *PMC*, premotor cortex; *SI*, primary sensory cortex; *SII*, secondary somatosensory cortex. (*Modified from Casey KL, Tran TD. Cortical mechanisms mediating acute and chronic pain in humans. Handb Clin Neurol. 2006;81:159-177.*)

(Figure 14-9). Cortical areas can be organized according to their relative contribution to the sensory, affective, and cognitive components of pain.[41,48] The primary sensory cortex (SI) discriminates early sensory aspects of pain including its location, time course, and intensity. The secondary somatosensory cortex (SII) integrates discriminative information from SI with noxious input directly received from subcortical structures. SII acts as a relay to other cortical areas (e.g., insula) that analyze noxious signals. The anterior portion of the insula (INC) is in close proximity to SII and mediates early aspects of pain including its anticipation. Connections with the entorhinal cortex (ERC) in the temporal lobe are critical, since anticipation requires past experiences. The inferior parietal lobule (IPL) plays a role for fostering attention to noxious stimuli and lack of function may result in maladaptive behavior. The dorsolateral prefrontal cortex (DLPFC) is involved in shifting attention between tasks and can thereby modulate pain. Activity in the DLPFC has been correlated with the magnitude of the placebo response.[49] The anterior cingulate cortex (ACC) serves multiple functions, including the execution of motor responses to noxious stimuli,

the association of negative affects with noxious input, and the acquirement of information to architecture learned responses to pain. The posterior cingulate cortex (PCC) also processes sensory and behavioral aspects of pain. The premotor cortex (PMC) assists the orchestration of motor responses to pain but might also contribute to stimulus recognition. The insular cortex (INC) acts as the neuronal interface between the somatosensory cortex and limbic cortical structures that modulate affective components of pain (e.g., ACC and ERC). Activities in the mid- and posterior portions of the INC are associated with the recognition of the emotional and biologic significance of noxious input. The orbitofrontal cortex (OFC) plays a critical role for attaching emotional meaning to sensory input, which in turn guides behavior. The medioprefrontal cortex (MPFC) engages in the longer term evaluation of pain and the development of cognitive adaptive strategies. The hippocampus (HIP) and entorhinal cortex (ERC) are part of the cortical network that stores and retrieves sensory information and participate in elaborating the experience of pain based on emotional state, expectations, and past experiences.

DESCENDING PATHWAYS

The significance of descending control mechanisms in modulating pain was first recognized and incorporated into a neurophysiologic model called the "gate theory" by Melzack and Wall in 1965.[50] According to their theory, a gate built by primary afferent fibers, interneurons, and neurons descending from supraspinal sites controlled and modulated nociceptive traffic. While many of the neurophysiologic details turned out to be incorrect, the model was correct in principle.

As proposed by Melzack and Wall, spinal synaptic transmission is modulated by descending inhibitory and excitatory pathways originating in the brainstem. Supraspinal modulation of spinal nociceptive processes as well as autonomic and motor responses is critical for orchestrating an integrated and meaningful response to injury and pain.[51] Descending control mechanisms either attenuate or augment nociceptive and non-nociceptive signaling contingent on overall biologic needs.[52] For example, if a "fight-or-flight" response is most meaningful in the context of an injury, descending control mechanisms typically dampen spinal nociceptive processes. Alternatively, if a "guarding-and-heeling" behavior is most beneficial, descending facilitatory pathways can enhance spinal nociceptive processes (e.g., central sensitization and hyperalgesia associated with tissue injury).[53] Accordingly, the balance between inhibitory and facilitatory descending influences is highly dynamic and changes over the course of acute and chronic injuries.[54]

Under baseline conditions, descending inhibitory control mechanisms dominate and dampen spinal nociceptive signaling. Acute nociceptive input can enhance such activity to suppress sensory input from heterotopic body regions. This leads to the perceptional accentuation of the nociceptive signal and attracts increased attention to the affected body site (diffuse noxious inhibitory control).

The neuroanatomic architecture of the descending control system reflects its multidimensional role (Figure 14-10). Central to the system is the rostral ventral medulla (RVM), which integrates input from several supraspinal structures and acts as the major relay between supraspinal and spinal sites. Some of the same structures exert both inhibitory and excitatory influences.

Structural Components

The best studied components are the periaqueductal gray (PAG) and the rostral ventromedial medulla (RVM), a system rich in opioid receptors and critical for mediating endogenous analgesia.[55,56] Several pontine and medullary noradrenergic nuclei including the locus coeruleus build a second important complex.[57] Other supraspinal regions contribute to descending control mechanisms. While most act via the PAG-RVM axis, some project directly to the dorsal horn (e.g., parabrachial nucleus and dorsal reticular nucleus).

Both the PAG and RVM receive direct input from the spinal dorsal horn and several supraspinal sites. The PAG projects to the RVM, which in turn projects profusely via the dorsolateral funiculus to superficial and deep laminae in the dorsal horn. The PAG-RVM system is tonically active and exerts its spinal control by presynaptic inhibition of primary afferents, postsynaptic inhibition of spinal projection neurons,

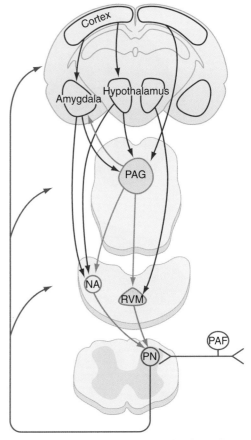

Figure 14-10 Major structural components exerting descending nociceptive control. The interrelationship of major neuroanatomical components exerting descending nociceptive control is shown. The periaqueductal gray (PAG) and rostral ventral medulla (RVM) are strategically located to integrate input from cerebral structures and relay processed information to the spinal dorsal horn. Noradrenergic pontine and medullary nuclei (NA) constitute a second important structure directly projecting to the dorsal horn. Presynaptic and postsynaptic mechanisms modulate nociceptive information that is transmitted from primary afferents (PAF) to spinal projection neurons (PN). Alternatively, indirect actions are exerted via inhibition or excitation of spinal interneurons. Cortical areas, the amygdala and the hypothalamus are among the cerebral structures exerting top-down control. These structures are relevant for the modulation of pain by stress, emotion, and cognition. *(Modified from Millan MJ. Descending control of pain. Prog Neurobiol. 2002;66:355-474.)*

inhibition or activation of interneurons that act on projection neurons, and nonsynaptic release of mediators that diffuse within the dorsal horn (volume transmission). The PAG-RVM axis is critical for generating an orchestrated response to nociceptive barrage and stress. Not surprisingly it is a central site of action for many analgesic drug classes, including opioids, cyclooxygenase inhibitors, and cannabinoids.[58]

The PAG receives input from multiple supraspinal structures, including the prefrontal cortex, hypothalamus, and amygdala. This top-down control of the PAG-RVM axis is important for the modulation of pain by cognitive influences, emotional factors, and stress. For example, projections from the amygdala and hypothalamus are relevant for hypoalgesia associated with intense fear or stress. Similarly, projections from the prefrontal cortex that are relayed via the cingular cortex have been implicated in placebo-mediated analgesia.[59]

Inhibition of Nociception   Facilatation of Nociception

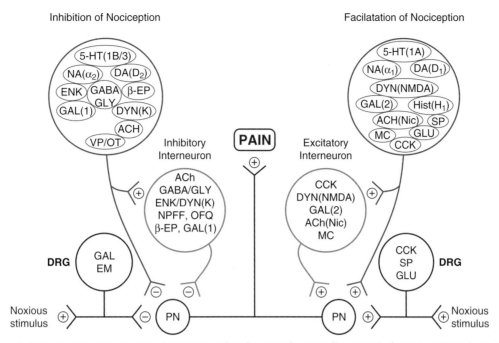

Figure 14-11 Major biochemical components exerting descending nociceptive control. Descending control of spinal nociceptive processes is exerted by multiple neurotransmitters. Transmitters contributing to inhibition of nociceptive signaling are depicted on the left, while transmitters enhancing nociceptive signaling are depicted on the right. This physical separation serves didactic reasons and has no anatomical foundation. Transmitters are contained in descending pathways, in inhibitory or excitatory interneurons, and in primary afferent terminals. Only principal transmitter locations are shown (subtypes are indicated in parentheses). *ACH*, Acetylcholine; *β-EP*, β-endorphin; *CCK*, cholecystokinin; *DA*, dopamine; *DRG*, dorsal root ganglion; *DYN*, dynorphin; *EM*, endomorphin; *ENK*, enkephalin; *GABA*, γ-hydroxy-butyric acid; *GAL*, galanin; *GLU*, glutamate; *GLY*, glycine; *Hist*, histamine; *5-HT*, serotonin; *MC*, melanocortin; *NA*, noradrenaline; *NMDA*, N-methyl-D-aspartate; *NPFF*, neuropeptide FF; *OFQ*, orphanin FQ; *OT*, oxytocin; *PN*, projection neuron; *SP*, substance P; *VP*, vasopressin. *(Modified from Millan MJ. Descending control of pain.* Prog Neurobiol. *2002;66:355-474.)*

The RVM includes the nucleus raphe magnus and adjacent reticular formation. The RVM is functionally defined as the pontomedullary area in which electrical stimulation and microinjection of opioids produce behavioral analgesia. Conversely, injection of the neuropeptides cholecystokinin or neurotensin causes an exaggerated pain response. Reflective of the dual function of structures involved in descending control, the RVM can exert inhibitory and facilitatory influences on spinal processes. The structural correlates of such bimodal action are different cell types, most importantly ON and OFF cells. OFF cells exert inhibitory control, while ON-cells exert facilitatory effects.[58] A shift toward ON-cell activity has been implicated in pronociceptive states associated with inflammation and nerve injury.

Pontine and medullary noradrenergic nuclei including the locus coeruleus project to the dorsal horn via the ventrolateral funiculus. These descending neurons are the primary source of spinal noradrenaline.[57] They receive supraspinal input from regions including the amygdala, hypothalamus, and parabrachial nucleus. In addition, the PAG exerts some descending control via projections to noradrenergic nuclei. The noradrenergic system displays low tonic activity that becomes significantly enhanced with tissue or nerve injury. This might explain why spinally administered α-adrenergic agonists are particularly potent for attenuating pain associated with significant inflammation or nerve injury. The noradrenergic pathway also plays an important role in mediating stress-induced analgesia.

Neurochemistry

The biochemistry of descending control mechanisms is multifaceted and involves many mediators. Figure 14-11 provides an overview of relevant neurotransmitters and their predominant action on spinal nociceptive processes. Not all transmitters exert the same net effect on nociception at spinal and supraspinal sites. For example, histamine elicits pronociceptive effects when administered spinally but exerts antinociceptive effects at supraspinal sites by enhancing descending inhibitory control. Similarly, some transmitters exert pro- and anti-nociceptive effects at different supraspinal sites, such as GABA, dynorphin, and neurotensin. Major transmitter systems exerting descending control are the monaminergic, cholinergic, GABAergic, opioidergic, and glutamatergic systems. Additional transmitters include histamine, vasopressin, oxytocin, cholecystokinin, neurotensin, galanin, substance P, and cannabinoids.[51]

Monaminergic projection neurons are the only source of spinally released norepinephrine, dopamine, and serotonin. Monoamines exert dual inhibitory and excitatory functions contingent on the activated receptor subtype and receptor location on neuronal elements. For example, activation of spinal α1-adrenergic, dopamine D2 receptors augments pronociceptive signaling, while activation of spinal α2-adrenergic, dopamine D1, and $5HT_{1B}$ and $5HT_3$ receptors enhances antinociceptive activities. Other neurotransmitters generated at supraspinal sites and released into the dorsal horn via descending projection neurons include histamine, vasopressin, and oxytocin.

Cholinergic, GABAergic, and opioidergic transmitters are released by descending projection neurons but are also synthesized by dorsal horn neurons. Muscarinic cholinergic receptors are most relevant for acetylcholine-mediated spinal anti-nociceptive activity, while different nicotinic cholinergic receptor subtypes exert anti- or pro-nociceptive functions (e.g., α4β2 *versus* α4β3). GABA enhances anti-nociceptive processes in the dorsal horn via stimulation of both GABA$_A$ and GABA$_B$ receptor, while GABAergic actions at supraspinal sites are more complex. Glycine receptors are often colocalized with GABA receptors, reflecting the synergistic role of GABA and glycine in suppressing nociceptive signaling.

The μ-, δ-, and κ-opioid receptors are differentially stimulated by their endogenous ligands β-endorphin (μ), endomorphin (μ), enkephalin (μ, δ), and dynorphin (κ). Endomorphin and enkephalin elicit anti-nociceptive effects at spinal and supraspinal sites. However, dynorphin exerts dual actions. Activation of spinal κ-receptors attenuates nociceptive signaling, while non-opioidergic spinal actions of dynorphin (e.g., via the NMDA receptor) facilitate pro-nociceptive processes. At the supraspinal level activation of κ-receptors has bidirectional influence on descending control mechanisms. Other neurotransmitters released by descending projection and spinal neurons include melanocortin and orphanin FQ, neuropeptide FF, cholecystokinin, neurotensin, and galanin.

Substance P and glutamate are neurotransmitters not only released by primary afferent fibers but also by descending projection neurons. Finally, endogenous cannabinoids facilitate descending inhibition of spinal nociception via activation of cannabinoid type 1 (CB1) receptors. Spinal anti-nociceptive effects are also elicited by the local release of endogenous cannabinoids.

EMERGING DEVELOPMENTS

Nociceptors as Novel Drug Targets

Significant research efforts have advanced our understanding of the molecular biology of nociceptors and the discovery of new analgesic drug targets. Several compounds aiming at nociceptive signal transduction are currently under development. Among them are agonists and antagonists of the TRPV1 receptor, which will be discussed in more detail as in illustrative example. Other examples include subtype-specific antagonists of voltage-gated Na$^+$ channels (Na$_v$1.3, 1.7, and 1.8), purinergic receptors (P2X$_3$), TRP receptors (TRPV3 and TRPA1), and bradykinin receptors (B1). Considering the complexity of nociceptive signal transduction one might expect that different compounds will show preferential activity for certain types of pain and might not be suitable for systemic administration. Nevertheless, these development efforts are of significant interest and will hopefully broaden the armamentarium of analgesic drugs.

The TRPV1 receptor is an attractive drug target due to its integral role in nociceptive signal transduction and substantial preclinical evidence supporting its effectiveness in models of inflammatory, osteoarthritic, and cancer pain.[60] Agonists cause very short-lived activation of the TRPV1 receptor accompanied by a transient burning pain that is followed by longer term inactivation. Drug development efforts for agonists focus on their topical/local application, since systemic administration results in significant adverse effects. Recently, the Food and Drug Administration approved a capsaicin patch (Qutenza) for the topical treatment of pain in patients suffering from postherpetic neuralgia. Current phase 2/3 clinical trials examine the topical use of TRPV1 agonists for osteoarthritic pain (cream), cluster headache (nasal spray), and postsurgical pain following bunionectomy or inguinal hernia repair (local instillation).

A number of clinical trials have examined the efficacy of several TRPV1 antagonists for alleviating inflammatory pain. While effective as anti-hyperalgesic agents, many programs halted the clinical development of TRPV1 antagonists due to significant safety concerns. Two major problems evolved. First, administration of TRPV1 antagonists caused transient but marked hyperthermia. Second, study participants developed insensitivity to noxious heat posing a potential but significant risk for accidental injuries.[60,61] Both of the undesirable effects are mediated by the TRPV1 receptor. While topical administration of TRPV1 agonists is a promising adjuvant analgesic approach, the fate and potential clinical utility of systemic TRPV1 antagonists remains uncertain.

ROLE OF GLIA

Researchers have mainly focused on dissecting the neuronal mechanisms of pain. Glial cells have largely been viewed as structural components building the architectural frame necessary for supporting the topographic organization of neurons. However, during the past 2 decades glial cells have emerged as an active and integral component of the pain signaling system.[62] Gaining a better understanding of glial cells and their specific function will provide new insight into mechanisms of acute and chronic pain and reveal novel targets amenable to innovative analgesic strategies.

Among glial cells, microglia and astrocytes have received most attention. Microglial cells are macrophages that reside in the CNS and serve in immune surveillance and host defense. Quiescent at a basal state, microglia become quickly activated upon CNS perturbation. Along with their phagocytic function, microglia upregulate receptor expression (e.g., complement) and release proinflammatory mediators, including cytokines. Astrocytes are in close contact with neurons and surround the majority of synapses. Many CNS synapses are "tripartite" and consist of three structural elements that cross-communicate: presynaptic and postsynaptic neuronal structures, and surrounding astrocytes. In addition, astrocytes communicate among themselves via gap junctions and extracellular release of adenosine triphosphate (ATP), thereby building a signaling network that indirectly links neuronal events in neighboring synapses (Figure 14-12). Contrasting with microglia, astrocytes are active at basal conditions. They synthesize an array of transmitters and receptors, many of them also expressed by neurons. Examples include opioidergic, glutamatergic, GABAergic, cholinergic, purinergic, and noradrenergic receptors. However, astrocytes also bind chemokines, cytokines, and prostanoids.[63] Finally, there is cross-communication between microglia and astrocytes, with each cell type capable of activating the other cell type.

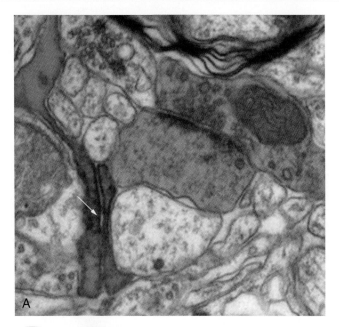

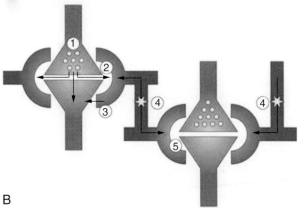

Figure 14-12 Tripartite synapses and neuroglial signaling network. The structural principles allowing neuroglial cross-communication are the tripartite synapse and gap junctions between astrocytes. **A,** The electron micrograph illustrates the two modes of communication. Synaptic communication occurs between pre- and postsynaptic neuronal elements (pink) that are in close contact with astrocytic processes (blue). Astrocytes communicate among themselves via gap junctions *(white arrow).* **B,** The neuroglial communications patterns are depicted schematically. Steps in this dynamic interaction involve the release of transmitters from presynaptic terminals (1), collateral transmitter action on receptors and transporters of astrocytes (2), release of glial transmitters that in turn influence neuronal activity (3), diffusion of transmitters to neighboring astrocytes via gap junctions (4), and subsequent release of glial transmitters at distant synapses (5). *(Modified from Giaume C, Koulakoff A, Roux L. Astroglial networks: a step further in neuroglial and gliovascular interactions. Nat Rev Neurosci. 2010;11:87-99.)*

Glial cells participate in modulating pain upon their activation by events such as tissue trauma and peripheral inflammation. Disruption of glial activation attenuates nociception in various animal models. This highlights the pronociceptive actions of neuroexcitatory products released by glial cells including proinflammatory cytokines and prostaglandins. Of particular interest are studies demonstrating that systemic administration of glial modulators (methotrexate and propentofylline) attenuate pain. Similarly, intrathecal injection of the antiinflammatory cytokine interleukin-10 results

in anti-nociceptive effects. Modulation of glial activity offers a promising new prospect for the management of pain.

GENETIC FACTORS

Patients demonstrate large interindividual differences in their susceptibility to pain as well as their response to analgesic drugs.[64] Genetic factors explain some of these differences and significant efforts are currently directed towards decoding the underlying molecular signatures (see Chapter 4). The availability of a "molecular thumbprint" holds the promise of identifying patients at risk for developing certain pain conditions (e.g., persistent postoperative pain) or experiencing aversive or ineffective drug responses. In addition, a better understanding of the genetics of pain might provide insight into novel analgesic drug targets.

A series of studies has identified several gene variants associated with variations in pain susceptibility.[65] For example, a variant of the gene coding for a subtype of a voltage-gated K^+ channel ($K_v1.9$; *KCNS1*) is associated with increased sensitivity to experimental pain stimuli as well as the propensity to develop chronic pain.[8] Similarly, a variant of a subtype of a voltage-gated Na^+ channel ($Na_v1.7$; *SCN9A*) is associated with increased acute and chronic pain.[9] These findings are consistent with some of the functions of these ion channels in the processing of pain and point to potential novel drug targets. However, future research will need to clarify whether these and other targets revealed by genetic approaches can successfully be exploited in a clinical setting. Similarly, it is not yet clear whether genotypic signatures will allow for the effective and selective use of preemptive strategies in patients at particular risk for developing certain pain conditions.

Several genetic variants have been linked to interindividual differences in analgesic drug responses. Best studied are the opioids. One specific variant of the gene coding for the µ-opioid receptor (A118G; *OPRM1*) has fairly consistently been linked to decreased analgesic opioid effects.[66] Other variants possibly affecting opioid-mediated analgesia are located on genes coding for the melanocortin 1 receptor *(MC1R)*, the 5-HT_{2A} receptor *(HT2A)*, a serotonin-transporter *(5-HTTLPR)*, catechol-O-methyltransferase, P-glycoprotein *(ABCB1)*, and G-protein-activated inwardly rectifying potassium channel subunit *(KCNJ6)*.[67-71]

The gene coding for MCR1 has received particular attention in the field of anesthesia based on a study reporting altered minimum alveolar concentration requirements for volatile anesthetics in redheaded women.[72] Subjects carrying inactivating variants of MCR1 possess a red-hair and fair-skin phenotype. Nonfunctional variants of MCR1 are associated with increased analgesic effects of µ-opioid agonists, and in women only of κ-opioid agonists (Figure 14-13).[73,74]

Any particular variant typically explains a relatively small fraction of differences observed between carriers of the major or minor alleles.[75] This is not surprising considering the polygenetic nature of pain and analgesic responses. Whether polygenetic signatures will be of utility to predict analgesic response profiles in individual patients is subject of future research. Nevertheless, the use of genetics tools for moving closer to personalized medicine is an exciting yet challenging prospect.

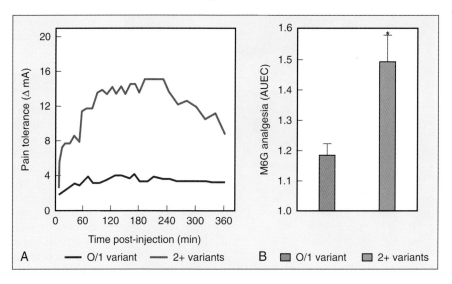

Figure 14-13 The efficacy of morphine-6-gluronide (M6G) for attenuating electrically induced experimental pain is increased in red-haired subjects carrying two nonfunctional variants of the gene encoding melanocortin-1 receptor (MCR1) compared with carriers of one or two functional variants. **A,** The maximum current (mA) evoking pain was significantly greater in redheads than in controls after administration of 0.3 mg/kg M6G. **B,** M6G mediated analgesic effects are expressed as the area under curve depicting increases of the maximum tolerated electrical current over time. Symbols and bars are mean ± SEM; *$P < .05$. *(From Mogil JS, Ritchie J, Smith SB, et al. Melanocortin-1 receptor gene variants affect pain and mu-opioid analgesia in mice and humans.* J Med Genet. *2005;42:583-587.)*

KEY POINTS

- The transduction of nociceptive signals in peripheral endings of nociceptors is a complex process involving a mosaic of receptors and ion channels that are directly or indirectly activated by multiple ligands.
- Nociception related signal transduction is highly interactive, redundant, tissue-specific, time dependent, and contingent on the type of injury. This complexity poses significant challenges, and opportunities, for identifying novel and broadly effective analgesic compounds.
- Most effective might be compounds targeting structures conveying information from multiple nociceptive processes, such as certain ion channels. Analgesic strategies might also be tailored towards specific indications such as pain conditions arising from certain types of tissue or injury.
- Anatomic and neurochemical details of dorsal horn neurocircuits processing nociceptive signals are still quite limited. Recent studies shed light on the synaptic connections between primary afferents, interneurons, and projection neurons, as well as on the receptors and ion channels involved.
- Comprehensive functional characterization of neuronal networks in the dorsal horn explains available analgesic therapies and should facilitate identification of novel analgesic drug targets.
- Descending control mechanisms regulating nociceptive traffic at the level of the dorsal horn involve both pro- and anti-nociceptive effects of some neurotransmitters contingent on release-site and available receptor subtypes. Interactions and redundancies of different neurotransmitter systems are subject to dynamic modulation by tissue or nerve injury.
- Descending control mechanisms are not restricted to nociception but also involve projections to spinal sites exerting autonomic and motor control. The simultaneous actions on nociceptive, autonomic and motor processes raise the possibility that compounds targeting this system might cause significant adverse effects.
- Multitarget strategies including agonist and antagonist approaches simultaneously exploiting mechanisms of descending inhibition and facilitation are promising for achieving clinically effective analgesia without exerting unacceptable side effects.
- The top-down control of spinal and supra-spinal nociceptive processes also provides a rational for nonpharmacologic approaches including behavioral therapies or brain stimulation techniques (e.g., magnetic or electrical).
- A complex network of cortical and subcortical structures is required to process and integrate pain at the conscious and subconscious level. Pain elicits integrated autonomic, endocrine, and motor responses at the subconscious level, as well as sensory, affective, and cognitive responses at the conscious level that are normally tailored to protection of the body, but can be pathologically activated in chronic pain states.
- Appreciation of the multifaceted nature of pain is critical to providing the multidimensional approaches required for its successful alleviation.

Key References

Melzack R, Wall PD. Pain mechanisms: a new theory. *Science.* 1965;150:971-979. This manuscript introduced the gate-control theory. This theory broke with the idea that pain signaling from peripheral tissue to the brain was a hard-wired process and consequently was the product of an invariant relationship between input intensity and response magnitude. Instead, Melzack and Wall proposed that nociceptive signals were modulated at the level of the spinal cord. (Ref. 50)

Melzack R. The McGill Pain Questionnaire: major properties and scoring methods. *Pain.* 1975;1:277-299. Melzack systematically analyzed the language used by patients to describe their pain, established the multidimensional character of pain, and built the basis for the definition of pain along the three experiential axes of sensation, affect, and cognition. An important consequence of this work was the insight that the multifaceted nature of pain requires a multidimensional approach for treatment including pharmacologic, behavioral, and cognitive strategies. (Ref. 41)

Reynolds DV. Surgery in the rat during electrical analgesia induced by focal brain stimulation. *Science.* 1969;164:444-445. This manuscript provided early proof for the existence of a powerful endogenous analgesic system. Electrical stimulation of midbrain structures in nonanesthetized rats allowed for surgical interventions without provoking nociceptive behaviors. Today, the critical role of the periaqueductal gray, the region stimulated by Reynolds, for controlling nociceptive signaling is well established. (Ref. 55)

Pert CB, Snyder SH. Opioid receptor: demonstration in nervous tissue. *Science.* 1973;79:1011-1014. This manuscript provided direct evidence for the expression of opioid receptors in the central nervous system and demonstrated their functional relevance in mitigating analgesia upon stimulation. This work clearly documented that opioids exert their analgesic actions via central mechanisms. (Ref. 56)

Woolf CJ. Evidence for a central component of postinjury pain hypersensitivity. *Nature.* 1983;306:686-688. Woolf demonstrated that hyperalgesia associated with tissue injury (increased sensitivity to pain) was partly due to the amplified processing of nociceptive signals at the level of the spinal cord. This early work documented that structures in the central nervous system can undergo plastic changes and become sensitized (central sensitization) in response to tissue injury. (Ref. 38)

References

1. Joshi GP, Ogunnaike BO. Consequences of inadequate postoperative pain relief and chronic persistent postoperative pain. *Anesthesiol Clin North America.* 2005;23(1):21-36.
2. Kehlet H, Jensen TS, Woolf CJ. Persistent postsurgical pain: risk factors and prevention. *Lancet.* 2006;367(9522):1618-1625.
3. Dolin SJ, Cashman JN, Bland JM. Effectiveness of acute postoperative pain management: I. Evidence from published data. *Br J Anaesth.* 2002;89(3):409-423.
4. Macrae WA. Chronic post-surgical pain: 10 years on. *Br J Anaesth.* 2008;101(1):77-86.
5. Lavand'homme P. Chronic pain after vaginal and cesarean delivery: a reality questioning our daily practice of obstetric anesthesia. *Int J Obstet Anesth.* 2010;19(1):1-2.
6. Hinrichs-Rocker A, Schulz K, Jarvinen I, et al. Psychosocial predictors and correlates for chronic post-surgical pain (CPSP)—a systematic review. *Eur J Pain.* 2009;13(7):719-730.
7. Diatchenko L, Slade GD, Nackley AG, et al. Genetic basis for individual variations in pain perception and the development of a chronic pain condition. *Hum Mol Genet.* 2005;14(1):135-143.
8. Costigan M, Belfer I, Griffin RS, et al. Multiple chronic pain states are associated with a common amino acid-changing allele in KCNS1. *Brain.* 2010;133(9):2519-2527.
9. Reimann F, Cox JJ, Belfer I, et al. Pain perception is altered by a nucleotide polymorphism in SCN9A. *Proc Natl Acad Sci U S A.* 2010;107(11):5148-5153.
10. De Kock M, Lavand'homme P, Waterloos H. 'Balanced analgesia' in the perioperative period: is there a place for ketamine? *Pain.* 2001;92(3):373-380.
11. De Kock M, Lavand'homme P, Waterloos H. The short-lasting analgesia and long-term antihyperalgesic effect of intrathecal clonidine in patients undergoing colonic surgery. *Anesthesia and Analgesia.* 2005;101(2):566-572.
12. Buvanendran A, Kroin JS, Della Valle CJ, et al. Perioperative oral pregabalin reduces chronic pain after total knee arthroplasty: a prospective, randomized, controlled trial. *Anesth Analg.* 2010;110(1):199-207.
13. Gold MS, Gebhart GF. Nociceptor sensitization in pain pathogenesis. *Nat Med.* 2011;16(11):1248-1257.
14. Birklein F, Schmelz M. Neuropeptides, neurogenic inflammation and complex regional pain syndrome (CRPS). *Neurosci Lett.* 2008;437(3):199-202.
15. Caterina MJ, Schumacher MA, Tominaga M, et al. The capsaicin receptor: a heat-activated ion channel in the pain pathway. *Nature.* 1997;389(6653):816-824.
16. Handwerker HO. Chapter 3 Nociceptors: neurogenic inflammation. *Handb Clin Neurol.* 2006;81:23-33.
17. Knowlton WM, Bifolck-Fisher A, Bautista DM, et al. TRPM8, but not TRPA1, is required for neural and behavioral responses to acute noxious cold temperatures and cold-mimetics in vivo. *Pain.* 2010;150(2):340-350.
18. Bautista DM, Jordt SE, Nikai T, et al. TRPA1 mediates the inflammatory actions of environmental irritants and proalgesic agents. *Cell.* 2006;124(6):1269-1282.
19. Yu FH, Catterall WA. Overview of the voltage-gated sodium channel family. *Genome Biol.* 2003;4(3):207.
20. Wood JN. Chapter 5 Molecular mechanisms of nociception and pain. *Handb Clin Neurol.* 2006;81:49-59.
21. Cox JJ, Reimann F, Nicholas AK, et al. An SCN9A channelopathy causes congenital inability to experience pain. *Nature.* 2006;444(7121):894-898.
22. Fertleman CR, Baker MD, Parker KA, et al. SCN9A mutations in paroxysmal extreme pain disorder: allelic variants underlie distinct channel defects and phenotypes. *Neuron.* 2006;52(5):767-774.
23. Boucher TJ, Okuse K, Bennett DL, et al. Potent analgesic effects of GDNF in neuropathic pain states. *Science.* 2000;290(5489):124-127.
24. Bayliss DA, Barrett PQ. Emerging roles for two-pore-domain potassium channels and their potential therapeutic impact. *Trends Pharmacol Sci.* 2008;29(11):566-575.
25. Noel J, Zimmermann K, Busserolles J, et al. The mechano-activated K+ channels TRAAK and TREK-1 control both warm and cold perception. *Embo J.* 2009;28(9):1308-1318.
26. Edvinsson L, Ho TW. CGRP receptor antagonism and migraine. *Neurotherapeutics.* 2010;7(2):164-175.
27. Lewin GR, Mendell LM. Nerve growth factor and nociception. *Trends Neurosci.* 1993;16(9):353-359.
28. Mantyh PW, Koltzenburg M, Mendell LM, et al. Antagonism of nerve growth factor-TrkA signaling and the relief of pain. *Anesthesiology.* 2011;115(1):189-204.
29. Lane NE, Schnitzer TJ, Birbara CA, et al. Tanezumab for the treatment of pain from osteoarthritis of the knee. *N Engl J Med.* 2010;363(16):1521-1531.
30. Hill R. NK1 (substance P) receptor antagonists—why are they not analgesic in humans? *Trends Pharmacol Sci.* 2000;21(7):244-246.
31. Indo Y, Tsuruta M, Hayashida Y, et al. Mutations in the TRKA/NGF receptor gene in patients with congenital insensitivity to pain with anhidrosis. *Nat Genet.* 1996;13(4):485-488.
32. Todd AJ. Neuronal circuitry for pain processing in the dorsal horn. *Nat Rev Neurosci.* 2010;11(12):823-836.
33. Todd AJ. Chapter 6 Anatomy and neurochemistry of the dorsal horn. *Handb Clin Neurol.* 2006;81:61-76.
34. Bice TN, Beal JA. Quantitative and neurogenic analysis of neurons with supraspinal projections in the superficial dorsal horn of the rat lumbar spinal cord. *J Comp Neurol.* 1997;388(4):565-574.
35. Uta D, Furue H, Pickering AE, et al. TRPA1-expressing primary afferents synapse with a morphologically identified subclass of substantia gelatinosa neurons in the adult rat spinal cord. *Eur J Neurosci.* 2010;31(11):1960-1973.
36. Scatton B. The NMDA receptor complex. *Fundam Clin Pharmacol.* 1993;7(8):389-400.
37. Sandkuhler J. Models and mechanisms of hyperalgesia and allodynia. *Physiol Rev.* 2009;89(2):707-758.

38. Woolf CJ. Evidence for a central component of post-injury pain hypersensitivity. *Nature.* 1983;306(5944):686-688.

39. Woolf CJ, Shortland P, Coggeshall RE. Peripheral nerve injury triggers central sprouting of myelinated afferents. *Nature.* 1992; 355(6355):75-78.

40. Neumann S, Doubell TP, Leslie T, et al. Inflammatory pain hypersensitivity mediated by phenotypic switch in myelinated primary sensory neurons. *Nature.* 1996;384(6607):360-364.

41. Melzack R. The McGill Pain Questionnaire: major properties and scoring methods. *Pain.* 1975;1(3):277-299.

42. Andrew D, Krout KE, Craig AD. Differentiation of lamina I spinomedullary and spinothalamic neurons in the cat. *J Comp Neurol.* 2003;458(3):257-271.

43. Dostrovsky JO. Chapter 10 Brainstem and thalamic relays. *Handb Clin Neurol.* 2006;81:127-139.

44. Neugebauer V. Chapter 11 Subcortical processing of nociceptive information: basal ganglia and amygdala. *Handb Clin Neurol.* 2006; 81:141-158.

45. Neugebauer V, Li W, Bird GC, et al. The amygdala and persistent pain. *Neuroscientist.* 2004;10(3):221-234.

46. Han JS, Li W, Neugebauer V. Critical role of calcitonin gene-related peptide 1 receptors in the amygdala in synaptic plasticity and pain behavior. *J Neurosci.* 2005;25(46):10717-10728.

47. Li W, Neugebauer V. Block of NMDA and non-NMDA receptor activation results in reduced background and evoked activity of central amygdala neurons in a model of arthritic pain. *Pain.* 2004; 110(1-2):112-122.

48. Casey KL, Tran TD. Chapter 12 Cortical mechanisms mediating acute and chronic pain in humans. *Handb Clin Neurol.* 2006;81:159-177.

49. Wager TD, Rilling JK, Smith EE, et al. Placebo-induced changes in FMRI in the anticipation and experience of pain. *Science.* 2004; 303(5661):1162-1167.

50. Melzack R, Wall PD. Pain mechanisms: a new theory. *Science.* 1965;150(699):971-979.

51. Millan MJ. Descending control of pain. *Prog Neurobiol.* 2002; 66(6):355-474.

52. Mason P. Chapter 15 Descending pain modulation as a component of homeostasis. *Handb Clin Neurol.* 2006;81:211-218.

53. Urban MO, Gebhart GF. Supraspinal contributions to hyperalgesia. *Proc Natl Acad Sci U S A.* 1999;96(14):7687-7692.

54. Terayama R, Dubner R, Ren K. The roles of NMDA receptor activation and nucleus reticularis gigantocellularis in the time-dependent changes in descending inhibition after inflammation. *Pain.* 2002; 97(1-2):171-181.

55. Reynolds DV. Surgery in the rat during electrical analgesia induced by focal brain stimulation. *Science.* 1969;164(878):444-445.

56. Pert CB, Snyder SH. Opiate receptor: demonstration in nervous tissue. *Science.* 1973;179(77):1011-1014.

57. Pertovaara A, Almeida A. Chapter 13 Descending inhibitory systems. *Handb Clin Neurol.* 2006;81:179-192.

58. Heinricher MM, Tavares I, Leith JL, et al. Descending control of nociception: specificity, recruitment and plasticity. *Brain Res Rev.* 2009;60(1):214-225.

59. Petrovic P, Kalso E, Petersson KM, et al. A prefrontal non-opioid mechanism in placebo analgesia. *Pain.* 2010;150(1):59-65.

60. Pal M, Angaru S, Kodimuthali A, et al. Vanilloid receptor antagonists: emerging class of novel anti-inflammatory agents for pain management. *Curr Pharm Des.* 2009;15(9):1008-1026.

61. Rowbotham MC, Nothaft W, Duan WR, et al. Oral and cutaneous thermosensory profile of selective TRPV1 inhibition by ABT-102 in a randomized healthy volunteer trial. *Pain.* 2011;152(5):1192-1200.

62. Watkins LR, Wieseler-Frank J, Milligan ED, et al. Chapter 22 Contribution of glia to pain processing in health and disease. *Handb Clin Neurol.* 2006;81:309-323.

63. Hansson E, Ronnback L. Astrocytic receptors and second messenger systems. *Adv Mol Cell Biol.* 2004;31:475-501.

64. Aubrun F, Langeron O, Quesnel C, et al. Relationships between measurement of pain using visual analog score and morphine requirements during postoperative intravenous morphine titration. *Anesthesiology.* 2003;98(6):1415-1421.

65. Lotsch J. Genetic variability of pain perception and treatment—clinical pharmacological implications. *Eur J Clin Pharmacol.* 2011; 67(6):541-551.

66. Walter C, Lotsch J. Meta-analysis of the relevance of the OPRM1 118A>G genetic variant for pain treatment. *Pain.* 2009;146(3):270-275.

67. Aoki J, Hayashida M, Tagami M, et al. Association between 5-hydroxytryptamine 2A receptor gene polymorphism and postoperative analgesic requirements after major abdominal surgery. *Neurosci Lett.* 2010;479(1):40-43.

68. Campa D, Gioia A, Tomei A, et al. Association of ABCB1/MDR1 and OPRM1 gene polymorphisms with morphine pain relief. *Clin Pharmacol Therapeut.* 2008;83(4):559-566.

69. Rakvag TT, Ross JR, Sato H, et al. Genetic variation in the catechol-O-methyltransferase (COMT) gene and morphine requirements in cancer patients with pain. *Mol Pain.* 2008;4:64.

70. Kosek E, Jensen KB, Lonsdorf TB, et al. Genetic variation in the serotonin transporter gene (5-HTTLPR, rs25531) influences the analgesic response to the short acting opioid Remifentanil in humans. *Mol Pain.* 2009;5:37.

71. Nishizawa D, Nagashima M, Katoh R, et al. Association between KCNJ6 (GIRK2) gene polymorphisms and postoperative analgesic requirements after major abdominal surgery. *PLoS One.* 2009;4(9): e7060.

72. Liem EB, Lin CM, Suleman MI, et al. Anesthetic requirement is increased in redheads. *Anesthesiology.* 2004;101(2):279-283.

73. Mogil JS, Ritchie J, Smith SB, et al. Melanocortin-1 receptor gene variants affect pain and mu-opioid analgesia in mice and humans. *J Med Genet.* 2005;42(7):583-587.

74. Mogil JS, Wilson SG, Chesler EJ, et al. The melanocortin-1 receptor gene mediates female-specific mechanisms of analgesia in mice and humans. *Proc Natl Acad Sci U S A.* 2003;100(8):4867-4872.

75. Lotsch J, Geisslinger G. A critical appraisal of human genotyping for pain therapy. *Trends Pharmacol Sci.* 2010;31(7):312-317.

Chapter 15

OPIOID AGONISTS AND ANTAGONISTS

Takahiro Ogura and Talmage D. Egan

HISTORICAL PERSPECTIVE

The white "latex" juice of the poppy plant is the source of more than 20 opiate alkaloids. *Opium*, a word derived from the Greek word for "juice," is the brownish residue observed after the poppy's juice is desiccated. *Opiate* is the older term classically used in pharmacology to mean a drug derived from opium. *Opioid*, a more modern term, is used to designate all substances, both natural and synthetic, that bind to opioid receptors (including antagonists).

Opium and its derivatives have been known for millennia to relieve pain. Laudanum, or tincture of opium (a mixture of opium and alcohol), was used as early as the 1600s as an analgesic. Sir Christopher Wren, the acclaimed English man of arts and letters, was the first to inject opium into a living organism using a hollow feather quill as the delivery system in 1659. Serturner, a German pharmacist, isolated morphine from opium in 1805. Having initially called morphine "somniferum" (after the Latin botanical name *Papaver somniferum*—the poppy that brings sleep), the name was later changed to *morphine*, alluding to Morpheus, the Greek god of dreams.

Opium and its derivatives have frequently been the basis of international conflict. The Opium Wars of the 1800s were fought between China and the Western powers in large part in response to Western importation of opium into China. The opium houses of 19th century China, where opium was freely available for sale and consumption, illustrated the frightening societal consequences of large scale drug abuse. Recognition of these problems in the United States eventually culminated in The Harrison Narcotics Act of 1914 that criminalized narcotic possession. The prevalence of addiction clinics and drug-related violence and crime in modern society emphasizes the chronicity of the societal difficulties that stem from this drug class and others.

Opioids play an indispensible role in the practice of medicine, especially anesthesiology, critical care and pain management. A sound understanding of opioid pharmacology, including both basic science and clinical aspects, is critical for the safe and effective use of these important drugs. This chapter focuses on intravenous opioids used perioperatively.

BASIC PHARMACOLOGY

Structure-Activity

The opioids of clinical interest in anesthesiology share many structural features. Morphine, the principal active compound derived from opium, is a *benzylisoquinoline* alkaloid; the benzylisoquinoline structural backbone is present in many important naturally occurring drugs, including papaverine, tubocurarine, and morphine. Morphine's benzylisoquinoline-based structure is shown in Figure 15-1. Many commonly used semisynthetic opioids are created by simple modification of the morphine molecule. Codeine, for example, is the 3-methyl derivative of morphine. Similarly, hydromorphone, hydrocodone, and oxycodone are also synthesized by relatively simple modifications of morphine. More complex alteration of the morphine molecular skeleton results in mixed agonist-antagonists like nalbuphine and even pure competitive antagonists like naloxone.

Some of the morphine derivatives have chiral centers and thus are typically synthesized as racemic mixtures of two enantiomers; only the levorotatory enantiomer is significantly

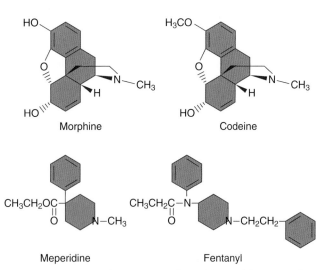

Figure 15-1 The molecular structures of morphine, codeine, meperidine, and fentanyl. Note that codeine is a simple modification of morphine (as are many other opiates); fentanyl and its congeners are more complex modifications of meperidine, a phenylpeperidine derivative.

active at the opioid receptor. The naturally occurring, stereospecific enzymatic machinery in the poppy plant produces morphine only in the levorotatory form.

The fentanyl series of opioids are chemically related to meperidine. Meperidine is the first completely synthetic opioid and can be regarded as the prototype clinical phenylpiperidine. As shown in Figure 15-1, fentanyl is a simple modification of the basic phenylpiperidine structure found within meperidine; the other commonly used fentanyl congeners like alfentanil and sufentanil are somewhat more complex versions of the same phenylpiperidine skeleton. Because these drugs have no chiral center and therefore exist in a single form, the pharmacologic complexities of stereochemistry do not apply.[1]

As outlined in Table 15-1, opioids share many physicochemical features in common, although some individual drugs have unique features. In general, opioids are highly lipid-soluble weak bases that are highly protein bound and largely ionized (protonated) at physiologic pH. Opioid physicochemical properties are thought to have important implications on their clinical behavior. For example, highly lipid-soluble, relatively unbound, un-ionized molecules like alfentanil and remifentanil have a shorter latency-to-peak effect after bolus injection, presumably due to their more rapid transfer across cellular membranes.

Mechanism

Opioids produce their main pharmacologic effects by interacting with opioid receptors. Investigation of opioid receptor genetics, structure, and function over the past several decades has greatly enhanced understanding of opioid pharmacology.

Cloning of the opioid receptors, first accomplished in rodents and subsequently in humans, was an important first step in eventually elucidating opioid receptor structure and function. Using the rat μ opioid receptor cDNA sequence as a guide, investigators were able to identify its human homolog, describing the amino acid sequence, strong binding affinity for an endogenous opioid ligand (i.e., enkephalin), and chromosomal assignment (i.e., chromosome 6).[2]

Opioid receptors are typical of the G-protein coupled family of receptors widely found in biology (e.g., β-adrenergic, dopaminergic). Like other G-protein coupled receptors, opioid receptors have seven transmembrane portions, intracellular and extracellular loops, an extracellular N-terminus,

Table 15-1. Selected Opioid Physicochemical and Pharmacokinetic Parameters

	MORPHINE	FENTANYL	SUFENTANIL	ALFENTANIL	REMIFENTANIL
pKa	8.0	8.4	8.0	6.5	7.1
% Un-ionized at pH 7.4	23	<10	20	90	67?
Octanol-H_2O partition coefficient	1.4	813	1778	145	17.9
% Bound to plasma protein	20-40	84	93	92	80
Diffusible fraction (%)	16.8	1.5	1.6	8.0	13.3
Vdc (L/kg)	0.1-0.4	0.4-1.0	0.2	1.1-0.3	0.06-0.08
Vdss (L/kg)	3-5	3-5	2.5-3.0	0.4-1.0	0.2-0.3
Clearance (mL/min/kg)	15-30	10.20	10-15	4-9	30-40
Hepatic extraction ratio	0.6-0.8	0.8-1.0	0.7-0.9	0.3-0.5	NA

From Bailey PL, Egan TD, Stanley TH. Intravenous opioid anesthetics. In: Miller RD, ed. *Anesthesia*. 5th ed. New York: Churchill Livingstone; 2000:312.
NA, Not applicable; *Vdc*, volume of distribution of central compartment; *Vdss*, volume of distribution at steady state.

and an intracellular C-terminus. There is considerable amino acid sequence homology among the various opioid receptor subtypes; most of the nonhomologous sequences occur in the extracellular portions of the protein. The extracellular domains are thought to be important in discriminating between the various receptor ligands.

Expression of cloned opioid receptors in cultured cells has facilitated analysis of the intracellular signal transduction mechanisms activated by opioid receptors.[3] As shown in Figure 15-2, binding of opioid agonists with the receptors leads to activation of the G-protein (actually three distinct G-protein subunits), producing effects that are primarily inhibitory (decreased cAMP production, decreased Ca^{2+} influx, increased K^+ efflux); these effects ultimately culminate

in membrane hyperpolarization of the cell and reduction of neuronal excitability.

Three classic opioid receptors have been identified using molecular biology techniques: μ, κ, and δ receptors. These receptors are also described by an international nomenclature scheme as MOP, KOP, and DOP (mu, kappa, and delta opioid peptide). More recently, a fourth opioid receptor, ORL1 (also known as NOP), has also been identified, although its function appears to be quite different than that of the classic opioid receptors. As shown in Table 15-2, each of these opioid receptors has a commonly employed experimental bioassay, associated endogenous ligands, a set of agonists and antagonists, and a spectrum of physiologic effects when the receptor is activated. Although the existence of opioid receptor

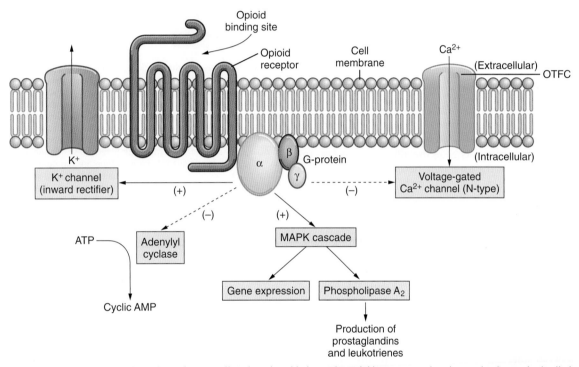

Figure 15-2 Opioid mechanisms of action. The endogenous ligand or drug binds to the opioid receptor and activates the G protein (3 distinct protein subunits), resulting in multiple effects that are primarily inhibitory. The activities of adenylate cyclase and the voltage dependent Ca^{2+} channels are depressed. The inwardly rectifying K^+ channels and mitogen activated protein kinase (MAPK) cascade are activated. *AMP*, Adenosine monophosphate; *ATP*, adenosine triphosphate; *OTFC*, oral transmucosal fentanyl citrate.

Table 15-2. A Summary of Selected Features of Opioid Receptors

	MU (μ)	DELTA (δ)	KAPPA (κ)
Tissue bioassay*	Guinea pig ileum	Mouse vas deferens	Rabbit vas deferens
Endogenous ligand	β-Endorphin	Leu-enkephalin	Dynorphin
	Endomorphin	Met-enkephalin	
Agonist prototype	Morphine	Deltorphin	Buprenorphine
	Fentanyl		Pentazocine
Antagonist prototype	Naloxone	Naloxone	Naloxone
Supraspinal analgesia	Yes	Yes	Yes
Spinal analgesia	Yes	Yes	Yes
Respiratory depression	Yes	No	Yes
Gastrointestinal effects	Yes	No	Yes
Sedation	Yes	No	Yes

From Bailey PL, Egan TD, Stanley TH. Intravenous opioid anesthetics. In: Miller RD, ed. *Anesthesia*. 5th ed. New York: Churchill Livingstone; 2000:312.
*Traditional experimental method to assess opioid receptor activity in vivo.

subtypes (e.g., μ-1, μ-2) has been proposed, it is not clear from molecular biology techniques that distinct genes code for them. Posttranscriptional and posttranslational modification of opioid receptors certainly occurs and could be responsible for conflicting data regarding opioid receptor subtypes. It is well known, for example, that the mRNA coding for the human μ receptor undergoes alternative splicing, resulting in subtle differences in the final receptor.[4]

As confirmed by autoradiographic and binding techniques, opioid receptors are widely expressed in the central nervous system (CNS). In the spinal cord, they are mainly localized to the substantia gelatinosa of the dorsal horn. In the brain, they are especially concentrated in the periaqueductal gray region, the limbic system, area postrema, thalamus, and cerebral cortex. Opioid receptors are also found outside the CNS in gastrointestinal, biliary, and other tissues. Action by agonists at these peripheral receptors accounts for some of the adverse effects of opioids such as constipation.

In accordance with the wide distribution of opioid receptors in the CNS, opioids appear to exert their therapeutic effects at multiple sites. Opioid agonism at the level of the spinal cord inhibits the release of substance P from primary sensory neurons in the dorsal horn, mitigating the transfer of painful sensations to the brain. Opioid actions in the brainstem modulate nociceptive transmission in the dorsal horn of the spinal cord through descending inhibitory pathways. Opioids are also thought to change the affective response to pain through actions in the forebrain; decerebration prevents opioid analgesic efficacy in rats.[5] Furthermore, functional magnetic resonance imaging studies in humans have demonstrated that morphine induces signal activity in reward structures in the brain.[6]

Studies in genetically altered mice have yielded important information about opioid receptor function. In μ opioid receptor knockout mice, morphine-induced analgesia, reward effect, and withdrawal effect are absent.[7,8] Figure 15-3 demonstrates the simple power of these site-directed mutagenesis techniques, confirming how μ opioid receptor (MOR) knockout mice exhibit no analgesic effect to morphine as assessed by measuring the time to jumping off a hot plate. Importantly, MOR knockout mice also fail to exhibit respiratory depression in response to morphine.[9] Confirming the importance of opioid receptor ligands in the biology of "endogenous" analgesia systems, β-endorphin knockout mice fail to show naloxone reversible, stress-induced analgesia but maintain a normal analgesic response to morphine.[10]

Metabolism

The intravenous opioids in common perioperative clinical use are transformed and excreted by a wide variety of metabolic pathways. In general, opioids are metabolized by the hepatic microsomal cytochrome P450 (CYP) system, although hepatic conjugation and subsequent excretion by the kidney are important for some drugs. For certain opioids, the specific metabolic pathway involved has important clinical implications in terms of active metabolites (e.g., morphine, meperidine) or an ultrashort duration of action (e.g., remifentanil). For other opioids, genetic variation in the metabolic pathway can drastically alter the clinical effects (e.g., codeine). These nuances are addressed in a subsequent section focused on individual drugs.

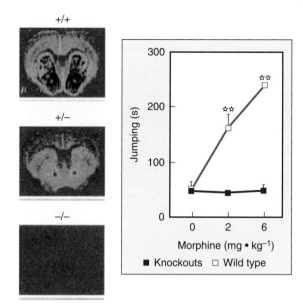

Figure 15-3 Receptor distribution and response to morphine in μ opioid receptor knockout mice. On the left side are computer enhanced color autoradiograms of coronal sections of mice brain demonstrating diminished μ opioid receptors in the heterozygotes (+/−) and complete absence of μ opioid receptors in the homozygotes (−/−) compared to wild type littermates (+/+). The right panel shows the antinociceptive responses to morphine administration during the "hot-plate" test in μ opioid receptor knockouts (−/−) and their wild type littermates. The knockouts are represented by the filled squares; the wild type are the open squares. The two stars indicate a highly significant difference between groups ($P < .01$). The knockouts exhibit no analgesic response to morphine. *(Adapted with permission from Matthes HW, Maldonado R, Simonin F, et al. Loss of morphine-induced analgesia, reward effect and withdrawal symptoms in mice lacking the mu-opioid-receptor gene.* Nature. *1996;383:819-823.)*

CLINICAL PHARMACOLOGY

Pharmacokinetics

Because in most respects opioids are pharmacodynamically similar, pharmacokinetic differences form the scientific foundation for the rational selection and administration of opioids in anesthesia practice. Key pharmacokinetic behaviors to consider are the latency-to-peak effect after bolus injection (i.e., bolus front-end kinetics), the time to offset of effect after bolus injection (i.e., bolus back-end kinetics), the time to steady-state after starting a continuous infusion (i.e., infusion front-end kinetics), and the time to offset of effect after stopping a continuous infusion (i.e., infusion back-end kinetics).

Applying opioid pharmacokinetic concepts to clinical anesthesiology requires recognition of several fundamental principles. First, a table of opioid pharmacokinetic parameters can rarely be instructive in terms of understanding how the pharmacokinetic behavior of the individual drugs compares (see Chapter 2). Understanding pharmacokinetic behavior is best achieved through computer simulation. Second, because opioid clinical behavior differs depending on whether the drugs are administered by bolus injection or continuous infusion, these two clinical conditions must be considered separately.[11] Third, the time course of drug levels predicted through pharmacokinetic simulation cannot be considered in a vacuum; pharmacokinetic information must be integrated with knowledge about the concentration-effect relationship and drug interactions (pharmacodynamics) in order to be clinically useful.

The latency-to-peak effect and the offset of effect after bolus injection of various opioids can be explored by predicting the time course of effect site concentrations after a bolus is administered. Because the opioids differ in terms of potency (and thus the required dosages), for comparison purposes the effect site concentrations must be normalized to the percent of peak concentration for each drug. Considering morphine, hydromorphone, fentanyl, sufentanil, alfentanil, and remifentanil as among the most commonly used intravenous opioids intraoperatively, Figure 15-4, *A*, illustrates how these opioids differ in terms of latency-to-peak effect (i.e., bolus front-end kinetics).

The simulation of a bolus injection (see Figure 15-4, *A*) has obvious clinical implications. For example, when a rapid onset of opioid effect is desirable, morphine may not be a good choice. Similarly, when the clinical goal is a brief pulse of opioid effect followed by a rapid dissipation of effect, remifentanil or alfentanil are preferred. Note how remifentanil's concentration has declined substantially before fentanyl's peak concentration has been achieved (bolus back-end kinetics). The simulation illustrates why the front-end kinetics of fentanyl make it a drug well suited for patient-controlled analgesia (PCA). In contrast to morphine, the peak effect of a fentanyl bolus is manifest before a typical PCA lockout period has elapsed, thus mitigating a "dose stacking" problem.

The latency-to-peak effect is governed by the speed with which the plasma and effect site come to equilibrium (the ke0 parameter). Drugs with a more rapid equilibration are thought to have a higher "diffusible" fraction (the proportion of drug that is un-ionized and unbound). It is important to emphasize that a substantial limitation of these latency-to-peak effect simulations is that a very large dose of any opioid can produce a rapid onset (because a supratherapeutic drug level in the effect site is reached even though the peak concentration comes later).

The time to steady-state after beginning a continuous infusion is also best explored through pharmacokinetic simulation. Again, because the potency of the various opioids differs, the predicted effect site concentrations must be normalized to the final steady-state concentrations in order to contrast the behavior of the drugs. Using the same prototypes, Figure 15-4, *B*, shows the time required to achieve steady-state effect site concentration (infusion front-end kinetics).

The simulation of simple, constant rate infusions has obvious clinical implications. First, it is clear that for most commonly used intravenous opioids, the time required to reach a substantial fraction of the ultimate steady-state concentration is very long in the context of intraoperative use. To reach a near steady-state more quickly requires a bolus be administered before the infusion is commenced (or increased). Remifentanil perhaps represents a partial exception to this general rule. Another extremely important clinical application of this simulation is that concentrations will rise for many hours after an infusion is commenced; thus, practitioners must be aware that concentrations are typically rising even though the infusion rate may have been the same for hours. That remifentanil achieves a near steady-state relatively quickly makes it an especially useful drug for total intravenous anesthesia because it is thus more "titratable."

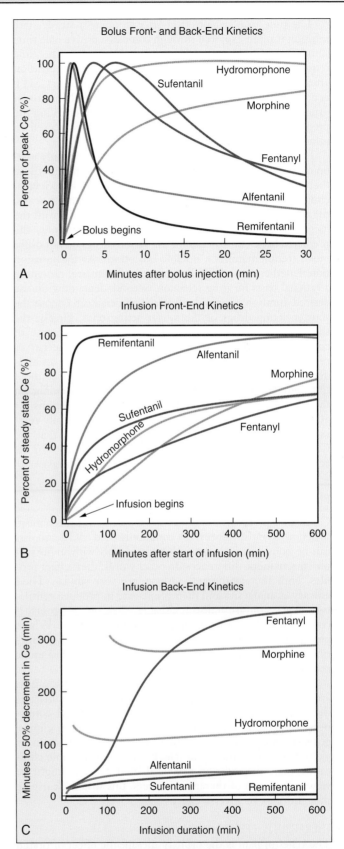

Figure 15-4 Opioid pharmacokinetics. Simulations illustrating front-end and back-end pharmacokinetic behavior after administration by bolus injection or continuous infusions for morphine, hydromorhpone, fentanyl, alfentanil, sufentanil, and remifentanil using pharmacokinetic parameters from the literature (see text). *(Data from references 39, 40, 92-96.)*

The time to offset of effect after stopping a steady-state infusion is often explored through context-sensitive half-time simulation (CSHT; see Chapter 2).[12] Defined as the time required to achieve a 50% decrease in plasma concentration after stopping a continuous, steady-state infusion, the CSHT is a means of normalizing the pharmacokinetic behavior of drugs so that rational comparisons can be made regarding the predicted offset of drug effect. The CSHT is thus focused on infusion back-end kinetics.

Figure 15-4, C, is a CSHT simulation for commonly used opioids (strictly speaking it is the 50% decrement time because the simulation is for effect-site concentrations).[13] Several clinically important points are obvious. First, for most drugs, the time to a 50% decrease in concentration changes with the length of the infusion. Thus, for very brief infusions, the predicted back-end kinetics for the various drugs do not differ much (remifentanil is a notable exception). As the infusion time lengthens, the CSHTs begin to differentiate, providing a rational basis for drug selection. Second, depending on the desired duration of opioid effect, the clinician can choose the shorter acting drugs or the longer acting ones. Finally, the shapes of these curves differ depending on the degree of concentration decline required; in other words, the curves representing the time required to achieve a 20% or an 80% decrease in concentration (e.g., the 20% or 80% decrement time simulations) are quite different.[11] Thus, depending on the anesthesia technique applied, the CSHT simulations (or 50% decrement time) are not necessarily the clinically relevant simulations. It is also important to recognize that the CSHT simulation for morphine does not account for its active metabolite (see later section on individual drugs).

Pharmacodynamics

Given that μ receptor agonists share a common mechanism of action, in most respects the commonly used MOR agonists can be considered pharmacodynamic equals with important pharmacokinetic differences. In other words, their effect profiles, both therapeutic and adverse, are very similar. Their efficacy as analgesics and their propensity to produce ventilatory depression are indistinguishable when one μ agonist is compared with another at equipotent concentrations. Where pharmacodynamic differences exist, they are typically a function of non-opioid receptor mechanisms, such as histamine release, among others.

Clinically important μ agonist pharmacodynamic effects are observed is many organ systems. Figure 15-5 summarizes the major pharmacodynamic effects of the fentanyl congeners. Depending on the clinical circumstances and clinical goals of treatment, some of these widespread effects can be viewed as therapeutic or adverse. For example, in some clinical settings, the sedation produced by μ agonists might be viewed as a goal of therapy; in others, this would clearly be thought of as an adverse effect.

THERAPEUTIC EFFECTS

The relief of pain is the primary therapeutic effect of opioid analgesics. Acting at spinal and brain μ receptors, opioids are thought to provide analgesia both by attenuating the nociceptive traffic from the periphery and by altering the affective response to painful stimulation centrally. The μ agonists are most effective in treating "second pain" sensations carried by

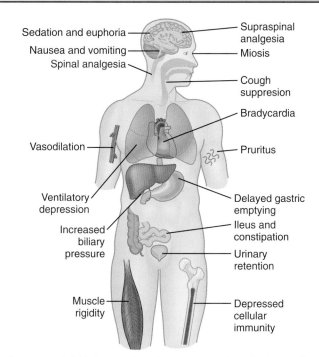

Figure 15-5 Opioid pharmacodynamics. A summary chart of selected effects of the fentanyl congeners (see text).

slowly conducting, unmyelinated C fibers; they are less effective in treating "first pain" sensations (carried by small, myelinated A-δ fibers) and neuropathic pain. A unique aspect of opioid-induced analgesia (in contrast to drugs like local anesthetics) is that other sensory modalities are not affected (e.g., touch, temperature).

Perioperatively (certainly intraoperatively), sedation produced by μ agonists is also one of the targeted effects. The brain is the anatomic substrate for the sedative action of μ agonists. With increasing doses, μ agonists eventually produce drowsiness and sleep (the relief of pain no doubt contributes to the promotion of sleep in uncomfortable patients both preoperatively and postoperatively, independent of the intrinsic sedative effect). With sufficient doses (higher than typically used clinically), the μ agonists produce pronounced δ wave activity on the electroencephalogram which resembles the pattern observed during natural sleep.

The μ agonists produce significant pain relief at doses that do not produce sleep; this is the basis of their clinical utility in the treatment of pain in ambulatory patients. On the other hand, the fact that increasing doses eventually produce drowsiness (and therefore the inability to request additional doses) is the essential scientific foundation for the safety of PCA devices. It is important to emphasize that μ agonists, even when given in very high doses, do not reliably produce unresponsiveness and amnesia; thus, they cannot be viewed as complete anesthetics when used alone.[14]

Suppression of the cough reflex is another important therapeutic effect of the μ agonists in the practice of anesthesia. This antitussive effect is mediated through the cough centers in the medulla. Attenuation of the cough reflex presumably makes coughing and struggling against an indwelling endotracheal tube less likely. This effect is particularly important during fiberoptic intubation of the trachea in an awake patient as an approach to the difficult airway. Curiously, dextrorotatory isomers of opioids (e.g., dextromethorphan) produce this effect even though they do not have analgesic activity. Opioids can sometimes be associated with a paradoxical increase in coughing, typically after a bolus dose is administered. This poorly understood phenomenon is often briefly observed during induction of anesthesia when opioids are used as part of the induction regimen.

ADVERSE EFFECTS

Depression of ventilation is the most significant adverse effect associated with μ agonist drugs. When the airway is secured and ventilation is controlled intraoperatively, opioid induced depression of ventilation is of little consequence. However, in the postoperative period, significant depression of ventilation associated with opioid analgesia can be a life-threatening complication and is a major source of morbidity and mortality, especially in high-risk populations such as obstructive sleep apnea patients.

The main anatomic substrate for depression of ventilation by the μ agonists is the ventilatory control center in the medulla. The μ agonists alter the ventilatory response to arterial carbon dioxide. That depression of ventilation is mediated by the MOR is supported by the observation that μ receptor knockout mice do not exhibit the effect when they receive morphine.[15]

The depression of ventilation is studied by artificially increasing inspired carbon dioxide while maintaining normal oxygen tension.[16] As shown in Figure 15-6, an increase in arterial carbon dioxide partial pressure dramatically increases the minute ventilation. Under the influence of opioid analgesics, the curve is flattened and shifted to the right such that at a given carbon dioxide partial pressure the minute ventilation is lower. More importantly, the "hockey stick" shape of the normal curve is lost such that under the influence of μ

agonists there may be a partial pressure of carbon dioxide below which the patient does not breathe (this point can be thought of as the "apneic threshold"). The μ agonists also depress the hypoxic drive to breathe, although this effect is less important clinically than the effect on carbon dioxide controlled ventilatory drive.[17]

The clinical signs of depressed ventilation are quite subtle with moderate opioid doses. Postoperative patients receiving opioid analgesic therapy can be awake and alert and yet sensitive testing will reveal significantly decreased minute ventilation. Moderate doses of μ agonists produce a decrease in the ventilatory rate (often associated with a slightly increased tidal volume). As the opioid concentration is increased, both ventilatory rate and tidal volume progressively decrease, eventually culminating in an irregular ventilatory rhythm and then complete apnea.

A variety of factors can increase the risk of opioid-induced ventilatory depression (Table 15-3). Clear risk factors include high opioid dose, advanced age, concomitant use of other CNS depressants, and renal insufficiency (for morphine). Natural sleep also appears to increase the ventilatory depressant effect of μ agonists.[18]

Opioids can alter cardiovascular physiology by a variety of mechanisms. Compared to many anesthetic drugs (e.g., propofol, volatile anesthetics), however, the cardiovascular effects of opioids, particularly the fentanyl congeners, are relatively mild (the unique cardiovascular effects of morphine and meperidine are discussed in the later section on individual drugs). In fact, in some clinical circumstances, such as when anesthetizing patients with ischemic heart disease, the cardiovascular effects of the fentanyl congeners can be viewed as therapeutic.

The fentanyl congeners produce a slowing of heart rate by directly increasing vagal nerve tone in the brainstem. In experimental animals this effect can be blocked by microinjection of naloxone into the vagal nerve nucleus or by peripheral vagotomy.[19,20] If the bradycardia is considered undesirable in patients, it can be readily treated with antimuscarinic drugs.

Opioids also produce vasodilation by depressing vasomotor centers in the brainstem (i.e., by decreasing central vasomotor tone) and to a lesser extent by a direct effect on vessels. This action affects both the venous and arterial vasculature, thereby reducing both preload and afterload. The resulting decrease in blood pressure, while typically mild in healthy patients, is much more pronounced in patients with elevated sympathetic tone such as patients with congestive heart failure or hypertension. At typical clinical doses, opioids do not appreciably alter myocardial contractility.

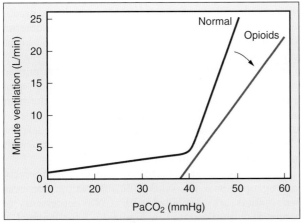

Figure 15-6 Opioid-induced ventilatory depression study methodology. The method characterizes the relationship between $PaCO_2$ and minute volume. The curve labeled "Normal" represents the expected response of minute volume to rising $PaCO_2$ levels in an awake human. Note the dramatic increase in minute volume as CO_2 tension rises. The curve labeled "Opioid" represents the blunted response of minute volume to rising CO_2 levels following administration of an opioid. Note that the slope of the curve decreases and the curve no longer has a "hockey-stick" shape; this means that at physiologic $PaCO_2$ levels, the patient receiving sufficient opioid may be apneic or severely hypoventilatory. (Adapted with permission from Gross JB. When you breathe IN you inspire, when you DON'T breathe, you...expire: new insights regarding opioid-induced ventilatory depression. Anesthesiology. 2003;99:767-770.)

Table 15-3. Factors Increasing the Magnitude and/or Duration of Opioid Induced Ventilatory Depression

High dose
Sleep
Central nervous system depressants
    Inhaled anesthetics, alcohol, barbiturates, benzodiazepines
Hyperventilation, hypocapnia
Respiratory acidosis
Decreased clearance
    Reduction of hepatic blood flow
    Renal insufficiency

Opioid-induced muscle rigidity is another potentially serious adverse effect of this drug class. Typically observed during the rapid administration of high bolus doses of the fentanyl congeners, opioid-induced muscle rigidity can make bag-and-mask ventilation during anesthesia induction impossible; the difficulty with bag-and-mask ventilation appears to be in large part a function of vocal cord rigidity and closure.[21] The rigidity tends to coincide with the onset of unresponsiveness.[22] Although the mechanism of opioid-induced muscle rigidity is unknown, it does not appear to be a direct action on muscle fibers because it can be prevented and treated with neuromuscular blockers.

In the perioperative setting, perhaps one of the most vexing (although not life threatening) adverse effects associated with the μ agonists is nausea and vomiting. Opioids stimulate the chemoreceptor trigger zone in the area postrema on the floor of the fourth ventricle (opioid receptors are expressed here) in the brain. This can lead to nausea and vomiting, an effect that is exacerbated by movement (this is perhaps why ambulatory surgery patients are more likely to be troubled by postoperative nausea and vomiting [PONV]). The use of postoperative opioids is a clear risk factor for the occurrence of PONV.[23] Numerous effective therapies exist for both the prophylaxis and treatment of PONV associated with opioids and other risk factors (see Chapter 29).[24]

Although it is of no clinical consequence in terms of patient safety or suffering, the pupillary constriction induced by μ agonists can be a useful diagnostic sign indicating some ongoing opioid effect. Opioids stimulate the Edinger-Westphal nucleus of the oculomotor nerve to produce miosis. Even small doses of opioid elicit the response and very little tolerance to the effect develops. Thus, miosis is a useful albeit nonspecific indicator of opioid exposure even in opioid tolerant patients. Opioid-induced pupillary constriction is naloxone reversible.

The μ agonists have important effects on gastrointestinal physiology. Opioid receptors are found throughout the enteric plexus of the bowel; their activation causes tonic contraction of gastrointestinal smooth muscle, thereby decreasing coordinated, peristaltic contractions. Clinically, this results in delayed gastric emptying and presumably higher gastric volumes in patients receiving opioid therapy preoperatively. Postoperatively, patients can develop opioid-induced ileus that can potentially delay the resumption of proper nutrition and discharge from the hospital. An extension of this acute problem is the chronic constipation associated with long-term opioid therapy.

Similar effects are observed in the biliary system, which also has an abundance of μ receptors. The μ agonists can produce contraction of the gallbladder smooth muscle and spasm of the sphincter of Oddi, potentially causing a falsely positive cholangiogram during gallbladder and bile duct surgery. These untoward effects are completely naloxone reversible and can be partially reversed by glucagon treatment. The mixed agonist-antagonists (e.g., butorphanol) appear to produce less pronounced biliary effects.[25]

In contrast to the gastrointestinal system, the urologic effects of opioids are regarded as minimal. Opioids can cause urinary retention by decreasing bladder detrusor tone and by increasing the tone of the urinary sphincter. These effects are at least in part centrally mediated, although peripheral effects are also likely given the widespread presence of opioid receptors in the genitourinary tract.[26,27] Although the urinary retention associated with opioid therapy is not typically pronounced, it can be troublesome in males, particularly when the opioid is administered intrathecally or epidurally.

The euphoria produced by μ agonists must be viewed as an adverse effect because it is the primary reason that this drug class is so widely abused. Opioid addicts experience a euphoria that drives a drug-seeking lifestyle that often ends tragically in death or incarceration. The physical tolerance and dependence that inevitably develop in chronic users result in an increased dose requirement and a withdrawal syndrome upon cessation of drug intake. The withdrawal syndrome is characterized by intense drug craving, restlessness, body aches and pains, runny nose, lacrimation, and perspiration. An acute withdrawal syndrome can be precipitated by the administration of opioid antagonists (e.g., naloxone) during routine clinical care to patients who are not openly known to be opioid addicts.

Although perhaps not typically thought of as an acute effect that would be relevant to perioperative practice, opioids are known to depress cellular immunity. This effect is particularly well documented for morphine, although data exist for other μ agonists as well. Morphine and the endogenous opioid β-endorphin, for example, inhibit the transcription of interleukin-2 in activated T cells, among other immunologic effects.[28] It appears that individual opioids (and perhaps classes of opioids) differ in terms of the exact nature and extent of their immunomodulatory effects. The clinical implications of opioid-induced impairment of cellular immunity are not well understood, but these effects might influence wound healing, perioperative infection risk, and cancer recurrence, among other outcomes. How this rapidly expanding knowledge will eventually impact clinical practice is evolving.

DRUG INTERACTIONS

Drug interactions can be based on two mechanisms: pharmacokinetic (i.e., wherein one drug influences the concentration of the other) or pharmacodynamic (i.e., wherein one drug influences the effect of the other). In anesthesia practice, while unintended pharmacokinetic interactions sometimes occur, pharmacodynamic interactions occur with virtually every anesthetic and are produced by design.

The most common pharmacokinetic interaction in opioid clinical pharmacology is observed when intravenous opioids are combined with propofol. Perhaps because of the hemodynamic changes induced by propofol and their impact on pharmacokinetic processes, opioid concentrations are expected to be modestly higher when given in combination with a continuous propofol infusion.[29]

The most important pharmacodynamic drug interaction involving opioids is the synergistic interaction that occurs when opioids are combined with CNS depressants (see Chapter 5).[30] As illustrated in Figure 15-7 for fentanyl and isoflurane, opioids dramatically reduce the minimum alveolar concentration (MAC) of a volatile anesthetic. Careful examination of "opioid-MAC reduction" data such as in Figure 15-7 reveals several clinically critical concepts. First, opioids synergistically reduce MAC. Second, the MAC reduction is substantial (depending on the dose, as much as 75% or more). Third, most of the MAC reduction occurs at moderate opioid levels (i.e., even modest opioid doses substantially reduce MAC). Fourth, the MAC reduction is not complete; that is, opioids are not complete anesthetics. The addition of the

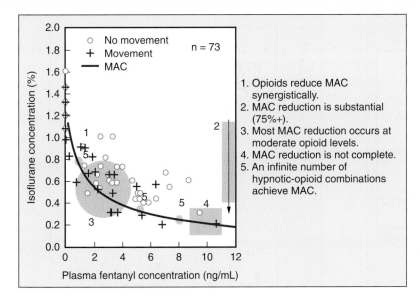

Figure 15-7 Volatile anesthetic minimum alveolar concentration (MAC) reduction by opioids: the prototype example of isoflurane and fentanyl. The solid curve is MAC; the dotted curves are the 95% confidence intervals (see text). *(Adapted with permission from McEwan AI, Smith C, Dyar O, et al. Isoflurane minimum alveolar concentration reduction by fentanyl. Anesthesiology. 1993;78:864-869.)*

opioid cannot completely eliminate the need for the other anesthetic. And fifth, there are an infinite number of hypnotic-opioid combinations that will achieve MAC (this implies that clinicians must choose the optimal combination based on the goals of the anesthetic and operation). As one might expect based on first principles, the synergistic interaction applies to both therapeutic and adverse effects such as depression of ventilation and hemodynamic variables.[31]

Because general anesthesia in the modern era is at least a two drug process consisting of a sedative and an opioid, these MAC reduction concepts form an important part of the scientific foundation of anesthesia clinical pharmacology. All of these concepts also apply when opioids are used in combination with propofol for total intravenous anesthesia (TIVA).[32] Recent work has advanced the understanding of opioid-sedative pharmacodynamic interactions by applying response surface analysis methods.[33] This approach enables the investigator to identify optimal target concentrations of the sedative and the opioid through simulation (see Chapters 2 and 5).

SPECIAL POPULATIONS
Hepatic Failure
Perhaps surprisingly, even though the liver is the metabolic organ primarily responsible for the biotransformation of most opioids, the degree of liver failure typically encountered in perioperative patients is usually not severe enough to have a major impact on opioid pharmacokinetics. The anhepatic phase of orthotopic liver transplantation is a notable exception to this general rule. With ongoing drug administration, concentrations of opioids that rely on hepatic metabolism are expected to rise significantly when the patient has no liver. Even after partial liver resection, a decrease in the ratio of morphine glucuronides to morphine is observed, indicating a decrease in the rate of morphine metabolism.[34] Because remifentanil's metabolism is completely unrelated to hepatic clearance mechanisms, its disposition is not affected during liver transplantation.[35]

Pharmacodynamic considerations can be important for opioid therapy in patients with severe liver disease. Patients with ongoing hepatic encephalopathy are thought to be particularly vulnerable to the sedative effects of opioids and thus this drug class must be used with caution in these patients.

Kidney Failure
Renal failure has implications of major clinical importance with respect to morphine and meperidine (see later section on individual drugs). For the fentanyl congeners, the clinical importance of kidney failure is much less marked, but nonetheless measurable. As with hepatic failure, remifentanil is also an exceptional case with respect to renal failure. Remifentanil's metabolism is not impacted by kidney disease (although the inactive acid metabolite does accumulate in such patients).[36]

Morphine is principally metabolized by conjugation in the liver; the resulting water-soluble glucuronides (i.e., morphine 3-glucuronide and morphine 6-glucuronide: M3G and M6G) are excreted via the kidney. The kidney also plays a role in the conjugation of morphine and may account for as much as half of its conversion to M3G and M6G.

M3G is inactive, but M6G is an analgesic with a potency rivaling morphine. Very high levels of M6G and life-threatening respiratory depression can develop in patients with renal failure as illustrated in Figure 15-8.[37] In view of these pharmacokinetic changes induced by renal failure, morphine may not be a good choice in patients with severely altered renal clearance mechanisms.

The clinical pharmacology of meperidine is also significantly altered by renal failure. Normeperidine, the main metabolite, has analgesic and excitatory CNS effects that range from anxiety and tremulousness to myoclonus and frank seizures. Because the active metabolites are subject to renal excretion, CNS toxicity secondary to accumulation of normeperidine is especially a concern in patients with renal failure. This shortcoming of meperidine has caused many hospital formularies to restrict its use or to remove it from the formulary altogether.

Gender
Recent data suggest that gender may have an important influence on opioid pharmacology. There is evidence, for example, that morphine is more potent in women than in men (i.e., that

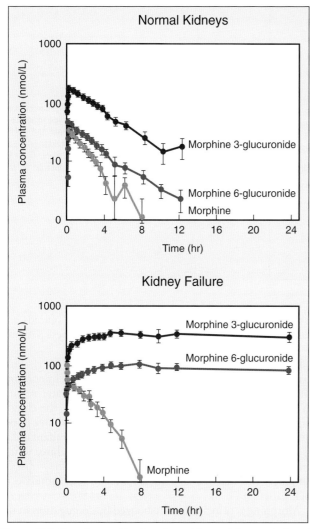

Figure 15-8 The pharmacokinetics of morphine and its metabolites in normal volunteers versus kidney failure patients. Note the significant accumulation of the metabolites in renal failure. *(Adapted with permission from Osborne R, Joel S, Grebenik K, et al. The pharmacokinetics of morphine and morphine glucuronides in kidney failure. Clin Pharmacol Ther. 1993;54: 158-167.)*

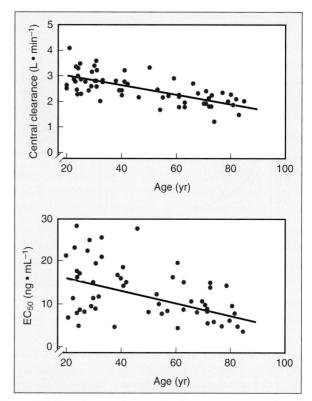

Figure 15-9 The influence of age on the clinical pharmacology of remifentanil. Although there is considerable variability, in general, older subjects have a lower central clearance and a higher potency (lower EC_{50}). EC_{50}, Effective concentration for 50% of maximal effect. *(Adapted with permission from Minto CF, Schnider TW, Egan TD, et al. Influence of age and gender on the pharmacokinetics and pharmacodynamics of remifentanil. I. Model development. Anesthesiology. 1997;86:10-23.)*

a lower concentration is required to produce comparable analgesia) and that it has a slower onset of action in women.[38] Although this information is clearly incomplete and emerging, some of these differences appear to be related to cyclic gonadal hormones.

Age

Advancing age is clearly an important factor influencing the clinical pharmacology of opioids. As shown in Figure 15-9, kinetic-dynamic model building studies in volunteers using the processed electroencephalogram as a surrogate measure of opioid effect have reproducibly shown that the fentanyl congeners are more potent in older patients.[39,40] Pharmacokinetic differences have also been described, including decreases in clearance and central distribution volume in older patients.

Although pharmacokinetic changes also play a role, pharmacodynamic differences are primarily responsible for the

decreased dose requirement in older patients (e.g., older than 65 years of age). These combined pharmacokinetic and pharmacodynamic changes mandate a reduction in remifentanil dosage by at least 50% or more in seniors. Similar dosage reductions are also prudent for other μ agonists.

Obesity

Although detailed information is unavailable for many commonly used opioids, evidence from the study of drugs introduced more recently suggests that body weight is an important factor influencing the clinical pharmacology of opioids. Opioid pharmacokinetic parameters, especially clearance, are more closely related to lean body mass than to total body weight. In practical terms, this means that morbidly obese patients do indeed require a higher dosage than lean patients in order to achieve the same target concentration, but the very obese patients do not need nearly as much as would be suggested by their total body weight.[41]

For example, as illustrated in the pharmacokinetic simulation shown in Figure 15-10, a total body weight (TBW) based dosing scheme in an obese patient results in excessive remifentanil effect-site concentrations compared to dosing calculation based on lean body mass (LBM).[42] In contrast, for lean patients, the concentrations that result from TBW based dosing regimens are not much greater than those based on lean body mass. It is likely that these concepts apply to other drugs as well.

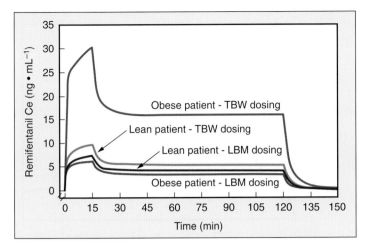

Figure 15-10 A pharmacokinetic simulation illustrating the consequences of calculating the remifentanil dosage based on total body weight (TBW) or lean body mass (LBM) in obese and lean patients (1 µg/kg bolus injection followed by an infusion of 0.5 µg/kg/min for 15 min and 0.25 µg/kg/min for an additional 105 min). Note that TBW-based dosing in an obese patient results in dramatically higher concentrations. Ce, Effect site concentration. (Adapted with permission from Egan TD, Huizinga B, Gupta SK, et al. Remifentanil pharmacokinetics in obese versus lean patients. Anesthesiology. 1998;89:562-573.)

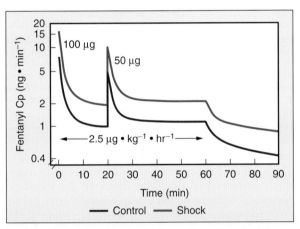

Figure 15-11 A pharmacokinetic simulation illustrating the influence of severe hemorrhagic shock on the disposition of fentanyl. Animals in shock achieve substantially higher blood concentration when receiving the same fentanyl dose. Cp, Plasma concentration. (Adapted with permission from Egan TD, Kuramkote S, Gong G, et al. Fentanyl pharmacokinetics in hemorrhagic shock: a porcine model. Anesthesiology. 1999;91:156-166.)

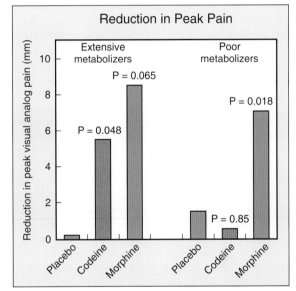

Figure 15-12 A volunteer study demonstrating that codeine is no more effective than placebo in patients who cannot convert codeine to morphine (i.e., poor metabolizers). Morphine retains its normal analgesic efficacy in such patients. Both codeine and morphine are effective in normal subjects (i.e., extensive metabolizers). The bars represent the median of the maximal reduction in peak pain as assessed by the cold pressor test using a visual analog scale. (Adapted with permission from Poulsen L, Brosen K, Arendt-Nielsen L, et al. Codeine and morphine in extensive and poor metabolizers of sparteine: pharmacokinetics, analgesic effect and side effects. Eur J Clin Pharmacol. 1996;51:289-295.)

Hemorrhagic

Although the data are from animal studies, it is clear that severe hemorrhage significantly alters the pharmacokinetic behavior of opioids. Both the clearance and distribution parameters are affected. As shown in the pharmacokinetic simulation presented in Figure 15-11, subjects experiencing severe hemorrhage can be expected to achieve blood concentrations that are approximately double those observed in control subjects when they receive identical doses.[43] Even a drug that does not require delivery to a metabolic organ like remifentanil is affected, although the effect is not as dramatic.[44] There is clear evidence from case reports that these observations apply to human pharmacology as well.[45]

UNIQUE FEATURES OF INDIVIDUAL AGENTS
Codeine
Codeine, while not commonly used intraoperatively, has special importance among opioids because of a well-characterized pharmacogenomic nuance associated with it. Codeine is actually a prodrug that is metabolized in part by O-demethylation into morphine, a metabolic process

mediated by the liver P450 isoform CYP2D6.[46] As demonstrated in Figure 15-12, patients who lack CYP2D6 because of deletion, frame shift, or splice mutations (approximately 10% of the Caucasian population) or whose CYP2D6 is inhibited (e.g., patients taking quinidine) do not respond normally to codeine even though they exhibit a normal response to morphine.[47,48]

Interestingly, Asians have less CYP2D6 activity and thus may be an ethnic group that are particularly resistant to codeine therapy.[49] Conversely, certain ethnic groups (e.g., Ethiopians) carry frequently duplicated, functional CYP2D6 genes, resulting in the ultra rapid conversion of codeine to morphine, and are thought to be particularly susceptible to the effects of codeine.[50] This gene duplication has recently been implicated in fatalities among infants breastfed by mothers who are ultrarapid metabolizers.[51]

Morphine

Morphine is the prototype opioid against which all newcomers are evaluated. Despite a century of opioid research, there is no evidence that any synthetic opioid is more effective in controlling pain than nature's morphine. Were it not for the histamine release mediated hypotension observed intraoperatively with high doses of morphine, it is conceivable that fentanyl would not have replaced morphine as the most commonly used opioid in anesthesia practice.

An important detail relating to morphine's clinical pharmacology is its slow onset time. Morphine's pKa renders it almost completely ionized at physiologic pH. This property, combined with its low lipid solubility, presumably accounts for morphine's prolonged latency-to-peak effect; morphine penetrates the CNS slowly. This feature has both advantages and disadvantages. The prolonged latency-to-peak effect (see Figure 15-4, A) means that morphine is less likely to cause acute respiratory depression after bolus injection of typical analgesic doses compared to the more rapid acting drugs because the relationship between minute ventilation and the partial pressure of carbon dioxide changes more slowly (thus there is more time for carbon dioxide to rise and sustain ventilatory drive). On the other hand, the slow onset time means that clinicians are more likely to inappropriately "stack" multiple morphine doses in a patient experiencing severe pain, thus creating the potential for a toxic "overshoot."[52]

Morphine's active metabolite, M6G, also has very important clinical implications. Although conversion to M6G accounts for only 10% of morphine's metabolism, M6G contributes to morphine's analgesic effects even in patients with normal renal function, particularly with longer term use. Because of morphine's high hepatic extraction ratio, the bioavailability of orally administered morphine is significantly lower than after parenteral injection. The hepatic first pass effect on orally administered morphine results in high M6G levels; in fact, it appears that M6G may be the primary active compound when morphine is administered orally.[53] Accumulation of M6G to potentially toxic levels in dialysis patients is another important implication of this active metabolite.

Methadone

Available in both intravenous and oral forms, racemic methadone has long been a mainstay in the treatment of opioid addicts because its long acting pharmacokinetic profile makes the development of an acute withdrawal syndrome less likely (i.e., methadone maintenance therapy). The N-methyl-D-aspartate (NMDA) receptor antagonism action of the dextrorotatory isomer of methadone may also serve to attenuate the effects of opioid tolerance and withdrawal syndrome.[54,55]

Methadone is also increasingly used in the treatment of chronic pain patients, particularly cancer-related pain.[56] Methadone's propensity to prolong the QT interval of the electrocardiogram by blocking the delayed rectifier potassium ion channel (IKr) may contribute to increased mortality in this patient population.[57]

Fentanyl

As the original fentanyl congener, its clinical application is well entrenched and highly diverse. Perhaps the most unique

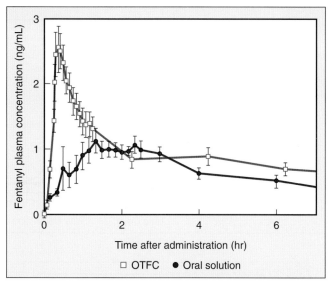

Figure 15-13 A volunteer study contrasting the bioavailability and peak plasma concentrations of an identical dose (15 μg/kg) of fentanyl delivered either orally or through the oral mucosa (i.e., oral transmucosal fentanyl [OTFC]). Note that the transmucosal approach yields higher peak concentrations earlier. *(Adapted with permission from Streisand JB, Varvel JR, Stanski DR, et al. Absorption and bioavailability of oral transmucosal fentanyl citrate. Anesthesiology. 1991;75:223-229.)*

aspect of fentanyl's clinical application is the numerous ways in which fentanyl is delivered. In addition to the intravenous method, fentanyl has also been delivered by transdermal, transmucosal, transnasal, and transpulmonary routes.

Oral transmucosal delivery of fentanyl citrate (OTFC) results in the faster achievement of higher peak levels than when the same dose is swallowed as seen in Figure 15-13.[58] It is the avoidance of the first pass effect through transmucosal absorption that results in this significantly greater bioavailability. That OTFC is noninvasive and rapid in onset has made it a successful therapy for breakthrough pain in opioid tolerant cancer patients, often in combination with a transdermal fentanyl patch.

Alfentanil

Alfentanil was the first opioid to be administered almost exclusively by continuous infusion. Because of its relatively short terminal half-life, alfentanil was originally thought to be an opioid with a rapid offset of effect after termination of a continuous infusion.[59] Subsequent advances in pharmacokinetic theory (i.e., the CSHT) proved this assertion to be false.[11] However, alfentanil is in fact a short-acting drug after a single bolus injection because of its high diffusible fraction; it reaches peak effect site concentrations quickly and then begins to decline (see Pharmacokinetics and Figure 15-4). Alfentanil illustrates how a drug can exhibit different pharmacokinetic profiles depending upon the method of administration (i.e., bolus versus continuous infusion). Relative to fentanyl and sufentanil, hepatic metabolism of alfentanil is more unpredictable because of the significant interindividual variability of hepatic CYP3A4, the primary enzyme responsible for alfentanil biotransformation. Because alfentanil has a relatively low hepatic extraction ratio compared to fentanyl, it is more vulnerable to variations in CYP3A4 activity.[60]

Sufentanil

Sufentanil's distinguishing feature is that it is the most potent opioid commonly used in anesthesia practice. Because it is more intrinsically efficacious at the opioid receptor, the absolute doses used are much smaller compared to other less potent drugs (1000-fold less than morphine).

Remifentanil

Remifentanil is a prototype example of how specific clinical goals can be achieved by designing molecules with specialized structure-activity (or structure-metabolism) relationships. As shown in Figure 15-14, the medicinal chemists responsible for the development of remifentanil sought to produce a potent opioid that would lose its μ receptor agonist activity upon ester hydrolysis, thereby creating an intravenous opioid with a very short-acting pharmacokinetic profile.[61] The perceived unmet need driving remifentanil's development was that the practice of anesthesia requires a degree of pharmacokinetic responsiveness unnecessary in most medical disciplines and that anesthetics (opioids included) therefore ought to be short-acting so that they can be titrated during the rapidly changing conditions of anesthesia and surgery.

Compared to the currently marketed fentanyl congeners, remifentanil's context sensitive half-time is short, on the order of about 5 minutes (see Figure 15-4, C).[62] Pharmacodynamically, remifentanil exhibits a short latency-to-peak effect similar to alfentanil and a potency slightly less than fentanyl (see Figure 15-4, A).[63]

Remifentanil's role in modern anesthesia practice is now relatively well established; its unique pharmacokinetic profile makes it possible to manipulate rapidly the degree of opioid effect in a way that could not be achieved with the previously

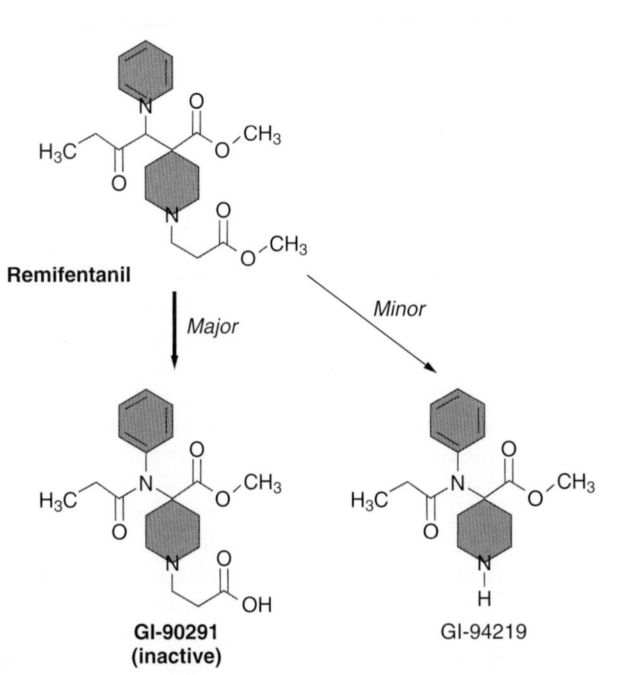

Figure 15-14 Remifentanil metabolic pathway. De-esterification (i.e., ester hydrolysis) by non-specific plasma and tissue esterases to an inactive acid metabolite (GI-90291) accounts for the vast majority of remifentanil's metabolism. *(Adapted with permission from Egan TD, Lemmens HJ, Fiset P, et al. The pharmacokinetics of the new short-acting opioid remifentanil (GI87084B) in healthy adult male volunteers. Anesthesiology. 1993;79: 881-892.)*

marketed fentanyl congeners. Remifentanil is therefore perhaps best suited for cases where its responsive pharmacokinetic profile can be exploited to advantage (e.g., when rapid recovery is desirable, when the anesthetic requirement rapidly fluctuates, when opioid titration is unpredictable or difficult, when there is a substantial danger to opioid overdose, or when a "high dose" opioid technique is advantageous but the patient is not going to be mechanically ventilated postoperatively).[64] Today, remifentanil's most common clinical application is the provision of TIVA in combination with propofol. It is also commonly used by bolus injection when a brief pulse of opioid effect followed by rapid recovery is advantageous (e.g., in preparation for local anesthetic injection during monitored anesthesia care).

Naloxone (and Others)

Although it is an opioid antagonist, naloxone and related drugs are classified as opioids because they bind to the opioid receptor. Naloxone, a derivative of oxymorphone, is a competitive antagonist of all opioid receptor types, but its greatest affinity is for the μ receptor. When administered in typical doses in the absence of ongoing opioid therapy (or abuse), naloxone has no discernible pharmacodynamic effects. When opioid effects are present, naloxone given in sufficient doses can reverse all effects mediated by opioid receptors.

The most common clinical use of naloxone perioperatively is the reversal of excessive opioid induced ventilatory depression.[65] Other uses include the emergency reversal of ventilatory depression in neonates whose mothers received opioids for labor analgesia and in cases of accidental or intended opioid overdose (e.g., heroin) in the emergency department.

A few nuances of naloxone's clinical pharmacology are extremely important for safe use. Naloxone is rapidly metabolized in the liver and has a very high clearance; thus, its duration of action is nearly always shorter than that of the opioid whose effects it is intended to reverse. Patients who receive naloxone for the emergency reversal of life threatening ventilatory depression must be monitored for recurrence of the opioid effects. Also, rarely, naloxone administration has been complicated by severe adverse hemodynamic effects including pulmonary edema and even sudden death in previously healthy individuals (some tachycardia is to be expected).[66]

Several drugs closely related to naloxone have been developed for other purposes. The long-acting opioid antagonists naltrexone and nalmefene were developed for the maintenance treatment of previously detoxified opioid addicts. Methylnaltrexone and alvimopan, permanently charged opioid antagonists that do not easily enter the CNS, were developed for the prevention and treatment of opioid induced bowel dysfunction (see later).

Nalbuphine (and Others)

Like the complete antagonists, strictly speaking the "mixed" agonist-antagonist drugs are also considered opioids because they bind to the opioid receptor. This group of synthetic and semisynthetic opioids includes nalbuphine, pentazocine, and butorphanol; these drugs are partial agonists at the κ receptor and complete, competitive antagonists at the μ receptor. Both the analgesic and ventilatory depressant effects of these drugs exhibit a ceiling effect when compared to morphine and they do not reduce MAC as powerfully as morphine or fentanyl.[67,68]

As a class, these opioid agonist-antagonists (or "partial agonists") were developed with the hope that they would be effective analgesics but less subject to diversion and abuse. These drugs are indeed efficacious in the treatment of mild to moderate pain (and they do have less abuse potential), but the analgesic ceiling effect has limited their more widespread use. Perhaps their most common perioperative use is the reversal of excessive opioid induced ventilatory depression (μ antagonism) while maintaining some analgesic effect (partial κ agonism). As μ antagonists, these drugs will of course precipitate a withdrawal syndrome in opioid dependent patients and are thus sometimes used in the maintenance treatment of opioid addicts.[69] Buprenorphine is a related drug that is an antagonist at the κ receptor but a partial agonist at the μ receptor.

CLINICAL APPLICATION

Opioids play a vital role in virtually every area of anesthesia practice. In the treatment of postoperative pain, opioids are the primary therapeutic agent, whereas in most other settings in perioperative medicine, opioids are therapeutic adjuncts used in combination with other drugs.

Common Clinical Indications

Postoperative analgesia is the longest standing indication for opioid therapy in anesthesia practice and of course dates back to the earliest days of the specialty. In the modern era, opioid administration via PCA devices is perhaps the most common mode of delivery. In recent years, opioids are increasingly combined postoperatively with various other agents such as nonsteroidal anti-inflammatory drugs (NSAIDs) to increase efficacy and safety (see Chapter 16).

Internationally, the most common clinical indication for opioids in anesthesia practice is their use as part of what came to be known as "balanced anesthesia." The term connotes the use of multiple agents (e.g., inhalation agents, neuromuscular blockers, and opioids) in smaller doses to produce the state of anesthesia. With this technique, the opioids are primarily used for their MAC reduction effects. A basic assumption underlying this balanced anesthesia approach is that the drugs used in combination mitigate the disadvantages of the individual drugs (i.e., the inhaled agents) used in higher doses as monotherapy.

"High dose opioid anesthesia," a technique originally described for morphine in the early days of open heart surgery and later associated with the fentanyl congeners, is another common application of opioids.[70,71] The original scientific underpinning of this approach was that high doses of opioids enabled the clinician to reduce the volatile agent to a minimum, thereby avoiding the direct myocardial depression and other untoward hemodynamic effects associated with high concentrations of volatile anesthetics in patients whose cardiovascular systems were already compromised. That the fentanyl drugs often produce a relative bradycardia is also thought to be helpful in mitigating against myocardial ischemia. Currently, while the general concept is still applied, the opioid doses used today are more moderate. In this setting, opioids are also administered for their possible beneficial effects in terms of cardioprotection (i.e., preconditioning).

Total intravenous anesthesia (TIVA) is a more recently developed and increasingly popular indication for opioids in anesthesia practice. As the name implies, this technique relies entirely upon intravenous agents for the provision of general anesthesia. Most commonly, continuous infusions of remifentanil or alfentanil are combined with a propofol infusion. Both the opioid and the sedative are often delivered by TCI enabled pumps. A clear advantage of this technique, perhaps among others, is the enhanced patient well being in the early postoperative period, including less nausea and vomiting and often a feeling of euphoria.[72]

Rational Drug Selection and Administration

In articulating a scientific foundation for rational opioid selection, it is most important to recognize that pharmacokinetic considerations are paramount. Indeed, the μ agonists can be considered pharmacodynamic equals with important pharmacokinetic differences.[73] In other words, for practical purposes all μ agonists are essentially equally efficacious when equipotent concentrations are achieved, but they differ in terms of their pharmacokinetic behavior. Thus, rational selection of one μ agonist over another requires the clinician to identify the desired temporal profile of drug effect and then choose an opioid that best achieves it (within constraints such as pharmacoeconomic concerns).

In selecting the appropriate opioid, among the key questions to address are: How quickly must the desired opioid effect be achieved? How long must the opioid effect be maintained? How critical is it that opioid-induced ventilatory depression or sedation dissipate quickly (e.g., will the patient be mechanically ventilated postoperatively)? Is the capability to raise and lower the level of opioid effect quickly during the anesthetic critical? Will there be significant pain postoperatively that will require opioid treatment? All of these questions relate to the optimal temporal profile of opioid effect. The answers to these questions are addressed through the application of pharmacokinetic concepts.

For example, when a brief pulse of opioid effect followed by rapid recovery is desired (e.g., to provide analgesia for a retrobulbar block), a bolus of remifentanil or alfentanil might be preferred. When long-lasting opioid effect is desired, such as when there will be significant postoperative pain or when the patient's trachea will remain intubated, a fentanyl infusion is a prudent choice. In cases where it is critical that the patient be awake and alert shortly after the procedure is finished (e.g., a craniotomy in which the surgeons hope to perform a neurologic exam in the operating room immediately postoperatively), a remifentanil infusion might be advantageous.

The formulation of a rational administration strategy also requires the proper application of pharmacokinetic principles. An important goal of any dosing scheme is to reach and maintain a steady state level of opioid effect. In order to achieve a steady-state concentration in the site of action, opioids are frequently administered by continuous infusion. This is increasingly accomplished through the use of target controlled infusion technology (see later), which requires familiarity with the appropriate pharmacokinetic model for the opioid of interest. When these systems are not available, the clinician must remember that infusions must be preceded by a bolus in order to come to a near steady-state in a timely fashion.

EMERGING DEVELOPMENTS

Opioids and Cancer Recurrence

Recently, concerns have been raised that opioids administered as part of a general anesthetic for cancer surgery may have an adverse impact on cancer recurrence rates. This concern is supported by considerable *in vitro* and animal data demonstrating immunosuppressive and angiogenic effects of opioids (particularly morphine). Retrospective human studies also provide some support for the hypothesis that opioid administration perioperatively may increase the risk of cancer recurrence. For example, a retrospective study found higher prostate cancer recurrence rates in patients who received standard postoperative opioid analgesia *versus* patients who received postoperative epidural analgesia (Figure 15-15).[74]

Surgical treatment often represents the best chance for curing cancer, but an operation is presumably associated with systemic release of tumor cells. Moreover, it is assumed that micrometastatic disease often exists despite surgery. The body's natural anticancer defenses, in combination with adjunctive chemotherapy or radiation therapy, are relied upon to prevent the residual microscopic disease from proliferating into a frank cancer recurrence. In addition to opioid analgesia, the stress response to surgery and an independent effect of general anesthesia might also contribute to the impairment of cellular immunity that is thought to be responsible for the increased cancer recurrence risk. If this hypothesis is confirmed through prospective trials, it would presumably have a major impact on the anesthesia techniques applied to cancer surgery patients, including a more prominent role for regional postoperative analgesia techniques to reduce the overall opioid load. At this stage, this hypothesis is unproven and the data must be interpreted with caution until more definitive information is available.[75]

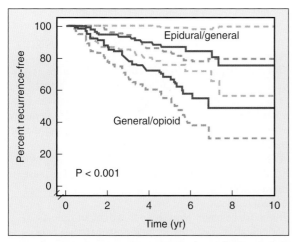

Figure 15-15 Kaplan-Meier recurrence-free survival estimates for patients given general anesthesia and postoperative opioids (general-opioid) and for patients given general anesthesia combined with epidural analgesia (epidural-general) during radical prostatectomy for prostate cancer; univariable *P* < .001. Vertical tick marks represent censored values. Blue dashed lines show 95% confidence intervals for the epidural-general group; brown dashed lines show 95% confidence intervals for the general-opioid group. *(Adapted with permission from Biki B, Mascha E, Moriarty DC, et al. Anesthetic technique for radical prostatectomy surgery affects cancer recurrence: a retrospective analysis.* Anesthesiology. *2008;109:180-187.)*

Computerized Delivery Methods

Advances in pharmacologic modeling and infusion pump technology have now made it possible to administer injectable anesthetics via a computer controlled infusion pump.[76] By coding a pharmacokinetic model into a computer program and linking it to an electronic pump modified to accept computerized commands, delivery according to a drug's specific pharmacokinetic parameters can be achieved. The physician operating a target-controlled infusion (TCI) system designates a target concentration to achieve rather than specifying an infusion rate. The TCI system then calculates the necessary infusion rates to achieve the targeted concentration. The system changes the infusion rates at frequent intervals (i.e., as often as every 10 seconds). Successful use of a TCI pump thus requires knowledge of the therapeutic concentrations appropriate for the specific clinical application.

Computer-controlled drug delivery in the operating room is an exciting area with well established clinical utility, although it is admittedly difficult to demonstrate obvious outcome improvements when compared to traditional delivery methods. TCI administration of opioids is common for all of the fentanyl congeners. Although TCI systems are widely used in North America for research purposes, they are not yet commercially available for routine clinical use (unlike much of the rest of the world).[77]

Opioid Antagonists for Ileus and Constipation Therapy

An important development in the treatment of opioid-induced adverse effects is the use of μ receptor antagonists to treat opioid induced postoperative ileus and constipation.[78,79] Methylnaltrexone and alvimopan are μ receptor antagonists whose physicochemical properties prevent them from crossing the blood-brain-barrier in appreciable amounts. These drugs thus block the μ receptors in the gut without antagonizing the therapeutic μ agonist effects that are mediated in the CNS. Controlled, randomized trials have demonstrated their efficacy in the prevention and treatment of postoperative ileus and the constipation associated with chronic opioid use.

Opioid-Induced Hyperalgesia and Acute Tolerance

It is well known that long-term exposure to opioids produces tolerance to opioid effects; huge opioid doses may be needed to provide adequate perioperative analgesia in patients receiving chronic, high dose opioid therapy.[80] However, recent evidence suggests that even brief exposure to opioids may result in an increased dose requirement.

Acute tolerance and opioid-induced-hyperalgesia are pharmacologically distinct phenomena that can both result in the need for a dose escalation to maintain adequate analgesia. In general pharmacologic terms, tolerance is a decrease in the response to a drug due to its continued administration. Hyperalgesia, in contrast, is an increased response to a stimulus that is normally painful.[81]

Considered in terms of the dose-response relationship, opioid tolerance shifts the curve to the right, whereas opioid-induced-hyperalgesia shifts the curve downward because of a change in pain sensitivity (Figure 15-16).[82] Both phenomena manifest clinically as a need for a higher dose to achieve the

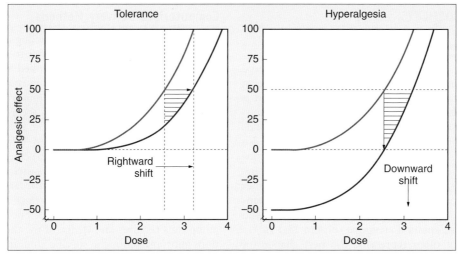

Figure 15-16 Tolerance versus opioid-induced-hyperalgesia in terms of the dose-effect relationship changes. Tolerance shifts the dose-response curve to the right (but does not alter pain sensitivity). Opioid-induced-hyperalgesia shifts the dose-response curve downward because of increased pain sensitivity. The stripped area represents the net increase in dose required to achieve 50% of the maximal analgesic effect. *(Adapted with permission from Chu LF, Angst MS, Clark D. Opioid-induced hyperalgesia in humans: molecular mechanisms and clinical considerations.* Clin J Pain. *2008;24:479-496.)*

same analgesic effect. Distinguishing between the two can be therapeutically important because tolerance calls for an increased dosage whereas opioid-induced-hyperalgesia may be more prudently addressed with non-opioid analgesics and other adjuncts, because opioids exacerbate the problem.

Whether acute tolerance and opioid-induced-hyperalgesia play important roles in the management of perioperative patients is controversial.[81] While numerous animal studies have demonstrated the occurrence of opioid-induced hyperalgesia, the data in humans are more ambiguous.[83-87] Current thinking suggests that both phenomena may coexist to some degree in certain perioperative settings.[81] Risk factors for their occurrence include high opioid dose, prolonged use, and perhaps inhalation anesthesia (i.e., propofol may mitigate risk).[88,89] There is increasing evidence that NMDA receptor antagonism mediated through drugs like ketamine may also mitigate the severity of opioid-induced-hyperalgesia.[90]

The mechanism of opioid-induced-hyperalgesia is unknown. It likely involves both central and peripheral nervous system adaptation including processes involving the NMDA receptor.[82] It is clear that endogenous opioid systems do not play a role in its pathogenesis.[91]

KEY POINTS

- Most of the clinically useful opioids are chemical modifications of morphine (e.g., hydromorphone, codeine, oxycodone) or meperidine (e.g., the fentanyl family of opioids).
- Opioids produce their primary effects by interacting with opioid receptors. Existing in three distinct types (i.e., μ, κ, and δ), these receptors are coupled with G-proteins that, when activated by drugs or endogenous ligands (e.g., β-endorphins), produce inhibitory effects that hyperpolarize the cell and thereby attenuate nociceptive impulses.
- For certain opioids, the metabolic pathway has very important clinical implications. M6G and normeperidine

are active metabolites that accumulate in renal failure, potentially causing toxicity. Remifentanil's high clearance because of esterase metabolism results in an extremely short duration of action.
- Opioids can be differentiated pharmacokinetically by their latency-to-peak effect after bolus administration, the time required to reach a steady-state after beginning an infusion, and the time required to achieve a specified level of drug concentration decline after stopping a continuous infusion (i.e., CSHT).
- Pharmacodynamically, the primary therapeutic effects for the perioperative use of opioids are analgesia and sedation. The most dangerous adverse effect in non-ventilated patients is depression of ventilation. Other opioid effects can be observed in virtually every organ system, in part because of the wide distribution of opioid receptors.
- The most important drug interaction for opioids is the synergism for both therapeutic and adverse effects that results when opioids are combined with sedatives (e.g., volatile anesthetics and propofol). These "MAC-reducing" effects are a fundamental concept underpinning modern anesthesia.
- When treating certain special populations (e.g., older adults, patients with severe hepatic or renal disease, morbid obesity, severe bleeding), significant dosage adjustments are necessary.
- The most common clinical applications of opioids in perioperative medicine include postoperative pain therapy, "balanced anesthesia," and total intravenous anesthesia.
- The rational selection of opioids for perioperative use focuses on pharmacokinetic considerations. The commonly used perioperative opioids can be considered pharmacodynamic equals with important pharmacokinetic differences (e.g., differences relating to the onset and offset of effect).

- The influence of perioperative opioid use on cancer recurrence after oncologic operations, target controlled opioid delivery via computerized pumps, the treatment and prevention of opioid induced ileus and constipation with poorly absorbable opioid antagonists, and the phenomena of acute tolerance and opioid-induced hyperalgesia are among the most important emerging developments in opioid pharmacology.

Key References

Egan TD, Lemmens HJ, Fiset P, et al. The pharmacokinetics of the new short-acting opioid remifentanil (GI87084B) in healthy adult male volunteers. *Anesthesiology*. 1993;79:881-892. This human volunteer study first described the unique pharmacokinetic profile of remifentanil, the esterase metabolized fentanyl congener that became the first true "ultra-short acting" opioid. In combination with propofol, remifentanil revolutionized the practice of TIVA and has become a mainstay of modern anesthesia practice, particularly in regions where intravenous anesthesia techniques are popular. (Ref. 62)

Matthes HW, Maldonado R, Simonin F, et al. Loss of morphine-induced analgesia, reward effect and withdrawal symptoms in mice lacking the mu-opioid-receptor gene. *Nature*. 1996;383:819-823. Using site directed mutagenesis techniques, these investigators demonstrated that μ receptor knockout mice failed to exhibit therapeutic effects to morphine but were otherwise phenotypically normal, confirming the importance of the μ receptor in opioid pharmacology. The μ receptor knockouts also showed no reward or withdrawal behavior or respiratory depression with morphine administration. (Ref. 7)

McEwan AI, Smith C, Dyar O, et al. Isoflurane minimum alveolar concentration reduction by fentanyl. *Anesthesiology*. 1993;78:864-869. This study quantitatively characterized the extent of isoflurane MAC reduction by fentanyl in humans, thus serving as a prototype pharmacodynamic drug interaction study. The concept of reducing the dose requirement of volatile anesthetics with opioids is one of the most important and widely applied concepts in anesthetic pharmacology. (Ref. 30)

Osborne R, Joel S, Trew D, et al. Morphine and metabolite behavior after different routes of morphine administration: demonstration of the importance of the active metabolite morphine-6-glucuronide. *Clin Pharmacol Ther*. 1990;47:12-19. This human volunteer study confirmed the importance of M6G as an active morphine metabolite, particularly after oral administration. Subsequent investigation has established M6G's role in patients with renal failure or in patients receiving longer term morphine therapy. (Ref. 53)

Poulsen L, Brosen K, Arendt-Nielsen L, et al. Codeine and morphine in extensive and poor metabolizers of sparteine: pharmacokinetics, analgesic effect and side effects. *Eur J Clin Pharmacol*. 1996;51:289-295. This human volunteer study demonstrated the importance of pharmacogenetic factors in determining the response to codeine, a prodrug of morphine. "Poor metabolizers" do not convert codeine to morphine in significant amounts and thus have no analgesic response to codeine, although they respond to morphine normally. This polymorphism relating to codeine metabolism is perhaps the best described pharmacogenetic issue in this area of therapeutics and serves as a prototype in understanding the potential clinical impact of these genetic nuances. (Ref. 46)

Shafer SL, Varvel JR. Pharmacokinetics, pharmacodynamics, and rational opioid selection. *Anesthesiology*. 1991;74:53-63. This simulation study demonstrated the importance of pharmacokinetic considerations in rational opioid selection for perioperative use. The context sensitive half-time was an outgrowth of this work. A key point of this paper is that opioid behavior is quite different for bolus administration compared to continuous infusion and that pharmacokinetic simulation is necessary to understand the implications of these pharmacokinetic differences. (Ref. 11)

References

1. Egan TD. Stereochemistry and anesthetic pharmacology: joining hands with the medicinal chemists. *Anesth Analg*. 1996;83:447-450.
2. Wang JB, Johnson PS, Persico AM, Hawkins AL, Griffin CA, Uhl GR. Human mu opiate receptor. cDNA and genomic clones, pharmacologic characterization and chromosomal assignment. *FEBS Lett*. 1994;338:217-222.
3. Minami M, Satoh M. Molecular biology of the opioid receptors: structures, functions and distributions. *Neurosci Res*. 1995;23:121-145.
4. Pan L, Xu J, Yu R, Xu MM, Pan YX, Pasternak GW. Identification and characterization of six new alternatively spliced variants of the human mu opioid receptor gene, Oprm. *Neuroscience*. 2005;133:209-220.
5. Matthies BK, Franklin KB. Formalin pain is expressed in decerebrate rats but not attenuated by morphine. *Pain*. 1992;51:199-206.
6. Becerra L, Harter K, Gonzalez RG, Borsook D. Functional magnetic resonance imaging measures of the effects of morphine on central nervous system circuitry in opioid-naive healthy volunteers. *Anesth Analg*. 2006;103:208-216.
7. Matthes HW, Maldonado R, Simonin F, et al. Loss of morphine-induced analgesia, reward effect and withdrawal symptoms in mice lacking the mu-opioid-receptor gene. *Nature*. 1996;383:819-823.
8. Sora I, Takahashi N, Funada M, et al. Opiate receptor knockout mice define mu receptor roles in endogenous nociceptive responses and morphine-induced analgesia. *Proc Natl Acad Sci U S A*. 1997;94:1544-1549.
9. Dahan A, Sarton E, Teppema L, et al. Anesthetic potency and influence of morphine and sevoflurane on respiration in mu-opioid receptor knockout mice. *Anesthesiology*. 2001;94:824-832.
10. Rubinstein M, Mogil JS, Japon M, Chan EC, Allen RG, Low MJ. Absence of opioid stress-induced analgesia in mice lacking beta-endorphin by site-directed mutagenesis. *Proc Natl Acad Sci U S A*. 1996;93:3995-4000.
11. Shafer SL, Varvel JR. Pharmacokinetics, pharmacodynamics, and rational opioid selection. *Anesthesiology*. 1991;74:53-63.
12. Hughes MA, Glass PS, Jacobs JR. Context-sensitive half-time in multicompartment pharmacokinetic models for intravenous anesthetic drugs [see comments]. *Anesthesiology*. 1992;76:334-341.
13. Youngs EJ, Shafer SL. Pharmacokinetic parameters relevant to recovery from opioids. *Anesthesiology*. 1994;81:833-842.
14. Hug CC Jr: Does opioid "anesthesia" exist? *Anesthesiology*. 1990;73:1-4.
15. Romberg R, Sarton E, Teppema L, Matthes HW, Kieffer BL, Dahan A. Comparison of morphine-6-glucuronide and morphine on respiratory depressant and antinociceptive responses in wild type and mu-opioid receptor deficient mice. *Br J Anaesth*. 2003;91:862-880.
16. Gross JB. When you breathe IN you inspire, when you DON'T breathe, you … expire: new insights regarding opioid-induced ventilatory depression. *Anesthesiology*. 2003;99:767-770.
17. Pattinson KT. Opioids and the control of respiration. *Br J Anaesth*. 2008;100:747-758.
18. Forrest WH Jr, Bellville JW. The effect of sleep plus morphine on the respiratory response to carbon dioxide. *Anesthesiology*. 1964;25:137-141.
19. Laubie M, Schmitt H, Vincent M. Vagal bradycardia produced by microinjections of morphine-like drugs into the nucleus ambiguus in anaesthetized dogs. *Eur J Pharmacol*. 1979;59:287-291.
20. Reitan JA, Stengert KB, Wymore ML, Martucci RW. Central vagal control of fentanyl-induced bradycardia during halothane anesthesia. *Anesth Analg*. 1978;57:31-36.
21. Bennett JA, Abrams JT, Van Riper DF, Horrow JC. Difficult or impossible ventilation after sufentanil-induced anesthesia is caused primarily by vocal cord closure. *Anesthesiology*. 1997;87:1070-1074.
22. Streisand JB, Bailey PL, LeMaire L, et al. Fentanyl-induced rigidity and unconsciousness in human volunteers. Incidence, duration, and plasma concentrations. *Anesthesiology*. 1993;78:629-634.
23. Apfel CC, Laara E, Koivuranta M, Greim CA, Roewer N. A simplified risk score for predicting postoperative nausea and vomiting: conclusions from cross-validations between two centers. *Anesthesiology*. 1999;91:693-700.
24. Apfel CC, Korttila K, Abdalla M, et al. A factorial trial of six interventions for the prevention of postoperative nausea and vomiting. *N Engl J Med*. 2004;350:2441-2451.

25. Radnay PA, Duncalf D, Novakovic M, Lesser ML. Common bile duct pressure changes after fentanyl, morphine, meperidine, butorphanol, and naloxone. *Anesth Analg.* 1984;63:441-444.

26. Dray A, Metsch R. Inhibition of urinary bladder contractions by a spinal action of morphine and other opioids. *J Pharmacol Exp Ther.* 1984;231:254-260.

27. Dray A, Metsch R. Spinal opioid receptors and inhibition of urinary bladder motility in vivo. *Neurosci Lett.* 1984;47:81-84.

28. Borner C, Warnick B, Smida M, et al. Mechanisms of opioid-mediated inhibition of human T cell receptor signaling. *J Immunol.* 2009;183:882-889.

29. Bouillon T, Bruhn J, Radu-Radulescu L, Bertaccini E, Park S, Shafer S. Non-steady state analysis of the pharmacokinetic interaction between propofol and remifentanil. *Anesthesiology.* 2002;97:1350-1362.

30. McEwan AI, Smith C, Dyar O, Goodman D, Smith LR, Glass PS. Isoflurane minimum alveolar concentration reduction by fentanyl. *Anesthesiology.* 1993;78:864-869.

31. Bailey PL, Pace NL, Ashburn MA, Moll JW, East KA, Stanley TH. Frequent hypoxemia and apnea after sedation with midazolam and fentanyl. *Anesthesiology.* 1990;73:826-830.

32. Vuyk J, Lim T, Engbers FH, Burm AG, Vletter AA, Bovill JG. The pharmacodynamic interaction of propofol and alfentanil during lower abdominal surgery in women. *Anesthesiology.* 1995;83:8-22.

33. Kern SE, Xie G, White JL, Egan TD. A response surface analysis of propofol-remifentanil pharmacodynamic interaction in volunteers. *Anesthesiology.* 2004;100:1373-1381.

34. Rudin A, Lundberg JF, Hammarlund-Udenaes M, Flisberg P, Werner MU. Morphine metabolism after major liver surgery. *Anesth Analg.* 2007;104:1409-1414.

35. Dershwitz M, Hoke JF, Rosow CE, et al. Pharmacokinetics and pharmacodynamics of remifentanil in volunteer subjects with severe liver disease. *Anesthesiology.* 1996;84:812-820.

36. Hoke JF, Shlugman D, Dershwitz M, et al. Pharmacokinetics and pharmacodynamics of remifentanil in persons with renal failure compared with healthy volunteers. *Anesthesiology.* 1997;87:533-541.

37. Osborne R, Joel S, Grebenik K, Trew D, Slevin M. The pharmacokinetics of morphine and morphine glucuronides in kidney failure. *Clin Pharmacol Ther.* 1993;54:158-167.

38. Sarton E, Olofsen E, Romberg R, et al. Sex differences in morphine analgesia: an experimental study in healthy volunteers. *Anesthesiology.* 2000;93:1245-1254.

39. Minto CF, Schnider TW, Egan TD, et al. Influence of age and gender on the pharmacokinetics and pharmacodynamics of remifentanil. I. Model development. *Anesthesiology.* 1997;86:10-23.

40. Scott JC, Stanski DR. Decreased fentanyl and alfentanil dose requirements with age. A simultaneous pharmacokinetic and pharmacodynamic evaluation. *J Pharmacol Exp Ther.* 1987;240:159-166.

41. Bouillon T, Shafer SL. Does size matter? *Anesthesiology.* 1998;89:557-560.

42. Egan TD, Huizinga B, Gupta SK, et al. Remifentanil pharmacokinetics in obese versus lean patients. *Anesthesiology.* 1998;89:562-573.

43. Egan TD, Kuramkote S, Gong G, Zhang J, McJames SW, Bailey PL. Fentanyl pharmacokinetics in hemorrhagic shock: a porcine model. *Anesthesiology.* 1999;91:156-166.

44. Johnson KB, Kern SE, Hamber EA, McJames SW, Kohnstamm KM, Egan TD. Influence of hemorrhagic shock on remifentanil: a pharmacokinetic and pharmacodynamic analysis. *Anesthesiology.* 2001;94:322-332.

45. Honan DM, Breen PJ, Boylan JF, McDonald NJ, Egan TD. Decrease in bispectral index preceding intraoperative hemodynamic crisis: evidence of acute alteration of propofol pharmacokinetics. *Anesthesiology.* 2002;97:1303-1305.

46. Poulsen L, Brosen K, Arendt-Nielsen L, Gram LF, Elbaek K, Sindrup SH. Codeine and morphine in extensive and poor metabolizers of sparteine: pharmacokinetics, analgesic effect and side effects. *Eur J Clin Pharmacol.* 1996;51:289-295.

47. Caraco Y, Sheller J, Wood AJ. Pharmacogenetic determination of the effects of codeine and prediction of drug interactions. *J Pharmacol Exp Ther.* 1996;278:1165-1174.

48. Eckhardt K, Li S, Ammon S, Schanzle G, Mikus G, Eichelbaum M. Same incidence of adverse drug events after codeine administration irrespective of the genetically determined differences in morphine formation. *Pain.* 1998;76:27-33.

49. Caraco Y, Sheller J, Wood AJ. Impact of ethnic origin and quinidine coadministration on codeine's disposition and pharmacodynamic effects. *J Pharmacol Exp Ther.* 1999;290:413-422.

50. Aklillu E, Persson I, Bertilsson L, Johansson I, Rodrigues F, Ingelman-Sundberg M. Frequent distribution of ultrarapid metabolizers of debrisoquine in an ethiopian population carrying duplicated and multiduplicated functional CYP2D6 alleles. *J Pharmacol Exp Ther.* 1996;278:441-446.

51. Madadi P, Ross CJ, Hayden MR, et al. Pharmacogenetics of neonatal opioid toxicity following maternal use of codeine during breastfeeding: a case-control study. *Clin Pharmacol Ther.* 2009;85:31-35.

52. Lotsch J, Dudziak R, Freynhagen R, Marschner J, Geisslinger G. Fatal respiratory depression after multiple intravenous morphine injections. *Clin Pharmacokinet.* 2006;45:1051-1060.

53. Osborne R, Joel S, Trew D, Slevin M. Morphine and metabolite behavior after different routes of morphine administration: demonstration of the importance of the active metabolite morphine-6-glucuronide. *Clin Pharmacol Ther.* 1990;47:12-19.

54. Price DD, Mayer DJ, Mao J, Caruso FS. NMDA-receptor antagonists and opioid receptor interactions as related to analgesia and tolerance. *J Pain Symptom Manage.* 2000;19: S7-S11.

55. Morgan RW, Nicholson KL. Characterization of the antinociceptive effects of the individual isomers of methadone after acute and chronic administrations. *Behav Pharmacol.* 2011;22:548-557.

56. Leppert W. The role of methadone in cancer pain treatment—a review. *Int J Clin Pract.* 2009;63:1095-1109.

57. Andrews CM, Krantz MJ, Wedam EF, Marcuson MJ, Capacchione JF, Haigney MC. Methadone-induced mortality in the treatment of chronic pain: role of QT prolongation. *Cardiol J.* 2009;16:210-217.

58. Streisand JB, Varvel JR, Stanski DR, et al. Absorption and bioavailability of oral transmucosal fentanyl citrate. *Anesthesiology.* 1991;75:223-229.

59. Stanski DR, Hug CC Jr. Alfentanil—a kinetically predictable narcotic analgesic. *Anesthesiology.* 1982;57:435-438.

60. Ibrahim AE, Feldman J, Karim A, Kharasch ED. Simultaneous assessment of drug interactions with low- and high-extraction opioids: application to parecoxib effects on the pharmacokinetics and pharmacodynamics of fentanyl and alfentanil. *Anesthesiology.* 2003; 98:853-861.

61. Egan TD. Remifentanil pharmacokinetics and pharmacodynamics. A preliminary appraisal. *Clin Pharmacokinet.* 1995;29:80-94.

62. Egan TD, Lemmens HJ, Fiset P, et al. The pharmacokinetics of the new short-acting opioid remifentanil (GI87084B) in healthy adult male volunteers. *Anesthesiology.* 1993;79:881-892.

63. Egan TD, Minto CF, Hermann DJ, Barr J, Muir KT, Shafer SL. Remifentanil versus alfentanil: comparative pharmacokinetics and pharmacodynamics in healthy adult male volunteers [published erratum appears in Anesthesiology 1996;85(3):695]. *Anesthesiology.* 1996;84:821-823.

64. Egan TD. The clinical pharmacology of remifentanil: a brief review. *J Anesth.* 1998;12:195-204.

65. Olofsen E, van Dorp E, Teppema L, et al. Naloxone reversal of morphine- and morphine-6-glucuronide-induced respiratory depression in healthy volunteers: a mechanism-based pharmacokinetic-pharmacodynamic modeling study. *Anesthesiology.* 2010;112:1417-1427.

66. Andree RA. Sudden death following naloxone administration. *Anesth Analg.* 1980;59:782-784.

67. Gal TJ, DiFazio CA, Moscicki J. Analgesic and respiratory depressant activity of nalbuphine: a comparison with morphine. *Anesthesiology.* 1982;57:367-374.

68. Murphy MR, Hug CC Jr. The enflurane sparing effect of morphine, butorphanol, and nalbuphine. *Anesthesiology.* 1982;57:489-492.

69. Strain EC, Preston KL, Liebson IA, Bigelow GE. Precipitated withdrawal by pentazocine in methadone-maintained volunteers. *J Pharmacol Exp Ther.* 1993;267:624-634.

70. Lowenstein E, Hallowell P, Levine FH, Daggett WM, Austen WG, Laver MB. Cardiovascular response to large doses of intravenous morphine in man. *N Engl J Med.* 1969;281:1389-1393.

71. Lunn JK, Stanley TH, Eisele J, Webster L, Woodward A. High dose fentanyl anesthesia for coronary artery surgery: plasma fentanyl concentrations and influence of nitrous oxide on cardiovascular responses. *Anesth Analg.* 1979;58:390-395.

72. Hofer CK, Zollinger A, Buchi S, et al. Patient well-being after general anaesthesia: a prospective, randomized, controlled

multi-centre trial comparing intravenous and inhalation anaesthesia. *Br J Anaesth*. 2003;91:631-637.

73. Mather LE. Pharmacokinetic and pharmacodynamic profiles of opioid analgesics: a sameness amongst equals? *Pain*. 1990;43:3-6.

74. Biki B, Mascha E, Moriarty DC, Fitzpatrick JM, Sessler DI, Buggy DJ. Anesthetic technique for radical prostatectomy surgery affects cancer recurrence: a retrospective analysis. *Anesthesiology*. 2008;109:180-187.

75. Bovill JG. Surgery for cancer: does anesthesia matter? *Anesth Analg*. 2010;110:1524-1526.

76. Egan TD. Target-controlled drug delivery: progress toward an intravenous "vaporizer" and automated anesthetic administration. *Anesthesiology*. 2003;99:1214-1219.

77. Egan TD, Shafer SL. Target-controlled infusions for intravenous anesthetics: surfing USA not! *Anesthesiology*. 2003;99:1039-1041.

78. Thomas J, Karver S, Cooney GA, et al. Methylnaltrexone for opioid-induced constipation in advanced illness. *N Engl J Med*. 2008;358:2332-2343.

79. Ludwig K, Enker WE, Delaney CP, et al. Gastrointestinal tract recovery in patients undergoing bowel resection: results of a randomized trial of alvimopan and placebo with a standardized accelerated postoperative care pathway. *Arch Surg*. 2008;143:1098-1105.

80. Davis JJ, Swenson JD, Hall RH, et al. Preoperative "fentanyl challenge" as a tool to estimate postoperative opioid dosing in chronic opioid-consuming patients. *Anesth Analg*. 2005;101:389-395.

81. Konopka KH, van Wijhe M. Opioid-induced hyperalgesia: pain hurts? *Br J Anaesth*. 2010;105:555-557.

82. Chu LF, Angst MS, Clark D. Opioid-induced hyperalgesia in humans: molecular mechanisms and clinical considerations. *Clin J Pain*. 2008;24:479-496.

83. Schmidt S, Bethge C, Forster MH, Schafer M. Enhanced postoperative sensitivity to painful pressure stimulation after intraoperative high dose remifentanil in patients without significant surgical site pain. *Clin J Pain*. 2007;23:605-611.

84. Guignard B, Bossard AE, Coste C, et al. Acute opioid tolerance: intraoperative remifentanil increases postoperative pain and morphine requirement. *Anesthesiology*. 2000;93:409-417.

85. Angst MS, Chu LF, Tingle MS, Shafer SL, Clark JD, Drover DR. No evidence for the development of acute tolerance to analgesic, respiratory depressant and sedative opioid effects in humans. *Pain*. 2009;142:17-26.

86. Cortinez LI, Brandes V, Munoz HR, Guerrero ME, Mur M. No clinical evidence of acute opioid tolerance after remifentanil-based anaesthesia. *Br J Anaesth*. 2001;87:866-869.

87. Lee LH, Irwin MG, Lui SK. Intraoperative remifentanil infusion does not increase postoperative opioid consumption compared with 70% nitrous oxide. *Anesthesiology*. 2005;102:398-402.

88. Shin SW, Cho AR, Lee HJ, et al. Maintenance anaesthetics during remifentanil-based anaesthesia might affect postoperative pain control after breast cancer surgery. *Br J Anaesth*. 2010;105:661-667.

89. Singler B, Troster A, Manering N, Schuttler J, Koppert W. Modulation of remifentanil-induced postinfusion hyperalgesia by propofol. *Anesth Analg*. 2007;104:1397-1403.

90. Joly V, Richebe P, Guignard B, et al. Remifentanil-induced postoperative hyperalgesia and its prevention with small-dose ketamine. *Anesthesiology*. 2005;103:147-155.

91. Chu LF, Dairmont J, Zamora AK, Young CA, Angst MS. The endogenous opioid system is not involved in modulation of opioid-induced hyperalgesia. *J Pain*. 2011;12:108-115.

92. Lotsch J, Skarke C, Schmidt H, Liefhold J, Geisslinger G. Pharmacokinetic modeling to predict morphine and morphine-6-glucuronide plasma concentrations in healthy young volunteers. *Clin Pharmacol Ther*. 2002;72:151-162.

93. Lotsch J, Skarke C, Schmidt H, Grosch S, Geisslinger G. The transfer half-life of morphine-6-glucuronide from plasma to effect site assessed by pupil size measurement in healthy volunteers. *Anesthesiology*. 2001;95:1329-1338.

94. Drover DR, Angst MS, Valle M, et al. Input characteristics and bioavailability after administration of immediate and a new extended-release formulation of hydromorphone in healthy volunteers. *Anesthesiology*. 2002;97:827-836.

95. Hill JL, Zacny JP. Comparing the subjective, psychomotor, and physiological effects of intravenous hydromorphone and morphine in healthy volunteers. *Psychopharmacology (Berl)*. 2000;152:31-39.

96. Hudson RJ, Bergstrom RG, Thomson IR, Sabourin MA, Rosenbloom M, Strunin L. Pharmacokinetics of sufentanil in patients undergoing abdominal aortic surgery. *Anesthesiology*. 1989;70:426-431.

Chapter 16

NON-OPIOID ANALGESICS

Shane Brogan, Srinand Mandyam, and Daniel A. Drennan

The term *non-opioid analgesics* seems to imply a motley group of agents self-consciously trying to establish their parity with their famously potent cousins: the opioid family. With contemporary understanding of the complexities of both acute and chronic pain, the importance of a multimodal approach to pain management pharmacotherapy has emerged, and the former outcasts have slowly been incorporated into the armamentarium of the anesthesiologist.

With the exception of the nonsteroidal antiinflammatory drugs, most non-opioid analgesics have stumbled awkwardly from other specialties like psychiatry and neurology into the field of pain medicine. As the specialty of pain medicine learned that opioids were not a panacea for all chronic pain conditions due to their long-term inefficacy, toxicities, and a propensity for misuse, greater emphasis was placed on non-opioid analgesics either as first-line treatment or as an adjunct to opioids.

Because of the pharmacologic heterogeneity of non-opioid analgesics, this chapter is broadly divided into two sections: one on nonsteroidal antiinflammatory drugs and one on drugs used for treatment of neuropathic pain.

NSAID HISTORY

Nonsteroidal antiinflammatory drugs (NSAIDs) have been used for millennia in the form of the prototypical agent, aspirin. Hippocrates wrote about using powdered willow bark for pain and fever in the fifth century BC. In the late 18th century, Stone isolated salicylic acid from willow, myrtle, and a number of other plants. However, it was not until early in the 20th century that Hoffmann, a chemist with Bayer Pharmaceuticals, discovered acetylsalicylic acid and marketed aspirin for fever, pain, and inflammation. It was not until later in the 20th century that aspirin became the generic name for this compound. Aspirin continues to be an important drug, but now more for its antiplatelet activity than for its original indications.

The newer NSAIDs were released in the 1960s, the first being indomethacin, closely followed by ibuprofen. Since then, several dozen agents have been released in the United States and elsewhere, competing for a lucrative commercial market. Over time, some of these agents have been withdrawn because of major toxicities, including hepatotoxicity, nephrotoxicity, and blood dyscrasias. The recent voluntary withdrawal of the blockbuster drug rofecoxib (Vioxx) generated considerable controversy and media coverage amidst concerns of increased cardiovascular risk.

Despite these controversies, NSAIDs remain very useful and widely used drugs for their analgesic and antipyretic effects. In the management of postoperative pain, NSAIDs are probably underused despite good evidence for their safety and efficacy.[1]

NONSTEROIDAL ANTIINFLAMMATORY DRUGS AND ACETAMINOPHEN

Basic Pharmacology

STRUCTURE-ACTIVITY RELATIONSHIPS
Nonsteroidal antiinflammatory agents are a diverse group of drugs broadly categorized into salicylates, acetic acid derivatives, propionic acid derivatives, oxicam derivatives, and the COX-2 selective agents (Figure 16-1). All act by blocking prostaglandin synthesis, both in the periphery and in the central nervous system (CNS).

Mechanism

Prostaglandins are lipid-based compounds derived enzymatically from fatty acids that have important physiologic functions including the mediation of the inflammatory response, the transduction of pain signals, and a central pyretic effect. The primary source of prostaglandins in humans is arachidonic acid, a 20-carbon polyunsaturated essential fatty acid that is, in turn, derived from cell membrane phospholipids. The NSAIDs act by inhibiting cyclooxygenase (COX) enzymes that catalyze the conversion of arachidonic acid to prostaglandins, thromboxanes, and prostacyclin (Figure 16-2).

The COX enzymes are now known to exist as three isoforms: COX-1, COX-2, and COX-3. COX-3 is a splice variant of COX-1, and is now recognized as the once elusive enzyme inhibited by acetaminophen.[2] However, controversy still exists about the existence of COX-3 inhibition in humans and the mechanism by which acetaminophen-mediated analgesia occurs. COX-1 and COX-2 are the isoforms targeted by the traditional NSAIDs, while the more selective COX-2 inhibitors preferentially block COX-2. COX-1 is considered to be the constitutive enzyme (often called the *housekeeping*

Propionic acid derivative – ibuprofen

Acetic acid derivative – indomethacin

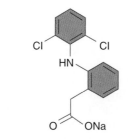
Fenamate NSAID – diclofenac

COX-2 selective NSAID – celecoxib

Enolic acid derivative (oxicam) – meloxicam

Salicylate – aspirin

Figure 16-1 Nonsteroidal antiinflammatory drugs (NSAIDs). Molecular structures of an agent from each class of NSAID. Note the disparate chemical structures between classes.

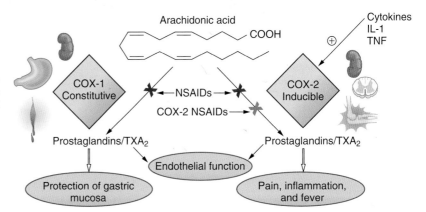

Figure 16-2 Mechanism of action of nonsteroidal antiinflammatory drugs, with comparison of cyclooxygenase (COX)-1 and COX-2 inhibition effects. COX-3 effects not shown.

enzyme), generating prostanoids involved in normal physiologic functioning such as gastrointestinal mucosal protection and hemostasis. COX-2, on the other hand, has low baseline expression but is inducible during physiologic stress by agents including proinflammatory cytokines, neurotransmitters, and growth factors.

However, this schema is acknowledged to be an oversimplification in that there are exceptions to this rule: for example, COX-2 is constitutively expressed in the kidney and CNS, and COX-1 can be induced by certain stress conditions in nerve tissue.[3] Although both enzymes are structurally similar and act basically in the same fashion, their respective gene expression profiles and selective inhibition can determine NSAID side effects and toxicity.

Metabolism

The primary mode of NSAID elimination is by hepatic biotransformation by cytochrome P450 (CYP 450) mediated oxidation or glucuronide conjugation. Renal excretion of unmetabolized drug is much less important, accounting for less than 10% of the administered dose. Biliary excretion has been described for certain NSAIDs, although this route plays a small role. Because NSAIDs share common metabolic pathways, nuances relating to metabolism are not a basis for therapeutic decisions regarding the appropriate NSAID for a given patient.

Clinical Pharmacology

PHARMACOKINETICS

NSAIDs are weak acids with pK_a values typically lower than 5, and therefore exist mostly in the ionized form at physiologic pH. NSAIDs, except aspirin, which is 50% to 80% bound, are highly bound to plasma proteins, primarily albumin. NSAID half-lives vary significantly between drugs (Table 16-1). Because oral NSAIDs are often prescribed for long-term use, a focus of modern NSAID development has been to design compounds that are relatively long-acting to facilitate improved patient compliance.

Most NSAIDs are rapidly absorbed following oral administration, with peak plasma concentrations generally reached within 2 to 3 hours. Factors affecting gastric emptying can

profoundly affect the time course of the clinical effects of NSAIDs. In part because of the variability in the time course of oral absorption, the use of rectal NSAIDs is popular in Europe for the management of postoperative pain and has the added advantage of being possible even when oral intake is not.[4] Ketorolac and ibuprofen are the only parenteral NSAIDs currently available in the United States, but an intravenous diclofenac and parecoxib are available elsewhere. Parenteral administration is advantageous in renal colic because of its more rapid onset than with oral administration, but it has demonstrated no obvious advantage over oral administration for any other indication.[5] Several other injectable NSAID dosage forms, such as diclofenac and ibuprofen, are in the later stages of development. Their role in pain and perioperative medical practice remain to be seen.

PHARMACODYNAMICS

Therapeutic Effects

NSAIDs are widely used for their analgesic properties, particularly when pain has an inflammatory component such as in certain rheumatologic conditions. Tissue trauma results in cell membrane disruption and release of arachidonic acid, the substrate for COX enzymes, and consequently a rise in local prostaglandin concentrations. These prostanoids, particularly PGE_2, result in sensitization of nociceptors to mechanical stimuli and other chemical mediators such as bradykinin, leading to increased nociceptor firing and pain perception. COX enzyme activity has also been identified in the CNS including the dorsal horn of the spinal cord, and it is postulated that COX inhibition also provides a central analgesic mechanism.[2]

The antipyretic effect of the NSAIDs is very predictable and has utility in the treatment of fever, both in adults and children. Perioperatively, NSAIDs are indicated in a multimodal analgesic approach, and the American Society of Anesthesiologists (ASA) recent practice guidelines for acute pain management in the perioperative setting encourage the use of NSAIDs unless contraindicated.[1] A less common NSAID indication (indomethacin is typically used) is in the prevention of ductus arteriosum closure when this would be detrimental in certain neonatal congenital heart conditions where an ongoing right-to-left shunt is desired before corrective surgery. Figure 16-3 provides an overview of the

Table 16-1. Summary of Nonsteroidal Antiinflammatory Drugs and Acetaminophen

DRUG	COMMON TRADE NAME	HALF-LIFE (HOURS)	PROTEIN BINDING, PERCENT	TYPICAL DAILY DOSE RANGE	TYPICAL DOSING SCHEDULE	TYPICAL PEDIATRIC DOSING, MG/KG/24 HR	NOTES
Acetaminophen/ paracetamol	Tylenol, Panadol Ofirmez (iv)	2	20-50	2-4 g	325-650 mg q4hr	10-15 mg/kg q6-8hr prn	No antiinflammatory effect
Propionic Acid Derivatives							
Fenoprofen	Nalfon	2-3	99	1.2-2.4 g	300-600 mg QID	900-1800 mg per body surface area in M²	
Flurbiprofen	Ansaid	2	99	200 mg	100 mg BID	NA	
Ibuprofen	Motrin, Advil, Brufen, others	6	99	1.2-2.4 g	400-800 mg QID	7.5-10 mg/kg QID	Higher doses sometimes used for inflammatory conditions; max dose 3200 mg/day
Ketoprofen	Orudis	2-4	99	225 mg	75 mg TID	NA	
Naproxen	Naprosyn	14	99	750-1000 mg	250-375 mg BID	5-10 mg/kg BID	
Naproxen Sodium	Alleve, Anaprox	14	99	550-1100 mg	275-550 mg BID	5-10 mg/kg BID	
Fenamates							
Diclofenac	Voltaren	1-2	99	150-200	50 mg TID 75 mg BID	2-3 mg/kg/24 hr	Hepatotoxicity rarely reported. Also has topical formulations
Tolmetin	Tolectin	5	99	800-2400 mg	400-800 mg TID	20-30 mg/kg/24 hr as 3-4 doses	
Ketorolac	Toradol	4-6	99	IV: 60 mg/day*	30 mg first dose; then 15 mg q6hr*	IV: 0.5 mg/kg/day, single dose only	*Half the dose if age >65 yr or weight <50 kg
Enolic Acid Derivatives (Oxicams)							
Meloxicam	Mobic	15-20	99	7.5-15	7.5-15 mg QD	NA	Higher dose typically used for rheumatoid arthritis Intermediate COX-1 and COX-2 selectivity
Piroxicam	Feldene	40-50	99	20 mg	10-20 mg QD	NA	
Nabumetone	Relafen	24	99	1000-1500 mg	500-750 mg BID	NA	
Acetic Acid Derivatives							
Etodolac	Lodine	7	99	400-1200 mg	200-400 mg TID/QID	15-20 mg/kg/24 hr	
Indomethacin	Indocin, others	2-5	90	100-200 mg	25-50 mg TID/QID	2-4 mg/kg/24 hr	
Sulindac	Clinoril	8-16	99	400 mg	150-200 mg	BID/TID	
COX-2 Selective NSAID							
Celecoxib	Celebrex	6-12	97	200 mg	100-200 mg QD/BID	3 mg/kg BID	400 mg/day used for acute pain

BID, Twice daily; *IV*, intravenous; *prn*, as needed; *q*, every; *QD*, every day; *QID*, four times daily; *TID*, three times daily.

pharmacodynamic effects of NSAIDs, including both therapeutic and adverse effects.

Adverse Effects

NSAIDs have a number of nonspecific adverse effects including rash and gastrointestinal upset (e.g., dyspepsia, abdominal pain, and diarrhea). The following paragraphs describe specific adverse effects.

CARDIOVASCULAR EFFECTS

All NSAIDs, and not just the COX-2 selective agents, can increase the risk of serious cardiovascular thrombotic events

such as myocardial infarction and stroke.[6,7] The mechanisms underlying these adverse effects are complicated but likely include an imbalance between the prothrombotic and vasoconstricting activity of thromboxane A_2 (TXA$_2$), and the antithrombotic and vasodilatory effects of prostacyclin (PGI$_2$), thereby favoring deleterious thromboxane effects.[8] In addition, NSAIDs increase blood pressure in a dose-dependent fashion, which may also be linked to the increased cardiovascular risks associated with their use.[9] Prolonged administration of COX-2 selective NSAIDs can cause adverse events through inhibition of PGI$_2$, including development of hypertension and the promotion of thrombus development in a ruptured plaque.[6] Recent reviews of both nonselective

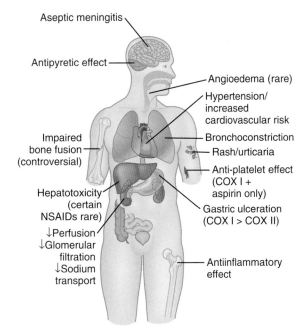

Figure 16-3 Overview of the common pharmacokinetic and pharmacody-namic effects of nonsteroidal antiinflammatory agents.

NSAIDs and COX-2 inhibitors have found that nonselective NSAIDs and celecoxib carry little risk of ischemic stroke, whereas rofecoxib and valdecoxib (both discontinued) are associated with significant risk.[10,11] However, the cerebrovascular safety of nonselective NSAIDs has been questioned in other studies, suggesting that all NSAIDs should be used with caution in patients with high risk for cerebrovascular disease.[7]

The perioperative administration of NSAIDs, especially the COX-2 selective agents for short-term use, has been subject to some controversy due to their possible role in increasing morbidity after cardiac surgery.[12,13] However, a recent metaanalysis of studies using parecoxib and valdecoxib compared with placebo in noncardiac surgery concluded that there were no differences in cardiovascular events between groups.[14]

In 2005, a consensus statement issued by the Food and Drug Administration (FDA) Arthritis Advisory Committee and the Drug Safety and Risk Management Advisory Committee concluded that COX-2 selective agents are important treatment options for pain management and that the preponderance of data demonstrates that the cardiovascular risk associated with celecoxib is similar to that associated with commonly used, older, nonselective NSAIDs. The committee also concluded that short-term use of NSAIDs does not appear to increase cardiovascular risk and that rigorous scientific studies are needed to characterize the longer term cardiovascular risks of these therapies. With respect to the longer term use of NSAIDs, a careful risk-benefit analysis should be performed, particularly in those already at risk for cardiovascular events.[15]

BONE HEALING
Bone healing is dependent on an inflammatory response involving numerous cytokines including interleukin (IL)-1,

IL-6, tumor necrosis factor, and fibroblast growth factor, so it is not surprising that agents that disrupt normal cytokine function can impair bone homeostasis and repair.[16] There are convincing animal data that nonselective and COX-2 inhibitor NSAIDs inhibit bone healing.[17-19] This inhibition of healing response has been used therapeutically to prevent heterotrophic bone formation after arthroplasty.[20] In a rat model of femoral fracture healing, celecoxib or rofecoxib delayed fracture healing compared to indomethacin.[21] At 8 weeks postoperatively, there was still evidence of the original fracture in these two groups.

However, human data on possible detrimental effect of NSAID use in the perioperative period is conflicted and controversial.[22] The issue of bone healing and NSAIDs has been addressed mostly in the spinal fusion literature. Successful spinal fusion surgery demands a robust bone healing process, so spine surgeons place great importance on mitigating all risk of nonunion with measures such as smoking cessation and NSAID avoidance. A retrospective analysis of 288 patients who underwent instrumented spinal fusion from L4 to the sacrum demonstrated a 5 times higher nonunion rate when ketorolac was used in the immediate postoperative period.[23] In contrast, another retrospective study found that, in 405 consecutive patients who underwent primary lumbar spinal fusion, a subset of patients who had ketorolac 30 mg intravenously every 6 hours for 2 days had similar fusion rates to a group that had no NSAIDs.[24] A recent metaanalysis of five retrospective studies explored the relation of ketorolac dose and successful spinal fusion rates, and concluded that high-dose ketorolac (>120 mg/day) might be associated with poor outcomes, whereas standard dose ketorolac (<120 mg/day) was not.[25] In the absence of any prospective or randomized studies, and realizing that bony nonunion is a high morbidity outcome, use of perioperative NSAIDs in spinal fusion cases should be considered carefully, particularly when other risk factors for poor bone healing (e.g., smoking) exist. In nonspine orthopedic surgery, there is good evidence of NSAID analgesic efficacy and no significant association with compromised bone healing.[22,26]

ALLERGY AND HYPERSENSITIVITY
All NSAIDs, including aspirin, can induce hypersensitivity reactions of two general types, both likely related to the inhibition of prostaglandin synthesis. Provocation of asthmatic attacks in patients with vasomotor rhinitis and nasal polyposis is likely related to inhibition of normal production of the bronchodilator PGE_2. NSAIDs also rarely induce the syndrome of urticaria and angioedema related to inhibition of prostaglandin effects that normally stabilize histamine stores in mastocytes and inhibit the inflammatory response.[27] In susceptible individuals, this unchecked inflammation can result in spontaneous degranulation of mastocytes with release of histamine in the respiratory tract and skin, which leads to bronchoconstriction and urticaria. This process is COX-1 mediated, and therefore COX-2 selective NSAIDs may be used, but with caution, in NSAID intolerant patients.[28,29]

GASTROINTESTINAL TOXICITY
The long-term use of oral NSAIDs inhibits production of prostaglandins that maintain normal gastrointestinal mucosal integrity, and results in gastric and colonic mucosal damage including erosion and ulceration. In addition, oral NSAIDs

can cause local irritation, and when erosion and/or ulceration is present, hemostasis is compromised by COX-1 inhibition. This constellation of physiologic derangements results in a spectrum of gastrointestinal problems, ranging from mild gastritis to peptic ulceration with perforation.

The morbidity and mortality of NSAID use is very significant, although it appears to be abating in recent years, likely due to the more widespread use of proton pump inhibitors, rather than the use of COX-2 inhibitors.[30] Risk factors identified for the development of NSAID-induced ulcers include advanced age, history of previous ulcer, concomitant use of corticosteroids, higher doses of NSAIDs (including the use of more than one NSAID), concomitant administration of anti-coagulation, serious systemic disorders, cigarette smoking, consumption of alcohol, and concomitant infection with *Helicobacter pylori*. Short term use of NSAIDs in the perioperative period carries little risk of mucosal injury, although intolerance or nausea can be an issue in patients given NSAIDs on an empty stomach.

HEMOSTATIC EFFECTS

Platelets, lacking a nucleus and the ability to generate new proteins like COX, are particularly susceptible to the effects of COX inhibitors. Aspirin irreversibly acetylates COX enzymes and inhibits platelet aggregation for the 10- to 14-day lifespan of the platelet. Other nonselective NSAIDs reversibly inhibit COX, causing only transient reduction in TXA_2 formation. Consequently, inhibition of platelet activation resolves after most of the drug is eliminated. For example, a single 300 to 900 mg dose of ibuprofen can inhibit platelet aggregation for 2 hours after administration, and the effect is largely dissipated by 24 hours. Overall, with the exception of aspirin, NSAIDs cause transient, dose-dependent, and modest bleeding time abnormalities, which often do not exceed normal limits.[8] However, clinical studies have revealed some significant issues with perioperative hemostasis and nonselective NSAID use. In total hip arthroplasty, patients taking nonselective NSAIDs had more intraoperative and postoperative blood loss than those who did not.[31] Despite concern on the part of many ear, nose, and throat surgeons regarding the use of NSAIDs for pain control after pediatric tonsillectomy, a thorough metaanalysis of studies addressing this concern failed to find any significant association between NSAIDs and perioperative bleeding requiring return to the operating room.[32] Importantly, the COX-2 enzyme has not been identified in platelets, so the COX-2 inhibitors are not thought to have deleterious anti-platelet effects.[33]

RENAL TOXICITY

Aspirin and all other NSAIDs, including COX-2 inhibitors, can transiently decrease renal function in selected patients, resulting in hypertension, edema, and even acute renal failure. These effects occur more often in patients with underlying renal disease and in those with intravascular volume depletion.[34] Renal perfusion and glomerular filtration are closely regulated by renal prostaglandin synthesis, particularly in the fluid depleted state. Inhibition of this system is the postulated mechanism of NSAID-induced Na^+ retention and renal dysfunction. In the perioperative setting, NSAIDs seldom cause clinically significant renal impairment, but should be withheld in patients who are significantly volume

depleted, have intraoperative oliguria, or have preexisting renal impairment.

OTHER TOXICITIES

Aspirin and diclofenac are the most potentially hepatotoxic NSAIDs, and should be avoided in patients with pre-existing hepatic failure.[35] NSAIDs have been implicated in hypersensitivity-induced aseptic meningitis, generally manifesting with meningeal signs commencing within weeks of starting therapy. It is a diagnosis of exclusion after ruling out an infectious cause of the meningeal irritation.

Drug Interactions

Hypoalbuminemia increases the free fraction of NSAIDs in the plasma, thus affecting their distribution and elimination. The high degree of serum protein binding increases interaction risk with other highly protein bound drugs. In clinical practice, however, this is rarely significant, and NSAIDs can be used safely in conjunction with other agents commonly used in perioperative practice. One exception is the potential for nephrotoxicity when NSAIDs are used concomitantly with other potentially nephrotoxic drugs such as the aminoglycosides, radiographic contrast media, and diuretics. Nonselective NSAIDs should be used with caution in patients who have been on other platelet-inhibiting drugs or anticoagulants.

Special Populations

RENAL FAILURE

In general, NSAIDs are avoided in patients with renal failure. The use of NSAIDs in patients with preexisting renal insufficiency can have deleterious effects as discussed earlier. Renal failure influences NSAID kinetics by reducing renal excretion of the drugs and metabolites normally eliminated in the urine and by affecting their distribution and biotransformation.[36] All NSAIDs are very highly bound to plasma proteins, and hemodialysis will not likely increase elimination of these agents. No dosage adjustments are therefore necessary for hemodialysis patients receiving NSAIDs.

LIVER DISEASE

The majority of NSAIDs have low hepatic clearance, so mild to moderate liver disease should theoretically not interfere with their oral bioavailability. Because NSAIDs are so avidly protein-bound, alteration of liver albumin synthesis would be expected to cause alterations in the unbound drug fraction in plasma. Diclofenac has been the agent most implicated with hepatic dysfunction and should be avoided in patients with liver disease.

OLDER AGE

Advanced age is an independent risk factor for both cardiovascular disease and NSAID gastropathy, so NSAIDs should be used with additional caution in this population. However, the opioid-sparing effects of NSAIDs in the postoperative period make NSAIDs an attractive pain management adjunct, particularly when concerns exist regarding oversedation, delirium, or respiratory depression in older patients receiving opioids. In older adults, the relatively high lipid solubility of NSAIDs, potentially decreased plasma protein levels, and reduced renal function all contribute to an increased likelihood of toxicity. Therefore, the lowest effective dose of NSAID should be administered, with frequent follow-up (sometimes including renal function tests) for assessment of side effects or toxicity.[37]

Unique Features of Individual Agents

MELOXICAM

Meloxicam, an NSAID of the enolic acid type, is unique in that it selectively blocks COX-2 over COX-1, and is therefore considered an intermediate between COX-2 selective agents and the nonselective NSAIDs. Consequently, meloxicam might have a better gastrointestinal tolerability profile compared with nonselective agents and can be considered if celecoxib is unavailable or contraindicated.[27]

KETOROLAC

Ketorolac, until recently, was the only parenteral NSAID available in the United States and was therefore used quite extensively in the perioperative period. Pharmacologically, it is a member of the pyrrolo-pyrrole group, and is avidly protein bound resulting in a low volume of distribution. Ketorolac is extensively conjugated in the liver and then excreted in the urine. Time to measurable effect is about 30 minutes, with a peak effect noted at 1 to 2 hours and a duration of action of 4 to 6 hours.

In the management of postoperative pain, ketorolac has proven to be very useful, with an opioid-sparing effect and efficacy similar to morphine in the treatment of moderate pain.[38,39] Concerns exist regarding the renal safety profile of ketorolac in the perioperative setting that have necessitated modifications of dosing guidelines. Previously, the drug was administered at a 60-mg initial dose followed by 30 mg every 4 hours, and cases of acute tubular necrosis were reported. Gastrointestinal bleeding and operative site bleeding have also been reported and are mostly associated with advanced patient age, duration of therapy beyond 5 days, and higher dosing regimens.[40] Subsequently, dosing recommendations were decreased by more than 50%. The ketorolac package insert now advises the following intravenous dosing protocol: for a single dose, 30 mg IV or 15 mg if patient age is greater than 65 or body weight less than 50 kg; for multiple dosing, patients should be commenced on 30 mg every 6 hours, not to exceed 120 mg in a 24-hour period; in those older than 65 years or weighing less than 50 kg, the dosing should be 15 mg every 6 hours, not to exceed 60 mg in 24 hours.[41] In no circumstance should dosing go beyond 5 days of therapy, and ketorolac is best avoided in patients with a history of peptic ulcer disease or renal impairment.

ACETAMINOPHEN

Acetaminophen, while strictly speaking not an NSAID, is generally grouped in this therapeutic class and plays a major role in analgesic therapy. Acetaminophen is a para-aminophenol derivative with analgesic and antipyretic properties similar to aspirin. The very useful antipyretic effect is thought to be a direct effect on the hypothalamic heat-regulating centers via inhibiting action of endogenous pyrogens. Recent reports suggest that acetaminophen acts via the serotonergic pathways, COX-3 inhibition, and/or endogenous cannabinoid potentiation to provide analgesia, but its mechanism of action remains poorly understood.[42-44] Although equipotent to aspirin in inhibiting central prostaglandin synthesis, acetaminophen has no significant peripheral prostaglandin synthetase inhibition and is therefore less useful than NSAIDs for painful inflammatory disorders.

Acetaminophen has few side effects in the usual dosage range; unlike NSAIDs, no significant gastrointestinal toxicity or platelet function inhibition occur. Acetaminophen has, however, been associated with the development of hypertension but has not yet been associated with increased cardiovascular risk.[45] Nephrotoxicity also can occur with acetaminophen but less frequently than it occurs with NSAIDs.[46]

Acetaminophen is completely and rapidly absorbed following oral administration, and peak serum concentrations are achieved within 2 hours. About 90% of acetaminophen is hepatically metabolized to sulfate and glucuronide conjugates for renal excretion with a small amount secreted unchanged in the urine. Minor metabolites are responsible for the hepatotoxicity seen in overdose.[47] CYP 450 enzyme system induction in the liver by any agent, including ethanol, increases the formation of toxic free radial metabolites and thereby increases hepatotoxicity. In the healthy individual, daily doses of 2.6 to 3.2 g are generally considered safe, and acetaminophen dosing should not exceed 4 g/day.[48,49] In patients with a history of ethanol abuse or liver disease, acetaminophen should generally be avoided.

The bioavailability of rectal acetaminophen is variable and is approximately 80% of that following oral administration. The rate of rectal absorption is slower, with maximum plasma concentration occurring 2 to 3 hours after administration. Doses of 40 to 60 mg/kg of rectal acetaminophen have been shown to have an opioid-sparing effect in the management of postoperative pain.[50] In Europe, an intravenous prodrug form of acetaminophen, propacetamol, and intravenous acetaminophen are available for clinical use and have been shown to reduce postoperative opioid consumption.[51,52] In 2011, an intravenous form of acetaminophen was introduced in the United States for the parenteral management of pain and fever.[53] Intravenous acetaminophen (1 g every 4 hours for 24 hours) was well tolerated, improved pain reporting, and decreased morphine consumption after orthopedic surgery.[54]

Oral NSAIDs

COMMON CLINICAL INDICATIONS

Postoperative Analgesia

While opioids continue to be the mainstay of analgesia during the perioperative period, NSAIDs and acetaminophen alone can be sufficient for the management of mild pain and are a very useful adjunct in the management of moderate to severe pain. The latest ASA practice guidelines for acute pain management in the perioperative setting encourage the use of NSAIDs and other adjuncts whenever possible.[1] The preoperative administration of oral COX-2 selective NSAIDs can reduce cerebrospinal fluid (CSF) and surgical site PGE_2 levels in humans during the perioperative period with an associated decrease in pain. In addition to reducing CSF PGE_2 levels, COX-2 selective NSAIDs decreased CSF IL-6 (a major pro-inflammatory cytokine) levels. The IL-6 modulation by COX-2 inhibitors is not well understood, but is likely to be related to the PGE_2 pathway.[55]

A recent metaanalysis examined the effect of adding acetaminophen, nonselective NSAIDs, or COX-2 selective NSAIDs to opioid patient-controlled analgesia. The results suggested that all three analgesic agents provided an opioid dose-sparing effect (25%-55%). Moreover, the addition of NSAIDs to morphine was associated with a decrease in the incidence of postoperative nausea and vomiting and sedation (Tables 16-2 and 16-3).[26] Clinical trials of COX-2 selective NSAIDs used preoperatively and into the postoperative period for patients undergoing both major surgery and minimally invasive surgery have demonstrated improved clinical outcomes, including reduction in postoperative pain, opioid use, and nausea.[26,56,57] A metaanalysis of clinical studies evaluating COX-2 inhibitors compared with nonselective NSAIDs (which do not differentiate between COX-1 and COX-2) for postoperative pain showed that the analgesic efficacy of COX-2 inhibitors in the 6 hours after surgery was similar to or better than ibuprofen.[58]

NSAIDs in Chronic Pain

Chronic pain has been defined as pain that extends beyond the expected period of healing or beyond a certain arbitrary period of time, or more specifically as pain that extends beyond 3 to 6 months from the original injury. The use of NSAIDs in chronic pain has an important role in selected conditions. Conditions with a predominant inflammatory component such as rheumatoid arthritis are likely to respond favorably to NSAIDs, whereas noninflammatory conditions such as peripheral neuropathic pain are unlikely to respond.[59] An advantage of NSAIDs in chronic pain is their ability to offer an opioid-sparing effect so that opioid doses can be minimized, thereby lowering any potential opioid-related

Table 16-2. 24-Hour Morphine Consumption (in Milligrams)

REGIMENS	# Patients With ACTIVE	# Patients With CONTROL	CHANGE IN MORPHINE REQUIREMENT	WMD [95% CI]
Acetaminophen				
Multiple dose	379	334		−8.31 [−10.9 to −5.72]
NSAIDs				
Single dose	553	496		−10.3 [−18.3 to −2.34]
Multiple dose	495	398		−19.7 [−26.3 to −13.0]
Continuous	276	253		−18.3 [−26.8 to −9.74]
COX-2 Inhibitors				
Single dose	70	69		−7.22 [−10.6 to −3.82]
Single dose	91	91		−27.8 [−44.3 to −11.4]
Multiple low dose	272	273		−9.99 [−13.4 to −6.58]
Multiple high dose	535	411		−13.3 [−17.8 to −8.81]

−40 −20 0 20
$WMD_{mg\ morphine}$

Reprinted with permission from Elia N, Lysakowski C, Tramer MR. Does multimodal analgesia with acetaminophen, nonsteroidal antiinflammatory drugs, or selective cyclooxygenase-2 inhibitors and patient-controlled analgesia morphine offer advantages over morphine alone? Meta-analyses of randomized trials. *Anesthesiology*. 2005;103:1296-1304.
A weighted mean difference (WMD) less than 0 indicates less morphine consumption with active compared with control. When the 95% confidence interval (CI) does not include 0, the difference is considered statistically significant. COX-2 inhibitor = 200 mg celecoxib, a 50 mg rofecoxib; multiple high dose = valdecoxib and parecoxib 40 mg/12 hr and parecoxib 40 mg/6 hr; multiple low dose = valdecoxib and parecoxib 20 mg/12 hr.
NSAID, Nonsteroidal antiinflammatory drug.

Table 16-3. Visual Analog Scale Score for Pain Intensity at Rest at 24 Hr (0-10 cm)

REGIMENS	# Patients With ACTIVE	# Patients With CONTROL	CHANGE IN PAIN SCORE	WMD [95% CI]
Acetaminophen				
Multiple dose	175	180		−0.29 [−0.71 to 0.14]
NSAIDs				
Single dose	390	369		−0.75 [−1.61 to 0.11]
Multiple dose	288	265		−1.00 [−1.25 to −0.75]
Continuous	225	201		−0.97 [1.37 to −0.57]

−2 −1 0 1
$WMD_{VAS\ pain\ intensity}$

Reprinted with permission from Elia N, Lysakowski C, Tramer MR. Does multimodal analgesia with acetaminophen, nonsteroidal antiinflammatory drugs, or selective cyclooxygenase-2 inhibitors and patient-controlled analgesia morphine offer advantages over morphine alone? Meta-analyses of randomized trials. *Anesthesiology*. 2005;103:1296-1304.
A weighted mean difference (WMD) less than 0 indicates less pain with active compared with control. When the 95% confidence interval (CI) does not include 0, the difference is considered statistically significant. Meta-analyses were performed when data from at least three trials or more than 100 patients could be combined; this was not the case for cyclooxygenase-2 inhibitors.
NSAID, nonsteroidal antiinflammatory drug.

toxicity. However, the long-term (possibly lifelong) use of NSAIDs is not without its own risk, particularly in patients at risk for NSAID toxicity, including older adults and those with preexisting renal or cardiac disease.

Data on the long-term efficacy of NSAIDs for chronic pain is limited, whereas the long-term risk has been better defined.[15] In a metaanalysis of NSAID efficacy in chronic back pain, there was a small benefit with NSAID therapy when sciatica was not present; with sciatica, no difference was found.[60]

As is the case with all pharmacotherapeutic options for the management of chronic pain, any analgesic agent should be introduced only after careful consideration of the condition being treated and patient comorbidities. In the case of NSAIDs, close follow-up is essential to screen for efficacy and toxicity; with discontinuation if they are inefficacious or poorly tolerated.

Rational Drug Selection

In general, NSAIDs have similar analgesic efficacy, and individual drug choice is more often determined by differences in tolerability, local availability, route of administration, and cost. In the perioperative setting, intravenous agents such as ketorolac and acetaminophen are often used for practical reasons, but thought should be given to alternative preoperative oral regimens that might significantly reduce cost. Many of the older nonselective NSAIDs can be purchased over-the-counter in the United States, whereas the COX-2 inhibitor celecoxib is available only by prescription. Celecoxib, due to the presence of a sulpha moiety, is contraindicated in patients who report a history of sulpha allergy.

A summary table of the most commonly used agents is presented in Table 16-1. This information constitutes the rational basis for drug selection of these agents.

Topical NSAID Preparations

Because NSAIDs are the drugs of choice for musculoskeletal pain and adverse events occur commonly with systemic NSAID therapy, formulation of topical dosage forms to limit systemic exposure was a logical pharmaceutical development. Topical formulations are those that are applied locally in proximity to the affected area and which provide effective concentrations at the local target tissues without producing the systemic levels that are associated with common adverse effects.[61] These differ from transdermal dosage forms that deliver full systemic levels of the drug through the skin into the circulation. In the United States, diclofenac is the only approved topical NSAID and comes in gel, patch, and ointment form. Topical NSAIDs produce high drug concentration in dermis, muscle, synovium, and joint cartilage, while plasma drug concentrations are less than 10% of those obtained after oral administration. However, substantial interindividual variability exists in transdermal drug penetration. While the anatomic site of application has little effect on systemic drug absorption, individual skin and connective tissue differences can alter topical absorption of drugs. For selected conditions, topical NSAIDs have been shown to be comparable in efficacy to the oral route (Figure 16-4).

The specific topical NSAID formulation can greatly impact its absorption and penetration through the skin. Differences in formulations are based on the dosage form (gel, solution,

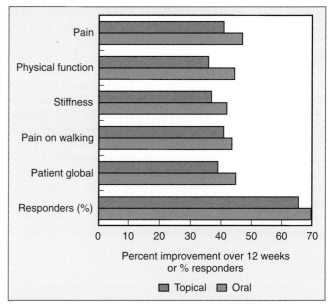

Figure 16-4 Efficacy of topical diclofenac is comparable to oral diclofenac for osteoarthritic knee pain at 12 weeks. These data illustrate that, compared to the oral route, topical administration of NSAIDs may be similarly efficacious in selected indications. *(Adapted from Simon LS, Grierson LM, Naseer Z, et al. Efficacy and safety of topical diclofenac containing dimethyl sulfoxide [DMSO] compared with those of topical placebo, DMSO vehicle and oral diclofenac for knee osteoarthritis. Pain. 2009;143:238-245.)*

or patch), different salts of the same molecule (diclofenac sodium, diclofenac potassium, or diclofenac epolamine), carrier-mediated transport (lipid emulsions or solid nanoparticles), and penetration enhancement methods, either chemical (addition of penetration enhancer like menthol or dimethylsulfoxide [DMSO]) or physical (heat-mediated penetration enhancement or electrical charge-mediated penetration enhancement such as iontophoresis).

The most common side effects reported in studies using topical NSAIDs are application site reactions, including dermatitis (reported in 7% of treated patients). Serious side effects are exceptionally rare.[62-64]

DRUGS USED FOR THE TREATMENT OF NEUROPATHIC PAIN

Introduction and Historical Perspective

The International Association for the Study of Pain (IASP) defines neuropathic pain as pain that results from a lesion or disease affecting the somatosensory system.[65] It has been traditionally thought that opioids are ineffective in the treatment of neuropathic pain, but this is not strictly true and is still considered controversial.[66,67] However, it is fair to say that opioids are generally *less* effective in the treatment of neuropathic pain compared to nociceptive pain and consequently are typically used as a second-line treatment after the typical neuropathic drugs have failed to provide satisfactory results. The medical management of patients with neuropathic pain is a challenge to the medical community and has largely been steered by guidelines and systematic reviews of numerous pharmacologic interventions.

The drugs with the best efficacy in neuropathic pain are the tricyclic antidepressants (TCAs), certain anticonvulsants, selective norepinephrine reuptake inhibitors, and topical agents. Duloxetine, a selective norepinephrine and serotonin reuptake inhibitor, also is used in the management of certain neuropathic pain conditions.

The TCAs were introduced in the 1950s as the first agents used in the pharmacologic treatment of depression. Before this, they were used as antipsychotics, presumably due to their marked sedative effects. However, it was noted that TCAs sometimes produced the opposite effect, elevating the mood and even inducing mania. This stimulating effect was later harnessed in the treatment of depression, with the first publication of imipramine as an antidepressant by the Swiss psychiatrist Ronald Kuhn in 1957.[68] While often effective, the TCAs were plagued by their unpleasant antihistaminergic and anticholinergic side effects. In 1974, the first selective serotonin reuptake inhibitors (SSRIs) were discovered, the most promising of which was fluoxetine. It was not until 1986 that fluoxetine (Prozac) was released on the Belgian market, and the following year it gained FDA approval in the United States. This promptly ended the use of TCAs for the management of depression, and Prozac rapidly became a blockbuster drug, with more than 22 million U.S. prescriptions written in 2007 alone. However, the TCAs continue to be used, albeit at much lower doses, for the management of neuropathic pain. Perhaps surprisingly, their efficacy, in terms of numbers needed to treat, is actually better than the aggressively marketed anticonvulsant agents discussed later.[69]

Gabapentin is an anticonvulsant initially approved for the treatment of partial seizures, but in 1995 was anecdotally noted to be helpful in the treatment of certain pain conditions, leading to clinical studies in neuropathic pain conditions where it was found to be clinically helpful. Gabapentin is confusingly named because it was originally designed to be a γ-aminobutyric acid (GABA) analogue, but it transpired that it had no significant GABA activity; instead, it was involved with voltage gated N-type calcium channels. In 2005, pregabalin (Lyrica), with almost identical receptor activity to gabapentin, was released on the U.S. market with specific indications for neuropathic pain. Two years later, the FDA approved pregabalin for the management of fibromyalgia.

TRICYCLIC ANTIDEPRESSANTS

Basic Pharmacology

TCAs are heterocyclic compounds that were previously used in the treatment of major depressive disorder before the development of SSRIs. Since the release of the first SSRI, fluoxetine (Prozac) in 1987, TCAs are rarely used in the management of depression due to a high burden of side effects at antidepressive doses, yet their low-dose use continues to have an important role in the treatment of chronic neuropathic pain.[69] The analgesic properties of TCAs are thought to be independent of their treatment effects on depression. TCAs are structurally related to phenothiazine antipsychotic agents and are named after their chemical structure comprised of two benzene rings joined to a seven-member ring containing nitrogen, oxygen, and carbon (Figures 16-5 and 16-6).[70]

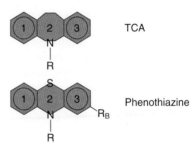

Figure 16-5 The figure at the top shows the prototypical three-ring structure of a tricyclic antidepressant (TCA). Notice its similarity to the structure of a phenothiazine-type antipsychotic drug pictured below. TCAs were originally modeled after this class of antipsychotic medications. R and R_B represent different side chains for the various phenothiazines.

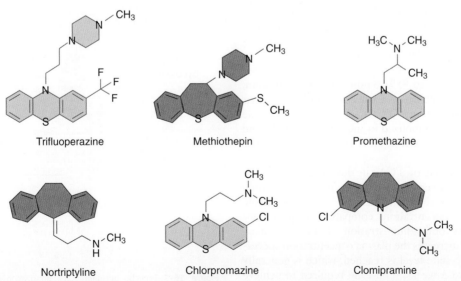

Trifluoperazine   Methiothepin   Promethazine

Nortriptyline   Chlorpromazine   Clomipramine

Figure 16-6 A comparison of the molecular structures of select phenothiazine-type medications (blue) and tricyclic antidepressants (red).

Mechanism of Action

The mechanism of action for the analgesic properties of TCAs is unknown but it is thought to be related to reuptake inhibition of serotonin and norepinephrine in the spinal cord and modulation of descending inhibitory pathways. In addition, many TCAs also have high affinity as *antagonists* at the 5-HT2 (5-HT2A and 5-HT2C), 5-HT6, 5-HT7, α1-adrenergic, and NMDA receptors. Sigma (σ1 and σ2) receptor (formally considered to be an opioid receptor) *agonism* is noted that may contribute to their efficacy as well as their side effects.[71-76]

Metabolism

The metabolism of tricyclics is dependent primarily on hepatic CYP 450 oxidative enzymes. Although the activities of some P450 isoenzymes are largely under genetic control, they may be influenced by patient variables, such as ethnicity and age, as well as the concomitant use of other medications or substances. Metabolism of TCAs, especially their hydroxylation, results in the formation of active metabolites, which contribute to both the therapeutic and the adverse effects of these compounds. Tertiary amines like amitriptyline and imipramine are demethylated to secondary amines, which retain clinical activity. Therefore, when parent compounds that generate active metabolites are prescribed, it is necessary to measure the total tricyclic concentration of clinically active substances in the when monitoring therapeutic concentrations.[77] The most important step in tricyclic metabolism involves forming inactive hydroxycompounds that are readily excreted in the urine. Renal clearance of TCA metabolites is reduced by normal aging, accounting for much of the increased risk of toxicity in older patients.[78]

Clinical Pharmacology

PHARMACOKINETICS

The most important factor influencing the pharmacokinetics of TCAs is their metabolism (discussed earlier). The pharmacokinetics of TCAs are characterized by substantial first-pass metabolism, a large volume of distribution, extensive protein binding, and an elimination half-life averaging about 1 to 3 days. The mean half-lives of amitriptyline and nortriptyline are about 21 and 32 hours, respectively, allowing for convenient once-daily dosing.[79] All of the tricyclic drugs are rapidly absorbed after oral administration and, at therapeutic plasma concentrations, are 90% to 95% bound to plasma albumin. They also bind to extravascular tissues, accounting for their large volumes of distribution.[80] TCAs are highly lipid-soluble drugs, are extensively metabolized in the liver, and are bound to tissues where their concentration is 10 to 20 times higher than plasma levels.[77]

Plasma concentrations of TCAs in the therapeutic range are thought to be between 50 and 300 ng/mL. Desipramine and nortriptyline, both secondary amines, have higher tissue and red blood cell concentrations compared to the tertiary amines.[80] Repetitive oral administration of TCAs at fixed doses and intervals increases the plasma concentration successively until a steady-state level is reached, which is generally attained within 1 to 3 weeks. The time required to achieve steady-state depends on the elimination rate and should be determined after five times the elimination plasma half-life. Individuals who metabolize TCAs very slowly ("slow hydroxylators") may require more than 3 weeks to reach steady-state plasma levels.[77]

PHARMACODYNAMICS

Therapeutic Effects

Numerous clinical trials have shown the efficacy of TCAs in treating chronic pain conditions. It is postulated that TCAs exert their therapeutic effects by increasing the levels of serotonin and norepinephrine in the spinal cord, enhancing the descending inhibitory pathways of pain modulation. The dorsolateral pontine tegmentum is the major source of noradrenergic neurons that project to the spinal dorsal horn, while the rostral ventromedial medulla is the primary source of serotonergic neurons that project to the spinal dorsal horn. Both norepinephrine and serotonin can inhibit nociceptive dorsal horn neurons when applied locally. Additional studies conclude that opioid analgesia is enhanced in the presence of antidepressant therapy.[81]

Adverse Effects

The pharmacodynamic effects of TCAs on norepinephrine and serotonin reuptake are complicated by their simultaneous activity at multiple other receptor types including muscarinic, α1-adrenergic, dopaminergic, and histamine H1 (Figure 16-7), resulting in the side effect profile listed in Table 16-4.

Common adverse effects of TCAs include sedation, urinary retention, gastrointestinal distress, dry mouth, and weight gain. Major adverse effects, typically only observed at higher doses, include Q-T prolongation, conduction abnormalities, cardiac arrest, hepatic failure, paralytic ileus, hyperthermia, orthostatic hypotension, decreased seizure threshold (see Figure 16-7 and Table 16-4).[82]

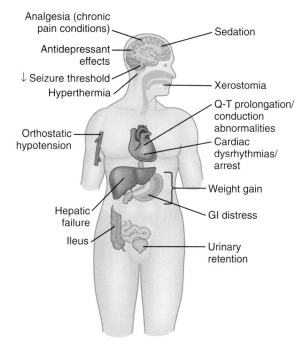

Figure 16-7 Tricyclic antidepressant pharmacodynamics: a summary of selected therapeutic and adverse effects.

Table 16-4. Common Side Effects Associated with Selected Tricyclic Antidepressants

	SEDATION	ANTICHOLINERGIC EFFECTS	HYPOTENSION	CARDIAC EFFECTS	SEIZURES	WEIGHT GAIN
Amitriptyline	+++	+++	+++	+++	++	++
Clomipramine	++	+++	++	+++	+++	+
Desipramine	0/+	+	+	++	+	+
Nortriptyline	+	+	+	++	+	+

Note marked differences in the toxicity of certain TCAs compared with others.
0/+, Minimal; *+*, mild; *++*, moderate; *+++*, moderately severe.

Toxic effects and fatalities are expected when TCA plasma concentrations reach approximately 1000 ng/mL, while the therapeutic concentration is in the 50 to 300 ng/mL range. Patients with plasma TCA concentrations greater than 450 ng/mL tend to develop CNS toxicity consisting of agitation, confusion, and memory impairment. Major toxicity and death is associated with concentrations above 1000 ng/mL.[80]

Drug Interactions

The degree of drug interactions with TCAs is largely dependent upon the specific tricyclic agent used and its relative inhibitory potential of hepatic CYP 450 oxidative enzymes. Desipramine and nortriptyline have the least drug interactions because they are weak CYP 450 2D6 inhibitors and are unlikely to be involved in clinically relevant interactions unless the serum levels are high, for example following overdose, or in "slow hydroxylators." Amitriptyline, imipramine, clomipramine, dothiepin, and doxepin, all tertiary amines, are more potent CYP 450 inhibitors and therefore are more problematic in terms of drug interactions.[80]

It is important to use extreme caution when prescribing TCAs in patients taking monoamine oxidase inhibitors (MAOIs), SSRIs, or other anticholinergics. Cimetidine, haloperidol, and phenothiazines can increase TCA plasma levels. Drugs such as carbamazepine, a CYP 450 inducer, may reduce plasma levels of tricyclics. Concomitant use of NSAIDs or warfarin can increase the risk of gastrointestinal bleeding due to the inhibitory effect of serotonin on platelet aggregation.[83-85]

TCAs are known to prolong the QTc interval so care should be taken with the concomitant use of other agents associated with QT prolongation, potentially proarrhythmic medications, sodium channel blockers, cardiac glycosides, and noradrenergic drugs, such as cocaine and amphetamines.

Special Populations

In patients with cardiovascular diseases (e.g., coronary artery disease, hypertension, arrhythmias), the previously discussed cardiovascular risks of tricyclics are compounded. Older patients receiving TCAs may be more predisposed to orthostatic hypotension and falls, and are more susceptible to the cognitive side effects due to factors such as altered renal metabolism and protein binding.[86] Selection of a less anticholinergic TCA, low initial dose, slow titration, and follow up of blood pressure (measured both when supine and standing) is recommended in older patients.[80] Observational studies showed increased mortality after myocardial infarction in patients using type 1A antiarrhythmic agents; therefore TCAs are contraindicated after a recent myocardial infarction.[87]

It is recommended that patients with liver disease have laboratory screening of serum electrolytes and liver function tests before initiation of TCA treatment with caution advised during dose titration.

TCAs should be used with caution in patients with renal dysfunction because metabolites are excreted in the urine. Chronic kidney disease affects TCA elimination by changing glomerular blood flow and filtration, tubular secretion and reabsorption, and renal bioactivation and metabolism. It is therefore recommended to reduce the drug dose and slowly titrate based upon serum drug concentration monitoring (including the active metabolites).[87]

Unique Features of Individual Agents

In general, TCAs are equally effective in their treatment of neuropathic pain and the choice of a particular agent is usually determined based upon the side effect profile.

Amitriptyline blocks the reuptake of both norepinephrine and serotonin, but it more potently blocks the reuptake of the former. It has a high affinity for histamine H1 and muscarinic M1 receptors; compared with other tricyclics, it is highly sedating and associated with weight gain and more anticholinergic side effects (Table 16-4).

Desipramine also blocks the reuptake of norepinephrine and serotonin, but it has more affinity for norepinephrine reuptake blockade. It has less affinity for histamine H1 receptors, thereby resulting in less sedation in comparison to other TCAs. It also has less affinity for muscarinic M1 receptors and therefore has less anticholinergic effects.

Doxepin, also FDA approved for anxiety disorders, has the highest affinity for histamine H1 receptors, is highly sedating, and is associated with weight gain.

Imipramine is similar to amitriptyline in terms of its ability to block norepinephrine and serotonin reuptake, but it also has strong affinities for α-adrenergic, histamine H1, and muscarinic M1 receptors. Hence, it is associated with orthostasis, sedation, weight gain, and anticholinergic side effects; however, the intensity of these symptoms is less than those of amitriptyline. Imipramine is demethylated in the liver to desipramine.

Nortriptyline, the active metabolite of amitriptyline, is similar to desipramine in that it has more affinity for blocking the reuptake of norepinephrine over serotonin. It has relatively less affinity for histamine H1 and muscarinic M1 receptors and therefore has a more favorable side effect profile.

Common Clinical Indications

TCAs are now rarely used for the management of depressive disorders but have become a mainstay in the treatment of several chronic pain syndromes. According to guidelines published by the IASP, low-dose TCAs are recommended as first line therapy in many neuropathic pain conditions including diabetic neuropathy, post-herpetic neuralgia, and central pain syndromes.[88]

Numerous studies show that TCAs are effective in treating chronic nonmalignant pain, including diabetic neuropathic pain, post-herpetic neuralgia, radicular pain, and pain originating from conditions such as human immunodeficiency virus (HIV), complex regional pain syndrome, and autoimmune disorders. TCAs have also been used in fibromyalgia, temporomandibular joint disorder, interstitial cystitis, phantom limb pain, premenstrual pain, and pelvic pain, and are a mainstay in preventive treatment of migraine and tension headaches. Mixed data support the efficacy of TCAs in surgical acute pain as an adjunctive medication in patients recovering from amputation and traumatic or surgical nerve injuries.[89,90]

Many prescribers take advantage of the sedating histaminergic side effects of tricyclics by prescribing them as sleep aids. In general, TCAs promote initiation and continuity of sleep while suppressing rapid eye movement sleep in a dose-dependent manner.[91]

Rational Drug Selection

As discussed earlier, the basic approach to prescribing TCAs is based on the side effect profiles in that they tend to vary from each drug in this class. In general, desipramine and nortriptyline have the most favorable side effect profiles. However, because they have more affinity for norepinephrine reuptake blockade as opposed to serotonin or histamine H1, they can be very activating and may not be suitable for use before bedtime.

Tricyclics (e.g., doxepin and amitriptyline) have more affinity to histamine H1 receptors, thereby possessing sedative qualities that can be useful in patients with insomnia.

GABAPENTIN AND PREGABALIN

Pharmacology

Neuropathic pain resulting from peripheral nerve sensitization and ectopic transmission of noxious stimuli can resemble the abnormal hyperexcitability of neuronal transmission seen in epileptic disorders. The use of anticonvulsant agents by the mainstream pain medicine community has a long history but evidence of their efficacy often came later, as practitioners first used these antiepileptic agents "off label" before rigorous scientific validation was achieved. Numerous anticonvulsants have been used in the treatment of neuropathic pain, including phenytoin, topiramate, carbamazepine, and sodium valproate. While some of these agents continue to be used for certain conditions (e.g., carbamazepine for trigeminal neuralgia) the newer anticonvulsants with FDA approval for the management of pain—gabapentin and pregabalin—have largely supplanted their role. These second generation antiepileptic medications, referred to as *gabapentinoids*, provide much better tolerability in terms of side effects and toxicity, and offer greater receptor selectivity than first generation drugs.[82]

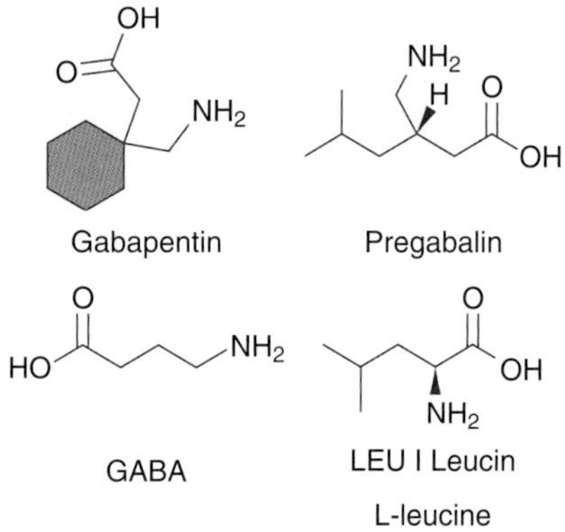

Figure 16-8 A comparison of the chemical structures of gabapentin, pregabalin, the neurotransmitter GABA, and the amino acid L-leucine.

Gabapentin and pregabalin are branched-chain amino acids and chemical analogues of the neurotransmitter GABA. Despite their name, neither drug has activity in the GABAergic neurotransmission system. They are functionally similar to the essential amino acid leucine in that they competitively bind $\alpha_2\delta$ calcium channel subunits (Figure 16-8).[86] Gabapentin is described as 1-(aminomethyl)cyclohexaneacetic acid ($C_9H_{17}NO_2$), while the chemical name of pregabalin is (S)-3-(aminomethyl)-5-methylhexanoic acid ($C_8H_{17}NO_2$).[92,93]

Mechanism

The mechanism of action for gabapentin and pregabalin is also uncertain, but both drugs have high binding affinities to the $\alpha_2\delta$-1 subunit of presynaptic voltage-gated calcium channels in the CNS.[94] Their analgesic effects may be related to calcium influx inhibition as well as inhibition of the release of excitatory neurotransmitters in spinal and supraspinal pathways.[82] It is hypothesized that conditions such as neuropathic pain and epilepsy may involve excessive formation of excitatory synapses. A recent study showed that by binding to this $\alpha_2\delta$-1 subunit, gabapentin prevents the binding of thrombospondin, a synaptogenic protein secreted by astrocytes, thereby impeding synapse formation between neurons.[95]

Animal studies using genetically modified mice show that selective binding to the $\alpha_2\delta$-1 subunit is necessary for these drugs to exert their antinociceptive, anticonvulsant, and anxiolytic effects.[96-98]

Metabolism

The metabolic profiles of gabapentin and pregabalin are very similar. Both drugs are metabolized to their corresponding N-methyl metabolite in dogs but undergo minimal metabolism in humans.[86]

Clinical Pharmacology

PHARMACOKINETICS

Gabapentin and pregabalin readily disintegrate after oral administration but there are some significant differences in the absorption of the two drugs related to the L-amino acid transporter (LAT) system that facilitates the absorption of large, neutral amino acids as well as the absorption of both gabapentin and pregabalin.[100] Preclinical data suggest that gabapentin is transported solely by the LAT1 transporter, which results in dose-limited absorption due to nearly maximal transporter saturation at a dose of 2400 to 2700 mg/day. The absorption of pregabalin is also facilitated by the LAT family of transporters but is also mediated by an additional pathway allowing almost complete, nonsaturable incorporation into the bloodstream.[101] Therefore pregabalin displays linear pharmacokinetics over its recommended oral dose range of 75 to 900 mg/day (Figure 16-9).[86,101] Gabapentin has an elimination half-life of 5 to 7 hours, and is primarily excreted unchanged in the urine with 10% to 23% excretion in the feces. The renal clearance of gabapentin does decrease in patients with kidney disease, and the drug is dialyzable.[99] Pregabalin has a mean elimination half-life of 6.3 hours, does not undergo any protein binding in the plasma, and has negligible metabolism. Approximately 98% of the dose is excreted unchanged in the urine. Pregabalin blood concentrations can be reduced by 50% by hemodialysis but a supplementary pregabalin dose of 25 to 100 mg after dialysis may be used to restore a therapeutic level.[99]

Peak plasma concentration after gabapentin absorption occurs 1.5 to 4 hours after administration of an oral dose and its oral bioavailability is dose dependent with minimal additional absorption achieved after a dose of 2700 mg/day. Pregabalin is rapidly absorbed after oral administration with 90% bioavailability and peak plasma concentrations seen after just 1 hour. Steady-state concentrations of pregabalin in plasma are seen after approximately 1 to 2 days of treatment.[99,101]

PHARMACODYNAMICS
Therapeutic Effects
Gabapentin and pregabalin bind the $\alpha_2\delta$-1 subunit of presynaptic voltage-gated calcium channels in the dorsal horn of the spinal cord and brain thereby preventing calcium influx and the release of excitatory neurotransmitters.[93] As stated earlier, the mechanism by which both drugs exert their analgesic

properties is unknown, and although both drugs are structural analogues of GABA, neither modify this neurotransmitter nor are they converted metabolically into GABA or a GABA agonist. In addition, neither drug inhibits GABA reuptake or degradation.[92]

Adverse Effects

With careful dosing, gabapentin and pregabalin are typically well tolerated medications. Dizziness and somnolence are the most commonly reported adverse effect of both drugs, and the latter is the most frequent reason for discontinuation. Other reported side effects include xerostomia, peripheral edema, angioedema, blurred vision, ataxia, dysarthria, tremor, lethargy, memory impairment, euphoria, constipation, decrease or loss of libido, and weight gain (Figure 16-10). The adverse effects of gabapentinoids are reversible and dose dependent.

Abrupt discontinuation and withdrawal of gabapentinoids may precipitate seizures, particularly in a patient with a preexisting seizure disorder. Anxiety, insomnia, nausea, pain, and sweating are the most frequently reported adverse events following abrupt discontinuation. It is recommended that these medications be gradually tapered over the course of at least 1 week to avoid these symptoms.[92,93]

Drug Interactions

Because gabapentin undergoes minimal metabolism, it is unlikely to have any interactions with other medications. Concomitant administration of other antiepileptic drugs including phenobarbital, carbamazepine, valproate, and phenytoin do not alter gabapentin pharmacokinetics.[100] Gabapentin does not induce or inhibit hepatic enzymes and therefore it does not appear to be affected by drugs that are

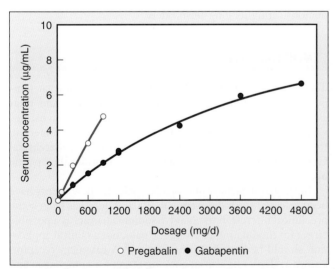

Figure 16-9 Mean steady-state minimum plasma drug concentration values in 33 healthy subjects given oral pregabalin or gabapentin every 8 hours. Note the more linear dose-to-serum concentration relationship of pregabalin compared with gabapentin. *(From Bockbrader HN, Wesche D, Miller R, et al. A comparison of the pharmacokinetics and pharmacodynamics of pregabalin and gabapentin. Clin Pharmacokinet. 2010;49:661-669.)*

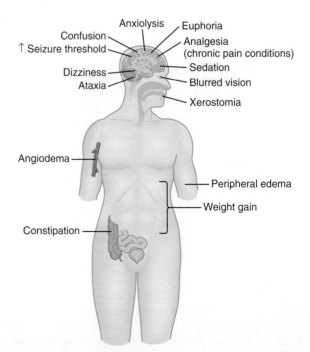

Figure 16-10 Gabapentinoid pharmacodynamics: a summary of selected therapeutic and adverse effects.

inducers or inhibitors of cytochrome P450 enzymes. The use of antacids aluminum hydroxide and magnesium hydroxide may reduce the bioavailability of gabapentin by up to 20%. It is therefore recommended that gabapentin should not be administered until at least 2 hours after antacid use. Agents that prolong the transit time of gabapentin in the small intestine could potentially increase its bioavailability. One study demonstrated that gabapentin's bioavailability was increased by 50% when a 600-mg dose was coadministered with oral morphine.[102] A statistically significant but clinically irrelevant decrease was reported in the oral clearance of gabapentin with the concurrent use of cimetidine.[100]

Pregabalin is also similarly unlikely to be associated with any pharmacokinetic drug interactions as it does not undergo hepatic metabolism and does not induce or inhibit cytochrome P450 enzyme systems. Studies in healthy volunteers as well as various other patient populations show that the pharmacokinetics of pregabalin were not significantly altered by simultaneous administration of lorazepam, oxycodone, alcohol, oral contraceptive drugs, antihyperglycemics, furosemide, and numerous other anticonvulsants. Concomitant use of pregabalin with oxycodone or alcohol had an additive effect on cognitive and gross motor functioning, but not respiration.[103] Furthermore, pregabalin does not demonstrate any changes in its bioavailability when administered with agents that reduce gastrointestinal transit time.

Special Populations

Gabapentinoids are excreted almost exclusively by the renal system and their clearance is directly related to creatinine clearance. Numerous studies have shown that serum levels of gabapentin and pregabalin increased with decreasing renal function, and that both drugs are readily dialyzable. Therefore, dosage adjustments based on creatinine clearance are necessary in patients with renal dysfunction or those on hemodialysis. The pharmacokinetics of both drugs are not affected by sex or race, but clearance is decreased in older patients secondary to age-related changes in renal function.[102-104]

Unique Features of Individual Agents

The slight differences in the chemical structure of gabapentin and pregabalin differentiate their pharmacokinetic and pharmacodynamic properties. Pregabalin is advantageous in that it possesses nonsaturable absorption at clinically relevant doses resulting in linear pharmacokinetics. Pregabalin also has a steeper dose response relationship than gabapentin (see Figure 16-9), and appears to achieve a greater treatment effect in post-herpetic neuralgia and epilepsy.[86]

Pregabalin has more selective binding to the $\alpha_2\delta$-1 subunit, has a more favorable side effect profile, and has a simpler, twice-a-day dosing regimen versus gabapentin, which must be dosed three times per day.

Common Clinical Indications

Gabapentin is currently FDA approved for post-herpetic neuralgia and partial seizures, while pregabalin is FDA approved for partial seizures, painful diabetic peripheral neuropathy, post-herpetic neuralgia, and fibromyalgia. Furthermore, recent guidelines published by the IASP recommend both

drugs as first-line therapy for these conditions as well as central pain syndromes such as central post-stroke pain and pain related to spinal cord injury and multiple sclerosis.[88]

Numerous studies show the efficacy of gabapentin in HIV-related neuropathic pain, pain associated with Guillain-Barré syndrome, neuropathic cancer pain, complex regional pain syndrome, phantom limb pain, and neuropathic pain in spinal cord injury patients. In addition to its FDA-approved indications, pregabalin has also been shown to be effective in treating generalized anxiety and social anxiety disorders.[105]

Newer studies that have investigated the role of gabapentinoids in managing postoperative pain have yielded mixed results. While some studies that looked at the administration of gabapentin to patients undergoing craniotomies, thoracotomies, and thyroidectomies showed favorable results in terms of controlling acute pain as well as preventing chronic pain, others show that it is an inferior as a single agent compared to numerous other drugs used in this setting.[106]

The same holds true for pregabalin, in that some studies show it may decrease perioperative opioid and epidural use in patients with more acute neuropathic pain than acute inflammatory pain, and it may also decrease the incidence of chronic pain when surgery involves a more neuropathic type acute pain process.[107] A large metaanalysis of numerous randomized controlled trials showed no clear beneficial effect of pregabalin in acute postoperative pain.[108]

Rational Drug Selection

For the most part, gabapentin and pregabalin have minimal drug interactions making them versatile drugs in combination with other neuropathic pain medications. Gabapentin is also relatively less expensive in that it is available in a generic form and available in most inpatient and outpatient settings.[92] Pregabalin has the advantage of high oral bioavailability that results in predictable dose-dependent responses, and has a short titration period that is better tolerated by patients. Because it is a newer drug, pregabalin is relatively expensive with no generic formulation, and there are limited studies demonstrating its long-term safety.[70]

EMERGING DEVELOPMENTS

The development of new NSAIDs has been somewhat tempered by the controversies surrounding NSAIDs and their associations with increased morbidity and mortality in cardiovascular disease. In perioperative medicine, practitioners in the United States do not yet have access to a parenteral COX-2 inhibitor and eagerly await this important therapeutic option.

In the battle against neuropathic pain, no new agents have been released since duloxetine in 2004. There has been some preclinical interest in the Nav1.7 sodium channel as a possible target for modulating neuropathic pain, but a clinical application should be considered futuristic.[109] A capsaicin receptor, known as TrpV1, is also an enticing target for antagonism and analgesia, but clinical trials of various TrpV1 antagonists have been discontinued due to unfavorable adverse effects.[110]

Ziconotide is a novel conopeptide isolated from the venom of the marine snail, *Conus magus*, and has shown analgesic efficacy in the treatment of refractory chronic pain.[111,112] The unique analgesic properties of ziconotide are mediated by blockade of N-type voltage-sensitive calcium channels, inhibiting depolarization-induced calcium influx and reducing neurotransmitter release from nociceptive afferents. Ziconotide is suitable for intrathecal use only, and no development of tolerance, respiratory depression, drug dependence, or withdrawal symptoms have been reported in numerous studies. Various other marine peptides have been isolated with often fascinating properties, but no analgesics have achieved clinical success since ziconotide was approved by the FDA in 2004.[113]

KEY POINTS

- NSAIDs inhibit the conversion of arachidonic acid to prostaglandins, thromboxane, and prostacyclin.
- NSAIDs are generally well tolerated, but distinct toxicities exist; patient comorbidities and the clinical scenario should be considered carefully when prescribing.
- Controversies exist regarding NSAIDs and perioperative hemostasis. While NSAIDs rarely cause clinically significant hemostatic derangement, they should be used with caution when other causes of coagulopathy exist.
- COX-2 inhibitors do not affect platelet function and should be considered when there are concerns regarding postoperative hemostasis.
- Gastrointestinal toxicity is rarely a problem with the short-term, perioperative use of NSAIDs, but is a significant cause of morbidity and mortality with long-term use.
- NSAIDs are safe and useful adjuncts in the management of noncardiac postoperative pain.
- COX-1 and COX-2 inhibitors should be avoided in patients with renal insufficiency.
- Topical NSAIDs can produce local therapeutic effects without significant systemic drug levels, therefore avoiding the adverse effects of oral agents.
- Acetaminophen, available in oral, rectal, and intravenous formulations, is useful for the management of mild to moderate pain, and at appropriate therapeutic doses lacks the toxicity associated with NSAIDs.
- The analgesic properties of TCAs are thought to be related to reuptake inhibition of serotonin and norepinephrine.
- TCA adverse side effects include QT prolongation, conduction abnormalities, orthostatic hypotension, anticholinergic effects, weight gain, and sedation.
- Gabapentinoids bind to the $\alpha_2\delta$-1 subunit of presynaptic voltage-gated Ca^{2+} channels in the CNS; their analgesic effects might be related to inhibition of Ca^{2+} influx and the release of excitatory neurotransmitters in spinal and supraspinal pathways.
- Gabapentinoids are structural analogues of GABA but have no GABA receptor effects.
- Dizziness and somnolence are the most commonly reported adverse effects of gabapentinoids.
- Gabapentin is approved for post-herpetic neuralgia and partial seizures. Pregabalin is approved for partial seizures, painful diabetic peripheral neuropathy, post-herpetic neuralgia, and fibromyalgia.
- There are mixed results regarding the efficacy of gabapentinoids in treating acute postoperative pain.

Key References

Bockbrader HN, Wesche D, Miller R, et al. A comparison of the pharmacokinetics and pharmacodynamics of pregabalin and gabapentin. *Clin Pharmacokinet*. 2010;49:661-669. This article presents an extensive head-to-head comparison of the pharmacokinetics of pregabalin and gabapentin while highlighting their differences in bioavailability and the rationale behind maximal dose titration. (Ref. 86)

Cardwell M, Siviter G, Smith A. Non-steroidal anti-inflammatory drugs and perioperative bleeding in paediatric tonsillectomy. *Cochrane Database Syst Rev*. 2005;(2):CD003591. This careful review concludes that perioperative use of NSAIDs does not result in an increased reoperation rate in pediatric tonsillectomy. (Ref. 32)

Egan KM, Wang M, Fries S, et al. Cyclooxygenases, thromboxane, and atherosclerosis: plaque destabilization by cyclooxygenase-2 inhibition combined with thromboxane receptor antagonism. *Circulation*. 2005;111:334-342. This paper provides an overview of the complex field of vascular endothelial homeostasis and how NSAIDs can potentially derange healthy function and result in cardiovascular morbidity. (Ref. 6)

Elia N, Lysakowski C, Tramer MR. Does multimodal analgesia with acetaminophen, nonsteroidal antiinflammatory drugs, or selective cyclooxygenase-2 inhibitors and patient-controlled analgesia morphine offer advantages over morphine alone? Meta-analyses of randomized trials. *Anesthesiology*. 2005;103:1296-1304. This is an important work that carefully analyzes the effects of non-opioid analgesics on various perioperative outcomes. (Ref. 26)

Gajraj NM. The effect of cyclooxygenase-2 inhibitors on bone healing. *Reg Anesth Pain Med*. 2003;28:456-465. This paper presents a balanced interpretation of the literature pertaining to NSAIDs and bone healing. (Ref. 22)

Gillman PK. Tricyclic antidepressant pharmacology and therapeutic drug interactions updated. *Br J Pharmacol*. 2007;151:737-748. This paper offers an updated review of the TCA pharmacology and drug interactions by incorporating new data resulting from assays using human cloned receptors (HCRs) which allow more accurate measurement of affinities at a range of CNS receptors. (Ref. 80)

McGettigan P, Henry D. Cardiovascular risk and inhibition of cyclooxygenase: a systematic review of the observational studies of selective and nonselective inhibitors of cyclooxygenase 2. *JAMA*. 2006;296:1633-1644. This carefully conducted review analyzed multiple studies in an attempt to classify different NSAIDs in terms of their cardiovascular risk. Their data confirmed the safety concerns of rofecoxib, but supported the relative cardiovascular safety of celecoxib and naproxen, and raised concerns about the safety of diclofenac. (Ref. 15)

Molnar G, Gupta RN. Plasma levels and tricyclic antidepressant therapy: Part 2 Pharmacokinetic, clinical and toxicologic aspects. *Biopharm Drug Dispos*. 1980;1:283-305. This is one of the first review articles to cover the clinically relevant aspects of TCA plasma levels and their relationship to biologic action with respect to pharmacokinetic factors, clinical correlation, and toxicology. (Ref. 77)

Moore RA, Straube S, Wiffen PJ, et al. Pregabalin for acute and chronic pain in adults. *Cochrane Database Syst Rev*. 2009;(3):CD007076. This is the first meta-analysis of double-blind randomized controlled trials that explored the analgesic effects of pregabalin with pain assessment as the primary or secondary endpoint. This confirmed a modest utility for chronic neuropathic pain, but showed a lack of efficacy for acute pain. (Ref. 108)

Samad TA, Sapirstein A, Woolf CJ. Prostanoids and pain: unraveling mechanisms and revealing therapeutic targets. *Trends Mol Med*. 2002;8:390-396. This is a very nice overview of the physiology of prostanoids and how nonsteroidal antiinflammatory agents modulate their function. A thorough understanding of this topic is essential to the understanding of both the therapeutic effects and toxicities of NSAIDs. (Ref. 2)

Schafer AI. Effects of nonsteroidal antiinflammatory drugs on platelet function and systemic hemostasis. *J Clin Pharmacol*. 1995;35:209-219. This useful paper gives a practical discussion of how aspirin and NSAIDs impact hemostasis. (Ref. 8)

Straube S, Derry S, Moore RA, et al. Single dose oral gabapentin for established acute postoperative pain in adults. *Cochrane Database Syst Rev*. 2010;(5):CD008183. This metaanalysis examined the efficacy and adverse effects of single dose oral gabapentin for established acute postoperative pain using methods that permit comparison with other analgesics evaluated in standardized trials using almost identical methods and outcomes. (Ref. 106)

References

1. Practice guidelines for acute pain management in the perioperative setting: an updated report by the American Society of Anesthesiologists Task Force on Acute Pain Management. *Anesthesiology*. 2004;100(6):1573-1581.
2. Samad TA, Sapirstein A, Woolf CJ. Prostanoids and pain: unraveling mechanisms and revealing therapeutic targets. *Trends Mol Med*. 2002;8(8):390-396.
3. O'Banion MK. Cyclooxygenase-2: molecular biology, pharmacology, and neurobiology. *Crit Rev Neurobiol*. 1999;13(1):45-82.
4. Montane E, et al. Analgesics for pain after traumatic or orthopaedic surgery: what is the evidence—a systematic review. *Eur J Clin Pharmacol*. 2006;62(11):971-988.
5. Tramer MR, et al. Comparing analgesic efficacy of non-steroidal anti-inflammatory drugs given by different routes in acute and chronic pain: a qualitative systematic review. *Acta Anaesthesiol Scand*. 1998;42(1):71-79.
6. Egan KM, et al. Cyclooxygenases, thromboxane, and atherosclerosis: plaque destabilization by cyclooxygenase-2 inhibition combined with thromboxane receptor antagonism. *Circulation*. 2005;111(3):334-342.
7. Kearney PM, et al. Do selective cyclo-oxygenase-2 inhibitors and traditional non-steroidal anti-inflammatory drugs increase the risk of atherothrombosis? Meta-analysis of randomised trials. *BMJ*. 2006;332(7553):1302-1308.
8. Schafer AI. Effects of nonsteroidal antiinflammatory drugs on platelet function and systemic hemostasis. *J Clin Pharmacol*. 1995;35(3):209-219.
9. Whelton A. COX-2-specific inhibitors and the kidney: effect on hypertension and oedema. *J Hypertens Suppl*. 2002;20(6):S31-S35.
10. Roumie CL, et al. Nonaspirin NSAIDs, cyclooxygenase 2 inhibitors, and the risk for stroke. *Stroke*. 2008;39(7):2037-2045.
11. Andersohn F. et al. Cyclooxygenase-2 selective nonsteroidal anti-inflammatory drugs and the risk of ischemic stroke: a nested case-control study. *Stroke*. 2006;37(7):1725-1730.
12. Nussmeier NA, et al. Complications of the COX-2 inhibitors parecoxib and valdecoxib after cardiac surgery. *N Engl J Med*. 2005;352(11):1081-1091.
13. Ott E, et al. Efficacy and safety of the cyclooxygenase 2 inhibitors parecoxib and valdecoxib in patients undergoing coronary artery bypass surgery. *J Thorac Cardiovasc Surg*. 2003;125(6):1481-1492.
14. Schug SA, et al. Cardiovascular safety of the cyclooxygenase-2 selective inhibitors parecoxib and valdecoxib in the postoperative setting: an analysis of integrated data. *Anesth Analg*. 2009;108(1):299-307.
15. McGettigan P, Henry D. Cardiovascular risk and inhibition of cyclooxygenase: a systematic review of the observational studies of selective and nonselective inhibitors of cyclooxygenase 2. *JAMA*. 2006;296(13):1633-1644.
16. Dunstan CR, et al. Systemic administration of acidic fibroblast growth factor (FGF-1) prevents bone loss and increases new bone formation in ovariectomized rats. *J Bone Miner Res*. 1999;14(6):953-959.
17. Seidenberg AB, An YH. Is there an inhibitory effect of COX-2 inhibitors on bone healing? *Pharmacol Res*. 2004;50(2):151-156.
18. Allen HL, Wase A, Bear WT. Indomethacin and aspirin: effect of nonsteroidal anti-inflammatory agents on the rate of fracture repair in the rat. *Acta Orthop Scand*. 1980;51(4):595-600.
19. Bo J, Sudmann E, Marton PF. Effect of indomethacin on fracture healing in rats. *Acta Orthop Scand*. 1976;47(6):588-599.
20. Fransen M, Neal B. Non-steroidal anti-inflammatory drugs for preventing heterotopic bone formation after hip arthroplasty. *Cochrane Database Syst Rev*. 2004;(3):CD001160.
21. Simon AM, Manigrasso MB, O'Connor JP. Cyclo-oxygenase 2 function is essential for bone fracture healing. *J Bone Miner Res*. 2002;17(6):963-976.
22. Gajraj NM. The effect of cyclooxygenase-2 inhibitors on bone healing. *Reg Anesth Pain Med*. 2003;28(5):456-465.
23. Glassman SD, et al. The effect of postoperative nonsteroidal anti-inflammatory drug administration on spinal fusion. *Spine*. 1998;23(7):834-838.
24. Pradhan BB, et al. Ketorolac and spinal fusion: does the perioperative use of ketorolac really inhibit spinal fusion? *Spine*. 2008;33(19):2079-2082.
25. Li Q, Zhang Z, Cai Z. High-dose ketorolac affects adult spinal fusion: a meta-analysis of the effect of perioperative nonsteroidal anti-inflammatory drugs on spinal fusion. *Spine*. 2011;36(7):E461-E468.
26. Elia N, Lysakowski C, Tramer MR. Does multimodal analgesia with acetaminophen, nonsteroidal antiinflammatory drugs, or selective cyclooxygenase-2 inhibitors and patient-controlled analgesia morphine offer advantages over morphine alone? Meta-analyses of randomized trials. *Anesthesiology*. 2005;103(6):1296-1304.
27. Szczeklik A, Gryglewski RJ, Czerniawska-Mysik G. Clinical patterns of hypersensitivity to nonsteroidal anti-inflammatory drugs and their pathogenesis. *J Allergy Clin Immunol*. 1977;60(5):276-284.
28. Bavbek S, et al. Safety of selective COX-2 inhibitors in aspirin/nonsteroidal anti-inflammatory drug-intolerant patients: comparison of nimesulide, meloxicam, and rofecoxib. *J Asthma*. 2004;41(1):67-75.
29. Dona I, et al. Response to a selective COX-2 inhibitor in patients with urticaria/angioedema induced by nonsteroidal anti-inflammatory drugs. *Allergy*. 2011;66(11):1428-1433.
30. Cryer B. NSAID-associated deaths: the rise and fall of NSAID-associated GI mortality. *Am J Gastroenterol*. 2005;100(8):1694-1695.
31. An HS, et al. Effects of hypotensive anesthesia, nonsteroidal anti-inflammatory drugs, and polymethylmethacrylate on bleeding in total hip arthroplasty patients. *J Arthroplasty*. 1991;6(3):245-250.
32. Cardwell M, Siviter G, Smith A. Non-steroidal anti-inflammatory drugs and perioperative bleeding in paediatric tonsillectomy. *Cochrane Database Syst Rev*. 2005;(2):CD003591.
33. Reiter R, Resch U, Sinzinger H. Do human platelets express COX-2? *Prostaglandins Leukot Essent Fatty Acids*. 2001;64(6):299-305.
34. Taber SS, Mueller BA. Drug-associated renal dysfunction. *Crit Care Clin*. 2006;22(2):357-374.
35. O'Connor N, Dargan PI, Jones AL. Hepatocellular damage from non-steroidal anti-inflammatory drugs. *QJM*. 2003;96(11):787-791.
36. Verbeeck RK. Pathophysiologic factors affecting the pharmacokinetics of nonsteroidal antiinflammatory drugs. *J Rheumatol Suppl*. 1988;17:44-57.
37. Chutka DS, Takahashi PY, Hoel RW. Inappropriate medications for elderly patients. *Mayo Clin Proc*. 2004;79(1):122-139.
38. Stouten EM, et al. Comparison of ketorolac and morphine for postoperative pain after major surgery. *Acta Anaesthesiol Scand*. 1992;36(7):716-721.
39. Cepeda MS, et al. Comparison of morphine, ketorolac, and their combination for postoperative pain: results from a large, randomized, double-blind trial. *Anesthesiology*. 2005;103(6):1225-1232.
40. Strom BL, et al. Parenteral ketorolac and risk of gastrointestinal and operative site bleeding. A postmarketing surveillance study. *Jama*. 1996;275(5):376-382.
41. Torodol Package Insert. 2009 [cited 2011 February]; available from: http://www.bedfordlabs.com/BedfordLabsWeb/products/inserts/Div-KRL-P05.pdf.
42. Chandrasekharan NV, et al. COX-3, a cyclooxygenase-1 variant inhibited by acetaminophen and other analgesic/antipyretic drugs: cloning, structure, and expression. *Proc Natl Acad Sci U S A*. 2002;99(21):13926-13931.
43. Pickering G, et al. Acetaminophen reinforces descending inhibitory pain pathways. *Clin Pharmacol Ther*. 2008;84(1):47-51.
44. Hama AT, Sagen J. Cannabinoid receptor-mediated antinociception with acetaminophen drug combinations in rats with neuropathic spinal cord injury pain. *Neuropharmacology*. 2011;58(4-5):758-766.
45. Gaziano JM. Nonnarcotic analgesics and hypertension. *Am J Cardiol*. 2006;97(9A):10-16.

46. Mazer M, Perrone J. Acetaminophen-induced nephrotoxicity: pathophysiology, clinical manifestations, and management. *J Med Toxicol*. 2008;4(1):2-6.

47. Steventon GB, Mitchell SC, Waring RH. Human metabolism of paracetamol (acetaminophen) at different dose levels. *Drug Metabol Drug Interact*. 1996;13(2):111-117.

48. Stewart DM, et al. Acetaminophen overdose: a growing health care hazard. *Clin Toxicol*. 1979;14(5):507-513.

49. Bertin P, Keddad K, Jolivet-Landreau I. Acetaminophen as symptomatic treatment of pain from osteoarthritis. *Joint Bone Spine*. 2004;71(4):266-274.

50. Cobby TF, et al. Rectal paracetamol has a significant morphine-sparing effect after hysterectomy. *Br J Anaesth*. 1999;83(2):253-256.

51. Cattabriga I, et al. Intravenous paracetamol as adjunctive treatment for postoperative pain after cardiac surgery: a double blind randomized controlled trial. *Eur J Cardiothorac Surg*. 2007;32(3):527-531.

52. Delbos A, Boccard E. The morphine-sparing effect of propacetamol in orthopedic postoperative pain. *J Pain Symptom Manage*. 1995;10(4):279-286.

53. Ofirmev, package insert. 2011 [cited 2011 October]; available from: http://www.ofirmev.com/pdf/OFIRMEVPrescribingInformation.pdf.

54. Sinatra RS, et al. Efficacy and safety of single and repeated administration of 1 gram intravenous acetaminophen injection (paracetamol) for pain management after major orthopedic surgery. *Anesthesiology*. 2005;102(4):822-831.

55. Buvanendran A, et al. Upregulation of prostaglandin E2 and interleukins in the central nervous system and peripheral tissue during and after surgery in humans. *Anesthesiology*. 2006;104(3):403-410.

56. Buvanendran A, et al. Effects of perioperative administration of a selective cyclooxygenase 2 inhibitor on pain management and recovery of function after knee replacement: a randomized controlled trial. *JAMA*. 2003;290(18):2411-2418.

57. Buvanendran A, et al. Anesthetic techniques for minimally invasive total knee arthroplasty. *J Knee Surg*. 2006;19(2):133-136.

58. Romsing J, Moiniche S. A systematic review of COX-2 inhibitors compared with traditional NSAIDs, or different COX-2 inhibitors for post-operative pain. *Acta Anaesthesiol Scand*. 2004;48(5):525-546.

59. Ramiro S, Radner H, van der Heijde D, et al. Combination therapy for pain management in inflammatory arthritis (rheumatoid arthritis, ankylosing spondylitis, psoriatic arthritis, other spondyloarthritis). *Cochrane Database Syst Rev*. 2011;(10):CD008886.

60. Roelofs PD, et al. Non-steroidal anti-inflammatory drugs for low back pain. *Cochrane Database Syst Rev*. 2008;(1):CD000396.

61. Haroutiunian S, Drennan DA, Lipman AG. Topical NSAID therapy for musculoskeletal pain. *Pain Med*. 2010;11(4):535-549.

62. Mason L, et al. Topical NSAIDs for acute pain: a meta-analysis. *BMC Fam Pract*. 2004;5:10.

63. Roelofs PD, et al. Nonsteroidal anti-inflammatory drugs for low back pain: an updated Cochrane review. *Spine (Phila Pa 1976)*. 2008;33(16):1766-1774.

64. Simon LS, et al. Efficacy and safety of topical diclofenac containing dimethyl sulfoxide (DMSO) compared with those of topical placebo, DMSO vehicle and oral diclofenac for knee osteoarthritis. *Pain*. 2009;143(3):238-245.

65. Treede RD, et al. Neuropathic pain: redefinition and a grading system for clinical and research purposes. *Neurology*. 2008;70(18):1630-1635.

66. Gilron I, et al. Morphine, gabapentin, or their combination for neuropathic pain. *N Engl J Med*. 2005;352(13):1324-1334.

67. Eisenberg E, McNicol ED, Carr DB. Efficacy and safety of opioid agonists in the treatment of neuropathic pain of nonmalignant origin: systematic review and meta-analysis of randomized controlled trials. *JAMA*. 2005;293(24):3043-3052.

68. Kuhn R. The treatment of depressive states with G 22355 (imipramine hydrochloride). *Am J Psychiatry*. 1958;115(5):459-464.

69. Sindrup SH, Jensen TS. Efficacy of pharmacological treatments of neuropathic pain: an update and effect related to mechanism of drug action. *Pain*. 1999;83(3):389-400.

70. Sinatra RS JJ, Watkins-Pitchford JM. Overview and use of antidepressant analgesics in pain management. In: *The Essence of Analgesia and Analgesics*. New York, NY: Cambridge University Press; 2011:338-346.

71. Branchek TA, Blackburn TP. 5-ht6 receptors as emerging targets for drug discovery. *Annu Rev Pharmacol Toxicol*. 2000;40:319-334.

72. Cusack B, Nelson A, Richelson E. Binding of antidepressants to human brain receptors: focus on newer generation compounds. *Psychopharmacology (Berl)*. 1994;114(4):559-565.

73. Narita N, et al. Interactions of selective serotonin reuptake inhibitors with subtypes of sigma receptors in rat brain. *Eur J Pharmacol*. 1996;307(1):117-119.

74. Sanchez C, Hyttel J. Comparison of the effects of antidepressants and their metabolites on reuptake of biogenic amines and on receptor binding. *Cell Mol Neurobiol*. 1999;19(4):467-489.

75. Sills MA, Loo PS. Tricyclic antidepressants and dextromethorphan bind with higher affinity to the phencyclidine receptor in the absence of magnesium and L-glutamate. *Mol Pharmacol*. 1989;36(1):160-165.

76. Stam NJ, et al. Human serotonin 5-HT7 receptor: cloning and pharmacological characterisation of two receptor variants. *FEBS Lett*. 1997;413(3):489-494.

77. Molnar G, Gupta RN. Plasma levels and tricyclic antidepressant therapy: Part 2 Pharmacokinetic, clinical and toxicologic aspects. *Biopharm Drug Dispos*. 1980;1(6):283-305.

78. Rudorfer MV, Potter WZ. Metabolism of tricyclic antidepressants. *Cell Mol Neurobiol*. 1999;19(3):373-409.

79. Sinatra RS JJ, Watkins-Pitchford JM. Tricyclic antidepressants. In: *The Essence of Analgesia and Analgesics*. New York: Cambridge University Press; 2011:347-350.

80. Gillman PK. Tricyclic antidepressant pharmacology and therapeutic drug interactions updated. *Br J Pharmacol*. 2007;151(6):737-748.

81. Wasan AD SM, Clark MR. Psychiatric illness, depression, anxiety, and somatoform pain disorders. In: Fishman SM, Rathmell JP, ed. *Bonica's Management of Pain, B.J.*. Lippincott Williams & Wilkins; 2010:393-417.

82. Sinatra RS JJ, Watkins-Pitchford JM. *The Essence of Analgesia and Analgesics*. New York: Cambridge University Press; 2011:292-294.

83. Dalton SO, et al. Use of selective serotonin reuptake inhibitors and risk of upper gastrointestinal tract bleeding: a population-based cohort study. *Arch Intern Med*. 2003;163(1):59-64.

84. Dalton SO, Sorensen HT, Johansen C. SSRIs and upper gastrointestinal bleeding: what is known and how should it influence prescribing? *CNS Drugs*. 2006;20(2):143-151.

85. de Abajo FJ, Rodriguez LA, Montero D. Association between selective serotonin reuptake inhibitors and upper gastrointestinal bleeding: population based case-control study. *BMJ*. 1999;319(7217):1106-1109.

86. Bockbrader HN, et al. A comparison of the pharmacokinetics and pharmacodynamics of pregabalin and gabapentin. *Clin Pharmacokinet*. 2010;49(10):661-669.

87. Haanpaa ML, et al. Treatment considerations for patients with neuropathic pain and other medical comorbidities. *Mayo Clin Proc*. 2010;85(3 Suppl):S15-S25.

88. Ballantyne JC, Cousins MJ, Giamberardino MA, et al. *Pharmacological Management of Neuropathic Pain, in Pain: Clinical Updates*. Seattle: IASP Press; 2010.

89. Kerrick JM, et al. Low-dose amitriptyline as an adjunct to opioids for postoperative orthopedic pain: a placebo-controlled trial. *Pain*. 1993;52(3):325-330.

90. Kalso E, Tasmuth T, Neuvonen PJ. Amitriptyline effectively relieves neuropathic pain following treatment of breast cancer. *Pain*. 1996;64(2):293-302.

91. Gursky JT, Krahn LE. The effects of antidepressants on sleep: a review. *Harv Rev Psychiatry*. 2000;8(6):298-306.

92. Sinatra RS, Jahr JS, Watkins-Pitchford JM. *Gabapentin, in The Essence of Analgesia and Analgesics*. New York: Cambridge University Press; 2011:294-297.

93. Sinatra RS, Jahr JS, Watkins-Pitchford JM. *Pregabalin, in The Essence of Analgesia and Analgesics*. New York: Cambridge University Press; 2011:298-301.

94. Luo ZD, et al. Injury type-specific calcium channel alpha 2 delta-1 subunit up-regulation in rat neuropathic pain models correlates with antiallodynic effects of gabapentin. *J Pharmacol Exp Ther*. 2002;303(3):1199-1205.

95. Eroglu C, et al. Gabapentin receptor alpha2delta-1 is a neuronal thrombospondin receptor responsible for excitatory CNS synaptogenesis. *Cell*. 2009;139(2):380-392.

96. Dooley DJ, et al. Ca2+ channel alpha2delta ligands: novel modulators of neurotransmission. *Trends Pharmacol Sci.* 2007;28(2):75-82.

97. Field MJ, et al. Identification of the alpha2-delta-1 subunit of voltage-dependent calcium channels as a molecular target for pain mediating the analgesic actions of pregabalin. *Proc Natl Acad Sci U S A.* 2006;103(46):17537-17542.

98. Taylor CP, Angelotti T, Fauman E. Pharmacology and mechanism of action of pregabalin: the calcium channel alpha2-delta (alpha2-delta) subunit as a target for antiepileptic drug discovery. *Epilepsy Res.* 2007;73(2):137-150.

99. Eisenberg E, et al. Antiepileptic drugs in the treatment of neuropathic pain. *Drugs.* 2007;67(9):1265-1289.

100. Hachad H, Ragueneau-Majlessi I, Levy RH. New antiepileptic drugs: review on drug interactions. *Ther Drug Monit.* 2002;24(1):91-103.

101. Piyapolrungroj N, et al. Mucosal uptake of gabapentin (neurontin) vs. pregabalin in the small intestine. *Pharm Res.* 2001;18(8):1126-1130.

102. Eckhardt K, et al. Gabapentin enhances the analgesic effect of morphine in healthy volunteers. *Anesth Analg.* 2000;91(1):185-191.

103. Lyseng-Williamson KA, Siddiqui MA. Pregabalin: a review of its use in fibromyalgia. *Drugs.* 2008;68(15):2205-2223.

104. Singh D, Kennedy DH. The use of gabapentin for the treatment of postherpetic neuralgia. *Clin Ther.* 2003;25(3):852-889.

105. Tassone DM, et al. Pregabalin: a novel gamma-aminobutyric acid analogue in the treatment of neuropathic pain, partial-onset seizures, and anxiety disorders. *Clin Ther.* 2007;29(1):26-48.

106. Straube S, et al. Single dose oral gabapentin for established acute postoperative pain in adults. *Cochrane Database Syst Rev.* 2010;(5):CD008183.

107. Durkin B, Page C, Glass P. Pregabalin for the treatment of postsurgical pain. *Expert Opin Pharmacother.* 2010;11(16):2751-2758.

108. Moore RA, et al. Pregabalin for acute and chronic pain in adults. *Cochrane Database Syst Rev.* 2009;(3):CD007076.

109. Liu M, Wood JN. The roles of sodium channels in nociception: implications for mechanisms of neuropathic pain. *Pain Med.* 2011;12(Suppl 3):S93-S99.

110. Knotkova H, Pappagallo M, Szallasi A. Capsaicin (TRPV1 Agonist) therapy for pain relief: farewell or revival? *Clin J Pain.* 2008;24(2):142-154.

111. Rauck RL, et al. A randomized, double-blind, placebo-controlled study of intrathecal ziconotide in adults with severe chronic pain. *J Pain Symptom Manage.* 2006;31(5):393-406.

112. Staats PS, et al. Intrathecal ziconotide in the treatment of refractory pain in patients with cancer or AIDS: a randomized controlled trial. *JAMA.* 2004;291(1):63-70.

113. Mayer AM, et al. The odyssey of marine pharmaceuticals: a current pipeline perspective. *Trends Pharmacol Sci.* 2010;31(6):255-265.

Chapter 17

LOCAL ANESTHETICS

Suzuko Suzuki, Andreas Koköfer, and Peter Gerner

HISTORICAL PERSPECTIVE

Cocaine, the first local anesthetic, was isolated from leaves of the coca plant, *Erythroxylum coca*, by Nieman in 1860. The medicinal use of coca had long been a tradition of Andean cultures and was introduced in Europe as a stimulant after the conquest of the Americas. Its first clinical use was investigated and described by Freud in his publication *Über Coca* in 1884. Freud's descriptions of the properties of cocaine prompted Koller, an Austrian ophthalmologist, to use cocaine as a topical anesthetic for ophthalmologic procedures, and subsequently the clinical application of cocaine became widespread.[1] However, the toxic and addictive properties of cocaine leading to many deaths among patients and staff were soon identified. Consequently, the injection of cocaine became obsolete, and the need arose for safer alternatives for cocaine.

Discovery of Novel Local Anesthetics

Clinical applications of local anesthetics range from local infiltration or application to allow painful procedures, to peripheral or neuraxial nerve blocks to relieve acute or chronic pain, to intravenous injection to treat cardiac arrhythmias or pain. The development of modern organic chemistry enabled the synthesis of the first analogue of cocaine, procaine (known today by its trade name Novocaine) in 1905. Procaine was not without problems, however, including a very long onset time, short duration, and low potency. Cocaine and procaine are both ester local anesthetics. A breakthrough came in the 1940s when the Swedish pharmaceutical company Astra introduced lidocaine (Xylocaine). This amide local anesthetic had fewer undesirable effects than procaine and provided deeper anesthesia. Many new amide local anesthetics were subsequently introduced with differences in speed of onset, potency, and duration of action. Bupivacaine was synthesized in 1957 and rapidly gained popularity because of its long duration of action. However, because of the association of bupivacaine with cardiac toxicity, a less toxic long-acting drug was sought. Bupivacaine is a racemic mixture of the (+) and (−) enantiomers, with lesser toxicity associated with the S-(−) form compared to the R-(+) form. This led to the development of levobupivacaine and ropivacaine. Today, many local anesthetic agents, including both ester and amide types, are available for specific administration routes and purposes.

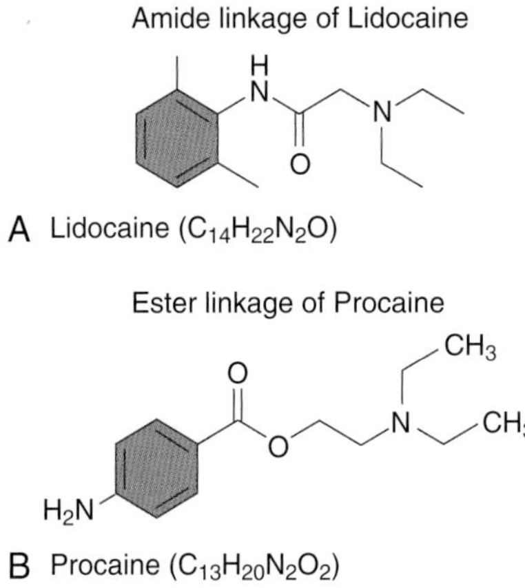

Amide linkage of Lidocaine

A Lidocaine ($C_{14}H_{22}N_2O$)

Ester linkage of Procaine

B Procaine ($C_{13}H_{20}N_2O_2$)

Figure 17-1 Local anesthetic structural classification. Amide linkage of lidocaine (**A**) and ester linkage of procaine (**B**).

CHEMICAL STRUCTURE AND FEATURES

All currently available local anesthetics consist of a lipophilic phenyl ring and a tertiary amine (Figure 17-1).

Ester versus Amide Type Local Anesthetics

Clinically used local anesthetics are often classified as amino-amides (lidocaine, prilocaine, bupivacaine) or amino-esters (procaine, chloroprocaine, tetracaine, cocaine). This classification is based on the type of chemical bond, amide or ester, linking the lipophilic phenyl ring with the hydrophobic tertiary amine (Figure 17-1). Amide and ester local anesthetics differ in their chemical stability, metabolism, and allergic potential. Amides are extremely stable, whereas esters are relatively unstable, particularly in neutral or alkaline solution. Amide compounds undergo enzymatic degradation in the liver, whereas ester compounds are hydrolyzed in plasma by esterase enzymes. Cocaine, an ester, is an exception, as it is metabolized predominantly by the liver. The metabolites of esters include *p*-aminobenzoic acid (PABA), which can occasionally induce allergic reactions. Allergies to amides are extremely rare.[2]

Chiral Forms

Local anesthetics are available either as single enantiomers or racemic mixtures. Enantiomers consist of two stereoisomers (left/sinister or right/dexter) that are mirror images of each other with respect to a specific chiral center. A racemic mixture contains equal amounts of the two enantiomers. The two forms can possess different pharmacologic properties that are of clinical importance. For example, bupivacaine, a commonly used amide type local anesthetic, is a racemic mixture, and levobupivacaine is the pure levorotatory enantiomer. Levobupivacaine demonstrates comparable potency and efficacy as bupivacaine but has significantly less cardiac and central nervous system toxicity likely related to reduced affinity for subtypes of Na^+ channels expressed in brain and cardiac tissues.[3,4] Racemic- or R(+)-bupivacaine produces faster and more potent blockade of Na^+ channels in swine ventricular cardiomyocytes than levobupivacaine. In addition, racemic or

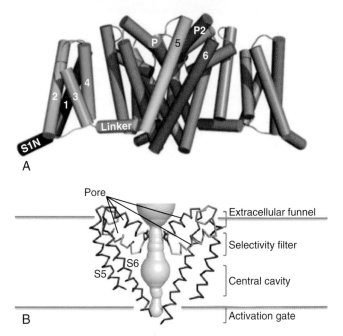

Figure 17-2 Structure of a bacterial voltage-gated sodium channel. **A,** The structure consists of four identical subunits; the voltage-sensing domain of one subunit (S-S4) has been removed for clarity. Each subunit contains six transmembrane segments folded in a complex to form the ion selective pore gated by voltage. One subunit (S1-6) is highlighted in color; the other three are in gray. Transmembrane segments S5 and S6 line the ion pore, the P loops form the selectivity filter, and S1-S4 form the voltage sensor. **B,** The transmembrane pore module, consisting of an outer funnel like vestibule, a selectivity filter, the central cavity, and the intracellular activation gate. Four lateral openings lead from the cellular membrane to the lumen of the pore, giving hydrophobic access to lipophilic drugs, which are able to penetrate through these pores. *(Modified from Payandeh J, Scheuer T, Zheng N, et al. The crystal structure of a voltage-gated sodium channel. Nature. 2011;475:353-358.)*

R(+)-bupivacaine produces a greater reduction of the maximum rate of depolarization in animal cardiomyocytes, suggestive of the difference in Na^+ conductance.[5]

Physiochemical Properties of Local Anesthetics and Their Clinical Implications

In general, with increasing length of the carbon backbone, local anesthetics exhibit greater lipid solubility, protein binding, potency, and duration of action. However, these relationships are not linear and are often influenced by multiple other factors. Local anesthetics must penetrate through the lipid-rich nerve sheaths and cell membrane in order to reach their targets, voltage-gated Na^+ channels (Na_v). The binding site of local anesthetics is located inside the channel pore and is not readily reachable from the extracellular side as inferred from pharmacologic studies. This concept has recently gained support from the atomic resolution structure of a bacterial voltage-gated Na^+ channel (Figure 17-2).[6] Therefore local anesthetics must cross the nerve membrane into the cell interior by diffusing through the lipid bilayer in order to reach their binding site. Consequently, the potency of each local anesthetic is closely related to its lipid solubility and its dependence on pH.[7]

The tertiary amine on the hydrocarbon backbone of local anesthetics is a weak base capable of accepting a hydrogen ion

Table 17-1. Different Nerve Types: Characteristics and Sensitivity to Local Anesthetics

FIBER	DIAMETER, μm	CONDUCTION SPEED, M/SEC	SENSITIVITY TO BLOCK	MYELINATION	ANATOMIC LOCATION	FUNCTION
A-α	15-20	80-120	++	+++	Afferent and efferent from muscles and joints	Motor, proprioception
A-β	8-15	80-120	++	+++	Afferent and efferent from muscles and joints	Touch, pressure, proprioception
A-γ, A-δ	3-8	4-30	+++	++	Efferent to muscle spindles, sensory roots, and afferent peripheral nerves	Pain, temperature, touch/motor
B	4	10-15	++++	+	Preganglionic sympathetic	Autonomic—preganglionic
C	1-2	1-2	++++	–	Postganglionic sympathetic, sensory roots, and afferent peripheral nerves	Pain, temperature, touch

Modified from De Jong RH. *Local anesthetics.* St. Louis: Mosby; 1994; and Goodman LS, Gilman A, Hardman JG, et al. *Goodman & Gilman's The Pharmacological Basis of Therapeutics.* 9th ed. New York: McGraw-Hill, Health Professions Division; 1996.

with low affinity to form a conjugated acid. Most local anesthetics have pKa values relatively close to but higher than physiologic pH (with some exceptions such as prilocaine that has a secondary amine and benzocaine that has a primary amine) (Table 17-1). Around physiologic pH (7.4), local anesthetics exist in these two forms,[7a] the positively charged conjugated acid and unprotonated neutral form, the ratio described by the Henderson-Hasselbach equation:

$$pKa = log([H+][B-]/[BH])$$

$$pKa = pH + log([B-]/[BH]) \qquad [1]$$

where B is the base form and BH is the conjugated acid.

Local anesthetics cross the lipid membrane much faster in their neutral lipophilic form than their cationic form. Alkalinization by sodium bicarbonate addition to local anesthetic solutions increases the pH and shifts the equilibrium in favor of the neutral base forms, which facilitates translocation of the local anesthetic into the cellular interior.[8,9] Once inside the cell, the lower pH shifts the equilibrium toward the positively charged protonated form. The charged form antagonizes Na^+ channels more potently than the neutral form.[9a,10]

The onset of action of local anesthetic action depends on the route of administration and the dose or concentration of drug. In the subarachnoid space where the nerves lack a sheath, local anesthetics are able to reach their targets more readily, leading to a more rapid onset of nerve block with a much smaller dose compared to peripheral nerves. In peripheral nerve blocks, deposition of local anesthetic is in the vicinity of the nerves and the amount of drug that reaches the nerve depends on the diffusion of the drug and the proximity of the injection to the nerve. For a given route of administration, increasing the concentration can accelerate onset.[11] For instance, chloroprocaine is much slower in onset than lidocaine at equal concentrations because its pKa of 9.1 favors the positively charged form at physiologic pH. However, a 3% solution is the typical concentration of chloroprocaine used clinically, which provides a much faster onset than other agents at their clinically used concentrations (e.g., 0.25% bupivacaine, 0.5% ropivacaine, or 1.5% mepivacaine) simply because there are more molecules present to diffuse into the nerve.

The duration of action of local anesthetics is determined primarily by their protein binding (see Table 17-4). Local anesthetics with a high affinity for protein remain bound to the nerve membrane longer. In other words, binding to Na^+

channels with higher affinity results in a channel blocking effect of longer duration. Duration of action is also influenced by the rate of vascular uptake of local anesthetic from the injection site. The duration of peripheral nerve blocks ranges from 30 to 60 minutes with short-acting agents such as procaine and chloroprocaine to nearly 10 hours with long-acting local anesthetics such as bupivacaine and tetracaine. The rate of vascular uptake significantly affects local anesthetic duration of action as local anesthetics provide their effect as long as they remain at the site of deposition. Therefore deposition of local anesthetics at a highly vascular site such as the intercostal space has a higher rate of vascular uptake. Vasoconstriction slows the rate of vascular absorption and thus prolongs the duration of action. For this purpose, vasoconstrictive agents such as epinephrine and phenylephrine are frequently added to local anesthetics as adjuvants to increase duration. The prolongation of nerve block with vasoconstrictors is more prominent with local anesthetics of intermediate durations such as lidocaine and prilocaine than with longer acting agents such as bupivacaine, possibly because the effect of long-acting local anesthetics outlasts that of vasoconstrictors. Local anesthetics themselves tend to have bimodal effects on vascular smooth muscle such that vasoconstriction results at lower doses while vasodilation predominates at higher concentrations with some minor differences between individual agents.[12]

Pharmacodynamics

ANATOMY OF NERVES

The surface of the nerve axon is formed by the lipid bilayer membrane that is embedded with various proteins including ion channels. Myelinated nerve axons are surrounded by Schwann cells. Schwann cells produce myelin that wraps around the axons to form the *myelin sheath*. When seen lengthwise, the myelin sheath is punctuated by gaps called *nodes of Ranvier*. Other axons such as postganglionic autonomic efferent and some of the nociceptive afferent fibers lack a myelin sheath (Figure 17-3). Nerve axons are further organized within three layers of connective tissue: the *endoneurium*, *perineurium*, and *epineurium* (see Figure 17-3). Nerve fibers are encased in endoneurium, loose connective tissue that consists of glial cells and fibroblasts along with blood capillaries. These fibers are grouped together by dense collagenous perineurium to form a unit called a *fascicle*. The fascicles are surrounded by a thicker layer of epineurium. The nerves are further encased in fascia. These are the structures that local anesthetics must penetrate in order to block effectively nerve conduction. Nerves are typically characterized by their degree of myelination, axonal diameter, and speed of impulse conduction (see Table 17-1). They are classified as A, B, and C fibers, which roughly corresponds to their

decreasing cross-sectional diameters. A and B fibers are myelinated, and C fibers are unmyelinated. A and C fibers are further divided into subclasses by their anatomic location and physiologic functions.

ELECTROPHYSIOLOGY OF NEURAL CONDUCTION

The lipid bilayer of the axonal membrane is relatively impermeable to sodium ions but selectively permeable to potassium ions. The ATP-dependent Na^+/K^+ pump (Na/K-ATPase) exports Na^+ and imports K^+ in a 3:2 ration to maintain a concentration gradient of these ions across the axonal membrane.[13] The higher concentration of K^+ in the intracellular space and the greater permeability of the membrane to K^+ lead to the relative negative electrochemical potential of the cell interior. Resting neural membranes have an electrochemical potential of around −70 mV. When Na^+ channels open, sodium ions rush inward down the concentration gradient. Other channels, including Ca^{2+} and K^+ channels are sensitive to the change in electrical potential and open in response to the depolarization. Neurons are activated by the transduction of chemical, molecular, or thermal stimuli into electrical potential via the influx of cations to raise the electrical potential. The conduction of electrochemical impulses in axons is an *all or none* phenomenon. When the depolarization is strong enough, the stimuli is conducted by sequential depolarization of the neural membrane along the axonal length via the opening of Na^+ channels and net inward movement of sodium ions. The sodium ions inside of the cell diffuse along the axon in both directions and passively depolarize the adjacent membrane thereby triggering the opening of additional Na^+ channels by reaching their activation threshold potential.[14] Because the upstream region of the membrane is already depolarized and in a refractory state, the electrical impulse can propagate only in an anterograde direction along the axon (Figure 17-4, *A*). In myelinated axons, the myelin sheath serves as insulation, and this local phenomenon takes place only at the nodes of Ranvier. Therefore the nerve impulse is able to "skip" the

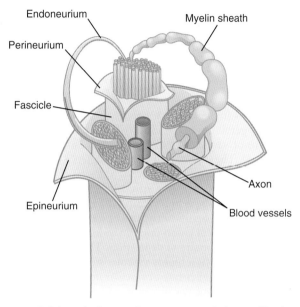

Figure 17-3 Schematic diagram of nerve structure. Each nerve fiber is surrounded by Schwann cells and encased within three layers of connective tissue: endoneurium, perineurium, and epineurium. Schwann cells wrap layers around some of the axon forming sequential units of myelin sheath with gaps in between each myelin unit. Unmyelinated fibers are simply embedded within the cytoplasm of Schwann cells. *(Modified from Schematic structure of a peripheral nerve. The peripheral nervous system and reflex activity. In: Marieb EN, Hoehn K, eds.* Human Anatomy and Physiology. *7th ed. San Francisco: Pearson Education, Inc; 2007. p. 498.)*

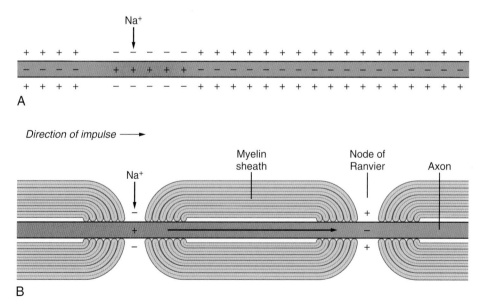

Figure 17-4 Action potential propagates along the axon unidirectionally. The upstream region of the axonal membrane is still in the refractory period and unable to achieve the threshold for depolarization. **A,** Action potential propagates continuously along the unmyelinated axon by sequential depolarization of the nerve membrane. **B,** In myelinated axon, the action potential is conducted only at the nodes of Ranvier, skipping the distance between adjacent nodes *(salutatory conduction)*.

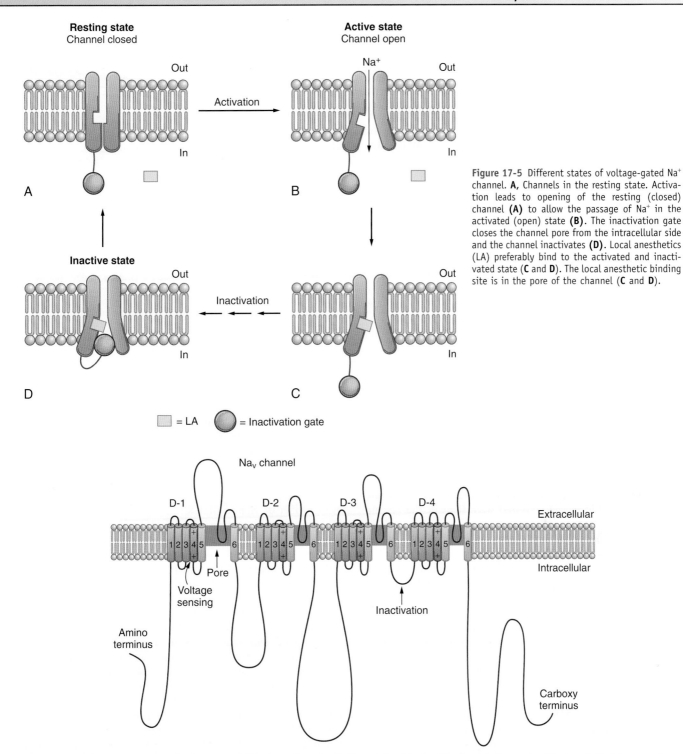

Resting state
Channel closed

Activation

Out

In

A

Active state
Channel open

Na⁺

Out

In

B

Inactive state

Out

In

D

Inactivation

Out

In

C

☐ = LA   ⬤ = Inactivation gate

Figure 17-5 Different states of voltage-gated Na⁺ channel. **A,** Channels in the resting state. Activation leads to opening of the resting (closed) channel **(A)** to allow the passage of Na⁺ in the activated (open) state **(B)**. The inactivation gate closes the channel pore from the intracellular side and the channel inactivates **(D)**. Local anesthetics (LA) preferably bind to the activated and inactivated state **(C** and **D)**. The local anesthetic binding site is in the pore of the channel **(C** and **D)**.

Na$_v$ channel

D-1   D-2   D-3   D-4

Extracellular

1 2 3 4 5 6   1 2 3 4 5 6   1 2 3 4 5 6   1 2 3 4 5 6

Intracellular

Pore

Voltage
sensing

Inactivation

Amino
terminus

Carboxy
terminus

Figure 17-6 Schematic structure of voltage-gated Na⁺ channel α-subunit. It contains four homologous domains, each with six α-helical transmembrane segments. The intracellular loops that connect S5 and S6 of each of the four domains (P loops) are positioned extracellularly and extend inward to form the narrowest point of the channel pore and provide its ion-selectivity.

length of myelin to the next node (saltatory conduction), making much faster conduction possible (see Figure 17-4, *B*).

VOLTAGE-GATED NA⁺ CHANNELS AND THEIR INTERACTION WITH LOCAL ANESTHETICS

Ion channels are multi-subunit transmembrane proteins that fold in a complex manner to form ion selective pores gated by voltage or ligands (see Figure 17-2). Ion channels can switch between different conformations in a voltage-dependent manner that determines pore opening (activation), closing (inactivation), and reactivation (to the resting state) (Figure 17-5). Voltage-gated Na⁺ channels consist of a single α-subunit and varying auxiliary β-subunits. The α subunit forms the ion-conducting pore of the channel and consists of four homologous domains, each with six α-helical transmembrane segments (Figure 17-6). The loops that connect the S5 and S6 segments of these α-helices of each of the four domains are positioned extracellularly and extend inward, which form the narrowest point of the channel pore and are thought to provide its ion-selectivity (see Figure 17-2). In the resting state, the ion pore of the Na⁺ channel is closed (see Figure 17-5, *A*). Depolarizing voltage changes lead to movement of the voltage sensor (S1-S4) due to outward movement of positive charges in the S4 segment, which in turn leads to the rearrangement of S6 segments that results in opening of the channel pore (see Figure 17-5, *B*). The activated channel is inactivated within milliseconds by another conformational change, resulting in the movement of the S6 segment and the S5-S6 linker acting as an inactivation gate (see Figure 17-5, *D*).

The inactivated state differs from the resting state in its molecular conformation as well as its interaction with local anesthetics, which selectively bind and stabilize the inactivated state. Local anesthetics dose-dependently decrease peak Na⁺ current through voltage-gated Na⁺ channels.[15] The binding site for local anesthetics is located interior of the ion-selective pore and can be approached via two different pathways: through the pore interior, or hydrophilic pathway, and laterally through the lipid membrane, or hydrophobic pathway (see Figure 17-2, *B*). When bound, local anesthetics stabilize the inactivated state and prevent further activation. They can also bind in the ion channel pore to prevent ion flux (open-state block). Local anesthetics have a higher affinity for Na⁺ channels in the activated (open) and inactivated (channel pore in open conformation but intracellularly closed by inactivation gate) state than those in the resting closed state (see Figure 17-5, *C-D*). The difference in the affinity is attributed to the difference in the availability of the two pathways for local anesthetics to reach their binding site. The binding site is more accessible in the activated state than in the resting state.

In the presence of local anesthetics, repeated depolarization results in an incremental decrease in Na⁺ current until it reaches a newer steady level of inhibition, which is termed *use-dependent* or *phasic inhibition*.[16] With repeated depolarization, a greater number of Na⁺ channels are in the active or inactivated state and are bound to local anesthetics. Furthermore the dissociation rate of local anesthetics from their binding site is slower than the rate of transition from inactivated to resting state. Therefore repeated stimulation results in accumulation of local anesthetic bound Na⁺ channels, which manifests as use-dependent inhibition or block (Figure 17-7).[16a]

Na⁺ CHANNEL DIVERSITY

There are multiple subtypes of voltage-gated Na⁺ channels arising from variation in the homologous α-subunit genes. The nine subtypes now known in mammals (Na$_v$1.1 through 1.9) are differentially expressed in various tissues with cell- and tissue-specific functions. Sodium channels such as Na$_v$1.8, Na$_v$1.9, and Na$_v$ 1.7 are expressed exclusively in peripheral neurons.[17-19] The Na$_v$1.7 subtype determines the ability of nociceptive neurons to transmit noxious stimuli. Rare loss-of-function mutations of Na$_v$1.7 are reported in patients with channelopathy-associated insensitivity to pain, in which patients have selective lack of pain and smell sensation.[20] On the other hand, several gain-of-function mutations of genes related to the regulation or function of Na$_v$1.7 result in overactivity of this channel and are associated with the congenital

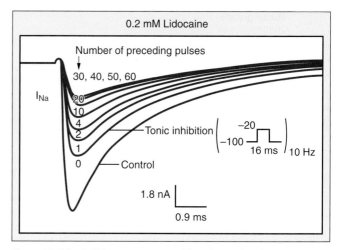

Figure 17-7 Ionic Na⁺ currents measured by voltage-clamping technique by depolarization applied infrequently ("tonic" test). After equilibration with 0.2 mM lidocaine, the currents measured tonically are reduced significantly compared to control currents. Application of repeated depolarizations results in a dynamic reduction of currents after each depolarization ("use-dependent" inhibition). *(Modified from Butterworth JF, Strichartz GR. Molecular mechanisms of local anesthesia: a review. Anesthesiology. 1990;72:711-734.)*

pain disorders erythermalgia (also termed *erythromelalgia*) and paroxysmal extreme pain disorder.[21] Na$_v$1.7 also appears to be involved in the development of inflammatory pain.[22] The observation that ProTX-II, a Na$_v$1.7-selective antagonist from spider venom, prevents propagation of action potentials in nociceptive fibers suggests that selective Na$_v$1.7 blockers might provide a novel target for analgesic therapy.[23]

MECHANISM OF NERVE BLOCK

Only a very small fraction (1%-2%) of local anesthetic reaches the nerve membrane even when placed in close proximity to the nerve.[24] The quality of nerve blockade is determined not only by the potency of the individual local anesthetic, but also by the concentration and volume of the local anesthetic. The potency of a local anesthetic can be expressed as the minimum effective concentration (MEC) at which complete nerve block is established. The volume of local anesthetic is also important as a sufficient length of axon must be blocked in order to prevent regeneration of the impulse in the adjacent node of Ranvier. This is understood by the phenomenon of decremental conduction whereby depolarization of the membrane decays with the distance away from the front of the action potential, and impulse propagation stops when the depolarization falls below the conduction threshold (Figure 17-8). If less than the critical length of the axon is blocked, the action potential can be regenerated in the proximal membrane segment or node when the decaying depolarization is still above threshold for Na⁺ channel activation.

OTHER MECHANISMS OF LOCAL ANESTHETIC ACTION

Local anesthetics block other ion channels besides Na⁺ channels including voltage-gated K⁺ channels and Ca²⁺ channels, but with lower potency compared to Na⁺ channels. Local anesthetics also bind intracellular G protein-coupled receptors and possibly influence the regulation of intracellular Ca²⁺.[25] The significance of these local anesthetic actions is still unclear.

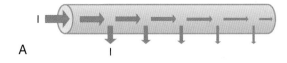

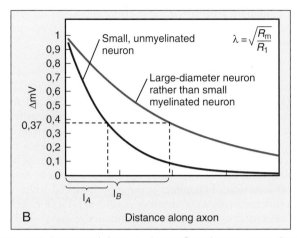

Figure 17-8 Decremental decay. **A,** Current flow along an axon, showing the flow across the membrane and within the cytoplasm gradually dissipating (*arrow* width is proportional to current flow). **B,** Depolarization of the nerve membrane is strongest at the site of activation and dissipates decrementally as an inverse first-order exponential with increasing distance from the site of activation. The length constant (λ) (which is the distance where the decrement is $1/e$, or 37% of the initial voltage change) depends on the ratio of the resistance of the axonal membrane (R_m) to the longitudinal resistance of the cytoplasm (R_l) and therefore to the diameter of the neuron.

Lidocaine, one of the most studied local anesthetics, has been shown to possess an antiinflammatory effect.[26] Lidocaine appears to inhibit the release of proinflammatory cytokines and prevent leukocyte adhesion. Clinically, some local anesthetics have also been shown to be effective in treatment of predominantly inflammatory conditions such as irritable bowel diseases (see Emerging Developments).

Difference Between Peripheral and Central Nerves

Peripheral nerves are covered by a nerve sheath while axial nerves are encased in three layers of meninges: the pia matter, arachnoid, and dura matter. The pia matter is adherent to the nerve itself and separated from arachnoid by cerebral spinal fluid that fills the space between the two layers. This space is called spinal or intrathecal space where the "naked" or exposed nerves float in cerebrospinal fluid. The dura matter further outlines the arachnoid membrane, forming a tough covering around the central neuraxis. These meninges taper off as the spinal nerve roots exit the vertebral column via the foramina and course through the epidural space. The presence of these meninges in the nerve roots in the epidural space requires ten times the dose of local anesthetic to produce complete nerve block compared to that required in the intrathecal space.

Differential Block

Different nerve types show varying susceptibility to nerve block. Table 17-1 displays the characteristics of different nerve types. Clinically, sensory functions are blocked before motor function. This differential nerve block was initially attributed to differences in axon size.[27] Nociceptive-selective nerve block (differential block) has been attempted with

concentrations of local anesthetics that are just high enough for only certain nerve fibers (smaller diameter, thinly myelinated Aδ or unmyelinated C-fibers), but not for others (larger diameter, myelinated nerves such as Aβ). Nevertheless, nerve block does not always follow this size principle in that Aγ is blocked at lower concentration than C fibers and myelinated fibers before unmyelinated fibers.[28] The latter can be explained by the need to block only the node in myelinated fibers compared to the whole critical length of the nerve membrane in unmyelinated fibers. Therefore complete pain relief is generally accomplished only with simultaneous low-threshold sensory sympathetic and motor blockade, leading to numerous adverse effects. Current efforts are to explore such nerve blocking mechanisms and develop agents that are more selective or exclusively pain-fiber selective than currently used local anesthetics.[29]

Pharmacokinetics

The plasma concentrations of local anesthetics are determined by intravascular absorption, distribution, biotransformation, and excretion. All of these are affected by patient factors such as age, body size, and organ function. Therefore clinical data must be synthesized with the pharmacology of the local anesthetics in order to predict overall pharmacokinetics in each individual.

ABSORPTION

The rate and extent of systemic absorption of local anesthetic depend on multiple factors: site of injection, dose, physiochemical properties of the drugs, and presence of vasoconstrictive or other adjuvants. Injection in a more vascular tissue results in higher plasma concentration of local anesthetic in a shorter time. Thus a given dose of local anesthetic that can be administered safely for one type of block can result in higher plasma levels and potential systemic toxicity in another type of block. Clinically, the order of decreasing rate of systemic absorption is intravenous, intercostal, caudal, epidural, brachial plexus, femoral, sciatic, and subcutaneous injections.[30] The plasma concentration of local anesthetic is generally directly proportional to the dose injected regardless of the concentration of the injectate or the speed of injection. Furthermore, the lipid solubility can influence absorption such that more lipid-soluble agents are absorbed more slowly than less lipid-soluble ones.[31] This is likely due to sequestration of local anesthetic in lipophilic tissue as well as direct vasoconstriction of vascular smooth muscles by more potent lipid-soluble agents at low doses.[32] The use of vasoconstrictors such as epinephrine reduces the rate of systemic absorption as mentioned earlier. The addition of epinephrine to bupivacaine and etidocaine significantly decreases the rate of absorption in brachial plexus block but the effect is minimal when used epidurally.[31]

DISTRIBUTION

Local anesthetics are distributed throughout the body but their concentrations vary between different tissue types with preference to more vascular tissues. The rate of distribution can typically be described by a two-compartment model with rapid and slow phases. The rapid phase involves uptake in highly perfused tissues reaching rapid equilibration. For example, lung is a major site of uptake for local anesthetic.

297

The slow phase depends on the slow equilibration of less perfused tissues and on specific properties of individual local anesthetics.

METABOLISM

The major difference between ester and amide type local anesthetics is their metabolism. Ester type local anesthetics undergo hydrolysis by plasma esterases. An exception to this is cocaine which is metabolized in the liver by carboxylesterase. One of the metabolites of ester type local anesthetics, PABA, can cause allergic reactions in susceptible individuals. Amide type local anesthetics undergo biotransformation mainly in the liver. The rate of metabolism varies between different agents such that degradation of lidocaine is faster than mepivacaine, whose metabolism is still faster than bupivacaine. The metabolites of amide type local anesthetics are excreted by the kidneys. Prilocaine can be metabolized in the kidney. About 5% of amide type local anesthetics is renally excreted unchanged. Therefore patients with decreased hepatic or renal functions eliminate amide type local anesthetics more slowly and are at increased risk for systemic toxicity. An exception is articaine, which is inactivated by plasma carboxylesterase. Table 17-2 displays the pharmacokinetic properties of selected local anesthetics.

Table 17-2. Pharmacokinetic Properties of Selected Local Anesthetics

	V_{DSS} (L/KG)	CLEARANCE (L/KG/H)	$T_{1/2}$ (H)
Chloroprocaine	0.5	2.96	0.1
Procaine	0.93	5.62	0.1
Lidocaine	1.30	0.85	1.6
Prilocaine	2.73	2.03	1.6
Mepivacaine	1.2	0.67	1.0
Bupivacaine	1.02	0.41	3.5
Levobupivacaine	0.9	0.3	3.5
Ropivacaine	0.84	0.63	1.9

Adapted from Rosenberg PH, Veering BT, Urmey WF. Maximum recommended doses of local anesthetics: a multifactorial concept. *Reg Anesth Pain Med.* 2004;29:564-574.

$t_{1/2}$, Elimination half time; V_{dss}, volume of distribution at steady state.

ADDITIVES

Various agents have been studied as additives to local anesthetics with the intent to improve the quality and duration of neuraxial and peripheral nerve blocks. Such agents include α-adrenergic agonists, sodium bicarbonate, opioids, NMDA type glutamate receptor antagonists (Table 17-3) for clinical use, and benzodiazepines, tramadol, and cholinesterase inhibitors for investigational use.

Adrenergic Agents

Epinephrine is used as a marker for detecting intravascular injection in both neuraxial (epidural) and peripheral nerve blocks. α-Adrenergic agents also prolong and intensify the nerve block.[33] This prolongation is due to local vasoconstriction, leading to decreased vascular absorption, making more local anesthetic available for nerve block. The extent of block prolongation depends on the specific local anesthetic and the site of injection. This effect is most pronounced when used with shorter acting local anesthetics such as lidocaine. Activation of central α_2-adrenergic receptors in the spinal cord also enhances analgesia by epinephrine and other α-adrenergic agonists.

α_2-Adrenergic Agonists

More selective α_2-adrenergic agonists such as clonidine and dexmedetomidine also produce analgesic effects mediated by supraspinal and spinal adrenergic receptors. Clonidine has been studied extensively; it prolongs block duration and decreases local anesthetic requirement in caudal block.[34] However, clonidine has considerable side effects such as hypotension, bradycardia, and sedation. These side effects can be beneficial or undesirable depending on the patient.

Opioids

Opioids are also used in neuraxial blocks either alone or in combination with local anesthetics. Intrathecal morphine (0.1-0.2 mg) provides analgesia up to 20 hours after cesarean section.[35] Fentanyl (10-25 μg) improves the spread and prolongs the block in spinal anesthesia in a dose-dependent manner.[36] Sufentanil (5 μg) produces an effect comparable to 0.2 mg morphine (although much shorter) with a lower incidence of pruritus.[35]

Table 17-3. Typically Used Additives to Local Anesthetics

AGENT	MAIN MECHANISM	COMMON INDICATION	COMMON DOSAGE FOR CERTAIN INDICATIONS
Epinephrine	Vasoconstriction α_2 adrenergic agonism	Peripheral nerve block Infiltration anesthesia Epidural anesthesia Marker for intravascular injection	3-5 μg/mL
Opioids	Opioid receptor agonism	Neuraxial block	Intrathecal morphine 100-200 μg Intrathecal sufentanil 5 μg Intrathecal fentanyl 10-25 μg Epidural fentanyl 2-10 μg/mL Epidural sufentanil 0.25-1 μg/mL Epidural hydromorphone 20 μg/mL
		Peripheral nerve block	Fentanyl 1-2 μg/mL Sufentanil 0.1 μg/mL Morphine 30 μg/mL
Ketamine	NMDA receptor antagonism Opioid receptors?	Intrathecal	Intrathecal 5-25 mg
Clonidine	α2 adrenergic agonism	Neuraxial block Peripheral nerve block	Epidural 25-75 μg Peripheral block 25-150 μg/mL

Epidural morphine used as an adjunct to bupivacaine or ropivacaine provides effective postoperative analgesia for orthopedic surgeries.[37] Morphine is also used in labor epidural analgesia after cesarean section to prolong postoperative analgesia. Respiratory depression is an undesired side effect that can last longer than the analgesic effect and thus mandates monitoring. Epidural fentanyl (2-10 µg/mL) is also used as an adjunct to local anesthetics or alone. Because there is substantial systemic absorption of the fentanyl congeners when injected epidurally, their analgesic effect is partially due to a systemic effect. Sufentanil, being even more lipophilic than fentanyl, provides similar plasma levels regardless of whether it is administered by an intravenous or epidural route.[38] Nevertheless, some authors suggest that sufentanil (0.75-1 µg/mL) is a valuable adjuvant for epidural analgesia with improved analgesia and decreased intravenous opioid requirement.[39] Hydromorphone (20 µg/mL), which is less lipophilic than fentanyl or sufentanil, is also an effective adjunct to local anesthetics.[40,41]

Evidence to support the use of opioids in peripheral nerve blocks is limited.[42] Use of buprenorphine (0.3 mg) along with 1% mepivacaine, 0.2% tetracaine, and epinephrine in brachial plexus block prolonged analgesia by 3-fold.[43,44] But, opioids are not widely used for this purpose.

Ketamine
Analgesia with ketamine is mainly due to NMDA receptor antagonism but might also involve other mechanisms such as opioid receptor agonism.[45,46] Intrathecal administration of ketamine along with bupivacaine shortens the onset of analgesia and decreases the duration of analgesia.[47,48] When used in peripheral nerve block, ketamine appears to prolong postoperative analgesia. Its role in epidural analgesia is unclear at this point.

Others
Other agents such as tramadol, neostigmine, and midazolam have also been used as adjuvants with favorable results, but data are extremely limited and they are not in routine clinical use.

Toxicity

The toxicity of local anesthetics is the limiting factor in their clinical applications. Local anesthetics are relatively safe if administered appropriately. However, significant systemic or localized toxicity can result from unintended intravascular, intrathecal, or intraneural injection or if excessive dos are administered resulting in major systemic absorption.[48a]

SYSTEMIC TOXICITY
Systemic toxicity manifests primarily in the cardiovascular and central nervous systems.

Cardiovascular System
Local anesthetics affect the cardiovascular system both directly by affecting cardiac myocytes and peripheral vascular smooth muscle cells, and indirectly by actions on the autonomic nervous system. The more potent, lipophilic local anesthetics such as bupivacaine, tetracaine, and etidocaine are more cardiotoxic than the less lipophilic agents such as procaine, prilocaine, and lidocaine (Table 17-4).[49] Local anesthetics act directly by decreasing the conduction in Purkinje fibers and cardiomyocytes by prolonging the recovery time. The dissociation of bound bupivacaine from the local anesthetic binding site is slower ("fast-in," "slow-out" of the bupivacaine block of the cardiac Na^+ channel).[50] Local anesthetics are also direct myocardial depressants via a mechanism related to reduced Ca^{2+} influx and release from the sarcoplasmic reticulum.[51,52] The action of local anesthetics on peripheral vascular smooth muscle is biphasic with vasoconstriction at low concentrations and vasodilation at higher concentrations.[12] The exception is cocaine, which produces vasoconstriction at any dose.

Indirect cardiovascular effects of local anesthetics are related to the use of neuraxial techniques and include hypotension, bradycardia, and cardiopulmonary collapse if not treated promptly. Mild to moderate symptoms are usually responsive to intravenous fluids and indirect or direct acting adrenergic agents such as ephedrine and phenylephrine. Severe symptoms and complications are associated with high dermatomal level blocks, use of sedatives, delayed recognition of unintentional subarachnoid or intravenous injection, and delayed treatment; these severe complications might require pharmacologic and even mechanical cardiopulmonary support.[53,54]

The severe cardiovascular toxicity associated with epidural use of 0.75% bupivacaine (and other local anesthetics) in the obstetric population in the late 1970s and early 1980s serves as a prototype example of the public health implications of local anesthetic systemic toxicity. The introduction of epidural analgesia for labor pain was accompanied by multiple reports of local anesthetic induced cardiac arrest and death in parturients. These tragic outcomes culminated in the relabeling of bupivacaine by the Food and Drug Administration (FDA), cautioning against the use of high concentrations in the obstetric population and the refinement of epidural test dosing techniques.[55] Continued concern about the complications associated with local anesthetic toxicity decades later has resulted in further advancements in treatment (e.g., lipid rescue; see later).[55-57]

Central Nervous System
Central nervous system toxicity manifests initially as anxiety, dizziness, circumoral numbness, lightheadedness, and tinnitus. Objective symptoms include shivering, muscle twitching, tremors, and eventually generalized tonic-clonic seizure. With a high dose intravascular injection, a brief period of early symptoms and seizure can be followed by respiratory depression and respiratory arrest. Factors that increase susceptibility to CNS toxicity include the use of more potent local anesthetics and the concomitant presence of respiratory or metabolic acidosis (by decreasing the convulsive threshold). Respiratory acidosis also reduces protein binding of local anesthetics, increasing local anesthetic availability for further toxic effects.[58,59] Elevated $PaCO_2$ leads to cerebral vasodilation and increased delivery of drug to the CNS. However, acidosis promotes amine protonation leading to less diffusion into nerve cells.

Treatment of Local Anesthetic Systemic Toxicity
When unintentional intravenous injection of local anesthetic is suspected or systemic toxicity is detected, benzodiazepine should be given prophylactically as an anticonvulsant.[60] The patient should be monitored closely for any early neurologic signs and symptoms. If the patient seizes, the airway must be

Table 17-4. Physiochemical Properties of Selected Local Anesthetics

	pKa	IONIZATION AT pH 7.4 (%)	PARTITION COEFFICIENT	PROTEIN BOUND (%)
Ester Type				
Procaine	8.9	97	100	6
Chloroprocaine	8.7	95	810	N/A
Tetracaine	8.5	93	5822	76
Amide Type				
Lidocaine	7.9	76	366	65
Prilocaine	7.9	76	129	55
Mepivacaine	7.6	61	130	78
Bupivacaine	8.1	83	3420	96
Levo-bupivacaine	8.1	83	3420	98
Ropivacaine	8.1	83	775	94

Modified from Liu SS. Local anesthetics and analgesia. In: Ashburn MA, Rice LJ, eds. *The Management of Pain*. New York: Churchill Livingstone; 1997:141-170.

protected to prevent aspiration and hypoventilation, and the seizure should be treated promptly with an intravenous anticonvulsant such as diazepam; sodium thiopental or propofol are acceptable alternatives. Appropriate monitoring should be applied to assess cardiovascular and pulmonary function. Hypoventilation and respiratory acidosis should be supported with supplemental oxygen or artificial airway and mechanical ventilation. Hypotension and bradycardia should be treated with intravenous fluids and chronotropes, inotropes, and vasoactive agents. Epinephrine is still considered the mainstay of immediate treatment and the use of vasopressin has also been suggested.[61] However, literature findings conflict as to their benefit, and further studies are warranted.[61] Intravenous administration of lipid emulsion has been used with immediate and successful resuscitation of patients with refractory local anesthetic induced cardiac toxicity, and is now a part of standardized treatment algorithms (see Emerging Developments).[60] Concern for epinephrine-induced arrhythmia has been raised; the use of vasopressin is supported by animal studies and may be considered.[62]

The role of antiarrhythmic drugs in local anesthetic induced ventricular arrhythmia is not established and the data are unclear. Sodium channel antagonists such as amiodarone should be theoretically avoided; however, its use is supported in one animal study.[62] Calcium channel blockers are contraindicated in that they can further depress myocardial function.

ALLERGIC REACTIONS
True allergy to local anesthetics is rare but occurs more commonly with ester local anesthetics than with amide local anesthetics.[63] The accepted explanation is that amino-esters are metabolized to PABA, which is immunogenic.[2] Some preparations of amino-amides contain methylparaben, which has a similar chemical structure as PABA and is a possible allergen in cases of allergic reaction with the use of amide local anesthetics.[64] Preservative-free preparations of local anesthetics are available to address the problems associated with methylparaben.

NEUROTOXICITY AND OTHER TISSUE TOXICITY
Direct neuronal tissue toxicity (e.g., transient neurologic symptoms [TNS] and cauda equina syndrome) has been described with multiple local anesthetics, but the incidence appears to be significantly higher with lidocaine and mepivacaine than bupivacaine, prilocaine, and procaine.[65] TNS is characterized by transient hyperalgesia or dysesthesia in the low back, buttocks, and lower extremities following seemingly uneventful spinal anesthesia but without permanent neurologic damage. Risk of TNS is associated with the use of lidocaine, lithotomy position, and ambulatory procedures. The risk increases with dose, but does not appear to correlate with the concentration of local anesthetic because there is no difference in the incidence of TNS with 0.5% and 5% lidocaine.[66] The etiology of TNS is unclear, but direct neurotoxicity can be demonstrated in vitro and in animal models.[67] Symptoms typically respond to nonsteroidal antiinflammatory drugs and trigger point injections. That the mechanism of neural toxicity is poorly understood is underscored by a recent study in patients demonstrating that intraneural injection of mepivacaine into the sciatic nerve is typically not associated with neural injury.[68]

The potential neurotoxic effects of local anesthetics came to the attention of public health officials in the United States after the introduction of microcatheters for spinal anesthesia in the late 1980s. Reports of cauda equina syndrome associated with typical "spinal" doses of local anesthetic solution injected through microcatheters appeared in the literature. Subsequent investigation using in vitro models of the subarachnoid space revealed that local anesthetic injection through the microcatheters resulted in maldistribution of the drug (i.e., pooling), exposing the nerve tissue to unusually high concentrations of local anesthetic.[69,70] The incidence of the problem was high enough to culminate in voluntary withdrawal of the microcatheters by the manufacturer.

SPECIFIC LOCAL ANESTHETICS

Tables 17-4 and 17-5 give an overview of the physicochemical properties of the local anesthetics described.

Amide Local Anesthetics
LIDOCAINE
Lidocaine was the first widely used local anesthetic, and is available for infiltration as well as peripheral (including Bier's block), spinal, and epidural blocks. Its use for spinal anesthesia has declined due to concerns about neurotoxicity and transient neurologic symptoms (TNS; see earlier).[65] It can be applied topically as an ointment or jelly, or nebulized as an aerosol to anesthetize the upper airway. Intravenous injection of lidocaine to achieve low plasma levels (<5 μg/mL) results in systemic analgesia, possibly not only due to an action in the CNS but also by affecting peripheral nerves or cutaneous nerve endings. Clinically, lidocaine has been administered as an infusion to treat chronic neuropathic pain and can predict efficacy for oral Na^+ channel blocking drugs such as mexiletine.

Lidocaine causes vasodilation at most concentrations; the addition of epinephrine can significantly reduce absorption of lidocaine by nearby vessels, allowing more of the initially administered dose to enter the neural compartment, thereby prolonging the duration of action by as much as 50%.[33] Experimentally, intravenous lidocaine profoundly suppresses both increased peripheral neuronal "firing" induced by injury and inflammation as well as central sensitization of wide dynamic range neurons in the spinal cord dorsal horn.[71-74]

PRILOCAINE
Prilocaine has a similar clinical profile as lidocaine and is used for infiltration, peripheral nerve blocks, and spinal and epidural anesthesia. Because prilocaine causes significantly less vasodilation than lidocaine, addition of epinephrine is not necessary to prolong the duration of action, which may be an advantage when epinephrine is contraindicated. Prilocaine shows the least systemic toxicity of all amide local anesthetics and is therefore useful for intravenous regional anesthesia. However, it causes methemoglobinemia (>500 mg dose) due to its metabolite o-toluidine, which has significantly limited its use.

MEPIVACAINE
The anesthetic profile of mepivacaine is also similar to lidocaine but with a slightly longer duration of action. However,

Table 17-5. Recommended Dosages of Selected Local Anesthetics

	ROUTE	ONSET	RECOMMENDED DOSE (MG/KG)	MAXIMUM DOSE (MG) WITH OR WITHOUT EPINEPHRINE		DURATION (HR)
				Plain	+ Epinephrine	
Ester type						
Procaine	Spinal	Fast	15	1000	–	0.5-1
Chloroprocaine	Subcutaneous	Fast	10	800	1000	0.5-1
	Peripheral block	Fast	10	800	1000	0.5-1
	Epidural	Fast	10	800	1000	0.5-1
Tetracaine	Topical	Fast	0.2	20	–	0.5-6
Amide type					–	
Lidocaine	Subcutaneous	Fast	4	300	500	0.5-3
	Intravenous	Fast	4	300		0.5-1
	Peripheral block	Fast	4	300	500	1-3
	Epidural	Fast	4	300	500	1-2
	Spinal	Fast	1.5	100	–	0.5-1
	Topical	Fast	4	300	–	0.5-1
Prilocaine	Subcutaneous	Fast	8	600	–	1-2
	Intravenous	Fast	8	600	–	0.5-1
	Peripheral block	Fast	8	600		0.5-3
	Epidural	Fast	8	600		1-3
Mepivacaine	Subcutaneous	Fast	5	400	500	1-4
	Peripheral block	Fast	5	400	500	2-4
	Epidural	Fast	5	400	500	1-3
	Spinal	Fast	1.5	100		1-2
Bupivacaine	Subcutaneous	Fast	2.5	175	225	2-8
	Peripheral block	Slow	2.5	175	225	4-12
	Epidural	Moderate	2	170	225	2-5
	Spinal	Fast	0.3	20	–	1-6
Levobupivacaine	Subcutaneous	Fast	2	150	–	2-8
	Peripheral block	Slow	2	150	–	14-17
	Epidural	Moderate	2	150	–	5-9
	Spinal	Fast	0.3	20	–	1-6
Ropivacaine	Subcutaneous	Fast	3	200	–	2-6
	Peripheral block	Slow	3.5	250	–	5-8
	Epidural	Moderate	3	200	–	2-6

Modified from Covino BG, Wildsmith JAW. Clinical pharmacology of local anesthetic agents. In: Cousins MJ, Bridenbaugh PO, eds. *Neural Blockade in Clinical Anesthesia and Management of Pain.* 3rd ed. Philadelphia: Lippincott-Raven; 1998:97-128; and Foster RH, Markham A. Levobupivacaine: a review of its pharmacology and use as a local anaesthetic. *Drugs.* 2000;59:551-579.

it is not as effective when applied topically. Although toxicity appears to be less than with lidocaine, metabolism of mepivacaine is prolonged in the fetus and newborn and is, therefore, not used for obstetric anesthesia. Vasodilation is mild, but adding epinephrine can significantly prolong action.

BUPIVACAINE

Bupivacaine (a racemic mixture of both the R and S enantiomers) provides prolonged and intense sensory analgesia, often outlasting the motor block. For epidural analgesia and anesthesia, bupivacaine is usually used at concentrations from 0.25% to 0.5%, with a 2- to 5-hour duration of action. Peripheral nerve blocks are also performed with these concentrations, depending on the amount of motor block sought. Peripheral blocks can last for 12 to 24 hours. Intrathecal use provides approximately 2 to 3 hours of anesthesia and 4 to 6 hours of analgesia. Other clinical uses include tissue infiltration and "trigger point" injections in treating myofascial pain. Epinephrine is sometimes added as a marker for intravascular injection and to prolong the duration of action due to decreased vascular absorption. However, as vasoconstriction has less impact on the duration of more hydrophobic agents, epinephrine is more commonly added to more hydrophilic agents such as lidocaine.

Reports of sudden cardiac arrest with bupivacaine injection were associated with considerable morbidity and mortality.

Its high affinity for Na^+ channels and high lipid solubility are probably the main cause. By consensus, the 0.75% concentration of bupivacaine is not used in obstetrics because of the associated mortality/toxicity (see earlier).

LEVOBUPIVACAINE

Levobupivacaine is a single enantiomer preparation consisting of the S-enantiomer of bupivacaine. Compared with racemic bupivacaine, levobupivacaine has considerably reduced CNS and cardiovascular toxicity, allowing a larger dose to be given. An animal model demonstration of the lower potential for cardiovascular toxicity associated with levobupivacaine compared with dextro-bupivacaine is shown in Figure 17-9. The clinical profile and potency of levobupivacaine appears to be similar to that of bupivacaine. Levobupivacaine is particularly useful when large doses are required, such as for plexus blocks that are performed without ultrasound guidance.

ROPIVACAINE

Concerns about the cardiotoxicity of bupivacaine led to the development of ropivacaine. Ropivacaine is structurally similar to bupivacaine but was developed as a single, less toxic enantiomer (as with levo-bupivacaine); it can be administered in larger doses than racemic bupivacaine before early signs of toxicity develop.[75] However, if equipotent concentrations/dosages are compared, the difference between bupivacaine

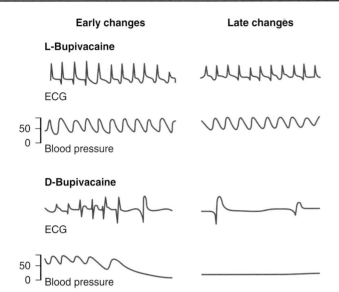

Early changes   Late changes

L-Bupivacaine

ECG

50
0
Blood pressure

D-Bupivacaine

ECG

50
0
Blood pressure

Figure 17-9 Representative changes in the electrocardiogram (lead II) and arterial blood pressure 2 to 3 seconds after infusion of levo-bupivacaine (L-bupivacaine) or D-bupivacaine (2 mg/kg) in an anesthetized rat. The changes of the rhythm and blood pressure are displayed. *(Modified from Denson DD, Behbehani MM, Gregg RV. Enantiomer-specific effects of an intravenously administered arrhythmogenic dose of bupivacaine on neurons of the nucleus tractus solitarius and the cardiovascular system in the anesthetized rat. Reg Anesth. 1992;17:311-316.)*

and ropivacaine becomes less clear. Overall the clinical profile of ropivacaine is similar to racemic bupivacaine, taking into account that it is less lipid soluble and less potent than bupivacaine. Epidural application can allow for even greater sensory block without significant motor block. An intrinsic vasoconstricting effect (also true for levo-bupivacaine) might augment the duration of action and reduce the incidence of cardiotoxicity.

Ester Local Anesthetics

PROCAINE

Procaine was used mainly for infiltration and spinal blocks in the early 20th century before lidocaine became popular. Low potency, slow onset (probably due to its high pK$_a$), and short duration of action limit the use of procaine. Allergic reactions are possible due to the production of the metabolite PABA.

CHLOROPROCAINE

Due to its relatively low potency and extremely low toxicity, relatively high concentrations of chloroprocaine can be used. It also has an extremely short plasma half-life because it is metabolized rapidly by plasma cholinesterase. Reports of CNS toxicity in the form of seizures are extremely unusual. It is thought to have the lowest CNS and cardiovascular toxicity of all agents in current use. Chloroprocaine is used commonly for epidural anesthesia. It is also used for peripheral blocks in combination with other long-acting, slow-onset local anesthetics for the combined effect of rapid onset and prolonged duration. In obstetrics, epidural chloroprocaine, with or without bicarbonate, is used to attain rapidly surgical levels of anesthesia in preparation for cesarean section. Another theoretical advantage in obstetrics is that there is virtually no transmission of chloroprocaine to the fetus.[76] Epidurally administered chloroprocaine can, however, interfere with the

action of subsequent administration of epidural amide anesthetics or opioids.[77]

Controversy exists regarding the use of chloroprocaine related to reports of persistent, serious neurologic deficits associated with accidental massive subarachnoid injection (i.e., adhesive arachnoiditis). Initially, the agent itself was implicated, but subsequent evaluation suggested that the preservative antioxidant bisulfite is responsible. However, after elimination of bisulfite a number of reports of back pain have appeared. Recently, a renewed interest has actually suggested that bisulfite may be neuroprotective in an animal model.[78]

TETRACAINE

Tetracaine is a slow onset, potent and intermediate to long acting ester-type local anesthetic. Even longer duration of action can be achieved when administered along with a vasoconstrictor such as epinephrine. However it is quite toxic, and has been suggested to cause neurotoxicity at high doses in animal studies resulting in cauda equina syndrome with repeated spinal dosing. It is used mainly topically or sometimes for spinal anesthesia. Tetracaine is highly lipid soluble and a significant amount can be absorbed when used in the mucous membrane or wounded skin.[79]

COCAINE

The only naturally occurring local anesthetic used clinically is also the only local anesthetic that causes intense vasoconstriction. Thus it is often used as a topical anesthetic, e.g., when anesthetizing the cornea or the nasal airway before endotracheal intubation. Cocaine inhibits the neuronal reuptake of catecholamines and can therefore cause hypertension, tachycardia, dysrhythmias, and other serious cardiac effects.

BENZOCAINE

Benzocaine has a slow onset, short duration of action and is both minimally potent and minimally toxic. Its clinical use is limited to topical anesthesia to anesthetize mucous membranes; for example to anesthetize the oral and pharyngeal mucosa before fiberoptic endotracheal intubation. Excessive use of benzocaine is associated with methemoglobinemia.

Mixture of Local Anesthetics

The rationale for the mixture of local anesthetics is an attempt to benefit from their respective pharmacokinetics (e.g., a quick onset with the short-lasting drug while maintaining the long duration of the long-acting drug). However, the beneficial effects of the use of mixtures of local anesthetic agents might be overstated. For example, bupivacaine provides clinically acceptable onset of action as well as prolonged duration of anesthesia. In addition, the use of catheter techniques for many forms of regional anesthesia makes it possible to extend the duration of action of rapid and short acting agents such as chloroprocaine or lidocaine. Most importantly, one should be cautioned against the use of maximum doses of two local anesthetics. Toxicities of these agents are independent and should be presumed to be additive.[80]

TOPICAL LOCAL ANESTHETICS
EMLA

EMLA cream is a eutectic mixture of the local anesthetics lidocaine and prilocaine, each at a concentration of 2.5%. It is a eutectic mixture because the mixture has a melting point below room temperature and therefore, exists as a viscous liquid, rather than a solid powder. EMLA should be applied to intact skin surfaces because application to breached skin surfaces can lead to unpredictably rapid absorption. It provides dermal analgesia by the release of the lidocaine and prilocaine from the cream into the skin, which leads to blockade of pain transmission originating from free nerve endings. The onset, quality, and duration of dermal analgesia are primarily dependent on the duration of skin application. Although there is considerable interpatient variation, EMLA cream should be applied under an occlusive dressing for about 1 hour to provide adequate analgesia for insertion of an intravenous catheter or the drawing of blood at roughly 2.5 g of the cream applied over a 25 cm^2 area of skin. Large application area, long duration of application, and impaired elimination can result in high blood concentrations of the local anesthetics. The maximum recommended duration of exposure is 4 hours, although exposures of up to 24 hours have not led to toxic plasma levels of local anesthetics. Caution must be taken in children or very small adults as plasma levels of lidocaine and prilocaine are dependent on patient size and rate of systemic drug elimination.

Lidocaine Patch (5%)

The lidocaine patch (Lidoderm) was approved by the FDA in 1999 for the treatment of pain associated with post-herpetic neuralgia, a severe chronic neuropathic pain condition. The patch is a topical delivery system intended to deliver low doses of lidocaine to superficially damaged or dysfunctional cutaneous nociceptors in an amount sufficient to produce analgesia without mechanosensory block. Its recommended dosing is an application of up to three patches to intact painful skin areas for 12 hours per day. Pharmacokinetic studies have demonstrated that clinically insignificant plasma levels are achieved with this formulation. The levels are $\frac{1}{10}$ of those required to produce cardiac effects and $\frac{1}{32}$ of those required to produce toxicity. However, patients often report pain relief even during the 12 hours between applications of a patch, despite the short plasma half-life of lidocaine, suggesting that some cumulative benefit results from prolonged local delivery of the drug.

EMERGING DEVELOPMENTS

Lipid Rescue

The first report showing that the infusion of soybean oil emulsion improved resuscitation after bupivacaine induced cardiovascular collapse in an animal model was published more than a decade ago.[81] Meanwhile, numerous case reports as well as experimental studies have shown the therapeutic effect of intravenous infusion of lipid emulsion in refractory systemic local anesthetic toxicity.[82] The mechanism behind lipid rescue is unclear. In cardiac myocytes, the preferred energy substrate is fatty acids and inhibition of fatty acid metabolism can lead to myocardial dysfunction. One of the postulated mechanisms of lipid rescue is attributed to the reversal of inhibitory effect on fatty acid metabolism produced by some of the potent local anesthetics such as bupivacaine. In isolated rat heart, infusion of lipid at a subtherapeutic dose produces positive inotropic effect.[83] Another hypothesis

is that the lipids sequester the local anesthetics. This can explain the similar antidote effect of lipid infusion for other lipophilic medications including calcium channel blockers, beta blockers, and antidepressants. There is a limited number of cases reporting adverse outcomes after lipid rescue, mainly recurrent cardiovascular instability. One of the theoretical complications of lipid infusion is pancreatitis induced by hyperlipidemia and hyperamylasemia. In addition, careful monitoring of patients for several hours after even successful treatment with lipid infusion is essential as there can be a return of cardiovascular instability as plasma levels of the lipids decline.[84]

Heat-Assisted Delivery

Controlled Heat-Assisted Drug Delivery (CHADD), a disposable oxygen-activated system that allows controlled release of heat to enhance the delivery of local anesthetics, has been used with lidocaine and tetracaine. The formulation is an emulsion in which the active ingredients are in oil phase as a eutectic mixture containing 70 mg of lidocaine and 70 mg of tetracaine in a ratio of 1:1 by weight.[85] Heat is generated using a mixture of iron powder, activated carbon, sodium chloride, wood flour, and water. The local anesthetics are packed in a shallow chamber below the CHADD patch and sealed in an airtight packet.[85] When applied to the skin, the CHADD patch gets heated spontaneously and increases the temperature of the skin, thereby enhancing the permeation of the drugs through the epidermis. The heating element produces a temperature of 39°C to 41°C for 2 hours and reduces the duration of onset of action of local anesthetics compared to other topically applied local anesthetics such as lidocaine/prilocaine combination.[86,87]

Ultrasound Guidance to Deliver Local Anesthetics

With improvement in the image quality generated by newer ultrasound equipment, use of ultrasound guidance in procedures is increasing in various aspects of clinical practice. High-resolution ultrasound can provide direct real-time imaging of peripheral nerves and identify tissue planes that permit favorable local anesthetic distribution for conduction block and catheter placement. For safe and successful ultrasound-guided neural blockade, one must be familiar with the relevant cross-sectional anatomy and the coordination of the imaging probe with the block needle. The real-time and continuous visualization of the procedure needle and the relevant anatomy enhances the safety of needling through the structures and the quality of block by visualized guidance compared to the blind or nerve-stimulator guided techniques.[88-90] If desired, ultrasound guidance can be combined with nerve stimulation to further confirm proximity to neural structures. Nonetheless, the quality of ultrasound-guided procedures is operator dependent and requires manual dexterity and practice.

Local Anesthetics and the Inflammatory Response

Local anesthetics have been shown to possess antiinflammatory effects. They appear to affect mainly polymorphonuclear granulocytes (PMNs), but effects on macrophages and monocytes are also implicated.[91] Overactive inflammatory responses that destroy rather than protect are critical in the development of a number of peri-operative disease states, such as postoperative pain, adult respiratory distress syndrome, systemic inflammatory response syndrome, and multiorgan failure. Some local anesthetics (lidocaine or bupivacaine) reduce the formation of leukotriene B4 and IL-1. In particular, leukotriene B4 is a potent stimulator of PMNs that leads to their margination, degranulation, diapedesis, and superoxide release. It enhances vascular permeability and is also a potent chemotactic substance. Therefore preventing activation of PMNs is likely a strong basis to suppress the inflammatory process. Additionally, local anesthetics (ropivacaine and lidocaine) attenuate TNFα and Ca^{2+} dependent upregulation of the CD11b-CD18 complex, surface proteins that allow PMN adhesion to endothelium.[92] This is thought to be one of the key mechanisms for the therapeutic effect seen with low dose topical application of ropivacaine in ulcerative colitis.[93] Wound healing is another area of interest in relation to the local anesthetic inhibition of PMN adhesion. But studies have yielded contradictory results such that *in vivo* investigations have demonstrated delayed wound healing, no effects, or even improved wound healing after local anesthetic infiltration.[91]

Local anesthetics are also likely to be involved in yet another aspect of the inflammatory process. Various substances such as TNF, platelet-activation factor, IL-8, lipopolysaccharide, and certain colony stimulating factors "prime" PMNs for subsequent activation that leads to a potentiated response of PMNs. The mechanism of priming is not fully understood but might play a pivotal role in the overstimulation of inflammatory pathways. Lidocaine and other local anesthetics appear to block the priming of PMNs in a dose-dependent manner.[91] This could account for how local anesthetics can decrease tissue damage without significantly inhibiting PMN functions required for host defense.

Another immune modulating effect of local anesthetics involves impaired release of lysosomal enzymes with inhibition of free radical release from macrophages.[94] Macrophage functions of cytokine release, respiratory burst, and phagocytosis are sensitive to intracellular pH changes, and are regulated by vacuole-type H-translocating adenosine triphosphatase (H^+-ATPase) [note + is superscript] and the Na^+-H^+ exchanger. Local anesthetics inhibit these transporters in human PMNs *in vitro*.[95]

Liposomal Formulations

Liposomes are biocompatible microscopic lipid vesicles with a bilayer membrane structure that are used to deliver drugs over a longer period. However, tissue reaction to such formulations has been problematic as conventional local anesthetics are intrinsically myotoxic with increases in toxicity over extended durations of exposure. They are also myotoxic when released from a delivery system, even when the delivery systems themselves are minimally toxic.[96] In contrast, site 1 sodium channel blockers (like saxitoxin) do not cause myotoxicity or neurotoxicity which could make them desirable for an extended release formulation.[97] However, these substances, being very hydrophilic, are difficult to encapsulate effectively in polymeric particles. Recently a liposomal formulation using saxitoxin was shown to produce sciatic nerve blockade up to 7.5 days in rats with minimal systemic and local toxicity.[98]

KEY POINTS

- Local anesthetics are classified as ester or amide type based on the linkage between the lipophilic phenyl ring and the hydrophilic tertiary amine. This difference is reflected in their physiochemical and pharmacokinetic properties.
- Local anesthetics bind to voltage gated Na^+ channels and block depolarizing Na^+ current through these channels.
- Properties such as lipid solubility, protein binding, and pKa of individual local anesthetics affect their speed of onset, potency, and duration of action. Raising the pH of local anesthetic solution favors the membrane-permeable neutral form and accelerates onset of action.
- Voltage-gated Na^+ channels transition between resting, activated (open), and inactivated states via coordinated conformational changes. Local anesthetics have higher affinity for the activated and inactivated states than the resting state.
- There are multiple subtypes of voltage-gated Na^+ channels arising from expression of nine homologous α-subunit genes that are differentially expressed in various tissues. Some Na^+ channel subtypes such as $Na_v1.8$, $Na_v1.9$, and $Na_v 1.7$ are expressed exclusively on peripheral nerves and play important roles in nociception.
- The rate of systemic absorption decreases from intravenous, intercostal, caudal, epidural, brachial plexus, femoral and sciatic, and subcutaneous administration. The same dose of local anesthetic can result in higher plasma concentration and potential for systemic toxicity depending on the type of block.
- Ester type local anesthetics undergo mainly hydrolysis by plasma esterases. Decreased activity or absence of plasma cholinesterase can increase the risk for systemic toxicity with ester type local anesthetics.
- Amide type local anesthetics undergo biotransformation mainly in the liver. Their metabolites and about 5% of the unchanged drug are excreted by the kidneys. Patients with decreased hepatic or renal function have longer elimination times and are at increased risk for systemic toxicity.
- The systemic and local toxicity of local anesthetics are the limiting factors in their clinical use. Systemic toxicity manifests primarily in central nervous system and cardiovascular effects and local toxicity by nerve degeneration (neurotoxicity).
- Lipid emulsion infusion and avoidance of hypoxia and acidosis are recognized as crucial in the treatment of local anesthetic toxicity. Lipid emulsion should be available whenever local anesthetics are administered in large doses such as during placement of peripheral nerve and neuraxial blocks.

Key References

Courtney KR, Kendig JJ, Cohen EN. Frequency-dependent conduction block: the role of nerve impulse pattern in local anesthetic potency. *Anesthesiology*. 1978;48:111-117. The phenomenon of use-dependent block was shown in vivo (sciatic nerve fiber studies). (Ref. 16)

Heavner JH. Cardiac toxicity of local anesthetics in the intact isolated heart model: a review. *Reg Anesth Pain Med.* 2002;27:545-555. This comprehensive review on local anesthetic cardiac toxicity, the most dreaded complication of this group of drugs, concisely summarizes the literature findings on this topic, including biochemical and physicochemical aspects that are relevant to clinicians and researchers. (Ref. 49)

Ritchie JM, Greengard P. On the active structure of local anesthetics. *J Pharmacol Exp Ther.* 1961;133:241-245. Studies showing that, contrary to former beliefs, the charged form of local anesthetics is responsible for blocking impulse conduction. (Ref. 9a)

Rosenberg PH, Veering BT, Urmey WF. Maximum recommended doses of local anesthetics: multifactorial concept. *Reg Anesth Pain Med.* 2004;29:564-574. This is an excellent overview on relevant concepts put in a clinical context. (Ref. 48a)

Scholz A. Mechanisms of (local) anaesthetics on voltage-gated sodium and other ion channels. *Br J Anaesth.* 2002;89:52-61. This is a valuable reference for readers looking for a comprehensive overview of the mechanisms of local anesthetic interactions with ion channels. (Ref. 16a)

Strichartz GR, Sanchez V, Arthur R, et al. Fundamental properties of local anesthetics. II. Measured octanol: buffer partition coefficients and pKa values of clinically used drugs. *Anesth Analg.* 1990;71:158-170. Important work elucidating fundamental characteristics of local anesthetics. (Ref. 7a)

Weinberg GL, VadeBoncouer T, Ramaraju GA, et al. Pretreatment or resuscitation with a lipid infusion shifts the dose-response to bupivacaine-induced asystole in rats. *Anesthesiology.* 1998;88:1071-1075. This milestone article led the foundation of what is now known as lipid rescue. (Ref. 81)

References

1. Ruetsch YA, Boni T, Borgeat A. From cocaine to ropivacaine: the history of local anesthetic drugs. *Curr Top Med Chem Aug.* 2001;1(3):175-182.
2. Eggleston S, Lush L. Understanding allergic reactions to local anesthetics. *Ann Pharmacother.* 1996;30:851-857.
3. Knudsen K, Suurkula MB, Blomberg S, et al. Central nervous and cardiovascular effects of I.V. infusions of ropivacaine, bupivacaine and placebo in volunteers. *Br J Anaesth.* 1997;78:507-514.
4. Nau C, Wang SY, Strichartz GR, et al. Block of human heart hH1 sodium channels by the enantiomers of bupivacaine. *Anesthesiology.* 2000;93:1022-1033.
5. Mather LE, Chang DH. Cardiotoxicity with modern local anaesthetics: is there a safer choice? *Drugs.* 2001;61:333-342.
6. Payandeh J, Scheuer T, Zheng N, et al. The crystal structure of a voltage-gated sodium channel. *Nature.* 2011;475:353-358.
7. Hemmings HC, Greengard P. Positively active: how local anesthetics work. *Anesthesiology.* 2010;113:250-252.
7a. Strichartz GR, Sanchez V, Arthur R, et al. Fundamental properties of local anesthetics. II. Measured octanol: buffer partition coefficients and pKa values of clinically used drugs. *Anesth Analg.* 1990;71:158-170. Important work elucidating fundamental characteristics of local anesthetics.
8. Hille B. The pH-dependent rate of action of local anesthetics on the node of Ranvier. *J Gen Physiol.* 1977;69:475-496.
9. Ohki S, Gravis C, Pant H. Permeability of axon membranes to local anesthetics. *Biochimica Biophys Acta.* 1981;643:495-507.
9a. Ritchie JM, Greengard P. On the active structure of local anesthetics. *J Pharmacol Exp Ther.* 1961;133:241-245. Studies showing that, contrary to former beliefs, the charged form of local anesthetics is responsible for blocking impulse conduction.
10. Chernoff DM, Strichartz GR. Tonic and phasic block of neuronal sodium currents by 5-hydroxyhexano-2′,6′-xylide, a neutral lidocaine homologue. *J Gen Physiol.* 1989;93:1075-1090.
11. Cousins MJ, Bridenbaugh PO. *Neural Blockade in Clinical Anesthesia and Management of Pain.* 3rd ed. Philadelphia: Lippincott-Raven; 1998.
12. Johns RA, DiFazio CA, Longnecker DE. Lidocaine constricts or dilates rat arterioles in a dose-dependent manner. *Anesthesiology.* 1985;62:141-144.
13. Hille B. *Ion Channels of Excitable Membranes.* 3rd ed. Sunderland, Mass: Sinauer; 2001.
14. Hodgkin AL. *The Conduction of the Nervous Impulse.* Springfield, Ill,: C C Thomas; 1964.
15. Ulbricht W. Sodium channel inactivation: molecular determinants and modulation. *Physiol Rev.* 2005;85:1271-1301.
16. Courtney KR, Kendig JJ, Cohen EN. Frequency-dependent conduction block: the role of nerve impulse pattern in local anesthetic potency. *Anesthesiology.* 1978;48:111-117.
16a. Scholz A. Mechanisms of (local) anaesthetics on voltage-gated sodium and other ion channels. *Br J Anaesth.* 2002;89:52-61. This is a valuable reference for readers looking for a comprehensive overview of the mechanisms of local anesthetic interactions with ion channels.
17. Akopian AN, Sivilotti L, Wood JN. A tetrodotoxin-resistant voltage-gated sodium channel expressed by sensory neurons. *Nature.* 1996;379:257-262.
18. Black JA, Dib-Hajj S, McNabola K, et al. Spinal sensory neurons express multiple sodium channel alpha-subunit mRNAs. *Brain Res Mol Brain Res.* 1996;43:117-131.
19. Dib-Hajj SD, Binshtok AM, Cummins TR, et al. Voltage-gated sodium channels in pain states: role in pathophysiology and targets for treatment. *Brain Res Rev.* 2009;60:65-83.
20. Cox JJ, Reimann F, Nicholas AK, et al. An SCN9A channelopathy causes congenital inability to experience pain. *Nature.* 2006;444:894-898.
21. Jarecki BW, Sheets PL, Jackson JO, et al. Paroxysmal extreme pain disorder mutations within the D3/S4-S5 linker of Nav1.7 cause moderate destabilization of fast inactivation. *J Physiol.* 2008;586:4137-4153.
22. Nassar MA, Stirling LC, Forlani G, et al. Nociceptor-specific gene deletion reveals a major role for Nav1.7 (PN1) in acute and inflammatory pain. *Proc Natl Acad Sci U S A.* 2004;101:12706-12711.
23. Schmalhofer WA, Calhoun J, Burrows R, et al. ProTx-II, a selective inhibitor of NaV1.7 sodium channels, blocks action potential propagation in nociceptors. *Molecular Pharmacol.* 2008;74:1476-1484.
24. Popitz-Bergez FA, Leeson S, Strichartz GR, et al. Relation between functional deficit and intraneural local anesthetic during peripheral nerve block. A study in the rat sciatic nerve. *Anesthesiology.* 1995;83:583-592.
25. Xiong Z, Bukusoglu C, Strichartz GR. Local anesthetics inhibit the G protein-mediated modulation of K+ and Ca++ currents in anterior pituitary cells. *Mol Pharmacol.* 1999;55:150-158.
26. Giddon DB, Lindhe J. In vivo quantitation of local anesthetic suppression of leukocyte adherence. *Am J Pathol.* 1972;68:327-338.
27. Gasser HS, Erlanger J. The role of fiber size in the establishment of a nerve block by pressure or cocaine. *Am J Physiol* 1929;581-591.
28. Gokin AP, Philip B, Strichartz GR. Preferential block of small myelinated sensory and motor fibers by lidocaine: in vivo electrophysiology in the rat sciatic nerve. *Anesthesiology.* 2001;95:1441-1454.
29. Gerner P, Binshtok AM, Wang CF, et al. Capsaicin combined with local anesthetics preferentially prolongs sensory/nociceptive block in rat sciatic nerve. *Anesthesiology.* 2008;109:872-878.
30. Wildsmith JA, Tucker GT, Cooper S, et al. Plasma concentrations of local anaesthetics after interscalene brachial plexus block. *Br J Anaesth.* 1977;49:461-466.
31. Tucker GT, Mather LE. Clinical pharmacokinetics of local anaesthetics. *Clin Pharmacokin.* 1979;4:241-278.
32. Johns RA, Seyde WC, DiFazio CA, et al. Dose-dependent effects of bupivacaine on rat muscle arterioles. *Anesthesiology.* 1986;65:186-191.
33. Sinnott CJ, Cogswell III LP, Johnson A, et al. On the mechanism by which epinephrine potentiates lidocaine's peripheral nerve block. *Anesthesiology.* 2003;98:181-188.
34. Gabriel JS, Gordin V. Alpha 2 agonists in regional anesthesia and analgesia. *Curr Opin Anaesth.* 2001;14:751-753.
35. Karaman S, Kocabas S, Uyar M, et al. The effects of sufentanil or morphine added to hyperbaric bupivacaine in spinal anaesthesia for caesarean section. *Eur J Anaesth.* 2006;23:285-291.
36. Liu S, Chiu AA, Carpenter RL, et al. Fentanyl prolongs lidocaine spinal anesthesia without prolonging recovery. *Anesth. Analg.* 1995;80:730-734.
37. Axelsson K, Johanzon E, Essving P, et al. Postoperative extradural analgesia with morphine and ropivacaine. A double-blind comparison between placebo and ropivacaine 10 mg/h or 16 mg/h. *Acta Anaesth Scand.* 2005;49:1191-1199.

38. Miguel R, Barlow I, Morrell M, et al. A prospective, randomized, double-blind comparison of epidural and intravenous sufentanil infusions. *Anesthesiology*. 1994;81:346-352.

39. Kampe S, Weigand C, Kaufmann J, et al. Postoperative analgesia with no motor block by continuous epidural infusion of ropivacaine 0.1% and sufentanil after total hip replacement. *Anesth Analg*. 1999;89:395.

40. Liu S, Carpenter RL, Mulroy MF, et al. Intravenous versus epidural administration of hydromorphone. Effects on analgesia and recovery after radical retropubic prostatectomy. *Anesthesiology*. 1995;82:682-688.

41. Mulroy MF. Epidural hydromorphone: a step closer to the view from the top. *Reg Anesth Pain Med*. 2010;35:333-334.

42. Murphy DB, McCartney CJ, Chan VW. Novel analgesic adjuncts for brachial plexus block: a systematic review. *Anesth Analg*. 2000;90:1122-1128.

43. Candido KD, Franco CD, Khan MA, et al. Buprenorphine added to the local anesthetic for brachial plexus block to provide postoperative analgesia in outpatients. *Reg Anesth Pain Med* 2001;26:352-356.

44. Candido KD, Winnie AP, Ghaleb AH, et al. Buprenorphine added to the local anesthetic for axillary brachial plexus block prolongs postoperative analgesia. *Reg Anesth Pain Med*. 2002;27:162-167.

45. Sarton E, Teppema LJ, Olievier C, et al. The involvement of the mu-opioid receptor in ketamine-induced respiratory depression and antinociception. *Anesth Analg*. 2001;93:1495-1500.

46. Hirota K, Okawa H, Appadu BL, et al. Stereoselective interaction of ketamine with recombinant mu, kappa, and delta opioid receptors expressed in Chinese hamster ovary cells. *Anesthesiology*. 1999;90:174-182.

47. Togal T, Demirbilek S, Koroglu A, et al. Effects of S(+) ketamine added to bupivacaine for spinal anaesthesia for prostate surgery in elderly patients. *Eur J Anaesth*. 2004;21:193-197.

48. Kathirvel S, Sadhasivam S, Saxena A, et al. Effects of intrathecal ketamine added to bupivacaine for spinal anaesthesia. *Anaesthesia*. 2000;55:899-904.

48a. Rosenberg PH, Veering BT, Urmey WF. Maximum recommended doses of local anesthetics: multifactorial concept. *Reg Anesth Pain Med*. 2004;29:564-574. This is an excellent overview on relevant concepts put in a clinical context.

49. Heavner JE. Cardiac toxicity of local anesthetics in the intact isolated heart model: a review. *Reg Anesth Pain Med*. 2002;27:545-555.

50. Clarkson CW, Hondeghem LM. Mechanism for bupivacaine depression of cardiac conduction: fast block of sodium channels during the action potential with slow recovery from block during diastole. *Anesthesiology*. 1985;62:396-405.

51. Herzig S, Ruhnke L, Wulf H. Functional interaction between local anaesthetics and calcium antagonists in guineapig myocardium: 1. Cardiodepressant effects in isolated organs. *Br J Anaesth*. 1994;73:357-363.

52. Chamberlain BK, Volpe P, Fleischer S. Inhibition of calcium-induced calcium release from purified cardiac sarcoplasmic reticulum vesicles. *J Biol Chem*. 1984;259:7547-7553.

53. Lee LA, Posner KL, Cheney FW, et al. Complications associated with eye blocks and peripheral nerve blocks: an American Society of Anesthesiologists closed claims analysis. *Reg Anesth Pain Med*. 2008;33:416-422.

54. Lee LA, Posner KL, Domino KB, et al. Injuries associated with regional anesthesia in the 1980s and 1990s: a closed claims analysis. *Anesthesiology*. 2004;101:143-152.

55. Moore DC, Batra MS. The components of an effective test dose prior to epidural block. *Anesthesiology*. 1981;55:693-696.

56. Morishima HO, Pedersen H, Finster M, et al. Bupivacaine toxicity in pregnant and nonpregnant ewes. *Anesthesiology*. 1985;63:134-139.

57. Albright GA. Cardiac arrest following regional anesthesia with etidocaine or bupivacaine. *Anesthesiology*. 1979;51:285-287.

58. Apfelbaum JL, Shaw LM, Gross JB, et al. Modification of lidocaine protein binding with CO2. *Can Anaesth Soc J*. 1985;32:468-471.

59. Burney RG, Difazio CA, Foster JA. Effects of pH on protein binding of lidocaine. *Anesth Analg*. 1978;57:478-480.

60. Neal JM, Bernards CM, Butterworth JF, et al. ASRA practice advisory on local anesthetic systemic toxicity. *Reg Anesth Pain Med*. 2010;35:152-161.

61. Wolfe JW, Butterworth JF. Local anesthetic systemic toxicity: update on mechanisms and treatment. *Curr Opin Anaesthesiol*. 2011;24:561-566.

62. Weinberg GL. Current concepts in resuscitation of patients with local anesthetic cardiac toxicity. *Reg Anesth Pain Med*. 2002;27:568-575.

63. Sidhu S, Shaw S, Lush L. A 10-year retrospective study on benzocaine allergy in the United Kingdom. *Am J Contact Derm*. 1999;10:57-61.

64. Larson CE. Methylparaben—an overlooked cause of local anesthetic hypersensitivity. *Anesth Progress* 1977;24:72-74.

65. Zaric D, Pace NL. Transient neurologic symptoms (TNS) following spinal anaesthesia with lidocaine versus other local anaesthetics. *Cochrane Rev*. 2009:CD003006.

66. Pollock JE, Liu SS, Neal JM, et al. Dilution of spinal lidocaine does not alter the incidence of transient neurologic symptoms. *Anesthesiology*. 1999;90:445-450.

67. Drasner K, Sakura S, Chan VW, et al. Persistent sacral sensory deficit induced by intrathecal local anesthetic infusion in the rat. *Anesthesiology*. 1994;80:847-852.

68. Sala-Blanch X, López AM, Pomés J, et al. No clinical or electrophysiologic evidence of nerve injury after intraneural injection during sciatic popliteal block. *Anesthesiology*. 2011;115:589-595.

69. Rigler ML, Drasner K, Krejcie TC, et al. Cauda equina syndrome after continuous spinal anesthesia. *Anesth Analg*. 1991;72(3):275-281.

70. Rigler ML, Drasner K. Distribution of catheter-injected local anesthetic in a model of the subarachnoid space. *Anesthesiology*. 1991;75:684-692.

71. Kirillova I, Teliban A, Gorodetskaya N, et al. Effect of local and intravenous lidocaine on ongoing activity in injured afferent nerve fibers. *Pain*. 2011;152:1562-1571.

72. Puig S, Sorkin LS. Formalin-evoked activity in identified primary afferent fibers: systemic lidocaine suppresses phase-2 activity. *Pain*. 1996;64:345-355.

73. Biella G, Sotgiu ML. Central effects of systemic lidocaine mediated by glycine spinal receptors: an iontophoretic study in the rat spinal cord. *Brain Res*. 1993;603(2):201-206.

74. Sotgiu ML, Lacerenza M, Marchettini P. Effect of systemic lidocaine on dorsal horn neuron hyperactivity following chronic peripheral nerve injury in rats. *Somatosens Mot Res*. 1992;9:227-233.

75. McClure JH. Ropivacaine. *Br J Anaesth*. 1996;76:300-307.

76. Abboud TK, Khoo SS, Miller F, et al. Maternal, fetal, and neonatal responses after epidural anesthesia with bupivacaine, 2-chloroprocaine, or lidocaine. *Anesth Analg*. 1982;61:638-644.

77. Karambelkar DJ, Ramanathan S. 2-Chloroprocaine antagonism of epidural morphine analgesia. *Acta Anaesthesiol Scand*. 1997;41:774-778.

78. Taniguchi M, Bollen AW, Drasner K. Sodium bisulfite: scapegoat for chloroprocaine neurotoxicity? *Anesthesiology*. 2004;100:85-91.

79. Miller II KJ, Rao YK, Goodwill SR, et al. Solubility and in vitro percutaneous absorption of tetracaine from solvents of propylene glycol and saline. *Int J Pharmaceut*. 1993;98:101-111.

80. de Jong RH, Bonin JD. Toxicity of local anesthetic mixtures. *Toxicol Appl Pharmacol*. 1980;54:501-507.

81. Weinberg GL, VadeBoncouer T, Ramaraju GA, et al. Pretreatment or resuscitation with a lipid infusion shifts the dose-response to bupivacaine-induced asystole in rats. *Anesthesiology*. 1998;88(4):1071-1075.

82. Jamaty C, Bailey B, Larocque A, et al. Lipid emulsions in the treatment of acute poisoning: a systematic review of human and animal studies. *Clin Toxicol (Phila)*. 2010;48:1-27.

83. Stehr SN, Ziegeler JC, Pexa A, et al. The effects of lipid infusion on myocardial function and bioenergetics in l-bupivacaine toxicity in the isolated rat heart. *Anesth Analg*. 2007;104:186-192.

84. Marwick PC, Levin AI, Coetzee AR. Recurrence of cardiotoxicity after lipid rescue from bupivacaine-induced cardiac arrest. *Anesth Analg*. 2009;108:1344-1346.

85. Tadicherla S, Berman B. Percutaneous dermal drug delivery for local pain control. *Ther Clin Risk Manag*. 2006;2:99-113.

86. Friedman PM, Mafong EA, Friedman ES, et al. Topical anesthetics update: EMLA and beyond. *Dermatol Surg*. 2001;27:1019-1026.

87. Sawyer J, Febbraro S, Masud S, et al. Heated lidocaine/tetracaine patch (Synera, Rapydan) compared with lidocaine/prilocaine cream (EMLA) for topical anaesthesia before vascular access. *Br J Anaesth*. 2009;102:210-215.

88. Marhofer P, Schrogendorfer K, Wallner T, et al. Ultrasonographic guidance reduces the amount of local anesthetic for 3-in-1 blocks. *Reg Anesth Pain Med*. 1998;23:584-588.

89. Williams SR, Chouinard P, Arcand G, et al. Ultrasound guidance speeds execution and improves the quality of supraclavicular block. *Anesth Analg*. 2003;97:1518-1523.

90. Gray AT. Ultrasound-guided regional anesthesia: current state of the art. *Anesthesiology*. 2006;104:368-373.

91. Hollmann MW, Durieux ME. Local anesthetics and the inflammatory response: a new therapeutic indication? *Anesthesiology*. 2000;93:858-875.

92. Ohsaka A, Saionji K, Sato N, et al. Local anesthetic lidocaine inhibits the effect of granulocyte colony-stimulating factor on human neutrophil functions. *Exp Hematol*. 1994;22:460-466.

93. Martinsson T, Oda T, Fernvik E, et al. Ropivacaine inhibits leukocyte rolling, adhesion and CD11b/CD18 expression. *J Pharmacol Exp Ther*. 1997;283:59-65.

94. Peck SL, Johnston RB Jr, Horwitz LD. Reduced neutrophil superoxide anion release after prolonged infusions of lidocaine. *J Pharmacol Exp Ther*. 1985;235:418-422.

95. Haines KA, Reibman J, Callegari PE, et al. Cocaine and its derivatives blunt neutrophil functions without influencing phosphorylation of a 47-kilodalton component of the reduced nicotinamide-adenine dinucleotide phosphate oxidase. *J Immunol*. 1990;144:4757-4764.

96. Padera R, Bellas E, Tse JY, et al. Local myotoxicity from sustained release of bupivacaine from microparticles. *Anesthesiology*. 2008;108:921-928.

97. Rodriguez-Navarro AJ, Berde CB, Wiedmaier G, et al. Comparison of neosaxitoxin versus bupivacaine via port infiltration for postoperative analgesia following laparoscopic cholecystectomy: a randomized, double-blind trial. *Reg Anesth Pain Med*. 2011;36:103-109.

98. Epstein-Barash H, Shichor I, Kwon AH, et al. Prolonged duration local anesthesia with minimal toxicity. *Proc Natl Acad Sci U S A*. 2009;106:7125-7130.

Chapter 18

NEUROMUSCULAR PHYSIOLOGY AND PHARMACOLOGY

Edward A. Bittner and J.A. Jeevendra Martyn

The neuromuscular junction (NMJ) is among the most studied of all synapses and serves as a prototype for understanding communication between neurons and effector cells within the central and peripheral nervous systems. Although a complete understanding of its development and function in normal and pathologic states is lacking, the introduction of new and powerful research techniques has revealed detailed information about the mechanics of neuromuscular transmission.[1] Recent discoveries suggest a more complex signaling system with adaptive receptor physiology and a multifaceted action-response scheme. These discoveries, although adding complexity, help align experimentally derived findings with clinical observations of therapeutic effects and side effects of drugs acting on the cholinergic system.

The physiology and pharmacology of the NMJ is pivotal to many areas of anesthetic practice including perioperative management and critical care. Despite the central role of the NMJ, in many clinical circumstances our ability to manipulate the NMJ to the patient's advantage is deficient. This is best illustrated by the ongoing problem of residual neuromuscular paralysis recorded after general anesthesia, despite the use and availability of intermediate-acting neuromuscular blocking agents (NMBAs), better monitors for assessment of paralysis, and availability of drugs for reversal of paralysis (see Chapter 19).[2,3]

The complexities of normal neuromuscular function are altered by many pathologic states not originally thought to involve the NMJ. For example, an unexpected consequence of improved survival after a critical illness, such as sepsis or acute respiratory distress syndrome (ARDS), is the "unmasking" of profound disease of the nerve, NMJ, and muscle causing substantial morbidity and mortality.[4,5]

This chapter reviews salient features of the structure and function of the NMJ relevant to understanding the clinical effects of NMBAs, neuromuscular monitoring, and the management of disorders of the neuromuscular system in anesthesia and critical care. A detailed discussion of NMBAs and drugs that reverse the effects of NMBAs is provided in Chapter 19.

OVERVIEW OF NEUROMUSCULAR TRANSMISSION

The classic model of neuromuscular transmission is straightforward. The nerve synthesizes acetylcholine (ACh), which is stored in small uniformly sized membrane vesicles called *synaptic vesicles.* When the distal motor nerve is stimulated by an action potential, it causes voltage-gated Ca^{2+} channels to open, giving rise to an abrupt, rapid, transient increase in nerve terminal Ca^{2+} concentration.[6] The elevated Ca^{2+} concentration triggers fusion of ACh-containing synaptic vesicles to the presynaptic membrane, where they release ACh into the synaptic cleft that separates the nerve from the muscle.[6] ACh released into the cleft binds to nicotinic AChRs on the surface of the post-junctional muscle membrane. These heteropentameric ligand-gated ion channels are nonselective cation channels in the postjunctional membrane that allow influx of Na^+, resulting in endplate depolarization and muscle contraction.[6] Much of the released ACh is instantaneously hydrolyzed by synaptic acetylcholinesterase present in the cleft and never reaches its target. The excess release of ACh contributes to a margin of safety that ensures successful neurotransmission.[7]

STRUCTURE AND FUNCTION OF THE NEUROMUSCULAR JUNCTION

The structure and function of the NMJ can be conveniently divided into presynaptic, synaptic cleft, and postsynaptic entities (Figure 18-1).

Presynaptic Structure and Function

The presynaptic portion of the NMJ is responsible for neurotransmitter (ACh) synthesis, uptake and storage of neurotransmitter into synaptic vesicles, ACh release and reuptake of choline after its hydrolysis, and control of ion flow across the nerve terminal cell membrane. Each motor neuron represents a large myelinated axon that extends from the ventral horn of the spinal cord or medulla to the NMJ. As it approaches the target muscle, the myelinated motor axon divides into 20 to 100 unmyelinated fibers, each of which innervates a single muscle fiber.[8] The functional group of terminal nerve fibers and the muscle fibers they serve is called a *motor unit.* The terminal myelin-free portion of the nerve axon is encapsulated by a Schwann cell. The Schwann cells are not primarily involved in neuromuscular transmission but support the connection between nerve and muscle and promote maintenance of the nerve terminal (see Figure 18-1).[9,10]

Synaptic Cleft Structure and Function

The junctional or synaptic cleft is the gap (approximately 50 nm) between the nerve terminal ending and the muscle membrane.[11] The cleft contains a basal lamina composed of a

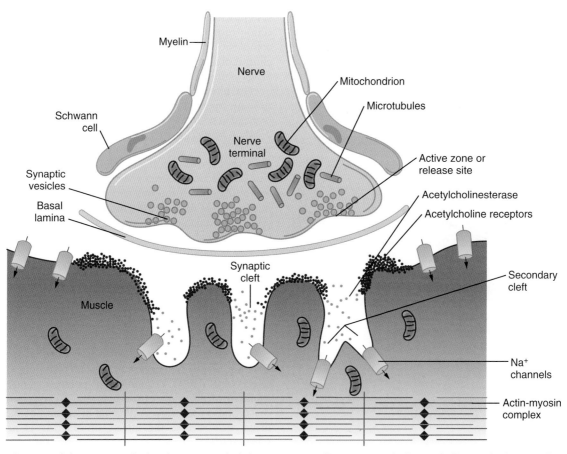

Figure 18-1 Structure of the neuromuscular junction, composed of the motor neuron (i.e., nerve terminal), muscle fiber, and Schwann cell. As the nerve approaches the muscle fibers it loses its myelin sheath and divides into branches that innervate many individual muscle fibers. The motor nerve without myelin is covered by the Schwann cell. The nerve terminal contains vesicles clustered about membrane thickenings, the active zones, at the synapse, and mitochondria and microtubules further from the synapse. A synaptic gutter or cleft, made up of a primary and many secondary clefts, separates the nerve from the muscle. The muscle surface is corrugated, and dense areas on the shoulders of each fold contain acetylcholine receptors. Sodium channels are present at the bottom of the clefts and throughout the muscle membrane. Acetylcholinesterase, as well as other proteins and proteoglycans that stabilize the neuromuscular junction, are present in the synaptic clefts.

variety of cell and other adhesion macromolecules that modulate neuromuscular signaling processes. These molecules include acetylcholinesterase, α- and β-laminin, and collagen.

After release from the nerve terminal, ACh diffuses the short distance across the synaptic cleft to the postsynaptic membrane. The high concentration of ACh in combination with the short distance between the site of release and the postsynaptic membrane ensure rapid transmission. Approximately 50% of the released ACh is either degraded by acetylcholinesterase or diffuses out of the cleft before it reaches its target.[8] Acetylcholinesterase is anchored to the basal lamina where it degrades ACh into acetate and choline, thereby terminating the activity of the transmitter. Choline is then taken up into the presynaptic terminal by a specific transporter for resynthesis of ACh within the nerve terminal.

Postsynaptic Membrane

The muscle membrane is highly corrugated with deep invaginations representing primary (shallower) and secondary (deeper) clefts such that the total surface area of each endplate is very large (see Figure 18-1). The depths of these folds vary between muscle types and species. The shoulders of the folds contain high densities of AChRs (approximately 5 million in each junction) anchored into the muscle cell membrane by a complex system of cytoskeletal proteins. AChRs are sparse in the depths between the folds which contain a high density of voltage-gated Na+ channels for amplification of AChR-induced depolarization.

The perijunctional zone is the area of muscle that lies immediately beyond the junctional area. It serves the critical function of transducing the signal from the junction into deeper regions of the muscle cell. The perijunctional zone contains a high density of Na+ channels that promote amplification of the transduced signal, culminating in muscle contraction. The density of Na+ channels in the perijunctional zone is greater than in more distal parts of the muscle membrane.[12] Furthermore, specific isoforms of AChRs and Na+ channels are expressed in the perijunctional area at different stages of life and during pathologic conditions that decrease nerve activity. Mutations in AChRs and Na+ and Ca2+ channels in this area have been identified.[13,14] For example, in hypokalemic periodic paralysis, characterized by episodes of severe flaccid muscle paralysis, the muscle fiber membrane becomes electrically inexcitable, which can be precipitated by low serum K+ levels. This pathologic state is the archetypal skeletal muscle channelopathy caused by dysfunction of specific sarcolemmal Na+ or Ca2+ ion channels.[15] These variations in receptors and channels contribute to differences in response to neuromuscular drugs observed in different age groups and pathologic conditions.[16,17]

QUANTAL THEORY OF NEUROMUSCULAR TRANSMISSION

Synaptic vesicles containing neurotransmitter are clustered along thickened, electron-dense patches of membrane in the terminal portion of the nerve referred to as *active zones*. High-resolution scanning microscope imaging reveals small protein particles arranged between vesicles in the active zone that are believed to be voltage-gated Ca2+ channels. These channels permit Ca2+ to enter the nerve and initiate the process that ultimately triggers vesicle release. The close proximity of voltage-gated Ca2+ channels to the vesicle fusion apparatus is believed to contribute to the rapidity with which ACh is released (~200 ns).[6]

The number of quanta of ACh released by a stimulated nerve is strongly influenced by the concentration of extracellular ionized Ca2+ and its influx into the nerve. Doubling extracellular Ca2+ concentration results in a 16-fold increase in quantal release.[18] The effect of increasing Ca2+ in the nerve ending is seen clinically as the phenomenon of posttetanic potentiation. This can occur after the nerve of a patient paralyzed with a nondepolarizing NMBA is stimulated at high tetanic frequencies. With each stimulus, Ca2+ enters the nerve, but because it cannot be excreted as quickly as the nerve is stimulated, it accumulates during the tetanic period. The nerve ending contains an elevated amount of Ca2+ for some time after the tetanic stimulation, and if another stimulus is applied during this time, it increases the amount of ACh that is released. The increased amount of ACh released antagonizes the nondepolarizing NMBA and results in the characteristic increase in twitch size observed after tetanic stimulation (posttetanic potentiation).

The amount of ACh released by each nerve impulse is large, at least 200 quanta, consisting of about 5000 ACh molecules each, and about 500,000 AChRs are activated.[19] The ions (mainly Na+ and some Ca2+) that flow through the AChR channels cause maximal depolarization of the endplate, resulting in an endplate potential that exceeds the threshold for stimulation of the muscle. This produces a biologic advantage. By releasing more molecules of transmitter than actually are needed and evoking a greater response than needed while using only a small fraction of the vesicles and receptors available, neurotransmission has a substantial margin of safety and at the same time has substantial capacity in reserve.[20]

SYNAPTIC VESICLES AND RECYCLING

Two major pools of vesicles are involved in ACh release: a readily releasable pool (sometimes called V2) and a reserve pool (sometimes called V1).[21,22] The readily releasable pool is smaller and is confined to an area very close to the nerve membrane where the vesicles are bound to the active zones. These are the vesicles that are normally available to release neurotransmitter. The reserve pool contains the majority of synaptic vesicles which are tethered to the cytoskeleton in a filamentous network composed mainly of actin, synapsin, synaptotagmin, and spectrin.

The larger reserve pool (V1) can be mobilized to the readily releaseable store when there is increased demand, such as when the nerve is stimulated at high frequencies or for long periods of time. Under such high demand conditions, increases in Ca2+ concentration penetrate more deeply than normal into the nerve or might enter via L-type Ca2+ channels (see later). This probably activates Ca2+-dependent enzymes that break the links with synapsin that hold the reserve vesicles to the cytoskeleton, thereby allowing mobilization of vesicles to release sites. Repeated stimulation of the nerve requires replenishment of the nerve ending with synaptic vesicles, a process known as *mobilization*.

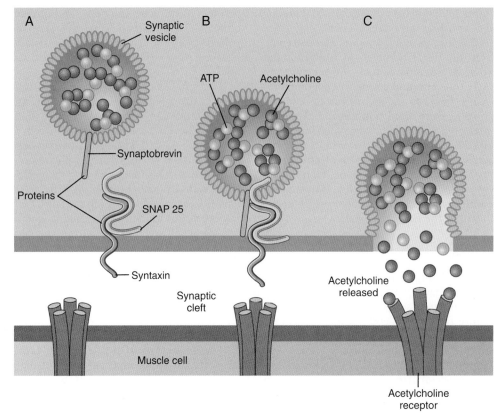

Figure 18-2 Membrane fusion and exocytosis of acetylcholine vesicles from the motor nerve terminal. **A,** Acetylcholine is stored in synaptic vesicles. Its release is mediated by SNARE proteins. SNAP-25 and syntaxin are nerve terminal membrane SNARE proteins. **B,** During depolarization and Ca²⁺ entry through voltage-gated Ca²⁺ channels, SNARE proteins on the vesicle (synaptobrevin) and on the membrane (SNAP-25 and syntaxin) interact and the vesicle is attached to the membrane. **C,** Upon depolarization and Ca²⁺ entry, Ca²⁺ binding to the Ca²⁺ sensor synaptotagmin triggers fusion of the vesicle to the nerve membrane at the active zone to release its contents, acetylcholine.

The aggregate process is involved in maintaining the capacity of the nerve ending to release neurotransmitter. This process encompasses everything from uptake of choline and synthesis of acetate to the movement of vesicles to release sites. The rate-limiting steps of this process appear to be the uptake of choline and the activity of choline acetyltransferase, the enzyme that synthesizes acetylcholine.[23]

The complex process of docking, fusion, and release of neurotransmitter from synaptic vesicles is called *exocytosis*. Three proteins, synaptobrevin, syntaxin, and SNAP-25, within the group of soluble N-ethylmaleimide-sensitive factor attachment receptor (SNARE) proteins have key roles in the process of exocytosis (Figure 18-2).[24] A complex of syntaxin and SNAP-25 is attached to the plasma membrane. After initial contact, synaptobrevin on the vesicle forms a ternary complex with syntaxin and SNAP-25 that consists of a zippered helical bundle. This complex forces the vesicle close to the nerve terminal membrane at the active zone (release site). Synaptotagmin, a protein on the vesicular membrane that acts as the Ca²⁺ sensor, localizes the vesicles to synaptic zones rich in Ca²⁺ channels and stabilizes the vesicles in the docked state.[25] After fusion and exocytosis, the used vesicle and membrane parts are recycled through an active process into the nerve terminal; there they are reused to form new vesicles (endocytosis), filled with ACh, and then transported to the active sites for release.

NERVE TERMINAL ACTION POTENTIAL

During the nerve action potential, Na⁺ from outside the nerve flows down its electrochemical gradient across the cell membrane and the resulting depolarizing voltage opens voltage-gated Ca²⁺ channels, which permit Ca²⁺ to enter the nerve down its electrochemical gradient, triggering the release of ACh. Of the several subtypes of Ca²⁺ channels, four voltage-gated Ca²⁺ channels are important for spontaneous and evoked release of ACh: P-, N-, L-, and R-type channels. P-type channels are found only in nerve terminals immediately adjacent to the active zones and are probably the major type responsible for the normal release of neurotransmitter.[26] They are voltage-gated and open and close in response to changes in the membrane voltage caused by the nerve action potential.

During the nerve action potential, the Ca²⁺ current persists until the channels inactivate and outward fluxes of K⁺ from inside the nerve return the membrane potential to normal. As with Ca²⁺ channels on the nerve terminal, there are several forms of K⁺ channels including voltage-gated and Ca²⁺-activated K⁺ channels. These K⁺ channels limit the duration of nerve terminal depolarization and thereby Ca²⁺ entry and release of neurotransmitter.[27]

In the absence of an action potential, small spontaneous depolarizing potentials can be recorded at the postsynaptic

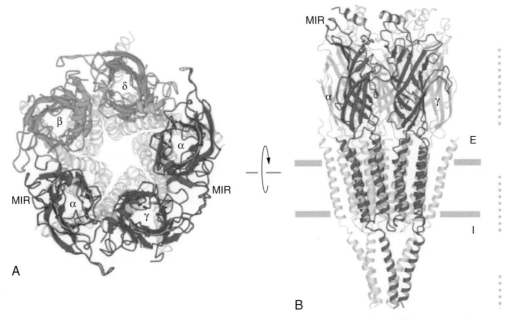

Figure 18-3 Ribbon diagrams of the nicotinic acetylcholine receptor, as viewed from above the synaptic cleft **(A)** and parallel with the plasma membrane plane **(B)**. For clarity, only the ligand-binding domain is highlighted in **A** and only the front two subunits are highlighted in **B**) (α, red; β, green; γ, blue; δ, light blue). The main immunogenic region (MIR), where antibodies against the receptor in myasthenia gravis patients bind, is very close to the acetylcholine binding site. The membrane is indicated by horizontal bars (*E*, extracellular; *I*, intracellular). The dotted lines on the right denote the three main zones of subunit contacts during folding and formation of the receptor channel. *(Reproduced from Unwin N. Refined structure of the nicotinic acetylcholine receptor at 4A resolution.* J Mol Biol. *2005;346:967-989.)*

muscle membrane. These miniature endplate potentials (MEPPs) are the result of the spontaneous release of a small number of ACh-containing vesicles. They have only $\frac{1}{100}$th the amplitude of the evoked potential produced when the motor nerve is stimulated. Statistical analysis has led to the conclusion that there is a minimum size for MEPPs and that the size of all MEPPs is equal to or a multiple of this minimum size, equivalent to the fusion of a single synaptic vesicle.[28] Consequently, it was deduced that MEPPs are produced by these uniform sized packages or *quanta* of released transmitter in the absence of stimulation. Stimulation-evoked endplate potential depolarization is the additive effect produced by several hundred vesicles synchronously discharging quanta of neurotransmitter. Except for the reduced amplitude, MEPPs resemble the endplate potential in their time course and their sensitivity to drugs.

ACETYLCHOLINESTERASE

Acetylcholinesterase is a type-B carboxylesterase enzyme located primarily in the synaptic cleft with a smaller concentration in the extrajunctional area. Acetylcholinesterase is secreted by the muscle and remains attached to it by collagen fastened to the basal lamina. ACh molecules that do not bind immediately with a receptor or those released after reacting with a receptor are hydrolyzed almost instantly (in less than 1 ms) by acetylcholinesterase. Approximately 50% of the released ACh is hydrolyzed into choline and acetate before reaching the receptor.[6] Choline is taken up by the nerve terminal and reused for synthesis of ACh.

ACETYLCHOLINE RECEPTORS

Structure

Nicotinic AChRs belong to the cys-loop superfamily of pentameric ligand-gated ion channels that share a common architecture, with five subunits surrounding a central ion-conducting pore. Each subunit is built upon four transmembrane segments with the second transmembrane segment lining the pore (Figure 18-3).[29] Each subunit is composed of approximately 400 to 500 amino acids. The AChRs are synthesized in muscle cells and anchored to the endplate membrane by the 43-kDa protein rapsyn. Four subtypes of muscle membrane AChRs are of clinical importance: α3β2 presynaptically; 2α1β1δε or 2α1β1δγ and α7 AChRs postsynaptically (Figure 18-4). The α-subunits contain two adjacent cysteines essential for ACh binding and the non–α subunits contribute to the specificity and stability of each receptor isoform.[30]

Neuronal AChRs include homomeric and heteromeric isoforms, with α7-9-subunits forming homomeric (formed of same subunit) AChRs and heteromeric AChRs formed by a combination of α2-6- and β2-4-subunits with a stoichiometry of 2 α and 3 β. Compared with muscle AChRs, which have two distinct agonist binding sites—one high affinity between α1 and δ and a lower affinity site between α1 and δ—neuronal AChR agonist binding sites vary based on the subunit composition. This variation contributes to the pharmacologic specificity of each receptor isoform. Heteromeric neuronal AChRs have two α-subunit binding sites between the α- and β-subunits, while the homomeric isoforms (e.g., α7) have five potential binding sites, although the number of bound agonists required for receptor activation is not known.

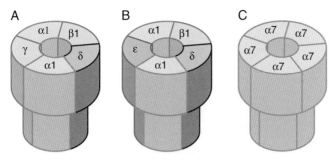

Figure 18-4 Diagram of postsynaptic nicotinic acetylcholine receptors on the muscle membrane. They are pentameric proteins. The mature junctional receptor **(B)** is composed of 2α1-subunits, and one each of β1-, δ-, and ε-subunits. In the immature or fetal receptor **(A)**, which is mostly extra-junctional, the ε-subunit is absent and is replaced by the γ-subunit, while all other subunits are the same as the mature receptor. The α7-acetylcholine receptor **(C)** is a homomeric receptor formed of five α7 subunits.

Although many potential receptors are possible by combining different subunits, only a few have been found to be of biologic importance. In the NMJ, the α3β2 (neuronal) subtype is found in the presynaptic nerve ending. The 2α1β1δγ and α7 AChRs are found postsynaptically during development and denervation, and in other acquired pathologic states (e.g., immobilization and burns).[6] NMBAs and their metabolites can block ACh-mediated effects on neuronal AChRs in vitro.[31] Small amounts of NMBA do cross the blood-brain barrier, but larger amounts most likely cross in critical illness where the blood-brain barrier is more permeable. The long-term effects of NMBAs on AChRs in the central nervous system are unclear, although inadvertent acute direct administration is known to cause seizures. Interestingly, NMBAs decrease hypoxic ventilatory response in partially paralyzed humans; the mechanism for this response might be inhibition of neuronal AChRs within the carotid body.[32]

Electrophysiology

The electrophysiologic technique of patch clamping has provided valuable insight into the functioning of prejunctional and postjunctional AChRs. With patch clamping, a glass micropipette is pressed onto the lipid membrane to form a seal. The pipette is filled with an ionic solution and conducts electric current to an amplifier. Depending on the configuration of the patch, the composition of the pipette or external solution can be changed to include drugs such as ACh, an NMBA, or other drugs to study the ion channels under different conditions and the current or voltage monitored. Using these methods it is possible to determine how alterations in subunit composition, environment, or drugs change receptor electrophysiology.

Under normal conditions, the ion-conducting pore of the AChR is closed by the approximation of the pore gate. When an agonist such as ACh occupies both binding sites, a conformational change occurs, opening a channel through which ions flow along a concentration gradient. Both α-subunits must be occupied simultaneously by agonist; if only one is occupied, the channel remains closed. The NMBAs bind to one or more of the α-subunits, thus preventing ACh from binding and opening the ion channel. This interaction between ACh and NMBAs is competitive and the outcome—neuromuscular transmission or block—depends on the relative concentration and binding characteristics of the agonist (ACh) and antagonist (NMBA).

The AChR ion channel accommodates many cations and electrically neutral molecules but excludes anions. The resulting depolarizing current measured by patch clamp recording through each open channel is miniscule (only a few picoamperes). However, each nerve terminal action potential releases enough ACh to open about 500,000 channels simultaneously, and the total current is more than adequate to depolarize the endplate and produce muscle contraction.

In addition to open or closed states, receptor channels are capable of a variety of other conformational current-passing states.[33,34] They alter the amount of time that they remain open, open and close more slowly than usual, open briefly and repeatedly, or allow passage of fewer or more ions than they usually do (conductance). Receptor channels are dynamic structures that are influenced by a variety of drugs and changes in external milieu, including membrane fluidity, temperature, electrolyte balance, and chemical and physical factors.[34,35] The net effect of these channel influences is ultimately reflected in the strength of neuromuscular transmission and muscle contraction.

Receptor Types

POSTSYNAPTIC RECEPTORS

The trophic function of the nerve and the associated electrical activity are vital for the development, maturation, and maintenance of the NMJ.[36,37] During the late embryonic stage, the motor nerve axons grow into the developing muscle and release growth factors, including agrin and neuregulins (NRβ1 and NRβ2) essential to the maturation of myotubules to muscle. Agrin, a nerve derived protein, stimulates postsynaptic differentiation by activating a muscle-specific tyrosine kinase (MuSK). Agrin, together with neuregulins and other trophic factors, induces the clustering of AChRs and other essential muscle-derived proteins including MuSK, rapsyn, and Erbβ, all of which are necessary for maturation and stabilization of AChRs at the NMJ.

During development (fetus) and at birth, postsynaptic AChRs are composed mainly of 2α1β1δγ and α7 AChRs (see Figure 18-4). Just before birth and shortly thereafter, the 2α1β1δγ AChRs (also called *immature AChRs*) are replaced by mature receptors with a subunit composition of 2α1β1δε. The immature receptors expressed in the fetus are more sensitive to depolarization by ACh, and this increased sensitivity might play a role in directing the nerve bud to muscle. The mechanism of the change from immature to mature receptors is unknown; however, the neuregulin NRβ1 (also called *ARIA*), which binds to one of the Erbβ receptors, seems to play a role. In the rodent, it takes about 2 weeks for complete conversion of immature to mature AChRs, while in humans this process takes longer.[6] The mechanism and time course for disappearance of α7 AChRs in muscle of the newborn is unknown.

PRESYNAPTIC

Compared with postsynaptic AChRs, the structure and function of presynaptic AChRs are not as well understood. Differences exist between presynaptic and postsynaptic AChRs in their ability to bind toxins, as well as agonists and antagonists. Presynaptic AChRs are autoreceptors responsible for increased release of ACh into the synaptic cleft by means of a positive feedback system.[38] This positive feedback system is further regulated by a negative feedback system that senses when the concentration of transmitter in the synaptic cleft has increased to appropriate levels and shuts down further release. Targeted inhibition of presynaptic $\alpha 3\beta 2$ receptors during high-frequency repetitive stimulation results in typical tetanic fade (i.e., the decrease of twitch height during repetitive nerve-stimulated muscle contraction).[39] This tetanic fade during experimental conditions equates to the train-of-four (TOF) fade seen clinically during neuromuscular monitoring after nondepolarizing NMBAs and is used as an indicator of the presence of relaxant-induced residual muscle weakness (see Chapter 19).[40] In contrast to block of presynaptic $\alpha 3\beta 2$ receptors produced by clinically used nondepolarizing NMBAs, the depolarizing agent succinylcholine (SCh) does not inhibit $\alpha 3\beta 2$ receptors.[41] This explains why TOF fade is absent during SCh-induced block.[38] Fade, however, is not always a prejunctional phenomenon, exemplified by the disease myasthenia gravis (MG), a postjunctional disease that shows fade during repetitive stimulation. Fade in MG is due to decrease of postjunctional AChRs, reflecting decreased margin of safety. Thus from a practical point of view, fade observed during repetitive nerve stimulation reflects decreased margin of safety rather than a prejunctional or postjunctional phenomenon.

MATURE AND IMMATURE POSTJUNCTIONAL RECEPTORS

Mature postjunctional AChRs are composed of five subunits consisting of two $\alpha 1$-subunits and one each of the $\beta 1$, δ, and ϵ-subunits (see Figure 18-4). Although the innervated NMJ only synthesizes the mature form of AChR, expression of other receptor isoforms can be induced with decreased neural influence or activity, as seen for example in the fetus before innervation or in adult patients after denervation such as occurs with upper or lower motor neuron injury, or after burn injury and immobilization. In these conditions, immature receptors consisting of $2\alpha 1\beta 1\delta\gamma$ AChRs together with $\alpha 7$ receptors are re-expressed (Figure 18-5). The immature heteromeric AChR is structurally similar to the mature AChR but with a γ-subunit replacing the ϵ-subunit. The immature receptors are also referred to as extrajunctional because they are expressed mostly, but not exclusively, in the extrajunctional region of the muscle membrane. The $\alpha 7$ AChRs are homomeric composed of five $\alpha 7$-subunits. These AChRs have been demonstrated in fetal and denervated muscle and seem to be reexpressed in conditions such as immobilization and burns and possibly in other pathologic states of upregulation of AChRs (see later).

The immature $2\alpha 1\beta 1\delta\gamma$ receptors have a smaller conductance per channel and a longer mean channel open time (2- to 10-fold longer) compared with mature receptors. The difference in subunit composition can alter the sensitivity or affinity of the receptor for certain ligands. For example, ACh and the agonist SCh depolarize this isoform of the immature receptor more easily, requiring only $\frac{1}{10}$th to $\frac{1}{100}$th the dose necessary to depolarize mature receptors. Notably, the $\alpha 7$ AChR can be activated not only by ACh and SCh but also by their metabolites, succinylmonocholine and choline. Thus, the depolarization of the upregulated immature and $\alpha 7$ AChRs with SCh or its metabolites has the potential to cause massive efflux of K^+ to the extracellular fluid causing hyperkalemia (Figure 18-6). Conversely, the potency of the nondepolarizing

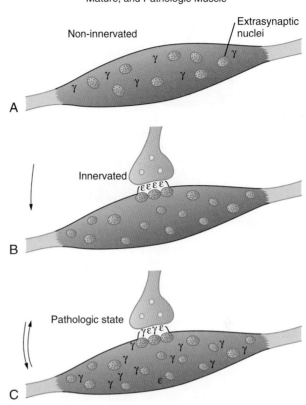

Distribution of AChRs in Developing, Mature, and Pathologic Muscle

Figure 18-5 Distribution of acetylcholine receptors in the fetal or denervated muscle membrane, mature neuromuscular junction and in acquired pathological states. **A,** In the fetus or in denervation, the AChRs are distributed throughout the muscle membrane. These receptors express γ- or $\alpha 7$-subunit containing AChRs. **B,** After birth, with innervation and maturation, AChRs cluster at the junctional area and contain the ϵ-subunit containing AChRs. **C,** In some pathologic states (e.g., burns, immobilization), despite the absence of denervation, AChRs spread throughout the muscle membrane and behave as if denervated, expressing γ and $\alpha 7$ subunits, as well as ϵ-subunits. (The topologic distribution of $\alpha 7$ AChRs on the muscle membrane in pathologic states is unknown, and therefore not depicted on Figure 18-5, **C.**) (See Figure 18-4 for detailed description of composition of postjunctional AChRs.)

NMBAs is decreased with immature receptors as documented by the resistance to these agents in patients with burns, denervation, and immobilization.[17] This resistance might be related to decreased affinity of the $2\alpha 1\beta 1\delta\gamma$ or $\alpha 7$ AChRs for nondepolarizing NMBAs and to upregulation of receptors in the perijunctional area.

UPREGULATION AND DOWNREGULATION OF RECEPTORS

A mechanism for the increased or decreased sensitivity to agonists and antagonist drugs suggests that *decreased* exposure to an agonist results in an increase in the number of receptors (upregulation), while *increased* exposure to an agonist can result in a decrease in the number of receptors (downregulation).[60] Consequently, diseases associated with decreased nerve-mediated contraction (e.g., stroke, spinal cord injury, immobility) result in upregulation of AChRs in skeletal muscle. At the NMJ, this upregulation of AChRs is complicated by the potential for three isoforms of AChRs to coexist. For example, after denervation, there is increased

Innervated muscle

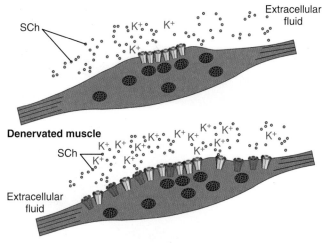

Denervated muscle

Figure 18-6 Response to succinylcholine (SCh) in innervated and denervated muscle. In innervated muscle, SCh-induced depolarization occurs only in the junctional area with limited efflux of K^+ from the cell to the extracellular space. In conditions of upregulated and extrajunctional AChRs, systemically administered SCh comes into contact with all the AChRs throughout the muscle membrane, causing massive efflux of K^+ into the extracellular fluid with potentially lethal hyperkalemia. This occurs because AChRs conduct both Na^+ and K^+, although they are more selective for Na^+.

expression of $2\alpha1\beta1\delta\gamma$ and $\alpha7$ AChRs at the junctional and extrajunctional sites, each of which have their own pharmacologic characteristics. Disease-induced receptor isoform changes and upregulation of AChRs play a role in the resistance to nondepolarizing NMBAs and hyperkalemia in response to SCh. The classic theory on the interaction of agonists and antagonists on upregulated and downregulated receptors is useful for understanding the responses observed with agonists and competitive antagonists of AChRs. In conditions associated with upregulation of AChRs (e.g., denervation), sensitivity to agonists increases whereas sensitivity to antagonists decreases. This is observed clinically by increased requirements for nondepolarizing NMBAs in patients with upregulation of AChRs (see later). Conversely, downregulation of AChRs leads to increased requirement for agonists and increased sensitivity to antagonists, as seen in MG.

RE-EXPRESSION OF IMMATURE RECEPTORS AFTER DENERVATION OR OTHER PATHOLOGIC STATES

After upper or lower motor neuron injury or in certain other pathologic states such as immobilization, burns, infection/inflammation, and critical illness, $2\alpha1\beta1\delta\gamma$ and $\alpha7$ AChRs are re-expressed, extending beyond the NMJ area (see Figure 18-5). In other words, AChR expression in the muscle membrane reverts to the form seen in the fetus or following denervation, despite the absence of overt anatomic denervation. In all of these conditions of AChR proliferation, there is also associated insulin resistance and muscle wasting as in denervation. The role of decreased anabolic signaling in the upregulation of AChRs is unclear. Electrical stimulation of denervated muscle can prevent reexpression of immature AChRs. It has been suggested that entry of Ca^{2+} into the muscle during activity prevents reexpression of immature receptors and possibly $\alpha7$ AChRs. Synthesis of immature receptors is initiated

within hours of inactivity, but it takes several days for full proliferation of receptors on the muscle membrane. With severe and prolonged injury the entire muscle surface, including the perijunctional area is densely covered with immature receptors. The junctional nuclei also continue to make mature receptors, which results in a mix of mature and immature receptors at the endplates. The change in receptor composition alters electrophysiologic, pharmacologic, and metabolic characteristics of the NMJ.

PLASTICITY OF THE NEUROMUSCULAR JUNCTION

Classically, transmission of an impulse from the motor nerve to muscle by the mature NMJ was viewed as a "static" relay form of transmission associated with limited plasticity for nerve outgrowth or formation of new synaptic contacts. More recently, it has emerged that adult NMJs are constantly undergoing structural remodeling and that the NMJ reflects a dynamic equilibrium between growth and regression.[42] This equilibrium can be influenced by a variety of factors including drugs, toxins, aging, disuse, and injury. In addition to the continuous remodeling that occurs at the adult NMJ under normal conditions, extended periods of increased or decreased neuromuscular activity stimulate more extensive remodeling. For example, voluntary exercise can significantly alter neuromuscular morphology, resulting in an increase in area measurements of both the presynaptic and postsynaptic components of the NMJ with the effect depending on the muscle type (fast or slow twitch), age, and type of exercise (endurance or resistance training).[42,43]

A reduction in neuromuscular activity also causes structural alterations in the NMJ. Total disuse resulting either from denervation or synaptic blockade by drugs (NMBAs) or toxins (botulinum or tetanus-clostridial, or tetrodotoxin-puffer fish poisoning) prevents impulse conduction between the nerve and muscle and leads to significant degenerative effects including reduction in endplate area with more shallow primary grooves and a reduced density of secondary folds.[44] Additionally, denervation results in migration of AChRs out of the folds and into the perisynaptic and extrasynaptic regions, resulting in reduced density of receptors at the endplate.[42] Denervation also affects presynaptic morphology with sprouting extending from the motor nerve terminals. Chronic disuse can also cause the presynaptic terminals to release increased amounts of ACh in response to nerve stimulation and increased spontaneous release of ACh quanta.

AGE-ASSOCIATED CHANGES IN THE NEUROMUSCULAR JUNCTION

Accumulating evidence points to age-associated degeneration of the NMJ as a key event leading to functional denervation, muscle wasting, and weakness.[45,46] Anatomic changes involve increased preterminal branching and axonal branching within individual NMJ with or without changes in the total area of the NMJ. The amount of postsynaptic endplate membrane that is *not* in contact with the nerve terminal also increases. The result is a decline in the trophic interaction of nerve and muscle and stimulus transmission. Coupled with the morphologic changes in the NMJ that occur with aging, functional changes in neurotransmission in older adults have been reported, including increased quantal content of neurotransmitter release and more rapid rundown of endplate potential strength during continuous stimulation of the preterminal neuron.[45] In addition, age-related alterations in axonal transport, which could affect the availability of trophic factors, have been reported. Despite these structural and functional changes associated with aging, it appears that an adequate margin of safety for transmission is generally maintained.

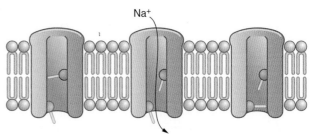

Figure 18-7 Diagram of the voltage-gated sodium channel. The bars represent parts of the protein that act as gates. The upper and lower bars represent voltage-dependent and time-dependent (inactivation) gates, respectively. Left side represents the resting state. Once activated by a change in voltage, Na⁺ moves into the cell (middle figure). Shortly after, the time-dependent inactivation gate closes with block of further influx of Na⁺ despite the voltage gate being open. (See text for further details.)

CLINICAL IMPLICATIONS—ACTIONS OF NEUROMUSCULAR BLOCKING DRUGS

Depolarizing Agents

Depolarizing NMBAs act, at least initially, by mimicking the effect of ACh and therefore can be considered agonists, although they block neurotransmission after initial stimulation. SCh, the only clinically used depolarizing NMBA, binds to the receptor, thereby opening AChR and allowing ion flow that results in endplate depolarization. In contrast to ACh, which has a brief duration of action (~1 ms or less) as a result of its rapid degradation by acetylcholinesterase, SCh is not susceptible to hydrolysis by acetylcholinesterase. Therefore, SCh remains in the synaptic cleft until the plasma concentration of SCh decreases or disappears due to breakdown by plasma pseudocholinesterase (butyrylcholinesterase) or elimination by the kidney. Thus SCh remains available for sustained AChR stimulation causing prolonged channel opening and depolarization of the endplate. SCh exerts a biphasic action on muscle: an initial contraction, observed as fasciculation, followed by relaxation lasting minutes to hours. The time required to hydrolyze or eliminate the drug from the body is the principal determinant of the duration of block (paralysis).

The biphasic action of SCh from initial excitation to eventual block of transmission results from the continuous depolarization of the endplate and inactivation of Na⁺ channels located at the edge of the endplate. Sodium channels have three major conformational states and can transition from one state to another (see Chapter 17). When the Na⁺ channel is in its resting state, the inactivation gate is open but the voltage-dependent gate is closed, and Na⁺ cannot pass. When the channel is subjected to a sudden change in voltage by depolarization, the voltage gate opens and Na⁺ flows through the channel. However, shortly after the voltage gate opens, the time-dependent inactivation gate closes, stopping the flow of ions. The inactivation gate cannot reopen until the voltage gate closes. When depolarization of the endplate stops, the voltage gate closes, the inactivation gate opens, and the channel returns to the resting state (Figure 18-7).

Depolarization of the endplate by SCh results in opening of voltage gates in adjacent Na⁺ channels, causing a wave of depolarization to sweep across the muscle, producing muscle contraction (fasciculation). Shortly after the voltage gates open, the inactivation gates close. Since the depolarizing SCh is not rapidly removed from the cleft, the endplate continues to be depolarized. As a result, the voltage gates of Na⁺ channels adjacent to the endplate remain open and the inactivation gates stay closed and Na⁺ cannot flow. Because the flow of ions through Na⁺ channels in the perijunctional area is stopped, the perijunctional zone does not depolarize and the channels beyond the perijunctional zone are freed from the depolarizing influence. The perijunctional zone, in effect, acts as a buffer that shields the rest of the muscle from the events at the endplate. In other words, the muscle membrane is divided into three zones: the endplate, which is depolarized by SCh (or ACh); the perijunctional muscle membrane, in which the Na⁺ channels exist in an inactivated state; and the rest of the muscle membrane, in which the Na⁺ channels remain in the resting state. Neuromuscular transmission is blocked because ACh release from the nerve cannot overcome the inactivated Na⁺ channels in the perijunctional zone. This phenomenon is called *accommodation*. During accommodation, neuromuscular transmission via ACh release is blocked; however, direct electrical stimulation of muscle can cause muscle contraction because the Na⁺ channels beyond the junctional area are in the resting excitable stable.

Nondepolarizing Agents

Nondepolarizing NMBAs block neuromuscular transmission predominantly by competitive antagonism of ACh at the postjunctional receptor. The effect of this competitive antagonism depends on the relative concentrations of NMBA and ACh and the comparative affinities of each for the AChR. Under normal conditions, acetylcholinesterase rapidly destroys ACh in the synaptic cleft thereby improving the competitive advantage of the NMBA to bind to the receptor. If an inhibitor of acetylcholinesterase is added to the mix, the concentration of ACh in the cleft remains high and there is a shift in favor of ACh binding to the receptor. The NMBAs compete with ACh at the two binding sites of the AChR. Therefore only one molecule of NMBA is needed to prevent activation of the receptor, whereas two ACh molecules are needed for activation. This biases the competition strongly in favor of the antagonist (NMBA) drug.

Reversal (Antagonism) of Neuromuscular Blocking Drugs

Since the nondepolarizing NMBAs block neuromuscular transmission primarily by competitive antagonism of ACh at the post-junctional receptor, the most straightforward way to overcome the effects of the blockade is to increase the competitive position of ACh by increasing the number of molecules available at the junctional cleft. By doing so, the probability is increased that agonist rather than antagonist molecules will occupy the available receptor sites. Normally, only about 500,000 of the 5 million available receptors are activated by a single nerve impulse. This leaves a large number of unoccupied receptors available to be occupied. Another means of increasing the competitive position of ACh is by increasing the length of time that ACh remains in the cleft. The nondepolarizing NMBAs bind to the receptor for slightly less than 1 ms, which is longer than the normal lifespan of ACh. Under normal conditions, the hydrolysis of ACh by acetylcholinesterase takes place so quickly that most of it is destroyed before a significant number of antagonist molecules can be dissociated from the receptor. Use of an acetylcholinesterase inhibitor prolongs the length of time that ACh remains in the junction and allows the ACh to bind to receptor when the antagonist dissociates. The recently developed γ-cyclodextrin sugammadex can bind directly to steroidal NMBAs reversing their action without altering concentrations of ACh at the junction (described further in Chapter 19).

Nonclassic Actions of Drugs Acting at the Neuromuscular Junction

Classic NMBAs interfere with neurotransmission directly by interacting with the agonist-binding sites on the AChR, but other drugs such as procaine, ketamine, or inhaled anesthetics can alter the opening and closing characteristics of the AChR ion channel and/or Na^+ channels through other mechanisms including α receptor desensitization and direct channel block.

DESENSITIZATION

Under normal conditions, the binding of two agonist molecules to the α-subunits of the AChR results in a conformational change that opens the channel and allows ions to flow. However, receptors continuously bound by agonists undergo a time-dependent conformational change that results in channel closure, known as desensitization. These receptors are no longer sensitive to the channel opening actions of agonists, analogous to inactivation of voltage-gated channels. Certain antagonists can bind to desensitized receptors trapping them in the desensitized state. This action of antagonists is not competitive with ACh but can be augmented by ACh if the latter promotes the change to the desensitized state. The mechanism by which desensitization occurs is not fully understood although some evidence suggests that phosphorylation of a tyrosine unit in the receptor plays a role.[47]

In addition to NMBAs, a number of commonly used drugs promote the transition of receptors from the sensitized to desensitized state or cause allosteric inhibition, thereby weakening neuromuscular transmission by reducing the margin of safety and by increasing the capacity of NMBAs to block transmission (Table 18-1). These actions are independent of the classic competitive inhibition of ACh. The net effect of desensitized receptors is that fewer receptor channels are open to allow passage of the transmembrane current, the efficacy of neuromuscular transmission is decreased, and the system is more susceptible to block by conventional antagonists such as NMBAs.

Table 18-1. Drugs That Can Promote Desensitization or Allosteric Inhibition of Nicotinic Cholinergic Receptors

Acetylcholinesterase inhibitors
  Neostigmine
  Pyridostigmine
  Difluorophosphate
  Edrophonium
Agonists
  Acetylcholine
  Decamethonium
  Carbachol
  Succinylcholine
Alcohols
  Ethanol
  Butanol
  Octanol
  Propanol
Antibiotics
  Aminoglycosides, polymyxins
Antiepileptics
  Carbamazepine (acute)
  Phenytoin (acute)
Calcium channel blockers
Cocaine
Local anesthetics
Phencyclidine (ketamine)
Phenothiazines
  Chlorpromazine
  Trifluoperazine
  Prochlorperazine
Volatile anesthetics

CHANNEL BLOCK

Drugs that prevent the flow of ions through channels by blocking the pore are referred to as channel-blocking drugs. Two major types of channel block can occur, open-channel block and closed channel block.[48] In closed channel block, certain drugs occupy the mouth of the channel and prevent ions from passing through the channel thereby preventing depolarization of the endplate. In open channel block a drug enters the open channel and binds within it. In both open and closed channel block, the normal flow of ions through the channel is prevented resulting in weaker or blocked neuromuscular transmission. Because the site of action of channel blocking drugs is not at the ACh recognition site, the effect is *not* reversed by increasing the synaptic concentration of ACh and therefore is not relieved by acetylcholinesterase inhibitors. In fact, increasing the concentration of ACh can increase channel blockade by causing the channels to be open more often and consequently to be more susceptible to open-channel block. There is evidence that cholinesterase inhibitors such as physostigmine and pyridostigmine can act as channel blocking drugs in this manner.[49] Channel block is believed to play a role in altered neuromuscular function associated with a variety of drugs, including some antibiotics, local anesthetics, tricyclic antidepressants, naloxone, and naltrexone (see Table 18-1). NMBAs cannot only bind to the ACh recognition site but also occupy the channel in high doses. Hence the difficulties in reversing deep neuromuscular block with anticholinesterases.

PHASE II BLOCK

Phase II block is a complex phenomenon that results when AChRs are continuously exposed to depolarizing agents (e.g.,

SCh). The NMJ is depolarized by the initial exposure to the depolarizing agent, but the membrane potential gradually recovers even though the NMJ is still exposed to the agonist. Neuromuscular transmission is prevented during phase II block by several processes: The repeated opening and closing of channels with influx of Na^+ and efflux of K^+ causes an electrolyte imbalance that distorts the function of the junctional membrane. Ca^{2+} entry into the muscle through the open channels causes disruption of receptors and sub-endplate structures.

NEUROMUSCULAR JUNCTION IN DISEASE AND INJURY

Important morphologic and physiologic changes in the NMJ occur in response to injury or disease. The common defect of all disorders of the NMJ is impairment of the margin of safety for neuromuscular transmission. Neurotransmission can fail at any point from the nerve terminal to the muscle endplate. If the endplate potential fails to reach the threshold for the muscle fiber, an action potential is not generated, the muscle fiber does not contract, and neuromuscular transmission fails. Failure to generate endplate potentials prevents muscle contraction and produces clinical weakness.

NMJ disorders can be classified as inherited and acquired or anatomically as presynaptic, synaptic, or postsynaptic. The etiology of the dysfunction can also be classified as autoimmune, congenital, pharmacologic, toxic, or traumatic. Most disorders of the NMJ are complex, and multiple mechanisms of failure coexist (Table 18-2).

Neuromuscular Junction in Disease

CONGENITAL MYASTHENIC SYNDROMES

Congenital myasthenic syndromes (CMS) are the most diverse group of inherited disorders of NMJ. They arise from mutations in essential presynaptic, synaptic, or postsynaptic proteins of the NMJ.[50,51] The majority are inherited recessively. Presynaptic defects are associated with abnormalities of quantal release of ACh or ACh resynthesis (mutation in choline acetyltransferase). Synaptic defects can be due to mutations in the endplate acetylcholinesterases and result in a deficiency of neurotransmission at the NMJ due to AChR downregulation as a result of sustained excess in synaptic ACh concentration. Postsynaptic defects, which comprise 75% of CMS, are due to mutations in AChR subunits that alter the kinetics of AChR ion channels or reduce channel density at the endplate. The most common mutations are in the ε-subunit of the AChR. The immature γ-subunit can substitute for the ε-subunit but with less efficient neuromuscular transmission. Mutation of the protein rapsyn, which is involved in AChR clustering, represents another frequent cause of CMS. Mutation of Dok-7, another postsynaptic protein involved in AChR clustering, has recently been linked with a limb-girdle pattern of weakness.[52] Many of these disorders present in the perinatal period with hypotonia and weakness, feeding or breathing difficulties, ptosis, ophthalmoplegia, and in some cases, life-threatening episodes of apnea. Some CMS disorders only become evident during adolescence and some even in adult life. Clinical features along with electrophysiologic and molecular criteria are used to distinguish the CMS subtype. Although at least 10 genes have been identified as sites of CMS mutations, others are likely to be identified. For this reason the diagnosis of CMS is sometimes made on the basis of clinical and electrophysiologic features alone.

Myasthenia Gravis

MG, the most common and well studied postsynaptic neuromuscular transmission disorder, is caused by antibody-mediated reduction in the number of functioning postsynaptic AChRs.[50,53] This complement-mediated destruction is caused by a variety of actions including antibodies directed against the AChR. The antibody binds to extracellular receptor epitopes, cross-linking adjacent AChRs resulting in enhanced receptor turnover (downregulation), and even allosteric interference with the ACh-AChR interaction. The morphologic result of this antibody-mediated destruction is loss of postsynaptic folds and voltage-gated Na^+ channels at the NMJ. Consequently, fewer AChRs are opened by each quantum of ACh release, and the amplitude of the MEPP is reduced. As a result there is marked reduction in the margin of safety and compromised neuromuscular transmission. The NMJ can partially compensate for the loss of AChRs by increasing neurotransmitter release from the nerve terminal.

Clinically, MG is characterized by a fluctuating fatigable weakness of the skeletal muscles. Early in the course of the disease, the weakness can be mild and is often confined to the ocular muscles. In more severe disease, extraocular, bulbar, and proximal muscles are involved. In severe cases, all skeletal muscles including those involved in ventilation can be affected. The diagnosis of MG depends on clinical features, the presence of autoantibodies, and electrophysiologic evidence of disordered neuromuscular transmission. Fade can be observed during repetitive nerve stimulation, even in the absence of NMBA, confirming the decreased margin of safety. Up to 20% of patients with clinical and electrodiagnostic evidence of MG do not have detectable levels of AChR antibodies. Of these "seronegative" MG patients, approximately 40% have serologic evidence of antibodies to muscle-specific kinase (MuSK), a postsynaptic transmembrane protein at the

Table 18-2. Neuromuscular Junction Disorders: Classification by Location of Failure

LOCATION OF DYSFUNCTION	DYSFUNCTION	EXAMPLE
Presynaptic	Choline acetyltransferase deficiency	
	↓ACh molecules/quanta	CMS-defect in ACh synthesis
	Dysfunction in quantal release mechanism	LEMS, botulism
Synaptic	Dysfunction of endplate acetylcholinesterase	CMS-endplate cholinesterase deficiency
Postsynaptic	Reduced AChR expression AChR mutations	Myasthenia gravis
	AChR kinetic abnormality	CMS-slow channel
	Na^+ channel mutations	CMS-fast channel

Ach, Acetylcholine; *AChR,* acetylcholine receptor; *CMS,* congenital myasthenic syndrome; *LEMS,* Lambert-Eaton myasthenic syndrome.

neuromuscular junction.[53] MuSK plays a key role during muscular development in the pathway leading to AChR clustering and formation of the NMJ.

Lambert-Eaton Myasthenic Syndrome

Lambert-Eaton myasthenic syndrome (LEMS) is an acquired presynaptic disorder of neuromuscular transmission caused by autoantibodies directed against voltage-gated Ca^{2+} channels in the motor nerve terminal resulting in down-regulation by endocytosis.[50,53] This reduces Ca^{2+} entry into the nerve terminal during an action potential and thus leads to a reduction in the number of quanta (amount of ACh) released. Morphologically, there is a reduction in the number and size of active zones. The disease is characterized by muscle weakness and fatigability of proximal limb muscles during activity. Oropharyngeal and ocular muscles are usually spared but respiratory muscle weakness can occur, giving rise to respiratory failure. Autonomic function is also abnormal in most patients with LEMS. It is associated with a number of malignancies as a paraneoplastic syndrome. This is most commonly seen with small cell lung cancer in which tumor cells express Ca^{2+} channels that resemble those found on the nerve terminal. Autoantibodies produced in response to the tumor cells also bind to the Ca^{2+} channels on the nerve terminal. In contrast to MG, where there is weakness or fade with repetitive stimulation of nerve, in LEMS with sustained muscle activity there is a transient increase in muscle strength from the initial low level. This is likely a consequence of temporary Ca^{2+} buildup in the nerve terminal and results in increased neuromuscular transmission. The diagnosis is based on detection of antibodies directed against voltage-gated Ca^{2+} channels and characteristic electromyographic findings. The majority of patients with LEMS respond to treatment with oral 3,4-diaminopyridine, which blocks voltage-gated K^+ channels, resulting in prolongation of the action potential and increased quantal release.[54] Treatment of the underlying malignancy can also improve the clinical situation. Patients with LEMS not associated with malignancy often respond to immunosuppressive treatment. Patients with LEMS are sensitive to both nondepolarizing and depolarizing NMBAs. They are significantly more sensitive to NMBAs than patients with MG.

Botulism

A number of naturally occurring toxins act in various ways to inhibit neuromuscular transmission. Botulinum neurotoxin is one of the most potent and lethal substances known and serves as a model for neurotoxic action at the NMJ. Botulism is the clinical syndrome caused by the anaerobic gram-positive organism *Clostridium botulinum*. Seven different serotypes of the organism have been identified, each producing antigenically distinct toxins. The different toxins target different proteins (e.g., toxin types A and E target the SNAP-25 protein of the SNARE complex) at the presynaptic region of the NMJ, resulting in block of release of ACh with ensuing denervation and accompanying muscle paralysis and atrophy.[55] Clinically, botulism generally presents with symptoms of fatigability of the bulbar and ocular muscles and in severe cases weakness of neck, extremities, and trunk, producing a generalized paralysis. Botulism can be fatal by causing respiratory failure and cardiac arrest. Long-term neuromuscular changes result from botulinum exposure in a dose-dependent manner.[56] The incidence of *Clostridium botulinum* infection appears to

be increasing, especially in patients with traumatic injuries, drug abusers, and tissue allograft recipients.[56] Botulinum toxin targeting the prejunctional SNARE proteins (see Figure 18-2) is used therapeutically to treat spasticity or spasm in certain neurologic diseases (e.g., torticollis) and cosmetically to treat wrinkles. In effect, botulinum toxin causes a chemical denervation, resulting in the correction of muscle spasm or wrinkles. Local injection for therapeutic purposes generally results in localized paresis, although systemic effects have been reported.[57]

Neuromuscular Junction in Acquired Pathologic States

STROKE AND SPINAL CORD INJURY

Dysfunction of central motor neurons due to spinal cord trauma or stroke is associated with muscle weakness or paralysis. This causes a reduction in evoked ACh that leads to upregulation of immature AChRs.[60] Upregulation of immature AChRs results in susceptibility to SCh-induced hyperkalemia (see Figure 18-6). The onset of vulnerability is not well defined, but on the basis of several case reports it ranges from 1 week to several months after injury and can persist for years or indefinitely depending on the degree of denervation.[58] These uncertainties warrant the avoidance of SCh in these patients.

BURNS/TRAUMA/CRITICAL ILLNESS

Thermal injury, direct muscle trauma, and infection are all associated with increased AChR expression, especially at sites proximate to the injury.[59] The concomitant presence of disease-induced immobilization can contribute to increased AChR expression and altered sensitivity to muscle relaxants. Chronic treatment with NMBAs commonly used in the intensive care unit to facilitate mechanical ventilation also upregulates AChRs, not only because of immobilization but also as a result of antagonism of the receptor itself. Infections that invariably produce upregulation of AChRs are those by clostridial species that produce toxins that cause paralysis by inhibiting the release of ACh. Infection with other pathogenic microorganisms can also lead to upregulation of AChRs. In all these conditions there is not only an increase in the number of AChRs but also a change in receptor isoforms. The duration of AChR upregulation in critically ill, burn or trauma patients has not been defined, but eventually it reverts to normal with recovery.

IMMOBILITY

Prolonged immobility is associated with muscle atrophy due to disuse. Although motor neurons remain intact, immobility results in a relative increase in $2\alpha1\beta1\gamma$ and $\alpha7$ AChRs. The result is a resistance to nondepolarizing NMBAs and increased sensitivity to depolarizing SCh. Resistance to nondepolarizing NMBAs has been reported to emerge as early as 4 days after immobilization and hyperkalemic cardiac arrest after the administration of SCh as early as 5 days after immobilization.[60,61] After remobilization, these abnormalities should revert to normal but the duration of the restorative process can take months and depends on the severity of the illness.[4] Based on these findings it is prudent to avoid SCh in patients who have been immobilized for more than 48 to 72 hours.

EMERGING DEVELOPMENTS

Disruption of signaling at the NMJ is both a planned intention of the anesthesiologist as well as an unintentional consequence of a myriad of drugs, toxins, and concurrent illness. Despite the central role of the NMJ in perioperative care, our understanding of and skill at manipulating the NMJ is deficient. Through the introduction of new and powerful research techniques, a more detailed understanding of neuromuscular transmission is emerging. Following are several examples of emerging developments in our understanding of neuromuscular physiology, monitoring, and the role of muscle relaxants in critical illness.

Train-of-Four Fade and Monitoring of Neuromuscular Function

An important study had suggested that during repetitive nerve stimulation, prejunctional AChRs ($\alpha3\beta2$) enhance further mobilization of ACh by a positive feedback mechanism to maintain twitch tension, and that block of prejunctional nicotinic AChRs by nondepolarizing NMBAs attenuates this enhanced mobilization of ACh, which results in fade.[62] Subsequent studies using specific antagonists indicated that blocking prejunctional $\alpha3\beta2$ AChRs decreases ACh release by the nerve, but fade was not observed concomitantly. However, fade was manifested when the $\alpha3\beta2$ blocker was administered together with high Mg^{2+} concentration in the extracellular fluid.[63] Higher Mg^{2+} levels, by itself, can decrease the margin of safety of neurotransmission, resulting in fade. Consistently botulinum toxin, which also decreases ACh release by a prejunctional mechanism, causes no fade, although it decreases twitch tension.[56] In contrast, the cobra snake venom, α-bungarotoxin, which binds exclusively to postjunctional AChRs, causes TOF fade. Similarly, fade is observed during repetitive nerve stimulation of patients with MG, a disease with decreased functional postjunctional AChRs.[64] Thus fade observed during TOF stimulation and neuromuscular monitoring can be due to prejunctional and/or postjunctional factors, and reflects decreased margin of safety or efficiency of neurotransmission that requires intervention.

Postoperative residual paralysis, reflected by TOF less than 0.90, is a risk factor for postoperative pulmonary complications.[2] However, anesthesiologists in the United States and the European Union do not routinely monitor neuromuscular block using TOF responses despite its utility to prevent postoperative residual curarization. Some authors strongly advocate that perioperative monitoring of evoked neuromuscular responses that assesses reversal from paralysis should be the standard of care.[65] Although European experts seem to agree on this statement, there does not seem to be a consensus in the United States. A survey of the current management of neuromuscular block suggests a lack of agreement among anesthesia providers about the best way to monitor neuromuscular function.[66] It is now well established that tactile or visual evaluation of TOF evaluation is prone to error.[65] Muscle function returns to normal when the TOF is more than 0.90 with or without reversal drugs. The accepted gold standard for neuromuscular monitoring is mechanomyography. However, its application and use is almost exclusively for research purposes. There is no consensus, however, whether objective measures using acceleromyography, kinemyography, or electromyography are equally effective. Important limitations of these latter devices for routine monitoring of residual paralysis is that they are cumbersome in the clinical setting and are sometimes unreliable because of external factors. Significant postoperative residual paralysis continues to be a clinical problem (see Chapter 19).

Muscle Relaxants in Critical Illness

Muscle relaxants are used in the intensive care unit (ICU) to produce effective synchronous mechanical ventilation, decrease energy expenditure, and prevent high intrathoracic or intracranial pressure during coughing and suctioning.[17,67,68] Several reports, however, implicate severe muscle weakness with the use of muscle relaxants in the ICU.[69,70] Muscle relaxants produce a state of complete immobilization leading to disuse atrophy and even a denervation-like state, evidenced by the upregulation of AChRs throughout the muscle membrane.[71] Thus immobilization (disuse) produced by muscle relaxants can aggravate systemic disease-induced muscle wasting in critically ill patients.

Despite the reported deleterious effects of muscle relaxants on muscle function, some reports validate the beneficial effects of muscle relaxants on oxygenation, survival, and/or increased time off the ventilator without increasing muscle weakness.[72,73] Synchronous ventilation with the use of small tidal volumes and limitation of end-inspiratory lung stretch with reduced plateau pressure might account for these improved benefits.[74] Thus the use of muscle relaxants in ICU can have beneficial or deleterious effects; guidelines for the appropriate use of muscle relaxants in perioperative period need consensus and refinement.

KEY POINTS

- Neuromuscular transmission in skeletal muscle occurs when a quantum of acetylcholine from the nerve ending is released and binds to nicotinic acetylcholine receptors (AChRs) on the postjunctional muscle membrane. These AChRs on the endplate respond by opening channels for the influx of sodium ions and subsequent endplate depolarization leads to muscle contraction. Activation is terminated when acetylcholine immediately dissociates from its receptor and is hydrolyzed by acetylcholinesterase.

- Neuromuscular transmission is a complex and dynamic process in which the effects of drugs are composites of actions that vary with drug, dose, activity in the junction and muscle, time after administration, presence of anesthetics or other drugs, and the age and condition of the patient.

- Classically, transmission of an impulse from the motor nerve to muscle by the mature neuromuscular junction was viewed as a "static" relay associated with limited plasticity for nerve growth or formation of new synaptic contacts. More recently, it has emerged that adult neuromuscular junctions constantly undergo structural remodeling influenced by a variety of factors including endogenous mediators/hormones, age, disuse, and injury.

Continued

KEY POINTS—cont'd

- Age-associated degeneration of the neuromuscular junction is a key event leading to functional denervation, muscle wasting, and weakness. Despite these structural and functional changes associated with aging, it appears that an adequate margin of safety for transmission is generally maintained.
- Neuromuscular junction disorders can be classified as inherited and acquired, or anatomically as presynaptic, synaptic, or postsynaptic. The etiology of the dysfunction can also be classified as autoimmune, congenital, pharmacologic, toxic, or traumatic.
- The common defect of all disorders of the neuromuscular junction is a decrease in the margin of safety for neuromuscular transmission, which can fail at any point from the nerve terminal to the muscle endplate or muscle. If the endplate potential fails to reach the threshold for the muscle fiber, an action potential is not generated, the muscle fiber does not contract, and neuromuscular transmission fails.
- The complexities of normal neuromuscular function are altered by many pathologic states not originally thought to involve the neuromuscular junction such as sepsis or acute respiratory distress syndrome, causing substantial morbidity and mortality.
- In some pathologic states such as denervation, burns, immobilization, inflammation, and sepsis, there is upregulation of immature AChRs, resulting in susceptibility to succinylcholine-induced hyperkalemia.

Key References

Campagna JA. Development of the neuromuscular junction. *Int Anesthesiol Clin.* 2006;44:1-20. This article provides an overview of the development of the neuromuscular junction and highlights recent advances that have a significant impact on the clinical practice of anesthesia. (Ref. 36)

Wilson MH, Deschenes MR. The neuromuscular junction: anatomical features and adaptations to various forms of increased, or decreased neuromuscular activity. *Int J Neurosci.* 2005;115:803-828. This review provides new insights into mature neuromuscular junction as a dynamic entity which continually undergoes remodeling under normal conditions and how the remodeling process is amplified with alterations in neuromuscular activity. (Ref. 42)

Fagerlund MJ, Eriksson LI. Current concepts in neuromuscular transmission. *Br J Anesth.* 2009;103:108-111. This review focuses on recent findings of clinical importance concerning neuromuscular transmission for understanding of the effects of neuromuscular blocking agents, neuromuscular monitoring and the management of disorders of the neuromuscular system within anesthesia and intensive care. (Ref. 11)

Martyn JA, Fukushima Y, Chon JY, et al. Muscle relaxants in burns, trauma, and critical illness. *Int Anesthesiol Clin.* 2006;44:123-143. Burned, trauma, and critically ill patients have the potential to exhibit aberrant responses to neuromuscular blocking drugs. This clinically focused overview describes the etiologic factors and molecular mechanisms responsible for these aberrant responses. (Ref. 17)

Martyn JA, Richtsfeld M. Succinylcholine-induced hyperkalemia in acquired pathologic states: etiologic factors and molecular mechanisms. *Anesthesiology.* 2006;104:158-169. This review focuses on recent findings concerning the etiologic factors and molecular mechanisms responsible for succinylcholine-induced hyperkalemia in acquired pathologic states. (Ref. 16)

Martyn JAJ, Fagerlung MJ, Eriksson LI. Basic principles of neuromuscular transmission. *Anaesthesia.* 2009;64(Suppl 1):1-9. This article provides a review of the structure and function of the neuromuscular junction in normal and pathologic states, which is important for understanding the mechanism of neuromuscular blocking drugs. (Ref. 6)

Newsom-Davis J. The emerging diversity of neuromuscular junction disorders. *Acta Myologica.* 2007;26:5-10. Historic overview of the remarkable diversity of disorders of the neuromuscular junction that have been discovered over the years with emerging research revealing the pathological processes that underlie these disorders. (Ref. 50)

O'Neill GN. Acquired disorders of the neuromuscular junction. *Int Anesthesiol Clin.* 2006;44:107-121. This review describes the major groups of acquired disorders of the NMJ with relevance to anesthetic practice including myasthenia gravis, Lambert Eaton Myasthenic syndrome, acquired "denervation" syndromes and drug-associated NMJ disorders. (Ref. 58)

O'Neill GN. Inherited disorders of the neuromuscular junction. *Int Anesthesiol Clin.* 2006;44:91-106. This article provides an overview of the major groups inherited disorders that affect the anatomy and/or function of the neuromuscular junction including the muscular dystrophies and congenital myasthenic syndromes. (Ref. 51)

References

1. Hughes BW, Kusner LL, Kaminski HJ. Molecular architecture of the neuromuscular junction. *Muscle Nerve.* 2006:33:445-461.
2. Murphy GS, Brull SJ. Residual neuromuscular block: lessons unlearned. Part I: definitions, incidence, and adverse physiologic effects of residual neuromuscular block. *Anesth Analg.* 2010;111:120-128.
3. Brull SJ, Murphy GS. Residual neuromuscular block: lessons unlearned. Part II: methods to reduce the risk of residual weakness. *Anesth Analg.* 2010;111:129-140.
4. Herridge MS, Tansey CM, Matté A, et al. Functional disability 5 years after acute respiratory distress syndrome. *N Engl J Med.* 2011;364:1293-1304.
5. Ali NA, O'Brien JM Jr, Hoffmann SP, et al. Acquired weakness, handgrip strength, and mortality in critically ill patients. *Am J Respir Crit Care Med.* 2008;178:261-268.
6. Martyn JAJ, Fagerlung MJ, Eriksson LI. Basic principles of neuromuscular transmission. *Anaesthesia.* 2009;64(Suppl 1):1-9.
7. Wood SJ, Slater CR. Safety factor at the neuromuscular junction. *Prog Neurobiol.* 2001;64:393-429.
8. Hirsch NP. Neuromuscular junction in health and disease. *Br J Anesth.* 2007;99:132-138.
9. Koirala S, Reddy LV, Ko CP. Roles of glial cells in the formation, function, and maintenance of the neuromuscular junction. *J Neurocytol.* 2003;32:987-1002.
10. Sugiura Y, Lin W. Neuron-glia interactions: the roles of Schwann cells in neuromuscular synapse formation and function. *Biosci Rep.* 2011;31:295-302.
11. Fagerlund MJ, Eriksson LI. Current concepts in neuromuscular transmission. *Br J Anesth.* 2009;103:108-111.
12. Betz WJ, Caldwell JH, Kinnamon SC. Increased sodium conductance in the synaptic region of rat skeletal muscle fibres. *J Physiol.* 1984;352:189-202.
13. Engel AG, Shen XM, Selcen D, Sine SM. What have we learned from the congenital myasthenic syndromes. *J Mol Neurosci.* 2010;40:143-153.
14. Kullmann DM, Waxman SG. Neurological channelopathies: new insights into disease mechanisms and ion channel function. *J Physiol.* 2010;588:1823-1827.
15. Matthews E, Hanna MG. Muscle channelopathies: does the predicted channel gating pore offer new treatment insights for hypokalaemic periodic paralysis? *J Physiol.* 2010;588:1879-1886.
16. Martyn JA, Richtsfeld M. Succinylcholine-induced hyperkalemia in acquired pathologic states: etiologic factors and molecular mechanisms. *Anesthesiology.* 2006;104:158-169.

17. Martyn JA, Fukushima Y, Chon JY, Yang HS. Muscle relaxants in burns, trauma, and critical illness. *Int Anesthesiol Clin.* 2006;44:123-143.

18. Wang X, Engisch KL, Li Y, Pinter MJ, Cope TC, Rich MM. Decreased synaptic activity shifts the calcium dependence of release at the mammalian neuromuscular junction in vivo. *J Neurosci.* 2004;24:10687-10692.

19. Peper K, Bradley RJ, Dreyer F. The acetylcholine receptor at the neuromuscular junction. *Physiol Rev.* 1982;62:1271-1340.

20. Rich MM. The control of neuromuscular transmission in health and disease. *Neuroscientist.* 2006;12:134-142.

21. Südhof TC. Synaptic vesicles: an organelle comes of age. *Cell.* 2006;127:671-673.

22. Lang T, Jahn R. Core proteins of the secretory machinery. *Hndbk Exp Pharmacol.* 2008;184:107-127.

23. Kelly RB. The cell biology of the nerve terminal. *Neuron.* 1988;1:431-438.

24. Engel AG. The neuromuscular junction. *Handb Clin Neurol.* 2008;91:103-148.

25. Heidelberger R. Neuroscience: sensors and synchronicity. *Nature.* 2007;450:623-625.

26. Uchitel OD, Protti DA, Sanchez V, Cherksey BD, Sugimori M, Llinás R. P-type voltage-dependent calcium channel mediates presynaptic calcium influx and transmitter release in mammalian synapses. *Proc Natl Acad Sci U S A.* 1992;89:3330-3333.

27. Naguib M, Flood P, McArdle JJ, Brenner HR. Advances in neurobiology of the neuromuscular junction: implications for the anesthesiologist. *Anesthesiology.* 2002;96:202-231.

28. Standaert FG. Release of transmitter at the neuromuscular junction. *Br J Anaesth.* 1982;54:131-145.

29. Zouridakis M, Zisimopoulou P, Poulas K, Tzartos SJ. Recent advances in understanding the structure of nicotinic acetylcholine receptors. *IUBMB Life.* 2009;61:407-423.

30. Luetje CW, Patrick J. Both alpha- and beta-subunits contribute to the agonist sensitivity of neuronal nicotinic acetylcholine receptors. *J Neurosci.* 1991;11:837-845.

31. Chiodini F, Charpantier E, Muller D, Tassonyi E, Fuchs-Buder T, Bertrand D. Blockade and activation of the human neuronal nicotinic acetylcholine receptors by atracurium and laudanosine. *Anesthesiology.* 2001;94:643-651.

32. Jonsson M, Wyon N, Lindahl SG, Fredholm BB, Eriksson LI. Neuromuscular blocking agents block carotid body neuronal nicotinic acetylcholine receptors. *Eur J Pharmacol.* 2004;497:173-180.

33. Albuquerque EX, Pereira EF, Alkondon M, Rogers SW. Mammalian nicotinic acetylcholine receptors: from structure to function. *Physiol Rev.* 2009;89:73-120.

34. Karlin, DiPaola M, Kao PN, Lobel P. Functional sites and transient states of the nicotinic acetylcholine receptor. In: Hille B, Fambrough DM, eds. Proteins of excitable membranes. *Society of General Physiologists Series.* 1987;41:43-45.

35. Arias HR. Positive and negative modulation of nicotinic receptors. *Adv Protein Chem Struct Biol.* 2010;80:153-203.

36. Campagna JA. Development of the neuromuscular junction. *Int Anesthesiol Clin.* 2006;44:1-20.

37. Witzemann V. Development of the neuromuscular junction. *Cell Tissue Res.* 2006;326:263-271.

38. Bowman WC, Prior C, Marshall IG. Presynaptic receptors in the neuromuscular junction. *Ann N Y Acad Sci.* 1990;604:69-81.

39. Faria M, Oliveira L, Timóteo MA, Lobo MG, Correia-De-Sá P. Blockade of neuronal facilitatory nicotinic receptors containing alpha 3 beta 2 subunits contribute to tetanic fade in the rat isolated diaphragm. *Synapse.* 2003;49:77-88.

40. Jonsson M, Gurley D, Dabrowski M, Larsson O, Johnson EC, Eriksson LI. Distinct pharmacologic properties of neuromuscular blocking agents on human neuronal nicotinic acetylcholine receptors: a possible explanation for the train-of-four fade. *Anesthesiology.* 2006;105:521-533.

41. Jonsson M, Dabrowski M, Gurley DA, et al. Activation and inhibition of human muscular and neuronal nicotinic acetylcholine receptors by succinylcholine. *Anesthesiology.* 2006;104:724-733.

42. Wilson MH, Deschenes MR. The neuromuscular junction: anatomical features and adaptations to various forms of increased, or decreased neuromuscular activity. *Int J Neurosci.* 2005;115:803-828.

43. Deschenes MR, Tenny KA, Wilson MH. Increased and decreased activity elicits specific morphological adaptations of the neuromuscular junction. *Neuroscience.* 2006;137:1277-1283.

44. Labovitz SS, Robbins N, Fahim MA. Endplate topography of denervated and disused rat neuromuscular junctions: comparison by scanning and light microscopy. *Neuroscience.* 1984;11:963-971.

45. Jang YC, Van Remmen H. Age-associated changes in the neuromuscular junction. *Exp Gerontol.* 2011;46:193-198.

46. Deschenes MR. Motor unit and neuromuscular junction remodeling with aging. *Curr Aging Sci.* 2011;4:209-220.

47. Plested CP, Tang T, Spreadbury I, Littleton ET, Kishore U, Vincent A. AChR phosphorylation and indirect inhibition of AChR function in seronegative MG. *Neurology.* 2002;59:1682-1688.

48. Maelicke A, Coban T, Storch A, Schrattenholz A, Pereira EF, Albuquerque EX. Allosteric modulation of Torpedo nicotinic acetylcholine receptor ion channel activity by noncompetitive agonists. *J Recept Signal Transduct Res.* 1997;17:11-28.

49. Maelicke A, Coban T, Schrattenholz A, et al. Physostigmine and neuromuscular transmission. *Ann N Y Acad Sci.* 1993;681:140-154.

50. Newsom-Davis J. The emerging diversity of neuromuscular junction disorders. *Acta Myologica.* 2007;26:5-10.

51. O'Neill GN. Inherited disorders of the neuromuscular junction. *Int Anesthesiol Clin.* 2006;44:91-106.

52. Palace J, Lashley D, Newsom-Davis J, et al. Clinical features of the DOK7 neuromuscular junction synaptopathy. *Brain.* 2007;130:1507-1515.

53. Conti-Fine BM, Milani M, Kaminski HJ. Myasthenia gravis: past, present, and future. *J Clin Invest.* 2006;116:2843-2854.

54. Wirtz PW, Titulaer MJ, Gerven JM, Verschuuren JJ. 3,4-diaminopyridine for the treatment of Lambert-Eaton myasthenic syndrome. *Expert Rev Clin Immunol.* 2010;6:867-874.

55. Rosales RL, Bigalke H, Dressler D. Pharmacology of botulinum toxin: differences between type A preparations. *Eur J Neurol.* 2006;13(Suppl 1):2-10.

56. Frick CG, Richtsfeld M, Sahani ND, Kaneki M, Blobner M, Martyn JA. Long-term effects of botulinum toxin on neuromuscular function. *Anesthesiology.* 2007;106:1139-1146.

57. Lange DJ, Rubin M, Greene PE, et al. Distant effects of locally injected botulinum toxin: a double-blind study of single fiber EMG changes. *Muscle Nerve.* 1991;14:672-675.

58. O'Neill GN. Acquired disorders of the neuromuscular junction. *Int Anesthesiol Clin.* 2006;44:107-121.

59. Ibebunjo C, Martyn J. Disparate dysfunction of skeletal muscles located near and distant from burn site in the rat. *Muscle Nerve.* 2001;24:1283-1294.

60. Martyn JA, White DA, Gronert GA, Jaffe RS, Ward JM. Up-and-down regulation of skeletal muscle acetylcholine receptors. Effects on neuromuscular blockers. *Anesthesiology.* 1992;76:822-843.

61. Hansen D. Suxamethonium-induced cardiac arrest and death following 5 days of immobilization. *Eur J Anaesthesiol.* 1998;15:240-241.

62. Bowman WC, Marshal IG, Gibb AJ, Harborne AJ. Feedback control of transmitter release at the neuromuscular junction. *Trends Pharmacol Sci.* 1988;9:16-20.

63. Faria M, Oliveira L, Timoteo MA, Lobo MG, Correia-De-Sa P. Blockade of neuronal facilitatory nicotinic receptors containing alpha 3 beta 2 subunits contribute to tetanic fade in the rat isolated diaphragm. *Synapse.* 2003;49:77-88.

64. Nitahra K, Sugi Y, Higa K, Shono S, Hamada T. Neuromuscular effects of sevoflurane in myasthenia gravis patients. *Br J Anaesth.* 2007;98:337-341.

65. Viby-Mogensen J, Claudius C. Evidence-based management of neuromuscular block. *Anesth Analg.* 2010;111:1-2.

66. Naguib M, Kopman AF, Lien CA, Hunter JM, Lopez A, Brull SJ. A survey of current management of neuromuscular block in the United States and Europe. *Anesth Analg.* 2010;111:110-119.

67. McCall M, Jeejeebhoy K, Pencharz P, Moulton R. Effect of neuromuscular blockade on energy expenditure in patients with severe head injury. *JPEN J Parenter Enteral Nutr.* 2003;27:27-35.

68. Norwood S, Myers MB, Butler TJ. The safety of emergency neuromuscular blockade and orotracheal intubation in the acutely injured trauma patient. *J Am Coll Surg.* 1994:646-652.

69. Segredo V, Caldwell JE, Matthay MA, Sharma ML, Gruenke LD, Miller RD. Persistent paralysis in critically ill patients after long-term administration of vecuronium. *N Engl J Med.* 1992;327:524-528.

70. Larsson L, Xiaopeng L, Edstrom L, et al. Acute quadriplegia and loss of muscle myosin in patients treated with nondepolarizing neuromuscular blocking agents and corticosteroids: mechanisms at the cellular and molecular levels. *Crit Care Med*. 2000;28:34-44.

71. Ibebunjo C, Martyn JAJ. Fiber atrophy, but not changes in acetylcholine receptor expression, contributes to the muscle dysfunction after immobilization. *Crit Care Med*. 1999;27:275-285.

72. Gainnier M, Roch A, Forel J-M, et al. Effect of neuromuscular blocking agents on gas exchange in patients presenting with acute respiratory distress syndrome. *Crit Care Med*. 2004;32:113-119.

73. Papazian L, Forel J-M, Gacouin A, et al. Neuromuscular blockers in early acute respiratory distress syndrome. *N Engl J Med*. 2010;363:1107-1116.

74. Slutsky AS. Neuromuscular blocking agents in ARDS. *N Engl J Med*. 2010;363:1176-1180.

Chapter 19

NEUROMUSCULAR BLOCKERS AND REVERSAL DRUGS

Cynthia A. Lien and Matthias Eikermann

HISTORICAL PERSPECTIVE

The nondepolarizing neuromuscular blocking agent (NMBA) d-tubocurarine has been used for 500 years as a paralyzing poison. In the 16th century Sir Walter Raleigh reported that hunters in South America were using darts and arrows dipped in curare to paralyze their living targets. Curare, the poison of the plant *Strychnos toxifera*, and its active component, d-tubocurarine, were isolated in the 1930s.[1] d-Tubocurarine was introduced into clinical practice in 1942 to induce neuromuscular block.[2] It was not widely used until the second half of the last century, when maintenance of neuromuscular blockade during surgery became widely accepted. Clinical utility of these agents includes improvement of surgical conditions and facilitating tracheal intubation and mechanical ventilation. Recent data suggest that this class of drugs has the potential to improve the outcome of patients with severe respiratory distress.[3] The use of NMBAs has now become quite common. In 2010, more than 100 million patients received NMBAs throughout the world, 80% of them nondepolarizing NMBAs.

Although the use of NMBAs has allowed the development of modern anesthesia and surgery, their use is not without risk.[4-8] Shortly after the introduction of NMBAs into clinical practice, Beecher and Todd reported an increased mortality in patients who had received NMBAs as part of their anesthetic.[5] Although their conclusions regarding cause and effect have been criticized, residual effects of NMBAs can adversely impact patient outcome.[8] As reported by Beecher, unrecognized residual paralysis negatively affects ability to breathe and airway protection. With the introduction of the intermediate-acting NMBAs rocuronium, vecuronium, and cisatracurium into clinical practice in the early 1990s, the incidence of residual neuromuscular blockade became less common.[7]

NEUROMUSCULAR BLOCKING AGENTS

Clinical Utility

Administration of NMBAs for tracheal intubation minimizes the chance of tissue trauma, which in turn decreases the incidence of postoperative upper airway trauma related symptoms.[8,9] Administration of NMBAs improves intubating conditions and reduces the incidence of vocal cord injury and postoperative hoarseness. Neuromuscular blockade also facilitates surgical exposure and minimizes potentially delete-rious complications of intraoperative patient movement.[10] However, it is not possible to guarantee the absence of patient movement throughout a surgical procedure by focusing only on maintenance of deep neuromuscular block, because patients can move even when their response to neuromuscular stimulation is significantly reduced (one or two responses to train-of-four [TOF] stimulation). Neuromuscular block is not a substitute for adequate anesthesia. Additionally, maintaining deep neuromuscular block throughout the course of a surgical procedure, such as ocular surgery or laparoscopic surgery, might not allow enough time at the conclusion of the pro-cedure for complete recovery of neuromuscular function. Therefore it has been argued that NMBAs are not always required to optimize surgical conditions during anesthesia.[11]

EFFECTS IN DIFFERENT MUSCLE GROUPS

The measured effects of NMBAs on muscle strength depend on the techniques used to measure neuromuscular transmis-sion. Additionally, the effects of NMBAs are different in dif-ferent groups of muscles due to their physiologic differences (see Chapter 18). The diaphragm is less susceptible to the effects of NMBAs compared with both peripheral muscles and pharyngeal upper airway dilator muscles. Following administration of an intubating dose of a competitive NMBA, recovery of diaphragmatic function occurs more rapidly than recovery in muscles of the extremity, such as the adductor pollicis, which is the muscle commonly used in clinical prac-tice for monitoring depth of neuromuscular block. The resis-tance of the diaphragm to neuromuscular blockade can be explained by a greater number of both acetylcholine-containing vesicles being released from presynaptic terminals with neural stimulation and postjunctional nicotinic acetyl-choline receptors than in peripheral muscles.[12]

In clinical practice, the response of the adductor pollicis muscle to stimulation of the ulnar nerve is typically monitored and its response is assessed by either visual or tactile evalua-tion. Other superficially located neuromuscular units can also be monitored. When the arms are tucked and not available for monitoring, the posterior tibial nerve that innervates the plantar muscles of the foot or the facial nerve that innervates the mimetic muscles of the face can be used for monitoring neuromuscular transmission. Different neuromuscular units have different sensitivities to NMBAs and different time courses of onset of and recovery from neuromuscular block (Figure 19-1).[13,14] This has been attributed to different blood flow to these different muscles.[15] These differences must be considered when dosing is based on monitoring at different sites. The mimetic muscles recover more quickly than those of the periphery, and the depth of block in response to a dose of NMBA is less profound than that in the arm or the leg. While different sites can be monitored, dosing recommenda-tions for NMBAs are based on the response of the adductor pollicis to stimulation of the ulnar nerve.

MONITORING NEUROMUSCULAR FUNCTION

The degree of interpatient variability in the effects of NMBAs and the potential adverse consequences of their residual

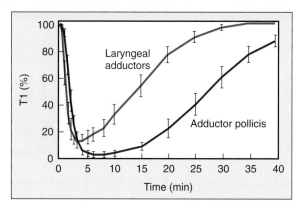

Figure 19-1 Onset of and recovery from vecuronium-induced neuromuscular block (0.07 mg/kg) at the larynx and the adductor pollicis. The larynx is relatively resistant to neuromuscular blockade. *(Adapted from Donati F, Meistelman C, Plaud B. Vecuronium neuromuscular blockade at the adductor muscles of the larynx and adductor pollicis.* Anesthesiology. *1991;74: 833-837.)*

effects at the conclusion of anesthesia underlie the importance of adequately monitoring their effects in clinical practice. Unfortunately, it is not possible to detect residual neuromus-cular block reliably with clinical tests of muscle strength or with commonly used qualitative monitors of neuromuscular function.[16-18]

Reduced strength of contraction during repetitive stimula-tion of a peripheral nerve is observed both with neuromuscu-lar transmission failure, as in myasthenia gravis, and with recovery from nondepolarizing neuromuscular block.[19] Proper muscle function requires different degrees of reserve in terms of neuromuscular transmission, depending on the test chosen. The ability of a test to measure the effects of an NMBA increases with the force of output required to pass the test. Assessment of fade during a supramaximal 100-Hz tetanic stimulation can detect subtle effects of NMBAs, whereas twitch height after low-frequency stimulation (e.g., 0.1-1 Hz) decreases only after blockade of 90% of acetylcho-line receptors.[20] This is clinically important, in that clinicians typically assess neuromuscular function using nontetanic stimulation of peripheral skeletal muscles, usually TOF or double-burst stimulation (DBS). Even though tetanus detects more subtle degrees of neuromuscular block, tetanic stimula-tion is exceptionally uncomfortable for the patient who is not deeply anesthetized. Additionally, interpretation of the sig-nificance of fade in the response to tetanic stimulation is difficult and the degree of fade has not been correlated with the TOF response.

Modes of Stimulation

TRAIN-OF-FOUR
The technique of TOF monitoring was introduced into clini-cal practice in 1970.[21,22] For measurement of the TOF response, muscle contraction is induced by stimulation of the corre-sponding motor nerve four times with a frequency of 2 Hz. Any superficial neuromuscular unit can be monitored in this fashion. In response to TOF stimulation, the TOF-ratio (TOFR) is the ratio of the amplitude of the fourth response to the first response.[21] If neuromuscular transmission is intact, TOF stimulation causes four twitches with identical

amplitudes, with a TOFR of 1. In contrast, after complete relaxation, TOF stimulation does not result in any muscle contraction and the TOF count (number of responses to TOF stimulation) is zero. Return of the first twitch is described as a TOF count of 1. This is followed by consecutive recovery of the second, third, and fourth twitch (TOF count 2, 3, and 4, respectively). Once the fourth twitch has returned, the fade between the first and the fourth twitch responses can be measured as the TOFR. For example, if the amplitude of the fourth twitch is 50% of the amplitude of the first twitch, the TOFR is 0.5. TOF count can also be used to estimate the recovery of the first twitch in the TOF to baseline values. When the first response in the TOF returns, strength of the first response is 10% of baseline values. Similarly, return of the second, third, and fourth responses corresponds to recovery of the first twitch in the TOF to approximately 20%, 35%, and 45% of baseline values.[23]

DOUBLE BURST

DBS was developed to improve detection of residual neuromuscular block.[24] Fade in the strength of the second response relative to the first response is used to determine whether residual neuromuscular block is present. Fade in the response to stimulation is equivalent to fade as detected with TOF stimulation; however, the reliability of qualitative monitoring with DBS is improved over that of TOF monitoring. DBS allows detection of fade when the second response is 60% of the first response. This occurs because the presence of the second and third responses to TOF stimulation makes the comparison of the strength of the fourth response to that of the first response more difficult. With TOF monitoring, only fade greater than 60% (the fourth response is 40% of the first response) can be reliably detected.[25] With DBS, either two or three short bursts of high-frequency tetanic stimuli are administered followed by a second series of two or three short bursts of tetanic stimuli, each resulting in a single muscular contraction. With full recovery from neuromuscular block, two equal responses occur with DBS.

Typically NMBA doses of two times the ED$_{95}$ (the dose required to cause on average 95% suppression of single twitch height) or greater are administered to facilitate tracheal administration. While recovery is monitored with TOF or DBS, onset and potency are typically determined with response to single twitch stimuli. For this pattern of stimulation, supramaximal stimuli are applied at a frequency of 0.1 Hz, or once every 10 seconds. Onset of neuromuscular block is defined as the fade in twitch response with each subsequent stimulus. With larger doses of NMBA, onset of 100% neuromuscular block is quicker and is more likely to develop in all patients.[26] Doubling the dose of rocuronium from 0.6 to 1.2 mg/kg shortens the average onset time from 1.5 minutes to just under 1 minute. When monitoring the effect of NMBAs administered to facilitate tracheal intubation, monitoring at the muscles of the face more accurately indicates adequacy of neuromuscular block in the upper airway.[27] When lower doses of NMBAs are administered, depth of block cannot be guaranteed because onset is quite variable between patients.[28] As shown in Figure 19-2, patients developed up to 80% neuromuscular block following administration of 0.1 mg/kg rocuronium.[29] Just as onset of block is variable with small doses of NMBAs, recovery is quite variable following administration of larger doses (see Figure 19-2).[30] This emphasizes the importance of monitoring depth of neuromuscular block throughout surgery to avoid overdosing.

Even though the most commonly used monitors of depth of neuromuscular block are qualitative monitors, quantitative monitors of depth of block are also available.[31] Without using these quantitative devices, clinicians can reliably detect only severe residual neuromuscular block (TOFR < 0.4), because twitch height at TOFR between 0.5 and 1 is perceived as four responses that are similar.[18] Optimally, quantitative methods for measurement of the evoked muscular response should be used. Commercially available techniques include mechanomyography, electromyography, kinemyography, and acceleromyography.

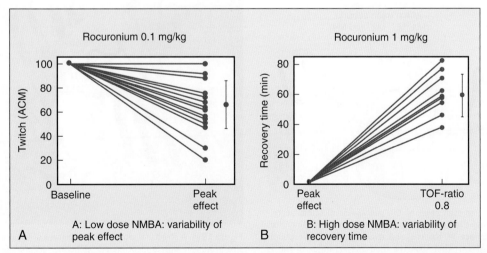

Figure 19-2 Variability of peak effect and recovery times determined with mechanomyography in response to low-dose (**A**) or high-dose (**B**) rocuronium in 20 children aged 2 to 8 years. In one child, rocuronium 0.1 mg/kg did not decrease muscle strength, whereas muscle strength was almost completely abolished in another. After rocuronium 1 mg/kg, recovery of a TOF-ratio to 0.9 varied from 30 to 85 minutes. *(Adapted from Eikermann M, Hunkemoller I, Peine L, et al. Optimal rocuronium dose for intubation during inhalation induction with sevoflurane in children. Br J Anaesth. 2002;89:277-281.)*

STRUCTURE-ACTIVITY RELATIONSHIPS

Neuromuscular Blocking Activity

Structure-activity relationships of NMBAs can affect neuromuscular blocking activity, pharmacokinetic properties, and side effect profiles. Since the early classification of NMBAs as rigid bulky molecules with amine functions incorporated into ring structures, much has changed in modern understanding of the relationships between their structures and function as neuromuscular blockers.[32]

The postjunctional nicotinic acetylcholine receptor is a pentameric member of the superfamily of ligand-gated ion channels. This mature form consists of five subunits: two alpha (α), one delta (δ), one beta (β), and one epsilon (ε) (Figure 19-3). In the immature (fetal) form, the ε subunit is replaced by a gamma (γ) subunit. The N- and C-terminal ends of each subunit are extracellular, with the protein transversing the lipid bilayer membrane four times, creating four transmembrane domains (M1, M2, M3, and M4). The M2 domain of each subunit creates the central ion pore (see Figure 19-3).

The agonist binding sites of the acetylcholine receptor are located at the interface of the α-δ and α-ε subunits where the N-terminus of each subunit interacts with that of the other to form the acetylcholine binding site. In order for the central pore of the receptor to open, allowing for influx of Na^+ and Ca^{2+} and efflux of K^+, two agonist molecules must be bound to the receptor. The two binding sites are not identical (the δ-subunit contributes to one receptor and the ε-subunit contributes to the other). These differences lead to varying affinity at each of the sites for agonists and competitive antagonists.[33-35] The fetal α-γ binding site is generally more sensitive than the mature α-ε one.[35] The α-γ binding site has up to a 500-fold greater affinity for d-tubocurarine than does the α-δ binding site.[36] In mature receptors, the α-δ binding site appears to be more important than the α-ε site in determining receptor affinity for pancuronium, vecuronium, and cisatracurium. It does not appear to play a significant role in determining the sensitivity to either metocurine or d-tubocurarine.[37]

The complexity of fitting large molecules, such as neuromuscular blocking agents, into acetylcholine receptor agonist binding sites (Figure 19-4) implies that conformational changes in the NMBA are required.[38] While these compounds are large, they can bend and fold and will seek a conformation requiring minimal energy. Interaction of the γTyr117 with the 2-N and 13' positions of d-tubocurarine suggests that allosteric changes in either the antagonist or receptor occur with binding.[39] Several different sites of interaction in the binding site are involved in binding the agonist or antagonist.[39] Different affinities at each of these sites might account for some of the synergism observed when different NMBAs are administered to the same patient.[40]

In addition to opening of the ion channel of postjunctional acetylcholine receptors, neuromuscular transmission is modulated by a population of prejunctional cholinergic receptors. These prejunctional nicotinic and muscarinic receptors on the motor nerve endings are involved in the modulation of the release of acetylcholine into the neuromuscular junction. Prejunctional nicotinic receptors are activated by acetylcholine and function in a positive feedback control system that serves to maintain the availability of acetylcholine when demand is high. They are involved in mobilization of synaptic vesicles containing acetylcholine toward the release sites in the presynaptic membrane of the motor nerve terminal, but not the actual process of acetylcholine release. These receptors are morphologically different than those at the postjunctional membrane and consist of three α subunits and two β subunits. All NMBAs tested, including mivacurium, atracurium, cisatracurium, d-tubocurarine, pancuronium, rocuronium, and vecuronium, inhibit presynaptic nicotinic acetylcholine receptors in a concentration-dependent fashion with concentrations causing 50% inhibition of response (IC_{50}) in the micromolar range.[41] Vecuronium and d-tubocurarine are the most potent inhibitors of this receptor subtype, and mivacurium the least

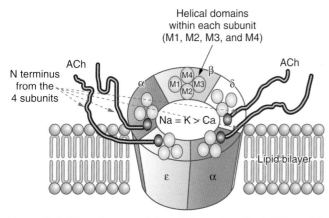

Figure 19-3 Schematic representation of the pentameric nicotinic acetylcholine receptor spanning the lipid bilayer. The acetylcholine binding sites are located at the interface of the α-ε and α-δ subunits. Each subunit contains four domains (M1-4) that span the lipid bilayer. Influx of Na^+ is the same as efflux of K^+, which is greater than the influx of Ca^+. *ACh:* Acetylcholine; *Na:* Na^+; *K:* K^+; *Ca:* Ca^{2+}. *(Adapted from Naguib M, Flood P, McArdle JJ, et al. Advances in neurobiology of the neuromuscular junction: implications for the anesthesiologist. Anesthesiology. 2002;96:202-231.)*

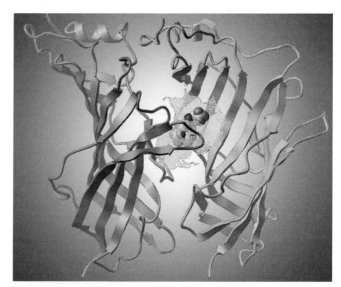

Figure 19-4 A structural model of the interface of the acetylcholine binding site in human muscle nicotinic acetylcholine receptor. Each binding site in the acetylcholine receptor has different affinities for neuromuscular blocking agents. *(From Dilger JP. Roles of amino acids and subunits in determining the inhibition of nicotinic acetylcholine receptors by competitive antagonists. Anesthesiology. 2007;106:1186-1195.)*

Table 19-1. Intubating Doses of Neuromuscular Blocking Agents

NEUROMUSCULAR BLOCKING AGENT	APPROXIMATE ED$_{95}$ (MG/KG)	INTUBATING DOSE ($\times$ ED$_{95}$)
Pancuronium	0.07	1-1.5
Rocuronium	0.30	2-4
Vecuronium	0.05	2-4
Atracurium	0.25	2
Cisatracurium	0.05	3-5

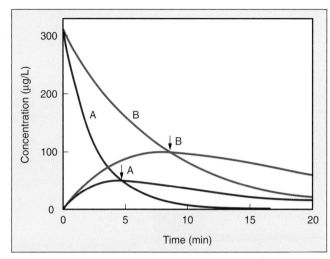

Figure 19-5 Theoretic changes following a bolus dose of neuromuscular blocking agent (NMBA) in its concentration in plasma (*blue and purple lines*) and in the biophase (*brown and red lines*) over time. The concentration of the NMBA in plasma decreases as a result of its clearance from plasma (*curve A*). The concentration in the biophase increases because of transfer of NMBA from plasma to the biophase. When the concentrations in plasma and biophase are similar (*arrow A*), the maximum concentration in the biophase is reached and the peak effect is obtained. The time required for equilibration between plasma and the biophase determines the onset time. If the NMBA is administered in the same dose but has a reduced clearance (*curve B*), equilibration occurs later (*arrow B*) and at a higher maximum concentration in the biophase. Onset time is prolonged and the peak effect is greater. (*Adapted from Beaufort TM, Nigrovic V, Proost JH, et al. Inhibition of the enzymic degradation of suxamethonium and mivacurium increases the onset time of submaximal neuromuscular block. Anesthesiology. 1998;89:707-714.*)

potent. Inhibition of this presynaptic receptor by NMBAs is primarily competitive, but d-tubocurarine and vecuronium also produce noncompetitive inhibition. The effects of blockade on these presynaptic receptors during periods of stress, such as TOF or tetanic stimulation likely accounts for the fade observed in the TOF response with small doses of NMBA, such as those administered before succinylcholine to decrease the incidence and severity of fasciculations of NMBAs.[42,43]

Onset of Block

Onset of neuromuscular block is proportional to the dose, usually described in terms of multiples of ED$_{95}$ (the dose causing 95% suppression of twitch response). The dose used for tracheal intubation is typically twice the ED$_{95}$ or more (Table 19-1), but lower doses of neuromuscular blocking agents that do not cause complete suppression of twitch response can improve intubating conditions during induction of anesthesia. Use of high doses is limited for a number of reasons that include increases in the duration of action (the time required from administration to recovery of twitch height to 25% of baseline, which increases with increasing dose), more frequent and severe side effects, and the limited benefit of increasing the dose beyond a certain point.[26,44,45]

Potency is inversely related to onset of neuromuscular block; the more potent a compound, the slower its onset of effect. Agents of lower potency are administered at a higher dose providing a higher concentration, and therefore a greater driving force for diffusion down their concentration gradient to the acetylcholine receptors of the neuromuscular junction. This has been found for the aminosteroid compounds, a series of tetrahydroisoquinolinium chlorofumarates, with three structurally unrelated compounds, and with compounds of different durations of action and structure.[46-49] Pharmacokinetic modeling with a fixed number of acetylcholine receptors shows that there is a set requirement for the number of antagonist molecules needed to establish block; an ED$_{95}$ > 0.1 mg/kg is necessary for a rapid onset of effect.[50]

In order to exert its effect, an NMBA must get into the neuromuscular junction, which is facilitated by its lipophilicity. The concentration of rapacuronium, a nondepolarizing NMBA with a rapid onset of effect, equilibrates between the plasma and the neuromuscular junction in approximately one-half the time required for equilibration of rocuronium and one-third the time required for equilibration of vecuronium. This is likely due to the more lipophilic nature of rapacuronium compared to rocuronium or vecuronium.[51]

The speed of onset of neuromuscular block after administration of an NMBA is also related to the speed of recovery of neuromuscular function.[52] This appears to be due to the more rapid equilibration between the plasma and effect compartment with drugs that are metabolized or redistributed more quickly (Figure 19-5).[52,53] Thus, in patients who are homozygous for atypical cholinesterase, equipotent doses of mivacurium or succinylcholine have a slower onset of effect.[54,55]

Understanding some of the factors impacting onset of neuromuscular block has led to the development of agents with faster onset. Structural changes in the steroidal NMBAs have yielded compounds with a rapid onset of effect (Figure 19-6). In clinical practice, these structural changes provide a real alternative to succinylcholine when intubation within 60 seconds is required. Rocuronium at 1 to 1.2 mg/kg provides rapid onset of block and is effectively used in this scenario.[26] While no longer clinically available because of inhibition of muscarinic receptors and resultant chest wall rigidity, rapacuronium also provided a rapid onset of neuromuscular block.[57]

Recovery from Neuromuscular Block

In developing a replacement for succinylcholine, short duration and rapid onset of effect are important. Rapacuronium was a promising candidate for fulfilling these requirements due to its rapid onset and duration of effect, which is shorter than that of mivacurium, the only other agent available at that time with a comparable recovery profile (Table 19-2).[56-58] Current research is aimed at enhancing recovery from neuromuscular block in addition to developing NMBAs with shorter durations of effect. Sugammadex, a selective relaxant binding

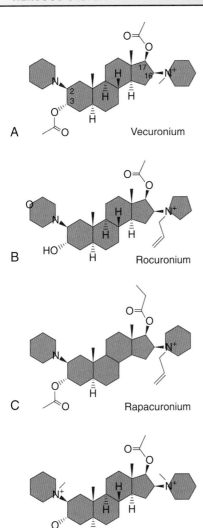

A Vecuronium

B Rocuronium

C Rapacuronium

D Pancuronium

Figure 19-6 The chemical structures of vecuronium, rocuronium, rapacuronium, and pancuronium. The acetyl ester in the steroid nucleus of vecuronium is absent in rocuronium. Substitutions made at positions 2 and 16 of vecuronium, including replacement of the methyl group at the quaternary nitrogen with an allyl group, reduces the potency of rocuronium 6-fold when compared with vecuronium. In rapacuronium, the acetoxy group present at position 17 of rocuronium has been replaced with an aceloxy group. This change further decreases potency of the NMBA so that rapacuronium is 10 times less potent than vecuronium.

Table 19-2. Pharmacodynamics of Rapacuronium Compared to Succinylcholine and Mivacurium

NEUROMUSCULAR BLOCKING AGENT	DOSE (MG/KG)	MINUTES TO MAXIMAL ONSET OF EFFECT	MINUTES TO RECOVERY TO A TOFR = 0.7
Succinylcholine	1.0	1.1	N/A
Rapacuronium	1.5	1.4	24.1
Mivacurium	0.15	3.3	28.9
	0.2	2.5	30.8
	0.25	2.3	32.2
	0.3	1.9	31.6

TOFR, Train-of-four ratio.

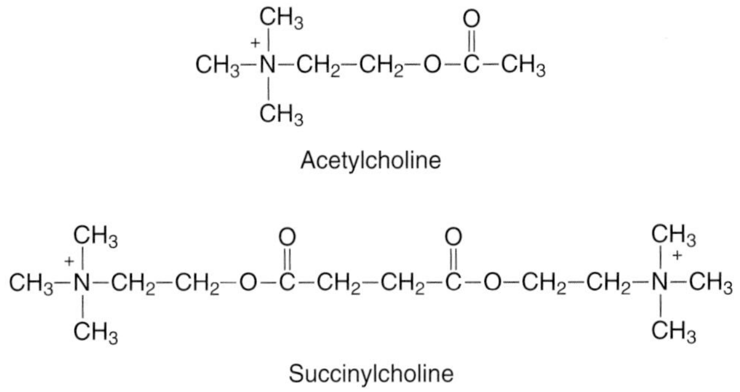

Acetylcholine

Succinylcholine

Figure 19-7 The chemical structure of succinylcholine. It is comprised of two molecules of acetylcholine groups bound together at their acetate methyl groups.

agent, is a cyclodextrin that encapsulates steroidal NMBAs (see Antagonism of Residual Neuromuscular Block). The duration of action of the fumarates is shortened by administration of L-cysteine (see Emerging Developments).

NEUROMUSCULAR BLOCKING AGENTS

Depolarizing Neuromuscular Blocking Agents: Succinylcholine

STRUCTURE AND METABOLISM
Succinylcholine is comprised of two molecules of acetylcholine bound at their acetate methyl groups (Figure 19-7). This structural similarity to acetylcholine allows it to stimulate acetylcholine receptors as an agonist, causing muscle depolarization. Unlike acetylcholine it is not a substrate for the acetylcholinesterase found at the neuromuscular junction that terminates normal neuromuscular transmission (see Chapter 18). Rather its neuromuscular blocking activity is terminated by diffusion out of the neuromuscular junction into plasma where it is hydrolyzed by butyrylcholinesterase (also known as plasma cholinesterase) to succinylmonocholine and choline. While succinylmonocholine is also a depolarizing agent, it is less potent than its parent compound, succinylcholine. The hydrolysis of succinylcholine by butyrylcholinesterase accounts for its short elimination half-life, which is estimated to be less than 1 minute.[59]

PHARMACODYNAMICS
The ED_{95} of succinylcholine is 0.3 to 0.63 mg/kg.[60] Because of its mechanism of action, rapid clearance and relative lack of potency ($ED_{95} > 0.1$ mg/kg), its onset of effect is faster than that of any other available neuromuscular blocking drug. A dose of 1 mg/kg results in complete block in 1 minute and recovery to a twitch height of 90% in 13 minutes or less.[61,62]

Recovery of neuromuscular function after administration of succinylcholine is prolonged by a decreased concentration of butyrylcholinesterase or decreased butyrylcholinesterase activity. Reduced butyrylcholinesterase, whether because of malnutrition, chronic disease, pregnancy, or medications, prolongs the duration of action of succinylcholine.[62,63] Since spontaneous recovery occurs faster than with any available nondepolarizing NMBA, the increased duration of action is not usually appreciated in the clinical setting. Significant decreases in butyrylcholinesterase activity can double the time required to full recovery of 100% twitch response from 10 to 22 minutes.[62] In contrast, patients who are homozygous for atypical butyrylcholinesterase metabolize succinylcholine much more slowly such that the depolarizing NMBA becomes a long-acting neuromuscular blocking agent.

The dibucaine number is used to identify individuals who have an atypical genotype for butyrylcholinesterase. Dibucaine inhibits normal butyrylcholinesterase more than it does the abnormal enzyme. It inhibits normal butyrylcholinesterase activity by about 80%; in individuals who are homozygous for the atypical variant, dibucaine inhibits the activity by only 20%. The enzyme activity of individuals who are heterozygous for atypical butyrylcholinesterase is inhibited by approximately 50%.

Clinical management of patients homozygous for atypical butyrylcholinesterase who have received succinylcholine involves conservative management with ventilator support and continued sedation until spontaneous recovery. Prolonged block with succinylcholine, based on monitoring of neuromuscular function, appears similar to that of a nondepolarizing agent with fade in the TOF response. Administration of an anticholinesterase to facilitate recovery of neuromuscular function is unlikely to be effective because it will also inhibit butyrylcholinesterase, further slowing hydrolysis of the compound.[64]

ADVERSE EFFECTS

Complications associated with administration of succinylcholine are more numerous than would likely be tolerated in any NMBA considered for human use today. However, because of a rapid onset and ultrashort duration of effect, it is frequently used in clinical practice. Most of its adverse effects (Table 19-3) are due to its depolarizing action. Because it also stimulates cholinergic autonomic receptors, all types of arrhythmias from tachycardia and bradycardia to junctional rhythms and ventricular dysrhythmias can be observed. To some extent, cardiac dysrhythmias following succinylcholine administration are dose related. Large doses can cause tachycardia, and in adults second doses administered within a few minutes of the first can cause bradycardia or a nodal rhythm.[65,66] Succinylcholine also lowers the threshold for arrhythmias induced by circulating catecholamines and increases circulating catecholamine levels.[67]

Because it activates acetylcholine receptors, which causes opening of the perijunctional voltage-gated Na^+ channels, allowing generation of a muscle response to neural stimulation (see Chapter 18), succinylcholine causes influx of Na^+ into muscle cells and the efflux of K^+. In normal patients, this typically results in an increase of 0.5 mEq/L of plasma K^+. In patients with significant burns, hemiparesis, or any other pathologic process that causes proliferation of extrajunctional receptors, the response to succinylcholine can be exaggerated, potentially resulting in hyperkalemic dysrhythmias and cardiac arrest.[68-70] The exaggerated efflux of K^+ is due to α^7 receptors as well as extrajunctional nicotinic receptors.[71]

The mechanisms of increases in intragastric, intracranial, and intraocular pressure have not been fully elucidated but include muscular contraction due to activation of acetylcholine receptors and cortical neuronal activation by stretch receptors. The observed increases can be attenuated by prior administration of small doses of nondepolarizing NMBAs such as 3 mg d-tubocurarine, 1 mg pancuronium, or 1 mg vecuronium, 2 to 3 minutes before administration of succinylcholine.[72-74]

When administered together with volatile anesthetics to patients who are susceptible, succinylcholine can trigger malignant hyperthermia although it is a weak trigger alone. A recent review article describes the pharmacology of triggering agents in malignant hyperthermia (see Chapter 6).[75]

Nondepolarizing Neuromuscular Blocking Agents

BENZYLISOQUINOLINIUM COMPOUNDS

There are currently two NMBAs of this class available in the United States: atracurium and cisatracurium. Both are intermediate-acting compounds, with a clinical duration of action of 20 to 50 minutes.

Atracurium

Atracurium (Figure 19-8), a bisquaternary ammonium benzylisoquinoline compound, is relatively potent, with an ED_{95} of 0.2 to 0.25 mg/kg and an intermediate duration of action.[76] Following administration of two times the ED_{95}, maximal block occurs in 2.5 minutes, recovery to 10% of baseline twitch amplitude (approximately 1 twitch in the TOF) occurs in 40 minutes, and complete spontaneous recovery of neuromuscular function occurs in about 60 minutes.[76,77]

Atracurium was the first NMBA introduced into clinical practice that does not require elimination by enzyme-catalyzed hydrolysis or excretion by the kidneys or liver. Chemical degradation to inactive products by Hofmann elimination (see Figure 19-8) is primarily responsible for its inactivation; enzymatic ester hydrolysis and renal elimination have lesser roles.[78] Other studies have found that ester hydrolysis can be responsible for metabolism of as much as 66% of an atracurium dose and that renal elimination can have a larger role in the pharmacokinetics of atracurium than initially appreciated.[79,80]

Hofmann elimination is a spontaneous, base-catalyzed, nonenzymatic chemical reaction by which atracurium is cleaved into two molecules.[78] Alkalosis increases resistance to atracurium-induced neuromuscular block, while hypothermia slows the temperature-dependent breakdown so that less atracurium is required to maintain a given depth of neuromuscular block.[79,81] The ester hydrolysis involved in atracurium metabolism is catalyzed by a nonspecific esterase distinct from the butyrylcholinesterase responsible for hydrolysis of succinylcholine and mivacurium.

Because recovery from atracurium-induced neuromuscular block occurs by nonsaturable chemical degradation rather than metabolism or redistribution, there is little to no cumulative effect with repeat doses or continuous infusion.[76,82,83] Thus sequential doses administered at the same point in

Table 19-3. Adverse Effects of Succinylcholine

Cardiac dysrhythmias
Hyperkalemia
Myalgias
Masseter spasm
Increased intracranial pressure
Increased intragastric pressure
Increased intraocular pressure

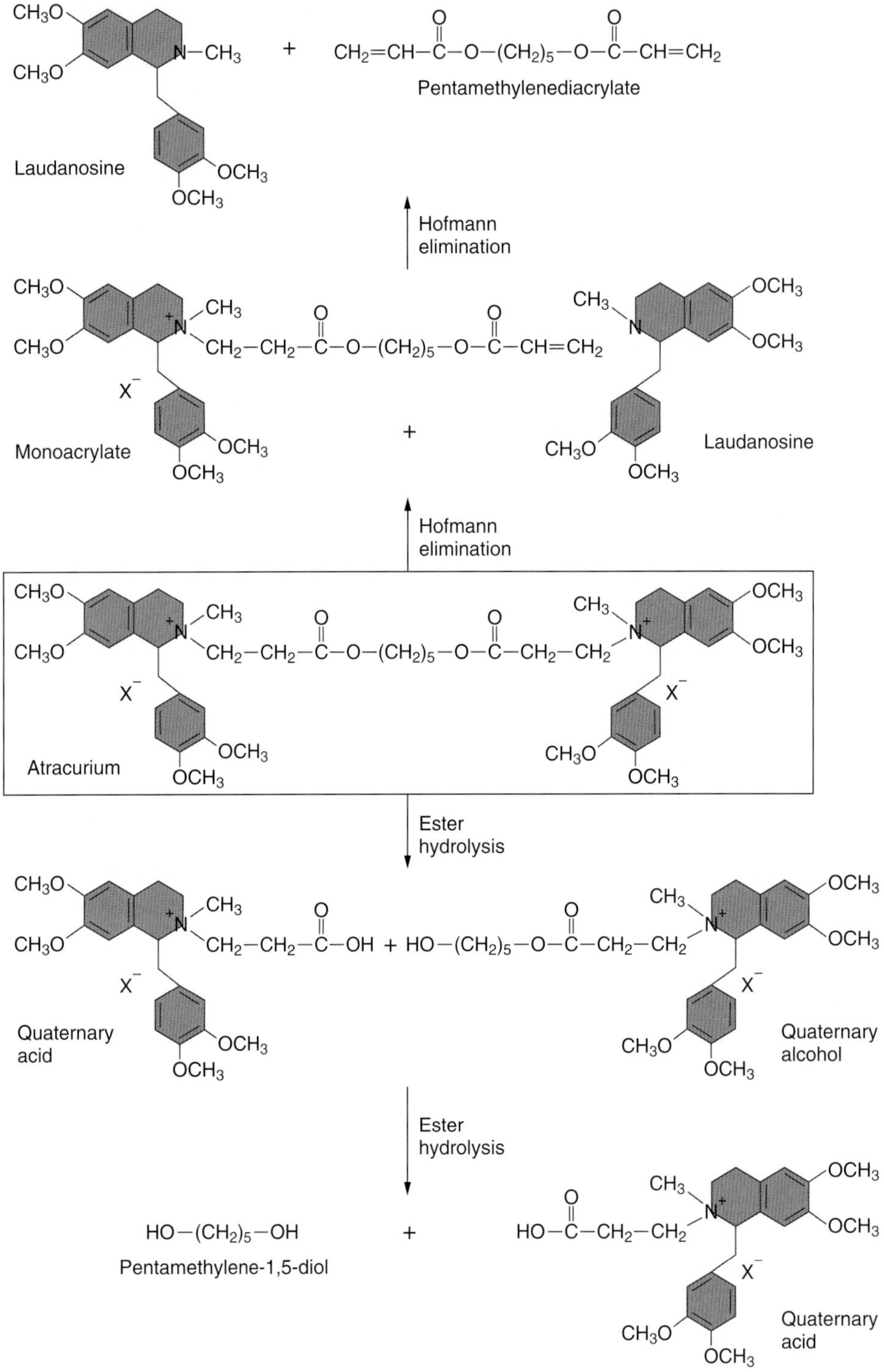

Figure 19-8 Degradation and inactivation of atracurium. Atracurium undergoes either Hofmann elimination to yield a monoacrylate and laudanosine or ester hydrolysis to yield a quaternary alcohol and a quaternary acid. Laudanosine, the major product, is excreted in urine and bile. *(Adapted from Basta SJ, Ali HH, Savarese JJ, et al. Clinical pharmacology of atracurium besylate [BW 33A]: a new non-depolarizing muscle relaxant. Anesth Analg. 1982;61:723-729.)*

spontaneous recovery have the same recovery characteristics as the preceding dose. With continuous infusion, no dosing revisions are required to maintain a stable depth of neuromuscular block, even with prolonged infusions.[84,85]

During prolonged infusions of atracurium, the elimination half-life is about 20 minutes with a clearance of 4.5 to 10 mL/kg/min, greater than that of long-acting NMBAs.[85] Because

of the relative lack of renal or hepatic elimination of atracurium compared to steroidal NMBAs, the pharmacokinetics and duration of action of atracurium are not affected by renal disease.[86-88] Similarly, its elimination half-life is not prolonged in patients with cirrhosis.[89]

Normal aging is accompanied by a number of physiologic changes that include decreases in hepatic and renal blood flow

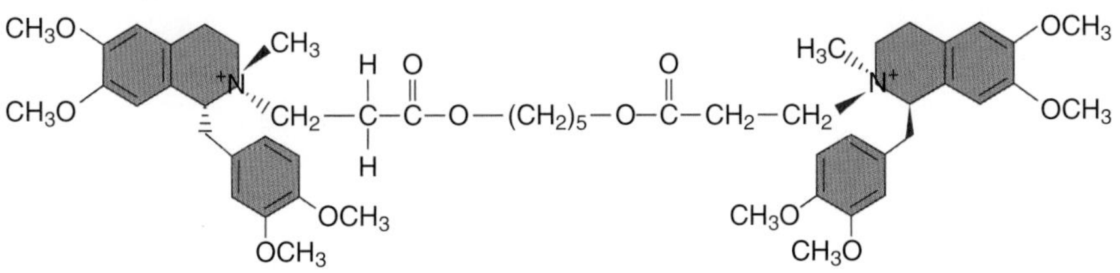

Figure 19-9 Chemical structure of cisatracurium. It is the 1 R-cis 1' R-cis stereoisomer, one of 10 stereoisomers comprising atracurium.

and function, as well as changes in the anatomy and function of the neuromuscular junction.[90] Despite these changes at the neuromuscular junction, the depth of block at a given plasma concentration of NMBA is the same in young and older individuals.[91] It appears that observed differences in the effects of NMBAs associated with aging are due to altered pharmacokinetics. As expected, prolongation of the effect of NMBAs in older adults is either less pronounced or not apparent for compounds that rely less on the kidney and liver for their elimination. For example, the duration of block with atracurium is not increased with advanced age.[92] Subsequent studies have shown that, even though the clearance of atracurium is similar in older and young patients, elimination half-life is prolonged in these patients.[93,94] Clearance remains constant because, while elimination through the renal pathway is decreased in older adults, clearance through non–end-organ–dependent pathways is increased.[93]

Cisatracurium

Cisatracurium (Figure 19-9) is the 1 R-cis 1'R-cis stereoisomer of the 10 stereoisomers that comprise atracurium and has been available since 1995. Its innovative development involved isolation and testing of individual stereoisomers from the parent mixture, with selection and further development of the one with reduced side effects. It is approximately threefold more potent than atracurium (ED_{95} of 0.05 mg/kg) and, like atracurium, has an intermediate duration of action.[95] Because of its greater potency, however, its onset of effect is considerably slower.[95] For this reason, doses of three to five times the ED_{95} are recommended for endotracheal intubation.[96] In contrast to atracurium, administration of such large doses is not associated with histamine release, and resultant hypotension or tachycardia.[97]

Like atracurium, cisatracurium undergoes Hofmann elimination. Clearance, elimination half-life, and volume of distribution are the same when doses of the ED_{95} or twice the ED_{95} are administered.[98] The clinical duration of action (the time required from administration of a dose to recovery of 25% T1 height) defines the earliest time that reversal of residual neuromuscular block is recommended. The duration of action of 0.1 mg/kg cisatracurium ($2\times ED_{95}$) is 45 minutes. Doubling the dose to $4\times ED_{95}$ increases it to 68 minutes and doubling it again to $8\times ED_{95}$ increases it by another 23 minutes, equivalent to the elimination half-life of the compound.[95]

Hofmann elimination accounts for 77% of total clearance of cisatracurium and renal elimination 16%.[99] The slight dependence on renal elimination likely contributes to the increase in elimination half-life of 14% and decrease in clearance of 13% observed in patients with renal failure.[100] Despite these pharmacokinetic changes in patients with renal dysfunction, no prolongation of the duration of action is found following a bolus dose.[101] As with atracurium, both volume of distribution and clearance of cisatracurium are increased in patients with hepatic failure.[102] Elimination half-life is unchanged, and thus the clinical duration of action and 25% to 75% recovery interval (the time required to recover from 25% to 75% of baseline twitch height) is unchanged in patients with liver failure.[102]

Recovery from cisatracurium-induced neuromuscular block occurs over the same time course in older surgical patients as it does in young adults.[103] An increase in its volume of distribution and no change in its clearance in older adults likely account for a prolongation of elimination half-life by up to 28%.[103] The decrease in renal function that occurs with normal aging could account for these pharmacokinetic differences. The prolonged elimination half-life of cisatracurium in the geriatric patient does not affect recovery from neuromuscular block induced with a bolus dose of the NMBA.

STEROIDAL COMPOUNDS

Pancuronium

Pancuronium (see Figure 19-6) is the only available NMBA with a long duration of action. It was the first of the steroidal agents introduced into clinical practice (1968). While once widely used, its utility since the introduction of shorter-acting compounds has become increasingly infrequent. Doses of 0.08 and 0.1 mg/kg used for tracheal intubation have durations of action of 86 and 100 minutes, respectively.[104] Its long duration of action is due to its primary elimination through the kidney, while it undergoes some deacetylation in the liver.[105]

Patients with liver disease due to either cholestasis or cirrhosis have an increase in volume of distribution for pancuronium, which might be responsible for the relative resistance of these patients to pancuronium-induced block.[106,107] However, clearance of pancuronium in these patients is decreased, and elimination half-life and duration of action are prolonged.[106,107]

As would be predicted, the clearance of pancuronium is decreased and elimination half-life prolonged in patients with renal failure.[108] Similarly, clearance is decreased and duration of action of pancuronium is prolonged in patients of advanced age.[109] With an increase in duration of action of about 30 minutes from 44 minutes to 73 minutes, there is an appreciable increase in the dosing interval required to maintain stable depth of block in older individuals.[109]

Vecuronium

Vecuronium (see Figure 19-6) was the first nondepolarizing NMBA with a shorter duration of action to be introduced into clinical practice. With an intermediate duration of action and lack of hemodynamic side effects, it set a standard against which all subsequent NMBAs have been compared. Vecuronium is a potent NMBA (ED_{95} is 0.05 mg/kg) with a

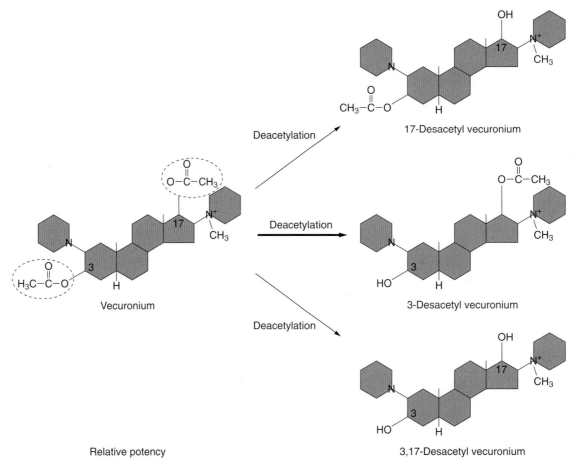

Relative potency

Figure 19-10 Metabolism of vecuronium. Metabolism in the liver leads to the primary metabolite, 3-desacetyl vecuronium, which is almost as potent as vecuronium and is cleared more slowly from the plasma. *(From Agoston S, Seyr M, Khuenl-Brady KS, et al. Use of neuromuscular blocking agents in the intensive care unit. Anesthesiol Clin North Am. 1993;11:345-360.)*

duration of action of 40 minutes.[26,110] Typically twice the ED_{95} is administered to facilitate tracheal intubation. Doses of five to six times the ED_{95} can be administered for more rapid onset of effect[111] without significant hemodynamic side effects.[111,112]

Vecuronium is the 2-desmethyl derivative of pancuronium. The lack of one methyl group at the quaternary ammonium of the 2 position increases its lipid solubility and significantly alters its degree of metabolism. While it undergoes more hepatic metabolism than pancuronium, it is primarily eliminated unchanged in the urine and bile. As much as 40% is cleared through the bile and 20% to 30% is eliminated in the urine.[113,114] The remainder of the compound is metabolized by the liver to 3-desacetylvecuronium, 17-desacetylvecuronium, and 3,17-desacetylvecuronium (Figure 19-10).[115] The 3-desacetyl metabolite has neuromuscular blocking activity.[116,117] Only 5% is excreted in the urine as the 3-desacetyl metabolite. Even so, the prolonged duration of action of vecuronium in critically ill patients with renal failure has been attributed to accumulation of this metabolite.[118]

There is a tendency for elimination half-life and duration of action to be increased with renal failure.[119-121] Changes in elimination half-life and clearance, though, are not as consistent in patients with renal failure who receive pancuronium. This is likely because the liver is the primary route of clearance of vecuronium from the plasma. Decreased vecuronium infusion rates are required to maintain a stable depth of block and maintenance doses have an increased duration of action in patients with renal failure.[122,123] Although vecuronium can be used safely in patients with renal failure, monitoring of depth of block is essential to guide dosing.

The impact of hepatic failure on the dose requirement of vecuronium is more predictable due to its dependence on the liver for its elimination. Volume of distribution is increased, clearance is decreased, and elimination half-life prolonged in patients with hepatic failure due to either cholestasis or cirrhosis.[124,125] Accordingly, the duration of action of vecuronium in increased in this patient population.[124,126]

In elderly patients, the clearance of vecuronium is decreased by 30% to 55% and elimination half-life is increased by 60%.[127,128] This results in a three-fold prolongation of the 25% to 75% recovery interval of vecuronium following either a bolus dose of 0.1 mg/kg or an infusion to maintain 90% suppression of twitch height for 90 minutes.[127,129] When dosed as an infusion to maintain a stable depth of block of 70% to 80% twitch depression, there was no difference in recovery intervals between groups.[128]

Rocuronium

Rocuronium (see Figure 19-6) has an intermediate duration of action with an ED_{95} of 0.3 mg/kg, making it about six times less potent than vecuronium and faster in onset than either vecuronium or atracurium.[26,130-133] At a dose of two times the ED$_{95}$, rocuronium has an onset of less than 2 minutes and a clinical duration of less than 40 minutes.[26] Increasing the dose to speed onset of neuromuscular block increases the duration of action.[26]

Rocuronium, like vecuronium, is eliminated primarily through the liver.[134] Because only 10% is eliminated through the kidneys, it is even less dependent on renal elimination than vecuronium.[135] It is not metabolized to any significant degree.

In patients with renal failure, the clearance of rocuronium is marginally decreased or unchanged, volume of distribution is increased, and elimination half-life is prolonged.[136,137] The duration of action of single and repeat doses of rocuronium can be prolonged in patients with hepatic failure.[138,139] This is due to a decrease in its clearance and an increase in its volume of distribution.[138-140]

Advanced age impacts the pharmacokinetics and duration of action of rocuronium. The duration of effect of repeat doses is prolonged and the clinical duration of 0.6 mg/kg is almost doubled.[141,142] Clearance of the compound is significantly decreased in this patient population.[142]

POSTOPERATIVE RESIDUAL NEUROMUSCULAR BLOCK

Postoperative residual neuromuscular block is not uncommon after anesthetic cases in which NMBAs are administered.[7,143,144] More than 30 years ago, a classic study evaluated neuromuscular transmission in patients following surgery and found residual paralysis (TOFR < 0.7) in 42% of patients who had received gallamine, pancuronium, or d-tubocurarine.[145] Intermediate-acting NMBAs were not available when that study was done. More recent studies report that residual block from intermediate-acting NMBAs can be present in one third to two thirds of patients following anesthesia.[7,146,147] The frequency of residual block depends on the time of assessment of depth of neuromuscular block, the manner in which depth of block is monitored, and the approaches used to reverse neuromuscular block at the conclusion of procedures.[145,148,149]

It has been known for decades that pulmonary function, as defined by respiratory rate, tidal volume, forced expiratory volume, and forced vital capacity, recovers, on average, at a TOFR of at least 0.6 measured at the adductor pollicis muscle. Based on this information, a TOFR of 0.6 was thought to be adequate recovery from the effects of NMBAs. Recent data suggest that lesser degrees of neuromuscular blockade can adversely affect respiratory function, airway patency, and airway protective reflexes (i.e., coughing and swallowing).

Respiratory Effects

A summary of the effects of subtle degrees of residual neuromuscular block on respiratory function and pharyngeal patency is presented in Table 19-4. In volunteers, even slight neuromuscular block, as reflected by a TOFR at the adductor pollicis muscle of 0.8 to 0.9, impairs the hypoxic ventilatory response and increases the risk of upper airway collapse.[150-154] A TOFR of 0.8, and potentially even 0.9, is associated with alterations in upper airway closing pressure (P$_{crit}$), upper airway dilatory muscle function, and airway volume during

Table 19-4. Pharmacodynamics of G-1-64 and TAAC3 Compared to Rocuronium and Mivacurium

NEUROMUSCULAR BLOCKING AGENT	ED$_{50}$ (µMOL/KG)	ONSET (MIN)	25%-75% RI (MIN)
G-1-64	0.13	1.3	4.6
TAAC3	0.1	0.9	0.7
Rocuronium	0.06	1.9	2.4
Mivacurium	0.011	3.2	3.5

ED$_{50}$, The dose causing 50% suppression of neuromuscular response to stimulation; 25%-75% RI, the recovery interval defined by the recovery from 25% of baseline muscle strength to 75% of baseline muscle strength.

inspiration.[150] Of note, tidal volume, vital capacity, and lung volume are typically normal at this low level of residual neuromuscular block. Thus, residual neuromuscular block can be present in the muscles of the upper airway at levels of block at which the respiratory muscles are unaffected.[155] These effects are difficult to measure and can go undetected by the clinician.

Risk of Airway Collapse

To maintain upper airway patency during inspiration, the forces generated by the respiratory "pump" muscles, which decrease intraluminal upper airway pressure and therefore tend to collapse the airway, have to be balanced by reflex dilating forces of the pharyngeal musculature. In the absence of neuromuscular block, this stability is maintained in part by the genioglossus muscle, the activity of which almost quadruples, at negative pharyngeal pressures. This compensatory increase in the activity of the genioglossus muscle with inspiration, which helps to maintain a patent airway, is markedly impaired during minimal neuromuscular block (TOF ratio 0.8) (Figure 19-11). This leads to an increase in airway collapsibility and a decrease in airflow with inspiration.[150,152] Partial paralysis markedly increases upper airway closing pressure (P$_{crit}$) to less negative values so that the airway collapses more easily during inspiration.[150] The relationship between the decrease in genioglossus activity caused by neuromuscular block and its effects on upper airway closing pressure (P$_{crit}$) and air flow are shown in Figure 19-11. As a result of the susceptibility of the upper airway to collapse during inspiration with minimal degrees of neuromuscular block, forced inspiratory volume in 1 second (FIV$_1$) is markedly impaired, while forced expiratory volume is maintained during partial paralysis.

In addition to maintenance of airway patency, the genioglossus muscle has an integral role in swallowing. Genioglossus activity during swallowing and maximum voluntary tongue contraction are impaired during residual neuromuscular block (Table 19-5).[150,153] An increased incidence of misdirected swallowing and a decreased upper esophageal sphincter resting tone occur with minimal neuromuscular blockade (TOF ratio 0.5-1) and persists even with recovery of the TOFR to unity.[153-155]

Difficulty swallowing can lead to aspiration.[153,154] With partial neuromuscular blockade there is reduced upper esophageal sphincter tone, while the pharyngeal constrictor muscle is minimally affected. The greater vulnerability of the upper

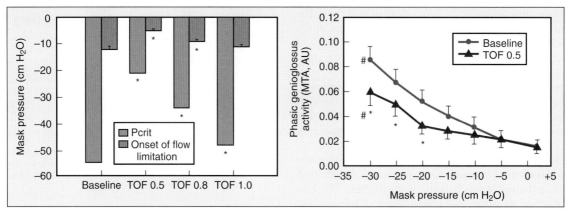

Figure 19-11 Effects of neuromuscular blockade on upper airway patency. The panel on the left displays the upper airway critical closing pressure (P_{crit}) and the airway pressure associated with the beginning of flow limitation during inspiration in awake healthy volunteers at baseline before neuromuscular blockade, with impaired neuromuscular transmission at train-of-four (TOF) ratios of 0.5 and 0.8, and after recovery of the TOF ratio to unity. Upper airway closing pressure *(blue bars)* significantly increases during partial neuromuscular blockade and is still abnormal once the TOF ratio recovers to unity. Evidence of flow limitation *(red bars)* is first observed at an average pressure of −12 cm H_2O. With a TOF ratio of 0.5 or 0.8, flow limitation occurs at significantly less negative values of mask pressure, indicating impairment of airway integrity. *$P < 0.05$ versus baseline. The panel on the right shows genioglossus muscle activity as a function of negative mask pressure without *(circles)* and with *(triangles)* partial neuromuscular blockade at a TOF ratio of 0.5. Genioglossus activity increases markedly as negative pressure is applied, but this effect is attenuated with partial neuromuscular block. *$P < 0.05$ versus baseline (same mask pressure); #$P < 0.05$ versus mask pressure + 5 cm H_2O (same level of neuromuscular function). *MTA,* Moving time average; *AU,* arbitrary units. *(Adapted from Eikermann M, Vogt FM, Herbstreit F, et al. The predisposition to inspiratory upper airway collapse during partial neuromuscular blockade. Am J Respir Crit Care Med. 2007;175:9-15.)*

Table 19-5. Effects of Partial Neuromuscular Block on Respiration

| | Monitoring of Adductor Pollicis Muscle | | |
VENTILATORY FUNCTION	TOFR = 0.5	TOFR = 0.8	TOFR = 1.0
Tidal volume	Normal	Normal	Normal
Forced vital capacity	↓↓	Normal	Normal
Pharyngeal function (swallowing)	↓↓↓	↓↓	↓
Upper airway patency (closing pressure)	↓↓↓	↓↓	↓
Hypoxic respiratory response	↓↓↓	↓↓	Normal

TOFR, Train-of-four ratio; ↓↓↓, consistently impaired; ↓↓, frequently impaired; ↓, usually normal.
Data from references 150, 151, 153, and 154.

airway muscles to NMBAs cannot be explained by a higher density of nicotinic acetylcholine receptors, differences in fiber size, or differences in fiber-type composition.[156,157] Some evidence suggests that the sensitivity of the airway dilator muscles to the effects of NMBAs might be explained by the high firing rate of the motor neurons innervating the muscle. Neuromuscular blocking drugs produce a progressive failure of neuromuscular transmission with increasing rates of stimulation. The TOF stimulation that is typically used to test the strength of the adductor pollicis utilizes a stimulation rate of 2 Hz. In contrast, the firing frequency of the genioglossus muscle during quiet breathing is significantly higher. It is also greater than that of the diaphragm (diaphragm 8-13 Hz, genioglossus 15-25 Hz).[158] This might account for the greater sensitivity of the genioglossus muscle to NMBAs and the greater susceptibility of the genioglossus muscle to NMBAs than the adductor pollicis as assessed by stimulation at 2 Hz.

Sensitivity of the Musculature of the Airway to Residual Block

There is a growing body of evidence that postoperative residual block results not only in physiologic impairment, but also in increased perioperative risk and health care–related costs.[147,149,154,159] The symptoms of residual neuromuscular block are difficult to recognize, and the subtle effects of NMBAs can have clinically significant consequences.[160,161] The incidence of critical respiratory events, including hypoxemia, hypoventilation, or upper airway obstruction following anesthesia increases with both the dose and duration of action of an NMBA.[162] Minimal neuromuscular block, defined by a TOFR of 0.7 or 0.8, is associated with an increased incidence of adverse respiratory events, including airway obstruction, moderate to severe hypoxemia, and development of atelectasis and pneumonia.[147,163,164] In addition to the effects of propofol and other anesthetics on airway tone, even very low levels of residual block can impair skeletal muscle strength and increase patient discomfort after an anesthetic, which can delay readiness for discharge after an ambulatory surgical procedure.[155,165,166]

Residual neuromuscular block can also have economic consequences. Length of stay in the postanesthesia care unit is significantly longer in patients with a TOFR less than 0.9 compared to patients with a greater degree of recovery of neuromuscular transmission.[159] This results in delayed discharge and substantially increases the chance that other patients will have to wait to enter the recovery area because of lack of available of space.

USE OF NEUROMUSCULAR BLOCKING AGENTS IN CRITICAL CARE

In the intensive care unit (ICU) the most common indications for NMBAs are facilitation of mechanical ventilation

Table 19-6. Undesirable Effects of Neuromuscular Blocking Agents in Critically Ill Patients

EFFECT	MECHANISM
	Persistent failure of neuromuscular transmission
Muscle weakness	Critical illness polyneuropathy
	Immobilization-induced atrophy of diaphragm
Impairment of ventilation-perfusion distribution	Spontaneous breathing abolished
Decreased right ventricular end-diastolic volume	
Posttraumatic stress syndrome	Awareness during paralysis

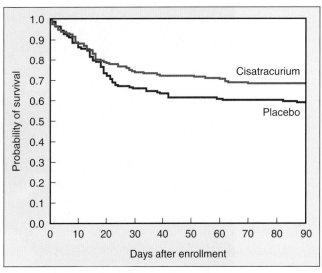

Figure 19-12 Probability of survival through day 90 in patients with acute respiratory distress syndrome receiving cisatracurium to facilitate mechanical ventilation compared to those not receiving a neuromuscular blocking agent. *(Adapted from Papazian L, Forel JM, et al. Neuromuscular blockers in early acute respiratory distress syndrome. N Engl J Med. 2010;363:1107-1116.)*

during respiratory failure, reduction of oxygen consumption, prevention of shivering, and control of intracranial hypertension.[165] However, the use of NMBAs in critically ill patients is associated with side effects as summarized in Table 19-6. ICU-acquired muscle weakness frequently occurs in critically ill patients and affects their long-term outcome.[166] Inflammation and immobilization are the main contributing mechanisms. Some data suggest that an association exists between ICU-acquired muscle weakness and the use of NMBAs, which is likely related to their skeletal muscle immobilizing effect.[167,168] In critically ill patients, immobility predicts long ICU and hospital length of stay as well as mortality, and neuromuscular blocking agents exacerbate immobilization-induced muscle weakness.[169,170]

Prolonged weakness has been reported following the use of all NMBAs and occurs in 20% of patients receiving NMBAs for more than 6 days.[171] Administration of corticosteroids increases the incidence to as much as 40%.[168] Minimizing these adverse events requires administering NMBAs only to those patients who require them and allowing intermittent recovery of neuromuscular function ("drug holidays").

In addition to contributing to myopathy, prolonged immobility results in the upregulation of acetylcholine receptors.[71] Administration of NMBAs to critically ill patients contributes to the upregulation of acetylcholine receptors.[172] This increase in acetylcholine receptors renders patients increasingly susceptible to hyperkalemia after succinylcholine administration and cardiac arrest. It may also manifest as an increasing requirement for NMBA in order to maintain the same depth of neuromuscular block.[173]

Short-term use of NMBAs in the ICU for treatment of severe acute respiratory distress syndrome (ARDS) can be of some benefit (Figure 19-12).[3] The mechanisms underlying this beneficial effect are unknown, but it is possible that lower transpulmonary pressures are associated with reduced barotrauma. However, reduction in transpulmonary pressure can also be achieved using sedative agents that lack the adverse effects of NMBAs. The benefits and risks of the use of NMBAs in critically ill patients must be considered when deciding on their use. For example, lack of spontaneous ventilation might decrease the incidence of barotrauma but, in patients with ARDS, breathing spontaneously with ventilator support improves matching of ventilation and perfusion. Additional data suggest that NMBAs exacerbate mechanical ventilation-induced diaphragmatic dysfunction.[174]

ANTAGONISM OF RESIDUAL NEUROMUSCULAR BLOCK

There are several possible means of enhancing recovery of neuromuscular function. These include increasing acetylcholine concentration at the neuromuscular junction or decreasing plasma concentrations of the NMBA through either encapsulation of the NMBA or increased metabolism (Figure 19-13).

Anticholinesterases

Anticholinesterases used for reversal of neuromuscular blockade inhibit acetylcholinesterase at the neuromuscular junction, which increases the concentration of acetylcholine at the motor endplate to overcome the NMBA-induced competitive block.[175,176] Cholinesterase inhibitors are the principal drugs used for reversal of NMBAs and, in the United States and some other countries, they remain the only option.

There is significant variation in the practice of antagonism of residual neuromuscular blockade. In contrast to most European countries, where routine antagonism is not typical, the majority of anesthesiologists in the United States commonly antagonize the residual effects of nondepolarizing NMBAs at the end of surgery. This is accomplished through the combined administration of a cholinesterase inhibitor (e.g., neostigmine) and an antimuscarinic agent, such as glycopyrrolate.[16] Routine antagonism of neuromuscular block is recommended by some anesthesiologists to ensure complete recovery in all patients regardless of whether depth of block was monitored objectively.[143,177,178] This practice, however, is not without risk, in that cholinesterase inhibitors can themselves induce muscle weakness when given in the absence of residual of neuromuscular blockade. Administering an anticholinesterase does not facilitate elimination of the NMBA from the body. Neostigmine blocks acetylcholine

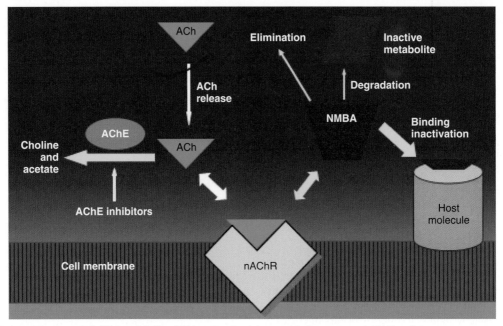

Figure 19-13 Pathways to increase available acetylcholine (ACh) at the nicotinic acetylcholine receptor (nAChR) and decrease neuromuscular blocking agent (NMBA). Acetylcholine and NMBA compete for the same binding sites in the receptor at the neuromuscular junction. Possible means to increase acetylcholine concentration include inhibiting acetylcholinesterase (AChE) to decrease its metabolism to choline and acetate. To decrease the NMBA at the neuromuscular junction, its plasma concentration has to decrease. This happens through its elimination in the urine or bile, its metabolism to inactive compounds—as occurs with atracurium, cisatracurium, mivacurium, and gantacurium—and its encapsulation by a host molecule such as sugammadex (a selective relaxant binding agent).

receptors, and excessive acetylcholine can cause both a depolarizing block and an open-channel block.[179-181]

DETERMINANTS OF SPEED AND ADEQUACY OF RECOVERY

Antagonism of nondepolarizing neuromuscular block with anticholinesterases requires varying amounts of time that are determined by several factors. Time from administration to peak effect varies with presynaptic acetylcholine reserve, as well as the spontaneous rate of recovery from neuromuscular blockade. The rate of spontaneous recovery depends on the NMBA used, the dose administered, patient temperature, the presence of metabolic abnormalities, such as hypokalemia, and concomitant medications. Anticholinesterases are typically given only once spontaneous recovery of neuromuscular function has begun. Under these circumstances, recovery of neuromuscular transmission is the function of primarily two processes: ongoing spontaneous recovery of neuromuscular function as the NMBA is eliminated from the neuromuscular junction and the increase in acetylcholine at the neuromuscular junction due to the effect of the anticholinesterase.

It takes longer to antagonize profound neuromuscular block than it does moderate neuromuscular block.[182] Additionally, recovery of muscle strength after administration of anticholinesterase depends on the rate of spontaneous recovery from the NMBA.[183] Anticholinesterase-facilitated recovery from neuromuscular block induced with an intermediate-acting compound occurs more quickly than that induced with a long-acting compound. Speed of recovery also depends on the anticholinesterase used for reversal. Recovery from a moderate depth of block occurs more quickly following the administration of edrophonium than neostigmine.[184]

If the NMBA is not metabolized more quickly than the anticholinesterase, neuromuscular block can recur (known as *recurarization*). Both neostigmine and edrophonium antagonize 90% neuromuscular block induced with d-tubocurarine for a period of 1 to 2 hours, after which neuromuscular block recurs if the NMBA has not been completely metabolized or eliminated.[185]

There is a ceiling effect in the reversal of neuromuscular block by anticholinesterases in that profound neuromuscular blockade cannot be reversed. Once the maximum dose of neostigmine (0.05-0.07 mg/kg) has been administered, additional anticholinesterase will not produce greater antagonism.[183]

ADVERSE EFFECTS

The effects of anticholinesterases are not limited to the motor-endplate. Administration also causes increases in acetylcholine beyond the neuromuscular junction. The muscarinic and nicotinic acetylcholine receptors in the parasympathetic system can also be activated, which causes pronounced vagal effects such as bradycardia, prolonged QT-interval, and asystole.[186] Other muscarinic parasympathetic side effects of anticholinesterases include bronchospasm, increased bronchial and pharyngeal secretions, miosis, and increased intestinal tone. Therefore anticholinesterases are typically administered in combination with antimuscarinic drugs, such as glycopyrrolate or atropine. These compounds block muscarinic but not nicotinic receptors so that neuromuscular block can be antagonized while muscarinic effects are minimized. Antimuscarinic compounds increase the risk of tachyarrhythmias and other side effects resulting from muscarinic receptor antagonism such as urinary retention, blurred vision, photophobia, mydriasis, xerostomia, dry skin, constipation, nausea, urinary retention, insomnia, and dizziness.

Unnecessary administration of anticholinesterases can cause muscle weakness.[187] Weakness of the airway dilator muscle genioglossus can lead to upper airway collapse during inspiration. Unnecessary administration of neostigmine (0.03 mg/kg) can also cause diaphragmatic dysfunction.[188] In humans, administration of even a moderate dose of anticholinesterase (neostigmine 0.03 mg/kg IV with glycopyrrolate 0.0075 mg/kg) given to healthy volunteers after complete spontaneous recovery from neuromuscular block increased airway collapsibility to a degree found with a TOF ratio = 0.5, and reduced compensatory genioglossus activity in response to negative airway pressure.[189]

DOSING

The optimal dose for antagonism of neuromuscular block depends on the depth of block, the duration of action of the NMBA used, the timing of the last dose of NMBA relative to administration of the anticholinesterase, and the monitoring technique used. Figure 19-14 summarizes current recommendations for dosing of anticholinesterases.[16] Ideally, anticholinesterases should be administered only when necessary (i.e., in the presence of residual paralysis). Without objective monitoring of neuromuscular function, it is not possible to discriminate between TOFR values of 0.4 and 0.9. Thus patients who have completely recovered from NMBAs occasionally receive unwarranted anticholinesterase, putting them at risk for anticholinesterase-induced muscle weakness. The administration of anticholinesterases should optimally be guided by evaluation of the TOF ratio. The typical dose of neostigmine for antagonism of profound neuromuscular block (a TOF count of 2) is 0.05 mg/kg and 0.015 to 0.025 mg/kg for antagonism of lesser degrees of neuromuscular block (a TOF count of 4 with no fade).[16,190] Profound block with a TOF count below 2 should not be antagonized by neostigmine because of the risk of inadequate recovery of neuromuscular function.[191] No anticholinesterase is required if TOFR is greater than 0.9 using a quantitative monitor of neuromuscular function.

PHARMACOKINETICS AND PHARMACODYNAMICS

Bolus doses of either neostigmine or edrophonium result in peak plasma concentrations within 5 to 10 minutes that decrease rapidly, followed by a slower decline that corresponds to the elimination phase.[185,192] A two-compartment analysis finds results that are similar for both drugs. The volume of distribution of these anticholinesterases is 0.7 to 1.4 L/kg and their elimination half-lives are 60 to 120 minutes. Clearance is 8 to 16 mL/kg/min, which is greater than the glomerular filtration rate because anticholinesterases are actively secreted. Therefore, in patients with renal failure, in whom the duration of action of NMBAs is likely to be increased, clearance of anticholinesterases is also reduced and elimination half-life increased. This makes dose adjustment of anticholinesterases in patients with renal dysfunction unnecessary.

The anticholinesterases have markedly different onset characteristics, possibly due to the different potency of each agent. Neostigmine is more potent than edrophonium and smaller doses are required to antagonize residual neuromuscular block. During a steady-state infusion of NMBA the onset of action of edrophonium is 1 to 2 min and that of neostigmine is 7 to 11 minutes.[185,192] Similar results have been obtained with neostigmine as an antagonist of either pancuronium or vecuronium or edrophonium as an antagonist of metocurine. Edrophonium has approximately one-twelfth the potency of neostigmine. Potency increases as spontaneous recovery from neuromuscular block occurs.[185]

Sugammadex

Sugammadex is a cyclodextrin that binds selectively to the steroidal neuromuscular blocking agents rocuronium, vecuronium, and pancuronium. Sugammadex encapsulates and inactivates the NMBA in the plasma, rendering it

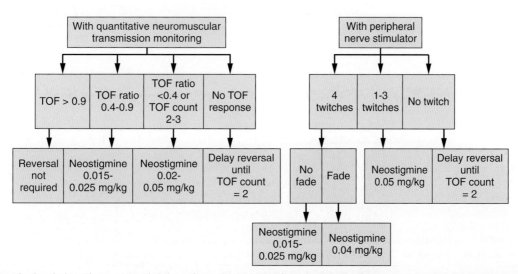

Figure 19-14 Neostigmine dosing. The recommended dose of neostigmine depends on how depth of neuromuscular block is monitored and on the degree of recovery. As little as 0.015 to 0.025 mg/kg of neostigmine is required at a train-of-four (TOF) count of 4 with no fade, whereas 0.04 to 0.05 mg/kg is needed at a TOF count of 2 or 3. If no twitch or only a single twitch can be evoked, neostigmine will not reverse neuromuscular block, and antagonism is best delayed until a TOF count of 2 is achieved. *(Adapted from Kopman AF, Eikermann M. Antagonism of non-depolarising neuromuscular block: current practice. Anaesthesia. 2009;64[Suppl 1]:22-30.)*

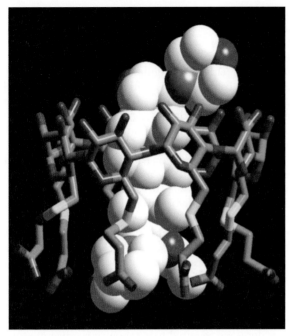

Figure 19-15 Interaction of the cyclodextrin, sugammadex, with the steroidal neuromuscular blocking agent (NMBA) rocuronium. Hydrophobic portions of the NMBA are located within the cyclodextrin ring. Hydrophilic portions remain exposed to plasma.

incapable of binding with acetylcholine receptors (Figure 19-15). Neuromuscular block produced by steroidal NMBAs can be rapidly and completely reversed without the side effects of anticholinesterases (Figure 19-16).[193] The complex of the cyclodextrin and steroidal NMBA is of high affinity and does not dissociate readily. In contrast to neostigmine, a reversal dose of sugammadex administered after complete recovery of neuromuscular function does not affect either genioglossus muscle activity or normal breathing.[194] Sugammadex provides a rapid and dose-dependent reversal of profound neuromuscular blockade induced by high-dose rocuronium (1.0 or 1.2 mg/kg) in adult surgical patients.[195,196] Sugammadex is indicated for reversal of rocuronium- and vecuronium-induced neuromuscular block in adults, and for routine reversal of rocuronium-induced neuromuscular blockade in children (2-17 years of age).

EMERGING DEVELOPMENTS

Tropane Derivatives

Research is ongoing with two different classes of neuromuscular blocking agents. The bisquaternary tropine and tropane derivatives provide a rapid onset of and recovery from

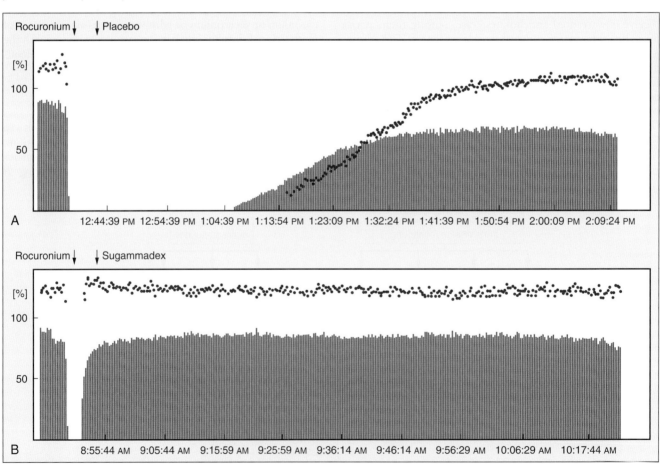

Figure 19-16 The speed of antagonism of rocuronium-induced block with sugammadex. In **A**, a placebo was administered 3 minutes after rocuronium 0.6 mg/kg. Recovery of twitch height is indicated by the blue lines and the train-of-four ratio (TOFR) by the red dots. In **B**, sugammadex, 8 mg/kg, was administered 3 minutes following the same dose of rocuronium. One minute after administration of sugammadex, the TOFR was 0.9. *(Adapted from Gijsenbergh F, Ramael S, Houwing N, et al. First human exposure of Org 25969, a novel agent to reverse the action of rocuronium bromide. Anesthesiology. 2005;103: 695-703.)*

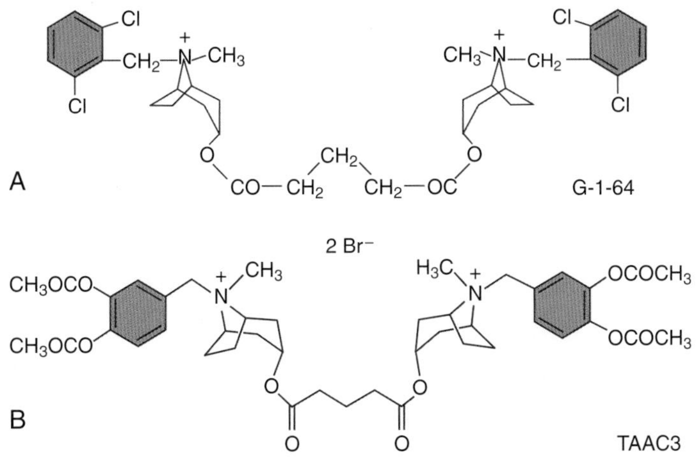

Figure 19-17 The chemical structures of G-1-64 and TAAC3.

neuromuscular block (see Table 19-4). These compounds consist of dimers of two tropine or tropane structures connected through their 3-hydroxy groups by different dicarboxylic acid ester linkages. Of the more than 250 of these compounds, G-1-64 and TAAC3 (Figure 19-17), have been most extensively studied.[197,198] Onset of effect for both is faster than for rocuronium in primates.[199] Both the rapid onset and short duration of block with TAAC3 have been attributed to its rapid destruction, which involves hydrolysis of nonspecific carboxyesterases on the diester linking group as well as esterase catalyzed removal of the quaternary group.

Fumarates

A different class of NMBAs, the fumarates, share some structural elements with mivacurium. Like mivacurium, they have three methyl groups between the quaternary nitrogen and the most proximal oxygen at each end of the carbon chain. This structural feature is different from either atracurium or cisatracurium, each of which has two methyl groups in this position. In contrast to benzylisoquinoliniums, the chlorofumarates have four chiral centers, two of which are quaternary ammoniums. Additionally, the head groups of these compounds are distinct.[77] Primate studies have shown that onset of these compounds is inversely related to potency. While the chlorofumarates are potent (ED$_{95}$ < 0.2 mg/kg), they have rapid onsets and very short durations of action.[200] One of the chlorofumarates, gantacurium, has been administered to human volunteers.[45] Maximal onset of block at the adductor pollicis and laryngeal adductors following doses approximating two and three times the ED$_{95}$ were comparable to onset of block following administration of succinylcholine (Table 19-7).[201] Large-scale intubation trials with this compound are necessary to determine its potential clinical utility.

As with atracurium and cisatracurium, the fumarates were chosen for development because of, in addition to their pharmacodynamic profile, their unique means of elimination from plasma.[200,202] Gantacurium is broken down by two different pathways; one is a slow, pH-sensitive hydrolysis, and the other is adduction of the naturally occurring amino acid cysteine (addition of a cysteine molecule to the NMBA, rendering a

Table 19-7. Comparison of Onset of Block by Gantacurium and Succinylcholine

| | | Minutes to Maximal Block | |
NEUROMUSCULAR BLOCKING AGENT	DOSE (MG/KG)	LARYNGEAL ADDUCTORS	ADDUCTOR POLLICIS
Gantacurium	0.36	1.1 ± 0.3	1.7 ± 0.2
	0.54	0.9 ± 0.2	1.5 ± 0.3
Succinylcholine	1.0	0.8 ± 0.3	1.5 ± 0.2

Note that the laryngeal muscles are blocked faster than the thumb.

new compound) (Figure 19-18).[203] This adduction reaction replaces the chlorine and saturates the fumarate double bond. The resultant product is structurally different than gantacurium and can no longer interact with the acetylcholine receptor. This unique means of inactivation likely accounts for its ultrashort duration of effect.[45] It also provides a novel means of shortening recovery from chlorofumarate-induced neuromuscular block.[204] L-cysteine has an elimination half-life of 1 to 2 hours. Exogenous cysteine administered to dogs during the early phases of spontaneous recovery of neuromuscular function or 1 minute after administration of gantacurium significantly shortens the time required to complete recovery compared to either spontaneous recovery or edrophonium-facilitated recovery. In Rhesus monkeys, doses of eight times the ED$_{95}$ of gantacurium have a duration of action of approximately 14 minutes. Administration of L-cysteine (10 mg/kg) 1 minute after administration of gantacurium results in return of complete neuromuscular function within 1 to 2 minutes. The rapid reversal of fumarate-induced neuromuscular block by administration of L-cysteine has the potential to decrease the frequency of residual neuromuscular block.[202]

Two analogues of the asymmetrical fumarate gantacurium, CW002 and CW011, have been synthesized to undergo slower L-cysteine adduction, yielding compounds with intermediate durations of action.[205] Volunteer trials are required to determine whether onset, recovery, and ease of antagonism are improved over that provided by compounds that are currently available.

341

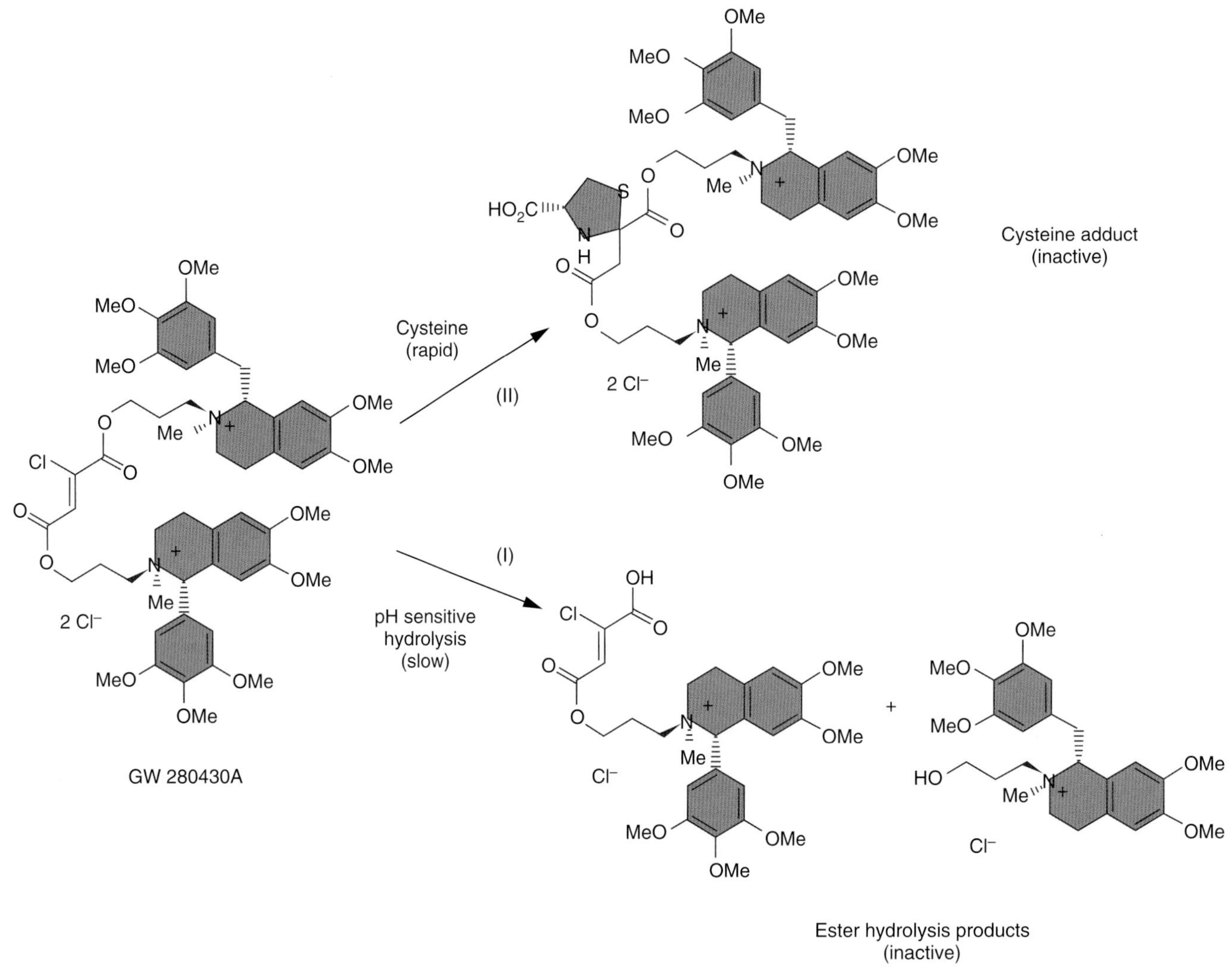

Figure 19-18 Degradation and inactivation of gantacurium (GW 280430A), an asymmetrical chlorofumarate. Gantacurium is inactivated by two pathways: rapid adduction of cysteine to yield an inactive cysteine adduct and a slower pH sensitive hydrolysis to yield ester hydrolysis products. *(From Savarese JJ, Belmont MR, Hashim MA, et al. Preclinical pharmacology of GW280430A [AV430A] in the rhesus monkey and in the cat: a comparison with mivacurium. Anesthesiology. 2004;100:835-845.)*

KEY POINTS

- Quantitative monitoring is the only way to ensure adequacy of neuromuscular function recovery at the conclusion of anesthesia and should be used to guide dosing of neuromuscular blocking agents.
- A TOF ratio less than 0.9 constitutes inadequate recovery of neuromuscular function. Inadequate recovery of neuromuscular function results in postoperative respiratory complications and delayed discharge from the postanesthesia care unit.
- Anticholinesterases are associated with significant adverse effects, have delayed onset, and do not guarantee adequate recovery of neuromuscular function.
- Development of newer drugs to facilitate recovery of neuromuscular function, such as the selective relaxant binding agent sugammadex, might decrease the incidence of postoperative residual neuromuscular block.
- The effect of neuromuscular blocking agents that are extensively metabolized can be rapidly antagonized by increasing their metabolism.

- Upper airway collapse occurs with subtle degrees of neuromuscular block.
- Administering neuromuscular blocking agents to mechanically ventilated patients in the ICU can improve their outcome.

Key References

Donati F, Meistelman C, Plaud B. Vecuronium neuromuscular blockade at the adductor muscles of the larynx and adductor pollicis. *Anesthesiology*. 1991;74:833-837. In this study, time to maximal effect of and recovery from vecuronium-induced neuromuscular block, 0.4 or 0.7 mg/kg, was determined at the adductor pollicis and the laryngeal adductors in 20 adult patients. While vecuronium had a more rapid effect in the laryngeal adductors, maximal depth of block was less profound than it was at the adductor pollicis. Recovery occurred more quickly in the larynx than at the adductor pollicis. (Ref. 13)

Eikermann M, Fassbender P, Malhotra A, et al. Unwarranted administration of acetylcholinesterase inhibitors can impair genioglossus and diaphragm muscle function. *Anesthesiology*.

2007;107:621-629. Administration of neostigmine to rats that had completely recovered from vecuronium-induced neuromuscular block resulted in impaired function of the genioglossus muscle and the diaphragm. With administration of the largest dose of neostigmine (1.2 mg/kg), tidal volume was significantly reduced and respiratory rate increased so that minute ventilation was unchanged from baseline. (Ref. 188)

Fuchs-Buder T, Meistelman C, Alla F, et al. Antagonism of low degrees of atracurium-induced neuromuscular blockade: dose-effect relationship for neostigmine. *Anesthesiology*. 2010;112:34-40. Administration of 10, 20, or 30 μg/kg neostigmine at TOFR of 0.4 or 0.6, when fade is likely not palpable in the TOF response, results in effective antagonism of residual atracurium-induced block. Neostigmine, 20 μg/kg will restore the TOFR to 0.9 or more within 10 minutes. Administration of these small doses of neostigmine does not augment existing neuromuscular block. (Ref. 190)

Kopman AF, Klewicka MM, Kopman DJ, et al. Molar potency is predictive of the speed of onset of neuromuscular block for agents of intermediate, short, and ultrashort duration. *Anesthesiology*. 1999;90:425-431. Times to peak effect of equipotent doses of five different neuromuscular blocking agents, succinylcholine, mivacurium, cisatracurium, vecuronium, and rocuronium, with different durations of action, structures, and mechanisms of action were studied. The less potent NMBAs, regardless of structure or duration of action were found to have the more rapid onsets of effect. This relationship had previously been demonstrated for long-acting NMBAs. (Ref. 49)

Koscielniak-Nielsen ZJ, Bevan JC, Popovic V, et al. Onset of maximum neuromuscular block following succinylcholine or vecuronium in four age groups. *Anesthesiology*. 1993;79:229-234. Subparalyzing doses of NMBAs were used to determine maximal onset of effect of patients of four different age groups: 1 to 3 years, 3 to 10 years, 20 to 40 years, and 60 to 80 years. Older subjects had slower onsets of maximal effect of NMBA. When large doses of NMBAs are administered to facilitate endotracheal intubation, time to onset of maximal effect cannot be appreciated. (Ref. 28)

Martyn JA, Richtsfeld M. Succinylcholine-induced hyperkalemia in acquired pathologic states: etiologic factors and molecular mechanisms. *Anesthesiology*. 2006;104:158-169. A review article describing the molecular mechanisms for hyperkalemia following administration of succinylcholine. The nicotinic α^7 acetylcholine receptor, which is activated by choline, acetylcholine, and succinylcholine, has a prolonged depolarization in the presence of agonist and may, in clinical situations wherein there is upregulation of acetylcholine receptors, have a significant role in the hyperkalemic response to succinylcholine. (Ref. 71)

Matteo RS, Backus WW, McDaniel DD, et al. Pharmacokinetics and pharmacodynamics of d-tubocurarine and metocurine in the elderly. *Anesth Analg*. 1985;64:23-29. This study of the pharmacokinetic and pharmacodynamics of metocurine and d-tubocurarine in elderly patients was the first to document that, while clearance was decreased, elimination half-life was prolonged, and recovery was slower in older patients, the plasma concentration-response relationships for these two NMBAs were the same in young adults and older adults. These findings indicate that, in older adults, it is decreased clearance rather than changes in the neuromuscular junction that causes the prolonged duration of effect of NMBAs. (Ref. 91)

Murphy GS, Szokol JW, Marymont JH, et al. Residual neuromuscular blockade and critical respiratory events in the postanesthesia care unit. *Anesth Analg*. 2008;107:130-137. An assessment of critical respiratory events in almost 7500 patients who had received general anesthesia. Just under 1% of patients had a critical respiratory event within 15 minutes of admission to the postanesthesia care unit. The majority of patients with a critical respiratory event (74%) had a TOFR of less than 0.7. Seventeen percent had a TOFR between 0.7 and 0.9. (Ref. 147)

Papazian L, Forel JM, Gacouin A, et al. Neuromuscular blockers in early acute respiratory distress syndrome. *N Engl J Med*. 2010;363:1107-1116. A multicenter trial of more than 300 intensive care patients with recent onset ARDS requiring mechanical ventilation. Patients were randomly assigned to receive either placebo or cisatracurium. Patients receiving cisatracurium had an improved 90-day survival and more time without ventilatory support. (Ref. 3)

Sundman E, Witt H, Olsson R, et al. The incidence and mechanism of pharyngeal and upper esophageal dysfunction in partially paralyzed humans: pharyngeal videoradiography and simultaneous manometry after atracurium. *Anesthesiology*. 2000;92:977-984. A volunteer trial demonstrating that pharyngeal dysfunction occurred with increased incidence at TOFR equal to 0.6, 0.7, and 0.8. Pharyngeal coordination was decreased at TOFR equal to 0.6 and 0.7, and partial neuromuscular block was associated with as much as a fivefold increase in misdirected swallows. (Ref. 154)

References

1. Cill RC. *White waters and black magic*. New York: Henry Holt and Co.; 1940.
2. Griffith HR, Johnson GE. The use of curare in general anesthesia. *Anesthesiology*. 1942;3:412-420.
3. Papazian L, Forel JM, Gacouin A, et al. Neuromuscular blockers in early acute respiratory distress syndrome. *N Engl J Med*. 2010;363:1107-1116.
4. Foldes FF, McNall PG, Borrego-Hinojosa JM. Succinylcholine, a new approach to muscular relaxation in anesthesiology. *N Engl J Med*. 1952;247:596-600.
5. Beecher HK, Todd DP. A study of the deaths associated with anesthesia and surgery: based on a study of 599, 548 anesthesia in ten institutions 1948-1952, inclusive. *Ann Surg*. 1954;140:2-35.
6. Abajian J, Arrowood JG, Barrett RH, et al. Critique of "A Study of the Deaths Associated with Anesthesia and Surgery". *Ann Surg*. 1955;142:138-141.
7. Bevan DR, Smith CE, Donati F. Postoperative neuromuscular blockade: a comparison between atracurium, vecuronium and pancuronium. *Anesthesiology*. 1988;69:272-276.
8. Mencke T, Echternach M, Kleinschmidt S, et al. Laryngeal morbidity and quality of tracheal intubation: a randomized controlled trial. *Anesthesiology*. 2003;98:1049-1056.
9. Mencke T, Echternach M, Plinkert PK, et al. Does the timing of tracheal intubation based on neuromuscular monitoring decrease laryngeal injury? A randomized, prospective, controlled trial. *Anesth Analg*. 2006;102:306-312.
10. Goldberg M. Complications of anesthesia for ocular surgery. *Ophthalmol Clin North Am*. 2006;19:293-307.
11. Alfille PH, Merritt C, Chamberlin NL, Eikermann M. Control of perioperative muscle strength during ambulatory surgery. *Curr Opin Anaesthesiol*. 2009;22:730-737.
12. Nguyen-Huu R, Molgo J, Servent D, Duvaldestin P. Resistance to D-tubocurarine of the rat diaphragm as compared to a limb muscle: influence of quantal transmitter release and nicotinic acetylcholine receptors. *Anesthesiology*. 2009;110:1011-1015.
13. Donati F, Meistelman C, Plaud B. Vecuronium neuromuscular blockade at the adductor muscles of the larynx and adductor pollicis. *Anesthesiology*. 1991;74:833-837.
14. D'Honneur G, Guignard B, Slavov V, Ruggier R, Duvaldestin P. Comparison of the neuromuscular blocking effect of atracurium and vecuronium on the adductor pollicis and the geniohyoid muscle in humans. *Anesthesiology*. 1995;82:649-654.
15. Bragg P, Fisher DM, Shi J, et al. Comparison of twitch depression of the adductor pollicis and the respiratory muscles. *Anesthesiology*. 1994;80:310-319.
16. Kopman AF, Eikermann M. Antagonism of non-depolarising neuromuscular block: current practice. *Anaesthesia*. 2009;64:22-30.
17. Fruergaard K, Viby-Mogensen J, Berg H, el-Mahdy AM. Tactile evaluation of the response to double burst stimulation decreases, but does not eliminate, the problem of postoperative residual paralysis. *Acta Anaesthesiol Scand*. 1998;42:1168-1174.
18. Viby-Mogensen J, Jensen NH, Engbaek J, Ording H, Skovgaard LT, Chraemmer-Jørgensen B. Tactile and visual evaluation of the response to train-of-four nerve stimulation. *Anesthesiology*. 1985;63:440-443.
19. Shorten GD. Postoperative residual curarisation: incidence, aetiology and associated morbidity. *Anaesth Intens Care*. 1993;21:782-789.

20. Waud BE, Waud DR. The relation between tetanic fade and receptor occlusion in the presence of competitive neuromuscular block. *Anesthesiology*. 1971;35:456-464.
21. Ali HH, Utting JE, Gray TC. Quantitative assessment of residual neuromuscular block. I. *Br J Anaesth*. 1971;43:473-477.
22. Ali HH, Utting JE, Gray TC. Quantitative assessment of residual antidepolarizing block. II. *Br J Anaesth*. 1971;43:478-485.
23. Lien CA, Belmont MR, Abalos A, Hass D, Savarese JJ. The nature of spontaneous recovery from mivacurium-induced neuromuscular block. *Anesth Analg*. 1999;88:648-653.
24. Engbaek J, Ostergaard D, Viby-Mogensen J. Double burst stimulation (DBS): a new pattern of nerve stimulation to identify residual neuromuscular block. *Br J Anaesth*. 1989;62:274-278.
25. Drenck NE, Ueda N, Olsen NV, et al. Manual evaluation of residual curarization using double burst stimulation: a comparison with train-of-four. *Anesthesiology*. 1989;70:578-581.
26. Magorian T, Flannery KB, Miller RD. Comparison of rocuronium, succinylcholine, and vecuronium for rapid-sequence induction of anesthesia in adult patients. *Anesthesiology*. 1993;79:913-918.
27. Lee HJ, Kim KS, Jeong JS, Cheong MA, Shim JC. Comparison of the adductor pollicis, orbicularis, oculi, and corrugator supercilii as indicators of adequacy of muscle relaxation for tracheal intubation. *Br J Anaesth*. 2009;102:869-874.
28. Koscielniak-Nielsen ZJ, Bevan JC, Popovic V, Baxter MRN, Donati F, Bevan DR. Onset of maximum neuromuscular block following succinylcholine or vecuronium in four age groups. *Anesthesiology*. 1993;79:229-234.
29. Eikermann M, Hunkemoller I, Peine L, et al. Optimal rocuronium dose for intubation during inhalation induction with sevoflurane in children. *Br J Anaesth*. 2002;89:277-281.
30. Debaene B, Plaud B, Dilly MP, Donati F. Residual paralysis in the PACU after a single intubating dose of nondepolarizing muscle relaxant with an intermediate duration of action. *Anesthesiology*. 2003;98:1042-1048.
31. Naguib M, Kopman AF, Lien CA, Hunter JM, Lopez A, Brull SJ. A survey of current management of neuromuscular block in the United States and Europe. *Anesth Analg*. 2010;111:110-119.
32. Bovet D. Some aspects of the relationship between chemical constitution and curare-like activity. *Ann N Y Acad Sci*. 1951;54:407-437.
33. Prince RJ, Sine SM. Epibatidine binds with unique site and state selectivity to muscle nicotinic acetylcholine receptors. *J Biol Chem*. 1998;273:7843-7849.
34. Blount P, Merlie JP. Molecular basis of the two nonequivalent ligand binding sites of the muscle nicotinic acetylcholine receptor. *Neuron*. 1989;3:349-357.
35. Neubirg RR, Cohen JB. Equilibrium binding of [3H]tubocurarine and [3H]acetylcholine by torpedo postsynaptic membranes: stoichiometry and ligand interactions. *Biochemistry*. 1979;18:5464-5475.
36. Paul M, Kindler CH, Fokt RM, Dressner MJ, Dipp NC, Yost CS. The potency of new muscle relaxants on recombinant muscle-type acetylcholine receptors. *Anesth Analg*. 2002;94:597-603.
37. Dilger JP. Roles of amino acids and subunits in determining the inhibition of nicotinic acetylcholine receptors by competitive antagonists. *Anesthesiology*. 2007;106:1186-1195.
38. Lee C. Structure, conformation, and action of neuromuscular blocking drugs. *Br J Anaesth*. 2001;87:755-769.
39. Willcockson IU, Hong A, Whisenant RP, et al. Orientation of d-tubocurarine in the muscle nicotinic acetylcholine receptor-binding site. *J Biol Chem*. 2002;277:42249-42258.
40. Liu M, Dilger JP. Synergy between pairs of competitive antagonists at adult human muscle acetylcholine receptors. *Anesth Analg*. 2008;107:525-533.
41. Jonsson M, Gurley D, Dabrowski M, Larsson O, Johnson EC, Eriksson LI. Distinct pharmacologic properties of neuromuscular blocking agents on human neuronal nicotinic acetylcholine receptors. *Anesthesiology*. 2006;105:521-533.
42. Engbaek J, Howardy-Hansen P, Ording H, Viby-Mogensen J. Precurarization with vecuronium and pancuronium in awake, healthy volunteers: the influence on neuromuscular transmission and pulmonary function. *Acta Anaesth Scand*. 1985;29:117-120.
43. Howardy-Hansen P, Moller J, Hansen B. Pretreatment with atracurium: the influence on neuromuscular transmission and pulmonary function. *Acta Anaesth Scand*. 1987;31:642-644.
44. Savarese JJ, Wastila WB. The future of benzylisoquinolinium relaxants. *Acta Anaesth Scand*. 1995;106:91-93.
45. Belmont MR, Lien CA, Tjan J, et al. Clinical pharmacology of GW280430A in humans. *Anesthesiology*. 2004;100:768-773.
46. Bowman WC, Rodger IW, Houston J, Marshall RJ, McIndewar I. Structure: action relationships among some desacetoxy analogues of pancuronium and vecuronium in the anesthetized cat. *Anesthesiology*. 1988;69:57-62.
47. Boros EE, Mook RA, Boswell GE, Wisowaty JC, Savarese JJ. Structure-activity relationships of the asymmetrical mixed-onium chlorofumarate neuromuscular blocker GW280430A and some congeners in rhesus monkeys. *Anesthesiology*. 1999;91:A1022.
48. Kopman AF. Pancuronium, gallamine, and d-tubocurarine compared: is speed of onset inversely related to drug potency? *Anesthesiology*. 1993;70:915-920.
49. Kopman AF, Klewicka MM, Kopman DJ, Neuman GG. Molar potency is predictive of the speed of onset of neuromuscular block for agents of intermediate, short, and ultrashort duration. *Anesthesiology*. 1999;90:425-431.
50. Donati F, Meistelman C. A kinetic-dynamic model to explain the relationship between high potency and slow onset time for neuromuscular blocking drugs. *J Pharmacokinet Biopharm*. 1991;19:537-552.
51. Wright PMC, Brown R, Lau M, Fisher D. A pharmacodynamics explanation for the rapid onset/offset of rapacuronium bromide. *Anesthesiology*. 1999;90:16-23.
52. Beaufort TM, Nigrovic V, Proost JH, Houwertjes MC, Wierda JM. Inhibition of the enzymic degradation of suxamethonium and mivacurium increases the onset time of submaximal neuromuscular block. *Anesthesiology*. 1998;89:707-714.
53. Wright PM, Brown R, Lau M, Fisher DM. A pharmacodynamic explanation for the rapid onset/offset of rapacuronium bromide. *Anesthesiology*. 1999;90:16-23.
54. Vanlinthout LE, Bartels CF, Lockridge O, Callens K, Booij LH. Prolonged paralysis after a test dose of mivacurium in a patient with atypical cholinesterase. *Anesth Analg*. 1998;87:1199-1202.
55. Hickey DR, O'Connor JP, Donati F. Comparison of atracurium and succinylcholine for electroconvulsive therapy in a patient with atypical plasma cholinesterase. *Can J Anesth*. 1987;34:280-283.
56. Andrews JI, Kumar N, van den Brom RH, Olkkola KT, Roest GJ, Wright PM. A large simple randomized trial of rocuronium versus succinylcholine in rapid-sequence induction of anaesthesia along with propofol. *Acta Anaesthesiol Scand* 1999;43:4-8.
57. Wierda JM, van den Broek L, Proost JH, Verbaan BW, Hennis PJ. Time course of action and endotracheal intubating conditions of Org 9487, a new short-acting steroidal muscle relaxant; a comparison with succinylcholine. *Anesth Analg*. 1993;77:579-584.
58. Savarese JJ, Ali HH, Basta SJ, et al. The clinical neuromuscular pharmacology of mivacurium chloride (BW B1090U). A short-acting nondepolarizing ester neuromuscular blocking drug. *Anesthesiology*. 1988;68:723-732.
59. Torda TA, Graham GG, Warwick NR, Donohue P. Pharmacokinetics and pharmacodynamics of suxamethonium. *Anaesth Intensive Care*. 1997;25:272-278.
60. Szalados JE, Donati F, Bevan DR. Effect of d-tubocurarine pretreatment on succinylcholine twitch augmentation and neuromuscular blockade. *Anesth Analg*. 1990;71:55-59.
61. Curran MJ, Donati F, Bevan DR. Onset and recovery of atracurium and suxamethoium induced neuromuscular blockade with simultaneous train-of-four and single twitch stimulation. *Br J Anaesth*. 1987;59:989-994.
62. Viby-Mogensen J. Correlation of succinylcholine duration of action with plasma cholinesterase activity in subjects with the genotypically normal enzyme. *Anesthesiology*. 1980;27:242-249.
63. Ryan DW. Preoperative serum cholinesterase concentration in chronic renal failure. *Br J Anaesth*. 1977;49:945-949.
64. Lien CA, Belmont MR, Wray Roth DL, Okamoto M, Abalos A, Savarese JJ. Pharmacodynamics and the plasma concentration of mivacurium during spontaneous recovery and neostigmine-facilitated recovery. *Anesthesiology*. 1999;91:119-126.
65. Goat VA, Feldman SA. The dual action of suxamethonium on the isolated rabbit heart. *Anaesthesia*. 1972;27:149-153.
66. Stoelting RK, Peterson C. Heart-rate slowing and junctional rhythm following intravenous succinylcholine with and without

intramuscular atropine preanesthetic medication. *Anesth Analg.* 1975;54:705-709.

67. Derbyshire DR. Succinylcholine-induced increases in plasma catecholamine levels in humans. *Anesth Analg.* 1984;63:465-467.

68. Gronert GA. Succinylcholine hyperkalemia after burns. *Anesthesiology.* 1999;91:320-322.

69. Hansen D. Suxamethonium-induced cardiac arrest and death following 5 days of immobilization. *Eur J Anaesthesiol.* 1998;15:240-241.

70. Larach MG, Rosenberg H, Gronert GA, Allen GC. Hyperkalemic cardiac arrest during anesthesia in infants and children with occult myopathies. *Clin Pediatr (Phila).* 1997;36:9-16.

71. Martyn JA, Richtsfeld M. Succinylcholine-induced hyperkalemia in acquired pathologic states: etiologic factors and molecular mechanisms. *Anesthesiology.* 2006;104:158-169.

72. Minton MD, Grosslight K, Stirt JA, Bedford RF. Increases in intracranial pressure from succinylcholine: prevention by prior nondepolarizing blockade. *Anesthesiology.* 1986;65:165-169.

73. Miller RD, Way WL. Inhibition of succinylcholine-induced increased intragastric pressure by nondepolarizing muscle relaxants and lidocaine. *Anesthesiology.* 1971;34:185-188.

74. Miller RD, Way WL, Hickey RF. Inhibition of succinylcholine-induced increased intraocular pressure by non-depolarizing muscle relaxants. *Anesthesiology.* 1968;29:123-126.

75. Hopkins PM. Malignant hyperthermia: pharmacology of triggering. *Br J Anaesth.* 2011;107:48-56.

76. Basta SJ, Ali HH, Savarese JJ, et al. Clinical pharmacology of atracurium besylate (BW 33A): a new non-depolarizing muscle relaxant. *Anesth Analg.* 1982;61:723-729.

77. Caldwell JE, Heier T, Kitts JB, Lynam DP, Fahey MR, Miller RD. Comparison of the neuromuscular block induced by mivacurium, suxamethonium or atracurium during nitrous oxide-fentanyl anaesthesia. *Br J Anaesth.* 1989;63:393-399.

78. Merrett RA, Thompson CW, Webb FW. In vitro degradation of atracurium in human plasma. *Br J Anaesth.* 1983;55:61-66.

79. Stiller RL, Cook DR, Chakravorti S. In vitro degradation of atracurium in human plasma. *Br J Anaesth.* 1985;57:1085-1088.

80. Fisher DM, Canfell PC, Fahey MR, et al. Elimination of atracurium in humans: contribution of Hofmann elimination and ester hydrolysis versus organ-based elimination. *Anesthesiology.* 1986;65:6-12.

81. Flynn PJ, Hughes R, Walton B, Jothilingam S. Use of atracurium infusions for general surgical procedures including cardiac surgery with induced hypothermia. *Br J Anaesth.* 1983;55:135S-138S.

82. Fisher DM, Rosen JI. A pharmacokinetic explanation for increasing recovery time following larger or repeated doses of nondepolarizing muscle relaxants. *Anesthesiology.* 1986;65:286-291.

83. Ali HH, Savarese JJ, Basta SJ, Sunder N, Gionfriddo M. Evaluation of cumulative properties of three new nondepolarizing neuromuscular blocking drugs BW A444U, atracurium and vecuronium. *Br J Anaesth.* 1983;55:107S-111S.

84. Eagar BM, Flynn PJ, Hughes R. Infusion of atracurium for long surgical procedures. *Br J Anaesth.* 1984;56:447-452.

85. Martineau RJ, St-Jean B, Kitts JB, et al. Cumulation and reversal with prolonged infusions of atracurium and vecuronium. *Can J Anaesth.* 1992;39:670-676.

86. Fahey MR, Rupp SM, Fisher DM, et al. The pharmacokinetics and pharmacodynamics of atracurium in patients with and without renal failure. *Anesthesiology.* 1984;61:699-702.

87. Ward S, Boheimer N, Weatherly BC, Simmonds RJ, Dopson TA. Pharmacokinetics of atracurium and its metabolites in patients with normal renal function, and in patients with renal failure. *Br J Anaesth.* 1987;59:697-706.

88. Hunter JM, Jones RS, Utting JE. Use of atracurium in patients with no renal function. *Br J Anaesth.* 1982;54:1251-1258.

89. Parker CJ, Hunter JM. Pharmacokinetics of atracurium and laudanosine in patients with hepatic cirrhosis. *Br J Anaesth.* 1989;62:177-183.

90. Naguib M, Flood P, McArdle JJ, Brenner HR. Advances in neurobiology of the neuromuscular junction: implications for anesthesiologists. *Anesthesiology.* 2002;96:202-231.

91. Matteo RS, Backus WW, McDaniel DD, Brotherton WP, Abraham R, Diaz J. Pharmacokinetics and pharmacodynamics of d-tubocurarine and metocurine in the elderly. *Anesth Analg.* 1985;64:23-29.

92. d'Hollander AA, Luyckx C, Barvais L, De Ville A. Clinical evaluation of atracurium besylate requirement for a stable muscle relaxation during surgery: lack of age-related effects. *Anesthesiology.* 1983;59:237-240.

93. Kitts JB, Fisher DM, Canfell PC, et al. Pharmacokinetics and pharmacodynamics of atracurium in the elderly. *Anesthesiology.* 1990;72:272-275.

94. Kent AP, Parker CJ, Hunter JM. Pharmacokinetics of atracurium and laudanosine in the elderly. *Br J Anaesth.* 1989;63:661-666.

95. Belmont MR, Lien CA, Quessy S, et al. The clinical neuromuscular pharmacology of 51W89 in patients receiving nitrous oxide/opioid/barbiturate anesthesia. *Anesthesiology.* 1995;82:1139-1145.

96. Bluestein LS, Stinson Jr LW, Lennon RL, Quessy SN, Wilson RM. Evaluation of cisatracurium, a new neuromuscular blocking agent, for tracheal intubation. *Can J Anaesth.* 1996;43:925-931.

97. Lien CA, Belmont MR, Abalos A, et al. The cardiovascular effects and histamine-releasing properties of 51W89 in patients receiving nitrous oxide/opioid/barbiturate anesthesia. *Anesthesiology.* 1995;82:1131-1138.

98. Lien CA, Schmith VD, Belmont MR, Abalos A, Kisor DF, Savarese JJ. Pharmacokinetics of cisatracurium in patients receiving nitrous oxide/opioid/barbiturate anesthesia. *Anesthesiology.* 1996;84:300-308.

99. Kisor DF, Schmith VD, Wargin WA, Lien CA, Ornstein E, Cook DR. Importance of the organ-independent elimination of cisatracurium. *Anesth Analg.* 1996;83:1065-1071.

100. Eastwood NB, Boyd AH, Parker CJR, Hunter JM. Pharmacokinetics of 1 R-cis 1'R-cis atracurium besylate (51W89) and plasma laudanosine in health and chronic renal failure. *Br J Anaesth.* 1995;75:431-435.

101. Boyd AH, Eastwood NB, Parker CJR, Hunter JM. Pharmacodynamics of the 1 R-cis 1'R-cis isomer of atracurium (51W89) in health and chronic renal failure *Br J Anaesth.* 1995;74:400-404.

102. De Wolf AM, Freeman JA, Scott VL, et al. Pharmacokinetics and pharmacodynamics of cisatracurium in patients with end-stage liver disease undergoing liver transplantation. *Br J Anaesth.* 1996;76:624-628.

103. Ornstein E, Lien CA, Matteo RS, Ostapkovich ND, Diaz J, Wolf KB. Pharmacodynamics and pharmacokinetics of cisatracurium in geriatric surgical patients. *Anesthesiology.* 1996;84:520-525.

104. Miller RD, Agoston S, Booij LHDJ, Kersten UW, Crul JF, Ham J. The comparative potency and pharmacokinetics of pancuronium and its metabolites in anesthetized man. *J Pharmacol Exp Ther.* 1978;207:539-543.

105. Agoston S, Vermeer GA, Kertsten UW, Meijer DK. The fate of pancuronium bromide in man. *Acta Anaesthesiol Scand.* 1973;17:267-275.

106. Somogyi AA, Shanks CA, Triggs EJ. Disposition kinetics of pancuronium bromide in patients with total biliary obstruction. *Br J Anaesth.* 1977;49:1103-1108.

107. Duvaldestin P, Agoston S, Henzel D, Kersten UW, Desmonts JM. Pancuronium pharmacokinetics in patients with liver cirrhosis. *Br J Anaesth.* 1978;50:1131-1136.

108. McLeod K, Watson MJ, Rawlins MD. Pharmacokinetics of pancuronium in patients with normal and impaired renal function. *Br J Anaesth.* 1976;48:341-345.

109. Duvaldestin P, Saada J, Berger JL, D'Hollander A, Desmonts JM. Pharmacokinetics, pharmacodynamics, and dose-response relationships of pancuronium in control and elderly subjects. *Anesthesiology.* 1982;56:36-40.

110. Agoston S, Salt P, Newton D, Bencini A, Boomsma P, Erdmann W. The neuromuscular blocking action of ORG NC 45, a new pancuronium derivative, in anaesthetized patients. A pilot study. *Br J Anaesth.* 1980;52:53S-59S.

111. Lennon RL, Olson RA, Gronert GA. Atracurium or vecuronium for rapid sequence endotracheal intubation. *Anesthesiology.* 1986;64:510-513.

112. Morris RB, Cahalan MK, Miller RD, Wilkinson PL, Quasha AL, Robinson SL. The cardiovascular effects of vecuronium (ORG NC45) and pancuronium in patients undergoing coronary artery bypass grafting. *Anesthesiology.* 1983;58:438-440.

113. Bencini AF, Scaf AH, Sohn YJ, Kersten-Kleef UW, Agoston S. Hepatobiliary disposition of vecuronium bromide in man. *Br J Anaesth.* 1986;58:988-995.

114. Bencini AF, Scaf AH, Agoston S, Houwertjes MC, Kersten UW. Disposition of vecuronium bromide in the cat. *Br J Anaesth*. 1985; 57:782-788.

115. Agoston S, Seyr M, Khuenl-Brady RS, Henning RH. Use of neuromuscular blocking agents in the intensive care unit. *Anesthesiol Clin North Am*. 1993;11:345-360.

116. Marshall IG, Gibb AJ, Durant NN. Neuromuscular and vagal blocking actions of pancuronium bromide, its metabolites, and vecuronium bromide (Org NC45) and its potential metabolites in the anaesthetized cat. *Br J Anaesth*. 1983;55:703-714.

117. Caldwell JE, Szenohradszky J, Segredo V, et al. The pharmacodynamics and pharmacokinetics of the metabolite 3-desacetylvecuronium (ORG 7268) and its parent compound, vecuronium, in human volunteers. *J Pharmacol Exp Ther*. 1994; 270:1216-1222.

118. Segredo V, Caldwell JE, Matthay MA, Sharma ML, Gruenke LD, Miller RD. Persistent paralysis in critically ill patients after long-term administration of vecuronium. *N Engl J Med*. 1992;327: 524-528.

119. Bencini AF, Scaf AH, Sohn YJ, et al. Disposition and urinary excretion of vecuronium bromide in anesthetized patients with normal renal function or renal failure. *Anesth Analg*. 1986;65:245-251.

120. Lynam DP, Cronnelly R, Castagnoli KP, et al. The pharmacodynamics and pharmacokinetics of vecuronium in patients anesthetized with isoflurane with normal renal function or with renal failure. *Anesthesiology*. 1988;69:227-231.

121. Fahey MR, Morris RB, Miller RD, Nguyen TL, Upton RA. Pharmacokinetics of Org NC45 (norcuron) in patients with and without renal failure. *Br J Anaesth*. 1981;53:1049-1053.

122. Bevan DR, Donati F, Gyasi H, Williams A. Vecuronium in renal failure. *Can Anaesth Soc J*. 1984;31:491-496.

123. Lepage JY, Malinge M, Cozian A, Pinaud M, Blanloeil Y, Souron R. Vecuronium and atracurium in patients with end-stage renal failure. A comparative study. *Br J Anaesth*. 1987;59:1004-1010.

124. Lebrault C, Duvaldestin P, Henzel D, Chauvin M, Guesnon P. Pharmacokinetics and pharmacodynamics of vecuronium in patients with cholestasis. *Br J Anaesth*. 1986;58:983-987.

125. Lebrault C, Berger JL, D'Hollander AA, Gomeni R, Henzel D, Duvaldestin P. Pharmacokinetics and pharmacodynamics of vecuronium (ORG NC 45) in patients with cirrhosis. *Anesthesiology*. 1985;62:601-605.

126. Hunter JM, Parker CJ, Bell CF, Jones RS, Utting JE. The use of different doses of vecuronium in patients with liver dysfunction. *Br J Anaesth*. 1985;57:758-764.

127. Lien CA, Matteo RS, Ornstein E, Schwartz AE, Diaz J. Distribution, elimination, and action of vecuronium in the elderly. *Anesth Analg*. 1991;73:39-42.

128. Rupp SM, Castagnoli KP, Fisher DM, Miller RD. Pancuronium and vecuronium pharmacokinetics and pharmacodynamics in younger and elderly adults. *Anesthesiology*. 1987;67:45-49.

129. d'Hollander A, Massaux F, Nevelsteen M, Agoston S. Age-dependent dose-response relationship of ORG NC 45 in anaesthetized patients. *Br J Anaesth*. 1982;54:653-657.

130. Booij LH, Knape HT. The neuromuscular blocking effect of Org 9426. A new intermediate-acting steroidal non-depolarising muscle relaxant in man. *Anaesthesia*. 1991;46:341-343.

131. Lambalk LM, De Wit AP, Wierda JM, Hennis PJ, Agoston S. Dose-response relationship and time course of action of Org 9426. A new muscle relaxant of intermediate duration evaluated under various anaesthetic techniques. *Anaesthesia*. 1991;46:907-911.

132. Wierda JM, Proost JH. Structure-pharmacodynamic-pharmacokinetic relationships of steroidal neuromuscular blocking agents. *Eur J Anaesthesiol*. 1995;11:45-54.

133. Bartkowski RR, Witkowski TA, Azad S, Lessin J, Marr A. Rocuronium onset of action: a comparison with atracurium and vecuronium. *Anesth Analg*. 1993;77:574-578.

134. Proost JH, Roggeveld J, Wierda JM, Meijer DK. Relationship between chemical structure and physicochemical properties of series of bulky organic cations and their hepatic uptake and biliary excretion rates. *J Pharmacol Exp Ther*. 1997;282:715-726.

135. Khuenl-Brady K, Castagnoli KP, Canfell PC, Caldwell JE, Agoston S, Miller RD. The neuromuscular blocking effects and pharmacokinetics of ORG 9426 and ORG 9616 in the cat. *Anesthesiology*. 1990;72:669-674.

136. Cooper RA, Maddineni VR, Mirakhur RK, Wierda JM, Brady M, Fitzpatrick KT. Time course of neuromuscular effects and pharmacokinetics of rocuronium bromide (Org 9426) during isoflurane anaesthesia in patients with and without renal failure. *Br J Anaesth*. 1993;71:222-226.

137. Szenohradszky J, Fisher DM, Segredo V, et al. Pharmacokinetics of rocuronium bromide (ORG 9426) in patients with normal renal function or patients undergoing cadaver renal transplantation. *Anesthesiology*. 1992;77:899-904.

138. Khalil M, D'Honneur G, Duvaldestin P, Slavov V, De Hys C, Gomeni R. Pharmacokinetics and pharmacodynamics of rocuronium in patients with cirrhosis. *Anesthesiology*. 1994;80:1241-1247.

139. van Miert MM, Eastwood NB, Boyd AH, Parker CJ, Hunter JM. The pharmacokinetics and pharmacodynamics of rocuronium in patients with hepatic cirrhosis. *Br J Clin Pharmacol*. 1997;44: 139-144.

140. Magorian T, Wood P, Caldwell J, et al. The pharmacokinetics and neuromuscular effects of rocuronium bromide in patients with liver disease. *Anesth Analg*. 1995;80:754-759.

141. Bevan DR, Fiset P, Balendran P, Law-Min JC, Ratcliffe A, Donati F. Pharmacodynamic behaviour of rocuronium in the elderly. *Can J Anaesth*. 1993;40:127-132.

142. Matteo RS, Ornstein E, Schwartz AE, Ostapkovich N, Stone JG. Pharmacokinetics and pharmacodynamics of rocuronium (Org 9426) in elderly surgical patients. *Anesth Analg*. 1993;77:1193-1197.

143. Viby-Mogensen J. Postoperative residual curarization and evidence-based anaesthesia. *Br J Anaesth*. 2000;84:301-303.

144. Hayes AH, Mirakhur RK, Breslin DS, Reid JE, McCourt KC. Postoperative residual block after intermediate-acting neuromuscular blocking drugs. *Anaesthesia*. 2001;56:312-318.

145. Viby-Mogensen J, Chraemmer Jorgensen B, Ording H. Residual curarization in the recovery room. *Anesthesiology*. 1979;50:539-541.

146. Baillard C, Gehan G, Reboul-Marty J, Larmignat P, Samama CM, Cupa M. Residual curarization in the recovery room after vecuronium. *Br J Anaesth*. 2000;84:394-395.

147. Murphy GS, Szokol JW, Marymont JH, Greenberg SB, Avram MJ, Vender JS. Residual neuromuscular blockade and critical respiratory events in the postanesthesia care unit. *Anesth Analg*. 2008;107: 130-137.

148. Kopman AF, Klewicka MM, Neuman GG. The relationship between acceleromyographic train-of-four fade and single twitch depression. *Anesthesiology*. 2002;96:583-587.

149. Murphy GS, Szokol JW, Marymount JH, et al. Intraoperative acceleromyographic monitoring reduces the risk of residual neuromuscular blockade and adverse respiratory events in the postanesthesia care unit. *Anesthesiology*. 2008;109:389-398.

150. Eikermann M, Vogt FM, Herbstreit F, et al. The predisposition to inspiratory upper airway collapse during partial neuromuscular blockade. *Am J Respir Crit Care Med*. 2007;175:9-15.

151. Eriksson LI, Sato M, Severinghaus JW. Effect of a vecuronium—induced partial neuromuscular block on hypoxic ventilatory response. *Anesthesiology*. 1993;78:693-699.

152. Herbstreit F, Peters J, Eikermann M. Impaired upper airway integrity by residual neuromuscular blockade: increased airway collapsibility and blunted genioglossus muscle activity in response to negative pharyngeal pressure. *Anesthesiology*. 2009;110:1253-1260.

153. Eriksson LI, Sundman E, Olsson R, et al. Functional assessment of the pharynx at rest and during swallowing in partially paralyzed humans: simultaneous videomanometry and mechanomyography of awake human volunteers. *Anesthesiology*. 1997;87:1035-1043.

154. Sundman E, Witt H, Olsson R, Ekberg O, Kuylenstierna R, Eriksson LI. The incidence and mechanism of pharyngeal and upper esophageal dysfunction in partially paralyzed humans: pharyngeal videoradiography and simultaneous manometry after atracurium. *Anesthesiology*. 2000;92:977-984.

155. Eikermann, M, Gerwig M, Hasselmann C, Fiedler G, Peters J. Impaired neuromuscular transmission after recovery of the train-of-four ratio. *Acta Anaesthesiol Scand*. 2007;51:226-234.

156. Sundman E, Yost CS, Margolin G, Kuylenstierna R, Ekberg O, Eriksson LI. Acetylcholine receptor density in human cricopharyngeal muscle and phyryngeal constrictor muscle. *Acta Anaesthesiol Scand*. 2002;46:999-1002.

157. Sundman E, Ansved T, Margolin G, Kuylenstierna R, Eriksson LI. Fiber-type composition and fiber size of the human cricophyryngeal muscle and the pharyngeal constrictor muscle. *Acta Anaesthesiol Scand*. 2004;48:423-429.

158. Saboisky JP, Gorman RB, De Troyer A, Gandevia SC, Butler JE. Differential activation among five human inspiratory motoneuron pools during tidal breathing. *J Appl Physiol.* 2007;102:772-780.

159. Butterly A, Bittner EA, George E, Sandberg WS, Eikermann M, Schmidt U. Postoperative residual curarization from intermediate-acting neuromuscular blocking agents delays recovery room discharge. *Br J Anaesthesia.* 2010;105:304-309.

160. Eikermann M, Groeben H, Bunten B, Peters J. Fade of pulmonary function during residual neuromuscular blockade. *Chest.* 2005;127:1703-1709.

161. Lunn, JN, Hunter AR, Scott DB. Anaesthesia-related surgical mortality. *Anaesthesia.* 1983;38:1090-1096.

162. Pedersen T, Viby-Mogensen J, Ringsted CL. Anaesthetic practice and postoperative pulmonary complications. *Acta Anaesthesiol Scand.* 1992;36:812-818.

163. Berg H, Viby-Mogensen J, Roed J, et al. Residual neuromuscular block is a risk factor for postoperative pulmonary complications. A prospective, randomized, and blinded study of postoperative pulmonary complications after atracurium, vecuronium and pancuronium. *Acta Anaesthesiol Scand.* 1997;41:1095-1103.

164. Murphy GS, Szokol JW, Franklin M, Marymont JH, Avram MJ, Vender JS. Postanesthesia care unit recovery times and neuromuscular blocking drugs: a prospective study of orthopedic surgical patients randomized to receive pancuronium or rocuronium. *Anesth Analg.* 2004;98:193-200.

165. Pinot RM. Neuromuscular blockade studies of critically ill patients. *Intensive Care Med.* 2002;28:1735-1741.

166. Herridge MS, Cheung AM, Tansey CM, et al, Canadian Critical Care Trials Group. One-year outcomes in survivors of the acute respiratory distress syndrome. *N Engl J Med.* 2003;348:683-693.

167. Tsukagoshi H, Morita T, Takahashi K, et al. Cecal ligation and puncture peritonitis model shows decreased nicotinic acetylcholine receptor numbers in rat muscle: immunologic mechanisms? *Anesthesiology.* 1999;91:448-460.

168. Shee CD. Risk factors for hydrocortisone myopathy in acute severe asthma. *Respir Med.* 1990;84:229-233.

169. Kasotakis G, Schmidt U, Perry D, et al. The surgical intensive care unit optimal mobility score predicts mortality and length of stay. *Crit Care Med.* 2011. [Epub ahead of print].

170. Testelmans D, Maes K, Wouters P, et al. Rocuronium exacerbates mechanical ventilation-induced diaphragm in rats. *Crit Care Med.* 2006;34:3018-3023.

171. Op de Coul AA, Lambregts PC, Koeman J, et al. Neuromuscular complications in patients given Pavulon (pancuronium bromide) during artificial ventilation. *Clin Neurol Neurosurg.* 1985;87:17-22.

172. Dodson BA, Kelly BJ, Braswell LM, Cohen NH. Changes in acetylcholine receptor number in muscle from critically ill patients receiving muscle relaxants: an investigation of the molecular mechanisms of prolonged paralysis. *Crit Care Med.* 1995;23:815-821.

173. Coursin DB, Klasek G, Goelzer SL. Increased requirements for continuously infused vecuronium in critically ill patients. *Anesth Analg.* 1989;69:518-521.

174. Putensen C, Mutz NJ, Putensen-Himmer G, Zinserling J. Spontaneous breathing during ventilatory support improves ventilation-perfusion distributions in patients with acute respiratory distress syndrome. *Am J Respir Crit Care Med.* 1999;159:1241-1248.

175. Barrow ME, Johnson JK. A study of the anticholinesterase and anticurare effects of some cholinesterase inhibitors. *Br J Anaesth.* 1966;38:420-431.

176. Bevan DR, Donati F, Kopman RF. Reversal of neuromuscular blockade. *Anesthesiology.* 1992;77:785-805.

177. Eriksson LI. Evidence-based practice and neuromuscular monitoring: it's time for routine quantitative assessment. *Anesthesiology.* 2003;98:1037-1039.

178. Arbous MS, Meursing AEE, van Kleef JW, et al. Impact of anesthesia management characteristics on severe morbidity and mortality. *Anesthesiology.* 2005;102:257-268, quiz 491-492.

179. Nagata K, Huang CS, Song JH, Narahashi T. Direct actions of anticholinesterases on the neuronal nicotinic acetylcholine receptor channels. *Brain Res.* 1997;769:211-218.

180. Legendre P, Ali DW, Drapeau P. Recovery from open channel block by acetylcholine during neuromuscular transmission in zebra fish. *J Neurosci.* 2000;20:140-148.

181. Drapeau P, Legendre P. Neuromuscular transmission on the rebound. *Receptors Channels.* 2001;7:491-496.

182. Rupp SM, McChristian JW, Miller RD, Taboada JA, Cronnelly R. Neostigmine and edrophonium antagonism of varying intensity neuromuscular blockade induced by atracurium, pancuronium, or vecuronium. *Anesthesiology.* 1986;64:711-717.

183. Beemer GH, Bjorksten AR, Dawsom PJ, Dawson RJ, Heenan PJ, Robertson BA. Determinants of the reversal time of competitive neuromuscular block by anticholinesterases. *Br J Anaesth.* 1991;66:469-475.

184. Engbaek J, Ording H, Ostergaard D, Viby-Mogensen J. Edrophonium and neostigmine for reversal of the neuromuscular blocking effect of vecuronium. *Acta Anaesthesiol Scand.* 1985;29:544-546.

185. Miller RD, Van Nyhuis LS, Eger II EI, Vitez TS, Way WL. Comparative times to peak effect and durations of action of neostigmine and pyridostigmine. *Anesthesiology.* 1974;41:27-33.

186. Gottlieb JD, Sweet RB. The antagonism of curare: the cardiac effects of atropine and neostigmine. *Can Anaesthetists Soc J.* 1963;10:114-121.

187. Caldwell JE. Reversal of residual neuromuscular block with neostigmine at one to four hours after a single intubating dose of vecuronium. *Anesth Analg.* 1995;80:1168-1174.

188. Eikermann M, Fassbender P, Malhotra A, et al. Unwarranted administration of acetylcholinesterase inhibitors can impair genioglossus and diaphragm muscle function. *Anesthesiology.* 2007;107:621-629.

189. Herbstreit F, Zigrahn D, Ochterbeck C, Peters J, EIkermann M. Neostigmine/Glycopyrrolate administered after recovery from neuromuscular block increases upper airway collapsibility by decreasing genioglossus muscle activity in response to negative pharyngeal pressure. *Anesthesiology.* 2010;113:1280-1288.

190. Fuchs-Buder T, Meistelman C, Alla F, Grandjean A, Wuthrich Y, Donati F. Antagonism of low degrees of atracurium-induced neuromuscular blockade: dose-effect relationship for neostigmine. *Anesthesiology.* 2010;112:34-40.

191. Bartkowski RR. Incomplete reversal of pancuronium neuromuscular blockade by neostigmine, pyridostigmine, and edrophonium. *Anesth Analg.* 1987;66:594-598.

192. Cronnelly R, Morris RB, Miller RD. Edrophonium: duration of action and atropine requirement in humans during halothane anesthesia. *Anesthesiology.* 1982;57:261-266.

193. Caldwell JE, Miller RD. Clinical implications of sugammadex. *Anaesthesia.* 2009;64:66-72.

194. Eikermann M, Zaremba S, Malhotra A, Jordan AS, Rosow C, Chamberlin NL. Neostigmine but not sugammadex impairs upper airway dilator muscle activity and breathing. *Br J Anaesth.* 2008;101:344-349.

195. Puhringer FK, Rex C, Sielenkamper AW, et al. Reversal of profound, high-dose rocuronium-induced neuromuscular blockade by sugammadex at two different time points: an international, multicenter, randomized, dose-finding, safety assessor-blinded, phase II trial. *Anesthesiology.* 2008;109:188-197.

196. Gijsenbergh F, Ramael S, Houwing N, van Iersel T. First human exposure of Org 25969, a novel agent to reverse the action of rocuronium bromide. *Anesthesiology.* 2005;103:695-703.

197. Gyermak L, Lee C, Nguyen N. Pharmacology of G-1-64, a new nondepolarizing neuromuscular blocking agent with rapid onset and short duration of action. *Acta Anaesthesiol Scand.* 1999;43:651-657.

198. Gyermak L, Lee C, Cho Y-M, Nguyen N, Tsai SK. Neuromuscular pharmacology of TAAC3, a new nondepolarizing muscle relaxant with rapid onset and ultrashort duration of action. *Anesth Analg.* 2002;94:879-885.

199. Gyermak L, Lee C. The development of ultrashort acting neuromuscular relaxant tropane derivatives. *J Crit Care.* 2009;24:58-65.

200. Boros EE, Bigham EC, Boswell E, et al. Bis- and mixed-tetrahydroisoquinolinium chlorofumarates: new ultra-short-acting nondepolarizing neuromuscular blockers. *J Med Chem.* 1999;42:206-209.

201. Lien CA, Savard P, Belmont M, Sunaga H, Savarese JJ. Fumarates: unique nondepolarizing neuromuscular blocking agents that are antagonized by cysteine. *J Crit Care.* 2009;24:50-57.

202. Savarese JJ, McGilvra JD, Sunaga H, et al. Rapid chemical antagonism of neuromuscular blockade by L-cysteine adduction to and inactivation of the olefinic (double-bonded) isoquinolinium diester compounds gantacurium (AV430A), CW 002, and CW 011. *Anesthesiology.* 2010;113:58-73.

203. Savarese JJ, Belmont MR, Hashim MA, et al. Preclinical pharmacology of GW 280430A (AV 430A) in the rhesus monkey and in the cat. *Anesthesiology*. 2004;100:835-845.

204. Sunaga H, Malhotra JK, Yoon E, Savarese JJ, Heerdt PM. Cysteine reversal of the novel neuromuscular blocking drug CW002 in dogs: pharmacodynamics, acute cardiovascular effects, and preliminary toxicology. *Anesthesiology*. 2010;112:900-999.

205. Heerdt PM, Malhotra JK, Pan BY, Sunaga H, Savarese J. Pharmacodynamics and cardiopulmonary side effects of CW002, a cysteine-reversible neuromuscular blocking drug in dogs. *Anesthesiology*. 2010;112:910-916.

Chapter 20

CARDIOVASCULAR PHYSIOLOGY: CELLULAR AND MOLECULAR REGULATION

Paul M. Heerdt and George J. Crystal

The human heart beats billions of times during the course of a normal life span, with each beat representing the amalgamation of electrical, biochemical, and mechanical events that occur over milliseconds. This chapter reviews the cellular and molecular processes that initiate and maintain blood pressure and blood flow to provide a framework for understanding concepts central to pharmacologic manipulation of the cardiovascular system.

HISTORICAL PERSPECTIVE

While many aspects of cardiovascular function have been known for thousands of years, it was not until the classic treatise by William Harvey in 1623 that the sequential relationship of the heart and vasculature was systematically characterized. Subsequent observation in both animals and man provided considerable insight into hemodynamics, particularly work by Stephen Hales who in the 1730s measured blood pressure in horses and man, determined cardiac output, and had such a sophisticated appreciation of anatomy and fluid dynamics that he proposed regulation of vascular resistance by the microcirculation. At the subcellular level, technologic advances over the past 25 years have clearly had a profound effect on modern understanding of the molecular processes involved with cardiovascular function. Nonetheless, beginning in the mid-1800s, and using relatively crude methodologies, scientists developed a remarkably detailed understanding of the cardiac action potential, the central role of Ca^{2+} in excitation-contraction coupling, and neurohormonal regulation of blood vessels.[1]

CARDIAC EXCITATION

General Concepts

The contraction of the heart follows from the spontaneous generation of an impulse (automaticity) that is routed through the anatomic conduction system, and ultimately to cardiomyocyte shortening. The path and speed of impulse conduction is dictated by the electrical characteristics of different cell types constituting the conduction system, which synchronizes contraction. The heart exhibits three main "electrical" characteristics that are regulated by the autonomic nervous

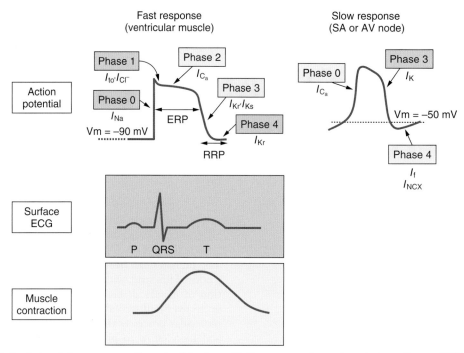

Figure 20-1 Representative fast and slow response action potentials along with the corresponding surface electrocardiogram (ECG) and the relative timing of cardiomyocyte contraction. Individual phases of the action potentials are depicted along with the predominant ion currents contributing to each phase. I_{Na}, Inward Na^+ current; I_{to}, transient outward current; I_{Cl}, inward chloride current; I_{Ca}, Ca^{2+} entry current; I_K, delayed rectifier K^+ current; I_{Kr}, rapid component of delayed rectifier K^+ current; I_{Ks}, slow component of delayed rectifier K^+ current; I_{K1}, inward rectifier potassium current; I_{NCX}, Na^+-Ca^{2+} exchange current; I_f, hyperpolarization activated funny current. *(Adapted with permission from: Balser JR, Thompson A. Cardiac electrophysiology. In: Hemmings H, Hopkins P, eds. Foundations of Anesthesia: Basic and Clinical Sciences. 2nd ed. London: Mosby; 2007:485-497).*

system: *chronotropy* (rhythm of automaticity), *bathmotropy* (cellular excitability), and *dromotropy* (impulse conduction). Pathologic abnormalities (both congenital and acquired), as well as a wide variety of drugs, can alter cellular automaticity, excitability, and the velocity and path of impulse conduction.

The fundamental process underlying all electrical activity in the heart is the action potential, which is an integrated movement of ions back and forth across the cell surface that results in rapid and reproducible changes in the electrical potential of the cell membrane (Figure 20-1). The characteristics and interactions among the various ion channels contributing to the action potential are complex and are reviewed more extensively in Chapter 24. For the current discussion, a definition of basic terms and concepts is presented below:

1. *Membrane potential:* Determined by the relative permeability of the cell membrane to specific ions, and forces both *chemical* (concentration gradient) and *electrostatic* (imparted by ion charge) that drive movement of ions across the membrane.

2. *Conductance:* An expression of how easily an ion flows across a membrane either through active pumps located in the membrane or ion channels; when specific ion channels open, conductance (*g*) for that ion increases.

3. *Resting membrane potential:* In cardiac cells, the conductance to K^+ is high at rest, primarily due to diffusion out of the cells via selective K^+ channels along a concentration gradient; intracellular K^+ ($[K^+]_i$) is ~150 mEq/L whereas extracellular K^+ ($[K^+]_o$) is ~5 mEq/L. The membrane is relatively impermeable to large anions such as proteins. Because these anions cannot follow K^+ out of the cell, the

inside of the cell becomes negatively charged relative to the outside, and the resting membrane potential of myocytes is ~-90 mV. While there is some movement of other ions across the cell membrane at rest, conductance is very low relative to K^+, so the resting membrane potential is close to the equilibrium potential for K^+ (E_K) of approximately -94 mV as calculated using the Nernst equation:

$$E_K = -61.5 \log([K^+]_i/[K^+]_o) \qquad [1]$$

Unlike K^+, myocyte conductance to Na^+ is low at rest because voltage-gated Na^+ channels that allow Na^+ entry into the cell are closed. Nonetheless, because the concentration of extracellular Na^+ is much higher than intracellular (~145 mM vs. 10 mM) and the cell interior is negatively charged, both chemical and electrostatic forces drive some Na^+ ions across the membrane. This movement is minimal, and only slightly increases the membrane potential above the E_K (i.e., from -94 to -90 mV). However, the slow Na^+ current could eventually depolarize the cell. Maintenance of the Na^+/K^+ gradient across the cell membrane is therefore critical and is actively achieved by expenditure of energy to move ions against an electrochemical gradient by the Na^+/K^+- ATPase. Also known as the "sodium pump," this protein extrudes 3 Na^+ ions for every two K^+ ions taken in, with ATP serving as the energy source; the pump is electrogenic in that charge movement across the membrane is unbalanced. Because of the central role of the Na^+/K^+- ATPase in maintaining membrane potential and its multiple downstream effects, the protein is the focus of extensive research.[2,3] Myocytes also express Ca^{2+}

channels that permit Ca^{2+} to enter the cells along its electrochemical gradient, that is, extracellular $[Ca^{2+}] \gg$ intracellular $[Ca^{2+}]$. Sarcolemmal Na^+/Ca^{2+} exchangers (NCX) use the inward gradient for Na^+ to drive the extrusion of Ca^{2+} ions and prevent intracellular accumulation. As with the Na^+/K^+-ATPase, the sarcolemmal NCX remains widely studied in regard to its role in cardiac pathology and as a target for pharmacologic manipulation.[4]

4. *Threshold potential:* The membrane potential at which inward currents exceed outward currents due to voltage-gating of Na^+ and Ca^{2+} channels, and depolarization becomes self-sustained. At this point, the action potential is initiated.

5. *Fast vs. slow response tissues (see Figure 20-1):* Fast response tissues depend upon the opening of voltage-gated Na^+ channels to initiate depolarization. These tissues include the atria and ventricles, along with the specialized infranodal conducting system (bundle of His, fascicles and bundle branches, terminal Purkinje fibers). In contrast, depolarization in slow response tissues, such as the sinoatrial (SA) and atrioventricular (AV) nodes, is initiated by movement of Ca^{2+} *through long lasting (L-type) voltage-gated Ca^{2+} channels.* Fast and slow response tissues also differ with regard to the magnitude and stability of their resting membrane potential (the basis for automaticity), and the amplitude of the action potential.

The Action Potential

In addition to differences in how depolarization is initiated between fast and slow tissues, there are fundamental differences in the subsequent action potential, underscoring how each tissue can exhibit different sensitivities to disease or drugs. The following comparison starts with the action potential phase during which depolarization begins for each tissue.

FAST RESPONSE TISSUE
Phase 0—Rapid Depolarization
When the membrane potential reaches threshold, *voltage-gated Na^+ channels open* leading to a rapid Na^+ entry along both a marked concentration gradient (chemical force), and the electrostatic force provided by charge difference across the membrane. Na^+ channels have the ability to automatically inactivate within a few milliseconds after opening, which self limits the influx of Na^+ ions. The Na^+ channels remain in this so-called fast-inactivated state until the membrane potential becomes more negative, at which time they return to their resting (ready-to-go) state. Before this can occur, however, the membrane potential becomes positive for a period of time (overshoot); although there is no longer an electrostatic drive for Na^+ to enter the cell, a concentration gradient still exists to push Na^+ across the membrane. During depolarization, *voltage-gated Ca^{2+} channels (VGCC)* also open but the inward flux is much slower than for Na^+.

Phase 1—Early Repolarization
With termination of the *inward Na^+ current (I_{Na})* resulting from Na^+ channel fast-inactivation and the positive membrane potential, both chemical and electrostatic forces promote K^+ efflux from the cell, described as a *transient outward current (I_{to})*, and a modest inward chloride current (I_{Cl}) to elicit a decline in membrane potential.

Phase 2—Plateau
A continued slow Ca^{2+} *entry current (I_{Ca})* offsets the electrical effect of K^+ loss secondary to opening of voltage-gated K^+ channels. The plateau voltage is sufficient to maintain Na^+ channels in the closed, fast-inactivated state.

Phase 3—Final Repolarization
This phase begins when the efflux of K^+ exceeds the influx of Ca^{2+}, and the I_{Ca} current ends. The *delayed rectifier K^+ current (I_K)* in phase 3 has both rapid (I_{Kr}) and slow (I_{Ks}) components that lead to repolarization and return to the resting potential.[5]

Phase 4—Resting Membrane Potential
The Na^+/K^+-ATPase extrudes Na^+ that entered during depolarization and restores the K^+ lost during repolarization. Once the resting potential is stabilized, Na^+ channels return to their resting state and are ready for the next depolarization.

During a single cardiac cycle (i.e., one action potential), the voltage-gated Na^+ channel exists in three different states: (1) resting, (2) active (open) during phase 0 depolarization, and (3) inactive at positive potentials (end of phase 0), and with marked depolarization (phase 2 plateau).[6,7] Even though Na^+ cannot pass through the channel when in the resting or inactivated conformations, these two states are physiologically distinct. In the resting state, achieving the threshold potential opens the channel. In contrast, once the Na^+ channel is inactivated, it cannot be activated again until it cycles back to the resting membrane potential, which brings it into the resting state. Most drugs, including various antiarrhythmic compounds, preferentially bind to the inactivated state of the Na^+ channel. These distinctions can be clinically important.

SLOW RESPONSE TISSUE
Phase 4—Slow Spontaneous Depolarization
When the membrane potential reaches its maximum negative point after repolarization (about −60 mV), slow, inward (depolarizing) Na^+ currents are activated. Referred to as *funny currents (I_f)*, because unlike most currents they are activated by hyperpolarization not depolarization, the I_f causes the membrane potential to begin a slow *spontaneous depolarization*.[8] When the membrane potential reaches about −50 mV, transient or *T-type Ca^{2+}* channels open, allowing Ca^{2+} to enter the cell along its electrochemical gradient and further depolarize the membrane. When the potential reaches about −40 mV, voltage-gated *L-type Ca^{2+}* channels (VGCC) open to further depolarize the cell until an action potential threshold is reached (between −40 and −30 mV). A slow decline in the outward movement of K^+ also occurs during phase 4 as the K^+ channels responsible for repolarization during phase 3 continue to close.

While funny currents have come to be known as the "membrane voltage clock" that dictates spontaneous membrane depolarization, recent studies have suggested that automaticity is more complex. Spontaneous, rhythmic release of Ca^{2+} into the cytoplasm from storage sites within the sarcoplasmic reticulum (SR) occurs during phase 4 and leads to activation of another depolarizing ionic current through the NCX (I_{NCX}), known as the "subsarcolemmal calcium clock."[9]

Phase 0—Depolarization
The I_f and T-type Ca^{2+} currents decline as their respective channels close, and depolarization is primarily caused by

increased Ca^{2+} conductance through the L-type Ca^{2+} channels that begins toward the end of phase 4. Movement of Ca^{2+} through these channels is not rapid, so the slope of phase 0 (the rate of depolarization) is much slower than found in fast response tissues. However, it is possible for fast response tissues to be converted to slow response tissues by tissue damage and electrolyte imbalance. Under these circumstances, Na^+ channels can become inactivated, with depolarization then dependent upon the slow Ca^{2+} channels.

Phase 1—plateau: None for slow response tissue.

Phase 2: None for slow response tissue.

Phase 3: K^+ channels open, thereby increasing outwardly directed, hyperpolarizing K^+ currents. At the same time, there is inactivation and closure of L-type Ca^{2+} channels, decreasing Ca^{2+} conductance and inward depolarizing Ca^{2+} currents.

Impulse Propagation and Conduction

When a slow action potential develops in a membrane, current flows from this membrane to adjacent areas. Ions can then flow from one cell to another via low-resistance *gap junctions*, and if the current flow is sufficient, cause sequential depolarization from cell to cell. The gap junctions are dynamic structures, opening and closing in response to changes in pH, Ca^{2+}, and under some circumstances, voltage.[10,11] Impulse propagation can also be affected by the orientation of myofibers and of the collagen matrix in which the fibers reside.

In order for an impulse to be conducted from cell to cell, or more globally to be spread throughout the heart, *cells in the path must be excitable (bathmotropy)*. The characteristics of excitability for a cell depend upon whether it exhibits fast or slow action potentials. Within fast response tissues, the membrane potential is not affected by an electrical impulse from the beginning of phase 0 to a midpoint in the repolarization process in phase 3 (the *effective refractory period*; see Figure 20-1). When the membrane potential recovers below −50 mV, enough of the fast Na^+ channels have transitioned from the inactivated to resting state to allow for the membrane to again depolarize. However, because not all fast channels have recovered, the slope and amplitude of any resulting action potentials will not be normal until the membrane potential has been allowed to stabilize at its more negative values at the end of phase 3 when the Na^+ channels have entirely recovered from fast inactivation (Figure 20-2). This represents the *relative refractory period*. In contrast, within slow response tissues the relative refractory period persists even after the membrane has fully repolarized, a characteristic known as *post-repolarization refractoriness*. Importantly, under most circumstances the heart rate—either spontaneous or paced within a physiologic range—provides a cycle length (beat-to-beat duration in milliseconds) that is longer than the refractory period thus allowing for full recovery of the action potential. However, *duration of the action potential is affected by cycle length*. For example, measurements obtained from canine Purkinje fibers show that at a cycle length of 630 ms (heart rate of 95 beats/min) the action potential duration was 180 ms while at 400 ms (heart rate of 150) action potential duration was shortened to 140 ms, although the amplitude was maintained, that is, the membrane was not in a relative refractory period.[12] This phenomenon appears to primarily reflect changes in K^+ conductance through delayed rectifier K^+ channels.[13]

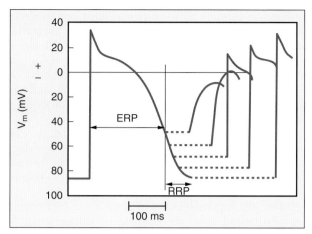

Figure 20-2 Relationship between action potential amplitude and the point at which stimulation occurs within the previous action potential. As stimulation occurs after the end of the effective refractory period (ERP) and progressively later in the relative refractory period (RRP), action potential amplitude increases. *(Adapted with permission from: Levy MN, Pappano AJ. Excitation: the cardiac action potential. In Levy MN, Pappano AJ, Cardiovascular Physiology. 9th ed., Mosby Elsevier, Philadelphia, 2007:13-32).*

The velocity at which an impulse is conducted *(dromotropy)* is largely determined by the resting membrane potential, the amplitude of the action potential, and the rate of change in membrane potential during phase 0 (dV_m/dt). These characteristics are affected by autonomic nervous system regulation, and pathologic or pharmacologic inactivation of Na^+ channels by hyperkalemia or ischemia-induced acidosis, direct damage to cardiomyocytes, or the effect of chemicals, particularly antiarrhythmic drugs. Accordingly, regional variations in conduction velocity can be dynamic and profound. Slow conduction in the atrioventricular (AV) and sinoatrial (SA) nodes range from 0.02 to 0.1 m/sec, fast conduction in cardiomyocytes range from ~0.3 to 1 m/sec, and those in specialized conducting fibers are even more rapid (~1 to 4 m/sec).

The only normal path for impulse conduction from the atria to the ventricles is through the AV node. Consequently, this region of the heart represents a site for physiologic, pathologic, and pharmacologic alteration of rhythm. Although much of the basic information regarding structure-based electrophysiology of the AV node has come from animal studies, it appears that the AV node and the surrounding "perinodal area" are comprised of multiple cell types that are electrophysiologically distinct.[14] Three main types have been described and are localized to regions within or adjacent to the AV node: the atrionodal (AN), nodal (N), and nodal-His (NH) cells. The small, ovoid *N cells* are the primary site where impulse conduction is slowed and therefore modulated, representing a distinctly slow-response tissue with few gap junctions and reduced excitability compared with surrounding cells. The Ca^{2+} current-dependent upstroke of phase 0, a major determinant of conduction velocity, is relatively prolonged in slow-response tissue. In contrast, surrounding "transitional cells" have a greater density of Na^+ channels, with an action potential and conduction velocity more like fast-response tissue; variations in AV node conduction (i.e., fast and slow pathway conduction) have been described in which impulses are diverted through regions with different conduction velocities.[14,15]

In keeping with a critical regulatory role, the AV node is densely innervated by autonomic nerve fibers, and can also be affected by autocoids (adenosine) and local metabolic influences (hypoxia, acidosis). Direct or pharmacologic stimulation of sympathetic or parasympathetic nerves has profound, often counterbalancing, effects on the action potentials, and therefore conduction velocity, of both N and transitional cells. Sympathetic stimulation activates G protein–coupled β-adrenergic receptors (predominantly β_1) to activate adenylyl cyclase, and via multiple mechanisms increases the L-type calcium current, I_f, and the inward rectifying K$^+$ current. Ultimately, β_1 agonism enhances automaticity and excitability, along with increasing action potential amplitude and conduction velocity (positive chronotropy, bathmotropy, and dromotropy). *Parasympathetic stimulation* activates G protein–coupled M2-muscarinic receptors to decrease adenylyl cyclase activity, and reduce automaticity and excitability, increase refractoriness, and slow AV node conduction (negative chronotropy, bathmotropy, and dromotropy). In addition, AV nodal cells express surface receptors for adenosine (A1); agonist binding stimulates inhibitory G proteins that inhibit adenylyl cyclase. In addition, pathways downstream to both M2 and A1 receptors affect I_f and various K$^+$ currents.[16] Rate-related hyperpolarization of the nodal cell membrane also contributes to reduced excitability, increased refractoriness, and AV conduction slowing to the point of even complete block.

EXCITATION-CONTRACTION COUPLING

While the generation and propagation of electrical impulses in the heart provide a stimulus, it is the mechanical response to this stimulus—cardiomyocyte contraction—that generates the pressure actually driving cardiovascular function. Literally hundreds of years of research, using both intact hearts and isolated muscle, have yielded several essential principles for cardiac contraction:

1. Cardiac muscle contraction, unlike that of skeletal muscle, is an all or none response.
2. The magnitude and rate of cardiac contractile responses reflect cytoplasmic Ca^{2+} concentration or Ca^{2+} sensitivity of contractile proteins.
3. When stimulated with greater frequency, the heart normally contracts with greater force and relaxes more rapidly.
4. Cardiac muscle contractile force is length-dependent.

Modern experimental techniques involving molecular biology have provided considerable insight into phenomena at the subcellular level, and have challenged some traditional fundamental assumptions. Furthermore, increased understanding of cardiac pathophysiology has underscored the importance of molecular regulation of *lusitropy* (relaxation), in addition, to that of *inotropy* (contractility).

Membrane Depolarization and Activator Calcium

During phase 2 of the fast tissue action potential, the influx (extracellular to intracellular) of Ca^{2+} via VGCCs and, to a much lesser extent the NCX, functions as "activator Ca^{2+}," which stimulates the sarcoplasmic reticulum (SR) to release a larger amount of Ca^{2+}, a process known as *Ca^{2+}-induced Ca^{2+} release* (Figure 20-3). Storage and release of Ca^{2+} by the SR are relatively complex processes modulated by high capacity Ca^{2+}-binding proteins such as *calsequestrin* and the *ryanodine-sensitive Ca^{2+} release channel*, respectively. Calsequestrin is able to bind and store large amounts of Ca^{2+} with low affinity, thus reducing the amount of free Ca^{2+} in the SR and maintaining a low concentration gradient relative to the cytoplasm. Known as the *ryanodine receptor (RyR)*, the SR Ca^{2+} release channel exists in multiple isoforms, with type 2 (RyR2) predominantly found in the heart. When activated, RyR2 has a very high conductance for Ca^{2+}; as Ca^{2+} exits the SR, dissociation of Ca^{2+} from calsequestrin provides for continued high conductance, and cytosolic Ca^{2+} concentrations rise rapidly from ~10^{-7} M to 10^{-5} M. Recent evidence indicates that SR Ca^{2+} release is not initially a global event, but occurs as bursts or "sparks" in zones where L-type VGCC in T-tubles are in close proximity to the SR and RyR2 proteins.[17] Less well appreciated, and of less physiologic importance, is the fact that SR Ca^{2+} release can also be stimulated by the second messenger *inositol triphosphate (IP$_3$)* binding to the IP$_3$ receptor (IP$_3$R) on the SR membrane.[18,19] This is a relatively slow-onset process that has been linked to stimulation of α-adrenergic receptors on cardiomyocytes and to muscle remodeling.[20,21]

As with all muscle, the molecular stimulus for contraction of the cardiomyocyte is Ca^{2+} binding with contractile proteins (Figure 20-4). Within the sarcomere, the *troponin complex containing the subunits TnI (binds to actin), TnC (the Ca^{2+} binding component), and TnT (binds troponin to tropomyosin)* dictates the interaction between actin and myosin. In the relaxed state, tropomyosin blocks formation of myosin cross-bridges. When cytoplasmic Ca^{2+} reaches ~10^{-6} M, binding to TnC results in a conformational change in troponin, leading to changes in tropomyosin that facilitate formation of actin-myosin cross-bridges. The resulting force is determined by the number of cross-bridges formed, the rate at which this process occurs, and the duration of cross-bridge attachment. Each cross-bridge cycle consumes one molecule of ATP. A simplified two-stage model involving "on-time" and "off-time" for actin-myosin cross-bridges has been proposed as a means to help characterize inotropic regulation.[18] Within this model, during each cross-bridge cycle (and there are many during each cardiac contraction), the myosin head attaches to actin and rotates to produce a unitary force for that interaction that is maintained during the on-time. Dissociation of myosin results in a non-force producing state during the off-time. It is then the combination of on-time and the unitary force that determines the force-time integral for each cross-bridge, and ultimately the number of cross bridges attached per unit time that determines overall contractile force.

As soon as the stimulus to release Ca^{2+} is terminated, active reuptake into the SR, and, to a lesser extent, extrusion from the cell via the NCX, leads to a rapid decline in intracellular Ca^{2+}, thus facilitating dissociation of Ca^{2+} from TnC, and to relaxation. The reuptake of Ca^{2+} into the SR is a fast (time constant of ~100 ms), energy-dependent process involving the *sarcoplasmic endoreticular calcium ATPase* (SERCA) and its regulatory protein *phospholamban (PLN)*. As with RyR, SERCA is found throughout the body in different isoforms; the type 2a isoform (SERCA2a) predominates in the heart. Under resting conditions, SERCA2a does not function at maximal capacity due to an inhibitory influence of PLN. However, the inhibitory effect of PLN is lost when the protein is phosphorylated at one of two sites, each sensitive to different kinases (PKA and CaMKII).[22]

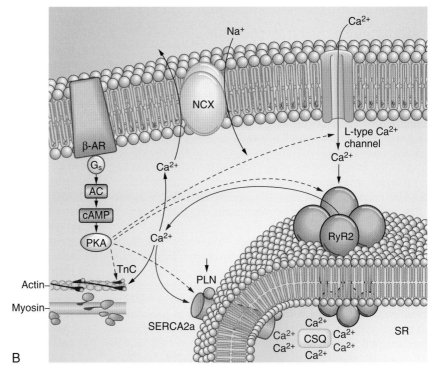

Figure 20-3 A, The sequence of events involved with excitation-contraction (EC) coupling in the cardiomyocyte. *1,* Membrane depolarization leads to an influx of "activator Ca^{2+}" via voltage-gated L-type Ca^+ channels. *2,* The relatively small amount of activator Ca^{2+} binds to the adjacent Ca^{2+} release channel, the ryanodine receptor subtype 2 (RyR2), on the sarcoplasmic reticulum (SR) and induces release of a large amount of Ca^+ stored within the SR on the binding protein calsequestrin (CSQ). *3,* Once in the cytoplasm, the released Ca^+ binds with troponin C (TnC) to produce muscle contraction. *4,* Cytoplasmic Ca^+ is then extruded from the cell via the sarcolemmal Na^+-Ca^{2+} exchanger (NCX) or taken back into the SR via the sarcoplasmic endoreticular Ca^{2+} ATPase subtype 2a (SERCA2a), activity of which is regulated by the phosphorylation state of the attendant protein phospholamban (PLN). **B,** Regulation of EC coupling by stimulation of β-adrenergic receptors (β-AR) on the cardiomyocyte (in red). Activation of adenylyl cyclase (AC) and ultimately of protein kinase A (PKA) leads to phosphorylation of L-type voltage-gated Ca^+ channel, RyR2, contractile proteins, and SERCA2a, resulting in increased Ca^+ influx, augmented Ca^+ release from the SR, altered TnC affinity for Ca^+, and increased Ca^+ reuptake into the SR by SERCA2a, respectively. *(Adapted with permission from: Vittone L, Mundina-Weilenmann C, Mattiazzi A. Phospholamban phosphorylation by CaMKII under pathophysiological conditions.* Front Biosci. *2008;13:5988-6005).*

Modulation of Excitation-Contraction Coupling

The interaction of Ca^{2+} with a variety of proteins plays a role in a wide range of cellular processes, in addition to muscle contraction and relaxation. Most proteins functioning as Ca^{2+} signaling targets or sensors share a specific Ca^{2+} binding motif referred to as *EF-hand.* Calmodulin (CaM) represents the prototypical Ca^{2+} sensor with four EF hands; proteins such as TnC and myosin light chain kinase in vascular smooth muscle originated from a prokaryotic CaM precursor via gene duplications and fusions.[23] Today, related proteins comprise one of the largest protein superfamilies known. Within the myocardium, the direct role of TnC is clear, but less apparent is the incorporation of CaM structure within both the L-type VGCC and RyR2. More recently, the S100 protein family has been linked to a wide range of Ca^{2+}-based intracellular functions.[23]

Because of the central role of Ca^{2+} in excitation-contraction coupling, changes in Ca^{2+} movement or binding can affect both inotropy and lusitropy (see Figure 20-3). For example,

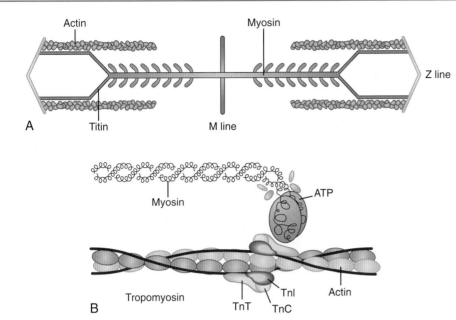

Figure 20-4 Schematic representation of the cardiac sarcomere **(A)** showing orientation of the structural elements (titin, M-line, Z-line) and contractile elements (actin and myosin). **B,** An expanded view of the site for actin-myosin interaction. In the absence of Ca^{2+}, tropomyosin prevents the interaction between the myosin head and actin. Binding of Ca^{2+} to the troponin C (TnC) component of a complex also containing troponin T (TnT) and troponin I (TnI) removes the inhibitory effect of tropomyosin allowing for actin-myosin interaction, ATP hydrolysis, and cross-bridge formation. *(Adapted with permission from: Nyhan D, Blanck TJJ. Cardiac physiology. In: Hemmings H, Hopkins P, eds.* Foundations of Anesthesia: Basic and Clinical Sciences. *2nd ed. London: Mosby; 2007:473-484).*

augmentation or inhibition of Ca^{2+} influx via L-type VGCC alters the activator Ca^{2+} entry and produces a positive or negative inotropic response, respectively. Similarly, physiologic, pathologic (i.e., dilated myopathy), or pharmacologic alterations in function of the RyR2 alter Ca^{2+} release from the SR and the subsequent contractile response.[18,24,25] In addition, physiologic, pathologic, or pharmacologic alterations in activity of SERCA2a, both directly and via PLN phosphorylation, affect the rapidity of Ca^{2+} reuptake into the SR. This influences both lusitropy and inotropy in that the amount of Ca^{2+} taken up during diastole influences how much can be released during the subsequent systole.[18,25,26] Changes in the Ca^{2+} sensitivity of TnC, and perhaps other regulatory proteins, represent a mechanism by which the cardiomyocyte can respond differently to the same amount of Ca^{2+}.[18]

The most prominent physiologic mechanism regulating cardiac Ca^{2+} dynamics and thus mechanical function (both inotropic and lusitropic) is the sympathetic nervous system.[27] Increased sympathetic stimulation acts largely via β-receptors, adenylyl cyclase, and PKA to alter a number of processes including (1) phosphorylation of L-type VGCC to increase channel open time and enhance RyR2 stimulation; (2) phosphorylation of PLN with subsequent "disinhibition" of SERCA2a and acceleration of SR Ca^{2+} uptake in diastole; (3) phosphorylation of TnI, which in turn leads to a reduction in the affinity of TnC for Ca^{2+}, allowing for more rapid dissociation and relaxation; (4) phosphorylation of RyR2 to augment SR Ca^{2+} release. In addition, secondary effects on a range of ion channels and regulatory proteins have been proposed.[28]

Autoregulation of Mechanical Function: Frequency and Length Dependence

FREQUENCY DEPENDENCE

In 1871, Bowditch observed that when an isolated frog heart was stimulated with greater frequency, it contracted with greater force. This "Bowditch effect," now more widely referred to as the *force-frequency relationship (FFR)*, has been

extensively studied in both isolated and intact muscle preparations. Modern experimental techniques have clearly established that the FFR is modulated by rapid adaptive alterations in intracellular Ca^{2+} cycling and as such represents true changes in both inotropy and lusitropy of the cardiomyocyte.[29] Because FFR is a fundamental property of cardiac muscle and an index of contractile reserve, it is widely used in assessing the response to conventional and emerging treatments for heart failure.[25,30] The FFR of human ventricular myocardium, and most other mammals, is normally positive, that is, increased stimulation frequency over a physiologic range augments contractile force, which occurs in association with an increase in the amplitude of Ca^{2+} transients. The FFR reflects an acute change in the integrated balance of the intracellular Ca^{2+} concentration, which is modulated primarily by increased SR Ca^{2+} load, and augmented Ca^{2+} flux through the sarcolemma via L-type VGCC and the Na^+-Ca^{2+} exchanger.[29] A key feature of the FFR appears to be activation of SERCA2a, at least in part due to PLN phosphorylation via activation of CaMKII.[22] Recent data also suggest a role for CaMKII phosphorylation of RyR2.[31]

In the setting of systolic heart failure, the FFR becomes negative—force declines with increasing stimulation rate—reflecting a pathologic loss of both inotropic and lusitropic reserve. Under these circumstances, Ca^{2+} cycling is impaired at multiple levels related to release from the SR, extrusion from the cell, and, most prominently, impaired SR reuptake by SERCA2a. Investigation has now established that activation (either pharmacologic or by mechanical unloading of the failing myocardium) and/or overexpression of SERCA2a can normalize the FFR.[18,25,30]

LENGTH DEPENDENCE

As discussed in Chapter 21, adaptation of the intact heart to increasing volume (preload) plays a critical role in maintaining cardiovascular homeostasis. Fundamentally, a progressive increase in muscle stretch results in a rapid progressive increase in contractile force *(Frank-Starling mechanism)*. This has been termed *heterometric autoregulation*, and does not reflect a change in Ca^{2+} cycling. Instead, there is formation of an increased number of acto-myosin cross bridges as the sarcomere lengthens, with maximal tension achieved when the sarcomere length is ~2.2 microns. Work with single myocytes has confirmed that the length-tension relationship is indeed an intrinsic property of individual cells, not the product of a "network effect" produced by the interaction of multiple linked myocytes.[32] While increasing length augments *contractile force*, it does not augment *contractility*, which by definition is independent of load. Using the concepts of on-time, off-time, and force-time integral as described earlier, an increase in myocyte length increases the number of cross-bridges, each with a unitary force, but not necessarily the on/off time and force-time integral for each cross-bridge. As described in Chapter 21, a change in contractility is defined as change in myocardial shortening at any given preload. Accordingly, if a muscle is progressively stretched in the presence of a β-adrenergic agonist, the force produced at any length will be greater than that measured in the absence of the β-agonist.

In 1960, Sarnoff observed in isolated dog hearts that, in addition to the rapid response, there is a slow, secondary response to muscle stretch, whereby contractile force continues to rise despite maintenance of a relatively fixed preload, a process he termed *homeometric autoregulation*.[33] Subsequent investigation by other investigators has established that this "second slow phase" (now commonly known as the *slow force response*) is modulated by a progressive rise in the peak Ca^{2+} transient.[32] Ultimately, the Frank-Starling relationship seems to have at least two cellular/molecular mechanisms: an acute change in myofilament cross-bridging and a secondary, late change in Ca^{2+} cycling. Recent work has focused on autocrine/paracrine mechanisms and downstream signaling processes associated with the slow force response, not necessarily for the mechanical response, but as a component in the maladaptive myocardial remodeling.[34]

VASCULAR REGULATION

While it is the function of the heart to provide a pulsatile, hydromotive source for moving blood into and through the circulation, it is the role of vessels to effectively disperse the pressure and flow generated both during systole and diastole. As such, blood vessels are structurally and functionally adapted to both facilitate global hemodynamics, i.e., elastic recoil of the aorta providing diastolic flow, and meet the differing needs of the various tissues. Central to vascular physiology is dynamic regulation of wall tension and cross sectional area by vascular smooth muscle (VSM).

Principles and Caveats

As with the myocardium, regulation of VSM can be simplified as reflecting changes in intracellular free Ca^{2+} concentration ($[Ca^{2+}]i$) and/or myofilament Ca^{2+} sensitivity. These processes are subject to a wide array of local, neural, and humoral mechanisms. Modern advances in molecular and analytical techniques have permitted elucidation of the downstream subcellular signaling pathways underlying adjustments of vascular tone. The highly complex, multilayered nature of these pathways helps explain why VSM responses can vary with vessel size and location.

In light of the critical importance of vasoregulation in the maintenance of blood pressure and flow, it is not surprising that considerable redundancy exists among signaling pathways and that pathways promoting vasorelaxation are closely intertwined with those promoting vasoconstriction to provide a system of checks and balances. It is important to keep in mind that pharmacologic interventions that raise or lower blood pressure initiate secondary compensatory events, such as the arterial baroreceptor reflex, that are not the direct result of a drug's primary effect on vascular tone. Most clinicians are aware that the integrated action of autonomic nervous tone, circulating chemicals, and local release of substances from the vascular endothelium is important in maintaining "stable" blood pressure. Less well appreciated, however, is the intrinsic *myogenic response* central to regional autoregulation, and the intriguing processes of *vasomotion*, a rhythmic, spontaneous variation in VSM tone within certain vascular beds.[35,36] Furthermore, it is becoming increasingly apparent that changes in VSM tone induced at one level of the circulation can be electrically propagated to others in what has been termed *conducted responses* modulated by gap junctions.[37] Gap junctions between endothelial cells and VSM cells facilitate direct, nonchemical interactions based upon propagated effects on resting membrane potential.[38,39]

Vascular Smooth Muscle Structure

The structure of VSM (smooth muscle) is distinctly different than that of cardiac muscle (striated muscle); while VSM also contains actin and myosin, the filaments are not organized into distinct bands to transmit force as in cardiac muscle.[40] Instead, there is a network of intermediate filaments, dense bodies in the myoplasm, and dense areas along the sarcolemma. In addition, VSM does not have troponin on the actin filaments (Figure 20-5), reflecting a profound, fundamental difference in how muscle activity is regulated (see later). *Relative to cardiac muscle, VSM is more dependent upon extracellular*

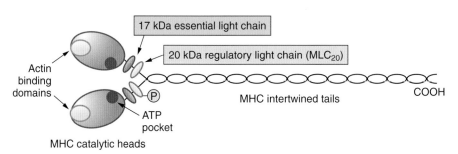

Figure 20-5 Vascular smooth muscle myosin comprised of intertwined myosin heavy chain (MHC) tails, the 17-kDa and 20-kDa light chains (with the 20-kDa unit representing the regulatory component MLC$_{20}$), and the catalytic heads that bind actin. *(Adapted with permission from: Cole WC, Welsh DG. Role of myosin light chain kinase and myosin light chain phosphatase in the resistance arterial myogenic response to intravascular pressure. Arch Biochem Biophys. 2011;510(2):160-173).*

Actin binding domains

17 kDa essential light chain

20 kDa regulatory light chain (MLC$_{20}$)

P

MHC intertwined tails

COOH

ATP pocket

MHC catalytic heads

Ca^{2+}, contracts more slowly, develops greater force, and can function over a wider range of length. In addition, once at full tension, this effect can be maintained with relatively little energy expenditure despite a reduction in activation (the "latch phenomenon").[41] Finally, in contrast to cardiac muscle, relaxation can be actively initiated and maintained (i.e., vasodilation).

Modulation of Vascular Smooth Muscle Tone

The sequence of events involved with contraction of VSM is shown in Figure 20-6. In brief, increased $[Ca^{2+}]i$ from either an increased flux of Ca^{2+} into the cell (primarily via L-type VGCCs) or by release of Ca^{2+} from the SR binds CaM at its four EF hand Ca^{2+}-binding sites. Calcium-CaM then activates *myosin light chain kinase* (MLCK), an enzyme that phosphorylates a serine at position 19 of the 20-kDa regulatory *myosin light chain* (MLC_{20}). Located at the junction between the myosin heavy chain "tails" and the globular "heads" containing the actin-binding domains and ATP binding sites (see Figure 20-5), MLC_{20} regulates the interaction between actin and myosin; when dephosphorylated, MLC_{20} prevents actin-myosin interaction. Alternatively, with phosphorylation

of MLC_{20}, cross-bridge formation between the myosin heads and actin filaments ensues and the VSM contracts. Relaxation is produced when $[Ca^{2+}]i$ declines, inactivating MLCK and inducing dephosphorylation of MLC_{20} by *myosin light-chain phosphatase* (MLCP). Besides MLC_{20} phosphorylation, thin filament-associated proteins such as *caldesmon* and *calponin* also control actin-myosin interactions; when dephosphorylated, these proteins block myosin binding and/or inhibit acto-myosin ATPase activity.[42] *Despite the complexity of vasoregulation, VSM tone is ultimately dictated by the phosphorylation state of MLC_{20} and, to a lesser extent, regulatory proteins like caldesmon and calponin.* A third process involving structural changes in the cytoskeleton that facilitate force transmission appears most relevant in vascular remodeling.[42]

The balance between VSM contraction and relaxation or "tone" is determined by factors that can be broadly classified as (1) purely mechanical, reflecting an autoregulatory myogenic effect; (2) electrical, modulated by cellular depolarization or hyperpolarization; and (3) chemical, modulated by receptors on VSM cells and adjacent endothelium. A brief summary of endogenous modulators of vasomotor tone and the signaling pathways that evoke an effect on $[Ca^{2+}]_i$ and/or the sensitivity of contractile proteins is shown in Figure 20-7. It is important to recognize that, even though VSM cells are commonly lumped together as a singular entity, there is marked phenotypic diversity reflecting tissue differences in the response to specific stimuli.[43] For example, the vascular response to local hypoxia in the lung (vasoconstriction) is opposite that in the brain (vasodilation).

Mechanisms of Vasoconstriction

Unlike cardiac muscle, depolarization is not required for contraction of VSM; Ca^{2+} entry into the cytoplasm alone can produce a response. However, membrane depolarization does play a role in the response to some stimuli and in the maintenance of tone.

Increasing $[Ca^{2+}]_i$ by increased transsarcolemmal influx:

- Voltage-gated (or operated) calcium channels (VGCC). These include both L- and T-type VGCCs, with L-type representing the primary path for activating Ca^{2+} influx.
- Receptor-operated calcium channels (ROCC). These represent Ca^{2+}-permeable channels gated by binding of an agonist to G protein–coupled receptors or tyrosine kinase–coupled receptors. Subsequent Ca^{2+} entry into VSM produces contraction.
- Store-operated calcium channels (SOCC). When intracellular Ca^{2+} stores become depleted, the process of "capacitive Ca^{2+} entry" via these channels is activated. It has been postulated that there is release of a diffusible messenger by the depleted intracellular Ca^{2+} store that affects sarcolemmal Ca^{2+} channels.[44]

Increasing $[Ca^{2+}]_i$ by SR Ca^{2+} release:

- Inositol triphosphate receptors (IP_3R). With agonist activation of a variety of G protein–coupled receptors (see Figure 20-7), phospholipase C (PLC) is activated which, in turn, leads to the hydrolysis of phosphatidylinositol bisphosphate (PIP_2) and formation of 1,2-diacylglycerol (DAG) and IP_3. Ca^{2+} release from the SR is then stimulated by IP_3 binding to the IP_3R, a tetrameric polypeptide with a central aqueous channel that permits Ca^{2+} movement into the cytosol. This receptor has binding domains for both IP_3 and Ca^{2+}, and

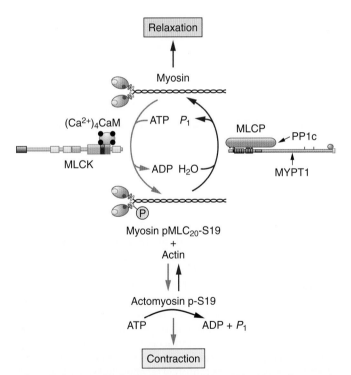

Figure 20-6 Events involved with contraction/relaxation of vascular smooth muscle. Calcium binds calmodulin (CaM) at its four EF hand Ca^{2+}-binding sites, and then activates myosin light chain kinase (MLCK) that, in turn, phosphorylates the 20-kDa regulatory myosin light chain (MLC_{20}). The interaction between actin and myosin is regulated by the phosphorylation state of MLC_{20}; with phosphorylation of MLC_{20} at serine 19 ($pMLC_{20}$-S19), cross-bridge formation between the myosin heads and actin filaments ensues with ATP hydrolysis and the vascular smooth muscle contracts. When $pMLC_{20}$-S19 is dephosphorylated by myosin light-chain phosphatase (MLCP), relaxation results. The MLCP complex has both phosphatase (PP1c) and regulatory components (MYPT1), and the dynamic interaction between Ca^{2+}-CaM, MLCK, and MLCP is influenced by a wide range of processes. *(Adapted with permission from: Cole WC, Welsh DG. Role of myosin light chain kinase and myosin light chain phosphatase in the resistance arterial myogenic response to intravascular pressure. Arch Biochem Biophys. 2011;510(2):160-173.)*

System	Stimulus	VSM transducer	Signal pathway	Response	Primary Effect
Neurohumoral	Angiotensin II	GPCR (All)	Primary: PLC activation Secondary: rho-kinase activation	Increase intracellular Ca^{2+}	Vasoconstriction
	Vasopressin	GPCR (V_1)			
	Histamine	GPCR (H_1)	Primary: AC activation Secondary: Endothelial H_1 stimulation, NO release	Decrease Ca^{2+} sensitivity Decrease intracellular Ca^{2+}	Vasodilation
	Epinephrine	GPCR (β_2)	AC activation		
Endothelial	Endothelin	GPCR (ET_A, ET_B)	PLC activation	Increase intracellular Ca^{2+}	Vasoconstriction
	Thromboxane A_2	GPCR (TXA_2)	PLC activation		
	PGH_2	GPCR (TXA_2/PGH_2)	PLC activation		
	Nitric oxide	Diffusion →	GC activation	Decrease Ca^{2+} sensitivity Decrease intracellular Ca^{2+}	Vasodilation
	Prostacyclin (PGI_2)	GPCR (IP_1)	AC activation		
	EDHF	? Diffusion	?	Hyperpolarize – decrease Ca^{2+} entry	
	Hydrogen sulfide	Diffusion	S-sulfhydration of K_{ATP} channel		
Local	Adenosine	GPCR (A_{2a})	Primary: AC activation Secondary: GC activation	Decrease Ca^{2+} sensitivity Hyperpolarization – decrease Ca^{2+} entry	Vasodilation
Mechanical	Decrease vessel wall tension	Membrane depolarization	Opening VGCC	Increase intracellular Ca^{2+}	Vasoconstriction
	Increase vessel wall tension	Membrane hyperpolarization	K^+ channels	Decrease Ca^{2+} entry	Vasodilation
Autonomic	Norepinephrine	GPCR (α_1)	Primary: PLC activation Secondary: rho-kinase activation	Increase intracellular Ca^{2+}	Vasoconstriction
	Acetylcholine	GPCR (muscarinic subtypes)			

Figure 20-7 *AC,* Adenylyl cyclase; *EDHF,* endothelium-derived hyperpolarizing factor; *GC,* guanylyl cyclase; *GPCR,* G protein–coupled receptor; *NO,* nitric oxide; *PLC,* phospholipase C; *VGCC,* voltage-gated calcium channel; *VSM,* vascular smooth muscle.

release of Ca^{2+} from the SR following binding to the IP_3R is biphasic (fast then slow).[42] As an example of integrative feedback, the IP_3R is regulated both by kinases involved with vasodilator pathways (i.e., PKA and PKG; see later), which inhibit Ca^{2+} release, and by high $[Ca^{2+}]_i$ (negative feedback).

- The ryanodine receptor (RyR). Although less important in VSM than cardiomyocytes, "calcium-induced calcium release" involving an RyR can provide rapid amplification of the Ca^{2+} signal induced by transsarcolemmal Ca^{2+} entry. Primary RyR isoforms in VSM are RyR2 and RyR3.

Increased myofilament sensitivity to $[Ca^{2+}]_i$:

- Inhibition of MLCP prevents dephosphorylation of MLC_{20} phosphorylation to augment the force developed by VSM at a fixed $[Ca^{2+}]_i$. MLCP is a holoenzyme (see Figure 20-6) composed of a type 1 protein phosphatase (PP1c) catalytic subunit, a large regulatory subunit (MYPT1), and a small subunit of unknown function. The MYPT1 subunit dictates activation of PP1c, and in targets myosin. Accordingly, inhibition of MLCP is accomplished by phosphorylation of MYPT1.[35]
- Regulation of thin filament-associated proteins. Caldesmon is an actin-binding protein located on actin filaments that blocks myosin binding. This effect is prevented by phosphorylation, primarily via mitogen-activated protein kinase (MAPK) and PKC. Calponin, another actin- and

calmodulin-binding protein that is relatively specific for VSM, is also located on actin filaments and inhibits acto-myosin ATPase and actin filament motility. Phosphorylation of calponin by PKC and CaMKII markedly decreases affinity for actin, which reduces its ability to inhibit acto-myosin ATPase.[42]

- Alteration in intracellular pH. Myofibrillar acto-myosin ATPase activity is pH-dependent, and increased by alkalinization. Intracellular pH can be rapidly increased by agonist-modulated activation of the Na^+/H^+ exchanger, an electroneutral transporter that mediates the 1:1 exchange of extracellular Na^+ for intracellular H^+, and is generally not activated in the basal state.[45] Activation of the Na^+/H^+ exchanger can be accomplished by phosphorylation through PKC- and Ca^{2+}-dependent pathways.

Mechanisms of Vasodilation

Decreasing $[Ca^{2+}]_i$ by decreasing entry:

- K^+ channels. These channels are critical to the establishment and regulation of membrane potential in VSM cells and thus a key regulator of inward Ca^{2+} via the VGCC. At least four different classes of K^+ channel exist, the most prominent being the: (1) ATP-sensitive (K_{ATP}); (2) large-conductance Ca^{2+}-activated (BK_{ca}); (3) voltage-activated (K_v); and (4) inward rectifier (K_{IR}). Opening of K^+ channels results in outward conductance, membrane hyperpolarization, reduced flux through VGCCs, and vasodilation. Again, as an example of integrative control, processes that induce *closure* of K^+ channels promote vasoconstriction.[46]

Decreasing [Ca^{2+}]$_i$ by increasing transsarcolemmal Ca^{2+} efflux:

- Plasma membrane Ca^{2+} ATPase (PMCA). The primary process for Ca^{2+} extrusion from the cell is active (energy-dependent) removal by PMCA. Activated by CaM, PMCA produces Ca^{2+} efflux from the cell in exchange for influx of $2H^+$. PMCA is regulated by multiple protein kinases in vasodilator pathways (PKA and PKG along with CaMKII all enhance PMCA affinity of Ca^{2+} and augment Ca^{2+} uptake).[47] In addition, the activity of PMCA is enhanced by some hormones and reduced by IP_3, another example of integrative control.

- The Na^+/Ca^{2+} exchanger. Unlike the PMCA that uses energy derived from ATP, the Na^+/Ca^{2+} exchanger utilizes energy from the electrochemical gradient for Na^+, transporting Na^+ into the cell while removing Ca^{2+} in a 3:1 ratio.

Decreasing [Ca^{2+}]$_i$ by enhanced SR Ca^{2+} reuptake:

- SERCA activity. As with cardiomyocytes, cytosolic Ca^{2+} is reduced by active SERCA reuptake into the SR using ATP as the energy source. This Ca^{2+} is then bound within the SR lumen primarily by calreticulin and calsequestrin to keep the free Ca^{2+} concentration relatively low, thus reducing the energy required to pump Ca^{2+} against a concentration gradient. Also, similar to the myocardium, VSM SERCA pumps are regulated by the phosphorylation state of PLB; when not phosphorylated, PLB inhibits SERCA activity (promoting VSM contraction). In contrast, when phosphorylated, SERCA inhibition by PLB is relieved, promoting Ca^{2+} reuptake and VSM relaxation.[48]

Modulators of decreased myofilament sensitivity to [Ca^{2+}]$_i$:

- Phosphorylation of MLCK. This is the main process by which desensitization of VSM occurs. Several kinases involved with vasodilatory pathways can phosphorylate MLCK to *reduce affinity for the Ca^{2+}-CaM complex*, resulting in decreased Ca^{2+} sensitivity of MLC_{20} for phosphorylation.

Vasoregulation Signaling Pathways

The processes described for regulating [Ca^{2+}]$_i$ or Ca^{2+} sensitivity are generally subject to upstream influences that activate, enhance, impede, or inhibit the response. Consistent with the wide range of local, neural, and humoral influences necessary for maintaining vascular homeostasis, the signaling pathways involved are complex and interconnected.

REGULATION OF [Ca^{2+}]$_i$

Three mechanisms are most prominent, with two being primarily associated with vasodilation (decreased [Ca^{2+}]$_i$), and the other with vasoconstriction (increased [Ca^{2+}]$_i$). However, inhibition of vasodilatory pathways promotes vasoconstriction, and vice versa.

Vasodilation: The G Protein-cAMP Pathway

Formation of cAMP following activation of adenylyl cyclase leads to *activation of PKA* and subsequent inhibition of Ca^{2+} mobilization at multiple levels, including inhibition of SR Ca^{2+} release, augmentation of SR Ca^{2+} reuptake, and inhibition of Ca^{2+} entry via VGCCs. In addition, PKA

phosphorylation of MLCK results in decreased myofilament Ca^{2+} sensitivity. *Adenylyl cyclase activity is stimulated via G_s protein activation (promoting VSM relaxation) or inhibited via G_i protein activation (promoting vasoconstriction).*

Vasodilation: Nitric Oxide-cGMP Pathway

Nitric oxide (NO) activates guanylyl cyclase to increase *formation of cGMP which, in turn, activates PKG*. Vasorelaxation is then produced by multiple mechanisms including phosphorylation of PLN and activation of SERCA, stimulation of the PMCA and Na^+/Ca^{2+} exchanger, inhibition of Ca^{2+} release from the SR by phosphorylation of the IP_3R, activation of K^+ channels, resulting in membrane hyperpolarization, and decreased Ca^{2+} entry via VGCCs.

Vasoconstriction: PLC-Phosphatidylinositol Pathway

Multiple endogenous modulators of vascular tone (norepinephrine, angiotensin II, endothelin-I) bind to G protein–coupled receptors that activate PLC to produce DAG and IP_3 (see Figure 20-7). As noted earlier, IP_3 binds to the IP_3R to evoke SR Ca^{2+} release, and DAG activates PKC, ultimately leading to phosphorylation of VGCCs and increased Ca^{2+} influx.

REGULATION OF MYOFILAMENT Ca^{2+} SENSITIVITY

Increased myofilament sensitivity to Ca^{2+}, with resultant augmentation of vasomotor tone, can be accomplished by phosphorylation of multiple proteins via three principal pathways.

1. rho Kinase. Agonist-induced Ca^{2+} sensitization is largely mediated by activation of the small GTPase (rho) via G protein–coupled receptors. Activated (rho) then interacts with rho kinase, leading to its activation, which, in turn, *can increase myofilament Ca^{2+} sensitivity* and promote contraction by both inhibition of MLCP and direct MLC_{20} phosphorylation.[49]

2. Protein kinase C. Activation of PKC via multiple mechanisms leads to *Ca^{2+} sensitization*. A variety of PKC-mediated mechanisms have been proposed: (1) PKC-dependent phosphorylation of caldesmon and calponin; (2) phosphorylation of MYPT-1 with resultant inhibition of MLCP; (3) phosphorylation of MLC_{20}; (4) activation of the Na^+/H^+ exchanger.

3. Tyrosine kinases. While having a number of independent functions, tyrosine kinases are also involved in the activation of rho and PKC, providing the basis for cross-talk among different kinase pathways involved in the *Ca^{2+} sensitization*. Both tyrosine kinases and phosphatases are present in large amounts in VSM, and influence other processes such as ion channel gating in addition to Ca^{2+} sensitization of the contractile process by phosphorylation of MLC_{20}.[50]

Regulation of Vascular Smooth Muscle by the Endothelium

The vascular endothelium is a single layer of thin cells lining the intimal surface of blood vessels. The last 20 years have seen a profound increase in the understanding of how VSM tone is regulated on a second to second basis by the vascular endothelium. With this understanding has come an appreciation of the critical role of the vascular endothelium in health and disease, which has made it an important target for drug development.[39,51]

Endothelial cells modulate VSM tone via synthesis and release of endothelium-derived relaxing factors and endothelium-derived contracting factors (see Figure 20-7). The relative balance is determined by anatomic location (i.e., relaxing factors predominate in most areas, but in peripheral veins and large cerebral arteries contracting factors are more prominent), and physiologic or pathologic stress.

ENDOTHELIUM-DERIVED RELAXING FACTORS
Nitric Oxide (NO)
Synthesized by endothelial nitric oxide synthase (eNOS), a Ca^{2+}-calmodulin-dependent enzyme, NO is the result of oxidation of L-arginine. *An increase in cytosolic Ca^{2+} in response to mechanical shear stress and/or a wide range of agonists with endothelial receptors (acetylcholine, bradykinin, serotonin, substance P, thrombin, vasoactive intestinal peptide) stimulates NO formation and release.* The molecule then diffuses into adjacent VSM cells and produces vasodilation via the cGMP pathway.

Prostacyclin (PGI₂)
Produced via the cyclo-oxygenase pathway for arachidonic acid metabolism, PGI_2 produces vasodilation via the cAMP pathway. As with NO, endogenous agonists (bradykinin, thrombin, serotonin, adenine nucleotides) induce *PGI_2 synthesis by triggering an increase in cytosolic Ca^{2+}.* PGI_2 also inhibits platelet adhesion to the vascular endothelium.

Endothelium-Derived Hyperpolarizing Factor (EDHF)
Initially described as a factor derived from endothelium that promotes vasodilation independent of NO and PGI_2, the precise molecular biology remains unclear; cellular effects of EDHF appear to reflect activation of K_{ATP} channels. Studies indicate that VSM can produce the gas hydrogen sulfide (H_2S) by metabolism of the amino acid L-cysteine and that H_2S promotes vasodilation. Recent data indicate that H_2S directly activates K_{ATP} channels, possibly by S-sulfhydration of cysteine residues, to produce membrane hyperpolarization and closure of VGCCs.[52] Ultimately, existing data suggest that H_2S is at least one of the EDHFs elaborated by the endothelium.

ENDOTHELIUM-DERIVED CONTRACTING FACTORS
Endothelin I (ET-1)
Although a family of endothelin isoforms exists (ET-1, -2, -3), the only one synthesized by endothelial cells is ET-1. Stimulated by angiotensin II, platelet-derived factors, thrombin, cytokines, reactive oxygen species, and local shear forces, an endothelin-converting enzyme cleaves a precursor protein to yield ET-1. Vasoconstriction by ET-1 is produced by binding to ETA and ETB receptors on VSM; these G protein–coupled receptors lead to IP_3 formation. ET-1 also binds to ETB receptors on endothelial cells to produce NO. The end result of vasoconstriction vs. vasodilation then reflects tissue type and receptor density.

Cyclooxygenase Products
Direct physical effects such as stretch along with local factors (i.e., hypoxia) and circulating hormones initiate formation of prostaglandin H_2 (PGH_2), thromboxane A_2 (TXA_2), and superoxide anions via the cyclooxygenase pathway. In the synthetic pathway, PGH_2 is upstream from TXA_2 but nonetheless retains biologic activity, with both substances producing vasoconstriction via the PLC-phosphatidylinositol pathway. In contrast, superoxide anions inactivate NO, thus removing a counterbalancing vasodilator effect.

Examples of Local, Autonomic, and Humoral Regulation of Vascular Smooth Muscle

LOCAL REGULATION
The *myogenic* response of small arteries and arterioles is characterized by intrinsic vasoconstriction after an increase of transmural pressure and by vasodilation following a decrease. It plays a critical role in the autoregulation of flow in different vascular beds and does not require the presence of an intact endothelium, although the factors released from the endothelium can modulate the response as can autonomic tone. As transmural pressure rises, membrane depolarization occurs with a subsequent rise in $[Ca^{2+}]_i$, largely via VGCC opening. However the mechanism of this depolarization, as well as the role of intracellular Ca^{2+} release in the myogenic response, remains controversial, and the contribution of various second messenger systems, along with the role of pulsatility and signals for adjacent vascular segments, remains unclear.[35,53]

Metabolites (e.g., adenosine, K^+) released locally as well as a decline in tissue oxygen tension will relax VSM. With increased metabolic rate (i.e., exercise), there is greater formation and release of metabolites, providing a mechanism to match oxygen supply with increased tissue demand. These effects are amplified by increased body temperature and decreased tissue pH.

AUTONOMIC REGULATION
Adrenergic
Both α- and β-adrenoceptors are present on VSM and endothelial cells. Norepinephrine release from sympathetic nerve terminals acts predominantly on postjunctional VSM α_1-adrenergic receptors to produce contraction. However, stimulation of α_2-receptors on endothelial cells induces NO release and vasodilation. In contrast, epinephrine is humoral and affects both α_1-receptors and β_2-receptors that mediate relaxation; the net result can vary among vascular beds, reflecting the distribution and affinity of different receptor subtypes.

Cholinergic
Muscarinic cholinergic receptors are also present on VSM and endothelial cells. While less prominent than sympathetic tone in vasoregulation, parasympathetic stimulation of muscarinic receptors evokes VSM contraction, primarily in the venous circulation. In the arterial circulation, stimulation of muscarinic receptors is primarily vasorelaxant via stimulation of endothelial cells to release EDRF.

HUMORAL
Vasopressin is formed in the hypothalamus and secreted by the posterior pituitary gland. In VSM, two main subtypes of G protein–coupled receptors for vasopressin are found (V1 and V2), with V1 agonism producing vasoconstriction and V2 stimulation producing vasodilation. The end response depends upon the regional circulation being studied. In addition to direct VSM effects, vasopressin also interacts with prejunctional and postjunctional adrenergic receptors to facilitate the effects of adrenergic agonists.

Angiotensin II is formed when the liver-derived precursor angiotensinogen is cleaved by renin (released by the kidney in response to decreased blood pressure or delivery of Na^+ and Cl^-), to produce angiotensin I, which is further cleaved by angiotensin converting enzyme to yield biologically active angiotensin II, a potent vasoconstrictor. Effects of angiotensin II are modulated by stimulation of a G protein–coupled receptor and activation of PLC.

Serotonin is derived from tryptophan and found primarily in the gastrointestinal tract and central nervous system. It is also found in platelets and contributes to both aggregation and local vasoconstriction via activation of 5-HT receptors. However, the vascular response to serotonin is complex, with the molecule producing vasodilation in some vascular beds. This effect appears to be influenced by both serotonin concentration and the relative density of receptor subtypes that modulate vasoconstriction or dilation.[54]

Primarily generated by mast cells and to a lesser extent basophils, when released into the circulation *histamine* causes local, and if intense enough systemic, vasodilation that can be profound. Multiple histamine G protein–coupled receptor subtypes exist, but smooth muscle responses appear to be more affected by which signaling pathways are linked to the receptor.[55] For example, in VSM, H1 receptors are primarily linked to the AC pathway to directly produce vasodilation, and this effect can be amplified by stimulation of H1 receptors on endothelial cells to release NO. In contrast, in bronchial smooth muscle, H1 receptors are linked to the DAG/IP_3 pathway and produce constriction.

KEY POINTS

- Action potentials vary within the heart and can be classified as fast or slow in nature. Characteristics of action potentials determine or contribute to cardiac automaticity, bathmotropy (cellular excitability), and dromotropy (impulse conduction).
- The normal heartbeat begins with spontaneous depolarization of cells within the sinoatrial node, and is the result of both a slow, inward Na^+ current (also known as a "funny" current) and spontaneous, rhythmic release of Ca^{2+} from the sarcoplasmic reticulum.
- Within the myocardium proper, fast action potentials occur and are initiated by rapid entry of Na^+ into the cell via voltage-gated Na^+ channels. These channels represent an important site for pharmacologic intervention.
- During phase 2 of the action potential, voltage-gated Ca^{2+} channels open and Ca^{2+} enters the cardiomyocyte. This small amount of activator Ca^{2+} induces release of a larger amount from the sarcoplasmic reticulum in what has been termed *calcium-stimulated calcium release*. As intracellular Ca^{2+} rises, binding to troponin C occurs, allowing interaction between actin and myosin and resulting in cardiomyocyte contraction. The amount of Ca^{2+} released during each beat along with the sensitivity of contractile proteins dictates myocardial inotropy (active relaxation).
- Relaxation ensues when Ca^{2+} is taken back into the sarcoplasmic reticulum or extruded from the cell. The rate at which Ca^{2+} is removed from the cytoplasm along

with how quickly it dissociates from the contractile proteins dictates myocardial lusitropy.
- When the myocardium is stimulated more frequently, adaptations occur within the cardiomyocyte causing Ca^{2+} to be cleared more quickly during diastole and released in larger amounts during systole. As a result, the myocardium exhibits increased inotropy (contractility) and lusitropy in what has been termed the *force-frequency relationship*.
- When the myocardium is stretched, the number of actin-myosin cross-bridges increases and the overall force of contraction increases. This represents the length-tension relationship, or Frank-Starling mechanism. Importantly, this effect initially does not involve an increase in Ca^{2+} release from the sarcoplasmic reticulum or a change in Ca^{2+} sensitivity of the contractile proteins, so although the force of contraction increases, myocardial inotropy does not. By definition, increased inotropy means an augmented ability to do work independent of muscle stretch.
- In contrast to the myocardium, Ca^{2+} entering vascular smooth muscle binds with calmodulin rather than troponin. The Ca^{2+}-calmodulin complex then activates myosin light chain kinase, which phosphorylates the 20-kDa regulatory myosin light chain, releasing inhibition of the actin-myosin interaction. Relaxation then ensues when the regulatory myosin light chain is dephosphorylated by myosin light chain phosphatase.
- Vascular smooth muscle tone is critical for maintaining blood pressure and proper distribution of tissue blood flow, and multiple levels of regulation exist. These encompass autonomic, humoral, and local processes as well as intrinsic myogenic responses to stretch that affect either the phosphorylation state of the regulatory myosin light chain or the sensitivity of contractile proteins.

Key References

Chen PS, Joung B, Shinohara T, et al. The initiation of the heart beat. *Circ J*. 2010;74:221-225. Presents current thought regarding how rhythmic changes in membrane voltage (the "membrane voltage clock") and spontaneous rhythmic sarcoplasmic reticulum Ca^{2+} release (the "calcium clock") both contribute to initiation of the heartbeat. (Ref. 16).

Cole WC, Welsh DG. Role of myosin light chain kinase and myosin light chain phosphatase in the resistance arterial myogenic response to intravascular pressure. *Arch Biochem Biophys*. 2011;510:160-173. Primarily focused upon the intrinsic capacity of vascular smooth muscle cells to contract and relax, this paper provides an excellent overview of the process of vasoregulation and provides a clear perspective on autoregulation. (Ref. 35).

Dora KA. Coordination of vasomotor responses by the endothelium. *Circ J*. 2010;74:226-232. Discusses emerging concepts of how the vascular endothelium interacts with vascular smooth muscle apart from just release of nitric oxide or endothelin. Emphasizes membrane hyperpolarization and processes that achieve this in both endothelial and smooth muscle cells. (Ref. 39).

Endoh M. Force-frequency relationship in intact mammalian ventricular myocardium: physiological and pathophysiological relevance. *Eur J Pharmacol*. 2004;500:73-86. Provides a clear discussion of frequency-dependent alterations of systolic and diastolic force in association with Ca^{2+} transients, and indicates the value of force-frequency analysis for evaluating the severity of cardiac contractile dysfunction, cardiac reserve capacity, and the effectiveness of therapeutic agents. (Ref. 29).

Hasenfuss G, Teerlink JR. Cardiac inotropes: current agents and future directions. *Eur Heart J*. 2011;32:1838-1845. Provides an excellent review of current concepts in myocardial inotropy as the basis for an in-depth discussion of emerging treatments for heart failure. (Ref. 18).

Kim HR, Appel S, Vetterkind S, et al. Smooth muscle signalling pathways in health and disease. *J Cell Mol Med*. 2008;12:2165-2180. An overview of smooth muscle in general with emphasis of concepts relevant to vasoregulation. (Ref. 42).

Remme CA, Bezzina CR. Sodium channel (dys)function and cardiac arrhythmias. *Cardiovasc Ther*. 2010;28:287-294. An overview of the structure and function of the cardiac Na+ channel along with the clinical and biophysical characteristics of inherited and acquired Na+ channel dysfunction. (Ref. 7).

Sarnoff SJ, Mitchell JH, Gilmore JP, et al. Homeometric autoregulation in the heart. *Circ Res*. 1960;8:1077-1091. A classic paper describing expanded understanding of the length-tension relationship. Includes an excellent historical perspective on the origins of the Frank-Starling mechanism. (Ref. 33).

Tomaselli GF, Marbán E. Electrophysiological remodeling in hypertrophy and heart failure. *Cardiovasc Res*. 1999;42(2):270-283. Nice review with excellent figures depicting the various ion channels and currents contributing to the myocardial action potential. (Ref. 5).

Zaugg M, Schaub MC. Cellular mechanisms in sympatho-modulation of the heart. *Br J Anaesth*. 2004;93:34-52. This review provides insights into the cellular and molecular mechanisms central to pharmacologic control of the sympathetic responses to surgical trauma and perioperative stress. (Ref. 28).

References

1. Granger HJ. Cardiovascular physiology in the twentieth century: great strides and missed opportunities. *Am J Physiol*. 1998;275 (Heart Circ Physiol 44):H1925-H1936.
2. Bers DM, Barry WH, Despa S. Intracellular Na+ regulation in cardiac myocytes. *Cardiovasc Res*. 2003;57(4):897-912.
3. Bers DM, Despa S. Na/K-ATPase–an integral player in the adrenergic fight-or-flight response. *Trends Cardiovasc Med*. 2009;19(4):111-118.
4. Bers DM, Despa S, Bossuyt J. Regulation of Ca2+ and Na+ in normal and failing cardiac myocytes. *Ann N Y Acad Sci*. 2006;1080:165-177.
5. Tomaselli GF, Marbán E. Electrophysiological remodeling in hypertrophy and heart failure. *Cardiovasc Res*. 1999;42(2):270-283.
6. Marban E, Yamagishi T, Tomaselli GF. Structure and function of voltage-gated sodium channels. *J Physiol*. 1998;508(Pt 3):647-657.
7. Remme CA, Bezzina CR. Sodium channel (dys)function and cardiac arrhythmias. *Cardiovasc Ther*. 2010;28(5):287-294.
8. Baruscotti M, Bucchi A, Difrancesco D. Physiology and pharmacology of the cardiac pacemaker ("funny") current. *Pharmacol Ther*. 2005;107(1):59-79.
9. Hesketh GG, Van Eyk JE, Tomaselli GF. Mechanisms of gap junction traffic in health and disease. *J Cardiovasc Pharmacol*. 2009;54(4):263-272.
10. Salameh A, Dhein S. Adrenergic control of cardiac gap junction function and expression. *Naunyn Schmiedebergs Arch Pharmacol*. 2011;383(4):331-346.
11. Singer DH, Ten Eick RE. Aberrancy: electrophysiologic aspects. *Am J Cardiol*. 1971;28(4):381-401.
12. Surawicz B. Role of potassium channels in cycle length dependent regulation of action potential duration in mammalian cardiac Purkinje and ventricular muscle fibres. *Cardiovasc Res*. 1992;26(11):1021-1029.
13. Meijler FL, Janse MJ. Morphology and electrophysiology of the mammalian atrioventricular node. *Physiol Rev*. 1988;68(2):608-647.
14. Munk AA, Adjemian RA, Zhao J, Ogbaghebriel A, Shrier A. Electrophysiological properties of morphologically distinct cells isolated from the rabbit atrioventricular node. *J Physiol (Lond)*. 1996;493:801-818.
15. Martynyuk AE, Zima A, Seubert CN, Morey TE, Belardinelli L, Dennis DM. Potentiation of the negative dromotropic effect of adenosine by rapid heart rates: possible ionic mechanisms. *Basic Res Cardiol*. 2002;97(4):295-304.
16. Chen PS, Joung B, Shinohara T, Das M, Chen Z, Lin SF. The initiation of the heart beat. *Circ J*. 2010;74(2):221-225.
17. Korzick DH. From syncytium to regulated pump: a cardiac muscle cellular update. *Adv Physiol Educ*. 2011;35(1):22-27.
18. Hasenfuss G, Teerlink JR. Cardiac inotropes: current agents and future directions. *Eur Heart J*. 2011;32(15):1838-1845.
19. Kockskämper J, Zima AV, Roderick HL, et al. Emerging roles of inositol 1,4,5-trisphosphate signaling in cardiac myocytes. *J Mol Cell Cardiol*. 2008;45(2):128-147.
20. Ruffolo RR Jr. The pharmacology of dobutamine. *Am J Med Sci*. 1987;294(4):244-248.
21. Zhang S, Lin J, Hirano Y, Hiraoka M. Modulation of ICa-L by alpha1-adrenergic stimulation in rat ventricular myocytes. *Can J Physiol Pharmacol*. 2005;83(11):1015-1024.
22. Vittone L, Mundina-Weilenmann C, Mattiazzi A. Phospholamban phosphorylation by CaMKII under pathophysiological conditions. *Front Biosci*. 2008;13:5988-6005.
23. Schaub MC, Heizmann CW. Calcium, troponin, calmodulin, S100 proteins: from myocardial basics to new therapeutic strategies. *Biochem Biophys Res Commun*. 2008;25;369(1):247-264.
24. Yano M, Yamamoto T, Kobayashi S, Matsuzaki M. Role of ryanodine receptor as a Ca2(+) regulatory center in normal and failing hearts. *J Cardiol*. 2009;53(1):1-7.
25. Kawase Y, Ladage D, Hajjar RJ. Rescuing the failing heart by targeted gene transfer. *J Am Coll Cardiol*. 2011;57(10):1169-1180.
26. Lipskaia L, Chemaly ER, Hadri L, Lompre AM, Hajjar RJ. Sarcoplasmic reticulum Ca(2+) ATPase as a therapeutic target for heart failure. *Expert Opin Biol Ther*. 2010;10(1):29-41.
27. Brodde OE, Bruck H, Leineweber K. Cardiac adrenoceptors: physiological and pathophysiological relevance. *J Pharmacol Sci*. 2006;100(5):323-337.
28. Zaugg M, Schaub MC. Cellular mechanisms in sympatho-modulation of the heart. *Br J Anaesth*. 2004;93(1):34-52.
29. Endoh M. Force-frequency relationship in intact mammalian ventricular myocardium: physiological and pathophysiological relevance. *Eur J Pharmacol*. 2004;500(1-3):73-86.
30. Heerdt PM, Holmes JW, Cai B, et al. Chronic unloading by left ventricular assist device reverses contractile dysfunction and alters gene expression in end-stage heart failure. *Circulation*. 2000;102(22):2713-2719.
31. Kushnir A, Shan J, Betzenhauser MJ, Reiken S, Marks AR. Role of CaMKIIdelta phosphorylation of the cardiac ryanodine receptor in the force frequency relationship and heart failure. *Proc Natl Acad Sci U S A*. 2010;107(22):10274-10279.
32. Campbell KS. Impact of myocyte strain on cardiac myofilament activation. *Pflugers Arch*. 2011;462(1):3-14.
33. Sarnoff SJ, Mitchell JH, Gilmore JP, Remensnyder JP. Homeometric autoregulation in the heart. *Circ Res*. 1960;8:1077-1091.
34. Cingolani HE, Ennis IL, Aiello EA, et al. Role of autocrine/paracrine mechanisms in response to myocardial strain. *Pflugers Arch*. 2011;462(1):29-38.
35. Cole WC, Welsh DG. Role of myosin light chain kinase and myosin light chain phosphatase in the resistance arterial myogenic response to intravascular pressure. *Arch Biochem Biophys*. 2011;510(2):160-173.
36. Aalkjær C, Boedtkjer D, Matchkov V. Vasomotion—what is currently thought? *Acta Physiol (Oxf)*. 2011;202(3):253-269.
37. Bagher P, Segal SS. Regulation of blood flow in the microcirculation: role of conducted vasodilation. *Acta Physiol (Oxf)*. 2011;202(3):271-284.
38. Schmidt VJ, Wölfle SE, Boettcher M, de Wit C. Gap junctions synchronize vascular tone within the microcirculation. *Pharmacol Rep*. 2008 ;60(1):68-74.
39. Dora KA. Coordination of vasomotor responses by the endothelium. *Circ J*. 2010;74(2):226-232.

40. Ding X, Murray PA. Vascular smooth muscle. In: Hemmings H, Hopkins P, eds. *Foundations of Anesthesia: Basic and Clinical Sciences.* 2nd ed. London: Mosby; 2007:461-469.

41. Murphy RA, Rembold CM. The latch-bridge hypothesis of smooth muscle contraction. *Can J Physiol Pharmacol.* 2005;83(10):857-864.

42. Kim HR, Appel S, Vetterkind S, Gangopadhyay SS, Morgan KG. Smooth muscle signalling pathways in health and disease. *J Cell Mol Med.* 2008;12(6A):2165-2180.

43. Fisher SA. Vascular smooth muscle phenotypic diversity and function. *Physiol Genomics.* 2010;42A(3):169-187.

44. Putney JW. Origins of the concept of store-operated calcium entry. *Front Biosci (Schol Ed).* 2011;3:980-984.

45. Wakabayashi I, Poteser M, Groschner K. Intracellular pH as a determinant of vascular smooth muscle function. *J Vasc Res.* 2006;43(3): 238-250.

46. Jackson WF. Potassium channels in the peripheral microcirculation. *Microcirculation.* 2005;12(1):113-127.

47. Oceandy D, Mamas MA, Neyses L. Targeting the sarcolemmal calcium pump: a potential novel strategy for the treatment of cardiovascular disease. *Cardiovasc Hematol Agents Med Chem.* 2007;5(4): 300-304.

48. Adachi T. Modulation of vascular sarco/endoplasmic reticulum calcium ATPase in cardiovascular pathophysiology. *Adv Pharmacol.* 2010;59:165-195.

49. Satoh K, Fukumoto Y, Shimokawa H. Rho-kinase: important new therapeutic target in cardiovascular diseases. *Am J Physiol Heart Circ Physiol.* 2011;301(2):H287-H296.

50. Rautureau Y, Paradis P, Schiffrin EL. Cross-talk between aldosterone and angiotensin signaling in vascular smooth muscle cells. *Steroids.* 2011;76(9):834-839.

51. Gielis JF, Lin JY, Wingler K, Van Schil PE, Schmidt HH, Moens AL. Pathogenetic role of eNOS uncoupling in cardiopulmonary disorders. *Free Radic Biol Med.* 2011;50(7):765-776.

52. Wang R. Signaling pathways for the vascular effects of hydrogen sulfide. *Curr Opin Nephrol Hypertens.* 2011;20:107-112.

53. Schubert R, Mulvany MJ. The myogenic response: established facts and attractive hypotheses. *Clin Sci (Lond).* 1999;96(4):313-326.

54. Calama E, Fernández MM, Morán A, et al. Vasodilator and vasoconstrictor responses induced by 5-hydroxytryptamine in the in situ blood autoperfused hindquarters of the anaesthetized rat. *Naunyn Schmiedebergs Arch Pharmacol.* 2002;366(2):110-116.

55. Simons FE. H1-Antihistamines: more relevant than ever in the treatment of allergic disorders. *J Allergy Clin Immunol.* 2003;112(4 Suppl):S42-S52.

Chapter 21

CARDIOVASCULAR PHYSIOLOGY: INTEGRATIVE FUNCTION

George J. Crystal and Paul M. Heerdt

A thorough understanding of basic principles of cardiovascular physiology is essential for effective and safe patient management in the perioperative period. This information provides a theoretical rationale for the use of drugs, intravenous infusions, and other therapeutic measures to maintain and optimize vital organ function.

The primary role of the circulation is to provide sufficient blood flow to satisfy the metabolic demands of body tissues. However, the circulation has additional functions, not considered here, including return of carbon dioxide to the lungs and other metabolic end products to the kidneys, supply of nutrients absorbed from the gastrointestinal tract to the tissues, regulation of body temperature, and distribution of hormones and other agents that regulate cellular function.

Tissue blood flow depends on activity of both the heart and blood vessels (Figure 21-1); arterial pressure, a major determinant of tissue blood flow, is the product of cardiac output and total peripheral resistance, while local vascular resistance, the other major determinant of tissue blood flow, is a function of local vasomotor tone.[1] The complex interplay of the relationships summarized in Figure 21-1 is the primary focus of this chapter.

CARDIAC PHYSIOLOGY

Basic Cardiac Anatomy

The atria are thin-walled structures that are similar in size and dimension on the right and left sides of the heart. However, the left and right ventricles (LV and RV) are quite different; the LV has an ellipsoidal-shape and is thick-walled whereas the RV is crescent-shaped (due to the concave free wall opposite the convex interventricular septum) and has a thin wall.[2] The mass of the LV is approximately six times that of the RV, which reflects their respective pressure loads (peak systolic aortic pressure > peak systolic pulmonary pressure). A high degree of interaction and interdependence exists between the ventricles because of their shared interventricular septum and the restraining influence of the surrounding pericardium.[3] The load on one ventricle is influenced by the filling of the other. Shifts of the septum can impair ventricular function by reducing diastolic filling secondary to reduced chamber compliance.

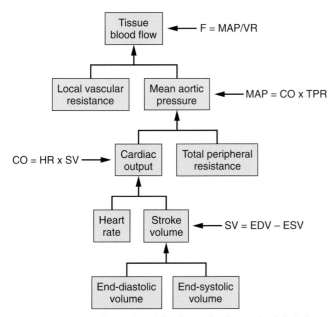

Figure 21-1 The cardiac and peripheral vascular factors (and their interrelationships) determining tissue blood flow. *CO,* Cardiac output; *EDV,* end-diastolic volume; *ESV,* end-systolic volume; *F,* flow; *HR,* heart rate; *MAP,* mean arterial pressure; *SV,* stroke volume; *TPR,* total peripheral resistance. *(Modified from Rothe CF. Cardiodynamics. Selkurt EE, ed. Physiology. Boston: Little, Brown and Company; 1971:321.)*

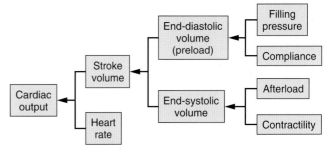

Figure 21-2 Determinants of cardiac output.

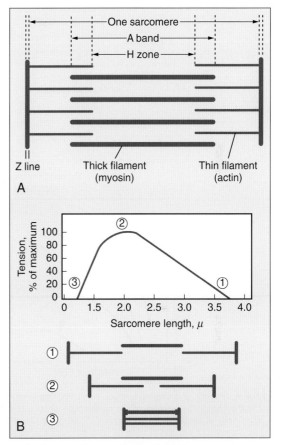

Figure 21-3 **A,** Contractile machinery and ultrastructure of the cardiac cell. **B,** Tension development as a function of sarcomere length. Myofilament overlap at three points in the length-tension curve is depicted below. *(Modified from Braunwald E, Ross J Jr, Sonnenblick EH. Mechanisms of Contraction of the Normal and Failing Heart. Boston: Little, Brown; 1968:77.)*

At the cellular level, the heart consists primarily of cells that contract (myocytes) or conduct impulses (Purkinje fibers). The myocardium proper is comprised of individual myocytes linked by specialized gap junctions to form a functional syncytium that allows rapid conduction of electrical charge, and intercalated discs that modulate force transmission during contraction. Cardiac cells display five basic characteristics: excitability (bathmotropy), conductivity (dromotropy), rhythmicity (chronotropy), contractility (inotropy), and relaxation (lusitropy).

Control of Cardiac Output

Cardiac output is the volume of blood pumped to body tissues per minute, and is equal to the product of heart rate and stroke volume (Figure 21-2). Normal values for cardiac output are 5 to 6 L/min in a 70-kg man, with a heart rate of 80 beats/min and a stroke volume of 60 to 90 mL/beat. Cardiac index is a normalized value for cardiac output based on body surface area, normally 2.5 to 3.5 L/min/m^2. Cardiac output varies in proportion to work requirement and oxygen demand.

Heart rate is normally determined by rhythmic spontaneous depolarizations of pacemaker cells in the sinoatrial (SA) node. The rate of these depolarizations is modulated by the autonomic nervous system. Sympathetic stimulation increases activity, whereas parasympathetic stimulation (vagus nerve) decreases activity of the SA node.

Stroke volume is the difference between end-diastolic volume and end-systolic volume (see Figure 21-2). It can be influenced by changes in end-diastolic volume (Starling's law), myocardial contractility, and afterload (see later).

The sarcomere is the basic functional unit of the myocardium (Figure 21-3, *A*).[4] The ultrastructural arrangement of the thick (myosin) and thin (actin) myofilaments within

the sarcomere and their interaction explain much of the mechanical behavior of cardiac muscle. Cardiac muscle contraction is initiated by an increase in intracellular Ca^{2+}, which results in the formation of cross-bridges between adjacent actin and myosin filaments. This process draws thin myofilaments and the Z lines toward the center of the sarcomere and is the fundamental mechanism for myocardial contraction.

The relation between resting sarcomere length and developed tension was originally defined in isolated skeletal muscle fibers (see Figure 21-3, *B*).[4] Developed tension is a direct function of the number of cross-bridges pulling in parallel, and thus on the amount of overlap between thin and thick filaments prior to activation. Subsequent work

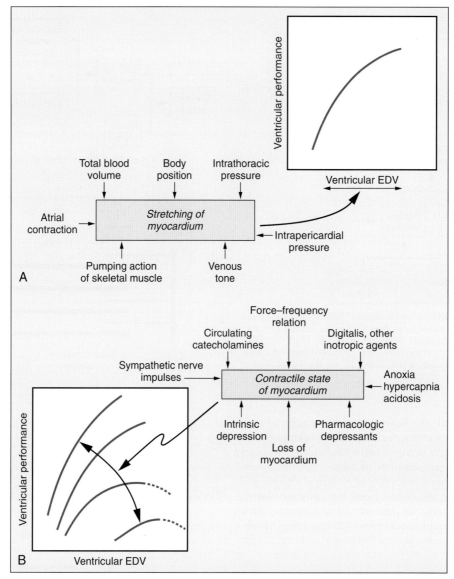

Figure 21-4 A, Diagram of a cardiac function curve, relating ventricular end-diastolic volume (EDV) to ventricular performance. *Bottom left:* Major factors determining the degree of stretching of the myocardium, that is, the magnitude of EDV. **B,** Diagram showing major factors affecting myocardial contractility. *Bottom left:* Family of cardiac function curves demonstrating the effect of contractility on cardiac performance. *(Reprinted with permission from Braunwald E, Ross J Jr, Sonnenblick EH. Mechanisms of Contraction of the Normal and Failing Heart. Boston: Little, Brown; 1968:275, 280.)*

extended this behavior to cardiac muscle. The length-tension relation provides the basis for Starling's law of the heart: the strength of contraction of the intact heart is proportional to the initial length of the cardiac muscle fiber, that is, end-diastolic volume (preload). This can be demonstrated using a cardiac function curve, which is a plot of ventricular performance (i.e., stroke volume), as a function of ventricular end-diastolic volume or an index thereof, such as ventricular end-diastolic pressure (Figure 21-4, *A*).[4] In vivo, cardiac muscle fibers are stretched by venous filling pressure. Normally, the volume in the ventricle before contraction (preload) sets the sarcomere to a suboptimal length; thus the active tension that can be developed is not maximal. Increases in end-diastolic volume due to enhanced venous return cause improvement in ventricular performance. Clinicians traditionally have equated filling pressure with preload, which assumes that the relationship between end-diastolic

pressure and end-diastolic volume (i.e., the compliance or distensibility) is constant. However, a fibrotic heart, hypertrophied heart, or aging heart has reduced compliance.

Venous return, hence cardiac filling, is augmented by conditions associated with reduced systemic vascular resistance. These include the opening of arteriovenous fistulae or conditions that mimic it, such as fever (marked dilation of cutaneous beds), pregnancy, and exercise (see Figure 21-4, *A*). Rapid, large reductions in total blood volume reduce venous return. At any given total blood volume, venous return is a function of the distribution of blood between the intrathoracic and extrathoracic compartments. For example, assumption of an upright posture, because of gravity, tends to increase extrathoracic volume at the expense of intrathoracic volume, thus reducing venous return. Elevation of intrathoracic pressure, as occurs during positive pressure ventilation or pneumothorax, has a similar effect. Sympathetic nerve stimulation produces

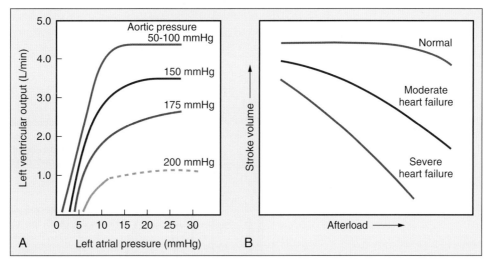

Figure 21-5 A, Left ventricular output as a function left atrial pressure, plotted at several aortic pressures (afterloads). Note that an increase in aortic pressure reduces left ventricular output at each filling pressure. **B**, Effect of increased afterload on stroke volume in normal and compromised hearts. *(A, Reprinted with permission from Sagawa K. Analysis of the ventricular pumping capacity as function of input and output pressure loads. In: Reeve EB, Guyton AC, eds.* Physical Bases of Circulatory Transport: Regulation and Exchange. *Philadelphia: WB Saunders; 1967;141-149. **B**, Modified from Cohn JN, Franciosa JA. Vasodilator therapy of cardiac failure.* N Engl J Med. *1977;297:27-31.)*

systemic venoconstriction, which augments cardiac filling, whereas drugs that interfere with adrenergic nerve function, such as ganglionic blockers or drugs that act directly to relax venous smooth muscle such as nitrates, have the opposite effect. Extravascular compression of veins by contracting muscle increases venous return during exercise. Atrial contraction normally makes a relatively minor contribution to ventricular filling, but it becomes more important at high heart rates, when the time available for passive ventricular filling is limited. Increases in pericardial pressure, as in cardiac tamponade, limit ventricular filling and stroke volume.

Contractility relates to the ability of the myocardium to perform mechanical work (i.e., to generate force and shorten), independently of changes in preload or afterload with heart rate fixed. Contractility can be illustrated graphically using a family of cardiac function curves (see Figure 21-4, *B*).[4] Changes in contractility can augment cardiac performance (positive inotropic effect), or depress it (negative inotropic effect). Movement of an entire curve upward (more work for a given preload) or downward (less work for a given preload) signifies a positive or negative inotropic effect, respectively. Examples of positive inotropic factors are circulating catecholamines and the cardiac sympathetic nerves; negative inotropic factors include severe anoxia or acidosis, and negative inotropes, such as most anesthetics.

Afterload is defined as the force opposing fiber shortening during ventricular ejection.[5] It is not synonymous with systemic arterial pressure, vasomotor tone, or vascular resistance. Instead, it should be thought of as the tension or stress in the ventricular wall during ejection. In accordance with the law of Laplace, afterload is directly related to intraventricular pressure and size and inversely related to wall thickness. Because of changing size, pressure, and wall thickness, afterload varies continuously during ventricular ejection. Thus it is difficult to quantify with precision. Despite the widespread use of aortic pressure for the left ventricle and pulmonary artery pressure for the right ventricle as indices of afterload *in vivo*, this approach should not be considered quantitative.

In isolated heart preparations, in which preload, inotropic state, and heart rate are controlled, increases in afterload cause reductions in left ventricular output (i.e., stroke volume; Figure 21-5, *A*).[6] In the intact circulation, this impairment in cardiac performance can be avoided by compensatory increases in contractility and/or venous return (preload). As demonstrated in Figure 21-5, *B*, there is no change in stroke volume when normal hearts are exposed to increased afterload (outflow resistance), but a decrease in stroke volume when failing hearts pump against similar conditions.[7]

The Cardiac Cycle

The events of the cardiac cycle are shown on Figure 21-6. The salient points are:
1. Atrial systole begins after the P wave of the electrocardiogram; ventricular systole begins near the end of the R wave and ends just after the T wave.
2. When ventricular pressure exceeds aorta pressure, the aortic valve opens, and ventricular ejection begins (at "O" in Figure 21-6).
3. The amount of blood ejected by the ventricle (stroke volume) is typically approximately 65% of end-diastolic volume (ejection fraction).
4. Most ventricular filling occurs prior to atrial systole.
5. Events on the right side of the circulation are similar to those on the left side, but are somewhat asynchronous. Right atrial systole precedes left atrial systole, and contraction of the RV typically begins after that of the LV. However, because pulmonary arterial pressure is less than aortic pressure, RV ejection precedes LV ejection.

Ventricular diastole is defined as the period in the cardiac cycle from the end of ejection until the onset of ventricular tension development of the succeeding beat and is comprised of four phases: isovolumic relaxation, early rapid filling, diastasis, and atrial systole.[8-12] Of these phases, only isovolumic relaxation is an active process that requires expenditure of energy by ventricular myocytes. Termed

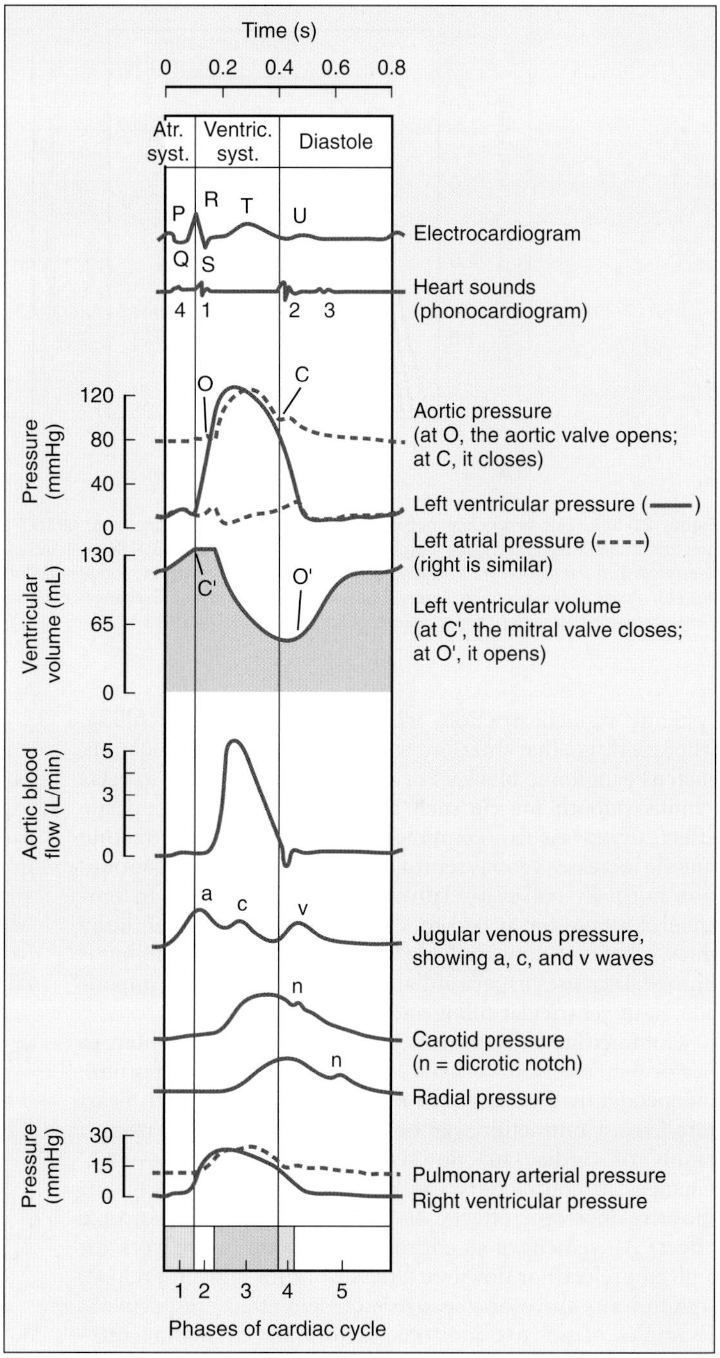

Figure 21-6 Events of a cardiac cycle. The phases of the cardiac cycle are identified at the bottom as follows: (1) atrial systole, (2) isovolumic ventricular contraction, (3) ventricular ejection, (4) isovolumic relaxation, (5) ventricular filling. *(Reprinted with permission from Ganong WF. Review of Medical Physiology. Norwalk, CT: Appleton & Lange; 1987:467.)*

ventricular lusitropy, this active process can be quantified most precisely as a time constant of the isovolumic pressure decline (the Greek letter tau, τ), calculated as the monoexponential decline of pressure during the isovolumic phase of the cycle. Relaxation is delayed, τ increased, and preload impaired in chronic processes such as hypertrophy or cardiomyopathy, or in acute processes such as ischemia or administration of negative inotropic drugs. In contrast, relaxation is generally enhanced, τ reduced, and preload facilitated by administration of positive inotropic drugs.

The phase of rapid early filling follows isovolumic relaxation and begins when ventricular pressure falls below atrial pressure. During this period, elastic recoil of the myocardium

in combination with continued relaxation create an atrial/ventricular pressure gradient (sometimes characterized as suction) that greatly facilitates ventricular filling. As the atrial/ventricular pressure gradient diminishes, the phase of diastasis (slow ventricular filling) begins, continuing until atrial systole. Early rapid filling normally accounts for 80% to 85% of ventricular end-diastolic volume; diastasis and atrial systole provide approximately 3% to 5% and 15% to 25%, respectively.[12] Multiple processes can alter diastolic filling dynamics, most notably ectopy arising from the atrioventricular node and ventricular pacing (no atrial systole), and reductions in ventricular compliance, such as concentric hypertrophy, ventricular interaction, and pericardial constraint.

The pattern of contraction differs for the left and right ventricles. The LV contracts in a relatively homogenous fashion with both the short and long axes shortening simultaneously. In contrast, the RV, which normally develops a pressure only 20% of that in the LV, contracts sequentially from the inflow tract to the outflow tract. The mechanical significance of this sequential pattern of contraction is unclear, but the process appears to reflect the different embryology of the inflow and outflow tracts, and is altered by sympathetic stimulation, positive inotropic drugs, autonomic blockade, and volatile anesthetics.

Indices of Cardiac Function

CARDIAC FUNCTION CURVES WITH THE PULMONARY ARTERY CATHETER

Introduction of the flow-directed pulmonary artery catheter in the late 1960s allowed measurements of cardiac output by thermodilution and of pulmonary capillary wedge pressure (PCWP), which was considered to reflect LV preload.[13-15] This made it possible for clinicians to construct ventricular function curves at the bedside and to use this information to guide treatment. The validity of this approach requires several conditions[16]:

1. Pressure from the left atrium (which is on average equal to LV end-diastolic pressure) must be reflected back through the pulmonary circulation; thus the tip of the pulmonary artery catheter must be wedged in a small pulmonary vessel so blood cannot flow beyond it.
2. Changes in the relationship between ventricular volume and pressure during diastole (compliance) must be taken into account. A stiff or noncompliant ventricle is evidenced by impaired diastolic filling and exaggerated pressure increases; this erroneously implies an increased preload, even though muscle stretch may be unaltered or even reduced. A stiff ventricle is characteristic of a variety of pathologic states, including myocardial ischemia, healing or healed myocardial infarction, myocardial hypertrophy, and constrictive pericarditis.
3. Afterload and heart rate must be constant when multiple cardiac function curves are used to assess changes in myocardial contractility, as reflected in stroke volume at a given preload.

ISOVOLUMIC CONTRACTION INDEX

One of the most common and useful indices of contractility is the maximal rate of change of the ventricular pressure pulse, so-called dP/dt max.[17] Interventions that acutely augment myocardial contractility, such as exercise and catecholamines, increase this index.[17,18] Values in the normal LV are approximately 1000 mm Hg/sec, whereas those in the RV average only 250 mm Hg/sec.[17] This difference has been attributed to the fact that peak dP/dt usually occurs at the instant of the opening of the semilunar valves and that developed pressure is substantially higher in the LV compared with the RV, and not to a difference in contractile state between ventricles.[13] Disadvantages of dP/dt max as an index of contractility include the need for high fidelity measurements of pressure, distortion by wall properties and valvular dysfunction, and dependence on loading conditions and heart rate. In order to correct for load dependency, the ratio of dP/dt to developed pressure or to a standard pressure has been employed.

EJECTION PHASE INDEX

The most frequently used clinical index of global contractile function is ejection fraction. Both invasive and noninvasive techniques have been used to determine ejection fraction from image-based volume measurements (echocardiography, angiography, magnetic resonance imaging, positron emission tomography scanning) or indicator dilution techniques. While ejection fraction provides useful information about systolic pump performance, it is heavily influenced by afterload. Such load-dependence is common to virtually all indices of contractility based upon ejection phase parameters. Another ejection phase index of contractility is the preload recruitable stroke work (PRSW) relationship.[19] To measure PRSW, venous return is decreased by inferior vena cava occlusion, resulting in a progressive reduction in ventricular end-diastolic volume. The area of the pressure-volume loop (which represents external work) is plotted for each beat as a function of end-diastolic volume (Figure 21-7). The slope of this relationship defines the work the ventricle can perform for a given preload and is a reflection of contractility; increased slope indicates increased contractility, and a fall in slope indicates decreased contractility. An advantage of PRSW is that it provides an index of overall ventricular performance, combining both systolic and diastolic components; however, it is not practical in the clinical environment.

Ventricular Pressure-Volume Loop: End Systolic Pressure Volume Relations

In 1898, Frank, using data from studies in isolated frog ventricles, presented the cycle of ventricular contraction as a loop defined by pressure (P) in the vertical axis and volume (V) in the horizontal axis.[20] Because of difficulties in measuring ventricular volume *in vivo*, research on pressure-volume relationships proceeded slowly during the first two thirds of the 20th century.[21] With the development of the isolated blood-perfused canine heart preparation, echocardiography, and ventriculography for studies in humans, there was a resurgence of activity in the 1970s and 1980s.[22-24] The use of pressure-volume analysis has been established as a powerful method to characterize ventricular pump properties throughout the cardiac cycle independent of loading conditions. However, the method is highly sophisticated, laborious, and requires specialized equipment and training.

The hemodynamic changes during a single cardiac cycle are displayed by plotting instantaneous ventricular pressure vs. volume (Figure 21-8, *A*).[21] Under steady-state conditions, this loop is repeated with each contraction. For a given cardiac cycle, there is a pressure-volume point that coincides with end-diastole (at the lower end of the loop). The increase in ventricular pressure during this period of filling, which ends when the mitral valve closes, reflects the compliance of the ventricular wall. During isovolumic contraction, pressure increases steeply while volume remains constant. Ventricular pressure rises to a level in excess of aortic pressure, the aortic valve opens, and blood is ejected. Ventricular ejection (systole) continues until ventricular pressure falls below aortic pressure and the aortic valve closes. The upper left hand corner of the loop coincides with end-systole. The period of isovolumic relaxation follows, which is characterized by a sharp decrease in pressure and no change in volume. The mitral valve then opens, thus completing one cardiac cycle. The area

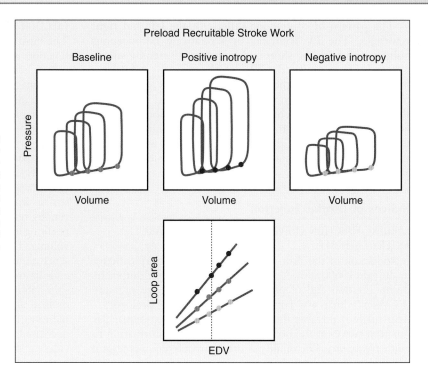

Figure 21-7 Use of the preload recruitable stroke work to assess inotropic state of the ventricle. Vena caval occlusion causes a progressive reduction in ventricular end-diastolic volume. The area of the pressure-volume loop is plotted for each beat as a function of the end-diastolic volume. The slope of this relationship defines how much work the ventricle can perform for a given preload and is a reflection of contractility, that is, a rise in the slope indicates increased contractility, and a fall in the slope indicates decreased contractility. *EDV,* End-diastolic volume.

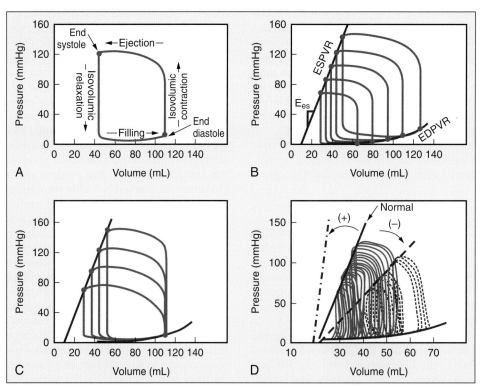

Figure 21-8 A, Pressure-volume loop of the left ventricle. **B,** Multiple pressure-volume loops generated by progressive reductions in preload. **C,** Multiple pressure-volume loops generated by progressive increases in afterload. **D,** Use of pressure-volume loops to provide a load-dependent index of myocardial contractility. An increase in end-systolic elastance (Ees) indicates an increase in the slope of end-systolic pressure-volume relationship (ESPVR) and an increase in myocardial contractility (positive inotropy), whereas a decrease in Ees indicates a decrease in the slope of ESPVR *(red loops)* and a decrease in myocardial contractility (negative inotropy) compared with normal *(blue loops)*. *ESPVR,* End-diastolic pressure-volume relationship. *(Reprinted with permission from Burkhoff D, Mirsky I, Suga H. Assessment of systolic and diastolic ventricular properties via pressure-volume analysis: a guide for clinical, translational, and basic researchers. Am J Physiol Heart Circ Physiol. 2005;289:H501-H512.)*

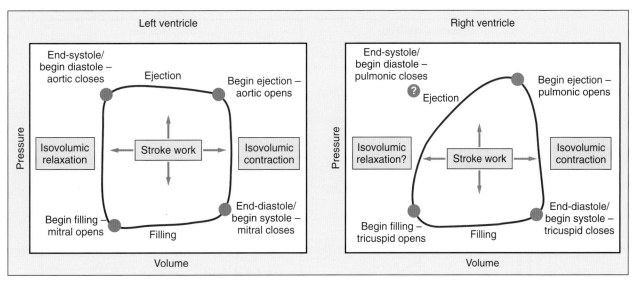

Figure 21-9 A comparison of the pressure-volume characteristics for the left and right ventricles.

within the pressure-volume loop represents the internal work of the ventricle, whereas external work is determined by the product of stroke volume and aortic pressure. An intervention that acutely changes loading conditions but has no effect on contractility, such as transient caval occlusion to reduce preload (see Figure 21-8, *B*) or administration of phenylephrine to increase afterload (see Figure 21-8, *C*), generates a family of loops.[21,22] The end-systolic points in the series of loops conform to a linear pressure-volume relationship, which defines the end-systolic pressure-volume relationship (ESPVR). End-systolic elastance (Ees) defines the slope of ESPVR and is a load-independent index of contractility. The diastolic pressure-volume points define a non-linear end-diastolic relationship (EDPVR). With a constant contractile state and afterload, the progressive reduction in preload causes the loops to shift toward lower volumes at end-systole and end-diastole, resulting in a decrease in stroke volume (see Figure 21-8, *B*). A selective increase in afterload causes narrowing and elongation of the loops, which results in a decrease in stroke volume (see Figure 21-8, *C*). The ESPVR responds to acute changes in myocardial contractility; an increase in its slope, Ees, indicates a positive inotropic intervention and a decrease in Ees indicates a negative inotropic intervention (see Figure 21-8, *D*).

The pressure-volume characteristics for the RV differ markedly from those of the LV (Figure 21-9).[25] Although clear in the pressure-volume loop of the LV, end-systole is not well defined in the normal RV. Due primarily to the sequential pattern of right ventricular free wall contraction, the low resistance of the pulmonary vascular bed, and the fact that blood ejected from the RV has inertia, the peak pressure within the RV normally occurs very early in systole and blood continues to leave via the pulmonic valve for an extended period. Consequently, the pressure-volume loop for the RV has a more triangular shape, with only a brief period of isovolumic relaxation. The prolonged low-pressure emptying of the RV renders this chamber very sensitive to changes in afterload. Because the RV does not demonstrate a defined end-systolic point, Ees analysis is not readily applicable, and PRSW is considered far superior for assessment of

contractility. With pulmonary hypertension, the pressure-volume loop in the RV is not triangular but resembles that of the LV, largely because of a change in both the magnitude and timing of peak RV pressure.[26]

HEMODYNAMICS AND SYSTEMIC VASCULAR CONTROL

Pressure Changes in Systemic and Pulmonary Circulations

Figure 21-10 compares the pressure changes as blood flows through the series-coupled components of the systemic and pulmonary circulations, from the large arteries to the arterioles, capillaries, and veins.[27] The normal pulmonary circulation is a low-pressure, low resistance circuit that accommodates the entire output of the RV.[28] This results in a smaller workload for the RV, which is in keeping with its much thinner wall. Although pressure in the ventricles falls nearly to zero during diastole, pressure is maintained in the large arteries. This is possible because a portion of the energy released by cardiac contraction during systole is stored in the distensible large arteries (the Windkessel effect). During diastole, the elastic recoil of the vessels converts this potential energy into forward blood flow, which ensures that capillary flow is continuous throughout the cardiac cycle. The most severe drop in pressure occurs in the arterioles; hence they are often termed resistance vessels. The diameter of arterioles is regulated by contractile activity of vascular smooth muscle. Variations in arteriolar diameter are an important determinant of local capillary blood flow and hydrostatic pressure. The summed effect of all the systemic resistance vessels, that is, the total peripheral resistance, is a major determinant, along with cardiac output, of arterial pressure, and thus of the driving force for tissue blood flow (see Figure 21-1).

Determinants of Blood Flow: Poiseuille's Law

Blood flow (F) is a function of arteriovenous pressure gradient (Pa − Pv) and local vascular resistance (R), according to the equation:

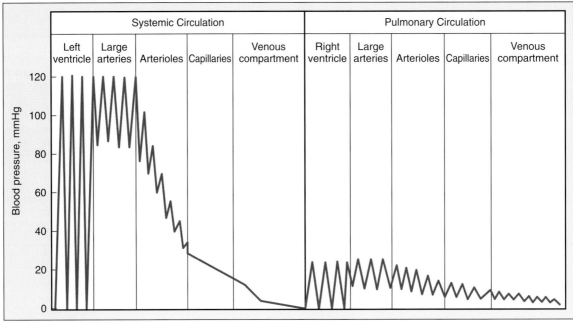

Figure 21-10 Blood pressure in the series coupled components of the systemic and pulmonary circulations. *(Modified from Folkow B, Neil E. Circulation. New York: Oxford University Press; 1971:6.)*

$$F = (Pa - Pv)/R \qquad [1]$$

This is analogous to Ohm's law in an electrical circuit. Because arterial and venous blood pressures are normally well maintained within narrow limits by homeostatic mechanisms, tissue blood flow usually varies inversely as a function of vascular resistance.

Poiseuille performed studies that yielded an equation describing resistance to flow in a straight, rigid tube of length (l) and radius (r):

$$R = \eta 8\,l\,/\,r^4 \qquad [2]$$

where η is the viscosity. Of note is that flow resistance varies inversely with tube radius raised to the fourth power. Thus small changes in tube radius cause large changes in resistance.

Because the length of blood vessels is relatively fixed, geometric changes in blood flow resistance occur by variations in vessel radius. These adjustments are primarily the result of contraction or relaxation of the smooth muscle investing the arterioles, which are the principal site of vascular resistance. However, in certain vascular beds (e.g., the left ventricular myocardium), extravascular compressive forces also play a role (see later). Chemical factors, which are linked to the metabolic activity of the tissue (e.g., adenosine) modulate vascular resistance so that blood flow (and oxygen delivery) is commensurate with local oxygen demands.

Blood Viscosity

Viscosity is the internal friction resulting from intermolecular forces operating within a flowing liquid. The term *internal friction* emphasizes that as a fluid moves within a tube, laminae in the fluid slip on one another and move at different speeds. The movement produces a velocity gradient in a direction

perpendicular to the wall of the tube termed the *shear rate*. Shear rate shows a direct correlation to rate of blood flow. Viscosity is defined as the factor of proportionality relating shear stress and shear rate for the fluid.

$$\text{Viscosity} = \text{shear stress/shear rate} \qquad [3]$$

Newton assumed that viscosity was a constant property of a particular fluid and independent of shear rate. Fluids that demonstrate this behavior are termed *Newtonian*. The units of viscosity are dynes per second per square centimeter, or *poise*.

The viscosity of blood varies as a direct function of hematocrit (Figure 21-11, *A*); the greater the hematocrit, the more friction there is between successive layers.[29] Plasma is a Newtonian fluid, even at high protein concentrations. However, because blood consists of erythrocytes suspended in plasma, it does not behave as a homogeneous Newtonian fluid; the viscosity of blood increases sharply with reductions in shear rate (see Figure 21-11, *A*). This non-Newtonian behavior of blood has been attributed to changes in the behavior of erythrocytes at low flow rates. At low flow, erythrocytes lose their axial position in the stream of blood, lose their ellipsoidal shape, form aggregates, and adhere to the endothelial walls of microvessels. The tendency toward erythrocyte aggregation appears dependent upon the plasma concentration of large proteins such as fibrinogen that form cell-to-cell bridges. Figure 21-11, *B*, demonstrates that non-Newtonian behavior is localized on the venous side of the circulation because of its lower shear rates, but that this behavior can be blunted or abolished by hemodilution.[30]

The tendency for increased hematocrit to increase blood viscosity is attenuated when blood flows through tubes of capillary diameter (see Figure 21-11, *C*).[31] This is because erythrocytes are normally very deformable, and with a diameter similar to that of the capillary, they can squeeze through

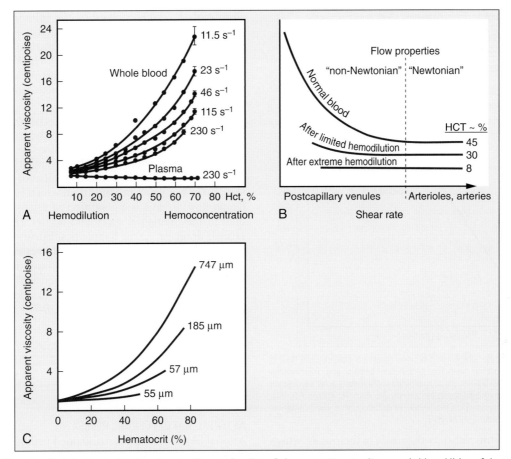

Figure 21-11 A, Viscosity of whole blood at various hematocrits as a function of shear rate. Hematocrit was varied by addition of dextran and packed red blood cells. Note that viscosity increases with hematocrit and that these increases are greatest at the lower shear rates. **B,** Graphic representation of the level of blood viscosity in the various vascular compartments. Under normal condition (hematocrit = 45%), viscosity increases in postcapillary venules because of reduced shear rate. Hemodilution can blunt or even completely eliminate this regional variation in viscosity. **C,** The effect of hematocrit on viscosity of blood in tubes of varying radii. In wide tubes, increasing hematocrit raises viscosity, whereas in narrow tubes it has no effect. *(A, Reprinted with permission from Messmer K. Hemodilution. Surg Clin N Am. 1975;55:659-678; B, Reprinted with permission from Messmer K, Sunder-Plassman L. Hemodilution. Prog Surg. 1974;12:208-245; C, Reprinted with permission from Feigl EO. Physics of cardiovascular system. In: Ruch TC, Patton HD, eds. Physiology and Biophysics II: Circulation, Respiration, and Fluid Balance. Philadelphia: WB Saunders; 1974:19.)*

the vessel lumen in single file with minimal extra force required. Thus the rate at which erythrocytes pass through the capillary has little influence on blood viscosity there.

Blood viscosity varies inversely with temperature. This is important during hypothermic cardiopulmonary bypass. After circulatory arrest, the shear stress required to reinitiate flow and to break up red cell aggregates is higher. Additional rheologic benefit may be gained by a further decrease in hematocrit.

Turbulent Flow

A principal condition of Poiseuille's law is that flow be laminar. Above a critical flow rate, the laminae break down into eddies that move in all directions. Such flow is said to be turbulent (Figure 21-12).[31] The tendency for turbulence is given by the Reynolds number (Re):

$$Re = v \, D\delta/\eta \qquad [4]$$

where v = linear velocity, D = diameter, δ = density, and η = viscosity. Re is dimensionless because it is the ratio of inertial

and cohesive forces. Inertial forces tend to disrupt the stream, whereas cohesive forces tend to maintain it. In long straight tubes, turbulence occurs when Re exceeds a value of approximately 2000. However, the critical Re is much less because of pulsatile flow patterns and complicated vascular geometries. When flow is turbulent, a greater portion of total fluid energy is dissipated as heat and vibration; thus the pressure drop is greater than predicted from the Poiseuille equation (see Figure 21-12). The vibrations associated with turbulent flow can often be heard by auscultation as a murmur.

Major Vessel Types: Structure and Function

The various vessel types have structural and geometric features (Figure 21-13, *A*) that determine their functional characteristics within the circulation (Figure 21-13, *B*).[32] The large conduit arteries are predominantly elastic structures, which allows them to convert intermittent cardiac output into continuous peripheral flow. Because the cross-sectional area of these vessels is small, the velocity of flow in them is high. The resistance to flow in the arteries is small, and thus the pressure drop is also small. The arterioles and the terminal

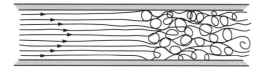

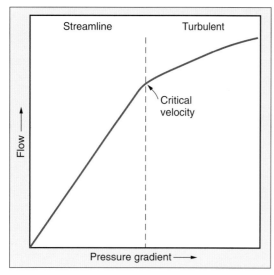

Figure 21-12 The linear relationship between pressure gradient and flow is shown. Beyond a critical velocity, turbulence begins and relationship between pressure and flow is no longer linear. *(Reprinted with permission from Feigl EO. Physics of cardiovascular system. In: Ruch TC, Patton HD, eds. Physiology and Biophysics II: Circulation, Respiration, and Fluid Balance. Philadelphia: WB Saunders; 1974:19.)*

arterioles have significant smooth muscle in their walls, which permits active changes in vascular diameter, and modulation of local vascular resistance and blood flow. Capillaries have a very large aggregate cross-sectional area (which decreases flow velocity) and a thin wall, both factors favoring blood-tissue gas exchange. The veins and venules have the greatest volume, which makes an appropriate site for blood storage.

FACTORS INFLUENCING THE BALANCE BETWEEN CAPILLARY FILTRATION AND ABSORPTION

Because the capillary wall is highly permeable to water and to almost all plasma solutes except plasma proteins; it acts like a porous filter through which protein-free plasma moves by bulk flow under the influence of a hydrostatic pressure gradient. Transcapillary filtration is defined as follows:

$$\text{Fluid filtration} = C_F[(P_{cap} - P_{IF}) - (\Pi_{cap} - \Pi_{IF})] \quad [5]$$

where C_F = capillary filtration coefficient; P_{cap} = capillary hydrostatic pressure; P_{IF} = interstitial fluid hydrostatic pressure; Π_{IF} = interstitial fluid oncotic pressure; Π_{cap} = capillary oncotic pressure. P_{cap} and Π_{IF} are forces of filtration. P_{cap} is determined by arterial pressure, venous pressure, and the ratio of postcapillary to precapillary resistance. Elevations of arterial pressure, venous pressure, or venous resistance/arterial resistance produce elevations of P_{cap}. P_{cap} is approximately 35 mm Hg at the arterial end of the capillaries and approximately 15 mm Hg at the venous end. Π_I is due to plasma proteins that have passed through the capillary wall and is normally very low compared with P_{cap}. Thus P_{cap} is normally the major force for filtration. P_{IF} and Π_{cap} are forces favoring

absorption. P_{IF} is determined by the volume of fluid and the distensibility of the interstitial space, and is normally nearly equal to zero. Π_{cap} is due to plasma proteins (predominantly albumin) and is approximately 25 mm Hg. Π_p is normally the major force for absorption. The direction and magnitude of capillary bulk flow is essentially a function of the ratio of P_{cap} to Π_{cap} (Figure 21-14).[33]

Filtered fluid that reaches the extravascular spaces is returned to the circulatory system via the lymphatic network. Under normal conditions (see Figure 21-14, *A*), filtration dominates at the arterial end of the capillary, and absorption at the venous end because of the gradient of hydrostatic pressure; there is a small net filtration, which is compensated by lymph flow. Edema is a condition of excess accumulation of fluid in the interstitial space and occurs when net filtration exceeds drainage via the lymphatics. Edema can be caused by (1) increased capillary pressure, (2) decreased plasma protein concentration, (3) accumulation of osmotically active substances in the interstitial space, (4) increased capillary permeability, or (5) inadequate lymph flow. Conditions resulting in edema are depicted in Figure 21-14, *B-D*.

MAJOR CARDIOVASCULAR REFLEXES

The salient features of the major cardiovascular reflexes are presented in Table 21-1.[34]

ARTERIAL BARORECEPTOR REFLEX
Arterial blood pressure is maintained within narrow limits by a negative feedback system called the arterial baroreceptor reflex.[35,36] Its major components of this system are (Figure 21-15, *A*): (1) an afferent limb composed of baroreceptors in the carotid artery and aortic arch and their respective afferent nerves, the glossopharyngeal and vagus nerves; (2) cardiovascular centers in the medulla that receive and integrate sensory information; and (3) an efferent limb composed of sympathetic nerves to the heart and blood vessels and the parasympathetic (vagus) nerve to the heart. Figure 21-15, *B*, presents the neural relationships of the arterial baroreceptor reflex.[37] Baroreceptors are stimulated by stretch of the vessel wall by increased transluminal pressure. Impulses originating in the baroreceptors tonically inhibit discharge of sympathetic nerves to the heart and blood vessels, and tonically facilitate discharge of the vagus nerve to the heart. A rise in arterial pressure reduces baroreceptor afferent activity, resulting in further inhibition of the sympathetic and facilitation of parasympathetic output. This produces vasodilation, venodilation, and reductions in stroke volume, heart rate, and cardiac output, which combine to normalize arterial pressure. A decrease in arterial pressure has opposite effects. The cardiovascular centers in the medulla are also under the influence of neural influences arising from the arterial chemoreceptors, hypothalamus, and cerebral cortex, and of local changes in PCO_2 and PO_2.

BEZOLD-JARISCH REFLEX
The Bezold-Jarisch reflex is a triad of responses (bradycardia, hypotension, and apnea) first observed following injection of *Veratrum* plant alkaloids in animals by von Bezold and Hirt in 1867.[29,38-40] Seventy years later, Jarisch and Richter[41,42] demonstrated that the receptor area was in the heart (not the great

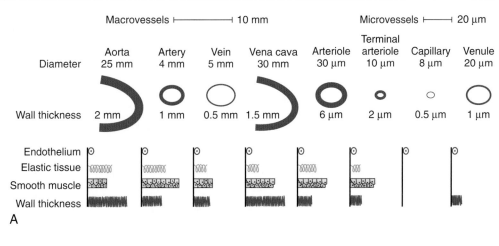

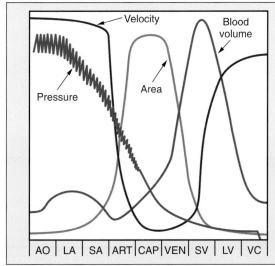

Figure 21-13 A, Dimensions and structural attributes of the various vessel types. **B,** Velocity, cross-sectional area, blood volume, and pressure within the various vessel types. *AO,* Aorta; *LA,* large arteries; *SA,* small arteries; *ART,* arterioles; *CAP,* capillaries; *VEN,* venules; *SV,* small veins; *LV,* large veins; *VC,* venae cavae. *(Modified from Berne RM, Levy MN. Principles of Physiology. St. Louis: CV Mosby; 1990:195.)*

vessels), the afferent pathway was in the vagus nerve, and the efferent pathway involved inhibition of sympathetic outflow to peripheral vessels and increased activity in the vagus nerve to the heart. The ventricular receptors underlying the Bezold-Jarisch reflex are nonencapsulated terminals of unmyelinated vagal C-fiber afferents in the walls of the ventricles.[43] Although *Veratrum* alkaloids are not normally present in animals, physiologic factors, including mechanical stimulation, can trigger the Bezold-Jarisch reflex.[44] The literature contains reports of "paradoxical" bradycardia during severe hemorrhage in humans.[45,46] Studies in a rabbit model demonstrated that this response is mediated by the ventricular receptors and by the ability of the Bezold-Jarisch reflex to override the arterial baroreceptor response.[47,48] During severe hemorrhage, the ventricular receptors can be excited by abnormal squeezing of the myocardium due to vigorous contraction around a nearly empty chamber.

BAINBRIDGE REFLEX

In 1915, Bainbridge demonstrated that intravenous infusion of saline or blood in the anesthetized dog produced tachycardia.[34,49] The elimination of the response following transection of the cardiac autonomic nerve supply and injection of the anticholinergic drug atropine demonstrated that the tachycardia was reflexive in origin, with the vagus nerves constituting the afferent limb and withdrawal of vagal tone the primary efferent limb. The increase in venous return is detected by stretch receptors in the right and left atria.[50,51] The Bainbridge reflex is present in primates, including man, but is much less prominent than in the dog, attributed to a more dominant arterial baroreceptor reflex in humans.[52] The Bainbridge reflex is obtunded or absent when the heart rate is high.[53] A "reverse" Bainbridge reflex has been proposed to explain decreases in heart rate observed under conditions in which venous return is reduced, such as during spinal and epidural anesthesia and controlled hypotension.[34]

TISSUE OXYGEN TRANSPORT

General Concepts

Oxygen serves as an electron acceptor in oxidative phosphorylation, enabling production of adenosine triphosphate (ATP) along efficient aerobic pathways. The high-energy phosphate bonds of ATP provide energy for functional and biochemical

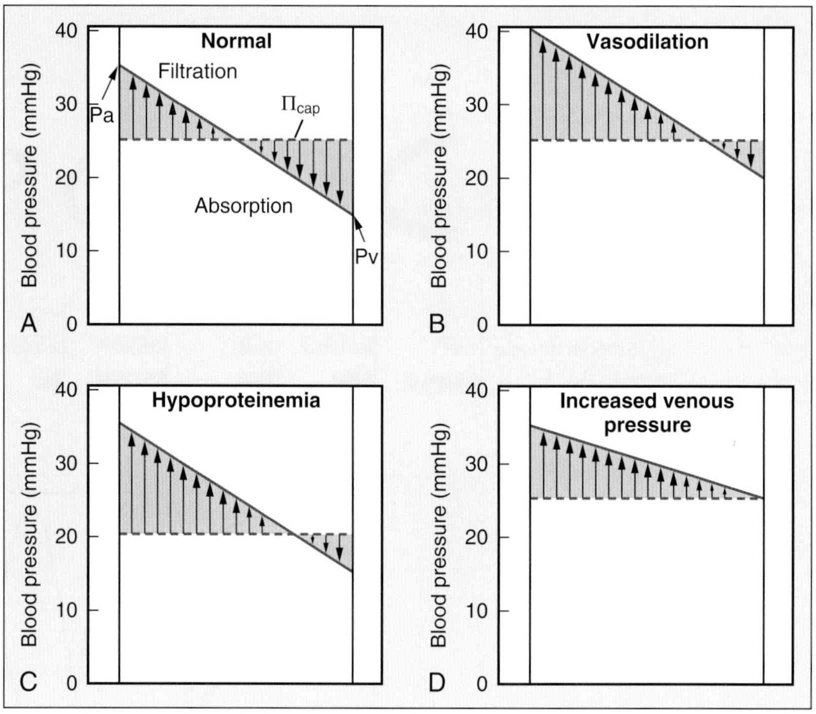

Figure 21-14 Capillary-tissue fluid exchange. See text for details. Π_{cap}, Capillary oncotic pressure; Pa, hydrostatic pressure at arterial end of capillary; Pv, hydrostatic pressure at venous end of capillary. (*Modified from Friedman JJ. Microcirculation. In: Selkurt EE. Physiology. Boston: Little, Brown; 1971:269.*)

Table 21-1. Major Cardiovascular Reflexes

REFLEX	RECEPTORS AND LOCATION	AFFERENT LIMB	EFFERENT LIMB AND RESPONSE
Arterial Baroreceptor Reflex	Stretch receptors in vessel wall of carotid sinus and aortic arch respond to changes in arterial blood pressure	Fibers in glossopharageal and vagus nerves to medulla	Homeostatic control of arterial blood pressure via changes in cardiac output and systemic vascular resistance mediated by the autonomic nervous system
Bezold-Jarisch Reflex	Mechanical and chemosensitive receptors in ventricular walls	Nonmyelinated vagal C-fibers to medulla	Inhibition of sympathetic outflow resulting in bradycardia, peripheral vasodilation, and hypotension
Bainbridge Reflex	Stretch receptors at junction of the vena cava and right atrium and at junction of the pulmonary vein and left atrium respond to changes in volume in central thoracic compartment	Fibers in vagus nerve to medulla.	Inhibition of vagal outflow and enhancement of sympathetic outflow to sino-atrial node causing tachycardia

Reprinted with permission from Crystal GJ, Salem MR. The Bainbridge and the "reverse" Bainbridge reflexes: history, physiology, and clinical relevance. *Anesth Analg.* 2012;114:520-532.

cellular processes within the cell, such as contraction of muscle proteins and ion transport.

The cardiovascular system acts in concert with the respiratory system in transporting oxygen to tissue mitochondria from its source in inspired air. Oxygen transport is comprised of a series of steps down a gradient in partial pressure, each associated with a PO_2 cost (Figure 21-16).[54] Normal oxygen delivery maintains PO_2 in the vicinity of mitochondria at 0.1 mm Hg, the optimal level required for unimpaired O_2 use (Figure 21-17).[55] The only effect of greater PO_2 values is to provide a gradient for diffusion of oxygen to mitochondria remote from capillaries.

The amount of oxygen carried from the lungs to tissues by circulating blood (i.e., convective systemic oxygen delivery – DO_2), is given by the equation:

$$DO_2 = CO \times CaO_2 \qquad [6]$$

where CO is cardiac output in L/min and CaO_2 is the arterial oxygen content in vol %.

Oxygen Transport in the Blood

CaO_2 is composed of oxygen bound to hemoglobin and dissolved in plasma. Oxygen bound is a function of hemoglobin concentration (Hb), oxygen carrying capacity for hemoglobin (1.39 mL O_2/g hemoglobin), and oxygen saturation of hemoglobin (SaO_2), according to the equation:

$$O_2 \text{ bound} = (Hb \times SaO_2 \times 1.39) \qquad [7]$$

Oxygen saturation of hemoglobin is a function of PO_2 as reflected in the oxyhemoglobin dissociation curve (Figure 21-18, *A*), a plot of oxyhemoglobin saturation as a function of PO_2.[56] At a PO_2 of 100 mm Hg, normal for arterial blood, hemoglobin saturation (SaO_2) is approximately 97%; at

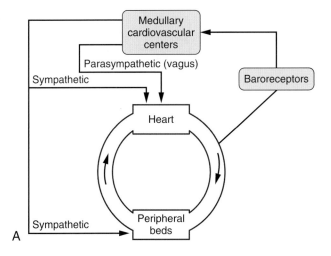

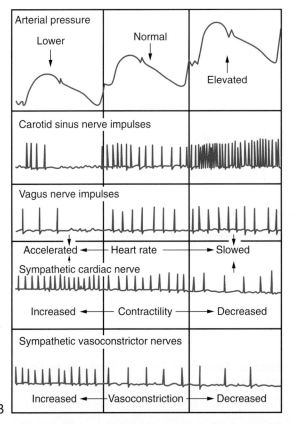

Figure 21-15 A, Diagram of arterial baroreceptor reflex loop. **B,** Effect of changes in arterial pressure on carotid sinus nerve discharge and impulse rate of efferent nerves. (*A, Modified from Rothe CF, Friedman JJ. Control of the cardiovascular system. In: Selkurt EE. Physiology. Boston: Little, Brown; 1971:372; B, Modified from Rushmer RF. Cardiovascular Dynamics. 3rd ed. Philadelphia: Saunders; 1970:165.*)

40 mm Hg, a typical value for mixed venous oxygen tension (PvO₂) in a resting person, the saturation is about 75%. The sigmoid shape of the curve reflects the fact that the four oxygen binding sites on the tetrameric hemoglobin molecule interact cooperatively with each other. When the first site binds a molecule of oxygen, the binding of the next site is facilitated, and so forth. The result is a curve that is steep up to PO₂ of 60 mm Hg and more shallow thereafter, approaching 100% saturation asymptomatically.

The shape of the oxyhemoglobin dissociation curve has important physiologic implications. The flatness of the curve above a PO₂ of 80 mm Hg assures a relatively constant oxyhemoglobin saturation for arterial blood despite wide variations in alveolar oxygen pressure. The steep portion of the curve between 20 and 60 mm Hg permits unloading of oxygen from hemoglobin at relatively high PO₂ values, which permits delivery of large amounts of oxygen into the tissue by diffusion.

The oxygen binding properties of hemoglobin are influenced by a number of factors, including pH, PCO₂, and temperature (see Figure 21-18, *B*).[57] These factors cause shifts of the oxyhemoglobin dissociation curve to the right or left without changing the slope. An increase in temperature or PCO₂, or a decrease in pH, all of which occur in active tissues, decreases the affinity of hemoglobin for oxygen, and shifts the oxyhemoglobin dissociation curve to the right. Thus a higher PO₂ is required to achieve a given saturation, which facilitates unloading of oxygen in the tissue. The extent of a shift in the oxyhemoglobin dissociation curve is quantified as the P_{50} PO₂ required for 50% saturation. The P_{50} of normal adult hemoglobin at 37°C and normal pH and PCO₂ is 26 to 27 mm Hg.

The metabolite 2,3-diphosphoglycerate (2,3-DPG) is an intermediate in anaerobic glycolysis (the biochemical pathway by which red blood cells produce ATP) that binds to hemoglobin. Increased erythrocyte 2,3-DPG concentration reduces the affinity of hemoglobin for oxygen (i.e., shifts the oxyhemoglobin dissociation curve to the right), whereas decreases have the opposite effect. Several factors influence red cell 2,3-DPG concentrations. For example, after storage in a blood bank for only 1 week, 2,3-DPG concentrations are one-third normal, resulting in a shift to the left in the oxyhemoglobin dissociation curve. On the other hand, conditions associated with chronic hypoxia (e.g., living at high altitude or chronic anemia) stimulate production of 2,3-DPG, which causes a rightward shift of the oxyhemoglobin dissociation curve.

Oxygen dissolved in blood is linearly related to PO₂. At 37°C it is defined by the equation:

$$O_2 \text{ dissolved} = 0.003 \text{ vol\%/mm Hg PO}_2 \quad [8]$$

Dissolved oxygen normally accounts for only 1.5% of total blood oxygen, but this contribution increases when the bound component is reduced during hemodilution. Because hemoglobin is essentially saturated at a PO₂ of 100 mm Hg, increases in arterial PO₂ (PaO₂) to above 100 mm Hg increase CaO₂ by raising the dissolved component.

Oxygen Supply and Consumption

For an individual with a hemoglobin concentration of 15 g/100 mL, PaO₂ of 100 mm Hg, PvO₂ of 40 mm Hg, and cardiac output of 5000 mL/min:

$$CaO_2 = (15 \times 0.97 \times 1.39) + (0.003 \times 100) = 20.5 \text{ vol\%}$$
$$DO_2 = (5000 \times 20.5/100) = 1025 \text{ mL} \times \text{min} \quad [9]$$
$$CvO_2 = (15 \times 0.75 \times 1.39) + (0.003 \times 40) = 15.8 \text{ vol\%}$$

and the arteriovenous oxygen content difference (CaO₂-CvO₂) = 20.5 − 15.8 = 4.7 vol%.

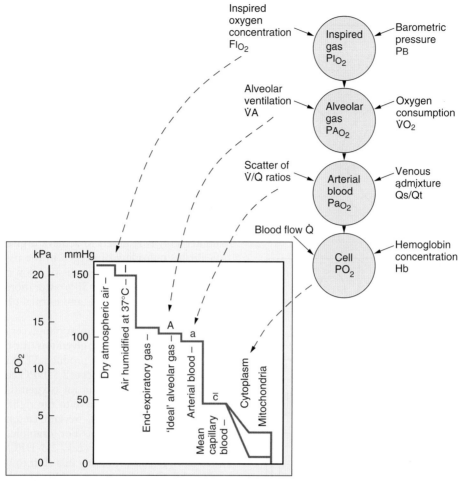

Figure 21-16 On the lower left is the oxygen cascade with PO_2 decreasing from the level in the ambient air down to the level in the mitochondria. On the right is listed the factors influencing PO_2 at various steps in the cascade. *(Reprinted with permission from Nunn JF. Nunn's Applied Respiratory Physiology. Oxford: Butterworth Heinemann; 1993:255.)*

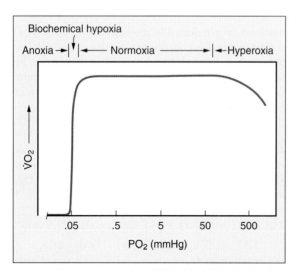

Figure 21-17 Oxygen consumption (VO_2) of isolated mitochondria as a function of PO_2. Oxygen consumption remains unchanged as long as PO_2 is above 0.5 mm Hg. *(Reprinted with permission from Honig CR. Modern Cardiovascular Physiology. Boston: Little, Brown and Company; 1981:185.)*

Diffusion of Oxygen to Tissues: Capillary to Cell Oxygen Delivery

The final step in the delivery of oxygen to tissue mitochondria is diffusion from the capillary blood. This process is determined by the capillary-to-cell PO_2 gradient and the diffusion parameters, capillary surface area, and blood-cell diffusion distance. In 1919, Krogh formulated the capillary recruitment model to describe the processes underlying oxygen transport in tissue, which was later expanded and refined.[58,59] Although Krogh's model is limited by multiple simplifying assumptions, it has value as a tool for appreciating the role of vascular control mechanisms in the transport of oxygen to tissue.

The model consists of a single capillary and the surrounding cylinder of tissue that it supplies (Figure 21-19).[55] Two interrelated oxygen gradients are involved: a longitudinal gradient within the capillary and a radial gradient extending into the tissue. Most oxygen in capillary blood is bound to hemoglobin and cannot leave the capillary. This bound oxygen is in equilibrium with the small amount of oxygen dissolved in the plasma. The consumption of oxygen by tissue creates a

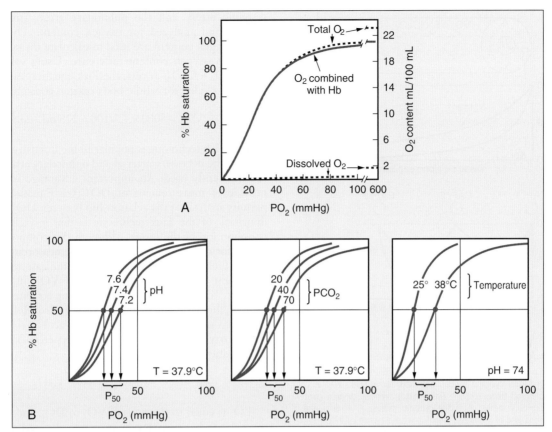

Figure 21-18 A, The oxyhemoglobin dissociation curve. The oxygen content of blood has two components: oxygen binding to hemoglobin (Hb) follows an S-shaped curve up to full saturation; the amount of oxygen in solution increases linearly with PO_2 without limit. **B,** Effects of variations in pH, PCO_2, and temperature on oxyhemoglobin dissociation curve. **(A,** Reprinted with permission from West JB. Respiratory Physiology: the Essentials. Baltimore: Williams & Wilkins; 1974; **B,** Reprinted with permission from Weibel ER. The Pathway for Oxygen. Cambridge, Mass: Harvard University Press; 1984:149.)

transcapillary gradient for oxygen. Diffusion of oxygen into tissue shifts the equilibrium between bound and dissolved oxygen so that more oxygen is released from hemoglobin. By this mechanism, oxygen dissociation from hemoglobin is controlled by tissue oxygen consumption.

The longitudinal oxygen gradient is created by extraction of oxygen by tissue as blood passes from the arterial to venous ends of the capillary. The arteriovenous oxygen difference is equivalent to the ratio of oxygen consumption to blood flow (Fick equation). An increase in oxygen consumption, a decrease in blood flow, or both, steepens the longitudinal oxygen gradient. Proportional changes in oxygen consumption and blood flow are required to maintain the longitudinal oxygen gradient constant.

A corresponding value for capillary PO_2 (PcO_2) can be estimated from the value for capillary O_2 content taking into account hemoglobin concentration and the oxyhemoglobin dissociation curve. The shape of the longitudinal gradient in PO_2 within the capillary is approximately exponential because of the influence of the oxyhemoglobin dissociation curve. The PcO_2 is the driving force for oxygen diffusion into tissue. Since PcO_2 is minimum at the venous end of the capillary, mitochondria in this region are most vulnerable to oxygen deficits.

The radial PO_2 gradient can be described by a value for mean tissue PO_2 (PtO_2) according to the equation:

$$\text{Mean } PtO_2 = PcO_2 - A \,(VO_2 \times r^2/4D) \qquad [10]$$

where PcO_2 is blood oxygen tension midway in the capillary, A is a constant related to the relationship between capillary radius and tissue cylinder radius, VO_2 is oxygen consumption of the tissue cylinder, r is the radius of the tissue cylinder ($\frac{1}{2}$ intercapillary distance), and D is the oxygen diffusion coefficient. r is determined by the number of capillaries perfused with red blood cells per volume of tissue and is controlled by precapillary sphincters. The favorable influence of capillary recruitment on tissue PO_2 is evident in Figure 21-19 (lower panel). If only capillaries "1" and "3" are open, diffusion distance is so large that PO_2 falls to zero toward the center of the tissue cylinder. The low tissue PO_2 causes relaxation of the precapillary sphincter controlling capillary "2." Perfusion of capillary "2" decreases diffusion distance and increases tissue PO_2 to an adequate level throughout the tissue.

Mean PtO_2 is a reflection of the overall balance between oxygen supply and demand within a particular tissue. An increase in blood flow without a change in oxygen demand (i.e., luxuriant perfusion) raises mean PtO_2 whereas reduction in blood flow without a change in oxygen demand lowers mean PtO_2. If mean PtO_2 falls below a critical level, tissue oxygen consumption is impaired. Measurements of mean PtO_2 have been obtained in laboratory animals in various tissues, including the myocardium and skeletal muscle, using a polarographic technique involving bare-tipped platinum electrodes.[60,61] The invasiveness of the technique has curtailed use of mean PtO_2 measurements in patients. Measurements

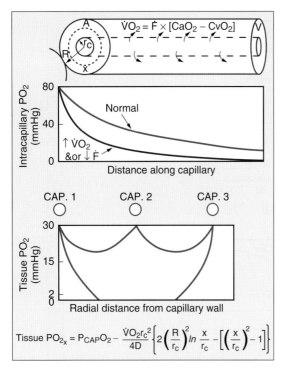

Figure 21-19 Longitudinal and radial oxygen gradients within tissue in accordance with Krogh cylinder model. See text for details. $\dot{V}O_2$, Oxygen consumption; F, blood flow; [$CaO_2 - CvO_2$], arteriovenous oxygen content difference; r_c, capillary radius; R, tissue cylinder radius; A, arterial end of capillary; V, venous end of capillary; x, point within tissue cylinder; $P_{CAP}O_2$, oxygen tension of capillary blood; D, diffusion coefficient for oxygen. *(Reprinted with permission from Honig CR. Modern Cardiovascular Physiology. Boston: Little, Brown; 1981:183.)*

of local venous PvO_2 provide an approximation for average end-capillary PO_2, and although they neglect the radial PO_2 gradient, they generally show a reasonable correlation to mean PtO_2.[62]

Oxygen Consumption

In a clinical setting, there are several methods to measure oxygen consumption (VO_2): oxygen loss or replacement into a closed breathing system, subtraction of expired from inspired volume of oxygen, and use of the Fick principle.[63,64]

Oxygen loss or replacement into a closed breathing system is the most fundamental method, is well validated, and has an accuracy well in excess of clinical requirements. However, it is cumbersome and requires meticulous attention to detail. The second method, subtraction of expired from inspired volume of oxygen, is a difficult and potentially inaccurate method since VO_2 is a small number that is calculated as the difference between two large numbers.

Under steady-state conditions, the Fick equation can be used to calculate systemic VO_2 as:

$$VO_2 = CO \times (CaO_2 - CvO_2) \qquad [11]$$

where ($CaO_2 - CvO_2$) is the systemic arteriovenous oxygen content difference expressed in vol %. In this approach, CO is usually measured by thermodilution using a pulmonary artery catheter. Samples of blood are collected from a

systemic artery and the pulmonary artery (mixed venous sample) and analyzed for oxygen content. The values for blood oxygen content are used to calculate the systemic arteriovenous oxygen content difference. Using values for CO and ($CaO_2 - CvO_2$) at rest, the Fick equation can be used to calculate a value for whole body oxygen consumption:

$$VO_2 = 5000 \times 4.7/100 = 228 \text{ mL/min} \qquad [12]$$

The Fick technique is popular in the intensive care setting because the necessary arterial and pulmonary artery catheters are frequently used. An important advantage is that it also provides a measurement of DO_2 (see Equation 6), which permits analysis of the relationship between DO_2 and VO_2. A drawback of the Fick technique is that it excludes oxygen consumption of the lungs. Although this component is negligible for normal lungs, simultaneous measurements of VO_2 by the Fick and gasometric methods indicate that it can be significant (as much as 20% of total VO_2) in critically ill patients.[65] The increased VO_2 in the lung is related to production of the superoxide and in turn hydroxyl free radicals, hydrogen peroxide, and hypochlorous acid.[66]

The oxygen extraction ratio (EO_2 in percent) is defined by the equation:

$$EO_2 = (CaO_2 - CvO_2)/CaO_2 \qquad [13]$$

EO_2 is equal to the ratio of VO_2 to DO_2, and thus reflects the balance between systemic oxygen demand and delivery. Measurements of EO_2, as well as of mixed venous oxygen saturation (SvO_2), are used clinically to assess overall adequacy of DO_2 in critically ill patients.[67-69]

A decrease in DO_2 can follow a significant reduction in any one of its major factors (Hb, SaO_2, or CO) or a smaller reduction in more than one of these factors, such as can occur in critical illness. If reduction in DO_2 is severe, it can produce tissue hypoxia (a fall in tissue PO_2 sufficient to limit mitochondrial VO_2 and to stimulate lactate production). Old terminology referred to the conditions of hypoxia resulting from reductions in Hb, SaO_2, and CO as anemic, hypoxic, and stagnant hypoxia, respectively.[70]

Critical Oxygen Delivery

DO_2 greatly exceeds VO_2 at rest (in the prior example, above 1025 compared with 228 mL/min) and thus EO_2 is relatively modest (25%), resulting in a substantial reserve for increased EO_2. This results in a biphasic relation between DO_2 and VO_2 (Figure 21-20).[71] At normal or high DO_2, VO_2 is constant and independent of DO_2 (see Figure 21-20, *A*). As DO_2 is gradually reduced, increased EO_2 maintains VO_2 (see Figure 21-20, *B*). Eventually a point is reached where EO_2 cannot increase sufficiently. Below this threshold, the so-called critical DO_2, VO_2 is limited by the supply of oxygen, about 10 mL/min/kg in anesthetized dogs.[72] A normal biphasic DO_2-VO_2 relationship exists in patients without respiratory failure undergoing coronary artery bypass surgery, whereas a direct linear relationship between DO_2 and VO_2 occurs in patients with acute respiratory distress syndrome, implying a pathologic impairment to tissue extraction of oxygen.[73-75]

Equations 6, 11, and 12 can be applied to individual tissues by substituting local blood flow for cardiac output and local venous oxygen measurements for mixed venous measurements. Body tissues vary widely with respect to the relation between baseline DO_2 and VO_2, and thus in their baseline EO_2 (Table 21-2). For example, in the left ventricle, baseline EO_2 is 70% to 75%, whereas in kidney it is only 5% to 10%. The high baseline EO_2 of the left ventricle renders it extremely dependent on changes in blood flow to maintain adequate oxygen transport.

DETERMINANTS OF MYOCARDIAL OXYGEN SUPPLY AND DEMAND

Control of Coronary Blood Flow

Blood flow to the myocardium, like that to other vascular beds, is a function of the arteriovenous pressure gradient and local vascular resistance (see Figure 21-1). Factors affecting coronary vascular resistance, and thus coronary blood flow, are presented in Figure 21-21.[76] In the left ventricular wall, coronary vascular resistance is determined by a throttling effect caused by extravascular compressive forces during systole (due to the high developed intracavitary pressure) and by active changes in the tone of arteriolar smooth muscle. The mechanical impediment to coronary blood flow is most prominent in the subendocardial layers of the LV wall such that blood flow in the left coronary circulation is maximal during diastole, rather than during systole as occurs in other tissues, including the right coronary circulation. The pressure gradient for blood flow in the LV wall is roughly the difference between aortic diastolic pressure and left ventricular end-diastolic pressure. Local metabolic mechanisms predominate in the active control of coronary vasomotor tone. These mechanisms ensure a close coupling between coronary blood

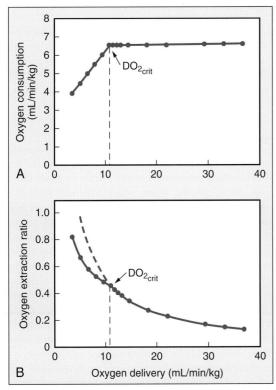

Figure 21-20 Changes in systemic oxygen consumption **(A)** and oxygen extraction ratio **(B)** during progressive reduction in oxygen delivery. An increased oxygen extraction ratio maintains oxygen consumption constant until oxygen delivery is lowered to a critical value (DO_{2crit}). The dashed line demonstrates the theoretical increase in oxygen extraction required to maintain oxygen consumption for levels of oxygen delivery below DO_{2crit}. *(Reprinted with permission from Schumacker PT, Cain SM. The concept of critical oxygen delivery. Intensive Care Med. 1987;13:223-229.)*

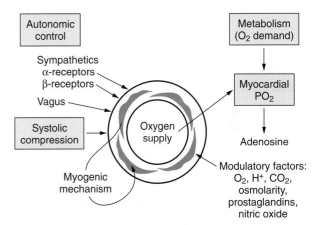

Figure 21-21 Factors influencing coronary vascular resistance. *(Reprinted with permission from Rubio R, Berne RM. Regulation of coronary blood flow. Prog Cardiovasc Dis. 1975; 18:105-122.)*

Table 21-2. Interorgan Variation in Baseline Values for Blood Flow, Oxygen Consumption, Arteriovenous Oxygen Difference, and Oxygen Extraction in the Average Human

ORGAN	BLOOD FLOW (ML/MIN/100 G)	OXYGEN CONSUMPTION (ML/MIN/100 G)	ARTERIOVENOUS O_2 DIFFERENCE (VOL %)	O_2 EXTRAOTION (%)
Left ventricle	80	8	14	70
Brain	55	3	6	30
Liver	55 }	2	6	30
Gastrointestinal tract	40			
Kidneys	400	5	1.3	6.5
Muscles	3	0.16	5	25
Skin	10	0.2	2.5	12.5
Rest of body	3	0.15	4.4	22

Adapted from Folkow B, Neil E. *Circulation*. New York: Oxford University Press; 1971:12.

flow and myocardial oxygen demand, which serves to maintain myocardial PO_2 (and coronary venous PO_2) nearly constant. Adenosine, a breakdown product of ATP, is a potent endogenous vasodilator that is thought to play a central role in metabolic regulation of coronary perfusion. However, other chemical factors also contribute, including carbon dioxide, oxygen, hydrogen ions, and nitric oxide released from the vascular endothelium.

Autoregulation refers to the intrinsic capability of the coronary circulation to maintain a relatively constant coronary blood flow over a wide range of perfusion pressures (about 60-120 mm Hg). This can be due to metabolic and/or myogenic mechanisms. A myogenic response refers to the intrinsic tendency of vascular smooth muscle to contract in response to increased distending pressure and to relax in response to decreased distending pressure. Higher tissue pressures in the subendocardium of the LV wall result in a reduced autoregulatory capability compared with the subepicardium. This contributes to greater vulnerability of that region to infarction during coronary insufficiency.

The coronary arterioles express both α- (constricting) and β_2- (dilating) adrenergic receptors and muscarinic receptors, and are supplied by sympathetic and parasympathetic (vagus) fibers. Stimulation of muscarinic receptors associated with the vascular endothelium causes production of nitric oxide that diffuses to underlying vascular smooth muscle cells, producing smooth muscle relaxation and vasodilation. Autonomic pathways normally play a subordinate role to local metabolic mechanisms in coronary vascular regulation.

Coronary Flow Reserve

Coronary flow reserve is the ratio of maximum coronary blood flow to resting coronary blood flow.[77] Local infusion of a vasodilating drug, such as adenosine or the reactive hyperemic response (the transient increase in blood flow that follows an interval of arterial occlusion), can be used to assess coronary flow reserve (Figure 21-22).[78] The temporal characteristics of the reactive hyperemic response have been explained by metabolites produced in ischemic tissue first dilating the resistance vessels and then washing out during reperfusion. Coronary occlusion of 60 seconds is usually required to maximally dilate the coronary circulation and thus to assess coronary reserve. Longer occlusions only increase the duration of the reactive hyperemic response. Coronary flow reserve in the normal right and left ventricular walls is appreciable (approximately 400%-500%), but is reduced in a variety of conditions, including left ventricular hypertrophy, coronary stenosis, and hemodilution (see Figure 21-22).[78] In the presence of coronary stenosis, dilation of downstream resistance vessels (i.e., recruitment of the coronary flow reserve) tends to maintain coronary blood flow (and myocardial oxygen supply) commensurate with myocardial oxygen demand. Coronary reserve is exhausted when the stenosis reaches about 90%, resulting in a decrease in resting blood flow.[79] Diminished coronary flow reserve renders the myocardium more vulnerable to ischemia secondary to increases in cardiac work or reductions in perfusion pressure. During exercise, turbulence can enhance the decrease in blood flow across a stenosis.

Myocardial Oxygen Demand

The heart is continuously active and normally depends almost exclusively on aerobic metabolism to meet its energy demands. Although the heart constitutes less than 0.5% of body weight, it accounts for about 7% of basal oxygen consumption. The most important determinants of myocardial oxygen demand are contractility, heart rate, and wall tension (Figure 21-23).[80,81] Wall tension is directly proportional to the pressure and radius of the heart and inversely proportional to wall thickness (law of Laplace). The area beneath the LV pressure pulse per minute, the time-tension index, bears a direct relationship to myocardial oxygen consumption. When external work (pressure × stroke volume) is considered, pressure work has a much greater oxygen cost than does flow work. Muscle shortening per se has only a small influence on myocardial oxygen consumption. Basal metabolism reflects ATP-requiring processes not directly related to contraction, such as activity of cell membrane Na,K-ATPase for maintaining the ionic environment, as well as other cellular processes such as protein synthesis. The oxygen cost of

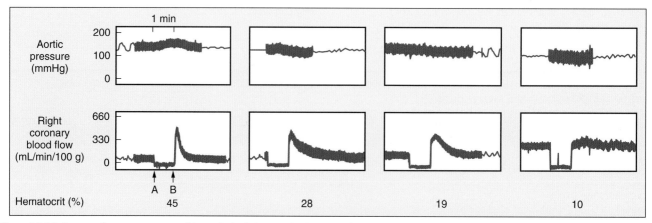

Figure 21-22 Coronary flow reserve assessed by analysis of the reactive hyperemic response in the right coronary circulation of a dog. Graded hemodilution was associated with a progressive diminution of this response. "A," begin occlusion of coronary artery; "B," release occlusion. (Reprinted with permission from Crystal GJ, Kim S-J, Salem MR. Right and left ventricular O_2 uptake during hemodilution and β-adrenergic stimulation. Am J Physiol. 1993;265:H1769-H1777.)

activation comprises two components: (1) electrical activation and (2) release and uptake of Ca^{2+} by the sarcoplasmic reticulum. The RV has a smaller baseline oxygen demand than the LV, consistent with a smaller pressure workload.[78,82]

Impaired Myocardial Oxygen Balance: Mechanisms of Myocardial Ischemia

Oxygen extraction in the LV is nearly maximal at baseline; thus increases in myocardial oxygen consumption are critically dependent upon proportional increases in coronary blood flow via locally produced vasodilating metabolites. If

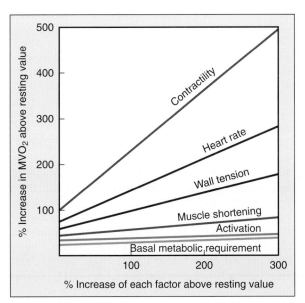

Figure 21-23 Determinants of myocardial oxygen consumption (MVO₂). It is noteworthy that the major determinants, contractility, heart rate, and wall tension, are hemodynamic variables that can be controlled by the anesthesiologist. *(Reprinted with permission from Marcus ML. The Coronary Circulation in Health and Disease. New York: McGraw-Hill; 1983:70.)*

coronary blood flow is insufficient to meet myocardial oxygen demand, compensatory mechanisms can be marshaled to preserve cell viability: an increase in the number of open capillaries, consumption of glycogen stores, and utilization of oxygen bound to tissue myoglobin.[80] However, these compensatory mechanisms are limited and can preserve cell viability in the presence of severe ischemia for only 20 min.[83]

When the vasodilator reserve of the coronary bed is compromised by a proximal stenosis (or by hypoxemia or anemia), the myocardium, especially the subendocardium, becomes vulnerable to ischemia (oxygen demand exceeding oxygen supply). Factors tending to promote this condition are presented in Figure 21-24. An increase in heart rate is detrimental to the oxygen supply/demand balance since it decreases myocardial oxygen supply by decreasing coronary blood flow (via shortening of the diastolic period), while also increasing myocardial oxygen demand. An increase in preload also reduces myocardial oxygen supply (by reducing the pressure gradient for coronary blood flow), and increases myocardial oxygen demand (via an increase in wall tension). An increase in aortic pressure increases myocardial oxygen supply by increasing coronary blood flow, but also increases myocardial oxygen demand via an increase in wall tension; its net effect depends on the balance between these factors. Under conditions of restricted coronary vasodilator reserve, the most favorable hemodynamic situation is characterized by low heart rate and preload, normal aortic pressure, and normal to moderate inotropic state.[84]

EMERGING DEVELOPMENTS

Understanding of cardiovascular physiology from a systems perspective has changed little in recent years. However, there have been substantial advances in the ability to apply these basic concepts at the bedside using minimally or entirely noninvasive technologies. For example, the improved accuracy and ease of use of noninvasive methods for beat-by-beat measurements of blood pressure has permitted evaluations of

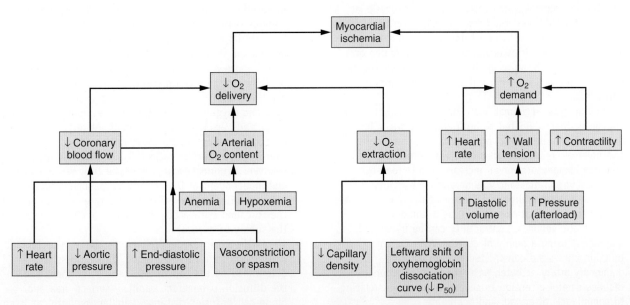

Figure 21-24 Conditions having detrimental influence on myocardial oxygen balance: mechanisms of myocardial ischemia.

autonomic responsiveness, in addition to continuous perioperative monitoring. Recent evidence suggests that loss of autonomic responsiveness due to age or chronic illness can have prognostic value.[85] Furthermore, noninvasive methods to quantify endothelial function have emerged, and data suggest that these assessments have prognostic significance.[86]

Extensive effort has been made toward developing and applying minimally or noninvasive methods for continuous measurement of cardiac output in patients who are not sufficiently compromised to justify the risk associated with insertion of a pulmonary artery catheter.[87] The new technologies to monitor cardiac output have fostered an awareness of the importance of fluid management in optimizing cardiac performance. These technologies also have the potential to provide objective information that can help guide perioperative fluid management and optimize cardiac performance. Studies showing improved outcome when goal-directed fluid administration algorithms are applied have provided the basis for the concept of "fluid responsiveness," which is essentially an assessment of where a patient's heart is in relation to the Starling curve.[88]

Continuous measurements of blood flow combined with measurements of hemoglobin concentration and oxygen saturation make it possible to calculate tissue oxygen delivery. Appreciation of the physiologic significance of this concept has provided the impetus for development of commercially available, noninvasive devices that assess oxygen saturation directly in various tissues, including skeletal muscle and brain, as a means to evaluate whether the circulation is providing sufficient oxygen to meet tissue metabolic demands.[89] Although the accuracy and interpretation of these measurements remain controversial, these devices have demonstrated potential utility and promise.

KEY POINTS

- Tissue blood flow depends on arterial pressure, which is the product of cardiac output and total peripheral resistance, and on local vascular resistance, which is a function of local vasomotor tone.
- The left and right ventricles have important functional and structural differences. These include lower developed pressure and workload, and a thinner wall for the right ventricle. The ventricles demonstrate a high degree of interdependence because of their shared interventricular septum and the restraining influence of the surrounding pericardium.
- Studies in isolated animal heart models show that stroke volume is directly related to both end-diastolic volume or preload (Starling's law) and myocardial contractility, and inversely related to afterload. The normal heart in vivo can compensate for an increase in afterload by increases in end-diastolic volume and contractility.
- A cardiac function curve is a plot of ventricular performance (e.g., stroke volume, as a function of end-diastolic volume). Contractility can be illustrated graphically using a family of curves. When cardiac function curves are constructed in vivo using a pulmonary artery catheter, accurate representation requires careful attention to several assumptions relating to compliance, afterload, and heart rate.

- Ventricular diastole is comprised of four phases: isovolumic relaxation, early rapid filling, diastasis, and atrial systole. Of these phases, only isovolumic relaxation is an active process that requires expenditure of energy by ventricular myocytes. Early rapid filling normally accounts for 80% to 85% of ventricular end-diastolic volume and diastasis and atrial systole provide approximately 3% to 5% and 15% to 25%, respectively.
- Ejection fraction is the most frequently used clinical index of global contractile function. It provides useful information about systolic pump performance, but is heavily influenced by afterload. Other more load-independent indices of contractility are preload recruitable stroke work index (PRSWI) and end-systolic elastance (Ees).
- The most severe drop in blood pressure occurs in the arterioles, hence they are often termed the *resistance vessels*. Arteriole diameter is regulated by the contractile activity of vascular smooth muscle. Variations in arteriolar diameter are an important determinant of local capillary blood flow and hydrostatic pressure.
- Viscosity is the internal friction resulting from intermolecular forces operating within a flowing liquid. Vascular resistance is directly related to blood viscosity and varies with hematocrit. Because of the presence of erythrocytes, blood is a non-Newtonian fluid (i.e., its viscosity increases sharply with reductions in shear rate).
- Hydrostatic pressure (P_{cap}) is normally the major force of filtration across the capillary wall. Oncotic pressure (Π_{cap}) is normally the major force of absorption. The direction and magnitude of capillary bulk flow is essentially a function of the ratio of P_{cap} to Π_{cap}. Under normal conditions, filtration dominates at the arterial end of the capillary, and absorption at the venous end. A small net filtration is usually observed, which is compensated for by lymph flow.
- The cardiovascular reflexes are neural feedback loops that regulate and modulate cardiac function and vascular tone. They are composed of an afferent (sensory) limb, integration in the medulla oblongata of the central nervous system, and an efferent (motor) limb.
- The arterial baroreceptor reflex is a primary homeostatic mechanism that maintains arterial blood pressure within narrow limits based on feedback from high-pressure stretch receptors in the aortic arch and carotid sinus.
- Systemic oxygen delivery (DO_2) is the product of cardiac output and arterial oxygen content. At rest, DO_2 greatly exceeds systemic oxygen consumption (VO_2), and thus the oxygen extraction ratio (EO_2) is relatively modest (~25%). At normal or high levels of DO_2, VO_2 is constant and independent of DO_2. As DO_2 is gradually reduced, increased EO_2 maintains VO_2 until a threshold is reached, the so-called critical DO_2, below which VO_2 is limited by the supply of oxygen.
- The final step in oxygen delivery to tissue mitochondria is diffusion from capillary blood. This process is determined by the capillary-to-cell PO_2 gradient and the diffusion parameters, capillary surface area and blood-cell diffusion distance. Capillary recruitment is an

important mechanism for maintaining tissue PO_2 at the level required for unimpaired oxidative metabolism.

- In a clinical setting, there are several methods to measure systemic VO_2: (1) oxygen loss or replacement into a closed breathing system, (2) the difference between expired and inspired volume of oxygen, and (3) use of the Fick principle, the most commonly used method. The oxygen extraction ratio (EO_2), defined as the arteriovenous oxygen difference divided by arterial oxygen content, reflects the balance between oxygen demand and delivery.

- In the left coronary circulation, extravascular compressive forces during systole (due to a high developed intracavitary pressure) result in blood flow occurring predominantly during diastole. The pressure gradient for blood flow in the left ventricular wall is approximated by the difference between aortic diastolic pressure and left ventricular end-diastolic pressure.

- Metabolic mechanisms coupling coronary blood flow to myocardial oxygen demand normally predominate in control of coronary vascular resistance, although parasympathetic (vasodilator) and sympathetic (vasoconstrictor) effects also play a role.

- Coronary flow reserve, the ratio of maximum coronary blood flow to resting coronary blood flow, is appreciable in the normal right and left ventricular walls (approximately 400% to 500%), but is reduced in a variety of conditions, including left ventricular hypertrophy, hemodilution, and coronary stenosis. Coronary reserve is exhausted when the stenosis reaches approximately 90%, resulting in a decrease in resting blood flow.

- The most important determinants of myocardial oxygen demand are contractility, heart rate, and wall tension. Wall tension is directly proportional to the pressure and radius of the heart and inversely proportional to wall thickness (Law of Laplace). When external work (pressure x stroke volume) is considered, pressure work has a much greater oxygen cost than does flow work.

- Oxygen extraction by the left ventricle is nearly maximal at baseline; thus increases in myocardial oxygen consumption critically depend on proportional increases in coronary blood flow via locally-produced vasodilating factors. When the vasodilator reserve of the coronary bed is compromised, for example, by a proximal stenosis, the myocardium becomes vulnerable to ischemia (oxygen demand > oxygen supply). With reduced coronary reserve, increases in heart rate and preload are detrimental, in that both these factors reduce oxygen supply (coronary blood flow) while increasing oxygen demand. An increase in aortic pressure augments myocardial oxygen supply by increasing blood flow, but it also increases myocardial oxygen demand by increasing wall tension.

Key References

Bradley AJ, Alpert JS. Coronary flow reserve. *Am Heart J.* 1991;122:1116-1128. Well-written discussion of the concept of coronary flow reserve: its physiologic underpinnings, measurement, and alterations by disease processes. (Ref. 77).

Braunwald E, Ross J, Jr, Sonnenblick EH. Control of myocardial oxygen consumption: physiologic and clinical considerations. *Am J Cardiol.* 1971;27:416-432. A classic paper summarizing the findings obtained in animal models describing factors regulating myocardial oxygen consumption. (Ref. 4).

Brutsaert DL, Sys SU. Relaxation and diastole of the heart. *Physiol Rev.* 1989;69:1228-1315. A critical assessment of the literature relating to events during diastole, the relaxation phase of the cardiac cycle in the normal heart as well in pathophysiologic scenarios. (Ref. 9).

Burkhoff D, Mirsky I, Suga H. Assessment of systolic and diastolic ventricular properties via pressure-volume analysis: a guide for clinical, translational, and basic researchers. *Am J Physiol Heart Circ Physiol.* 2005;289:H501-H512. A discussion of the use of pressure-volume analysis to assess the systolic and diastolic properties of the ventricle. The paper provides the theoretical basis of pressure-volume analysis and also practical information and simple guidelines for application and interpretation of pressure-volume data in preclinical and clinical studies. (Ref. 21).

Honig CR. *Modern Cardiovascular Physiology.* Boston: Little, Brown; 1981. A classic textbook covering a broad range of topics in cardiovascular physiology. It is distinguished by its attention to clinical applications of physiologic principles, and by its reliance on two themes: the concept of margin of safety or reserve of function and a systems-oriented approach. (Ref. 55).

Mebazaa A, Karpati P, Renaud E, Algotsson L. Acute right ventricular failure—from pathophysiology to new treatments. *Intensive Care Med.* 2004;30:185-196. A succinct and informative summary of right ventricular function under normal and pathophysiologic conditions. (Ref. 3).

Schumacker PT, Cain SM. The concept of a critical oxygen delivery. *Intensive Care Med.* 1987;13:223-229. Discusses the determinants of systemic oxygen delivery (DO_2) and how increases in oxygen extraction normally compensate for decreases in DO_2 to maintain oxygen consumption constant until a critical threshold is reached, the so-called critical oxygen delivery under normal and various pathologic conditions. (Ref. 71).

Summerhill EM, Baram M. Principles of pulmonary artery catheterization in the critically ill. *Lung.* 2005;183:209-219. Describes the indications, uses, limitations, and pitfalls in the use of the balloon-tipped pulmonary artery catheter to assess cardiac function and to guide fluid and vasoactive drug therapy in the care of critically ill patients. (Ref. 16).

References

1. Rothe CF. Cardiodynamics. In: Selkurt EE, ed. *Physiology.* Boston: Little, Brown; 1971:321-344.
2. Guarracino F, Cariello C, Danella A, et al. Right ventricular failure: physiology and assessment. *Minerva Anesthesiol.* 2005;71:307-312.
3. Mebazaa A, Karpati P, Renaud E, Algotsson L. Acute right ventricular failure—from pathophysiology to new treatments. *Intensive Care Med.* 2004;30:185-196.
4. Braunwald E, Ross J, Jr, Sonnenblick EH. *Mechanisms of Contraction of the Normal and Failing Heart.* Boston: Little, Brown; 1968:72-91, 269-291.
5. Lang RM, Borow KM, Neumann A, Janzen D. Systemic vascular resistance: an unreliable index of left ventricular afterload. *Circulation.* 1986;74:1114-1123.
6. Sagawa K. Analysis of the ventricular pumping capacity as function of input and output pressure loads. In: Reeve EB, Guyton AC, eds. *Physical Bases of Circulatory Transport: Regulation and Exchange.* Philadelphia: WB Saunders; 1967.
7. Cohn JN, Franciosa JA. Vasodilator therapy of cardiac failure. *N Engl J Med.* 1977;297:27-31.
8. Wiggers CJ. Studies on the duration of the consecutive phases of the cardiac cycle. I. The duration of the consecutive phases of the cardiac cycle and criteria for the precise determination. *Am J Physiol.* 1921; 56:415-438.
9. Brutsaert DL, Sys SU. Relaxation and diastole of the heart. *Physiol Rev.* 1989;69:1228-1315.

10. Zile MR, Brutsaert DL. New concepts in diastolic dysfunction and diastolic heart failure: Part I: diagnosis, prognosis, and measurements of diastolic function. *Circulation.* 2002;105:1387-1393.

11. Gibson DG, Francis DP. Clinical assessment of left ventricular diastolic function. *Heart.* 2003;89:231-238.

12. Villars PS, Hamlin SK, Shaw AD, Kanusky JT. Role of diastole in left ventricular function, I: Biochemical and biomechanical events. *Am J Crit Care.* 2004;13:394-405.

13. Scheinman MM, Abbott JA, Rapaport E. Clinical uses of a flow-directed right heart catheter. *Arch Intern Med.* 1969;124:19-24.

14. Swan HJ, Ganz W, Forrester J, Marcus H, Diamond G, Chonette D. Catheterization of the heart in man with use of a flow-directed balloon-tipped catheter. *N Engl J Med.* 1970;283:447-451.

15. Chatterjee K. The Swan-Ganz catheters: past, present, and future. A viewpoint. *Circulation.* 2009;119:147-152.

16. Summerhill EM, Baram M. Principles of pulmonary artery catheterization in the critically ill. *Lung.* 2005;183:209-219.

17. Mason DT. Usefulness and limitations of the rate of rise of intraventricular pressure (dp-dt) in the evaluation of myocardial contractility in man. *Am J Cardiol.* 1969;23:516-527.

18. Gleason WL, Braunwald E. Studies on the first derivative of the ventricular pressure pulse in man. *J Clin Invest.* 1962;41:80-91.

19. Schertel ER. Assessment of left-ventricular function. *Thorac Cardiovasc Surg.* 1998;46(Suppl 2):248-254.

20. Frank O. Zur Dynamic des Herzmuskels. *Z Biol.* 1895;32:370-447.

21. Burkhoff D, Mirsky I, Suga H. Assessment of systolic and diastolic ventricular properties via pressure-volume analysis: a guide for clinical, translational, and basic researchers. *Am J Physiol Heart Circ Physiol.* 2005;289:H501-H512.

22. Suga H, Sagawa K, Shoukas AA. Load independence of the instantaneous pressure-volume ratio of the canine left ventricle and effects of epinephrine and heart rate on the ratio. *Circ Res.* 1973;32:314-322.

23 Fortuin NJ, Pawsey CG. The evaluation of left ventricular function by echocardiography. *Am J Med.* 1977;63:1-9.

24. Dodge HT, Sandler H, Ballew DW, Lord JD, Jr. The use of biplane angiocardiography for the measurement of left ventricular volume in man. *Am Heart J.* 1960;60:762-776.

25. Redington AN, Gray HH, Hodson ME, Rigby ML, Oldershaw PJ. Characterisation of the normal right ventricular pressure-volume relation by biplane angiography and simultaneous micromanometer pressure measurements. *Br Heart J.* 1988;59:23-30.

26. Redington AN, Rigby ML, Shinebourne EA, Oldershaw PJ. Changes in the pressure-volume relation of the right ventricle when its loading conditions are modified. *Br Heart J.* 1990;63:45-49.

27. Folkow B, Neil E. *Circulation.* New York: Oxford University Press; 1971:6.

28. Salem MR, Crystal GJ. Pulmonary vascular tone and the anesthesiologist. *Middle East J Anesthesiol.* 2011;21:147-151.

29. Messmer K. Hemodilution. *Surg Clin N Am.* 1975;55:662.

30. Messmer K, Sunder-Plassman L. Hemodilution. *Prog Surg.* 1974;12:208.

31. Feigl EO. Physics of the cardiovascular system. In: Ruch TC, Patton HD, eds. *Physiology and Biophysics II: Circulation, Respiration, and Fluid Balance.* Philadelphia: WB Saunders; 1974:10-22.

32. Berne RM, Levy MN. *Principles of Physiology.* St. Louis: CV Mosby; 1990:195.

33. Friedman JJ. Microcirculation. In: Selkurt EE, ed. *Physiology.* Boston: Little, Brown; 1971:269.

34. Crystal GJ, Salem MR. The Bainbridge and the "reverse" Bainbridge reflexes: history, physiology, and clinical relevance. *Anesth Analg.* 2012;114:520-532.

35. Sagawa K. Baroreflex control of systemic arterial pressure and vascular bed, handbook of physiology. The cardiovascular system. Peripheral circulation and organ blood flow. *Am Physiol Soc.* 1983:453-496.

36. Dampney RA. Functional organization of central pathways regulating the cardiovascular system. *Physiol Rev.* 1994;74:323-364.

37. Rushmer RF. *Cardiovascular Dynamics.* 3rd ed. Philadelphia: Saunders; 1970:165.

38. Aviado DM, Guevara Aviado D. The Bezold-Jarisch reflex. A historical perspective of cardiopulmonary reflexes. *Ann N Y Acad Sci.* 2001;940:48-58.

39. Campagna JA, Carter C. Clinical relevance of the Bezold-Jarisch reflex. *Anesthesiology.* 2003;98:1250-1260.

40. Bezold AV, Hirt L. Uber die physiologischen Wirkungen des essigsauren Veratrine. *Unters Physiol Lab Wurzburg.* 1867;1:75-156.

41. Jarisch A, Richter H. Die afferenten bahnen des veratrine effektes in den herznerven. *Arch Exp Pathol Pharmacol.* 1939;193:355-371.

42. Jarisch A, Richter H. Die kreislauf des veratrins. *Arch Exp Pathol Pharmacol.* 1939;193:347-354.

43. Thoren PN. Characteristics of left ventricular receptors with non-medullated vagal afferents in cats. *Circ Res.* 1977;40:415-421.

44. Mark AL. The Bezold-Jarisch reflex revisited: clinical implications of inhibitory reflexes originating in the heart. *J Am Coll Cardiol.* 1983; 1:90-102.

45. Secher NH, Sander Jensen K, Werner C, Warberg J, Bie P. Bradycardia during severe but reversible hypovolemic shock in man. *Circ Shock.* 1984;14:267-274.

46. Secher NH, Jacobsen J, Friedman DB, Matzen S. Bradycardia during reversible hypovolaemic shock: associated neural reflex mechanisms and clinical implications. *Clin Exp Pharmacol Physiol.* 1992;19:733-743.

47. Oberg B, White S. The role of vagal cardiac nerves and arterial baroreceptors in the circulatory adjustments to hemorrhage in the cat. *Acta Physiol Scand.* 1970;80:395-403.

48. Oberg B, Thoren P. Increased activity in left ventricular receptors during hemorrhage or occlusion of caval veins in the cat. A possible cause of the vaso-vagal reaction. *Acta Physiol Scand.* 1972;85:164-173.

49. Bainbridge FA. The influence of venous filling upon the rate of the heart. *J Physiol.* 1915;50:65-84.

50. Goetz KL. Effect of increased pressure within a right heart cul-de-sac on heart rate in dogs. *Am J Physiol.* 1965;209:507-512.

51. Ledsome JR, Linden RJ. The effect of distending a pouch of the left atrium on the heart rate. *J Physiol.* 1967;193:121-129.

52. Boettcher DH, Zimpfer M, Vatner SF. Phylogenesis of the Bainbridge reflex. *Am J Physiol.* 1982;242:R244-R246.

53. Coleridge JC, Linden RJ. The effect of intravenous infusions upon the heart rate of the anaesthetized dog. *J Physiol.* 1955;128:310-319.

54. Nunn JF. *Nunn's Applied Respiratory Physiology.* Oxford: Butterworth Heinemann; 1993:255.

55. Honig CR. *Modern Cardiovascular Physiology.* Boston: Little, Brown; 1981:181-187.

56. West JB. *Respiratory Physiology: The Essentials.* Baltimore: Williams & Wilkins; 1974.

57. Weibel ER. *The Pathway for Oxygen.* Cambridge, Mass: Harvard University Press; 1984:149.

58. Krogh A. The number and distribution of capillaries in muscles with calculations of the oxygen pressure head necessary for supplying the tissue. *J Physiol.* 1919;52:409-415.

59. Kety SS. Determinants of tissue oxygen tension. *Fed Proc.* 1957;16:666-671.

60. Crystal GJ, Weiss HR. VO_2 of resting muscle during arterial hypoxia: role of reflex vasoconstriction. *Microvasc Res.* 1980;20:30-40.

61. Crystal GJ, Downey HF, Bashour FA. Small vessel and total coronary blood volume during intracoronary adenosine. *Am J Physiol.* 1981;241:H194-H201.

62. Tenney SM. A theoretical analysis of the relationship between venous blood and mean tissue oxygen pressures. *Respir Physiol.* 1974;20:283-296.

63. Nunn JF, Makita K, Royston B. Validation of oxygen consumption measurements during artificial ventilation. *J Appl Physiol.* 1989;67:2129-2134.

64. Makita K, Nunn JF, Royston B. Evaluation of metabolic measuring instruments for use in critically ill patients. *Crit Care Med.* 1990;18:638-644.

65. Smithies MN, Royston B, Makita K, Konieczko K, Nunn JF. Comparison of oxygen consumption measurements: indirect calorimetry versus the reversed Fick method. *Crit Care Med.* 1991;19:1401-1406.

66. Webster NR, Nunn JF. Molecular structure of free radicals and their importance in biological reactions. *Br J Anaesth.* 1988;60:98-108.

67. Astiz ME, Rackow EC, Kaufman B, Falk JL, Weil MH. Relationship of oxygen delivery and mixed venous oxygenation to lactic acidosis in patients with sepsis and acute myocardial infarction. *Crit Care Med.* 1988;16:655-658.

68. Pinsky MR. Assessment of adequacy of oxygen transport in the critically ill. *Appl Cardiopulm Pathophysiol.* 1990;3:271-278.

69. Levy PS, Chavez RP, Crystal GJ, et al. Oxygen extraction ratio: a valid indicator of transfusion need in limited coronary vascular reserve? *J Trauma.* 1992;32:769-774.

70. Barcroft J. On anoxaemia. *Lancet.* 1920;196:485-489.

71. Schumacker PT, Cain SM. The concept of a critical oxygen delivery. *Intensive Care Med.* 1987;13:223-229.

72. Cain SM. Oxygen delivery and uptake in dogs during anemic and hypoxic hypoxia. *J Appl Physiol.* 1977;42:228-234.

73. Shibutani K, Komatsu T, Kubal K, Sanchala V, Kumar V, Bizzarri DV. Critical level of oxygen delivery in anesthetized man. *Crit Care Med.* 1983;11:640-643.

74. Danek SJ, Lynch JP, Weg JG, Dantzker DR. The dependence of oxygen uptake on oxygen delivery in the adult respiratory distress syndrome. *Am Rev Respir Dis.* 1980;122:387-395.

75. Mohsenifar Z, Goldbach P, Tashkin DP, Campisi DJ. Relationship between O_2 delivery and O_2 consumption in the adult respiratory distress syndrome. *Chest.* 1983;84:267-271.

76. Rubio R, Berne RM. Regulation of coronary blood flow. *Prog Cardiovasc Dis.* 1975;18:105-122.

77. Bradley AJ, Alpert JS. Coronary flow reserve. *Am Heart J.* 1991;122:1116-1128.

78. Crystal GJ, Kim SJ, Salem MR. Right and left ventricular O_2 uptake during hemodilution and beta-adrenergic stimulation. *Am J Physiol.* 1993;265: H1769-H1777.

79. Gould KL, Lipscomb K. Effects of coronary stenoses on coronary flow reserve and resistance. *Am J Cardiol.* 1974;34:48-55.

80. Marcus ML. *The Coronary Circulation in Health and Disease.* New York: McGraw-Hill; 1983.

81. Braumwald E. Control of myocardial oxygen consumption: physiologic and clinical considerations. *Am J Cardiol.* 1971;27:416-432.

82. Kusachi S, Nishiyama O, Yasuhara K, Saito D, Haraoka S, Nagashima H. Right and left ventricular oxygen metabolism in open-chest dogs. *Am J Physiol.* 1982;243: H761-H766.

83. Jennings RB, Sommers HM, Smyth GA, Flack HA, Linn H. Myocardial necrosis induced by temporary occlusion of a coronary artery in the dog. *Arch Pathol.* 1960;70:68-78.

84. Hug CC Jr, Shanewise JS. In Miller RD, ed. *Anesthesia for Adult Cardiac Surgery. Anesthesia.* Churchill Livingstone; 1994:1757-1809.

85. Deschamps A, Denault A. Autonomic nervous system and cardiovascular disease. *Semin Cardiothorac Vasc Anesth.* 2009;13:99-105.

86. Hamburg NM, Benjamin EJ. Assessment of endothelial function using digital pulse amplitude tonometry. *Trends Cardiovasc Med.* 2009;19:6-11.

87. Funk DJ, Moretti EW, Gan TJ. Minimally invasive cardiac output monitoring in the perioperative setting. *Anesth Analg.* 2009;108: 887-897.

88. Wakeling HG, McFall MR, Jenkins CS, et al. Intraoperative oesophageal Doppler guided fluid management shortens postoperative hospital stay after major bowel surgery. *Brit J Anaesth.* 2005;95:634-642.

89. Krite Svanberg E, Wollmer P, Andersson-Engels S, Akeson J. Physiological influence of basic pertubations of assessed by non-invasive optical techniques in humans. *Appl Physiol Nutr Metab.* 2011;36: 946-957.

Chapter 22

VASOPRESSORS AND INOTROPES

Josh Zimmerman and Michael Cahalan

This chapter reviews the pharmacology of vasopressors and inotropes used commonly in acute care settings as well as comparable new drugs with promising clinical potential. It focuses on the pharmacodynamic properties of the drugs to a greater degree than their pharmacokinetic properties because most of these drugs have short half-lives, are administered by continuous infusion, and are titrated to clinical effect.

Relying on landmark studies from the past as well as recent findings, this chapter seeks to build the scientific foundation upon which the clinical use of these agents is based. Because their application to human pharmacology is unreliable, data derived exclusively from animal studies are not considered. Even when considering only human data, the effects of vasopressors and inotropes vary substantially due to patient factors. Clinicians know that when treating patients experiencing severe hypotension or cardiac failure, the effects of vasopressors and cardiotonic drugs depend on many associated factors including acid-base status, temperature, blood volume, and concomitant drug administration.[1]

HISTORICAL PERSPECTIVE

Vasoactive drugs have an extensive history and have been in clinical use for millennia. The early identification and isolation of vasoactive substances was based on extraction from plants and endocrine glands. For instance, ephedrine has been in clinical use as a diaphoretic and circulatory stimulant for more than 5000 years as the active component of the Chinese drug ma huang. Until the drug was finally isolated in 1887, it was extracted from the plant *Ephedra sinica*.[2]

Likewise foxglove had been in use for hundreds of years; William Withering published his historic book *An Account of the Foxglove, and Some of Its Medical Uses* in 1785.[3] This text detailed Withering's work with extracts of the plant *Digitalis purpurea* and described effects and side effects of the drugs now known as *digoxin* and *digitoxin*.

In the late 17th century, it was recognized that "an extract of the suprarenal glands caused contraction of the arteries and led to an increase in the beat of the auricles and ventricles," and that an extract of the pituitary gland possessed vasopressor activity. These substances would eventually be named *epinephrine* and *vasopressin*.[4,5]

While early medicinal chemistry work focused on developing progressively purer isolates of the active substances from natural sources, it eventually shifted to synthesizing drugs chemically. Dopamine was first synthesized in 1910 by Barger and Ewins, who immediately recognized its potency as a vasopressor.[6,7] Vasopressin was the first polypeptide hormone successfully synthesized, for which du Vigneaud won the Nobel Prize for Chemistry in 1955. Work by von Euler confirmed that norepinephrine helped mediate the activity of the sympathetic nervous system and contributed to his 1970 Nobel Prize.[8]

In the modern era, attempts were made to develop drugs with specific characteristics. Dobutamine was synthesized in the early 1970s for the specific purpose of providing a high level of inotropy without the vasodilatory limitations of isoproterenol.[9] Similarly, milrinone was developed in the early 1980s as an alternative to amrinone without the high incidence of fever and thrombocytopenia that limited the utility of amrinone.

The development of novel vasopressors and inotropes continues to this day. Levosimendan, for instance, entered clinical use in Europe as recently as 2000.

STRUCTURE-ACTIVITY RELATIONSHIPS

Many of the drugs in this chapter share structural similarities that affect their pharmacologic actions, although a few are chemically unrelated (Figure 22-1). Many sympathomimetics are derived from the parent compound β-phenylethylamine. Many of these drugs are also referred to as *catecholamines* due to the presence of hydroxyl substitutions on carbons 3 and 4 of the benzene ring of β-phenylethylamine. The most basic example of a catecholamine is dopamine, which is the 3,4-hydroxyl substituted form of β–phenylethylamine. It is the metabolic precursor to both norepinephrine and epinephrine as the substrate for dopamine β-hydroxylase. The addition of an N-substitution increases the activity at β-adrenergic receptors. Norepinephrine, like epinephrine, is derived from β-phenylethylamine, but the lack of N-substitution decreases its activity at the β receptors. The impact of the degree of amino substitution on β receptor activity is further reflected in the structures of isoproterenol and dobutamine. Both of these drugs have bulky side chains and as such have a high degree of β specificity.

Phenylephrine and ephedrine are not considered catecholamines, in that they are not hydroxylated on both the 3 and 4 carbons of their benzene ring (phenylephrine has a single substitution and ephedrine has none). This lack of hydroxylation prevents phenylephrine from effectively binding the β receptor despite the N-methyl substitution. Ephedrine's lack of hydroxylation substantially decreases its ability to stimulate directly adrenergic receptors. The presence of a methyl group on the α carbon of ephedrine blocks oxidation by monoamine oxidase and prolongs its action.

Milrinone, vasopressin, and levosimendan neither share structural similarities with the sympathomimetic drugs discussed, nor with one another. Milrinone is a bipyridine methyl carbonitryl derivative of amrinone. Vasopressin, as a nonapeptide hormone, consists of a sequence of nine amino acids (Cys-Tyr-Phe-Gln-Asn-Cys-Pro-Arg-Gly) while levosimendan is a pyridazone-dinitrile derivative.[10]

MECHANISMS

Although the drugs discussed in this chapter are applied in similar clinical settings, they do not all share a pharmacologic class or mechanism. They are perhaps best classified and considered based on their mechanism for increasing inotropy and vasoconstriction (see Chapter 20). Although the drugs that increase inotropy do so by different mechanisms, the common endpoint is positively influencing the interaction of Ca^{2+} with actin and myosin in the cardiac myocyte (Figure 22-2). Each of the β-agonists, phosphodiesterase inhibitors, cardiac glycosides, and calcium sensitizers accomplishes this in a different way.

Drugs that act on the β_1 receptor (such as epinephrine, dobutamine, dopamine, isoproterenol, and to a lesser extent ephedrine and norepinephrine) begin by stimulating the receptor on the cardiac myocyte sarcolemma with subsequent activation of the Gs protein. This protein activates adenylyl cyclase and enhances the formation of cyclic AMP (cAMP), which activates protein kinase A, thereby phosphorylating and increasing the open probability of voltage-gated Ca^{2+} channels. These channels allow Ca^{2+} influx to increase cytosolic Ca^{2+} concentration, which activates the coupling of actin and myosin in the myocyte. Protein kinase A also activates a Ca^{2+}-ATPase on the sarcoplasmic reticulum, leading to increased Ca^{2+} uptake in diastole and improved lusitropic function.

The inotropic effects of phosphodiesterase inhibitors (e.g., milrinone), like those of the adrenergic agonists, are mediated by cAMP. Unlike adrenergic agonists that increase cAMP by stimulating adenylyl cyclase, milrinone inhibits the breakdown of cAMP by phosphodiesterase type III (PDE3). Increased cAMP enhances Ca^{2+} release from the sarcoplasmic reticulum and increases the force generated by actin-myosin. The vasodilatory action of milrinone is also cAMP mediated. In vascular smooth muscle, cAMP inhibits myosin light chain kinase, the enzyme responsible for phosphorylating myosin light chains and causing smooth muscle contraction. Inhibition of PDE3 increases cAMP, thereby promoting vascular smooth muscle relaxation.

Digoxin increases cytosolic Ca^{2+} by inhibiting the action of a Na^+,K^+-ATPase on the cell membrane of cardiac myocytes. This leads to an increase in cytosolic Na^+, thereby decreasing the activity of Na^+-Ca^{2+} exchange and indirectly resulting in an increase in intracellular Ca^{2+} available to interact with actin and myosin.

Levosimendan, referred to as a *calcium sensitizer*, has a mechanism that is fundamentally different from the other inotropes discussed herein. Rather than increasing the content of intracellular Ca^{2+}, it acts to modulate the interaction of Ca^{2+}. It first binds the N-terminal lobe of cardiac troponin C (TnC), thereby stabilizing the Ca^{2+}-bound form of the protein. This serves to prolong the systolic interaction between actin and myosin and increase the force of contraction. Because binding of levosimendan to TnC is dependent on cytosolic Ca^{2+} concentration, it occurs almost exclusively during systole, leaving diastolic function relatively unaffected. Importantly, unlike other drugs discussed in this chapter, the increased inotropy is achieved without an increase in myocardial oxygen demand.[11]

The majority of drugs discussed herein exert their vasoconstrictive actions via α_1 receptors in the vasculature; the

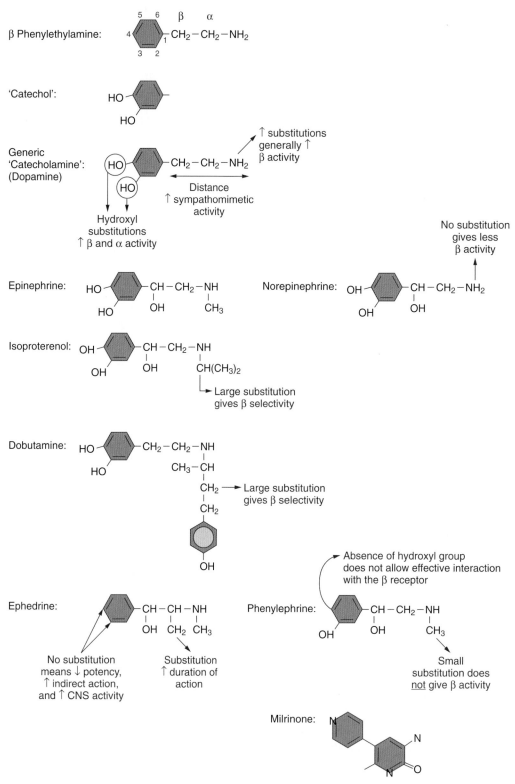

Figure 22-1 The chemical structures of selected sympathomimetic agents. Most are chemically related as catecholamines. Milrinone is a notable exception.

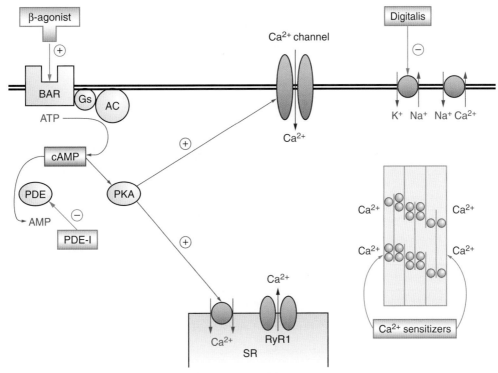

Figure 22-2 Mechanisms of action of selected positive inotropes indicating where the agents act in a cardiomyocyte. Ultimately cytosolic Ca^{2+} and its interaction with the actin-myosin complex causes myocyte contraction. The β-agonists and phosphodiesterase inhibitors accomplish this by increasing the activity of protein kinase A. The calcium sensitizers act directly by increasing Ca^{2+} affinity for troponin C at the actin-myosin complex. Digitalis compounds inhibit the Na^+, K^+-ATPase (Na^+ pump) indirectly increasing intracellular Ca^{2+}. *AC*, Adenylyl cyclase; *BAR*, β adrenergic receptor; *cAMP*, cyclic adenosine monophosphate; *PDE*, phosphodiesterase; *PDE-I*, phosphodiesterase inhibitor; *PKA*, protein kinase A; *SR*, sarcoplasmic reticulum.

exception is vasopressin that acts on the V1 receptor. Stimulation of α_1 or V1 receptors on vascular smooth muscle act (via separate G proteins) to stimulate phospholipase C (PLC), which hydrolyzes phosphatidylinositol bisphosphate (PIP_2) to generate inositol trisphosphate (IP_3) and diacylglycerol (DAG). IP_3 increases Ca^{2+} release from the sarcoplasmic reticulum, while DAG activates protein kinase C to increase Ca^{2+} influx via voltage-gated Ca^{2+} channels. This increase in cytosolic Ca^{2+} increases vascular smooth muscle tone.[12-14]

METABOLISM AND PHARMACOKINETICS

Vasopressors and inotropes generally have short half-lives and are rapidly metabolized, are administered by continuous infusion, and are titrated to clinical effect. This means that for practical purposes these drugs are pharmacokinetic equals; thus pharmacokinetic factors do not typically play an important role in rational drug selection of a specific inotrope or vasopressor. In general, these drugs exert their effects with an ongoing infusion; the effects rapidly decrease once the infusion is terminated. Levosimendan is a notable exception to this general rule.

The catecholamine class of drugs, which includes epinephrine, norepinephrine, dopamine, dobutamine, and isoproterenol, are all rapidly inactivated by methylation of a hydroxyl group of the catechol structure by catechol-*O*-methyltransferase (COMT). In addition, monoamine oxidase (MAO) catalyzes oxidative deamination of this group of compounds (with the exception of dobutamine). Approximately 25% of

dopamine is converted to norepinephrine in adrenergic nerve terminals; these nerve terminals also take up norepinephrine. Even though phenylephrine is not a catecholamine, it is nonetheless metabolized by MAO. Ephedrine and milrinone largely resist metabolism and are excreted in the urine, whereas vasopressin is metabolized by specific vasopressinases in the liver and kidney.

Levosimendan is unique in this group of drugs, in that it is metabolized to active compounds that are eliminated slowly. This results in clinical effects for up to a week after discontinuation of an infusion.[15]

PHARMACODYNAMICS AND DRUG INTERACTIONS

The pharmacodynamic profile of specific inotropes and vasopressors are a function of their relative receptor activities and mechanisms; an overview of receptor activities and physiologic effects is presented in Table 22-1. Adrenergic receptors have traditionally been divided into α and β, and have been subdivided into α_1, α_2, β_1, β_2, and β_3. Further subtyping has been performed, and several genetic variations have been described (see Pharmacogenetics).

The predominant location of α_1 receptors is on peripheral vasculature; stimulation results in vasoconstriction of the skin, muscles, and renal and mesenteric vasculature. There is some contribution of peripheral α_2 receptors to vasoconstriction, but agonism of α_2 receptors is not a major characteristic of drugs discussed here (for pharmacology of α_2 agonists, see Chapter 9).

Table 22-1. Receptor Activity and Physiologic Effects of Vasopressors and Inotropes

DRUG	α RECEPTOR	β₁ RECEPTOR	β₂ RECEPTOR	CARDIAC OUTPUT	HEART RATE	SVR	MAP	PVR
Epinephrine	++	++	++	↑	↑	↑	↑	0
Isoproterenol	0	+++	+++	↑	↑	↓	↓	0
Norepinephrine	+++	++	0	0	0	↑	↑	↑
Dopamine	++	++	0	↑	↑	↑	↑	0
Dobutamine	0	+++	+	↑	↑	↓	↓	↓
Milrinone	0	0	0	↑	0	↓	↓	↓
Phenylephrine	+++	0	0	0	↓	↑	↑	↑
Vasopressin	0	0	0	0	0	↑	↑	0
Ephedrine	+	+	+	↑	↑	↑	↑	0
Levosimendan	0	0	0	↑	0	↓	↓	↓

Effects vary significantly with dose and between individuals.
Increasing levels of stimulation of adrenergic receptors are represented by +, ++, +++.
MAP, Mean arterial pressure; *PVR*, pulmonary vascular resistance; *SVR*, systemic vascular resistance.

Table 22-2. Application, Dosing, and Interactions of Vasopressors and Inotropes

DRUG	DRUG OF CHOICE	BOLUS DOSE	INFUSION DOSE	RELEVANT DRUG INTERACTIONS
Epinephrine	Anaphylaxis; cardiac arrest	5-10 μg, up to 1 mg for cardiac arrest	0.02-0.3 μg/kg/min	Beta-blockers, MAO-I, pro-arrhythmic medications
Isoproterenol	Refractory bradycardia	No bolus dosing	0.01-0.2 μg/kg/min	No co-infusion with alkaline medications
Norepinephrine	Septic shock	No bolus dosing	0.05-0.5 μ/kg/min	MAO-I, TCA
Dopamine	Septic shock with systolic dysfunction	No bolus dosing	1-20 μg/kg/min	MAO-I, TCA, butyrophenones, phenothiazines, phenytoin
Dobutamine	Stress echocardiography	No bolus dosing	2-20 μg/kg/min	Co-administration with alkaline solutions can decrease activity
Milrinone	Weaning from cardiopulmonary bypass	Loading dose: 20-50 μg/kg over 10	0.2-0.75 μg/kg/min	Can precipitate with furosemide
Phenylephrine	Mild hypotension from general or regional anesthesia	50-200 μg	20-200 μg/min	MAO-I, TCA
Vasopressin	Post-cardiopulmonary bypass vasoplegia	0.5-2 units for mild hypotension, 20 units	0.1-0.4 μ/min	Carbamazapine, TCA, norepinephrine, lithium, heparin
Ephedrine	Mild hypotension from general or regional anesthesia	5-10 mg	No infusion dosing	MAO-I, TCA
Levosimendan	Unclear at this time	Loading dose: 12 μg/kg over 10 min	0.05-0.2 μg/kg/min	None yet identified

MAO-I, Monoamine oxidase inhibitors; *TCA*, tricyclic antidepressants; *SVR*, systemic vascular resistance; *MAP*, mean arterial pressure; *PVR*, pulmonary vascular resistance.

β₁ receptors are primarily located in the heart, where their stimulation results in increased inotropy, chronotropy, and lusitropy. β₂ receptors are widely distributed through the vasculature. Stimulation in peripheral vasculature results in dilation of muscular, splanchnic, and renal vessels. Bronchial smooth muscle has a high concentration of β₂ receptors, the activation of which causes bronchodilation. Additional effects include stimulation of glycogenolysis in the liver and a slowing of peristalsis. The β₃ receptor has been known for years to exist in adipose tissue, where its stimulation results in lipolysis. Its existence in the heart has been more recently recognized, and its role in normal physiology and disease, as well as the pharmacologic implications, is still being investigated. Current thinking suggests that β₃ receptor agonism in the heart causes a decrease in inotropy.

There is a potential interaction between monoamine oxidase inhibitors (MAOI) or tricyclic antidepressants (TCA) and several inotropes and vasopressors (Table 22-2.) Because MAO contributes to the metabolism of norepinephrine and TCAs inhibit its reuptake, patients taking either drug can have an exaggerated hypertensive response to norepinephrine, drugs that enhance norepinephrine release (ephedrine and dopamine), and drugs that are metabolized by MAO. This adverse pharmacokinetic drug interaction can have important implications in the perioperative and intensive care settings.

PHARMACOGENETICS

Although basic knowledge of the α and β adrenergic receptors forms the foundation for understanding the pharmacology of inotropes and vasopressors, recent research has unveiled considerable genetic complexity in the receptors.[16] There are at least nine distinct receptor subtypes (three subtypes of each α₁, α₂, and β) that are expressed in a variety of tissues. Many of these receptor subtypes also have well-described genetic variants. For example, 12 single nucleotide polymorphisms (SNPs) have been identified in the β₁ receptor and 19 in the β₂ receptor.[17,18] These are simple variations in the genetic code, but it is believed that they translate into clinically significant phenotypes. Polymorphisms have also been identified in the α_1 and α_2 receptors. There appears to be an association between some of these genotypes and the development of hypertension and heart failure.[19]

The majority of research on the impact of adrenergic receptor genetic variation has focused on its implications on the development and treatment of cardiovascular disease, as well as on the clinical outcomes after certain cardiac diagnoses (e.g., myocardial infarction). Little work has focused on the effects of vasopressors and inotropes in these different genotypes. It is reasonable to expect, however, that clinically significant differences seen in the response to receptor antagonists (e.g., β blockers) might also be observed for receptor agonists. Indeed, a polymorphism in the β_1 receptor affects the response to dobutamine, with a significantly greater heart rate and inotropic response.[20] Even though much work remains to be done in this area, it is likely that at least some of the large interindividual variability seen in the response to these drugs is a function of genetic variation.

INDIVIDUAL DRUGS

Epinephrine

Epinephrine is a naturally occurring sympathomimetic with nonselective adrenergic agonist activity. It is synthesized, stored, and released by the chromaffin cells of the adrenal medulla in response to physiologic stress. It binds to α, β_1 (the predominant β receptor in the heart), and β_2 (the predominant β receptor in the lungs and vasculature) receptors. Action at the β_3 receptor is not currently a target of clinical application of epinephrine.

Epinephrine is the drug of choice in two extreme clinical conditions: anaphylactic shock and cardiac arrest (Figure 22-3). In anaphylaxis, α receptor-mediated vasoconstriction of small arterioles and precapillary sphincters increases mean arterial pressure and decreases mucosal edema. Its β receptor-mediated effects cause bronchodilation and stabilization of mast cells. The latter decreases the release of histamine, tryptase, and other inflammatory mediators that perpetuate the pathophysiology of anaphylaxis. In cardiac arrest, epinephrine is given in large doses (1 mg every 3-5 minutes) to increase mean arterial pressure, thereby increasing cerebral perfusion pressure during chest compressions. The value and safety of its β receptor-mediated effects during cardiac arrest are controversial because they increase myocardial oxygen consumption. However, studies demonstrate better survival with epinephrine than without it.[21]

Other indications for epinephrine take advantage of specific subsets of its nonselective adrenergic agonism profile. Epinephrine is used to treat asthma (β_2-mediated bronchodilation), severe hypotension associated with bradycardia (β_1-mediated chronotropy) and/or low cardiac output (β_1-mediated inotropy), and to prolong the effects of local anesthetics (α-mediated vasoconstriction). Low doses of epinephrine (0.02-0.05 µg/kg/min) are used to increase depressed cardiac output after cardiopulmonary bypass; other catecholamines and inotropes have similar effects, but none has proven superior to epinephrine in terms of patient outcome. Epinephrine has also been studied as an alternative

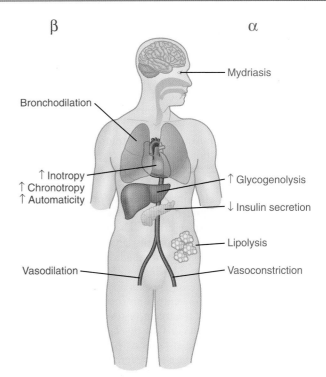

Figure 22-3 Summary of the effects of epinephrine mediated by α and β adrenergic receptor stimulation.

to other vasopressors in the treatment of vasodilatory shock from sepsis, even though the data do not yet support its use as a first-line therapy.[22]

Epinephrine's effects are route, time, and dose dependent. At low doses (0.01-0.05 µg/kg/min), the β receptor effects of epinephrine predominate, while at higher doses, α effects predominate (see Table 22-1). An intravenous bolus of epinephrine (5-15 µg) causes an initial increase in heart rate, systolic blood pressure, and systemic vascular resistance (from stimulation of α and β receptors), and a subsequent decrease in systolic and diastolic blood pressure and vascular resistance (from continued stimulation of β receptors with peripheral vasodilation).[23]

In healthy subjects, increasing rates of epinephrine infusion (0.01-0.2 µg/kg/min) progressively increase heart rate and systemic blood pressure. In general, at progressively higher continuous infusion rates, heart rate, blood pressure, systemic vascular resistance, and cardiac output increase while pulmonary artery pressure, central venous pressure, and pulmonary artery occlusion pressure remain unchanged.

Mast cell stabilization and bronchodilation via stimulation of β_2 receptors are the two most important nonhemodynamic, therapeutic effects of epinephrine. Epinephrine has numerous other nonhemodynamic effects that are potentially adverse. At doses typically administered for vasopressor and/or inotropic effects, these potentially adverse effects include:
- Hyperglycemia—due to increased liver glycogenolysis, reduced tissue uptake of glucose, and inhibition of pancreatic secretion of insulin.
- Hypokalemia—due to increased uptake of K^+ in skeletal muscle secondary to stimulation of β_2 receptors. Infusion of epinephrine at a rate of 0.1 µg/kg/min reduces plasma K^+ concentration by about 0.8 mEq/L.[24]

- Lactic acidosis—in theory due to inhibition of pyruvate dehydrogenase, causing pyruvate to be shunted to lactate.[25] Although the cause is not certain, epinephrine infusion results in lactic acidosis even in the absence of tissue hypoxia and might not signify a poor prognosis.[26]
- Myocardial ischemia—due to hypertension, tachycardia, and increased inotropy that increase myocardial oxygen demand.

Epinephrine is administered by continuous infusion, bolus, infiltration, or inhalation. Usual intravenous infusion doses are 0.02 to 0.3 μg/kg/min. Intravenous bolus doses range from 5 to 10 μg for moderate hypotension (mean arterial pressure 40-60 mm Hg) unresponsive to other vasopressors up to 1 mg as recommended by the American Heart Association Guidelines for cardiac arrest. The usual intramuscular dose is 0.3 mg administered into the lateral thigh (*vastus lateralis*), which produces significantly higher plasma concentrations than administration into the deltoid or subcutaneously. Subcutaneous administration results in delayed absorption and lower peak plasma concentrations than other routes. This is generally reserved for treatment of severe asthma in doses of 0.3 to 0.5 mg for adults or 0.01 mg/kg for children, when inhaled selective β_2 agonists cannot be administered.[27] In addition, epinephrine can be administered via an endotracheal tube during cardiac arrest if other routes are not available; the recommended dose is double the intravenous dose diluted with 10 mL of normal saline. Epinephrine is not effective orally due to rapid metabolism and does not cross the blood-brain barrier in sufficient amounts to directly affect the central nervous system.

Epinephrine should not be used in patients with acute cocaine intoxication due to the potential for exacerbation of myocardial ischemia and stroke. In patients with dynamic obstructions to ventricular outflow (e.g., tetralogy of Fallot and hypertrophic obstructive cardiomyopathy), epinephrine can worsen outflow obstruction and lower cardiac output. Administration of epinephrine with a β blocker can lead to significant α receptor stimulation without opposing β receptor-mediated vasodilation, which can result in severe vasoconstriction, hypertension, and heart failure. Care should also be taken when administering epinephrine with medications that predispose the heart to arrhythmia, particularly digitalis and halothane.

Isoproterenol

Isoproterenol was approved by the U.S. Food and Drug Administration (FDA) in 1947 and was used initially to treat asthma. Interestingly, it was the first drug for which the FDA required a package insert beginning in 1968. As the isopropyl derivative of norepinephrine, isoproterenol is a synthetic sympathomimetic with nonselective β adrenergic activity.

Stimulation of cardiac β_1 receptors by isoproterenol increases heart rate, inotropy, and lusitropy resulting in an increase in cardiac output and systolic blood pressure. Stimulation of β_2 receptors results in vasodilation of the muscle, kidney, skin, and splanchnic circulations thereby decreasing total peripheral vascular resistance and mean and diastolic blood pressure. The decrease in systemic blood pressure combined with increases in myocardial contractility and heart rate can precipitate myocardial ischemia in patients with significant coronary artery disease. At higher doses, palpitations, headache, and flushing can occur.

Isoproterenol was used initially via inhaler to treat asthma and bronchospasm, but has been replaced by β_2 selective bronchodilators. Currently isoproterenol is indicated in hemodynamically significant bradycardia until cardiac pacing can be established. In prior years, it was used immediately following cardiac transplantation to enhance inotropy and chronotropy without concomitantly increasing systematic vascular resistance. Currently other drugs are used in this setting more commonly (e.g., epinephrine, milrinone, and vasopressin with cardiac pacing as necessary).

Norepinephrine

Norepinephrine is a naturally occurring sympathomimetic with both α and β_1 receptor affinity. Its effects are comparable to epinephrine on β_1 receptors, but because of its greater affinity for α receptors and its near total inactivity at β_2 receptors, it is an intense vasoconstrictor. As the primary neurotransmitter of the sympathetic nervous system, it is released from postganglionic sympathetic nerve endings and comprises 10% to 20% of the catecholamine content of the adrenal medulla.

Norepinephrine causes an increase in systolic and diastolic blood pressures due primarily to an increase in systemic vascular resistance (see Table 22-1). Cardiac output does not increase, and can decrease due to increased resistance to ventricular ejection. Heart rate remains unchanged or decreases from compensatory baroreceptor-mediated vagal activity. Blood flow decreases in renal, mesenteric, splanchnic, and hepatic beds. Norepinephrine increases pulmonary vascular resistance, probably by α_1-mediated vasoconstriction.[28]

Norepinephrine is the drug of choice for septic shock when mean arterial pressure is less than 65 mm Hg despite adequate volume resuscitation.[29] Compared with dopamine in sepsis, norepinephrine is more likely to improve hypotension with fewer arrhythmias and tachycardia.[30-32] Norepinephrine is also used to treat hypotension following cardiopulmonary bypass. However, when used to treat hypotension associated with milrinone administration, norepinephrine is less effective in preserving a beneficial ratio of systemic and pulmonary vascular resistance than vasopressin.[33] Although norepinephrine increases pulmonary vascular resistance, its ability to substantially increase right ventricular perfusion pressure can make it a useful vasopressor in right heart failure.[34]

With regard to adverse effects, norepinephrine can cause severe hypertension with increased myocardial workload and cardiac ischemia. Systemic vasoconstriction can impair perfusion of the gut and other organs resulting in organ dysfunction and metabolic acidosis. Clinical studies, however, have not consistently shown a decrease in splanchnic perfusion or worsening organ function when septic patients are treated with norepinephrine.[35] In some cases a decrease in splanchnic perfusion is associated with improved gastrointestinal perfusion, suggesting a redistribution of blood flow in the gut.[36,37]

Dopamine

Dopamine is a naturally occurring catecholamine that stimulates β_1 and α_1 adrenergic receptors, as well as vascular D_1 dopamine receptors (primarily in mesenteric and renal vasculature). It is synthesized in the kidney and has both diuretic and natriuretic effects. In addition to its peripheral actions, it is an important neurotransmitter in the central nervous system (see Chapters 7 and 11).

At low plasma concentrations, dopamine acts primarily on the D_1 receptor in renal, mesenteric, and coronary vasculature (see Table 22-1) to produce vasodilation of these beds with a resultant increase in glomerular filtration rate, renal blood flow, Na^+ excretion, and urine output.[38] Low doses can also decrease systemic vascular resistance. Higher doses directly stimulate β_1 receptors and enhance release of norepinephrine from sympathetic nerve terminals to increase myocardial contractility, heart rate, systolic blood pressure, and pulse pressure. Diastolic blood pressure is minimally affected but pulmonary vascular resistance can increase.[39] At high doses, stimulation of α_1 receptors predominates resulting in generalized peripheral vasoconstriction.

It is commonly stated that doses of 0.5 to 3 µg/kg/min stimulate primarily DA1 receptors, 3 to 10 µg/kg/min stimulate primarily β_1 receptors, and greater than 10 µg/kg/min primarily stimulate α receptors, but clinically the hemodynamic effects of dopamine are difficult to predict based on these empirical dosing guidelines.[40] In healthy male volunteers, weight-based dopamine administration resulted in up to 75-fold intersubject variability in plasma concentrations.[41] However, no study has yet related plasma concentrations of dopamine with its effects. Therefore dosing should be titrated to physiologic effect, rather than being based on rigid concepts of relative receptor activity for a given dosage.

Dopamine has been recommended as first-line therapy in septic shock, particularly when accompanied by systolic dysfunction.[29] However, recent studies show worse outcome in septic patients treated with dopamine.[42] Comparison of dopamine with norepinephrine for treatment of shock showed a higher incidence of arrhythmias in all patients and higher mortality in patients with cardiogenic shock treated with dopamine.[32] Compared with dobutamine after cardiac surgery and in patients with chronic heart failure, dopamine resulted in less hemodynamic improvement.[43,44] When compared with dopexamine, it resulted in significantly more adverse cardiac events.[45]

Renal dose dopamine refers to an infusion of dopamine in low doses (usually 1-3 µg/kg/min) for treatment or prevention of acute renal failure with a goal of selective stimulation of D_1 receptors. It is a misleading phrase and outdated concept, as the effects of dopamine even in low doses are not exclusively limited to the kidneys. Even though low doses of dopamine increase renal blood flow, glomerular filtration, and urine output, numerous studies have failed to show a decreased incidence of renal failure with its use.[46]

Dopamine can cause tachycardia, tachyarrhythmias, and myocardial ischemia, and at high doses causes decreased splanchnic perfusion and gut ischemia.[35,47] In addition to its hemodynamic effects, dopamine reduces the ventilatory response to hypoxemia, consistent with its role as a neurotransmitter in the carotid bodies.[48] Dopamine infusions alter endocrine and immune function, including decreased secretion of growth hormone, prolactin, and thyroid stimulating hormone.[49] Like other vasoconstrictors, dopamine can cause skin necrosis and sloughing if extravasation occurs.

The renal and mesenteric vasodilating properties of low-dose dopamine are suppressed by dopamine receptor antagonists like butyrophenones and phenothiazines.[50,51] There are reports of dopamine causing hypotension and bradycardia in patients taking phenytoin.[52]

Dobutamine

Dobutamine is a direct-acting synthetic catecholamine and is the drug of choice for the noninvasive assessment of coronary disease (dobutamine stress echocardiography). Dobutamine is also used for short-term treatment of congestive heart failure and for low cardiac output after cardiopulmonary bypass. In patients with chronic low output cardiac failure, dobutamine was superior to dopamine in its ability to increase cardiac output without untoward side effects.[44] Likewise it is superior to dopamine in managing hemodynamically unstable patients after cardiac surgery, reducing cardiac filling pressures and pulmonary vascular resistance with less trachycardia.[39,43] Compared with milrinone after cardiac surgery, dobutamine was "comparable," producing a greater increase in cardiac output, blood pressure, and heart rate, but with a higher incidence of arrhythmias.[53]

In patients with congestive heart failure, the principal effect of dobutamine is an increase in myocardial contractility and ventricular ejection mediated by its β_1 effects. In contrast to epinephrine or dopamine, dobutamine generally reduces systemic vascular resistance (SVR) by a combination of direct vasodilation and a reflex decrease in sympathetic vascular tone. This might be offset by the increase in cardiac output, leading to no change or a decrease in mean arterial pressure. Dobutamine generally decreases cardiac filling pressures and pulmonary vascular resistance. Dobutamine has a variable effect on heart rate, but can significantly increase heart rate (particularly at the higher concentrations used in stress echocardiography).[9,54] After cardiopulmonary bypass the primary mechanism of increased cardiac output by dobutamine is an increase in heart rate (approximately 1.4 beats/min/µg/kg/min) with an increase in SVR.[55] The contrasting results of these studies reflect dobutamine's complex mechanisms of action, particularly with regard to the balance of α_1 stimulation and inhibition by its isomers, as well as patient factors.

Dobutamine can produce tachycardia, arrhythmias, and hypertension. Dobutamine can exacerbate myocardial ischemia in susceptible patients by increases in heart rate and contractility.

Milrinone

Milrinone is a phosphodiesterase type III inhibitor, and as such is a synthetic noncatecholamine inodilator. Milrinone increases cardiac index with reductions in arterial pressure, left ventricular end-diastolic pressure, and pulmonary vascular resistance. Heart rate can increase, although this is not a consistent response and bradycardia can also occur. Compared with dobutamine, milrinone produces less tachycardia with more pulmonary and systemic vasodilation.[56]

Milrinone significantly increases success in the first attempt at weaning from cardiopulmonary bypass with less need for catecholamine support but with a greater requirement for additional vasoconstrictors.[57,58] Milrinone might be preferable to adrenergic agonists in patients with chronic heart failure undergoing cardiopulmonary bypass as down-regulation of adrenergic receptors in this population can lead to decreased responsiveness to catecholamines. In addition, milrinone improves flow in internal mammary artery grafts and saphenous vein grafts.[59,60] Intravenous milrinone has also been used to reverse cerebral vasospasm after subarachnoid hemorrhage, while inhaled milrinone has been used to treat severe pulmonary hypertension and acute lung injury.[61-64]

Milrinone is attractive for use in right heart failure by increasing ventricular contractility and decreasing pulmonary vascular resistance. However, milrinone-induced decreases in SVR and arterial blood pressure might offset these benefits and worsen supply-demand balance in the failing right heart. For this reason, milrinone is often combined with norepinephrine or vasopressin in an attempt to offset peripheral vasodilation. Comparing these two combinations, adding low dose vasopressin to milrinone might be superior to adding norepinephrine in improving the ratio of systemic to pulmonary vascular resistances.[33]

The most common adverse effect of milrinone is arterial hypotension, though this is often a desired effect. Milrinone use is an independent risk factor for the development of atrial fibrillation after cardiac surgery, but the incidence is less than with dobutamine.[53,65] About 12% of patients given milrinone in phase 2 and 3 trials developed ventricular arrhythmias (primarily premature ventricular contractions).

Milrinone is given intravenously, but can also be nebulized. Intravenous dosing of milrinone is initiated with a loading dose of 20 to 50 μg/kg over 10 minutes, followed by an infusion of 0.2 to 0.75 μg/kg/min. Due to the high degree of renal clearance, the dose should be reduced in patients with reduced creatinine clearance.

Phenylephrine

Phenylephrine is a synthetic noncatecholamine α_1 agonist and produces dose-dependent vasoconstriction of cutaneous, muscular, mesenteric, splanchnic, and renal vasculature (see Table 22-1). Systemic arterial vasoconstriction increases systolic, diastolic, and mean arterial pressures, with reflex bradycardia. Phenylephrine can also cause pulmonary vasoconstriction and pulmonary hypertension.

Phenylephrine is the drug of choice for initial treatment of mild hypotension with normal or increased heart rate in the setting of general or regional anesthesia. The use of phenylephrine to support blood pressure during spinal anesthesia for cesarean section has long been discouraged due to concerns that vasoconstriction could have a deleterious effect on placental blood flow. Several recent studies have strongly contradicted this traditional teaching by documenting that phenylephrine does not worsen fetal outcome and might in fact be superior to ephedrine.[66,67] Phenylephrine is used to treat septic shock and vasodilatory shock after cardiopulmonary bypass. Even though its use as a first-line vasopressor in sepsis is not recommended, a study comparing phenylephrine to norepinephrine found no difference in adverse events or outcomes.[29,68] Phenylephrine has been used to increase right ventricular perfusion in pulmonary hypertension and right heart failure, though it can worsen right ventricular function and raise pulmonary artery diastolic pressures; norepinephrine appears to be more effective in this setting.[69,70] Phenylephrine is used topically as a nasal decongestant; as a mydriatic; and in ear, nose, and throat surgeries to constrict mucosa or control bleeding.

Severe bradycardia or even brief asystole can occur with higher doses of phenylephrine. With left ventricular dysfunction, the combination of bradycardia and increased afterload can significantly reduce cardiac output. Case reports document the risk of pulmonary edema, arrhythmias, cardiac arrest and death when phenylephrine is used topically in excessive doses during head and neck surgery to control bleeding.[71] Topical doses should be limited to no more than 0.5 mg in adults, and blood pressure and heart rate should be monitored. Severe hypertension can require treatment with an α_1 antagonist such as phentolamine or with a direct vasodilator such as hydralazine. β blockers or calcium channel blockers should not be administered in this setting because their cardiac depressant effects can result in acute heart failure.[71]

Vasopressin

Arginine vasopressin (AVP, vasopressin, also known as antidiuretic hormone) is a nonapeptide hormone synthesized in the magnocellular neurons of the paraventricular and supraoptic nuclei of the hypothalamus (see Chapter 30). It is stored and released from neurosecretory vesicles in the posterior pituitary gland (neurohypophysis).[14]

Vasopressin is typically given by continuous intravenous infusion. Previously recommended infusion rates for hypotension were from 0.01 to 0.04 units/min based on a study that suggested increased cardiac complications with doses above 0.04 units/min.[72] More recent studies, however, show that a dose of 0.067 units/min, compared to 0.03 units/min, resulted in better cardiovascular function with no apparent increase in side effects in patients with vasodilatory shock.[73,74] Further study will be required to identify the optimal doses for different clinical settings. Vasopressin can be given as a bolus of 1 to 2 units to treat intraoperative hypotension, although its effects are short-lived.

The hemodynamic effects of vasopressin are complex, and vary depending on the presence or absence of intact sympathetic and renin-angiotensin systems. Interestingly, the effect of vasopressin infusions in healthy volunteers appears to be minimal even at high plasma concentrations.[75] This paradoxical finding can be explained by the action of vasopressin on the area postrema of the central nervous system. The expected vasoconstrictive effect is effectively counterbalanced by an augmented baroreflex inhibition of efferent sympathetic activity.[76] In patients with septic shock, low dose vasopressin increases systemic arterial blood pressure and vascular resistance, but does not alter pulmonary vascular resistance or pressures, cardiac filling pressures, or cardiac index.[77] Heart rate can decrease, although this finding is not consistent.

Even though it is not considered a first-line therapy, vasopressin is used as an adjunct to catecholamines in the treatment of septic shock. Patients with septic shock have much lower plasma vasopressin concentrations than those with cardiogenic shock. This has been interpreted as a relative vasopressin deficiency caused by early depletion of hypothalamic stores or inhibition of vasopressin release.[78] The Vasopressin and Septic Shock Trial (VASST) compared norepinephrine with low-dose vasopressin to norepinephrine alone. There was no difference in overall mortality or adverse events, but mortality was reduced in patients with less severe sepsis who received vasopressin.[79]

Guidelines on the use of vasopressin in cardiopulmonary resuscitation are evolving. Endogenous vasopressin levels are higher in patients who are successfully resuscitated.[80] Studies have compared the use of vasopressin and epinephrine in cardiac arrest with variable outcomes.[81-84] It does not appear that vasopressin confers a significant benefit compared with epinephrine. The most recent American Heart Association guidelines state that vasopressin 40 U can replace either the first or second dose of epinephrine in adult cardiac arrest.[21]

Cardiopulmonary bypass is normally associated with a substantial increase in circulating vasopressin.[85] In some cases of post-bypass hypotension, plasma vasopressin concentrations are inappropriately low.[86] These patients frequently respond to low doses of vasopressin, as do some patients with vasodilatory shock after cardiac transplantation or left ventricular assist device placement.

Although not supported by specific studies, vasopressin is also used to treat intraoperative hypotension during general or epidural anesthesia. Clinical experience suggests that it might be useful in treating hypotension refractory to catecholamines in patients on long-term treatment with drugs that inhibit the renin-angiotensin system (angiotensin-converting enzyme inhibitors and angiotensin receptor blockers).[87]

In patients with septic shock, vasopressin reduces gastrointestinal mucosal perfusion and increases liver enzyme and total bilirubin concentrations.[88,89] In addition, it decreases platelet count (likely due to increased platelet aggregation) but does not significantly alter coagulation.[90]

Numerous drugs interact with vasopressin. Potentiation of its antidiuretic effect can be seen with carbamazepine, chlorpropamide, clofibrate, fludrocortisone, and tricyclic antidepressants. Inhibition of the antidiuretic effect can be observed in patients receiving demeclocycline, norepinephrine, lithium, heparin, and alcohol.

Ephedrine

Ephedrine is a synthetic noncatecholamine agonist at α, β_1, and β_2 receptors with both direct and indirect actions. Ephedrine is given as an intravenous bolus of 5 to 10 mg. It is effective in the same dose range when administered intramuscularly, albeit with slower onset and longer duration. When given in repeated doses, tachyphylaxis occurs, probably due to depletion of norepinephrine stores. Ephedrine causes an increase in systolic, diastolic, and mean arterial pressures. It increases myocardial contractility, heart rate, and cardiac output (see Table 22-1).

In the acute care setting, ephedrine is used primarily to treat mild hypotension and bradycardia associated with general or regional anesthesia. Previously, ephedrine was the first-line therapy for parturients with hypotension secondary to spinal or epidural anesthesia based on studies in pregnant ewes suggesting that ephedrine preserved uterine blood flow compared with other vasopressors.[91] These data have been challenged recently; phenylephrine appears to be as good or better in preserving uterine blood flow and does not cause or worsen maternal tachycardia.[92,93]

At higher doses, ephedrine causes hypertension and tachycardia. Because it crosses the blood-brain barrier, ephedrine can cause agitation and insomnia. In patients with prostatic hypertrophy, ephedrine can produce urinary retention. Because ephedrine causes release of norepinephrine, patients taking MAOIs can have an exaggerated hypertensive effect.

Digoxin

Digoxin, a cardiac glycoside, exerts its positive inotropic effects by inhibiting the plasma membrane Na^+,K^+-ATPase of cardiac myocytes. This leads to an increase in available Ca^{2+} as described above. While digoxin has been in clinical use for hundreds of years as an inotrope and to control heart rate in atrial fibrillation, it has largely been replaced by more effective medications with fewer side effects.

Digoxin is currently indicated (as a second or third line therapy) for ventricular rate control in atrial fibrillation and in the treatment of systolic heart failure.[94,95] Although it is effective in providing symptomatic relief for heart failure, it does so with a significant increase in mortality and its use should essentially be considered palliative.[96] It is likewise associated with increased mortality in atrial fibrillation patients, and while it is effective in decreasing ventricular rate at rest it does not prevent exercise-induced tachycardia, does not aid in conversion to sinus rhythm, and may be associated with conversion from sinus rhythm back to atrial fibrillation.[97]

In addition to concerns about increased mortality with the use of digoxin, its use is significantly limited by the high incidence of side effects. The therapeutic index of digoxin is very small requiring plasma concentration monitoring, and its use is frequently associated with a wide variety of cardiac arrhythmia including sinus bradycardia, sinus arrest, AV conduction delays, second- or third-degree heart block, and malignant ventricular arrhythmias. Digitalis toxicity is generally treated with digitalis binding antibody as well as lidocaine, magnesium, phenytoin, and correction of hypokalemia.

RATIONAL DRUG SELECTION

Rational selection of vasopressors and inotropes in clinical practice is founded on numerous factors including the targeted therapeutic goals and the adverse effects most critical to avoid. Because in most clinical scenarios there is not a clearly established evidence-based approach supported by outcome data, institutional protocols and physician experience often figure prominently in the formulation of a therapeutic plan. Once formulated, the plan is instituted as a therapeutic trial; the complexity and dynamic nature of circulatory physiology might necessitate a change in the initial regimen if the results are unsatisfactory or if conditions change.

In situations in which a variety of different drugs could potentially achieve the hemodynamic goals (and given the lack of class I evidence supporting the use of a particular drug), using a drug with which the practitioner has considerable experience is a reasonable approach. On the other hand, there are some clinical situations for which a particular drug might be preferable (see later). The overarching principle is that rational drug selection must match the physiologic state of the patient with the anticipated effects of the drugs under consideration; the clinician must periodically reassess both the patient's physiology and the drug choice to determine whether changes are necessary.

SEPTIC SHOCK

The pharmacologic management of septic shock has been the target of a huge volume of clinical research as well as the topic of published guidelines.[29] Norepinephrine is considered the drug of choice in septic shock when mean arterial pressure is less than 65 mm Hg despite volume resuscitation.

CARDIAC ARREST

The use of large doses of epinephrine (up to 1 mg every 3-5 minutes) is the treatment of choice in the pulseless patient while a definitive diagnosis is being sought.

Mild, Intraoperative Hypotension

Anesthesiologists are frequently faced with mild hypotension during the course of routine general and neuraxial anesthetics. As in all cases of hypotension, it is of paramount importance to identify the etiology in order to institute appropriate therapy. While the cause is being investigated, however, it is reasonable to administer small doses of ephedrine. Phenylephrine can also be used if low afterload is suspected and the patient has an adequate heart rate to tolerate the bradycardia associated with phenylephrine. It should be recognized, though, that the use of a vasoconstrictor can compromise cardiac output and organ perfusion in some cases.

HYPOTENSION IN THE PARTURIENT

Until recently, the conventional wisdom has been that phenylephrine is contraindicated in the hypotensive pregnant patient, and that ephedrine is the drug of choice. Recent literature, however, has contradicted that traditional teaching. In most routine circumstances, both ephedrine and phenylephrine are reasonable choices depending on the heart rate.

Right Heart Failure

In addition to identifying and treating reversible causes of elevated pulmonary vascular resistance, pharmacologic management is crucial in the critically ill patient with right heart failure. Guiding principles are to support myocardial contractility as well as perfusion of the ventricle. The combination of milrinone with vasopressin is an excellent choice in this situation. Milrinone provides inotropy as well as pulmonary vasodilation, while vasopressin supports perfusion of the right ventricle by increasing the systemic vascular resistance. In cases where milrinone proves inadequate to increase contractility adequately, the addition of epinephrine might be successful.

POST-BYPASS HYPOTENSION

Hypotension in the patient being weaned from cardiopulmonary bypass represents an extremely complex interplay of physiologic factors; no single drug or protocol can reasonably be expected to prove universally efficacious. A comprehensive discussion of this topic is beyond the scope of this chapter, but basic concepts guiding the therapeutic decisions are summarized in Figure 22-4.

Before treatment is initiated, the first step is to reach an underlying diagnosis. In contemporary cardiac anesthesia practice, transesophageal echocardiography is unparalleled as a diagnostic tool in this setting. A broad differential diagnosis in this situation often includes left and/or right ventricular systolic dysfunction, inappropriate vasodilation, hypovolemia, and inadequate heart rate, each of which alone and in combination requires a different pharmacologic approach.

The only drug that has been shown to improve ability to wean from cardiopulmonary bypass is milrinone. It provides excellent inotropic support, particularly in heart failure patients with downregulated autonomic receptors. Because its use is commonly associated with peripheral vasodilation and worsening hypotension, however, milrinone should generally be combined with vasopressin in this population. Epinephrine is also a common and appropriate choice in the hypotensive patient with decreased contractility of the right and/or left ventricle; its use is associated with an increase in cardiac output and blood pressure.

When pure vasodilation is the cause of post-cardiopulmonary bypass hypotension, vasopressin is an excellent choice as it acts independently of the adrenergic receptors and as such can be expected to be additive with catecholamines. However, its use in this setting is a relatively new approach. In contrast, dopamine, epinephrine and, to a somewhat lesser extent, norepinephrine have a long history of successful use in supporting hemodynamics following cardiopulmonary bypass.

EMERGING DEVELOPMENTS

Understanding the pharmacogenetic basis of the variability in response to vasopressors and cardiotonic drugs is a primary focus of contemporary research in this area. In the future, it is conceivable that vasopressor and inotropic therapy will be personalized to the individuals' genotype based on pretreatment testing. Combined with functional hemodynamic data allowing goal-directed therapy, it might eventually be possible to predict with accuracy and precision how an individual patient will respond to these drugs (see Chapter 4).[98]

Work continues as well in the area of drug development. For instance, the calcium sensitizer subclass of drugs has emerged in clinical practice only recently and is being compared to more conventional therapies. Levosimendan is currently the only clinically available calcium sensitizing inodilator. In patients with heart failure, it has been shown to cause an increase in stroke volume and cardiac output with little change in heart rate (see Table 22-1). Cardiac filling pressures and pulmonary artery pressure decrease as well.[15] Levosimendan is used in the treatment of acute decompensated heart failure, pulmonary hypertension, postpartum cardiomyopathy, and ventricular dysfunction after cardiac surgery. Several studies have compared levosimendan with dobutamine in acute decompensated heart failure with mixed results.[99-102] Nonetheless it represents a major advance in the development of new vasoactive drugs and exemplifies the continuing need for further research in the field.

HYPOTENSION AFTER CARDIOPULMONARY BYPASS

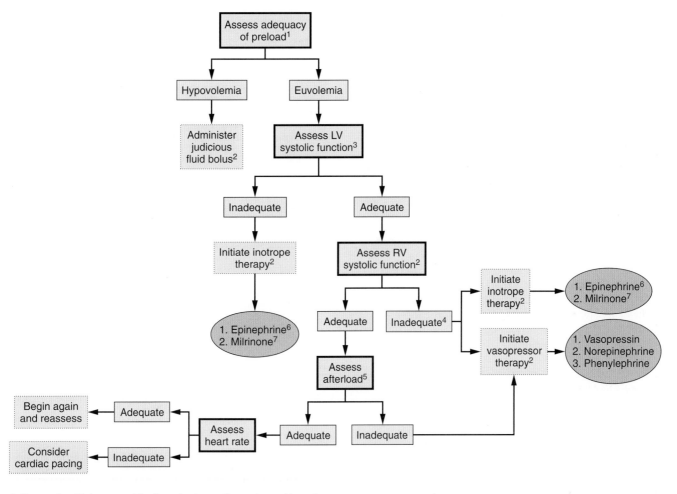

1. Generally utilizing a combination of echocardiography and invasive pressure measurements.

2. After each intervention, the clinical scenario should be reassessed to determine if patient has stabilized.

3. LV and RV systolic function is best evaluated with transesophageal echocardiography.

4. Causes of pulmonary vasoconstriction should be sought and corrected, and consideration should be given to instituting a pulmonary vasodilator such as nitric oxide or inhaled prostacyclin.

5. Low afterload (SVR) is indicated by adequate ventricular filling, a hyperdynamic ventricle, elevated cardiac output, and a low calculated SVR.

6. Dopamine could be considered in place if epinephrine, although epinephrine is usually considered the first-line drug.

7. The use of milrinone to support ventricular function in these patients will generally result in an increase in cardiac output, but in order to avoid worsening hypotension, it should be accompanied by the addition of vasopressin.

Figure 22-4 An approach to management of post-cardiopulmonary bypass hypotension.

KEY POINTS

- Vasoactive drugs have an extensive history and have been used clinically for more than 5000 years.
- Many inotropes and vasopressors are derivatives of β phenylethylamine; the nature and extent of the ethylamine side chain substitution determines their receptor specificity.
- While various inotropes and vasopressors exert their effects via different receptors and mechanisms, they generally increase the availability of calcium to interact with actin and myosin in either the cardiac myocyte or vascular smooth muscle.
- Catecholamines are primarily metabolized by catechol-O-methyl transferase and monoamine oxidase.
- Despite well-established profiles in selected populations, the effects of vasopressors and inotropes are difficult to predict in an individual, and thus these drugs should be titrated to effect rather than administered empirically.

Continued

KEY POINTS—cont'd

- A bolus of epinephrine can result in a transient increase in blood pressure from α receptor stimulation, followed by a drop below the previous baseline from unopposed β receptor stimulation. This serves as an example of the variable physiologic response to a given plasma concentration of a vasoactive agent.
- The use of low-dose dopamine as a means to preserve or improve renal function in critically ill patients is not supported by evidence despite extensive study and cannot be recommended.
- Phosphodiesterase inhibitors such as milrinone enhance cardiac function by inotropic and vasodilator actions. Their use can facilitate restoration of acceptable hemodynamic parameters following cardiopulmonary bypass.
- Contrary to longstanding dogma, either phenylephrine, an α-adrenergic agonist, or ephedrine, a mixed α- and β-adrenergic agonist, is an acceptable agent to treat hypotension in obstetric patients.
- Although once a mainstay inotrope in the treatment of heart failure, because of its low therapeutic index and frequent incidence of serious dysrhythmias, digoxin is no longer a first-line therapy.
- Treating an overdose of phenylephrine with beta-blockers or calcium channel blockers is contraindicated and can result in acute heart failure and death due to acute pulmonary edema.
- Description of the phenotypes associated with genetic variations in adrenergic receptors and development of calcium sensitizers are among important emerging developments in the field.

Key References

Dellinger R, Levy M, Carlet J, et al. Surviving Sepsis Campaign: international guidelines for management of severe sepsis and septic shock: 2008. *Intensive Care Med.* 2008;34:17-60. Best care of patients with sepsis as defined by a consensus of international experts. The evidence for use of various vasoactive drugs in addition to other medical and fluid management goals are discussed. (Ref. 29)

Doolan LA, Jones EF, Kalman J, et al. A placebo-controlled trial verifying the efficacy of milrinone in weaning high-risk patients from cardiopulmonary bypass. *J Cardiothorac Vasc Anesth.* 1997;11:37-41. Demonstrates the ability of milrinone, even a single dose, to improve the success of weaning high-risk patients from cardiopulmonary bypass. (Ref. 58)

Groudine SB, Hollinger I, Jones J, et al. New York State guidelines on the topical use of phenylephrine in the operating room. The Phenylephrine Advisory Committee. *Anesthesiology.* 2000;92:859-864. Highlights the severe complications of topical phenylephrine overdose as well as the potentially disastrous outcome when phenylephrine overdose is treated with negative inotropes (β blockers or calcium channel blockers). (Ref. 71)

Kellum JA, M Decker J. Use of dopamine in acute renal failure: a meta-analysis. *Crit Care Med.* 2001;29:1526-1531. Meta-analysis of 58 studies concluding that there is no justification for use of low-dose dopamine for treatment or prevention of acute renal failure. (Ref. 46)

Linton NW, Linton RA. Haemodynamic response to a small intravenous bolus injection of epinephrine in cardiac surgical patients. *Eur J Anaesthesiol.* 2003;20:298-304. Describes the hemodynamic response to small (5 μg) boluses of epinephrine, including an initial increase followed by a subsequent decrease in systemic

vascular resistance to less than 50% baseline. An excellent example of the response of adrenergic receptors to different plasma concentrations of agonist. (Ref. 23)

MacGregor DA, Smith TE, Prielipp RC, et al. Pharmacokinetics of dopamine in healthy male subjects. *Anesthesiology.* 2000;92:338-346. Shows up to 75-fold interpatient variability in plasma concentration when infusing dopamine. This highlights the importance of titrating to physiologic effect. (Ref. 41)

Ngan Kee WD, Khaw KS, Tan PE, et al. Placental transfer and fetal metabolic effects of phenylephrine and ephedrine during spinal anesthesia for cesarean delivery. *Anesthesiology.* 2009;111:506-512. Suggests that the balance of fetal oxygen supply and demand might be better achieved with phenylephrine than ephedrine. (Ref. 67)

Russell J, Walley K, Singer J, et al. Vasopressin versus norepinephrine infusion in patients with septic shock. *N Engl J Med.* 2008;358:877. Although vasopressin is not recommended as first-line therapy for patients with septic shock, when compared with norepinephrine in this population the outcomes are at least as good. In fact, patients with less severe sepsis have improved outcome with vasopressin. (Ref. 79)

Williams TD, Da Costa D, Mathias CJ, et al. Pressor effect of arginine vasopressin in progressive autonomic failure. *Clin Sci.* 1986;71:173-178. Demonstrates that vasopressin does not appreciably increase mean arterial pressure in healthy volunteers. This highlights the importance of underlying physiologic state when attempting to predict response to a vasoactive substance. (Ref. 75)

References

1. Levy B, Collin S, Sennoun N, et al. Vascular hyporesponsiveness to vasopressors in septic shock: from bench to bedside. *Intensive Care Med.* 2010;36(12):2019-2029.
2. Chen KK, Schmidt GF. The action of ephedrine, the active principle of the Chinese drug ma huang. *J Pharmacol Exp Ther.* 1924;24: 339-357.
3. Wilkins MR, Kendall MJ, Wade OL. William Withering and digitalis, 1785 to 1985. *Br Med J (Clin Res Ed).* 1985;290(6461):7-8.
4. Oliver G, Schafer EA. The physiological effects of extracts of the suprarenal capsules. *J Physiol.* 1895;18(3):230-276.
5. Oliver G, Schäfer EA. On the physiological action of extracts of pituitary body and certain other glandular organs: preliminary communication. *J Physiol (Lond).* 1895;18(3):277-279.
6. Barger G, Ewins A. CCXXXVII. Some phenolic derivatives of β-phenylethylamine. *J Chem Soc Trans.* 1910;97:2253-2261.
7. Barger G, Dale HH. Chemical structure and sympathomimetic action of amines. *J Physiol (Lond).* 1910;41(1-2):19-59.
8. Euler U. A specific sympathomimetic ergone in adrenergic nerve fibres (sympathin) and its relations to adrenaline and noradrenaline. *Acta Physiol Scand.* 1946;12:73-96.
9. Tuttle RR, Mills J. Dobutamine: development of a new catecholamine to selectively increase cardiac contractility. *Circ Res.* 1975; 36(1):185-196.
10. du Vigneaud V, Gish DT, Katsoyannis PG. A synthetic preparation possessing biological properties associated with argininevasopressin. *J Am Chem Soc.* 1954;76(18):4751-4752.
11. Ukkonen H, Saraste M, Akkila J, et al. Myocardial efficiency during levosimendan infusion in congestive heart failure. *Clin Pharmacol Ther.* 2000;68(5):522-531.
12. Salvi SS. Alpha1-adrenergic hypothesis for pulmonary hypertension. *Chest.* 1999;115(6):1708-1719.
13. Minneman KP. Alpha 1-adrenergic receptor subtypes, inositol phosphates, and sources of cell Ca2+. *Pharmacol Rev.* 1988;40(2): 87-119.
14. Barrett LK, Singer M, Clapp LH. Vasopressin: mechanisms of action on the vasculature in health and in septic shock. *Crit Care Med.* 2007;35(1):33.
15. Lilleberg J, Laine M, Palkama T, Kivikko M, Pohjanjousi P, Kupari M. Duration of the haemodynamic action of a 24-h infusion of levosimendan in patients with congestive heart failure. *Eur J Heart Fail.* 2007;9(1):75-82.
16. Ahlquist RP. A study of the adrenotropic receptors. *Am J Physiol.* 1948;153(3):586-600.

17. Leineweber K, Heusch G. Beta 1- and beta 2-adrenoceptor polymorphisms and cardiovascular diseases. *Br J Pharmacol*. 2009;158(1):61-69.

18. Von Homeyer P, Schwinn DA. Pharmacogenomics of β-adrenergic receptor physiology and response to β-blockade. *Anesth Analg*. 2011;113(6):1305-1318.

19. Sheppard R. Vascular tone and the genomics of hypertension. *Heart Fail Clin*. 2010;6(1):45-53.

20. Bruck H, Leineweber K, Temme T, et al. The Arg389Gly beta1-adrenoceptor polymorphism and catecholamine effects on plasma-renin activity. *J Am Coll Cardiol*. 2005;46(11):2111-2115.

21. Neumar RW, Otto CW, Link MS, et al. Part 8: adult advanced cardiovascular life support: 2010 American Heart Association Guidelines for Cardiopulmonary Resuscitation and Emergency Cardiovascular Care. *Circulation*. 2010;122(18 Suppl 3):S729-S767.

22. De Backer D, Creteur J, Silva E, Vincent J-L. Effects of dopamine, norepinephrine, and epinephrine on the splanchnic circulation in septic shock: which is best? *Crit Care Med*. 2003;31(6):1659-1667.

23. Linton NW, Linton RA. Haemodynamic response to a small intravenous bolus injection of epinephrine in cardiac surgical patients. *Eur J Anaesthesiol*. 2003;20(4):298-304.

24. Brown MJ, Brown DC, Murphy MB. Hypokalemia from β2-receptor stimulation by circulating epinephrine. *N Engl J Med*. 1983;309(23):1414-1419.

25. Totaro RJ, Raper RF. Epinephrine-induced lactic acidosis following cardiopulmonary bypass. *Crit Care Med*. 1997;25(10):1693-1699.

26. Cori CF, Cori GT. The mechanism of epinephrine action. IV. The influence of epinephrine on lactic acid production and blood sugar utilization. *J Biol Chem*. 1929;84:683-698.

27. Camargo CA, Rachelefsky G, Schatz M. Managing asthma exacerbations in the emergency department: summary of the National Asthma Education and Prevention Program Expert Panel Report 3 guidelines for the management of asthma exacerbations. *Proc Am Thorac Soc*. 2009;6(4):357-366.

28. Rudner XL, Berkowitz DE, Booth JV, et al. Subtype specific regulation of human vascular α1-adrenergic receptors by vessel bed and age. *Circulation*. 1999;100(23):2336-2343.

29. Dellinger R, Levy M, Carlet J, et al. Surviving Sepsis Campaign: international guidelines for management of severe sepsis and septic shock: 2008. *Intensive Care Med*. 2008;34(1):17-60.

30. Martin C, Papazian L, Perrin G, Saux P, Gouin F. Norepinephrine or dopamine for the treatment of hyperdynamic septic shock? *Chest*. 1993;103(6):1826-1831.

31. Meadows D, Edwards JD, Wilkins RG, Nightingale P. Reversal of intractable septic shock with norepinephrine therapy. *Crit Care Med*. 1988;16(7):663-666.

32. De Backer D, Biston P, Devriendt J, et al. Comparison of dopamine and norepinephrine in the treatment of shock. *N Engl J Med*. 2010;362(9):779-789.

33. Jeon Y, Ryu JH, Lim YJ, et al. Comparative hemodynamic effects of vasopressin and norepinephrine after milrinone-induced hypotension in off-pump coronary artery bypass surgical patients. *Eur J Cardiothorac Surg*. 2006;29(6):952-956.

34. Schreuder W, Schneider A, Groeneveld A, Thijs L. Effect of dopamine vs norepinephrine on hemodynamics in septic shock. Emphasis on right ventricular performance. *Chest*. 1989;95(6):1282-1288.

35. Marik PE, Mohedin M. The contrasting effects of dopamine and norepinephrine on systemic and splanchnic oxygen utilization in hyperdynamic sepsis. *JAMA*. 1994;272(17):1354-1357.

36. Nygren A, Thorén A, Ricksten S-E. Norepinephrine and intestinal mucosal perfusion in vasodilatory shock after cardiac surgery. *Shock*. 2007;28(5):536-543.

37. Nygren A, Thorén A, Ricksten S-E. Vasopressors and intestinal mucosal perfusion after cardiac surgery: norepinephrine vs. phenylephrine. *Crit Care Med*. 2006;34(3):722-729.

38. McDonald RH, Goldberg LI, Mcnay JL, Tuttle EP. Effect of dopamine in man: augmentation of sodium excretion, glomerular filtration rate, and renal plasma flow. *J Clin Invest*. 1964;43:1116-1124.

39. Salomon NW, Plachetka JR, Copeland JG. Comparison of dopamine and dobutamine following coronary artery bypass grafting. *Ann Thorac Surg*. 1982;33(1):48-54.

40. Goldberg LI, Rajfer SI. Dopamine receptors: applications in clinical cardiology. *Circulation*. 1985;72(2):245-248.

41. MacGregor DA, Smith TE, Prielipp RC, Butterworth JF, James RL, Scuderi PE. Pharmacokinetics of dopamine in healthy male subjects. *Anesthesiology*. 2000;92(2):338-346.

42. Sakr Y, Reinhart K, Vincent J-L, et al. Does dopamine administration in shock influence outcome? Results of the Sepsis Occurrence in Acutely Ill Patients (SOAP) Study. *Crit Care Med*. 2006;34(3):589-597.

43. Tarr TJ, Moore NA, Frazer RS, Shearer ES, Desmond MJ. Haemodynamic effects and comparison of enoximone, dobutamine and dopamine following mitral valve surgery. *Eur J Anaesthesiol Suppl*. 1993;8:15-24.

44. Loeb H, Bredakis J, Gunner R. Superiority of dobutamine over dopamine for augmentation of cardiac output in patients with chronic low output cardiac failure. *Circulation*. 1977;55(2):375.

45. Rosseel PM, Santman FW, Bouter H, Dott CS. Postcardiac surgery low cardiac output syndrome: dopexamine or dopamine? *Intensive Care Med*. 1997;23(9):962-968.

46. Kellum JA, M Decker J. Use of dopamine in acute renal failure: a meta-analysis. *Crit Care Med*. 2001;29(8):1526-1531.

47. Nevière R, Mathieu D, Chagnon JL, Lebleu N, Wattel F. The contrasting effects of dobutamine and dopamine on gastric mucosal perfusion in septic patients. *Am J Respir Crit Care Med*. 1996;154(6 Pt 1):1684-1688.

48. Ward DS, Bellville JW. Reduction of hypoxic ventilatory drive by dopamine. *Anesth Analg*. 1982;61(4):333-337.

49. Schenarts PJ, Sagraves SG, Bard MR, et al. Low-dose dopamine: a physiologically based review. *Curr Surg*. 2006;63(3):219-225.

50. Goldberg LI, Yeh BK. Attenuation of dopamine-induced renal vasodilation in the dog by phenothiazines. *Eur J Pharmacol*. 1971;15(1):36-40.

51. Yeh BK, McNay JL, Goldberg LI. Attenuation of dopamine renal and mesenteric vasodilation by haloperidol: evidence for a specific dopamine receptor. *J Pharmacol Exp Ther*. 1969;168(2):303-309.

52. Bivins BA, Rapp RP, Griffen WO, Blouin R, Bustrack J. Dopamine-phenytoin interaction. A cause of hypotension in the critically ill. *Arch Surg*. 1978;113(3):245-249.

53. Feneck RO, Sherry KM, Withington PS, Oduro-Dominah A, Group EMMT. Comparison of the hemodynamic effects of milrinone with dobutamine in patients after cardiac surgery. *J Cardiothorac Vasc Anesth*. 2001;15(3):306-315.

54. Leier CV, Webel J, Bush CA. The cardiovascular effects of the continuous infusion of dobutamine in patients with severe cardiac failure. *Circulation*. 1977;56(3):468-472.

55. Romson JL, Leung JM, Bellows WH, et al. Effects of dobutamine on hemodynamics and left ventricular performance after cardiopulmonary bypass in cardiac surgical patients. *Anesthesiology*. 1999;91(5):1318-1328.

56. Yamani MH, Haji SA, Starling RC, et al. Comparison of dobutamine-based and milrinone-based therapy for advanced decompensated congestive heart failure: hemodynamic efficacy, clinical outcome, and economic impact. *Am Heart J*. 2001;142(6):998-1002.

57. Lobato EB, Florete O, Bingham HL. A single dose of milrinone facilitates separation from cardiopulmonary bypass in patients with pre-existing left ventricular dysfunction. *Br J Anaesth*. 1998;81(5):782-784.

58. Doolan LA, Jones EF, Kalman J, Buxton BF, Tonkin AM. A placebo-controlled trial verifying the efficacy of milrinone in weaning high-risk patients from cardiopulmonary bypass. *J Cardiothorac Vasc Anesth*. 1997;11(1):37-41.

59. Lobato EB, Urdaneta F, Martin TD, Gravenstein N. Effects of milrinone versus epinephrine on grafted internal mammary artery flow after cardiopulmonary bypass. *J Cardiothorac Vasc Anesth*. 2000;14(1):9-11.

60. Arbeus M, Axelsson B, Friberg O, Magnuson A, Bodin L, Hultman J. Milrinone increases flow in coronary artery bypass grafts after cardiopulmonary bypass: a prospective, randomized, double-blind, placebo-controlled study. *J Cardiothorac Vasc Anesth*. 2009;23(1):48-53.

61. Fraticelli AT, Cholley BP, Losser M-R, Saint Maurice J-P, Payen D. Milrinone for the treatment of cerebral vasospasm after aneurysmal subarachnoid hemorrhage. *Stroke*. 2008;39(3):893-898.

62. Bueltmann M, Kong X, Mertens M, et al. Inhaled milrinone attenuates experimental acute lung injury. *Intens Care Med.* 2009;35(1):171-178.

63. Buckley MS, Feldman JP. Nebulized milrinone use in a pulmonary hypertensive crisis. *Pharmacotherapy.* 2007;27(12):1763-1766.

64. Lamarche Y, Perrault LP, Maltais S, Tétreault K, Lambert J, Denault AY. Preliminary experience with inhaled milrinone in cardiac surgery. *Eur J Cardiothorac Surg.* 2007;31(6):1081-1087.

65. Fleming GA, Murray KT, Yu C, et al. Milrinone use is associated with postoperative atrial fibrillation after cardiac surgery. *Circulation.* 2008;118(16):1619-1625.

66. Ngan Kee WD, Khaw KS, Lau TK, Ng FF, Chui K, Ng KL. Randomised double-blinded comparison of phenylephrine vs ephedrine for maintaining blood pressure during spinal anaesthesia for non-elective caesarean section. *Anaesthesia.* 2008;63(12):1319-1326.

67. Ngan Kee WD, Khaw KS, Tan PE, Ng FF, Karmakar MK. Placental transfer and fetal metabolic effects of phenylephrine and ephedrine during spinal anesthesia for cesarean delivery. *Anesthesiology.* 2009;111(3):506-512.

68. Morelli A, Ertmer C, Rehberg S, et al. Phenylephrine versus norepinephrine for initial hemodynamic support of patients with septic shock: a randomized, controlled trial. *Crit Care.* 2008;12(6):R143.

69. Rich S, Gubin S, Hart K. The effects of phenylephrine on right ventricular performance in patients with pulmonary hypertension. *Chest.* 1990;98(5):1102-1106.

70. Kwak YL, Lee CS, Park YH, Hong YW. The effect of phenylephrine and norepinephrine in patients with chronic pulmonary hypertension. *Anaesthesia.* 2002;57(1):9-14.

71. Groudine SB, Hollinger I, Jones J, DeBouno BA. New York State guidelines on the topical use of phenylephrine in the operating room. The Phenylephrine Advisory Committee. *Anesthesiology.* 2000;92(3):859-864.

72. Holmes CL, Patel BM, Russell JA, Walley KR. Physiology of vasopressin relevant to management of septic shock. *Chest.* 2001;120(3):989.

73. Luckner G, Mayr VD, Jochberger S, et al. Comparison of two dose regimens of arginine vasopressin in advanced vasodilatory shock. *Crit Care Med.* 2007;35(10):2280.

74. Torgersen C, Dünser MW, Wenzel V, et al. Comparing two different arginine vasopressin doses in advanced vasodilatory shock: a randomized, controlled, open-label trial. *Intensive Care Med.* 2010;36(1):57-65.

75. Williams TD, Da Costa D, Mathias CJ, Bannister R, Lightman SL. Pressor effect of arginine vasopressin in progressive autonomic failure. *Clin Sci.* 1986;71(2):173-178.

76. Hasser EM, Cunningham JT, Sullivan MJ, Curtis KS, Blaine EH, Hay M. Area postrema and sympathetic nervous system effects of vasopressin and angiotensin II. *Clin Exp Pharmacol Physiol.* 2000;27(5-6):432-436.

77. Tsuneyoshi I, Yamada H, Kakihana Y, Nakamura M, Nakano Y, Boyle WA. Hemodynamic and metabolic effects of low-dose vasopressin infusions in vasodilatory septic shock. *Crit Care Med.* 2001;29(3):487.

78. Landry DW, Levin HR, Gallant EM, et al. Vasopressin deficiency contributes to the vasodilation of septic shock. *Circulation.* 1997;95(5):1122-1125.

79. Russell J, Walley K, Singer J, et al. Vasopressin versus norepinephrine infusion in patients with septic shock. *N Engl J Med.* 2008;358(9):877.

80. Lindner KH, Haak T, Keller A, Bothner U, Lurie KG. Release of endogenous vasopressors during and after cardiopulmonary resuscitation. *Heart.* 1996;75(2):145-150.

81. Lindner KH, Dirks B, Strohmenger HU, Prengel AW, Lindner IM, Lurie KG. Randomised comparison of epinephrine and vasopressin in patients with out-of-hospital ventricular fibrillation. *Lancet.* 1997;349(9051):535-537.

82. Callaway CW, Hostler D, Doshi AA, et al. Usefulness of vasopressin administered with epinephrine during out-of-hospital cardiac arrest. *Am J Cardiol.* 2006;98(10):1316-1321.

83. Mukoyama T, Kinoshita K, Nagao K, Tanjoh K. Reduced effectiveness of vasopressin in repeated doses for patients undergoing prolonged cardiopulmonary resuscitation. *Resuscitation.* 2009;80(7):755-761.

84. Gueugniaud PY, David JS, Chanzy E, et al. Vasopressin and epinephrine vs. epinephrine alone in cardiopulmonary resuscitation. *N Engl J Med.* 2008;359(1):21.

85. Levine FH, Philbin DM, Kono K, et al. Plasma vasopressin levels and urinary sodium excretion during cardiopulmonary bypass with and without pulsatile flow. *Ann Thorac Surg.* 1981;32(1):63-67.

86. Argenziano M, Chen JM, Choudhri AF, et al. Management of vasodilatory shock after cardiac surgery: identification of predisposing factors and use of a novel pressor agent. *J Thorac Cardiovasc Surg.* 1998;116(6):973-980.

87. Boccara G, Ouattara A, Godet G, et al. Terlipressin versus norepinephrine to correct refractory arterial hypotension after general anesthesia in patients chronically treated with renin-angiotensin system inhibitors. *Anesthesiology.* 2003;98(6):1338-1344.

88. van Haren FMP, Rozendaal FW, van der Hoeven JG. The effect of vasopressin on gastric perfusion in catecholamine-dependent patients in septic shock. *Chest.* 2003;124(6):2256-2260.

89. Dünser MW, Mayr AJ, Ulmer H, et al. The effects of vasopressin on systemic hemodynamics in catecholamine-resistant septic and postcardiotomy shock: a retrospective analysis. *Anesth Analg.* 2001;93(1):7.

90. Dünser MW, Fries DR, Schobersberger W, et al. Does arginine vasopressin influence the coagulation system in advanced vasodilatory shock with severe multiorgan dysfunction syndrome? *Anesth Analg.* 2004;99(1):201-206.

91. Ralston DH, Shnider SM, DeLorimier AA. Effects of equipotent ephedrine, metaraminol, mephentermine, and methoxamine on uterine blood flow in the pregnant ewe. *Anesthesiology.* 1974;40(4):354-370.

92. Cooper DW, Carpenter M, Mowbray P, Desira WR, Ryall DM, Kokri MS. Fetal and maternal effects of phenylephrine and ephedrine during spinal anesthesia for cesarean delivery. *Anesthesiology.* 2002;97(6):1582-1590.

93. Lee A, Ngan Kee WD, Gin T. A quantitative, systematic review of randomized controlled trials of ephedrine versus phenylephrine for the management of hypotension during spinal anesthesia for cesarean delivery. *Anesth Analg.* 2002;94(4):920-926.

94. Association EHR, Surgery EAfC-T, Camm AJ, et al. Guidelines for the management of atrial fibrillation: the Task Force for the Management of Atrial Fibrillation of the European Society of Cardiology (ESC). *Eur Heart J.* 2010;31(19):2369-2429.

95. Jessup M, Abraham WT, Casey DE, et al. 2009 focused update: ACCF/AHA Guidelines for the Diagnosis and Management of Heart Failure in Adults: a report of the American College of Cardiology Foundation/American Heart Association Task Force on Practice Guidelines: developed in collaboration with the International Society for Heart and Lung Transplantation. *Circulation.* 2009;119(14):1977-2016.

96. Lindsay SJ, Kearney MT, Prescott RJ, Fox KA, Nolan J. Digoxin and mortality in chronic heart failure. UK Heart Investigation. *Lancet.* 1999;354(9183):1003.

97. Gjesdal K, Feyzi J, Olsson SB. Digitalis: a dangerous drug in atrial fibrillation? An analysis of the SPORTIF III and V data. *Heart.* 2008;94(2):191-196.

98. Giglio MT, Marucci M, Testini M, Brienza N. Goal-directed haemodynamic therapy and gastrointestinal complications in major surgery: a meta-analysis of randomized controlled trials. *Br J Anaesth.* 2009;103(5):637-646.

99. Delaney A, Bradford C, McCaffrey J, Bagshaw SM, Lee R. Levosimendan for the treatment of acute severe heart failure: a meta-analysis of randomised controlled trials. *Int J Cardiol.* 2010;138(3):281-289.

100. Follath F, Cleland JGF, Just H, et al. Efficacy and safety of intravenous levosimendan compared with dobutamine in severe low-output heart failure (the LIDO study): a randomised double-blind trial. *Lancet.* 2002;360(9328):196-202.

101. Mebazaa A, Nieminen MS, Filippatos GS, et al. Levosimendan vs. dobutamine: outcomes for acute heart failure patients on beta-blockers in SURVIVE. *Eur J Heart Fail.* 2009;11(3):304-311.

102. Bergh CH, Andersson B, Dahlström U, et al. Intravenous levosimendan vs. dobutamine in acute decompensated heart failure patients on beta-blockers. *Eur J Heart Fail.* 2010;12(4):40.

Chapter 23

ANTIHYPERTENSIVE DRUGS AND VASODILATORS

John W. Sear

Worldwide there are probably more than 1 billion people with raised blood pressure.[1] It is one of the most common chronic medical conditions internationally (U.S. National Center for Health Statistics, 2005), and occurs almost twice as often in African-Americans than in Caucasian-Americans. The incidence of hypertension increases with age, with a slightly greater incidence in men than in women.[2] In the United States, hypertension affects about 25% of all adults older than 40 years of age. More importantly, the prevalence of undiagnosed hypertension is about 1 in 15. In the United Kingdom, there are about 7.5 million patients suffering from raised blood pressure; but importantly 80% to 85% of these patients are either not treated or are being inadequately treated.

Blood pressure has been classified into four categories in the JNC VII Report (Joint National Committee on Prevention, Detection, Evaluation and Treatment of High Blood Pressure; 7th Report) based on systolic (left) and diastolic (right) pressures[3]:
- Normotension <120 and <80 mmHg
- Pre-hypertension 120-139 or 80-89 mmHg
- Stage I hypertension 140-159 or 90-99 mmHg
- Stage II hypertension >160 or ≥100 mmHg

In addition, patients with isolated systolic hypertension (ISH) are classified into ISH 1 (140-159/<90 mmHg) and ISH 2 (>160/<90 mmHg).

Many patients with hypertension have associated metabolic disorders (decreased high density lipoproteins; increased triglycerides; increased urates; and reduced glucose tolerance). These all contribute to the increased cardiovascular risk associated with high blood pressure, and to the possible development of type 2 diabetes mellitus. These additional comorbidities influence the choice of drug therapy for treatment of raised blood pressure.

In the United States, present strategies for treatment include initiation of treatment if blood pressure is more than 20 mmHg systolic or 10 mmHg diastolic above the target pressure. Many studies have shown monotherapy to be generally inadequate and to be associated with an increased incidence of cardiovascular events occurring early after starting treatment. The use of combination therapy is not new, in that it originates from the mid-1960s when studies showed the efficacy of fixed doses of reserpine, hydrochlorothiazide, and hydralazine.

HISTORICAL PERSPECTIVE

The causes of arterial hypertension are multiple, but can be divided into three distinct subgroups (Table 23-1). There are various ways of reducing the blood pressure and hence of treating hypertension. The history of the treatment of raised blood pressure shows how different drugs have been used to act on different effector sites or receptors. The dates of introduction of some of these early antihypertensive therapies are listed in Table 23-2.

One of the earliest treatments for hypertension was that described by Pauli using the sedative and hypotensive properties of sodium thiocyanate to obtain relief from the subjective symptoms of hypertension.[4] Another drug used for the treatment of malignant hypertension was sodium nitroprusside.[5,6] In the 1930s, the beneficial effects of extracts of *Rauwolfia serpentina* were first described with its first clinical use in 1955.[7,8] In the 1940s, sympathectomy was used to treat high blood pressure, often preceded by use of tetra-ethylammonium as a prognosticator to judge the likely success of the surgery, but was associated with a fairly high surgical mortality.

Real advances in management came with the introduction of ganglion blocking drugs (e.g., as mecamylamine, pempidine, hexamethonium, and pentolinium) in the 1950s. Other drugs introduced over the next decade included reserpine (a rauwolfia alkaloid) and hydralazine.[9] The combination of a ganglion blocker and general anesthesia resulted in the development of significant bradycardias and hypotension. Diuretics were also introduced for treatment of hypertension (initially chlorothiazide). The reduction in circulating fluid volume produced by the natriuresis enhanced the hypotensive effect of ganglion blocking agents and reduced some side effects of drugs such as reserpine. These synergistic interactions between drugs allowed a smaller dose of each drug and hence a less severe side-effect profile.

In the late 1950s and 1960s, two new important classes of drugs were introduced—adrenergic neuron blockers and the first generation of β-adrenoceptor blockers (see Chapter 13).

The antihypertensive effect of adrenergic neuron blockers (bretylium being the first) depends on inhibition of transmitter release from adrenergic nerve terminals in response to sympathetic nerve impulses. This results in a decrease in cardiac output, decrease in peripheral vascular resistance, and increase in venous capacitance. The main side effects of neuron blockade was postural hypotension, exertional hypotension, and hypotension in hot environments (all due to a failure of sympathetically mediated circulatory control).

α-Methyl DOPA (a false transmitter), introduced in 1961, reduces blood pressure by inhibition of norepinephrine synthesis. A slowly developing antihypertensive effect develops after repeated administration of small doses that do not exert a significant pressor effect. It is not established whether its hypotensive action is due to a peripheral effect (from impaired neuroeffector transmission) or to a central effect (involving the norepinephrine synapses in the medulla oblongata).

First-generation monoamine oxidase inhibitors (MAOIs), such as pargyline, were introduced in 1963. The antihypertensive effect of MAOIs has a slow onset that persists for a considerable period after cessation of treatment. In time, tolerance develops, probably due to fluid accumulation. The underlying mechanism for their antihypertensive effect is probably due to a change in composition of the monoamine stores of adrenergic neurons with a relative increase in amines other than norepinephrine (in particular, dopamine).

Other centrally acting drugs introduced in the 1960s include the α2adrenoceptor agonist clonidine and the second generation of adrenergic neuron blockers typified by bethanidine and debrisoquine. One of the first β-adrenergic blocking drugs introduced into clinical practice was pronethalol in 1962, followed by propranolol in 1965, alprenolol in 1967, and oxprenolol and practolol in 1968.

Table 23-1. Causes of Hypertension

Essential
Secondary
  Chronic kidney disease
  Coarctation of the aorta
  Cushing disease and other conditions leading to excess levels of glucocorticoid (including steroid therapy)
  Obstructive uropathy
  Pheochromocytoma
  Primary aldosteronism and other mineralocorticoid excess states
  Renovascular hypertension
  Sleep apnea
  Thyroid/parathyroid disease
Drugs
  Secondary to Na^+ and water retention, sodium salts of drugs, steroid treatment (mineralocorticoids, glucocorticoids, oral contraceptive pill); NSAIDs
  Vasoconstrictor drugs such as sympathomimetics
  Monoamine oxidase inhibitors through interaction with amines including dietary tyramine
  Rebound hypertension following acute withdrawal of clonidine, α-methyl DOPA, and β blockers

NSAIDs, Nonsteroidal anti-inflammatory drugs.

Table 23-2. Drugs Used in Treatment of Hypertension from Mid-1930s to 1966

1930s—Sedative drugs (barbiturates, bromides, cannabis preparations)
1940s—Surgical sympathectomy (bilateral thoracolumbar ganglionectomy)
1944—Salt-free diet (rice and fruit)
1945—Nitroprusside and thiocyanate salts
1950—Hexamethonium (the first of a series of improved ganglion-blocking drugs)
1952—Phenoxybenzamine and phentolamine (both used for treatment of hypertension, although introduced primarily for treatment of pheochromocytoma)
1953—Benefit of combination therapy recognized: pentolinium (ganglion blocker); hydralazine (vasodilator); reserpine and other rauwolfia alkaloids
1957—Mecamylamine (ganglion blocker) and chlorothiazide. Although chlorothiazide only had weak antihypertensive effects, its use was associated with a marked potentiation of the effect of other antihypertensive drugs
1959—Bretylium, the first adrenergic neuron blocker
1960—Guanethidine
1961—α-Methyl-DOPA (the first of the drugs that act through production of "false transmitters")
1962—Diazoxide (vasodilator)
1963—Monoamine oxidase inhibitors
1965—Propranolol, followed by oxprenolol and practolol; also bethanidine (second-generation adrenergic neuron blocker)
1966—Clonidine (centrally acting antihypertensive agent); desbrisoquine

At the same time, a major controversy and debate developed regarding whether antihypertensive drugs should be withdrawn from patients before anesthesia and surgery because of their effects in obtunding the normal mechanisms of cardiovascular control. The value of maintaining therapy was emphasized in a series of controlled studies of treated and untreated hypertensive patients.[10] Patients with well-controlled hypertension maintained on their drugs up to and including the morning of surgery experienced less cardiovascular instability than their untreated counterparts, especially in the postoperative period.

SITES AND MECHANISMS OF ANTIHYPERTENSIVE AND VASODILATOR DRUGS

The main center for neurogenic control of vascular tone and hence blood pressure is the vasomotor center in the midbrain. This affects both the sympathetic ganglia and parasympathetic nerves (Figure 23-1). There are two different central neural control systems involved in blood pressure regulation: neurogenic control (as outlined previously) and arterial baroreceptor reflexes.

Other humoral and endocrine control systems include the renin-angiotensin-aldosterone system; atrial natriuretic peptides; renal control of Na^+ and water excretion; eicosanoids; the kallikrein-kinin system; adrenal steroids (both glucocorticoids and mineralocorticoids); the endothelin system; and medullipin in patients with hypertension secondary to uremia and renal failure.

There are three main mechanisms by which drugs act in treatment of high blood pressure: (1) effects on the autonomic nervous system, (2) inhibition of the renin-angiotensin-aldosterone system, and (3) peripheral vasodilation. Based on these mechanisms, there are a number of potential sites of action for antihypertensive agents (Table 23-3).

Based on the three main antihypertensive mechanisms and the multiple sites at which drugs can act, there are different physiologic approaches to the reduction of blood pressure (Table 23-4).[11] Most drugs currently available do not act by a single mechanism. Within this physiologic approach to lowering blood pressure by vasodilation, the drugs available can be divided into three main subgroups (Table 23-5). Most of these vasodilator drugs act either on the arterial or venous circulations, with very few acting on both (Table 23-6).

BASIC PHARMACOLOGY AND MECHANISMS OF ACTION OF INDIVIDUAL DRUG CLASSES

Calcium Channel Blockers

These drugs have a direct, dose-related effect on three separate functions of the heart (conduction, contraction, and inotropy), and on peripheral and coronary vascular tone. When used to treat high blood pressure, the major effect of these drugs is arterial vasodilation by blockade of Ca^{2+} influx through L type voltage-gated Ca^{2+} channels in the smooth muscle cells of resistance vessels. They also reduce the increase in intracellular Ca^{2+} in response to membrane depolarization, and the secondary Ca^{2+}-induced Ca^{2+} release from intracellular stores. Some calcium channel blockers also reduce heart

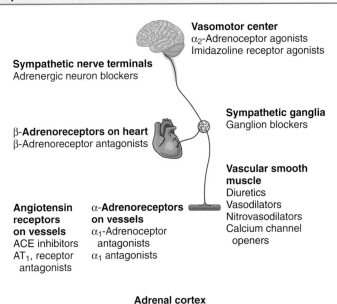

Figure 23-1 **A,** Sites of action within the body of drugs that can be used for the treatment of high blood pressure. **B,** Mechanisms of the neurogenic control of vascular tone via the vasomotor center. *EDRF,* Endothelial derived relaxing factor; *NO,* nitric oxide.

Table 23-3. Sites of Action of Antihypertensive Agents

Vasomotor center
Sympathetic nerve terminals
β adrenoceptor on heart
Sympathetic ganglia
Angiotensin receptors on vessels
α adrenoceptors on vessels
Vascular smooth muscle
Adrenal cortex
Kidney tubules
Juxtaglomerular cells that release renin

Table 23-4. Physiologic Strategies for Reduction of Blood Pressure

Decrease Systemic Vascular Resistance
Decreased sympathetic vascular motor tone
  Decreased central sympathetic activity
  Blockade of ganglionic transmission
  Impairment of vascular neuroeffector transmission
Decreased vascular reactivity
  Relaxation of vascular smooth muscle
  Decrease of Na^+ content of vascular tissue
Decreased humorally mediated vasoconstriction
  Inhibition of vasoconstrictor release
  Blockade of action of vasoconstrictors

Decrease Cardiac Output
Decreased sympathetic cardiac tone
  Decreased central sympathetic activity
  Blockade of sympathetic ganglionic transmission
  Impairment of cardiac neuroeffector transmission
Decreased cardiac reactivity
  Increased vagal activity
  Depression of myocardial reactivity directly
Decreased cardiac return
  Decreased venomotor tone (and thereby increased venous capacitance)
  Decreased circulating fluid volume

Adapted from Bowman WC, Rand MJ. *Textbook of Pharmacology.* 2nd ed. Oxford: Blackwell Scientific; 1980:23.26-23.

Table 23-5. Drugs and Their Physiologic Mechanisms for Lowering Blood Pressure

Neurogenically Acting Hypotensive Agents
  Central depression of catecholamines—rauwolfia alkaloids, alpha-methyl-DOPA, α_2 agonists, monoxidine
  Ganglion blockers—pentolinium, hexamethonium, trimetaphan
  Adrenergic nerve blockers—guanethidine, bethanidine, bretylium, monoamine oxidase inhibitors

Neurogenically Acting Vasodilators Acting on Adrenergic Receptors
  α_1 blockers—prazosin, indoramin, doxazosin, and related compounds
  α_1, α_2 blockers—phentolamine, phenoxybenzamine
  α_1, β_1 blockers—labetalol, carvedilol, nebivolol
  β_2 agonists—isoproterenol

Other Vasodilators
  Renin-angiotensin system antagonists—angiotensin-converting enzyme inhibitors, angiotensin II receptor antagonists, direct renin inhibitors
  Nitrovasodilators—nitric oxide, sodium nitroprusside, nitroglycerin, isosorbide dinitrate, isosorbide mononitrate
  Other vasodilators—hydralazine, minoxidil

Table 23-6. Sites of Action of Vasodilator Drugs

ARTERIOLAR	BOTH	VENODILATORS
Prazosin	Nitroprusside	Nitroglycerin
Phentolamine		
Phenoxybenzamine		
Tolazoline		
Hydralazine		
Diazoxide		
Calcium channel blockers		
Angiotensin-converting enzyme inhibitors		

Dihydropyridines (e.g., nifedipine and nicardipine) bind to the extracellular domain of the L-type voltage-gated Ca^{2+} channel (Ca_V1) in the cell membrane, so inhibiting Ca^{2+} influx.[10] These drugs primarily affect resistance vessels with minimal effects on veins due to the low density of L-type Ca^{2+} channels in capacitance vessels.

Phenylalkylamines (e.g., verapamil) act mainly on the heart where inhibition of voltage-gated Ca^{2+} channels is frequency-dependent. The phenylalkylamines probably enter the cell and bind internally to produce their effects.[12]

Benzothiazepines (e.g., diltiazem) bind on the extracellular side of the L-type channel.[13] Their effects are seen more on vascular compared with cardiac smooth muscle.

β Blockers

There are at least three distinct subtypes of β receptors (β_1, β_2, and β_3), each of which has different tissue distributions. Both β_1 and β_2 agonists mediate their cellular effects through increases in cyclic adenosine monophosphate (cAMP). β receptors are G protein–coupled receptors that traverse the lipid cell membrane seven times. The N-terminal end of the protein is extracellular and the C-terminal end intracellular. The region conferring β receptor coupling is thought to lie in the third cytoplasmic loop between the fifth and sixth transmembrane segments (for further detail of this receptor, see Chapter 1).

β_1 receptors are present mainly in heart muscle. The ligand-receptor complex is coupled to a Gs-protein, which in turn activates adenylyl cyclase to produce cAMP. The cAMP activates a protein kinase A, leading to enhanced influx of Ca^{2+} and, in turn, muscle contraction.

β_2 receptors exist in several sites. Some of these receptors can be identified in heart muscle (hence the rationale for use of salbutamol in some patients with low output states). However, they are more abundant in bronchial and peripheral vascular smooth muscle, where they lead to bronchodilation and vasodilation respectively.

β_3 receptors are present in adipose tissue and heart muscle. In contrast to β_1 and β_2 adrenoceptors, activation of β_3 leads to a *decrease* in inotropic state of the myocardium via a Gi protein–dependent pathway. Thus, as well as having an effect on thermogenesis, β_3 activation can lead to cardiodepressant effects.[14]

ACTION OF β BLOCKERS AT THE ADRENERGIC RECEPTOR
Administration of some β blockers restore receptor responsiveness to catecholamines after β receptor desensitization,

rate and myocardial contractility, which leads to decreased cardiac output and blood pressure.

There are three classes of calcium channel blockers. Difference in subunit structure of Ca^{2+} channels in vascular and cardiac tissues might explain the different selectivity of the drugs. The dihydropyridines act mainly on vascular smooth muscle of resistance vessels, while the non-dihydropyridines act on the myocardium. All three classes act on voltage-gated Ca^{2+} channels that are made up of five subunits (α_1, α_2, β, γ, and δ). The α_2 and δ subunit dimer and γ subunit are transmembrane, while the β unit is located intracellularly. The α_1 subunit forms the transmembrane ion channel.

leading to normal GRK2 activity (G protein–coupled receptor kinase 2; also known as BARK1, or β adrenoceptor kinase 1) and receptor protein subunit $G_{\alpha 1}$ levels. Other β blockers allow intracellular signaling to return toward normal despite concurrent catecholamine stimulation. A third class of β blockers (including metoprolol and carvedilol) have an additional property in reversing the effects of cardiac remodeling. These differences in action could explain why some β blockers protect myocytes more effectively than others, and why all are not equally effective in reducing perioperative ischemia, myocardial infarction, and cardiac mortality.[15,16]

β receptors can exist in three distinct activation states: stabilized and inactivated, nonstabilized and inactivated, or stabilized and activated. Normally there is a dynamic equilibrium between the activated and the two inactivated states. Drugs that stabilize the receptor in the activated state are either partial or full agonists; drugs that push the equilibrium toward the inactivated state are either full or partial agonists; drugs that block access to the receptor binding site without affecting the state of equilibrium are termed *neutral (competitive) antagonists* (see Chapter 1).

At the molecular level, some β blockers incompletely stabilize the activated state of the receptor, leading to a coupling of the receptor to the G intracellular protein (these are therefore partial agonists—bucindilol, xamoterol). They block the effects of potent agonists while generating low-level β adrenoceptor stimulation on their own. Other β blockers stabilize the receptor in the inactivated state, thus leading to receptor upregulation rather than the desensitization and downregulation seen with xamoterol. Such drugs are inverse agonists (metoprolol, nebivolol, sotalol). However, most of the β blockers are neutral or competitive antagonists, in that they bind to the β receptor without affecting its activation state.

These different molecular actions give rise to drugs with different clinical profiles. Thus the β_1 selective blockers (acebutolol, atenolol, bisoprolol, celiprolol, esmolol, xamoterol) diminish detrimental cardiac remodeling while preserving the protective effects of β_2 activation; the β_1, β_2, and α_1 blockers (e.g., bucinodilol, carvedilol, labetalol) decrease arterial vascular tone and serve as effective afterload reducing drugs, as well as blocking the deleterious effects of sympathetic hyperactivity. The partial inverse agonists (metoprolol and nebivolol) might reduce β receptor desensitization while maintaining functional β receptor responsiveness.

β adrenoceptor blocking drugs act as receptors by competitive antagonism. Their action to reduce blood pressure is by both decreasing cardiac output (through their effects on contractility and heart rate) and by inhibiting renin release from the kidneys. There are several ways of classifying the pharmacologic effects of the β adrenoceptor blockers, depending on their receptor specificity; the presence of either intrinsic sympathomimetic or vasodilator activity, and their lipophilicity or hydrophilicity (Table 23-7).

The *β_1 selective agents* such as atenolol, bisoprolol, and metoprolol are cardioselective, although this selectivity is reduced at higher doses. The pure β adrenoceptor blocking drugs do not cause vasodilation. These agents diminish the detrimental effects of myocardial remodeling while preserving the protective effects of β_2 activity.[17,18]

Nonselective (β_1 and β_2) agents have similar effects to the selective agents on blood pressure.

Table 23-7. Classification and Relative Potency of β Blockers Used for Treatment of Hypertension

ANTAGONISTS*	PARTIAL AGONISTS (ISA)*
Selective	
Atenolol (1)	Acebutolol
Metoprolol (3)	Practolol
Esmolol (0.02), landiolol	
Bisoprolol	
Nonselective	
Propranolol (1)	Oxprenolol (1)
Timolol (10)	Alprenolol
Nadolol	Pindolol (20)
Sotalol (0.1)	

*Number enclosed in parentheses indicates potency relative to propranolol at the β_1 receptor.
Vasodilators = labetalol (0.25), celiprolol, carvedilol, nebivolol.
ISA, Intrinsic sympathomimetic activity.

Partial agonists (pindolol) result in less resting bradycardia and some peripheral vasodilation.

Vasodilator activity is also produced by drugs with antagonist action at α receptors (labetalol, celiprolol, carvedilol), or by agents that promote endothelial nitric oxide production via the L-arginine-NO pathway (nebivolol).[19] The use of these drugs with vasodilatory properties can be advantageous when treating hypertension. One of the first drugs of this type (celiprolol) is formulated as a racemic mixture, is hydrophilic, and acts as a β_1 antagonist, mild β_2 agonist, and weak vasodilator.[20] Celiprolol also causes an increase in myocardial inducible NO synthase activity.

Angiotensin-Converting Enzyme Inhibitors and Angiotensin Receptor Antagonists

Renin is a protease synthesized in the kidney and catalyzes the production of angiotensin I from angiotensinogen (a 225 amino acid pro-hormone). Angiotensin-converting enzyme (ACE) then biotransforms angiotensin I to angiotensin II—the latter being a vasoconstrictor through action at angiotensin receptors. The molecular mechanism of action for angiotensin II is through coupling to the phospholipase C Gq protein–IP$_3$ transduction pathway. Angiotensin II also affects norepinephrine kinetics through facilitation of its release and prevention of its reuptake at sympathetic nerve terminals. The renin-angiotensin pathway can therefore be interrupted at two separate sites (both leading to vasodilation): direct inhibition of ACE and angiotensin receptor antagonism (Figure 23-2).

ACE inhibition occurs both in the plasma and in the vascular endothelium. Inhibition also has an effect to reverse arteriolar hypertrophy that occurs in hypertension, and reduce left ventricular hypertrophy. ACE inhibitors decrease conversion of angiotensin I to angiotensin II thereby reducing vasoconstrictor effects, aldosterone secretion, and sympathetic activation (all of which lead to hypertension). Angiotensin II acts on AT_1 receptors via Gq to activate phospholipase C. This has the effect of increasing intracellular diacyl glycerol (DAG) and IP$_3$, which increase Ca^{2+} release from the sarcoplasmic reticulum (SR) to cause vasoconstriction of the efferent arteriole.[21] Stimulation of the AT_2 receptor leads to

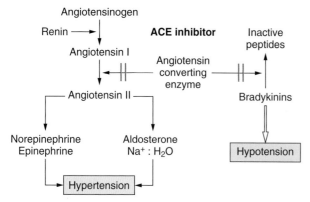

Figure 23-2 Mechanisms of action of angiotensin-converting enzyme inhibitors with inhibition of conversion of angiotensin I to angiotensin II, and inhibition of the breakdown of bradykinin to inactive peptides.

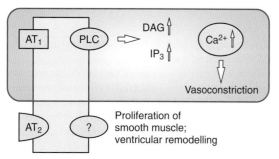

Figure 23-3 Mechanism of action of angiotensin II receptor blockers (at the AT1 and AT2 angiotensin receptors). *DAG,* Diacylglycerol; *IP3,* inositol trisphosphate; *PLC,* phospholipase C.

smooth muscle proliferation and ventricular remodeling (Figure 23-3).

Both ACE inhibitors and AT receptor antagonists produce arterial vasodilation not only by limiting the direct effects of angiotensin II on vascular smooth muscle but also by minimizing its ability to increase sympathetic vascular tone. Their action is also accompanied by an increase in parasympathetic tone. They also decrease the effect of aldosterone on the distal convoluted tubule of the nephron, so promoting salt and water loss. They also block breakdown of bradykinin, which, in turn, contributes to the vasodilator effects of the drugs.

ACE inhibitors prevent the breakdown of kinins, and the increased concentration of bradykinin is probably responsible for the unwanted side effects of cough and allergic reactions. Other side effects of ACE inhibitors include diarrhea. On the other hand, the angiotensin receptor antagonists prevent the vasoconstrictor effects of angiotensin II without affecting ACE activity.[10] So, in contrast to ACE inhibitors, they do not affect kinin production (and hence cough is not a prominent side effect of these drugs). These drugs act as selective blockers at the AT_1 receptors, with no effect on AT_2 receptors.

Diuretics

The action of diuretics to reduce blood pressure is twofold. First, they cause an initial decrease in intravascular volume, although compensatory mechanisms are activated and this effect is reduced over time. They have a secondary mechanism

to reduce blood pressure by direct arterial vasodilation. The exact mechanism involved is not clear but might be through a decrease in Ca^{2+} entry into smooth muscle cells and through stimulating local vasodilator prostaglandin formation. Although the decrease in intravascular volume and total body Na^+ occurs within weeks of the start of diuretic therapy, an increase in renin release causes them to return to normal. The antihypertensive effects of diuretics are not just related to their effects on Na^+ and water balance, because more effective diuretic agents (e.g., furosemide) are not very effective hypotensive agents.

There are three main classes of diuretics:

1. *Thiazides* inhibit Na^+/Cl^- co-transporters in the proximal diluting segment of the distal collecting tubule and early collecting duct. The diuretic effect of the thiazides (except metolazone and indapamide) is less effective in patients with renal impairment.[22] If used long term, thiazides inhibit maximal reabsorption of Na^+ to about 3% to 5% of the filtered load.

2. *Loop diuretics* have a short duration of action and hence are rarely used as first-line drugs for treatment of hypertension. They act on the medullary and cortical thick ascending limb segments of the nephron to prevent Na^+, Cl^-, and water reabsorption. There is some debate as to whether they also have other actions, such as systemic vasodilation and a reduction in left ventricular filling pressure secondary to preload reduction due to venodilation. However, they are useful if volume expansion contributes in part to the etiology of the hypertension (in patients with renal failure or from use of vasodilator drugs).

3. Of the *potassium-sparing diuretics*, both amiloride and triamterene have weak antihypertensive effects. However, spironolactone (an aldosterone antagonist) can be useful as an antihypertensive treatment in primary or secondary hyperaldosteronism, or if the hypertension is treatment-resistant. This class of diuretics has relatively weak natriuretic effects with a maximal excretion of only about 1% to 2% of filtered Na^+ load.[23]

Centrally Acting Agents

Most centrally acting antihypertensive drugs are no longer widely used. However, identifying their sites of action illustrates the diversity of approaches used to reduce blood pressure.

Reserpine acts to deplete neuronal stores of catecholamines both centrally and peripherally at the postganglionic neuron. Its mechanism of action is related to inhibition of norepinephrine and dopamine uptake into terminal synaptic vesicles, leading to increased breakdown of norepinephrine and reduced conversion of dopamine to norepinephrine. Although reserpine crosses the blood-brain barrier, this is probably not the site of its antihypertensive effect.

Bethanidine, guanethidine, and debrisoquin are selective postganglionic neuron blockers that act to inhibit release of norepinephrine from peripheral sympathetic nerve terminals. Although the exact mechanism of action of these drugs is not clear, there is evidence that the drugs must be actively taken up into neurons where they accumulate in synaptic vesicles, causing norepinephrine depletion. Their antihypertensive effects are through reduced adrenergic synaptic transmission.

α₂-Adrenoreceptor Agonists

α_2 Receptor agonists have several distinct pharmacologic effects—sedation, analgesia, and hypotension. The α_2 adrenoceptor is coupled to a Gi protein complex, which inhibits adenylyl cyclase, and Ca^{2+} and K^+ ion channels. The net result of α_2 agonist binding is reduced cAMP production, hyperpolarization, and decreased intracellular Ca^{2+}. α_2 Receptors occur both presynaptically and postsynaptically. Stimulation of presynaptic α_2 receptor decreases central sympathetic outflow. Agonist stimulation of postsynaptic α_2 receptors mediates the sedative and analgesic effects.[24]

Some of the earliest antihypertensive therapies were based on drugs acting on the control mechanisms in the central nervous system (CNS). There are α_2 adrenoceptors in the locus coeruleus in the floor of the fourth ventricle, where α_2 agonists act to cause sedation. The locus coeruleus also has afferent connections from the rostral ventrolateral medullary nuclei and efferent connections to noradrenergic fibers connecting to the thalamus and elsewhere. The α_2 agonists also block salivary gland secretion. Effects in the nucleus tractus solitarius lead to inhibition of sympathetic activity and reduce peripheral vasoconstriction. These drugs are no longer widely used in the treatment of hypertension, with the exception of α-methyl DOPA for treatment of preeclampsia of pregnancy.

Excessive hypotension secondary to α_2 agonist therapy can be reversed by vasopressors and inotropes. The use of ephedrine, phenylephrine, and dobutamine, but not norepinephrine, can be accompanied by an enhanced pressor response due to the β effects of these agents.

There are three main classes of α_2 agonists: (1) the phenylethylates (α-methyl DOPA, guanabenz), (2) the imidazolines (clonidine, dexmedetomidine, mivazerol), and (3) the oxaloazepines.

α-Methyl DOPA is converted in noradrenergic neurons to the false transmitter α-methyl norepinephrine, which is a potent α_2 agonist. It stimulates brainstem postsynaptic α_2 receptors to decrease sympathetic tone and systemic vascular resistance.

Clonidine acts as a presynaptic α_2 agonist on receptors in the brainstem, leading to reduction in sympathetic outflow and an increase in vagal activity. After intravenous dosing, there can be an initial transient hypertensive response due to peripheral vasoconstriction through α_1 and α_{2B} interactions. In contrast to α_2 agonists such as α-methyl DOPA, imidazoline compounds produce hypotension following direct intramedullary injection. This led to the proposal of the presence of nonadrenergic receptors in the lateral reticular nuclei of the ventrolateral medulla (VLM). Two types of nonadrenergic imidazoline receptors have been identified: I_1 receptors in brain and I_2 receptors in brain, pancreas, and kidney. A number of the α_2 agonists also have activity at I_1 receptors. It is likely that they mediate their effects through a G protein–coupled mechanism that results in an increase in arachidonic acid and the subsequent release of prostaglandins. This led to the development of two specific I_2 receptor agonists with more ideal hemodynamic profiles: monoxidine and rilmenidine. Both drugs have weaker affinity for central α adrenoceptors than α-methyl DOPA and clonidine. Other α_2 agonists include dexmedetomidine, which has a greater selectivity and specificity for α_2 receptors than clonidine ($\alpha_2:\alpha_1$ 1620:1

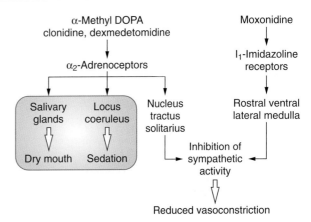

Figure 23-4 Mechanisms of action of α_2 adrenoreceptor agonists and I_1 imidazoline receptor agonists.

compared with 200:1); and mivazerol (119:1) (Figure 23-4). This latter sympatholytic drug has been examined for a role in myocardial protection, but there are no published studies examining its use in the treatment of perioperative hypertension.[25]

Monoxidine is a selective imidazoline receptor agonist that stimulates I_1 receptors in the VLM, thereby decreasing sympathetic outflow and lowering blood pressure. In contrast to some other drugs, its use is not associated with a reflex tachycardia.

α-Adrenoreceptor Antagonists

Agonists of the α_1 adrenoreceptor leads to an increased intracellular Ca^{2+}. The α_1 agonist-receptor interaction leads to activation of phospholipase C (linked to Gq), which increases hydrolysis of phosphatidylinositol bisphosphate (PIP_2) and increases synthesis of two second messengers: DAG and 1,4,5-inositol trisphosphate (IP_3). DAG activates protein kinase C while IP_3 increases the intracellular Ca^{2+} concentration by releasing Ca^{2+} from the SR. There is also evidence that IP_3 causes an increase in the Ca^{2+} sensitivity of the contractile proteins. The phosphorylated product of IP_3 (IP_4—1,3,4,5-inositol tetraphosphate) has been suggested as the messenger that enhances Ca^{2+} flux across the cell membrane, causing vasoconstriction.

The α_1 selective antagonists block α_1 receptors to prevent Ca^{2+} increases, thus leading to smooth muscle relaxation in arterioles and venous capacitance vessels.

There are two types of α_1 antagonists:
1. Selective α_1 antagonists: doxazosin, terazosin, prazosin, and indoramin
2. Nonselective α_1 antagonists: phentolamine and phenoxybenzamine

While the selective antagonists act in a competitive manner, phenoxybenzamine combines irreversibly with the α_1 receptors and so has a prolonged duration of effect. Phentolamine is a short-acting, reversible antagonist.

Nitrovasodilators

Nitric oxide (NO) was identified as the "endothelium-dependent relaxing factor" by Furchgott and Zawadski in

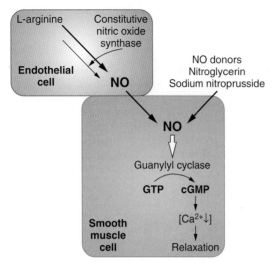

Figure 23-5 Mechanism of action of nitric oxide and nitric oxide donors on vascular smooth muscle. *cGMP*, cyclic guanosine monophosphate; *GMP*, Guanine monophosphate; *GTP*, guanine triphosphate; *NO*, nitric oxide.

1980,[26] and its mechanism defined by Palmer et al.[27] NO is an endogenous vasodilator that causes renal vasodilatation, leading to a diuresis and natriuresis and resulting in reduced blood pressure. There is some suggestion that deficiency in NO could contribute to the etiology of high blood pressure.

NO stimulates guanylyl cyclase to produce cyclic guanosine monophosphate (cGMP), which activates PKG (cGMP-dependent protein kinase). PKG then activates MLCP (myosin light chain phosphatase) to dephosphorylate myosin light chains, and hence produce vascular relaxation.[28] NO also activates sarcoplasmic and endoplasmic reticular Ca^{2+}-ATPase to enhance reuptake of Ca^{2+}, an effect that is cyclic GMP independent. NO might also activate K^+ channels, resulting in membrane hyperpolarization, thus closing voltage-gated Ca^{2+} channels (Figure 23-5).

There are a number of NO donors. Some vasodilators release NO spontaneously (sodium nitroprusside), while others (organic nitrates such as nitroglycerin) need active reduction of the nitrate radical by intracellular sulfhydryl groups. All NO donors are potentiated by phosphodiesterase-5 inhibitors that reduce hydrolysis of cyclic GMP (see later).[29]

Nitrites act as both arterial and venous dilators. They are usually associated with a reflex increase in heart rate; hence they are often coadministered with β blockers.

Sodium nitroprusside (SNP) is broken down in red cells with liberation of cyanide and NO. SNP has a rapid onset of action and is of short duration (1-2 minutes). While breaking down to form NO, SNP interacts with oxyhemoglobin to form cyan-methemoglobin and cyanide.[30] The latter is converted to thiocyanate through transsulfation by the liver enzyme rhodanase, with thiosulfate acting as the sulphur donor. There are still issues over the total safe dose of SNP. Prolonged administration leads to accumulation of thiocyanate and cyanide, with the development of venous hyperoxemia and metabolic acidosis.

Nitrates undergo denitration to produce NO, their active component. Denitration can involve reaction with sulfydryl groups or depends on the action of glutathione-S-transferase, cytochrome P450, and xanthine oxidoreductase. A stepwise

increase in the dose of infused nitrate leads to a reduction in venous tone and central venous pressure. This is accompanied by a gradual decrease in systemic pressure. Administration of bolus doses of nitrates cause significant and immediate decreases in arterial pressure.

Glyceryl trinitrate (GTN) or nitroglycerin acts as an NO donor, with a greater action on venous rather than arteriolar vessels. Its use can lead to tachyphylaxis due to a decrease in NO formation through generation of superoxide and peroxynitrite free radicals that inhibit aldehyde dehydrogenase. Without this enzyme, the conversion of organic nitrates and GTN to NO is impaired. In addition to decreasing blood pressure, GTN also reduces preload and myocardial oxygen demand. GTN is a coronary vasodilator (including relaxation of stenosed vessels) and brings about an increased collateral coronary flow, improved subendocardial perfusion, and improved diastolic function. Because nitroglycerin undergoes extensive first-pass metabolism after oral dosing, nitrates are administered orally as isosorbide dinitrate (ISDN) and its metabolite isosorbide mononitrate (ISMN). Although the main uses of GTN, ISMN, and ISDN are as antianginal drugs, they can also be used by titration for the control of blood pressure in the cardiac patient.

Adenosine stimulates purinergic receptors (P_1 and P_2) on endothelial cells to stimulate NO production. Adenosine also has direct effects on smooth muscle via a G protein–coupled pathway and activates ATP–sensitive K^+ channels, leading to membrane hyperpolarization and relaxation.[31,32] Adenosine receptor blockers prevent Ca^{2+} entry during phase 1 of the action potential, thus causing vascular relaxation. Although predominantly a coronary vasodilator, it can decrease blood pressure. It is not absorbed from the gut and is therefore given by the intravenous route. The half-life after intravenous dosing is less than 10 seconds. It is intracellularly phosphorylated to AMP and then deaminated to inosine, hypoxanthine, xanthine, and uric acid. Both theophylline and other xanthines are antagonists at both P_1 and P_2 receptors; hence their concurrent use increases dose requirements for adenosine. The uptake of adenosine into coronary endothelial cells is inhibited by dipyridamole.

Other Vasodilator

Minoxidil opens ATP-sensitive K^+ channels in vascular smooth muscle, hyperpolarizes the cell membrane, and closes voltage-gated Ca^{2+} channels, leading to smooth muscle relaxation and vasodilation.[33]

Hydralazine acts by promoting the influx of K^+ into vascular smooth muscle cells, thereby causing hyperpolarization and muscle relaxation.[34] It can also cause arterial vasodilation by promoting smooth muscle relaxation through activation of guanylyl cyclase, leading to an increase in cyclic GMP. Other mechanisms of action include inhibition of Ca^{2+} release from the SR, reduction in Ca^{2+} stores in the SR, and stimulation of NO formation by the vascular endothelium.

Diazoxide is chemically similar to thiazide diuretics but causes Na^+ retention. It is a powerful antihypertensive agent due to peripheral vasodilation secondary to opening K^+ channels.

Nicorandil promotes vasodilation of both systemic and coronary arteries by opening ATP-sensitive K^+ channels, hyperpolarization of the membrane, and reduced opening of voltage-gated Ca^{2+} channels and therefore vascular smooth muscle relaxation. This is enhanced by the local production of NO from a nitrate-like action that also causes venodilation.[35]

Ganglionic blockers formerly played a significant role in the modulation of blood pressure. Now only trimethaphan is used (rarely) in hypertensive emergencies or for the production of controlled hypotension during surgery. Ganglionic blockers act by inhibiting autonomic activity at both sympathetic and parasympathetic ganglia. The decrease in sympathetic outflow causes vasodilation.

Magnesium affects vascular tone by diverse mechanisms; it acts as a Ca^{2+} channel antagonist, stimulates production of vasodilator prostaglandins and NO, and alters the response of vascular endothelium to vasoactive agonists.[36]

Endothelin receptor antagonists reduce blood pressure by blocking the actions of endothelins. Endothelins act on both ET_A and ET_B receptors. Endothelin 1 (ET-1) causes vasoconstriction through activation of both types of receptor on vascular smooth muscle cells. The receptors are coupled to Gq, with activation leading to increased synthesis and release of IP_3 and Ca^{2+} release from the SR.[37,38] ET-1 synthesis and release is stimulated by a number of mediators: angiotensin II, arginine vasopressin, thrombin, cytokines, reactive oxygen species, and shear forces on the endothelium. Mixed ET-receptor antagonists lower arterial blood pressure and prevent vascular and myocardial hypertrophy. Use of these drugs has also been studied in the treatment of pulmonary hypertension.

Peripheral dopamine agonists cause selective vasodilation of a number of vascular beds (splanchnic, cerebral, and coronary circulations) and can therefore be used in the treatment of hypertension. There are two subtypes of peripheral DA receptors. DA_1 receptors are postsynaptic Gs protein-coupled receptors and cause vasodilation following increased intracellular cAMP and reduced intracellular calcium. The DA_2 receptor is presynaptic and is coupled to Gi protein, leading to reduced cyclic AMP, with membrane hyperpolarization and reduced norepinephrine release. The effects of dopamine on various catecholamine receptors are dose-dependent: DA_1 interactions occur at low doses, β_1 at moderate doses, and α_1 with high doses (see Chapter 22).

Fenoldopam is a selective DA_1 dopamine agonist without adrenergic receptor agonist properties. It is more potent than dopamine at DA_1 receptors and is useful for control of blood pressure. It also has no agonist effects at the DA_2 receptor. As such, it causes a decrease in blood pressure without increases in heart rate or contractility due to adrenergic effects. An advantage of the drug is that it does not cross the blood-brain barrier. It is available in the United States and some European countries, where it is recommended for acute or emergency control of blood pressure in the perioperative period.[39]

Phosphodiesterases catalyze the hydrolysis of cyclic nucleotides. Phosphodiesterase inhibitors (PDEIs) block the hydrolysis of cAMP or cGMP, so prolonging the effects on smooth muscle of signaling pathways involving these second messengers.[40,41] An increase in cAMP (or cGMP) leads to phosphorylation of myosin light chain kinase, leading to a reduction of its activity due to reduced affinity for the Ca^{2+}-calmodulin complex. The resulting reduced phosphorylation of myosin light chains leads to smooth muscle relaxation and vasodilatation. There are five subtypes of phosphodiesterase; PCE3 is

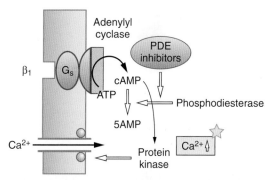

Figure 23-6 Mechanism of action of phosphodiesterase (PDE) inhibitors. β_1, β_1 Adrenoceptor; *Gs*, stimulatory subunit of the G protein complex; *cAMP*, cyclic adenosine monophosphate; *5AMP*, 5′ adenosine monophosphate.

inhibited by milrinone and enoximone, and PDE5 is inhibited by sildenafil and related compounds (see later).

PDE3 inhibition prevents the breakdown of cAMP. Specific phosphodiesterases also hydrolyze cGMP, which might contribute to the vasodilator effect of PDE5 inhibitors. As a result of the inhibition of cyclic nucleotide breakdown, PDEIs cause a decrease in systemic vascular resistance and a small but significant fall in arterial pressure (Figure 23-6).

Prostaglandins PGE_1 and PGI_2 (prostacyclin) have direct vasodilator actions via prostanoid receptors on vascular smooth muscle involving stimulation of cAMP. Although they decrease systemic vascular resistance (and therefore blood pressure), their main effect is on pulmonary vascular resistance (see later).

A number of other drugs are also vasodilators. These include ganglion-blocking neuromuscular blocking drugs (tubocurarine derivatives), general anesthetics, and histamine.

PHARMACOKINETICS, PHARMACODYNAMICS, AND ADVERSE EFFECTS

Calcium Channel Blockers

All calcium channel blockers are effective in reducing blood pressure, although there is some controversy over the adverse effects of short-acting drugs.[42] In general, they are all well tolerated and are becoming the first-line treatment for patients aged older than 55 years. The actions of the three classes of calcium channel blocking drugs differ. The relationship between vasodilation and negative inotropy is about 1:1 for both diltiazem and verapamil, 10:1 for nifedipine, and up to 1000:1 for the newer dihydropyridines.[43] In the same way, the side effects of calcium channel blockers differ according to the class of drug.

Verapamil (a phenylalkylamine) is a racemic mixture that is well absorbed orally and has high presystemic metabolism (about 85%; L-enantiomer >D-enantiomer). Metabolism is extensive by O-demethylation (25%) and N-dealkylation (40%) followed by conjugation. Some of the metabolites are active, especially nor-verapamil, which has about one-fifth to one-tenth the activity of the parent drug. Verapamil has a half-life of about 5 hours (range 2-7 hours), which can be prolonged in patients with liver disease. The clearance of L-verapamil is greater than that of the D-enantiomer,

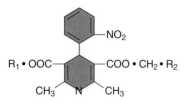

Figure 23-7 Structure of the dihydropyridine calcium entry blockers. R$_1$ and R$_2$ = side-chains at the 1 and 4 positions of the pyridine ring.

although the half-lives of the two enantiomers are similar. There is greater free fraction of L-verapamil, and hence it has a greater volume of distribution. Verapamil is excreted in the urine (70%; as metabolites and unchanged drug) and feces.

Diltiazem (a benzothiazepine) is well absorbed orally (>90%), but has a smaller fraction undergoing presystemic metabolism (about 50%). Diltiazem is extensively metabolized, and some of these metabolites are active.

All dihydropyridines (nifedipine, amlodipine, felodipine, isradipine, nicardipine, lacidipine, lercanidipine, nisoldipine) are well absorbed by the oral route (>90%), but because of their significant presystemic metabolism, sublingual dosing is preferable for some (e.g., nifedipine). Presystemic metabolism of nifedipine results in inactive metabolites with half-lives of about 9 hours, while that of the parent drug is about 2 to 6 hours, with plasma protein binding of more than 90% and a small volume of distribution (0.3-1.2 L/kg). Metabolites are excreted in both the urine (80%) and feces.

Chemical substitutions in nifedipine at the R1 position, with introduction of long side chains (as amlodipine), produce drugs with a longer duration of action and a half-life of up to 30 to 40 hours (felodipine 12-36 hours; isradipine 2-8 hours; nicardipine 3-12 hours; amlodipine 35-60 hours) (Figure 23-7). The dihydropyridines are metabolized by hepatic cytochrome P450 (mainly CYP 3A4), and hence there are many examples of drug-drug interactions either with CYP 3A4 inhibitors (the -azoles, -avirs, erythromycin, clarithromycin) or with other drugs competing for metabolism by the same isoform (e.g., midazolam, alfentanil, cyclosporin). Nifedipine shows a bimodal polymorphism of metabolism by CYP 3A4/5.

The calcium channel blockers all demonstrate age-related kinetics due to reduction in cardiac output (and liver blood flow), leading to increased bioavailability and decreased systemic clearance. Other side effects of dihydropyridine include vasodilation with flushing, headaches, ankle edema, and reflex tachycardia. The use of calcium channel blockers is contraindicated in patients with heart failure due to their negative inotropic effects (especially the non-dihydropyridines), and slowing of sinoatrial and atrioventricular node conduction, leading to bradycardia and heart block. Pronounced antihypertensive effects are mainly observed with the dihydropyridines. The decrease in blood pressure is accompanied by reflex tachycardia and increased myocardial oxygen utilization.

ADVERSE DRUG INTERACTIONS

Dihydropyridines increase plasma digoxin concentrations by inhibiting its tubular secretion by interaction with P-glycoprotein.

Verapamil can worsen cardiac failure in affected patients, causing hypotension due to both vasodilation and negative

inotropy. If verapamil is given in combination with a β blocker, patients can develop hypotension, asystole, and an increased incidence of arrhythmias.

Diltiazem reduces cardiac output and hepatic clearance of flow-limited drugs, such as propranolol and cyclosporin A. All non-dihydropyridines (diltiazem and verapamil) can cause bradycardia and heart block when administered in conjunction with β blockers. They can also exacerbate congestive heart failure through negative inotropic effects.

NEW CALCIUM CHANNEL BLOCKERS

Clevidipine (an intravenous dihydropyridine) is characterized by rapid onset of action, vascular selectivity and unique pharmacokinetics. Unlike other drugs in this class, it is not metabolized in the liver but undergoes breakdown of an ester-linkage in blood and extravascular tissues to produce inactive carboxylic acid metabolites. This leads to a rapid onset of effect (within 60 seconds) and short duration of action. It is highly protein bound (>99.5%) with a small volume of distribution (0.5-0.6 L/kg) and high clearance (0.105 L/kg/min). The rapid offset relates partly to its short elimination half-life (about 15 minutes). After infusions of up to 12 hours, the context-sensitive half-time of the drug is less than 2 minutes. Drug metabolism does not involve CYP enzymes, and hence its elimination is not affected by hepatic or renal disease, and there are no significant drug-drug interactions documented to date.[44] Clevidipine might be useful for emergency control of blood pressure by careful titration of an intravenous infusion.[45,46]

β Blockers

There are two main chemical structural types of β blockers: (1) amino-oxypropanol derivatives (propranolol, timolol, pindolol, metoprolol, atenolol, esmolol, and carvedilol) and hydroxyaminoethyl compounds (sotalol and labetalol). Although described in Table 23-7 as β1 selective blocking drugs, metoprolol, celiprolol, and bisoprolol all show β2 antagonism at high doses. Most β blockers are well absorbed when given orally, although atenolol and sotalol, being more polar, have lower oral absorption (about 50%). Carvedilol, metoprolol, and propranolol all undergo extensive presystemic metabolism; bisoprolol shows no presystemic metabolism and is only metabolized by about 50%. Both atenolol and sotalol are eliminated in urine mostly unchanged. The principal kinetics and dynamics of some commonly used β blocking agents for treatment of hypertension are summarized in Table 23-8.

Propranolol is a nonselective β-blocking drug (although β$_1$ activity >β$_2$ activity), with some membrane-stabilizing activity (MSA). It is highly lipid soluble and can therefore cross the blood-brain barrier, which can result in drug-induced depression. Propranolol undergoes extensive hepatic metabolism with less than 4% drug excreted unchanged in the urine and feces.

Oxprenolol is a β$_1$-selective blocker with intrinsic sympathomimetic activity (ISA) and MSA. Like propranolol, it is extensively metabolized with less than 5% excreted unchanged in the urine.

Metoprolol is a highly selective β$_1$ drug with no MSA and no ISA. Metoprolol shows polymorphism with regard to its metabolism; some of the metabolites (especially

Table 23-8. Pharmacokinetics and Pharmacodynamics of Common Beta Blockers

	ORAL ABSN (%)	BIOAVAIL ABILITY (%)	$T_{1/2}$ (HR)	PLASMA PROTEIN (%)	METABOLIC ROUTE	β_1 SELECTIVITY	ISA	MSA	VASODILATION	OTHER
Acebutolol	>50	30-50	3-6	26	100% H	Yes	Yes	Yes	No	Nil
Atenolol	40-50	>90	6-7	<3	10% H	Yes	No	No	No	Nil
Bisoprolol	>95	80-90	9-13	30	50% H	Yes	No	No	No	Nil
Carvedilol	25	R30; S15	7-10	98	H	No	No	Yes	Yes	Yes[1]
Celiprolol	30-70	>85	4-6	30	Minimal	Yes	No	No	Yes	Yes[2]
Labetalol	>95	15-90	3-4	50	90% H	Yes	No	No	Yes	Yes[3]
Metoprolol*	50-70	40-50	3-7*	5-10	90% H, gut	Yes	No	No	No	Nil
Nadolol	30-40	>95	17-24	30	Minimal	No	No	No	No	Nil
Nebivolol*	?	12-96	12-19*	?	Extensive H	Yes	No	No	Yes	Yes[4]
Oxprenolol	90	20-70	1-2	80	Extensive H	No	Yes	Yes	No	Nil
Pindolol	>95	85-90	3-4	40	H	No	Yes	Yes	No	Nil
Propranolol	>95	5-50	3-6	80-95	100% H	No	No	Yes	No	Nil
Timolol*	>95	50	2-5	80	80% H	No	No	No	No	Nil
Esmolol	N/A	N/A	0.14-0.18	55	Rbc-esterase	Yes	No	No	No	Nil

*, Drug showing polymorphism; *ABSN, absorption; H*, hepatic; *ISA*, intrinsic sympathomimetic activity; *MSA*, membrane stabilizing activity; *plasma protein (%)*, plasma protein binding; *Yes[1]*, α_1, β_2 antagonism; *Yes[2]*, β_2 agonism; *Yes[3]*, β_1 and β_2 antagonism, some ISA at β_2.

α-OH-metoprolol and *O*-desmethyl-metoprolol) are active at the β_1 receptor. There can also be extrahepatic metabolism.

Pindolol is excreted in the urine as both unchanged drug (40%) and metabolites following oxidation and glucuronide conjugation.

Atenolol has properties similar to those of metoprolol. It is eliminated by renal excretion (90%) as unchanged drug. Being hydrophilic, there are few central nervous system side effects due to minimal blood-brain barrier transfer.

Bisoprolol is a β_1-selective blocker that is well absorbed orally. Elimination is via the kidney (50% unchanged and 50% as an active metabolite) following hepatic biotransformation.

Nadolol is a (β_1-selective blocker that is eliminated solely by the kidney. Hence its use is contraindicated in patients with renal impairment.

Timolol is a nonselective β blocker that is eliminated by both hepatic metabolism and renal excretion (20% as unchanged drug).

Bextalol is a cardioselective blocker that is well absorbed and undergoes minimal presystemic metabolism. It has a half-life of 13 to 24 hours and is metabolized by hepatic hydroxylation with little conjugation. The hydroxyl-metabolite is excreted in the urine, together with 10% to 17% unchanged drug.

Acebutolol, carteolol, penbutolol, and pindolol are all nonselective agents with some ISA. Acebutolol is biotransformed by hydrolysis and N-acetylation in the liver to an active metabolite, diacetolol, which has a long half-life of 10 to 14 hours. There can also be some drug metabolism in the gut following oral dosing.

Celiprolol is a third-generation selective β_1 blocker with no MSA. This agent has some ISA at the β_2 receptor, manifest as weak bronchodilation and vasodilation.

ANTIHYPERTENSIVE EFFECT OF β BLOCKERS

The exact mechanism by which β blockers reduce blood pressure is unclear. They could act through reduction in cardiac output that is not compensated for by baroreflex mechanisms, and where there might be a resetting of the reflex. Some of the drugs (those that are lipophilic) can also have a central effect to reduce sympathetic outflow. Another antihypertensive effect can be through inhibition of renin release from the kidney.

NEW β BLOCKERS

Carvedilol (α_1, β_1, β_2 blocker) has a unique carbazole moiety. It is a nonselective agent that also blocks the α_1 receptor. Carvedilol has some MSA but no ISA. It exerts a greater clinical effect than other β blockers in the management of congestive cardiac failure and postmyocardial infarction. It is also an antioxidant with antiarrhythmic, antiapoptotic, and antiproliferative properties that influence carbohydrate and lipid metabolism.[47] Carvedilol is metabolized by CYP 2D6 to an active metabolite (a 4-hydroxy-phenol). Drug elimination is via the biliary route and excretion in the feces. Carvedilol has an elimination half-life of 7 to 10 hours.

Nebivolol is formulated as a racemic mixture. It is highly lipophilic and rapidly absorbed, with a peak effect of 0.5 to 2 hours. It has vasodilating properties that are mediated by stimulation of the L-arginine-NO pathway. It is only available as an oral preparation and undergoes extensive metabolism by glucuronidation, and N-dealkylation and oxidation by CYP P450 2D6 with less than 0.5% excreted unchanged. Because of genetic polymorphism of CYP 2D6, bioavailability varies from about 12% in fast metabolizers to 96% in poor metabolizers, and the terminal half-life from 11 hours to 30+ hours, respectively.[19,48,49] Both carvedilol and nebivolol reduce blood pressure through a decrease in systemic vascular resistance rather than the proposed decrease in cardiac output (see later).[47,49]

ADVERSE EFFECTS OF β BLOCKERS

Because of differences in pharmacologic profiles, different β adrenoceptor blockers have varied *side-effect profiles*, but there are some common features:

- All β blockers have negative inotropic effects and can cause acute left ventricular failure when given in large doses to patients with impaired left ventricular function.
- All β blockers can exacerbate intermittent claudication and Raynaud's phenomenon in patients with coexisting peripheral vascular disease.
- Large doses of β blockers can cause bradycardia leading to syncope.
- Nonselective β blockers that interact with β_2 receptors can result in bronchospasm in patients with asthma or chronic obstructive pulmonary disease due to blockade of β_2 receptors.
- β Blockade can cause significant blood lipid effects leading to increased triglycerides and decreased high-density lipoprotein cholesterol.
- Lipophilic β blockers that can cross the blood-brain-barrier can cause central nervous system effects leading to depression, sleep disturbances, vivid dreams, and hallucinations.
- Sudden withdrawal of β blockers results in increased catecholamine sensitivity; this upregulation can produce tachycardia, acute hypertension, and palpitations.

There are also important *drug interactions* involving β blockers:

- Cimetidine (a CYP inhibitor) decreases hepatic first-pass metabolism of propranolol and metoprolol, and the hepatic metabolism of bisoprolol.
- Carvedilol increases plasma concentrations of digoxin and the risk of toxicity.
- Concurrent administration of β blockers and verapamil increases risk of bradyarrhythmias and heart failure.
- Avoid use of sotalol in conjunction with other drugs that prolong the QT interval (e.g., amiodarone, disopyramide, procainamide, quinidine).
- All β blockers can potentiate the effects of insulin and other oral hypoglycemic drugs, and block the normal sympathetic responses to hypoglycemia. Some evidence suggests that this effect is more pronounced with nonselective β blockers.

Angiotensin-Converting Enzyme Inhibitors

Both captopril and enalapril are well absorbed orally, but absorption is decreased to 50% if taken in the presence of food. Captopril has limited presystemic metabolism (3%-14%), has a half-life of 1 to 2 hours, and has plasma protein binding of 30%. It undergoes both hepatic and renal elimination with 50% excreted unchanged and 50% transformed to inactive metabolites.

Enalapril is the orally administered prodrug of the active compound enalaprilat (available for intravenous use), which is formed when enalapril undergoes extensive presystemic metabolism. Enalapril has a half-life of less than 1 hour, but enalaprilat has a long half-life of 35 hours. Enalaprilat is excreted unchanged in urine.

Lisinopril shows slow and poor oral absorption (<25%) and is eliminated unchanged in the urine. It has a half-life of about 12 hours and low protein binding (3%-10%).

Ramipril is modestly well absorbed (about 60%), and undergoes some presystemic metabolism. Like enalapril, it is metabolized to the active form ramiprilat, which in turn undergoes partial excretion in the bile.

Other ACE inhibitor prodrugs include quinalopril and perindopril. The long half-lives of all the ACE inhibitors relate to their extensive binding to ACE in the plasma.

Angiotensin II Receptor Antagonists

Angiotensin II receptor antagonists act as competitive antagonists at the AT-1 receptor: currently they are only formulated as oral medications. Candesartan is rapidly and completely de-esterified during absorption of candesartan axetil. It is highly protein bound, and undergoes part metabolism, and part excretion in the bile. Unchanged drug is excreted in the urine. Candesartan has a half-life of about 10 hours, with a peak concentration at 3 to 4 hours.

Irbesartan is also rapidly and completely absorbed after oral dosing, and undergoes minimal presystemic metabolism. The drug is 90% bound to plasma proteins. It is metabolized by oxidation (CYP 2C9) and glucuronidation with a half-life of 12 hours. There are interactions between candesartan and other drugs metabolized by CYP 2CP in vitro, although no significant changes in disposition have been reported in vivo.

Losartan is well absorbed after oral administration, but undergoes extensive presystemic metabolism by CYP 2C9 and 3A4. The parent drug has a half-life of 2 hours, but there is an active metabolite (with a half-life of about 8 hours). Peak concentrations of drug and metabolite occur at about 1 and 4 hours respectively. Losartan is inactivated by further metabolism with two inactive metabolites excreted in the bile. Systemic bioavailability is double in patients with liver disease, but there is no change after oral dosing in patients with renal dysfunction.

Valsartan has a low systemic bioavailability (25%) reduced even further (to 15%) if administered with food. The drug is extensively protein bound (95%), and mostly excreted in the bile and feces (83%) with 13% eliminated in the urine. There is no effect of renal failure on valsartan disposition. It has a half-life of about 6 hours.

Other drugs of this class are mainly longer acting (due to longer elimination half-lives): eprosartan (5-9 hours), olmesartan (about 13 hours), and telmisartan (16-23 hours).

ADVERSE EFFECTS AND DRUG INTERACTIONS

Hypotension is associated with intravascular volume depletion due to accompanying diuretic therapy.

ACE inhibitors can cause renal impairment and hyperkalemia especially in patients with renal artery stenosis as perfusion of the affected kidney depends on the local production of angiotensin. Rashes are seen in about 10% of patients and can be accompanied by fever and eosinophilia. Rarely this is associated with episodes of angioneurotic edema.

Coadministration of NSAIDs (cyclooxygenase inhibitors) can reduce the hypotensive effects of ACE inhibitors. ACE inhibitors can inhibit the excretion of lithium, and can result in lithium toxicity. Angiotensin II receptor antagonists can cause hypotension if coadministered with diuretics. They should be used with caution in patients with renal failure, because they rarely lead to hyperkalemia.

Because these drugs do not affect the breakdown of kinins (as is seen with the ACE inhibitors), patients do not develop episodes of coughing, and rarely develop angioneurotic edema.

Diuretics

Diuretics are discussed in more detail in Chapter 34.

Thiazides are all absorbed when given orally and are excreted unchanged by the kidney. Half- lives range between 3 and 90 hours. Chlorthalidone is well absorbed (60%-70%) with negligible presystemic metabolism. Unlike some other thiazides, it has a long half-life (50-90 hours), with protein binding of 75%.

Loop diuretics act by inhibiting Na^+ and K^+ reabsorption in the ascending loop of Henle by inhibiting $Na^+/K^+/Cl^-$ co-transport. *Furosemide* is poorly absorbed (50%-65%), with poorer absorption in the presence of heart failure, is excreted mainly unchanged in the urine, has a plasma half-life of about 1 hour, and high protein binding (96%-98%). *Bumetanide* drug is well absorbed following oral administration (65%-95%). About 60% is excreted unchanged in the urine, with the rest being metabolized by the liver and excreted in urine and bile. Bumetamide has a half-life of 1.5 hours, volume of distribution of 9.5 to 35 L, and high protein binding (95%). As is seen with furosemide and the thiazides, bumetamide, in the presence of hypokalemia, potentiates the effects of glycosides and other antiarrhythmic drugs, thus increasing the incidence of arrhythmias.

Diazoxide is well absorbed orally (85%-95%), and has a long half-life (20-40 hours) and high protein binding (90%).

Amiloride shows poor oral absorption, with no presystemic metabolism. It has low protein binding, with a large volume of distribution (5 L/kg). Amiloride is almost completely excreted unchanged in urine and has a plasma half-life of 6 to 9 hours.

Spironolactone is an aldosterone antagonist that is well absorbed orally with a short half-life of 10 minutes. It is metabolized in the liver to the active compound canrenone, which has a half-life of 16 hours and is excreted by the kidney. Protein binding is high (98%). Because of the long half-life of its metabolite, spironolactone has a long duration of action with the maximum effect of the drug taking some days to be reached.

Triamterene undergoes incomplete (30%-83%) although rapid absorption from the gut. There is some presystemic metabolism, and it is extensively biotransformed in the liver before urinary excretion and variable biliary excretion. The elimination half-life is about 2 hours, with protein binding of 45%-70%.

ADVERSE EFFECTS AND DRUG INTERACTIONS

There are important side effects of all diuretics. Prolonged use of thiazides (especially in older adults) can lead to hyponatremia and hypokalemia, and an increased plasma uric acid concentration. Prolonged hypokalemia, in turn, leads to impaired glucose tolerance due to inhibition of insulin release, as well as enhancing digitalis toxicity. Whereas thiazides cause a reduction in Ca^{2+} excretion, the loop diuretics increase Ca^{2+} excretion.

Both groups of diuretics reduce clearance of lithium by the kidney (which increases the risk of toxicity as the latter has a narrow therapeutic range). Hypokalemia potentiates the effects of cardiac glycosides, as well as altering the effects of antiarrhythmic drugs, leading to ventricular arrhythmias (torsade de pointes).

All the potassium-sparing diuretics (amilioride, spironolactone, and triamterene) potentiate additively the potassium-sparing effects of ACE inhibitors, and therefore their coadministration can be dangerous. The potassium-sparing diuretics can also lead to hyperkalemia in patients also receiving potassium supplements or in patients with renal failure. These diuretics can also cause renal failure when coadministered to patients receiving NSAIDs. Spironolactone interferes with the assay of digitalis. Triamterene inhibits the urinary excretion of the antiparkinsonian drug amantadine.

α_2-Adrenoreceptor Agonists

There are no available data to suggest that α_2 agonists are useful for the rapid control of blood pressure in the perioperative period. They are used in special circumstances for treatment of chronic hypertension.

Clonidine is the archetypal drug of this group. It is moderately lipid soluble, shows complete absorption after oral dosing, but undergoes limited presystemic metabolism (up to 25%). Clonidine has a peak effect at 60 to 90 minutes and peak plasma concentration at 1 to 3 hours. Clonidine has a long half-life (12-24 hours), protein binding of 20% to 40%, and a large volume of distribution (2-4 L/kg). It is eliminated by both hepatic metabolism and renal excretion.

Dexmedetomidine was introduced into clinical practice more recently, although principally as a sedative rather than antihypertensive. It is the D-enantiomer of medetomidine. Dexmedetomidine has a volume of distribution of 100 L and clearance of about 40 L/hour. There is high protein binding to albumin and α_1 glycoprotein, and undergoes extensive hepatic biotransformation. Dexmedetomidine also has a weak inhibitory effect on CYP 2D6 mediated metabolism in vitro.

α-Methyl DOPA is incompletely absorbed following oral dosing and has variable (10%-60%) bioavailability. It has low protein binding (10%-15%), a half-life of 6 to 12 hours, and is eliminated through both the biliary tract and the kidney.

An important issue with these drugs is that all α_2 agonists have significant side-effect profiles. Central α_2 agonists (e.g., clonidine) cause decreased sympathetic activity, leading to postural or exertional hypotension. Other side effects include ejaculation failure and an effect on the central nervous system–mediated sedation and drowsiness. Significant side effects of α-methyl DOPA include orthostatic hypotension, dizziness, sedation, dryness of the mouth, nasal congestion, headaches, and impotence. Rebound hypertension can occur on withdrawal, but occurs less frequently than after cessation of clonidine. It can also cause a reversible positive Coombs test hemolytic anemia. I_1 receptor agonists (monoxidine) can cause dry mouth, nausea, fatigue, dizziness, and headaches.

α-Adrenoreceptor Antagonists

PHENTOLAMINE AND PHENOXYBENZAMINE

Phentolamine is a competitive nonselective antagonist of α_1 receptors, with a half- life of 3 to 13 hours and protein binding of 54%. Little more is known about its pharmacokinetics or metabolism, although it is excreted mainly unchanged by the kidney. Phentolamine has equal efficacy at α_1 and α_2 receptors, and is a 5-hydroxy-tryptamine (serotonin) antagonist.

Phenoxybenzamine is a haloalkylamine that acts as a noncompetitive, irreversible antagonist. The half-life is 18 to 24 hours, but the duration of effect depends on the cellular turnover of receptors—with evidence of drug action for 3 to 4 days. It is biotransformed probably in the liver. The slow onset of effect is due to the need for initial conversion of its ring structure to a reactive carbonium ion, which covalently binds to the α_1 receptor.

There are common adverse effects for both drugs (similar to those of other drugs that decrease sympathetic outflow), namely vasodilation leading to a reflex tachycardia, orthostatic hypotension secondary to venous pooling, nasal congestion, and ejaculatory failure. Headaches, lethargy, dizziness, nausea, and urinary frequency also occur.

Although labetalol is normally classified as a β-receptor antagonist, it also shows nonspecific α-receptor antagonist properties.

Prazocin, doxazocin, and *terazocin* are all absorbed orally (up to 65% for doxazocin), undergo some presystemic hepatic metabolism, and are then mostly broken down in the liver by dealkylation followed by conjugation. All three drugs have high protein binding (90%-98%).

Although the half-lives of the drugs vary (prazocin, 2-4 hours; doxazocin, 9-12 hours; terazocin, 11 hours), their therapeutic effects lasts longer (prazocin about 10 hours; doxazocin about 30 hours). Terazocin is eliminated unchanged in the urine and feces. There is need to reduce dosage of all three agents in patients with renal failure. This is not due to drug or metabolite accumulation but to increased drug sensitivity. The exact mechanism is unclear but may be due to increased absorption, decreased first-pass metabolism, altered drug binding, or decreased volume of drug distribution.

Indoramin is also well orally absorbed (>90%), but undergoes almost complete metabolism by presystemic metabolism. Indoramin has variable protein binding (72%-92%), a half-life of 2 to 10 hours, and might have active metabolites.

The antihypertensive effects of α_1 blocking drugs are enhanced by coadministration with other antihypertensive agents, especially diuretics and β blockers. α_1 Blockers should not be given in conjunction with MAOIs.

Vasodilators

HYDRALAZINE

Hydralazine is well absorbed orally, undergoes presystemic metabolism, and shows extensive metabolism (65%-90%) by acetylation (with a bimodal distribution). The half-life of hydralazine is 3 to 7 hours; because acetylation by NAT-2 occurs mainly during presystemic metabolism, the subsequent rate of drug clearance is not directly related to the rate of acetylation. There is a bimodal distribution of clearance; slow acetylators are at risk of developing a lupus-type condition. However, acetylator status does not appear to affect the half-life. Hydralazine has high protein binding (87%) and a large volume of distribution (3.6 L/kg).

The ratio of fast:slow acetylators in the population is racially determined. In Europe, the ratio is about 40:60; in Japan 85:15; and in the Inuit population 95:5. The consequences of this bimodal metabolic profile are twofold: first, slow acetylators can have an enhanced response to treatment; second, they can also have an increased risk of drug toxicity. The difference between fast and slow acetylators is not dependent on kinetic properties but rather on the amount of the NAT-2 isoform expressed. A reduced dose of hydralazine is indicated in the presence of renal and hepatic disease, regardless of the metabolic phenotype.

NICORANDIL

Nicorandil acts as a mixed vasodilator with part nitrate-like action and part K^+ channel opening effect.[50] After oral twice-daily dosing, steady-state concentrations are reached by 96 to 120 hours, although there is an onset of effect by 30 minutes after dosing. Nicorandil undergoes extensive hepatic metabolism to an inactive denitrated metabolite that is excreted in the urine and has a short half-life (1 hour) and high clearance (about 1.1 L/min).

Side effects associated with the use of nicorandil include headache in 25% to 50% of patients on starting the drug, as well as dizziness, nausea, and vomiting.

MINOXIDIL

Another arterial vasodilator (like hydralazine), *minoxidil* is well absorbed orally and has an elimination half-life of 3 to 4 hours. The duration of effect of a single dose is 8 to 12 hours. It is mainly prescribed in patients with resistant hypertension, but is often accompanied by significant side effects. These include hirsutism (therefore the drug is usually only prescribed in males), and peripheral edema due to fluid retention. Because it is a powerful vasodilator, other adverse effects include skin flushing, headache, reflex tachycardia, and associated palpitations. To overcome the edema and tachycardia, the drug is often coadministered with a β blocker and a diuretic.

NITRATES

Glyceryl trinitrate (or nitroglycerin) undergoes extensive hepatic presystemic metabolism when given orally, and is therefore usually given by the sublingual route, by which it is well absorbed and rapidly taken up into the circulation. Buccal administration has a similar effect, and this route is used for more prolonged action over a few hours. When given intravenously, there is drug breakdown by the cells of the vascular endothelium. Nitroglycerin is broken down (bioactivated) to 1,2 glyceryl nitrate and NO by hepatic mitochondrial aldehyde dehydrogenase. Tolerance develops over time as the enzyme is depleted by continuous exposure.

Isosorbide dinitrate (ISDN) is absorbed in the gut and extensively metabolized to active metabolites especially the mononitrate ISMN, which also shows good oral absorption but, in contrast to ISDN, has low presystemic metabolism. The half-lives of these nitrates are a few minutes for nitroglycerin, 1 hour for ISDN, and 4 hours for ISMN. Protein binding differs for the three agents (ISMN < 5%, for ISDN 30%, and nitroglycerin 60%). There are also differences in their volumes of distribution (ISMN 3 L/kg; ISDN 1-8 L/kg; nitroglycerin 0.7 L/kg).

Sodium nitroprusside is effective within 30 to 40 seconds of infusion, and offset is similarly rapid. It is broken down in the liver to cyanide and thiocyanate; together with the parent drug, both are excreted in the urine. Dose reduction is indicated for all nitrates in patients with renal or hepatic disease. There may be tolerance to vasodilatory effects of nitrates with prolonged dosing especially when given transdermally. The safe doses of nitroprusside are less than 1.5 µg/kg/min during hypotensive anesthesia and up to 8 µg/kg/min to treat hypertensive crises.

PHOSPHODIESTERASE INHIBITORS

The peripheral actions of the PDEIs are mediated by PDE3. There are two main chemical classes of inhibitors—the bipyridines (amrinone and milrinone) and the imidazolones (enoximone). These drugs cause vasodilation by increasing the intracellular cAMP in vascular smooth muscle, leading to activated outward Ca^{2+} transport and hence a decrease in intracellular Ca^{2+} concentration.

Amrinone has an elimination half-life of 2 to 4 hours, clearance of 4 to 9 mL/kg/min, and a small volume of distribution (1.3 L/kg). It has low protein binding (20%) and its elimination is not affected by renal disease. On the other hand, *milrinone* in healthy patients has an intermediate protein binding 70%, terminal half-life of 2 hours, clearance of 2 to 3 mL/kg/min, and volume of distribution of 0.4 to 0.5 L/kg; its terminal half-life is increased in patients with renal dysfunction. Enoximone has a higher clearance (10 mL/kg/min), protein binding (70%-85%), and longer terminal half-life of 6 to 7 hours. The action of enoximone is increased in renal failure due to the accumulation of the active sulfoxide metabolite.[51]

Other nonspecific PDEIs include the methylxanthines (e.g., theophylline and aminophylline) and the benzylisoquinoline, papaverine.

PHARMACOTHERAPY OF HYPERTENSION

Current first-line drugs for the treatment of high blood pressure are diuretics, ACE inhibitors and angiotensin II receptor blockers, and calcium channel blockers; the latter three groups of drugs potentiate the effect of the diuretics. Joint National Committee on Prevention, Detection, Evaluation and Treatment of High Blood Pressure 7th Report (JNC VII) indicates that thiazides are the first choice for treatment of uncomplicated hypertension, while combination therapy has greater efficacy than doubling of single drug dosage.[52] However, calcium channel blockers are an effective treatment in hypertensive patients for the prevention of stroke, but have little effect on the incidence of heart failure, major cardiovascular events, and cardiovascular and total mortality.[53]

β Blockers for the treatment of hypertension should be reserved for patients with associated coronary artery disease or tachycardia/tachyarrhythmias.[54-56] In comparisons with other treatments, β blockers show a greater ability to reduce the incidence of stroke (29% vs 17%) but no difference in prevention of coronary events and heart failure.[57] In patients with associated heart failure, thiazides, ACE inhibitors, aldosterone receptor blockers (spironolactone), and low-dose titrated β blockers are indicated. In patients with renal impairment, ACE inhibitors and angiotensin II receptor antagonists are the drugs of choice.[58]

A Cochrane Review of randomized trials of at least 1 year duration compared thiazides, β blockers, calcium channel blockers, ACE inhibitors, α_1 blockers, and angiotensin II receptor blockers as first-line therapies for patients with uncomplicated hypertension. The review concluded, "Low-dose thiazides reduced all cause mortality and morbidity (as stroke, coronary heart disease, cardiovascular events); ACE inhibitors and calcium channel blockers might be similarly effective but the evidence is less robust; and high-dose thiazides and β blockers are inferior to low-dose thiazides."[59]

HYPERTENSION AND ANESTHESIA

Present anesthetic practice dictates that all antihypertensive therapies (with the possible exception of high-dose ACE inhibitors and angiotensin II receptor antagonists) are maintained up to the time of surgery. Not all investigators agree that ACE inhibitors and angiotensin II receptor antagonists should be withheld.[60,61] However, preoperative evaluation for patients with hypertension should include the measurement of plasma K^+ concentrations, especially in patients receiving diuretics or renin-angiotensin system antagonists.

One of the present controversies is which groups of patients (if any) should the surgery be cancelled because of raised blood pressure? There are few data on the influence of coexisting hypertension on cardiovascular outcome following noncardiac surgery. None of the scoring systems used to categorize patient risk include hypertension as a factor. However, a recent study of outcome from Switzerland identified an increased incidence of cardiovascular complications (11.2% vs 4.6%; adjusted odds ratio 1.38 [1.27-1.49]) in the hypertensive subgroup.[62] These results are in keeping with the meta-analysis of Howell and colleagues[63] (odds ratio 1.35 [1.17-1.56]) for perioperative cardiovascular complications of cardiac mortality, myocardial infarction and heart failure, and arrhythmias.

The 2007 American College of Cardiology/American Heart Association (ACC/AHA) guidelines offer few substantive recommendations as to which hypertensive patients should be canceled to allow treatment before surgery, or how long such treatment should be continued before surgery.[64] Indeed the ACC/AHA Guidelines list "uncontrolled systemic hypertension" as a low-risk factor for cardiac complications. Observational data agree that stage 1 or 2 hypertension is not an independent risk factor for perioperative cardiovascular complications, and hence there is no scientific evidence to support postponing these patients in the absence of target organ damage. However, the case for stage 3 (SAP ≥ 180 and/or DAP ≥ 110 mmHg) hypertension is less clear. The ACC/AHA guidelines recommend control of blood pressure before surgery, but this is not supported by a large body of data relating exclusively to patients with these levels of blood pressure.

Based on clinical studies and practice, there is no evidence to cancel and treat hypertensive patients other than those with documented target organ damage. Blood pressure control should be optimized before surgery in patients in whom hypertension is associated with accompanying significant risk factors such as diabetes mellitus, coronary artery disease, peripheral vascular disease, impaired renal function, smoking, or hypercholesterolemia.[65,66]

Isolated systolic hypertension (ISH) is frequent in older adults. It is characterized by increased systolic pressure as well as pulse pressure due to increased large artery stiffness secondary to aging. There are also often associations with obesity and reduced physical activity. In nonsurgical patients with ISH, there is a clear association with increased prevalence of silent myocardial ischemia. The influence of ISH on perioperative outcomes has not been well studied, although a recent study (PROMISE—Perioperative Myocardial Ischemia in Isolated Systolic Hypertension) showed no increased incidence of myocardial ischemia in ISH patients.[67]

In patients with "white coat" hypertension, as many repeat blood pressures as possible should be obtained to inform clinical decisions. Starting a normally normotensive patient with white coat hypertension on inappropriate therapy can be dangerous. If surgery is to be deferred to allow white coat hypertension to be treated, it is unclear how long treatment should be given before surgery.

PULMONARY VASODILATORS

The pulmonary circulation is normally a low pressure, low resistance circuit (see Chapters 21 and 25). Pulmonary hypertension is defined as mean pulmonary artery pressure greater than 20 mmHg or systolic pulmonary artery pressure greater than 30 mmHg.

The causes of pulmonary hypertension are 50% idiopathic, and the remaining 50% is associated with connective tissue disorders, congenital heart disease, portal hypertension, infection with human immunodeficiency virus, or intake of appetite suppressant drugs such as fenfluramine or dexfenfluramine. The hypertension can be aggravated by hypoxic vasoconstriction and hence these patients should receive supplemental oxygen, while avoiding causative drugs.

Hypoxic pulmonary vasoconstriction (HPV; see Chapter 25) is mediated by the endothelium. The exact mechanism is not well defined, but the "redox theory" proposes the coordinated action of a redox sensor (within the proximal mitochondrial electron transport chain) that generates a diffusible mediator (probably a reactive oxygen species such as hydrogen peroxide) that regulates an effector protein (either a voltage-gated K^+ or Ca^{2+} channel). The subsequent inhibition of oxygen-sensitive K^+ $K_V1.5$ and $K_V2.1$ channels depolarizes pulmonary artery smooth muscle and activates voltage-gated Ca^{2+} channels. This leads to an influx of Ca^{2+} causing vasoconstriction.[68]

Hypoxic pulmonary vasoconstriction can be modulated by a number of variables. The reflex activity decreases with increases in pulmonary artery pressure, cardiac output, left atrial pressure, and central blood volume. Drugs also modulate the reflex and interfere with ventilation/perfusion matching (Table 23-9). Other perioperative conditions that impair the response include hypocapnia and hypothermia. When hypoxic pulmonary vasoconstriction is inhibited, there is an increase in alveolar-arterial oxygen gradient.

Until recently, the prognosis for patients with pulmonary hypertension was poor (with a survival of 5-6 years) even with treatment, and the only useful treatment was chronic calcium channel blockers. This has changed with the introduction of nitric oxide, prostacyclin analogs, PDEIs, and lung transplantation. Other useful therapies include inotropic drugs that can cause some right ventricular adaptation secondary to an increase in systolic function. Conversely these patients tolerate β adrenoceptor blockade poorly. Diuretics can also help by decreasing pericardial and pleural effusions, as well as improving right ventricular volumes and left ventricular diastolic function.

A classification of pulmonary vasodilators is shown in Table 23-10. There is no vasodilator that acts solely on the pulmonary vasculature. Adenosine, acetylcholine, nitroglycerin, and prostacyclin have the best ratio of pulmonary to systemic effects. Most drugs used to attempt a reduction in pulmonary blood pressure are not without significant side effects: systemic hypotension, pulmonary hypertension (drug-induced decrease in systemic blood pressure can increase pulmonary artery pressure by increasing cardiac output and sympathetic tone), decreased myocardial contractility, and hypoxemia. Because of these side effects, there have been a number of new treatments assessed since the mid-1990s.

Inhaled nitric oxide (iNO) readily diffuses from the alveoli to the vascular smooth muscle where it activates guanylyl cyclase to increase cGMP, causing pulmonary vasodilation. NO has little effect on the systemic circulation. It can be administered in doses ranging from 5 to 80 ppm. About 33% of patients with pulmonary hypertension show little or no response to iNO due to a nonreactive pulmonary circulation, rapid NO inactivation, abnormalities of the guanylyl cyclase system, or rapid breakdown of cGMP (although this can be inhibited by addition of dipyridamole). The main adverse effects of iNO are inhibition of platelet function, and rebound hypoxemia and pulmonary hypertension.

Prostanoid pulmonary vasodilators can be administered by a variety of different routes—intravenous (epoprostenol, treprostinil, iloprost); subcutaneous (treprostinil); inhalation (iloprost); oral (beraprost). Prostacyclin (PGI_2) is endogenously synthesized, predominantly by endothelial cells including the pulmonary vascular endothelium. Prostacyclin produces vasodilation in low-resistance beds such as the pulmonary circulation.[69] It not only stimulates the endothelial release of NO, but in turn, NO enhances PGI_2 synthesis in

---

Table 23-9. Effect of Vasoactive and Other Drugs on the Hypoxic Pulmonary Vasoconstrictor Reflex

DRUG	EFFECT
Hydralazine	None
Nifedipine	Inhibition
Verapamil	Inhibition
Nitroglycerin	Inhibition
Sodium nitroprusside	Inhibition
Nicardipine	None
Labetalol	None
Inhaled anesthetics	None to slight inhibition
Intravenous anesthetics ketamine and propofol	None
Thoracic epidural	No direct effect; but changes likely attributable to alterations in cardiac function

---

Table 23-10. Classification of Pulmonary Vasodilators

Direct-acting—hydralazine, nitroglycerin, sodium nitroprusside (through activation of guanylyl cyclase)
α-Adrenoceptor antagonists—tolazoline, phentolamine
β-Adrenoceptor agonists—isoproterenol (isoprenaline) (activation of adenylyl cyclase)
Calcium channel blockers—nifedipine, diltiazem
Prostaglandins—PGF_1 and prostacyclin
Adenosine
Endothelin receptor antagonists
Indirect-acting vasodilators—such as acetylcholine, which causes the release of nitric oxide

smooth muscle cells of the pulmonary artery. PGI_2 is spontaneously broken down by plasma hydrolysis to an inactive 6-keto metabolite, with a half-life of about 6 minutes. Animal studies show PGI_2 to have a high clearance (90-100 mL/kg/min), a volume of distribution of 357 mL/kg, and a half-life of 2.7 minutes.[70] Delivery of PGI_2 by aerosol causes minimal systemic effects, but dramatic and rapid improvement in arterial oxygenation and lowering of pulmonary artery pressure.

Phosphodiesterase Inhibitors.

Both NO and atrial natriuretic peptide (ANP) activate smooth muscle cell guanylyl cyclase to decrease intracellular Ca^{2+} with muscle relaxation, inhibition of cell proliferation, and activation of apoptosis. There is evidence that phosphodiesterase (PDE) is overexpressed in pulmonary hypertension, leading to an increased degradation of cGMP. There is also decreased expression on NO synthase. Hence therapy has focused on the efficacy of PDE5 inhibitors, which cause pulmonary vasodilation. PDE5 is located in the corpus cavernosus, vascular smooth muscle, and platelets.

Sildenafil reduces pulmonary vascular resistance. It has high oral bioavailability, with onset of effect within 15 minutes and peak hemodynamic effect at 2 hours. Sildenafil has a half-life of about 4 hours and is metabolized by two separate routes involving CYP 3A4 (major) and 2C9 (minor). Both pathways are influenced by CYP inhibitors and inducers. The drug is effective in reducing pulmonary artery pressure in both adults and children.

Tadalafil has a longer half-life and is hence viewed as a once-per-day drug.

For the effective treatment of pulmonary hypertension, combination therapies are often the most efficacious.

Novel Pulmonary Vasodilators.

A number of therapies are under evaluation in vitro and in animal models—these include potassium channel openers, antiproliferative drugs, rapamycin, and statins.

EMERGING DEVELOPMENTS

Direct Renin Inhibitors

Direct renin inhibitors are a new class of drugs that act as non–peptide renin inhibitors by binding competitively to renin and blocking the generation of angiotensin I from angiotensinogen. Direct renin inhibitors act on the juxtaglomerular cells of the kidney where the hormone is produced. They cause arterial and venous dilatation by blocking formation of angiotensin, and cause downregulation of sympathetic adrenergic activity and promotion of Na^+ and water excretion by the kidneys. Aliskiren can be used in patients when ACE inhibitors or angiotensin receptor antagonists (ARAs) are not tolerated. It has additive antihypertensive effects when combined with ARAs. Unlike ACE inhibitors and ARAs, they do not appear to cause a compensatory rise in plasma renin and produce a more complete block of the pathway.[71,72] They appear to possess fewer side effects than either ACE inhibitors or ARAs, and are recommended as a third-line treatment for hypertension (especially where resistant to other therapies).[73] There are few kinetic data available for the two currently available direct renin inhibitors, aliskiren and

remikiren. Both drugs are formulated for oral use only. *Aliskiren* is a piperidine derivative that is poorly absorbed, with an oral bioavailability of only 2.5%. Peak concentrations are seen at 1 to 3 hours. Aliskiren has a half-life of 24 to 40 hours, and protein binding of 47% to 51%. It is partly metabolized (about 19%) in the liver by CYP 3A4 to O-demethylated and carboxylic acid derivatives. The remainder of the drug is excreted unchanged in the feces.

Remikiren has a similar low bioavailability (<6%), a half-life of 1.5 hours, and clearance similar to hepatic blood flow. The effect lasts about 24 hours. It is recommended that the dose of both drugs be reduced in patients with renal impairment.[74,75] *Ivabradine* is a specific sinus node inhibitor that slows heart rate without having negative inotropic effects by inhibition of I_f ("funny channel") currents. The effects of ivabradine on heart rate also lead to an increased diastolic time and hence coronary flow. It is an alternative to β blocker or a heart rate-limiting calcium channel blocker and also has antianginal action when given with a β blocker. It has some antihypertensive effect through its action on heart rate. Use of ivabradine can be accompanied by the development of significant side effects: visual symptoms, blurring of vision, headache, dizziness, and bradycardia.[76]

Natriuretic Peptides

Natriuretic peptides (atrial and brain natriuretic peptides, ANP and BNP) act via transmembrane NP-receptors (NP-A, NP-B). Agonists binding to NP-A receptors cause vasodilation with increased glomerular filtration rate and enhanced Na^+ and water excretion, while NP-B receptor stimulation inhibits renin production. These peptides reduce blood pressure through vasodilation of both the arterial and venous systems (Figure 23-8). A number of new therapeutic approaches are being developed related to these peptides. These include neural endopeptidase (NEP) inhibitors (e.g., candoxatril), vasopeptidase inhibitors (e.g., omapatrilat, which inhibits both ACE and NEP), exogenous ANP and BNP (e.g., Nesiritide; recombinant BNP), and exogenous ANP as a coronary vasodilator.

Endothelin and Endothelin Blockade

Endothelins are vasoconstrictors found in endothelial cells that were first discovered in 1985 and identified in 1988.[77]

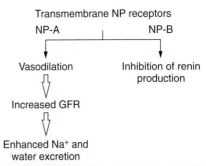

Figure 23-8 Possible mechanisms of action of natriuretic peptides (NP). Atrial and brain natriuretic peptides interact with NP-A and NP-B receptors to reduce blood pressure by vasodilation and enhanced salt and water excretion.

There are four distinct endothelin peptides (1, 2, 3, and 4). ET-1 and ET-3 are the endothelins present in vascular endothelial cells; ET-2 and ET-4 are found in the kidneys and intestines, and ET-3 is also found in the intestines, brain, lungs, and adrenal glands.

ET-1 is synthesized as a 212 residue precursor (prepro-ET) that undergoes cleavage by an atypical endopeptidase of the metalloprotease type to big ET-1 and subsequently ET-1. This latter cleavage occurs both intracellularly and on the surface of endothelial and smooth muscle cells. The stimuli to endothelin synthesis include the release of any of a series of noxious vasoconstrictor mediators—including activated platelets, endotoxins, thrombin, various cytokines, cell and tumor growth factors, angiotensin II, antidiuretic hormone, and adrenaline, as well as other stimuli such as hypoxia and insulin.

Inhibitors to synthesis include NO, natriuretic peptides, prostaglandins PGE_2 and PGI_2, and heparin. It is probable that endothelin-1 is stored as a preformed molecule in the endothelial cells, while the release mechanism is poorly understood. Endothelin-1 is a 21 amino acid peptide with vasoconstrictor and mitogenic properties, being a growth factor for both vascular smooth muscle and fibroblasts. The release of ET-1 appears to be stimulated by hypoxemia and inhibited by NO. There are two distinct endothelin receptors: ET-A and ET-B; both are G protein–coupled with ET-1 preferentially activating ET-A. This receptor is, in turn, coupled to three or more second messengers (including phospholipase C, protein kinase C, and IP_3). The mRNA for endothelin ET-A receptors is expressed in many human tissues, including vascular smooth muscle, heart, lungs, and kidney. Stimulation of ET-A receptors brings about vasoconstriction and cell proliferation, while ET-B stimulation causes release of NO and prostacyclin.[78] Patients with pulmonary hypertension can have enhanced pulmonary production and increased circulating levels of endothelin-1.[79,80]

There are two broad classes of blockers—selective to one or other receptor, and nonselective. All are undergoing evaluation in patients with pulmonary hypertension. They have beneficial effects in the management of the condition by reducing vascular resistance and altering vascular remodeling.[78]

Bosentan can be given as either a continuous infusion or as an oral preparation. The orally active preparation of this non-selective endothelin blocker has a half-life of about 7 hours. It is metabolized by CYP, and is an inducer of CYP 4AA and 2C9.[81]

Sitaxentan is an endothelin blocker with a specificity of A:B receptors of 6500:1 (this compares with a ratio of 20:1 for bosentan; a blocker is said to be selective if the ratio is greater than 100:1). Sitaxentan is also orally active and rapidly absorbed with a Tmax of 1 to 4 hours. Its elimination half-life is about 10 hours, and it is metabolized by CYP 2C9 and 3A4. The compound has also been shown to be a competitive inhibitor of CYP 2C9, 2C19, and 3A4/5.

Ambrisentan is another nonselective blocker with an A:B specificity of 77:1. It has a high oral bioavailability and a long half-life, therefore making it a once a day drug.

Darusentan is an endothelin A receptor antagonist that reduces both systolic and diastolic pressures. It might be a useful therapy in patients with refractory hypertension.

KEY POINTS

- Pharmacologic control of blood pressure can occur through central or peripheral actions, primarily effects on the sympathetic autonomic nervous system, or on the tone of the peripheral vasculature.
- Interactions with four classes of adrenergic receptors—α_1, α_2, β_1, and β_2—can modulate blood pressure. Antagonists at the α_1 receptor counteract the hypertensive effects of α_1 agonists, as well as reduce the vascular hypertrophy seen in hypertension. Antagonists at β_1 and β_2 receptors reduce heart rate and modulate sympathetic effects.
- β-adrenoceptor blockers include two classes—the aminooxypropanols (propranolol, metoprolol, esmolol, carvedilol) and the hydroxyaminoethyls (sotalol and labetalol). Pharmacologically there are three classes: partial agonists (bucindolol and xamoterol); inverse agonists (metoprolol, bisoprolol, nebivolol, sotalol) that stabilize the receptor in an inactive state; and neutral (competitive) antagonists (carvedilol, propranolol) that bind to the receptor without selectivity for active or inactive state. Further functional classification distinguishes antagonists as β_1 selective or nonselective, as having intrinsic sympathomimetic activity (ISA), or as having membrane stabilizing actions.
- Antagonists at β_1 receptors reduce myocardial remodeling while preserving β_2 mediated cardiac protection. Selective β_1 blockers also have negative inotropic and chronotropic effects.
- For the treatment of hypertension, β-adrenoceptor blockers with inverse agonist activity, or those with associated α_1 adrenceptor blocking activity (labetalol, carvedilol), might be preferred.
- Most peripheral vasodilators act through regulation of intracellular Ca^{2+} concentration in vascular smooth muscle. Vasodilators increase intracellular cAMP or cGMP, and bring about vasodilation by phosphorylation of phospholamban and promotion of increased uptake of Ca^{2+} into the sarcoplasmic reticulum.
- Calcium blockers block Ca^{2+} entry through L-type voltage-gated Ca^{2+} channels, leading to vasodilation. The three structural classes of blockers—phenylalkylamines (verapamil), benzothiazepines (diltiazem), and dihydropyridines (nifedipine)—have two main actions, vasodilation and negative inotropy.
- Nitrosovasodilators either cause spontaneous release of nitric oxide or undergo active reduction prior to nitric oxide release. Nitric oxide activates guanylyl cyclase to produce cGMP that activates protein kinase G and activates myosin light chain phosphatase, which dephosphorylates light chains to produce muscle relaxation.
- Inhibition of the renin-angiotensin system can occur through direct inhibition of angiotensin converting enzyme (ACE), angiotensin II receptor antagonism, or direct renin inhibition.
- Endothelins activate ET-A receptors to cause vasoconstriction and smooth muscle proliferation; endothelin antagonists mainly block the ET-A receptor to cause vasodilation.

- Potassium channel openers act by decreasing membrane potential through the efflux of K^+, thus reducing the activity of voltage-gated Ca^{2+} channels.
- Magnesium is a calcium channel blocker that also acts as an antihypertensive agent by stimulating production of prostaglandin E_1 and nitric oxide, and by altering the vascular smooth muscle response to vasoactive agents.
- The eicosanoids (prostaglandins E_1 and E_2; and prostaglandin I_2, known as prostacyclin) bind specific prostanoid receptors, leading to increased intracellular cAMP, activation of protein kinase A, and inhibition of smooth muscle contraction.
- Treatment options for pulmonary hypertension include calcium channel blockers; direct acting nitrovasodilators (e.g., nitroglycerin rather than nitroprusside); inhaled nitric oxide; endothelin blockers; prostanoids (prostacyclin); and phosphodiesterase 5 inhibitors (sildenafil and cogeners).

Key References

Chobanian AV, Bakris GL, Black HR, et al. Seventh Report of the Joint National Committee on Prevention, Detection, Evaluation and Treatment of High Blood Pressure. *Hypertension*. 2003;42:1206-1252. An updated report on the medical aspects of the prevention and management of hypertension. (Ref. 3)

Fleisher LA, Beckman JA, Brown KA, et al. AAC/AHA 2007 Guidelines on Perioperative Cardiovascular Evaluation and Care for Non-Cardiac Surgery. A report of the American College of Cardiology/American Heart Association Taskforce on Practice Guidelines. (Writing Committee to update the 2002 Guidelines on Perioperative Cardiovascular Evaluation for Non-Cardiac Surgery). *Circulation*. 2007;116:1971-1996. A set of guidelines for cardiovascular evaluation and care of the patient undergoing non-cardiac surgery. (Ref. 64)

Howell SJ, Foex P, Sear JW. Hypertension and perioperative cardiac risk. *Br J Anaesth*. 2004;92:570-583. Evidence for an association between hypertensive disease, elevated arterial pressure, and perioperative cardiac outcome are reviewed using a systematic review and metaanalysis of 30 observational studies. (Ref. 63)

Kirsten R, Nelson K, Kirsten D, et al. Clinical pharmacokinetics of vasodilators. Part I. *Clin Pharmacokin*. 1998;34:457-482. Part II. *Clin Pharmacokin*. 1998;35:9-36. Two review papers defining the mechanism of action and pharmacokinetic properties of vasodilator drugs used in the treatment of hypertension. (Refs. 10 and 40)

Kroen C. Does elevated blood pressure at the time of surgery increase perioperative cardiac risk? Proceedings of the 2nd Annual Cleveland Clinic Perioperative Medicine Summit. *Cleve Clinic J Med*. 2006;33:s5-s6. Elevated blood pressure by itself has not been shown to increase the incidences of perioperative cardiac events; however, target organ damage caused by chronic hypertension can confer increased cardiac risk. A useful review of some of those issues relating to the assessment and treatment of the patient with hypertension. (Ref. 65)

Law MR, Morris JK, Wald NJ. Use of blood pressure lowering drugs in the prevention of cardiovascular disease: metaanalysis of 147 randomised trials in the context of expectations from prospective epidemiological studies. *Br Med J*. 2009;338:b1665. doi: 10.1136/bmj.b1665. A meta-analysis of 147 randomized trials showing that all classes of blood pressure lowering drugs have a similar effect in reducing coronary heart disease events and stroke for a given reduction in blood pressure. (Ref. 57)

Sear JW. Perioperative control of hypertension: when will it adversely affect perioperative outcome? *Curr Hypertens Rep*. 2008;10:480-487. A review of the effects of increased blood pressure on perioperative outcomes. Only patients with a blood pressure ≥180/110 mmHg (stage II of JNC VII) or ≥140/90 mmHg plus target organ damage (stage I) need be canceled for institution of treatment before to noncardiac surgery. (Ref. 66)

Wright JM, Musini VM. First-line drugs for hypertension. *Cochrane Database Syst Rev*. 2009;8(3):CD0018419. This review sets out to quantify the benefits and harms of the major first-line antihypertensive drug classes: thiazides, β blockers, calcium channel blockers, ACE inhibitors, α blockers, and angiotensin II receptor blockers. First-line low-dose thiazides reduce all morbidity and mortality outcomes. First-line ACE inhibitors and calcium channel blockers might be similarly effective but the evidence is less robust. First-line high-dose thiazides and first-line β blockers are inferior to first-line low-dose thiazides. (Ref. 59)

References

1. Danaei G, Finucane MM, Lin JK, et al. National, regional and global trends in systolic blood pressure since 1980: systematic analysis of health examination surveys and epidemiological studies with 786 country-years and 5.4 million participants. *Lancet*. 2011;377:568-577.
2. Borzecki AM, Wong AT, Hickey EC, Ash AS, Berlowitz DR. Hypertension control: how well are we doing? *Arch Intern Med*. 2003;163:2705-2711.
3. Chobanian AV, Bakris GL, Black HR, et al. Seventh Report of the Joint National Committee on Prevention, Detection, Evaluation and Treatment of High Blood Pressure. *Hypertension*. 2003;42:1206-1252.
4. Pauli W. Ueber ionenwirkungen und ihre therapeutische verwendung. *Much Med Wschr*. 1903;50:153.
5. Johnson CC. The actions and toxicity of sodium nitroprusside. *Arch Int Pharmacodyn*. 1929;35:480.
6. Page IH, Corcoran AC, Dustan HP, Koppanyi T. Cardiovascular actions of sodium nitroprusside in animals and hypertensive patients. *Circulation*. 1955;11:188-198.
7. Sen G, Bose KC. Rauwolfia serpentina, a new Indian drug for insanity and high blood pressure. *Indian Med World*. 1931;2:194-201.
8. Vakil EJ. A clinical trial of rauwolfia serpentina in essential hypertension. *Br Heart J*. 1949;11:350.
9. Wilkinson EL, Beckman H, Hecht HH. Cardiovascular and renal adjustments to a hypotensive agent (1-hydrazinophthalazine: CIBA BA-5968; apresoline). *J Clin Invest*. 1952;31:872-879.
10. Kirsten R, Nelson K, Kirsten D, Heintz B. Clinical pharmacokinetics of vasodilators. Part I. *Clin Pharmacokin*. 1998;34:457-482.
11. Bowman WC, Rand MJ. The cardiovascular system. In: *Textbook of Pharmacology*. 2nd ed. Oxford: Blackwell Scientific; 1980:23.26-23.58.
12. Klockner U, Isenberg G. Myocytes isolated from porcine coronary arteries: reduction of currents through L-type Ca-channels by verapamil-type Ca-antagonists. *J Physiol Pharmacol*. 1991;42:163-179.
13. Kurokawa J, Adachi-Akahane S, Nagao T. 1,5-Benzothiazepine binding domain is located on the extracellular side of the cardiac L-type Ca2+ channel. *Mol Pharmacol*. 1997;51:262-268.
14. Skeberdis VA. Structure and function of beta3- adrenergic receptors. *Medicinia (Kaunus)*. 2004;40:407-413.
15. Groenning BA, Nilsson JC, Sondergaard l, et al. Anti-modeling effects on the left ventricle during beta-blockade with metoprolol in the treatment of chronic heart failure. *JACC*. 2000;36:2072-2080.
16. Udelson JE. Ventricular remodeling in heart failure and the effect of beta-blockade. *Am J Cardiol*. 2004;93:43b-48B.
17. Hjalmarson A, Goldstein S, Fagerberg B, et al. Effects of controlled-release metoprolol on total mortality, hospitalizations, and well-being in patients with heart failure: the Metoprolol CR/XL Randomized Intervention Trial in Congestive Heart Failure (MERIT-HF). *JAMA*. 2000;83:1295-1302.
18. Ahmet I, Krawczyk M, Zhu W, et al. Cardioprotective and survival benefits of long-term combined therapy with beta2 adrenoreceptor (AR) agonist and beta1 AR blocker in dilated cardiomyopathy post-myocardial infarction. *J Pharmacol Exp Ther*. 2008;325:491-499.
19. Prisant LM. Nebivolol: pharmacologic profile of an ultraselective, vasodilatory beta1-blocker. *J Clin Pharmacol*. 2008;48:225-239.
20. Milne RJ, Buckley M. Celiprolol—an updated review of its pharmacodynamic and pharmacokinetic properties, and therapeutic efficacy in cardiovascular disease. *Drugs*. 1991;41:941-969.

21. Carpenter CL. Actin cytoskeleton and cell signaling. *Crit Care Med.* 2000;28:(suppl 4):N94-N99.
22. Shimizu T, Yoshtomi K, Nakamura M, Imai M. Site and mechanism of actions of trichlormethiazide in rabbit distal nephron segments perfused in vitro. *J Clin Invest.* 1988;82:721-730.
23. Rose BD. Diuretics. *Kidney International.* 1991;39:336-352.
24. Maze M, Tranquilli W. Alpha2-adrenoceptor agonists: defining the role in clinical anesthesia. *Anesthesiology.* 1991;74:581-605.
25. Oliver MF, Goldman L, Julian DG, Holme I. Effect of mivazerol on perioperative cardiac complications during non-cardiac surgery in patients with coronary heart disease: the European Mivazerol Trial (EMIT). *Anesthesiology.* 1999;91:951-961.
26. Furchgott RF, Zawadski JV. The obligatory role of the endothelial cells in the relaxation of arterial smooth muscle by acetylcholine. *Nature.* 1980;288:373-376.
27. Palmer RM, Ferrige AG, Moncada S. Nitric oxide release accounts for the biological activity of endothelium-derived relaxing factor. *Nature.* 1987;327:524-526.
28. Cohen RA, Adachi T. Nitric-oxide-induced vasodilation: regulation by physiologic s-glutathionation and pathologic oxidation of the sarcoplasmic endoplasmic calcium ATPase. *Trends Cardiovasc Med.* 2006;16:109-114.
29. Yamamoto T, Bing RJ. Nitric oxide donors. *Proc Soc Exp Biol Med.* 2000;225:200-206.
30. Friederich JA, Butterworth JFT. Sodium nitroprusside: twenty years and counting. *Anesth Analg.* 1995;81:152-162.
31. Hein TW, Kuo L. cAMP independent dilation of coronary arterioles to adenosine: role of nitric oxide, G proteins and K(ATP) channels. *Circ Res.* 1999;85:634-642.
32. Sabouni MH, Hussain T, Cushing DJ, Mustafa SJ. G proteins subserve relaxation mediated by adenosine receptors in human coronary artery. *J Cardiovasc Pharmacol.* 1991;18:696-702.
33. Leblanc N, Wilde DW, Keef KD, Hume JR. Electrophysiological mechanism of minoxidil sulfate-induced vasodilation of rabbit portal vein. *Circ Res.* 1989;65:1102-1111.
34. Ellershaw DC, Gurne AM. Mechanisms of hydralazine induced vasodilation in rabbit aorta and pulmonary artery. *Br J Pharmacol.* 2001;134:621-623.
35. Simpson D, Wellington K. Nicorandil: a review of its use in the management of stable angina pectoris, including high-risk patients. *Drugs.* 2004;64:1941-1955.
36. Guerrero-Romero F, Rodriguez-Moran M. The effect of lowering blood pressure by magnesium supplementation in diabetic hypertensive adults with low serum magnesium levels: a randomized, double-blind, placebo controlled clinical trial. *Human Hypertens.* 2009;23:245-251.
37. Spieker LE, Noll G, Luscher TF. Therapeutic potential for endothelin receptor antagonists in cardiovascular disorders. *Am J Cardiovasc Drugs.* 2001;1:293-303.
38. Barton M, Yanagisawa M. Endothelin: 20 years from discovery to therapy. *Can J Physiol Pharmacol.* 2008;86:485-498.
39. Brogden RN, Markham A. Fenoldopam: a review of its pharmacodynamic and pharmacokinetic properties and intravenous potential in the management of hypertensive urgencies and emergencies. *Drugs.* 1997;54:634-650.
40. Kirsten R, Nelson K, Kirsten D, Heintz B. Clinical pharmacokinetics of vasodilators. Part II. *Clin Pharmacokin.* 1998;35:9-36.
41. Corbin JD, Francis SH. Cyclic GMP phosphdiesterase-5: target of silfenadil. *J Biol Chem.* 1999;274:13729-13732.
42. Furberg CD, Psaty BM, Meyer JV. Nifedipine. Dose-related increase in mortality in patients with coronary heart disease. *Circulation.* 1995;92:1326-1331.
43. Godfraind T, Salomone S, Dessy C, Verhelst B, Dion R, Schoevaerts JC. Selectivity scale of calcium antagonists in the human cardiovascular system based on in vitro studies. *J Cardiovasc Pharmacol.* 1992;20(suppl 5):S34-S41.
44. Peacock WF, Angeles JE, Soto KM, Lumb PD, Varon J. Parenteral clevidipine for the acute control of blood pressure in the critically ill patient: a review. *Ther Clin Risk Manag.* 2009;5:627-634.
45. Erikson AL, DeGrado JR, Fanikos JR. Clevidipine: a short-acting intravenous dihydropyridine calcium channel blocker for the management of hypertension. *Pharmacotherapy.* 2010;30:515-528.
46. Deeks ED, Keating GM, Keams J. Clevidipine: a review of its use in the management of acute hypertension. *Am J Cardiovasc Drugs.* 2009;9:117-134.
47. Stroe AF, Gheorghiaede M. Carvedilol: beta-blockade and beyond. *Rev Cardiovasc Med.* 2004;5:s18-s27.
48. Moen MD, Wagstaff AJ. Nebivolol: a review of its use in the management of hypertension and chronic heart failure. *Drugs.* 2006;66:1389-1409.
49. Munzel T, Gori T. Nebivolol: the somewhat-different beta-adrenergic receptor blocker. *J Am Coll Cardiol.* 2009;54:1491-1499.
50. Andersson KE. Clinical pharmacology of potassium channel openers. *Pharmacol Toxicol.* 1992;70:244-254.
51. Lehtonen LA, Antila S, Pentikäinen PJ. Pharmacokinetics and pharmacodynamics of intravenous inotropic agents. *Clin Pharmacokinet.* 2004;43:187-203.
52. Wald DS, Law M, Morris JK, Bestwick JP, Wald NJ. Combination therapy versus monotherapy in reducing blood pressure: meta-analysis on 11,000 participants from 42 trials. *Am J Med.* 2009;122:290-300.
53. Opie LH, Schall R. Evidence-based evaluation of calcium channel blockers for hypertension: equality of mortality and cardiovascular risk relative to conventional therapy. *J Am Coll Cardiol.* 2002;39:315-322. Erratum in: *J Am Coll Cardiol.* 2002;39:1409-1410.
54. De Caterina AR, Leone AM. The role of beta-blockers in first line therapy in hypertension. *Curr Atheroscler Rep.* 2011;13:147-153.
55. Ram CV. Beta-blockers in hypertension. *Am J Cardiol.* 2010;106:1819-1825.
56. Ong HT. Beta-blockers in hypertension and cardiovascular disease. *Br Med J.* 2007;334:946-949.
57. Law MR, Morris JK, Wald NJ. Use of blood pressure lowering drugs in the prevention of cardiovascular disease: meta-analysis of 147 randomised trials in the context of expectations from prospective epidemiological studies. *Br Med J.* 2009;338:b1665. doi: 10.1136/bmj.b1665.
58. Staessen JA, Wang J, Bianchi G, Birkenhäger WH. Essential hypertension. *Lancet.* 2003;361:1629-1641.
59. Wright JM, Musini VM. First-line drugs for hypertension. *Cochrane Database Syst Rev.* 2009;8(3):CD001841.
60. Sear JW, Jewkes C, Tellez J-C, Foex P. Does the choice of antihypertensive therapy influence haemodynamic responses to induction, laryngoscopy and intubation? *Br J Anaesth.* 1994;73:303-308.
61. Bertrand M, Godet G, Meersschaert K, Brun L, Salcedo E, Coriat P. Should the angiotensin II antagonists be discontinued before surgery? *Anesth Analg.* 2001;92:26-30.
62. Beyer K, Taffé P, Halfon P, et al. Hypertension and intra-operative incidents: a multicentre study of 125,000 surgical procedures in Swiss hospitals. *Anaesthesia.* 2009;64(5):494-502.
63. Howell SJ, Foex P, Sear JW. Hypertension and perioperative cardiac risk. *Br J Anaesth.* 2004;92:570-583.
64. Fleisher LA, Beckman JA, Brown KA, et al. AAC/AHA 2007 Guidelines on Perioperative Cardiovascular Evaluation and Care for Noncardiac Surgery. A report of the American College of Cardiology/American Heart Association Taskforce on Practice Guidelines. (Writing Committee to update the 2002 Guidelines on Perioperative Cardiovascular Evaluation for Non-Cardiac Surgery). *Circulation.* 2007;116:1971-1996.
65. Kroen C. Does elevated blood pressure at the time of surgery increase perioperative cardiac risk? Proceedings of the 2nd Annual Cleveland Clinic Perioperative Medicine Summit. *Cleve Clinic J Med.* 2006;33:s5-s6.
66. Sear JW. Perioperative control of hypertension: when will it adversely affect perioperative outcome? *Curr Hypertens Rep.* 2008;10:480-487.
67. Fayad AA, Yang HY, Ruddy TD, Waters JM, Wells GA. Perioperative myocardial ischemia and isolated systolic hypertension in non-cardiac surgery. *Can J Anesth.* 2011;58:428-435.
68. Archer SL, Wu XC, Thebaud B, et al. O2 sensing in the human ductus arteriosus: redox-sensitive K+ channels are regulated by mitochondria-derived hydrogen peroxide. *Biol Chem.* 2004;385:205-216.
69. Lowson SM, Doctor A, Walsh BK, Doorley PA. Inhaled prostacyclin for the treatment of pulmonary hypertension after cardiac surgery. *Crit Care Med.* 2002;30:2762-2764.
70. Vane JR, Botting RM. Pharmacodynamic profile of prostacyclin. *Am J Cardiol.* 1995;75:A3-A10.
71. Barrios V, Escobar C. Aliskiren in the management of hypertension. *Am J Cardiovasc Drugs.* 2010;10:349-358.

72. Duggan ST, Chwieduk CM, Curran MP. Aliskiren: a review of its use as monotherapy and as combination therapy in the management of hypertension. *Drugs.* 2010;70:2011-2049.

73. Oh BH, Mitchell J, Herron JR, Chung J, Khan M, Keefe DL. Aliskiren, an oral renin inhibitor, provides dose-dependent efficacy and sustained 24-hour blood pressure control in patients with hypertension. *J Am Coll Cardiol.* 2007;49:1157-1163.

74. Oparil S, Yarrows SA, Patel S, Zhang J, Satlin A. Dual inhibition of the renin system by aliskiren and valsartan. *Lancet.* 2007;370: 221-229.

75. Reboldi G, Gentile G, Angeli F, Verdecchia I. Pharmacokinetics, pharmacodynamics and clinical evaluation of aliskiren for hypertension treatment. *Exp Opinion Drug Metab Toxicol.* 2011;7:115-128.

76. Tardif JC, Ford I, Tendera M, Bourassa MG, Fox K. Efficacy of ivabradine, a new selective I_f inhibitor compared with atenolol in patients with chronic stable angina. *Europ Heart J.* 2005;26: 2529-2536.

77. Yanagisawa M, Kurihara H, Kimura S, et al. A novel potent vasoconstrictor peptide produced by vascular and endothelial cells. *Nature.* 1988;332:411-415.

78. Rich S, Mclaughlin W. Endothelin receptor blockers in cardiovascular disease. *Circulation.* 2003;108:2184-2190.

79. Stewart DL, Levy RD, Cernacek P, Langleben D. Increased plasma endothelin-1 in pulmonary hypertension: marker or mediator of disease. *Ann Int Med.* 1991;114:464-469.

80. Giaid A, Yanagisawa M, Langleban D, et al. Expression of endothelin-1 in the lungs of patients with pulmonary hypertension. *New Engl J Med.* 1993;328:1732-1739.

81. Yuan JX, Aldinger AM, Juhaszova M, et al. Dysfunctional voltage-gated K+ channels in pulmonary artery smooth muscle cells of patients with primary pulmonary hypertension. *Circulation.* 1998; 98:1400-1406.

Chapter 24

ANTIARRHYTHMIC DRUGS

Geoffrey W. Abbott and Roberto Levi

HISTORICAL PERSPECTIVE

The heart, and more specifically the heartbeat, has throughout history served as an indicator of well-being and disease, both to the physician and to the patient. Through one's own heartbeat, one can feel the physiologic manifestations of joy, thrills, fear, and passion; the rigors of a sprint or long-distance run; the instantaneous effects of medications, recreational drugs, or toxins; the adrenaline of a rollercoaster ride or a penalty shootout in a World Cup final. Although the complexities of the heart continue to humble the scientists and physicians who study it, the heart is unique in that, despite the complexity of its physiology and the richness of both visceral and romantic imagery associated with it, its function can be distilled down to that of a simple pump, the function and dysfunction of which we now understand a great deal (see Chapter 21). The history of development of pharmacologic agents to correct abnormalities in heart rhythm is, however, emblematic of drug development as a whole: major successes combined with paradoxes, damaging side effects, and the often frustrating intransigence of what would seem the most intuitive targets for antiarrhythmics—ion channels.[1,2]

In ancient Greek, Egyptian, and Chinese cultures, the pulse was recognized as a means to assess health, and for millennia it was the only measure of cardiac physiology and pathophysiology. In second-century Rome, Galen's work *De Pulsibus* became the first great treatise on the pulse as a window into human health and established Galen as the father of his discipline.[3] It was not for another 1500 years that the great physician, scientist, and naturalist William Harvey, of Folkstone in England, published his landmark (and then controversial) work *An Anatomical Exercise Concerning the Motion of the Heart and Blood in Animals*. This introduced the theory that blood circulates throughout the body, a hypothesis tested rigorously by Harvey with experiments on animals and the cadavers of executed criminals.[4] In the late 19th and early 20th centuries, Waller and Einthoven founded the field of electrocardiography, facilitating quantitative differential diagnoses of cardiac arrhythmias. This paved the way for modern cardiology and advances such as Wolff, Parkinson, and White's neurocardiac theory, the discovery of atrial fibrillation, and the increasingly sophisticated molecular genotype-phenotype correlations from which we benefit today.[5,6]

These latter advances also owe much to the work of molecular geneticists in the 1990s whose Herculean efforts (before routine high-throughput sequencing) helped identify the mutant ion channel genes underlying inherited arrhythmias such as long QT syndrome, working hand-in-hand with cellular electrophysiologists and physicians to exemplify the bedside-to-bench model of modern molecular medicine. Having said this, β blockers, the first antiarrhythmics of the modern era, were developed in the later 1950s to early 1960s not with ion channels in mind, but were a by-product of Sir James W. Black's desire to create improved therapies for angina and essentially "to stop the effects of adrenaline on the heart" following the death of his father after a myocardial infarction. The resulting class II antiarrhythmic drug, propranolol, ushered in a new era of drug development and proved effective in therapy of disorders including angina, arrhythmia, and hypertension.[7]

Despite the vast array of imaging, molecular, and electrocardiographic diagnostic tools available to cardiologists and other physicians, measurement of the pulse will likely be central to routine examination of the cardiac and holistic health of individuals for the foreseeable future. Timely, rhythmic beating of the heart is essential for health. When the heart develops sustained nonrhythmic beating, generally termed *arrhythmia*, the consequences can range from mild (e.g., syncope) to lethal (sudden cardiac death). Cardiac arrhythmias are treated by surgical ablation, electronic pacemaker, cardioversion, pharmacologic agents, or a combination of these, depending on the location and nature of the causal factor. For example, in the case of ventricular fibrillation—a life-threatening, chaotic tachycardia—electrical defibrillation is required immediately to prevent sudden cardiac death. Whereas, in many cases of atrial fibrillation, there is an underlying structural defect in the atria that can be successfully treated using radio-frequency catheter ablation, for example, to prevent the aberrantly conducting area from being an arrhythmogenic focus.

This chapter focuses on antiarrhythmic medications as frequently encountered in the perioperative and critical care settings. These are a broad class of drugs, incorporating numerous structural classes and modes of action, that are used based on the suspected or known molecular etiology of the arrhythmia to be treated. Recent advances in the understanding of the molecular basis for generation of electrical currents in the heart, and also the genetic basis of many cardiac arrhythmias, have contributed to the development and use of antiarrhythmic drugs. Furthermore, these advances have demonstrated the basis for the proarrhythmic action of some drugs; paradoxically, even some drugs that are classified and used as antiarrhythmics.

To fully understand the mechanism of action of antiarrhythmic drugs, one must understand both the underlying cause of the arrhythmia, and the molecular target of the antiarrhythmic; these may or may not be the same entity. Accordingly, this chapter includes not only a description of the basic and clinical pharmacology of the major classes of cardiac arrhythmias, but also a discussion of the mechanistic underpinnings of these arrhythmias.

Table 24-1. Singh-Vaughan Williams Classification of Antiarrhythmic Agents

CLASS	MECHANISM OF ACTION	DRUGS
Ia	Na+ channel blockade, prolonged repolarization	Procainamide, quinidine, disopyramide
Ib	Na+ channel blockade, shortened repolarization	Lidocaine, mexiletine, phenytoin, tocainide
Ic	Na+ channel blockade, repolarization unchanged	Encainide, flecainide, propafenone
II	Beta adrenoceptor antagonist	Esmolol, metoprolol, propranolol
III	Marked prolongation of repolarization	Amiodarone, bretylium, ibutilide, sotalol
IV	Calcium channel blockade	Diltiazem, verapamil

BASIC PHARMACOLOGY

Singh-Vaughan Williams Classification of Antiarrhythmic Drugs

Antiarrhythmic drugs include a wide range of structural and functional classes. While not perfect, a highly useful framework for their classification is that proposed by Singh and Vaughan Williams, usually referred to as the *Singh-Vaughan Williams (SVW) classification*. The SVW classification categorizes antiarrhythmic drugs into four classes (Table 24-1). Class I denotes sodium (Na+) channel blocking activity, with resultant delay in phase 0 depolarization and/or altered action potential duration. Class II agents counteract the effects of endogenous catecholamines (in particular epinephrine and norepinephrine) by antagonism of β adrenergic receptors, and hence are known as β blockers or β antagonists. Class III antiarrhythmics prolong the action potential and refractory period, acting primarily by potassium (K+) channel blockade. Class IV agents reduce heart rate, primarily by L-type calcium (Ca2+) channel blockade, which slows conduction through the sinoatrial (SA) and atrioventricular (AV) nodes.[8,9] (For a more detailed discussion of cardiac electrophysiology and myocyte depolarization, see Chapter 20.)

The primary reason that the SVW classification is to some extent imperfect is that many, if not most, antiarrhythmic drugs exhibit physiologically significant actions in more than one of the four classes. Typically, the classification is based upon the action that was first described for each drug, which is generally but not necessarily the most therapeutically significant mechanism of action for all types of arrhythmia for which the drug is prescribed. This discrepancy can occur because of nonspecificity of the drug, or because major metabolites of the drug exhibit different activity to that of the drug itself. Furthermore, some important antiarrhythmic drugs, including digoxin and adenosine, do not fit primarily into any of the four classes. However, the SVW classification is still the most useful framework for describing antiarrhythmic drugs, especially if one considers the net effect of each drug rather than all its specific molecular targets. The clinical pharmacology of the major antiarrhythmic drugs is summarized in Table 24-2.

Table 24-2. Antiarrhythmic Drugs

CLASS	MECHANISM	SPECIFIC DRUGS	CLINICAL USES	ADVERSE EFFECTS
Ia	Na^+ channel block (intermediate kinetics); K^+ channel block; repolarization prolonged	Quinidine Procainamide Disopyramide	Ventricular arrhythmias Prevention of paroxysmal recurrent atrial fibrillation Conversion of atrial flutter and fibrillation (quinidine, procainamide) Maintenance of sinus rhythm after conversion of atrial flutter and fibrillation Wolff-Parkinson-White syndrome (procainamide)	QTP/torsades de pointes, nausea, diarrhea, hepatotoxicity, myelosuppression Lethal ventricular arrhythmias, QTP/torsades de pointes, hypotension Lupus-like syndrome, blood dyscrasias Proarrhythmic, torsades de pointes, negative inotropy Parasympatholytic
Ib	Na^+ channel block (fast kinetics); repolarization shortened	Lidocaine Tocainide Mexiletine	Ventricular tachycardia/ fibrillation (lidocaine) Atrial fibrillation	Seizure, tremor, confusion/ delirium Ataxia, tremor
Ic	Na^+ channel block (slow kinetics); no effect on repolarization	Flecainide Propafenone	Prevention of paroxysmal atrial fibrillation Recurrent tachyarrhythmias of abnormal conduction system Contraindicated immediately post-myocardial infarction	Proarrhythmic, heart failure Proarrhythmic, nausea
II	β blockade Propranolol also shows class I effect	Nonselective Propranolol Nadolol β1 selective Esmolol Metoprolol Atenolol Bisoprolol Nonselective β/α blockade Carvedilol Labetalol	Reduce myocardial infarction mortality Prevention of recurrence of tachyarrhythmias Rate control	Bradycardia, hypotension, fatigue, depression
III	K^+ channel block Sotalol is also a β blocker Amiodarone and dronedarone have Class I, II, and III activity	Sotalol Ibutilide Dofetilide Amiodarone Dronedarone Bretylium (no longer available in U.S.)	Wolff-Parkinson-White syndrome Ventricular tachycardia/ fibrillation (sotalol bretylium, amiodarone) Conversion of atrial flutter and fibrillation (ibutilide, sotalol, dofetilide, amiodarone) Maintenance of sinus rhythm after conversion of atrial flutter and fibrillation (sotalol, dofetilide, amiodarone, dronedarone)	Proarrhythmic, QTP/torsades de pointes, bradycardia, heart failure Proarrhythmic, QTP/torsades de pointes Proarrhythmic, QTP/torsades de pointes Hypotension, bradycardia Pulmonary, neurologic, hepatic, dermatologic, ophthalmic, thyroid Increased mortality with heart failure Nausea, vomiting, diarrhea Proarrhythmic, hypotension
IV	Ca^{2+} channel block	Dihydropyridine (selective vasodilators) Nifedipine, nicardipine, amlodipine, isradipine Benzothiapine (less vasodilation; sinoatrial and atrioventricular node block) Diltiazem Phenylalkylamine (sinoatrial and atrioventricular node block) Verapamil	Hypertension Prevention of recurrent paroxysmal supraventricular tachycardia Reduce ventricular rate in atrial fibrillation Prevention of recurrent paroxysmal supraventricular tachycardia Reduce ventricular rate in atrial fibrillation	Bradycardia, hypotension, ankle swelling Bradycardia, hypotension, constipation
Other	Adenosine receptor activation Sodium pump inhibition Ca^{2+} channel block and other effects	Adenosine Digoxin Magnesium	Supraventricular arrhythmias Heart failure, atrial fibrillation Torsades de pointes	Bradycardia, nausea, vomiting, visual disturbances Hypotension, weakness

QTP, QT interval prolongation.

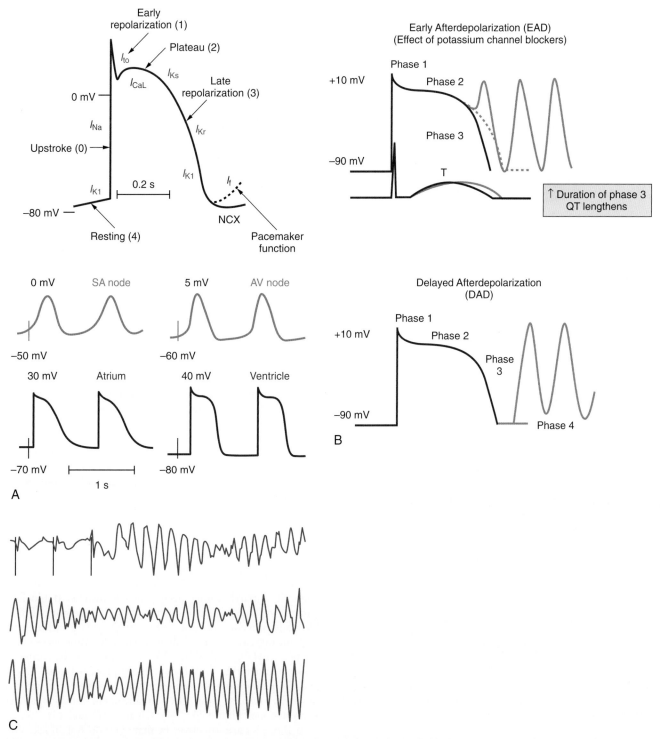

Figure 24-1 Cardiac action potentials and the electrocardiogram. **A,** *Upper,* a generic cardiac action potential illustrating the phases and major currents involved. NCX, sodium/calcium exchanger. *Lower,* comparison of nodal (SA, sinoatrial; AV, atrioventricular), atrial, and ventricular action potentials. **B,** *Upper,* ventricular action potential superimposed upon an electrocardiogram (ECG) showing the QT interval prolonging effects of potassium channel block and resultant early afterdepolarizations. *Lower,* delayed after-depolarizations. **C,** ECG showing torsades de pointes. *(Trace taken from Braunwald E, Zipes DP, Libby P, eds. Heart Disease. 6th ed. Philadelphia: WB Saunders; 2001:868.)*

Sodium Channels and Class I Antiarrhythmic Drugs

Voltage-gated Na^+ (Na_v) channels open in response to cell membrane depolarization to permit influx of Na^+, further depolarizing the cell. The predominant Na_v channel in human cardiac electrophysiology is $Na_v1.5$, which is encoded by the *SCN5A* gene. In most cardiac myocytes, $Na_v1.5$ activation mediates the upstroke in phase 0 of the action potential, in which the membrane potential is depolarized from around $-70\,mV$ to $+20\,mV$ due to Na^+ influx (Figure 24-1, *A*). $Na_v1.5$, like other mammalian Na_v channels, inactivates rapidly, which together with the transient outward K^+ current, I_{to}, shapes the

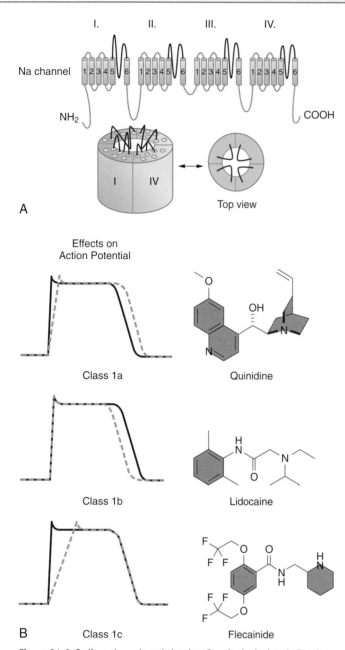

Figure 24-2 Sodium channels and the class I antiarrhythmics. **A,** Topology and subunit organization of the voltage-gated Na⁺ (Na$_v$) channel α subunit. The 24-transmembrane segments form four homologous domains (I-IV) that fold to create the ion pore. **B,** *Left,* effects of class Ia, Ib, and Ic antiarrhythmics *(dotted lines)* on cardiac myocyte action potentials *(purple lines)*. *Right,* exemplar class Ia *(Quinidine)*, Ib *(Lidocaine)*, and Ic *(Flecainide)* antiarrhythmics.

notch in phase 1 at the beginning of the human cardiac myocyte action potential.[10]

Class I antiarrhythmics exhibit Na$_v$ channel blocking activity. These drugs are often referred to as "membrane stabilizing agents" because by blocking cardiac Na$_v$ channels, which mediate myocyte depolarization, they reduce cellular excitability. Na$_v$ channels are composed of a 24-transmembrane-segment pore-forming α subunit that consists of four homologous domains (DI-DIV) also bears four voltage-sensing domains and one or more inactivation gates (Figure 24-2, *A*). The Na$_v$1.5 α subunits form cardiac ion channel complexes with single-transmembrane segment β subunits,

encoded by the *SCNxB* genes, which modify Na$_v$1.5 function and pharmacology.[11]

Class I antiarrhythmic drugs are thought to bind in the inner pore vestibule of Na$_v$ channels, with drugs from different structural classes including lidocaine, flecainide, and quinidine, and the anticonvulsant phenytoin, binding to an overlapping but nonidentical site influenced experimentally by mutations in the S6 transmembrane segment of domain IV.[12] Drugs in class I are subcategorized as Ia, Ib, or Ic depending on their effects on Na⁺ channel conduction and resultant effects on action potentials in cardiac myocytes expressing the predominant cardiac form of Na$_v$ channel, Na$_v$1.5 (see Figure 24-2, *B*).

Na$_v$1.5 is relatively insensitive to the canonical and lethal Na$_v$ channel antagonist tetrodotoxin (TTX), a nerve toxin present, among other animal sources, in the nerves, skin, and gonads of the Japanese puffer fish, *Fugu rubripes*. *F. rubripes* is saddled with the dual distinction of having the shortest known genome of any vertebrate organism and being a delicacy in Japan that must be prepared by certified chefs in order to decrease the chances of lethal doses of TTX being ingested by adventurous diners. Compared to its effects on Na$_v$1.5, TTX acts with up to 10³-fold higher potency on the predominantly neuronal Na$_v$ channel subtypes Na$_v$1.1-1.3 *(SCN1A-3A)* and the skeletal muscle-expressed channel Na$_v$1.4 *(SCN4A)*.[13] TTX, nicknamed "zombie powder" because its paralysis- and coma-inducing effects have led to its use in voodoo ceremonies (it does not cross the blood-brain barrier; those ingesting sublethal doses are potentially conscious while paralyzed), is therefore not a useful antiarrhythmic (owing to its inefficacy and lethality at low doses). However, TTX prolongs the local anesthetic effect of bupivacaine when the two are coadministered.[14] A recent high-resolution x-ray crystallographic structure of an Na$_v$ channel from *Arcobacter butzleri* has provided a first look at this class of proteins essential to function of nerve and muscle, and will likely enhance future class I antiarrhythmic development (see Chapter 17).[15]

β Receptors and Class II Antiarrhythmics

Class II antiarrhythmic drugs, also known as β blockers, antagonize the β adrenergic receptor (β receptor). This β blockade prevents activation of adenylyl cyclase and the consequent increase in intracellular cyclic adenosine monophosphate (cAMP), and thus also activation of its principal downstream target cAMP-dependent protein kinase (PKA), and the promotion of maximal myocardial performance that normally results from the enhancement of sympathetic nervous tone (Figure 24-3; see Chapters 12 and 13).

β Blockers are selective, in that they do not block other receptors, and specific, in that they do not antagonize cardiac stimulation and vasodilatation elicited by agents other than β agonists. All β blockers share the basic structure of β sympathomimetic side chain, which confers affinity for the receptor, along with an aromatic substituent, which determines potency; most are derivatives of the class-defining agent propranolol (see Figure 24-3, *B*). β Blockers are effective as antiarrhythmic agents because, by blocking the action of the sympathetic nervous system on the heart, they depress SA and AV node function, decrease conduction and automaticity, and prolong atrial refractory periods. β Blockers also reduce blood pressure, probably arising from a combination of reduced cardiac

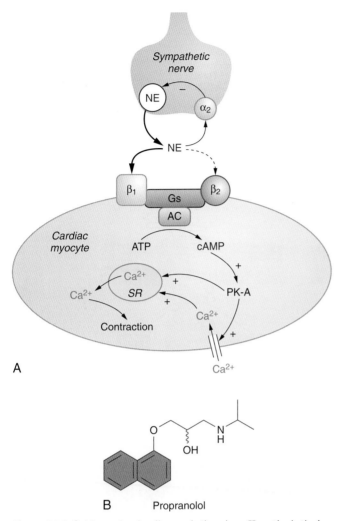

A

B   Propranolol

Figure 24-3 β-Adrenergic signaling and the class II antiarrhythmics. **A,** Schematic showing β-adrenergic signaling and its effects on cardiac function. *AC,* Adenylyl cyclase; *Gs,* G-stimulatory protein; *NE,* norepinephrine; *PK-A,* cAMP-dependent protein kinase; *SR,* sarcoplasmic reticulum. **B,** Structure of the canonical β blocker, propranolol.

output, renal renin release, and perhaps even effects within the central nervous system (see Chapter 23).[16,17] Inasmuch as an exaggerated increase in sympathetic tone typifies the deleterious reaction to congestive heart failure, β blockers, particularly the cardioselective ones, are used successfully also in the treatment of this ailment.[18] Propranolol is marketed as a *D,L*-racemic mixture (see Chapter 1 for a discussion of the pharmacologic implications of chirality), the reason being that the *L*-form is the β blocker while the *D*-form is a "membrane stabilizer," which adds antiarrhythmic effect to the β-blocking properties of the *L*-enantiomer.

Potassium Channels and Class III Antiarrhythmic Drugs

Class III antiarrhythmic drugs are defined by their ability to block K$^+$ channels. This activity increases action potential duration in cardiac myocytes and prolongs the refractory period, that is, extends the period during which the heart is refractory to premature electrical stimuli. Cardiac K$^+$ channels exhibit a much wider variety than other cardiac ion

channels, the two most physiologically and therapeutically important families of K$^+$ channels in the heart, based on current understanding, being the voltage-gated K$^+$ (K$_v$) channels and inward rectifier potassium (K$_{ir}$) channels.[19,20] Channels in both these families are predominantly involved in the repolarization phases of the cardiac myocyte action potential, because both K$_v$ and K$_{ir}$ channels only pass inward K$^+$ currents when the cell membrane potential is negative to the K$^+$ equilibrium potential, which is around −80 mV under physiologic conditions.

K$_v$ channels are each comprised of several subunit types. Similar to Na$_v$ channels, the pore-forming α subunits of K$_v$ channels are arranged in a 24-transmembrane-segment array forming an aqueous central pore with external voltage-sensing modules (Figure 24-4, *A*). However, in K$_v$ channels, this is composed of a tetramer of noncovalently-linked α subunits (each subunit having six transmembrane segments) rather than one contiguous α subunit with four homologous six-segment domains as in Na$_v$ and Ca$_v$ channels. In K$_v$ channel α subunits, the fourth transmembrane segment (S4) bears the basic residues that confer voltage sensitivity, while S6 lines the pore (see Figure 24-4, *A*). High-resolution X-ray crystallographic structures of bacterial and eukaryotic K$_v$ channels have revolutionized the study of these ubiquitous and essential proteins, including current understanding of drug binding sites.[21,22]

The most important K$_v$ α subunits in human ventricular repolarization are the *ether-à-go-go* related gene product (hERG; also named KCNH2) and KCNQ1. Tetramers of each of these coassemble with multiple single-transmembrane-domain ancillary or β subunits from the KCNE gene family. KCNQ1-KCNE1 complexes primarily generate the slowly activating I$_{Ks}$ current; hERG-KCNE2 complexes generate I$_{Kr}$; and each of the five KCNE proteins probably regulates these and other α subunits in the heart too.[23-26] I$_{Kr}$ and I$_{Ks}$ are crucial to phase 3 repolarization (see Figure 24-1, *A*); therefore, blocking these currents delays ventricular repolarization, which can be proarrhythmic or antiarrhythmic depending on the disease state, and other genetic and environmental factors.[27] hERG is particularly sensitive to drug block by a wide range of drugs, owing to its bearing an unusual array of hydrophobic residues, not conserved among other K$_v$ channels, in an internal pore cavity also predicted to be wider than in other K$_v$ channels (see Figure 24-4, *B*).[28]

Inhibitors of K$_v$ channels tend to bind in one of three distinct sites: the outer vestibule, the inner vestibule (drugs in these classes would be considered pore blockers), or on the voltage sensor, which is rarer among small molecules but is seen with some toxins from venomous animals, such as hanatoxin and SGTx from tarantula spiders.[29] The canonical inhibitors of hERG and KCNQ1 are E-4031 and Chromanol 293B, respectively, both of which bind in the inner vestibule and show relatively high specificity for their targets. Additionally, both drugs are sensitive to the presence of KCNE subunits in complex with the α subunits.[30] E-4031 will not be used in the future for antiarrhythmic therapy because pure hERG antagonists such as this cause dangerous repolarization delays. I$_{Ks}$ inhibitors are still being considered because it might be therapeutically useful to counteract the upregulation of I$_{Ks}$ during periods of high sympathetic activity associated with arrhythmia triggering. Other important K$_v$ channel targets of class III antiarrhythmic drugs include the K$_v$4 α

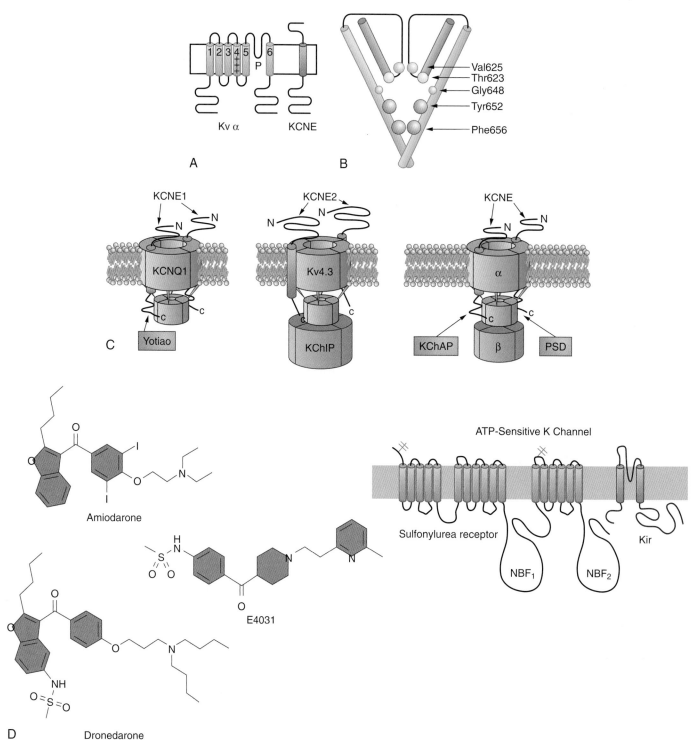

Figure 24-4 Potassium channels and the class III antiarrhythmics. **A,** Topology of a K$_v$ α subunit and a KCNE β subunit. **B,** Left, drug binding site within the hERG K$_v$ α subunit. Residues in red are crucial for binding of a variety of drugs, such as cisapride and terfenadine, and undergo π-bonding with the aromatic rings of methanesulfonanilides. Green and blue residues are less impactful on cisapride and terfenadine binding but important for methanesulfonanilide binding.[101] *Right,* structures of some class III antiarrhythmic drugs. **C,** Cartoons of some heteromeric K$_v$ channels containing α subunits, and both transmembrane and cytoplasmic β subunits. **D,** Topology of a K$_{ir}$ α subunit and an SUR subunit.

subunits that generate human ventricular I$_{to}$, (particularly active during phase 1 of the ventricular action potential), and K$_v$1.5, which generates the ultrarapidly activating K$^+$ current, I$_{Kur}$, important in atrial myocyte repolarization. K$_v$4 and K$_v$1.5 α subunits are also regulated by the KCNE subunits.[31,32] In addition, all the K$_v$ channels discussed herein are regulated by

a host of cytoplasmic β subunits and other regulatory proteins (see Figure 24-4, *C*), each of which can affect channel pharmacology either directly or indirectly, because changes in gating alter drug-binding kinetics.[30,33]

K$_{ir}$ channels do not possess a voltage sensor, but exhibit inward rectification because they are inhibited at more positive membrane potentials by intracellular constituents including Mg^{2+} and polyamines such as spermine. These channels are composed of a tetramer of α subunits, each with only two transmembrane segments, around a central, aqueous, K^+-selective pore (see Figure 24-4, D). The ventricular inward rectifier current I_{K1} is generated by $K_{ir}2$ family α subunits and contributes to stabilizing the cardiac potential, passing current at either end but less so when the myocyte is strongly depolarized (see Figure 24-1, A). The K_{ATP} channel, which also probably contributes to cardiac excitability, is an octamer of four $K_{ir}6$ α subunits and four membrane-spanning sulfonylurea receptor (SUR) subunits that render it ATP-sensitive.[19] A host of class III drugs, including amiodarone and dofetilide, inhibit K_{ir} channels by direct pore block within the inner vestibule.[34,35]

Calcium Channels and Class IV Antiarrhythmics

Class IV agents slow AV nodal conduction, primarily by L-type Ca^{2+} channel (LTCC) antagonism. LTCCs mediate the upstroke of nodal cell action potentials, unlike true atrial and ventricular myocyte action potentials in which the upstroke is mediated primarily by the faster activating and inactivating Na_v channel, $Na_v1.5$. Hence, nodal action potentials exhibit a much slower upstroke than that of typical atrial and ventricular myocytes (see Chapter 20). The transmembrane topology of voltage-gated Ca^{2+} channel (Ca_v) α subunits mirrors that of the Na_v channel α subunits: 24 transmembrane segments around an aqueous pore. LTCCs also incorporate a requisite array of ancillary subunits: the cytoplasmic β subunit, transmembrane δ and γ subunits, and extracellular α2 subunit (Figure 24-5, A). In cardiac muscle, the LTCC $Ca_v1.2$ α subunit is located in the T-tubules and is activated by cellular depolarization, via its voltage-sensing apparatus, which moves upon membrane depolarization and opens the discrete but connected pore. Ca^{2+} influx through $Ca_v1.2$, down the Ca^{2+} concentration gradient, helps depolarize the cell and increase cytosolic $[Ca^{2+}]$ directly, but also indirectly by activating the sarcoplasmic reticulum-located ryanodine receptor (RyR2 in cardiac muscle) through Ca^{2+}-activated Ca^{2+} release. In skeletal muscle, the mechanism is somewhat different: $Ca_v1.1$ is mechanically linked to RyR1 and acts as the latter's voltage sensor. Thus in skeletal muscle, RyR1 is activated primarily by membrane depolarization, with the $Ca_v1.1$ S4 domains acting as the RyR1 voltage sensors (see Figure 24-5, B).[36,37]

Most clinically relevant Ca_v channel blockers are in one of three chemical classes: the dihydropyridines, which are not generally indicated for arrhythmias; the phenylalkylamines, exemplified by verapamil; and the benzothiazepines, exemplified by diltiazem.[38] Diltiazem and verapamil (see Figure 24-5, C) are thought to bind overlapping but distinct sites within the S6 segments of repeats III and IV, and the Ca^{2+} selectivity filter of the α1 subunit of the cardiac LTCC $Ca_v1.2$.[39-41]

CLINICAL PHARMACOLOGY

Categories of Arrhythmogenic Mechanisms

The mechanistic bases for most, if not all, arrhythmias can be placed in one of three categories. These are discussed with the most common modes of treatment.[42-47]

AUTOMATICITY

Arrhythmias in this category arise from changes to the normal process of automaticity essential for cardiac rhythm (see Figure 24-1). They can be further separated into two sub-categories:

Normal automaticity arrhythmias are those that elicit speeding or slowing of the heartbeat, initially at least maintaining regular beating, although this is lost at some point, for example, at extremely high heart rates, due to an intrinsic inability of ion channels to function rapidly enough in concert. Arrhythmias in this category include sinus tachycardia and ventricular tachycardia (both being an increased heart rate). *The most common pharmacologic treatment of sinus tachycardia and ventricular tachycardia is with β blockers (class II antiarrhythmics).*

Abnormal automaticity arrhythmias are those in which regular activity is lost immediately and involve spontaneous impulse formation in partially depolarized cells (membrane potentials in the range of −40 to −60 mV). Examples of arrhythmias that can fall into this category include ventricular tachycardias and ectopic atrial tachycardias in the subacute phase (within 48 hours) following myocardial infarction, exercise-induced idiopathic ventricular tachycardias, and catecholamine-sensitive idiopathic ventricular tachycardias. *The most common pharmacologic treatment of idiopathic rhythms and ectopic atrial tachycardias is with Ca^{2+} channel blockers (class IV antiarrhythmics).*

Sinus rhythm is regulated by pacemaker channels (i.e., hyperpolarization-activated, cyclic nucleotide-gated monovalent cation-nonselective channels known as *HCN*), and to a greater or lesser extent, Ca^{2+} oscillations. Hence, human HCN4 mutation is associated with sinus-mediated pathologic slowing of the heart rate (sinus bradycardia).

TRIGGERED

Triggered arrhythmias are those in which a mistimed beat occurs before the previous beat is complete (see Figure 24-1, B). The ion channels involved in orchestrating each cardiac myocyte action potential must work in concert to generate rhythmic contraction of the heart. Because the various classes of ion channel each have distinct gating kinetics and refractory periods, if one type of ion channel dysfunctions, it can act asynchronously with the others, potentially causing triggered arrhythmias. Triggered arrhythmias can be separated into two main classes:

Early after-depolarizations (EADs) occur when myocardial repolarization is delayed sufficiently that the next action potential in a given cardiac myocyte begins before that myocyte is fully repolarized. A common clinical consequence is the arrhythmia referred to as *torsades de pointes* (TdP). TdP is so named because it appears on the electrocardiogram (ECG) as a twisted ribbon due to the variance in magnitude of the voltages associated with each heartbeat (see Figure 24-1, C). TdP most often occurs because of pharmacologic inhibition of specific ventricular myocyte K^+ channels, which results in a delay in ventricular myocyte repolarization and consequent prolongation of the QT interval on the ECG. A number of drugs inhibit these channels and can lead to TdP, including a number of drugs commonly used in anesthesia; some of the major QT interval prolonging drugs are summarized in Table 24-3. The QT interval represents the time from the onset of ventricular depolarization to the end of

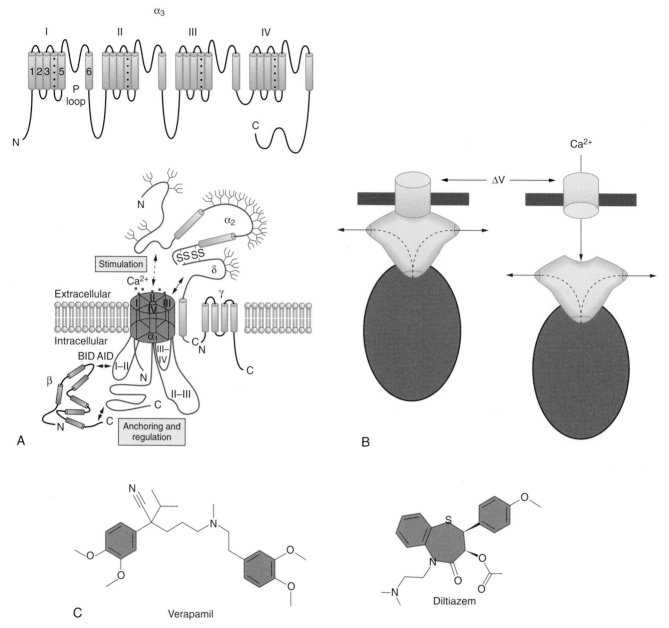

Figure 24-5 Calcium channels and the class IV antiarrhythmics. **A,** Upper, topology of a voltage-gated Ca^{2+} channel α subunit (Ca_v). Note similar structure to Na_v shown in Figure 24-2. *Lower,* heteromeric voltage-gated Ca^{2+} channel complex with $\alpha_2\delta$ accessory subunits. **B,** Juxtaposition of voltage-gated Ca^{2+} channel at the cell surface membrane *(blue)* and the SR-located ryanodine receptor in skeletal muscle *(left)* and cardiac muscle *(right)*. **C,** Structures of verapamil and diltiazem, key class IV antiarrhythmic drugs.

ventricular repolarization; prolongation of this interval can indicate long QT syndrome, of which there are now many well-defined subtypes with distinct molecular etiologies. When sufficiently long delays in repolarization occur, Na_v channels can recover from their refractory period and open before repolarization is complete, leading to an EAD in phase 2, 3, or 4 of the ventricular or atrial action potential (see Figure 24-1, *B*). *The most common pharmacologic treatment of TdP is with magnesium sulphate, β blockers (class II antiarrhythmics), and/or Ca^{2+} channel blockers (class IV antiarrhythmics).*

Delayed after-depolarizations (DADs) classically occur in digitalis toxicity. Digitalis toxicity can occur through a variety of mechanisms, but all serve to raise intracellular Ca^{2+}

concentration, generating a net depolarizing current that, together with the tendency of digitalis to increase vagal tone, leads to DADs (amongst other possible classes of arrhythmias). Unlike most EADs, DADs begin after repolarization, but before the next appropriately timed depolarization, that is, in phase 4 of the cardiac action potential (see Figure 24-1, *B*). *The most common pharmacologic treatment of DADs arising from digitalis toxicity is with Ca^{2+} channel blockers (class IV antiarrhythmics).*

CONDUCTION

Commonly arising from structural damage to the heart, but also from certain drug-ion channel interactions, localized

Table 24-3. Drugs Known to Prolong QT Interval

GENERIC NAME	CLASS	COMMENTS
Amiodarone	Antiarrhythmic	Females > males, TdP risk low
Arsenic trioxide	Anticancer	
Astemizole	Antihistamine	No longer available in U.S.
Bepridil	Antianginal	Females > males
Chloroquine	Antimalarial	
Chlorpromazine	Antipsychotic; antiemetic	
Cisapride	Gastrointestinal stimulant	No longer available in U.S.; available in Mexico
Citalopram	Antidepressant	
Clarithromycin	Antibiotic	
Disopyramide	Antiarrhythmic	Females > males
Dofetilide	Antiarrhythmic	
Domperidone	Antiemetic	Not available in U.S.
Droperidol	Sedative; antiemetic	
Erythromycin	Antibiotic; gastrointestinal stimulant	Females > males
Flecainide	Antiarrhythmic	
Halofantrine	Antimalarial	Females > males
Haloperidol	Antipsychotic	When given intravenously or at higher-than-recommended doses
Ibutilide	Antiarrhythmic	Females > males
Levomethadyl	Opioid agonist	Not available in U.S.
Mesoridazine	Antipsychotic	
Methadone	Opioid agonist	Females > males
Moxifloxacin	Antibiotic	
Ondansetron	Antiemetic	
Pentamidine	Antiinfective	Females > males
Pimozide	Antipsychotic	Females > males
Probucol	Antilipemic	No longer available in U.S.
Procainamide	Antiarrhythmic	
Quinidine	Antiarrhythmic	Females > males
Sevoflurane	Volatile anesthetic	
Sotalol	Antiarrhythmic	Females > males
Sparfloxacin	Antibiotic	
Terfenadine	Antihistamine	No longer available in U.S.
Thioridazine	Antipsychotic	
Vandetanib	Anticancer	

See www.azcert.org for more information.

slowed conduction within regions of the heart can cause re-entrant arrhythmias that can be categorized into two main types:

Reentrant circuits arise when one area of the heart contains a region of slowed ion conduction. When such regions occur, primarily due to the refractory period of Na_v channels arising from their rapid and extensive inactivation and its recovery, reentrant circuits are formed because normal conduction cannot proceed unidirectionally, but can proceed in a circle (Figure 24-6, *A*). They can be micro reentrant (involving a localized region within, e.g., one chamber of the heart) or macro reentrant, involving more than one chamber (see Figure 24-6, *B*). Such circuits are incompatible with normal cardiac rhythm because they disturb the (essentially)

unidirectional wave of depolarization/repolarization required for normal contraction to occur. These types of circuits cause atrial flutter, and ventricular and supraventricular tachycardias. *Monomorphic ventricular tachycardia is treated with class Ia Na_v channel blockers or K^+ channel blockers (class III antiarrhythmics). AV node reentrant tachycardias (supraventricular tachycardia or SVAT), which arise from reentry in the region of the AV junction, are treated with Ca^{2+} channel blockers (class IV antiarrhythmics) or adenosine.*

Fibrillation occurs when many micro reentrant circuits span an entire chamber of the heart. This is a different situation from a single macro reentrant circuit and is typically classified (according to the chambers in which it is occurring) as atrial fibrillation or ventricular fibrillation. The substrate for atrial fibrillation is probably most commonly structural heart disease, and while it is typically not acutely dangerous, it requires treatment. This is partly because it suggests an underlying defect and partly because a significant risk in atrial fibrillation is the formation of atrial thrombi that can result in launching of systemic emboli when sinus rhythm is reestablished. Approximately 2 to 3 million people in the United States suffer from atrial fibrillation, the majority in the aging population, and this number is expected to rise as the population ages. Another common cause of atrial fibrillation is major surgery such as open heart surgery or lung resection, with the underlying mechanism not being entirely clear. Hyperthyroidism can also cause atrial fibrillation; return to euthyroidism abrogates the atrial fibrillation in the majority of cases. *Atrial fibrillation is most commonly treated with Na_v channel blockers (class Ia antiarrhythmics) or K^+ channel blockers (class III antiarrhythmics).*

Ventricular fibrillation, in contrast, is acutely life-threatening because the heart in ventricular fibrillation cannot pump blood effectively. An estimated 300,000 people in the United States die annually of sudden cardiac death, with ventricular fibrillation being among the most common lethal arrhythmias. Ventricular fibrillation must be rapidly treated (within minutes) using DC shock. Cardiopulmonary resuscitation (CPR) can be used to keep the brain alive until defibrillation is possible, but CPR cannot restore normal cardiac rhythm. *Amiodarone is the first-line antiarrhythmic drug clinically demonstrated to increase return of spontaneous circulation in refractory ventricular fibrillation and pulseless ventricular tachycardia unresponsive to CPR, defibrillation, and vasopressor therapy. If amiodarone is unavailable, lidocaine can be considered as a second line drug with less evidence of efficacy compared with amiodarone. Magnesium sulfate is used for TdP associated with a long QT interval.*

CLINICAL APPLICATION

Class I—Sodium Channel Blockers

CLASS Ia Na_v CHANNEL BLOCKERS
The class Ia antiarrhythmics block ion conduction through $Na_v1.5$, the principal cardiac Na^+ channel; this delays and reduces the magnitude of peak depolarization in cardiomyocytes, and thus prolongs the action potential. Refractoriness is also increased in that Na_v channels require a greater hyperpolarization and longer time to recover from inactivation in the presence of class Ia agents. These effects can be

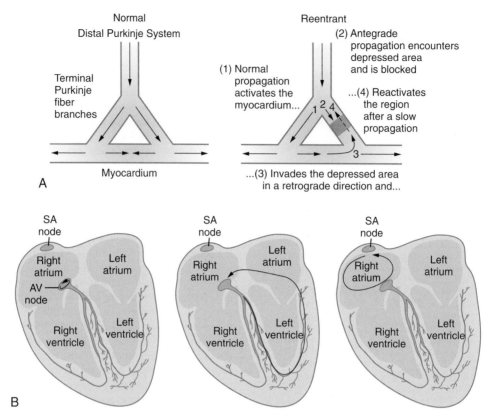

Figure 24-6 Reentrant circuits. **A,** Anatomy of a reentrant circuit. Depending on the relative speed of conduction and duration of refractory periods in two alternate longitudinal pathways, anterograde propagation can be blocked in one pathway whereas retrograde propagation progresses, creating a reentrant circuit. **B,** Examples of micro- and macro-reentrant circuits in the heart. *Left,* a micro-reentrant circuit in the AV node; *center,* a macro-reentrant circuit spanning the AV node and left atrium and ventricle; *right,* a micro-reentrant circuit in the right atrium.

therapeutic if the heart is beating too rapidly or in an uncoordinated fashion. Therefore, class Ia antiarrhythmics can be indicated for symptomatic premature ventricular beats, and ventricular and supraventricular tachyarrhythmias. They can also be used to prevent the acutely life-threatening condition ventricular fibrillation.

Quinidine exemplifies the advantages and potential drawbacks of class Ia antiarrhythmic drugs, and of the SVW classification itself. Aside from blocking $Na_v1.5$ channels in the activated state, which slows phase 0 depolarization (see Figure 24-2, *B*), quinidine also blocks certain voltage-gated K^+ channels, which in turn delays phase 3 repolarization and can in itself be proarrhythmic, prolonging the QT interval on the ECG (see Figure 24-1, *C*). It also widens the QRS complex through its effects on $Na_v1.5$. Quinidine can also decrease the slope of phase 4 depolarization in Purkinje fibers, thereby reducing automaticity. Because quinidine has antimuscarinic-based vagolytic properties that work against its direct action on the SA and AV nodes, it can actually increase conduction through these nodes. This presents problems because it can cause 1:1 conduction of atrial fibrillation, thereby increasing ventricular rate too. Thus, if used for atrial fibrillation, quinidine (and related class Ia agent, procainamide) must be accompanied by an AV node blocking agent to prevent this (e.g., class II or IV antiarrhythmics).

Quinidine is also a notable antimalarial: It kills the schizont parasite of *Plasmodium falciparum* and gametocyte parasite

stages of *Plasmodium* sp. Quinidine is associated with a number of contraindications and precautions aside from the AV conduction issues noted earlier: It can increase digoxin levels by decreasing renal and extrarenal clearance and can aggravate myasthenia gravis.[48]

Procainamide (only available in an intravenous formulation in the United States) is another important class Ia antiarrhythmic that can be used to treat atrial fibrillation in Wolff-Parkinson-White syndrome (WPWS). Other class Ia agents include ajmaline, lorajmaline, prajmaline, disopyramide, and sparteine.

CLASS Ib Na_v CHANNEL BLOCKERS

The class Ib antiarrhythmics have relatively little effect on conduction velocities and low proarrhythmic potential. They exhibit rapid Na_v channel binding kinetics and their main actions are to decrease the duration of the ventricular myocyte action potential and the refractory period (see Figure 24-2, *B*). Class Ib drugs have little effect on atrial myocyte action potentials, and therefore on atrial tissue, since they are, at baseline, relatively short compared to ventricular action potentials. Thus these drugs are primarily used to treat ventricular arrhythmias.[49]

Lidocaine (see Figure 24-2, *B*) is the archetypal class Ib antiarrhythmic. Like all class Ib drugs, its rapid binding and unbinding rates (endowing it with use-dependency or frequency-dependency) greatly diminish its effects at low heart rates, and exaggerate its effects at high heart rates. Lidocaine selectively targets the open and inactivated states of $Na_v1.5$, with low affinity for the deactivated (closed or resting) state. For this reason, lidocaine and other class Ib drugs can be efficacious in the therapy of rapid heart rate conditions including ventricular tachycardia and ventricular fibrillation prevention, and also in cases of symptomatic premature ventricular beats. Other notable class Ib drugs include mexiletine (which is metabolized to lidocaine), phenytoin, and tocainide.[47]

CLASS Ic Na$_v$ CHANNEL BLOCKERS

Class Ic antiarrhythmics exhibit relatively slow Na$_v$ channel binding kinetics, and can be used to treat both atrial and ventricular arrhythmias. Drugs in this class are indicated for treatment of nonsustained ventricular tachycardias, but are contraindicated when there is underlying heart disease such as myocardial infarction or left ventricular hypertrophy.[50] Class Ic agents typically slow Na$_v$ channel conduction, delaying the peak depolarization and somewhat prolonging the QT interval (see Figure 24-2, B).

Flecainide (see Figure 24-2, B), an important class Ic antiarrhythmic, displays little end-organ toxicity but can exhibit significant proarrhythmic effects. Interestingly, flecainide is now thought to also inhibit Ca^{2+} release from the cardiac sarcoplasmic reticulum Ca^{2+} release channel, ryanodine receptor 2 (RyR2), endowing it with therapeutic activity in individuals with catecholaminergic polymorphic ventricular tachycardia (CPVT).[51] The more well-recognized, class Ic action of flecainide confers its effectiveness in prevention of paroxysmal atrial fibrillation and flutter, paroxysmal supraventricular tachycardias, and sustained ventricular tachycardias.[52]

Class II—β Blockers

β-Adrenoceptor antagonists, also known as β blockers, are pharmacologic agents that competitively antagonize the β effects of catecholamines on the heart, blood vessels, bronchi, and so on (see Chapters 12 and 13). Propranolol was introduced in 1965 as the first therapeutically useful β blocker and more than 20 analogs are available today. They are used not only as antiarrhythmics, but also as antianginals and antihypertensives, in that they limit cardiac oxygen consumption and lower plasma renin activity. Depending on their relative β receptor affinities, β blockers are classified as nonselective (or "blanket" β blockers) when they block both β$_1$ and β$_2$ receptor subtypes like propranolol, or cardioselective (i.e., β1-selective), such as metoprolol, atenolol, and nebivolol. Third-generation β blockers endowed with vasodilating properties are also available, such as pindolol and carvedilol, which are therapeutically used in congestive heart failure.

Duration of action varies among the various analogs, esmolol being the shortest (T$_{1/2}$ ~9 minutes) and nadolol the longest-acting drug (T$_{1/2}$~24 hours), allowing once daily dosing. Lipid/water solubility of the various β blockers influences the route of elimination: the more lipid-soluble are eliminated primarily by the liver (e.g., propranolol and metoprolol), and the more water-soluble are eliminated primarily by the kidney (e.g., atenolol and nadolol). Thus hepatic cirrhosis and renal failure can prolong the action of lipid- and water-soluble β blockers, respectively.

Adverse effects of β blockers are due mainly to β$_2$-blocking effects. Among these, bronchospasm in patients with bronchial asthma or chronic obstructive pulmonary disease can cause severe dyspnea. Peripheral vasoconstriction can also occur with blockade of vascular β$_2$-receptors, as shown by a relatively rare worsening of symptoms of peripheral vascular disease (e.g., intermittent claudication, Raynaud phenomenon). Excessive β$_1$-blockade on the other hand can cause bradycardia, hypotension, and AV node conduction block.

β-Adrenoceptor stimulation enhances I$_{Ca-L}$ and I$_{Ca-T}$ currents and slows Ca^{2+} channel inactivation. It also increases sinus rate by increasing the I$_f$ pacemaker current and increases Ca^{2+} storage in the SR leading to DAD (see Figure 24-1, B). By inhibiting all of these effects, β blockers exert an antiarrhythmic action that is particularly effective whenever sympathetic activity is increased, such as in stressful conditions, acute myocardial infarction, and CPR following cardiac arrest. Bradycardia and slowing of AV nodal conduction (prolongation of the PR interval) are typically observed. Therefore, β blockers are valuable in terminating reentrant arrhythmias that include the AV node, and also in controlling ventricular rate in atrial fibrillation or flutter.

Overall, β blockers are effective in treating or preventing arrhythmias that share as a common denominator increased sympathetic activity. These include paroxysmal atrial tachycardia due to exercise or emotion, exercise-induced ventricular arrhythmias, arrhythmias associated with pheochromocytoma, arrhythmias associated with myocardial infarction, and all the arrhythmias accompanied by angina or hypertension.[17,53]

Class III—Potassium Channel Blockers

K$_v$ channels are the primary target for class III antiarrhythmics. By blocking K$_v$ channels, class III agents prolong the action potential and, therefore, increase refractoriness (see Figure 4-4, B). These drugs can thus be highly efficacious in the treatment of a variety of tachyarrhythmias, both ventricular and atrial. One of the great paradoxes of arrhythmia therapy is that action potential prolongation can be either therapeutic or life-threatening depending on the nature of the genetic, electrical, and/or structural defect in the patient. While K$_v$ channel blockade can help control dangerous tachycardia, it can also precipitate TdP due to its QT-prolonging effects; this in turn can lead to lethal ventricular fibrillation.

The problem with many class III agents is that they inhibit the hERG K$_v$ channel (which generates I$_{Kr}$ as explained earlier) in a reverse use-dependent manner that does not increase block with heart rate, but rather does the opposite. This impairs the crucial I$_{Kr}$ repolarization current, delaying phase 3 repolarization, most aggressively in bradycardia and less so in tachycardia, which can lead to a dangerously proarrhythmic tendency.

Two significant advances in the field of class III antiarrhythmic development are overcoming these problems. The first advance is exemplified by amiodarone (see Figure 24-4, B), a drug that actually has actions in all four SVW classes, but the major therapeutic effect of which is thought to result from its class III effects.[54] The big advantage of amiodarone over earlier agents (although it was first described in 1961, it was only approved for use in the United States in 1985) is that it inhibits both I_{Kr} and I_{Ks}. I_{Ks} is generated by a heteromer of the KCNQ1 K_v α subunit and most commonly the KCNE1 β subunit, and is the primary slow-activating component of the delayed rectifier K^+ current acting in phase 3 repolarization. I_{Ks} rises to prominence, in terms of its role in repolarization, at higher heart rates because KCNQ1-KCNE1 channels accumulate in the activated state, and conversely at these rates I_{Kr} is less effective at ventricular repolarization, hence the reverse use-dependence of "pure" I_{Kr} blockers. I_{Ks} probably acts as a safety factor, or repolarization reserve, to compensate for the relative impotency of I_{Kr} at high heart rates. Amiodarone, by blocking both I_{Kr} and I_{Ks}, exhibits a safer and more efficacious action on phase 3 repolarization. A related drug, dronedarone, lacks the iodine that is associated with some side effects of amiodarone, including skin photosensitivity and ocular abnormalities, and the former is therefore safer (although less efficacious) and still has the dual action of I_{Kr} and I_{Ks} antagonism, as does azimilide.[55-57] Azimilide, however, and tedisamil (which inhibits I_{Kr}, I_{to} and the ATP-sensitive inwardly rectifier K^+ current I_{KATP}) have proven marginally efficacious and also torsadogenic, leading to doubts about their ultimate usefulness in atrial fibrillation therapy.[58,59] Their key problem is that they do not present a big enough therapeutic window to reverse atrial tachyarrhythmias without causing an unsafe delay in ventricular repolarization; that is, they lack atrial specificity.

The majority of atrial fibrillation cases are linked to underlying disorders including structural heart disease, chronic alcohol use, hyperthyroidism, and pulmonary embolism. Most individuals with atrial fibrillation exhibit a chronic, sustained atrial arrhythmia, and the clinical manifestations range from palpitations to heart failure. Perhaps as many as a third of atrial fibrillation patients have "lone" atrial fibrillation, in which underlying heart or extracardiac disease is either occult or absent. Of these patients, some harbor ion channel mutations thought to be the substrate for atrial fibrillation. The KCNQ1 K_v channel gene is again involved. A key step in atrial fibrillation is thought to be shortening of the atrial effective refractory period; therefore, it is intuitive that, as with short QT syndrome, gain-of-function mutations in *KCNQ1* are linked to AF, in that they have the capacity to hasten repolarization. In addition, mutations in several members of the KCNE gene family of β subunits are associated with atrial fibrillation by increasing currents through the respective KCNQ1-KCNE channel complex.[60-62] Inherited mutations in *KCNA5*, which encodes the atrially expressed $K_v1.5$ potassium channel α subunit, also associate with AF. Nonchannel genes associated with AF include renin-angiotensin system genes, probably in combination with environmental agents that elevate blood pressure.[63,64]

Therapeutic approaches to AF involve not just lengthening of the atrial effective refractory period (pharmacologically or by electrical cardioversion), but also surgery to prevent recurrence and anticoagulation for stroke prevention. With respect to pharmacologic intervention to control the heart in atrial fibrillation, control of rhythm appears to offer no significant advantage in terms of mortality or stroke risk compared to controlling the rate, that is, returning the heart rate to somewhere between 60 and 100 beats per minute. However, rhythm control is desirable in newly diagnosed atrial fibrillation, and in other cases dictated by patient-specific factors,

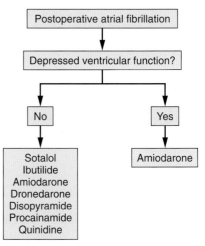

Figure 24-7 Rhythm control for postoperative atrial fibrillation. Given the side effect profile of amiodarone, it is generally reserved for use when other drugs are ineffective, contraindicated, or not well-tolerated. Dronedarone is contraindicated in patients with acutely decompensated heart failure. Sotolol may be used with caution in selected patients with mild to moderate reduction in left ventricular ejection fraction. *(Modified from Martinez EA, Bass EB, Zimetbaum P, et al. Control of rhythm: American College of Chest Physicians Guidelines for the prevention and management of postoperative atrial fibrillation after cardiac surgery. Chest. 2005;128 [Suppl 2]:48S-55S.)*

and remains the strategy of choice. For pharmacologic rate control, β blockers and Ca^{2+} channel blockers are most often employed, whereas for pharmacologic rhythm control, Na^+ channel blockers or K^+ channel blockers are used. The pharmacologic control of postoperative atrial fibrillation is summarized in Figure 24-7.

This introduces the second significant recent advance in class III antiarrhythmic development. The dependency of the human heart for hERG-mediated ventricular repolarization is problematic in an increasingly medicated population owing to the predilection of hERG for nonspecific drug block. In addition, hERG protein folding (part of the process that ensures that hERG channels reach the cell surface and pass K^+ ions) is highly sensitive to both drugs and inherited single amino acid substitutions. This incredibly unfortunate combination of circumstances is due in part to the fact that, for the majority of human evolution, drugs have not been an environmental factor and thus have not impacted natural selection.[65]

However, nature has provided a fortuitous solution to the hERG targeting conundrum. In human atrium, the ultra-rapidly activating K_v current, I_{Kur}, is generated by the $K_v1.5$ (gene name *KCNA5*) K_v channel α subunit, but $K_v1.5$ is not significantly functionally expressed in human ventricles. Pharmacologic inhibition of $K_v1.5$ can lengthen the atrial refractory period enough to be of therapeutic benefit in AF. Crucially, because it does not contribute to ventricular repolarization, specific $K_v1.5$ inhibition does not delay ventricular repolarization and therefore is not torsadogenic.

There are some caveats vis-à-vis $K_v1.5$ blockers. While Kv1.5 is in a different α subunit subfamily, it has been difficult to develop selective $K_v1.5$ antagonists that do not also inhibit hERG therapeutic concentrations. Interestingly, the most promising $K_v1.5$-blocking class III agents appear to be the less specific drugs that block $K_v1.5$, hERG, $K_v4.3$ (which generates to in human heart), and $Na_v1.5$. These drugs, exemplified by AVE0118 and RSD1235, inhibit $K_v1.5$ more effectively than the other channels, and the hERG block appears to be "balanced" by $Na_v1.5$ block (thus both ventricular repolarization and depolarization). Furthermore, $Na_v1.5$ inhibition by AVE0118 is use-dependent and therefore more efficacious the faster the atrium is fibrillating. In summary, as with many antiarrhythmics, nonspecificity can be tolerated and can even be desirable, depending on the targets and their location, the nature of the action on those targets, and the relative affinity for each target.[66-69]

Class IV—Calcium Channel Blockers

The class IV antiarrhythmics block voltage-gated Ca^{2+} channels, the primary target with respect to arrhythmias being the cardiac LTCC, $Ca_v1.2$. While in atrial and ventricular myocytes the primary role of Ca^{2+} is signaling in muscular excitation-contraction coupling, in nodal cells its primary role is electrical conduction of a depolarizing signal. By lowering ventricular myocyte intracellular $[Ca^{2+}]$, some class IV antiarrhythmics decrease the force of contraction of the heart, an effect referred to as *negative inotropy*. By slowing conduction through nodal cells, some class IV drugs reduce the heart rate, an effect referred to as *negative chronotropy* (see Chapter 21).

The dihydropyridines (e.g., nifedipine) are used to treat increased systemic vascular resistance but are not generally indicated for arrhythmias. The phenylalkylamines, exemplified by verapamil, are relatively myocardial-specific and cause negative inotropy with minimal vasodilation or reflex tachycardia. Verapamil is indicated for angina, with two probable main modes of action: dilatation of the main coronary arteries and arterioles, inhibiting coronary vasospasm, and reduction of oxygen utilization via unloading of the heart achieved by relaxing the peripheral arterioles. As an antiarrhythmic, verapamil is highly effective at slowing ventricular contraction rate in patients with atrial flutter or atrial fibrillation because it slows AV node conduction in a rate-dependent manner. This rate dependence also accounts for the fact that verapamil generally is much less effective at reducing already normal AV conduction rates—a desirable property—although it can occasionally induce AV node block in the absence of preexisting conduction defects. Verapamil is effective in reducing the frequency of episodes of paroxysmal supraventricular tachycardia, but can also induce ventricular fibrillation in patients with atrial flutter or fibrillation and a coexisting AV accessory pathway.[70-72]

The benzothiazepines, exemplified by diltiazem, exhibit myocardial specificity intermediate between the dihydropyridines and phenylalkylamines. Diltiazem causes excitation-contraction uncoupling, relaxation of coronary vascular smooth muscle and dilatation of coronary arteries, but has relatively modest negative inotropic effects. Diltiazem is typically prescribed for angina and hypertension, and is quite effective in lowering blood pressure in hypertensive individuals, with little effect on normotensives. It is also reportedly as effective as verapamil in the treatment of supraventricular tachycardias, and is also indicated for atrial flutter and atrial fibrillation. Its negative dromotropic effect (slowing of

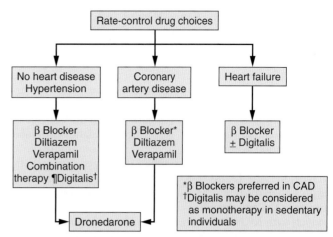

Figure 24-8 Selection of rate-control drug therapy is based on the presence or absence of underlying heart disease and other comorbidities. Combination therapy might be required. *CAD,* Coronary artery disease. *(Modified from Gillis AM, Verma A, Talajic M, et al. Canadian Cardiovascular Society Atrial Fibrillation Guidelines 2010: rate and rhythm management. Can J Cardiol. 2011;27:47-59.)*

conduction through the AV node) reduces oxygen consumption by increasing the time required for each heartbeat.[73,74] The rational selection of drugs for controlling heart rate is summarized in Figure 24-8.

EMERGING DEVELOPMENTS

Molecular Genetics of Arrhythmias

A combination of molecular genetics, recombinant DNA technology and physiologic techniques are revealing the secrets of many cardiac arrhythmias; intuitively, the majority of the genes linked thus far to abnormal cardiac rhythm are those that express ion channel proteins.[27] Many of these same ion channels are targets for clinically important antiarrhythmic and proarrhythmic drugs. An understanding of the precise molecular basis for an individual's arrhythmia can remove some of the uncertainty about how best to treat the arrhythmia, and facilitates genetic or other forms of testing of family members, permitting early diagnosis and preventive measures to avoid potentially lethal cardiac events.

LONG QT SYNDROME

A delay in ventricular myocyte repolarization can prolong the QT interval on the ECG and lead to TdP and even ventricular fibrillation. The most common inherited causes of this phenomenon are loss-of-function mutations in ventricular, voltage-gated K_v channels, which are primarily responsible for ventricular myocyte repolarization by virtue of K^+ efflux to restore a negative membrane potential (see Figure 24-1, *A*). Around 45% of individuals diagnosed with inherited long QT syndrome (LQTS) whose DNA has been sequenced have loss-of-function mutations in the *KCNQ1* gene. *KCNQ1* encodes the K_v channel pore-forming (α) subunit of the same name. *KCNQ1* mutations underlie long QT syndrome type 1 (LQT1), which is further divided into the autosomal dominant Romano Ward syndrome (RWS) and the recessive cardioauditory Jervell Lange-Nielsen syndrome (JLNS). Individuals with loss-of-function mutations in both KCNQ1 alleles (i.e., JLNS) exhibit both LQTS and profound sensorineural deafness. KCNQ1, in protein complexes with KCNE1, a single-transmembrane segment ancillary (β) subunit, generates the slowly activating ventricular repolarization current, I_{Ks}.[75]

I_{Ks} is important for phase 3 repolarization in the ventricular action potential, particularly when the dominant ventricular repolarization K^+ current, I_{Kr} (see later), is compromised, or during sustained exercise or other prolonged sympathetic activation. The KCNQ1-KCNE1 potassium channel is also expressed in the inner ear, where it is responsible for K^+ secretion into the endolymph (hence the deafness in JLNS). Individuals with KCNE1 mutations (1%-2% of sequenced LQTS cases) are classified as having LQT5; they exhibit RWS or JLNS with similar symptoms as LQT1 patients, indicating the KCNE1 β subunit is important for I_{Ks}.

I_{Kr} is generated by the human *ether-à-go-go* related gene product (hERG), the voltage-gated K^+ channel α subunit encoded by the *KCNH2* gene, probably in complexes with the KCNE2 β subunit and perhaps others. *KCNH2* loss-of-function mutations (LQT2) account for ~40% of known LQTS cases, *KCNE2* mutations (LQT6) ~1%.

The third most commonly linked LQTS gene is *SCN5A*, which encodes the $Na_v1.5$ cardiac voltage-gated Na^+ channel that underlies the upstroke in phase 0 of the cardiac myocyte action potential (see Figures 24-1, *A* and 24-2). $Na_v1.5$, like all voltage-gated Na^+ channels, inactivates rapidly, which together with the transient outward K^+ current, I_{to}, cause the notch at the beginning of the human ventricular myocyte action potential. Gain-of-function mutations in *SCN5A*, particularly those that increase Na^+ influx during phases 2-3 when the majority of $Na_v1.5$ channels are normally inactivated, delay repolarization because they produce persistent depolarizing force (Na^+ influx). *SCN5A* mutations account for 5% to 10% of LQTS cases and are categorized as LQT3. $Na_v1.5$ is an important antiarrhythmic target, with many drugs known to alter its inactivation kinetics.[76,77]

The remaining molecularly defined inherited LQTS cases are relatively rarer and are spread among other genes encoding K^+ channel subunits, Ca^{2+} channel subunits, and channel-associated proteins.

SHORT QT SYNDROME

Shortening of the QT interval, indicating premature ventricular repolarization, can also be pathogenic, further illustrating the importance of timely electrical activity in the heart. The majority of sequenced short QT syndrome (SQTS) cases are, intuitively, associated with *KCNQ1* or *KCNH2* gain-of-function mutations. SQT1 is associated with *KCNH2* mutation; SQT2 with *KCNQ1*; and the inward rectifier K^+ channel gene *KCNJ2* with SQT3. SQTS is characterized by a corrected QT interval (QTc) of less than 300 ms, and manifests as palpitations, syncope, and sudden cardiac death; patients with a QTc of up to 330 ms are also diagnosed with SQTS if they have had an arrhythmic event such as ventricular fibrillation, syncope or resuscitated sudden cardiac death. Also associated with an increased risk of both atrial and ventricular fibrillation, SQTS has been found to respond to hydroquinidine, whereas class IC and III antiarrhythmics were unable to prolong the QT interval in this context.

However, the current therapy of choice is an implantable cardioverter-defibrillator (ICD).[78-80]

BRUGADA SYNDROME

In contrast to the long and short QT syndromes, the majority of sequenced Brugada syndrome (BrS) cases (perhaps representing 30% of all BrS cases) have been linked to loss-of-function mutations in the *SCN5A* voltage-gated Na^+ channel gene that encodes $Na_v1.5$. BrS is an autosomal dominant, idiopathic form of ventricular fibrillation that manifests on the ECG as persistent ST-segment elevation in the right precordial leads, together with complete or incomplete right bundle branch block. BrS patients are strongly predisposed to life-threatening ventricular fibrillation even with a structurally normal heart, and BrS was recently found to be clinically and genetically the same disorder as sudden unexplained nocturnal death syndrome (SUNDS/SUDS) described in Southeast Asia, where BrS is endemic and is often mistaken for a supernatural curse by poorly educated people.

In BrS patients, the transient outward K^+ current that forms a notch at the start of the ventricular action potential is inadequately balanced by the voltage-gated Na^+ current due to loss of function in $Na_v1.5$, which is considered a trigger for ventricular tachycardia and fibrillation. Accordingly, a gain-of-function mutation in the KCNE3 β subunit, which regulates the K^+ channel underlying I_{to} ($K_v4.3$), was also recently associated with BrS. An ICD is again the treatment of choice for BrS patients, but quinidine can be used to inhibit I_{to}, and isoproterenol and cilostazol can bolster the voltage-gated Ca^{2+} current to the same end, that is, reduction of the action potential notch that provides a substrate for potentially catastrophic ventricular micro-reentry circuits.[81,82]

OTHER INHERITED ARRHYTHMIA SYNDROMES

Other inherited arrhythmia syndromes include cardiac conduction disease, Wolff-Parkinson-White syndrome (WPWS), catecholaminergic polymorphic ventricular tachycardia (CPVT), and various sinus node disorders.[75,83]

Lev-Lenègre syndrome, a progressive cardiac conduction disease, has been linked to SCN5A loss-of-function gene variants, and is characterized by slowed conduction, pathologic slowing of cardiac rhythm, and conduction system fibrosis. A pacemaker or ICD is the most common therapeutic strategy, although pharmacologic intervention can also be indicated.

WPWS, in its rare familial form, is linked to mutations in the *PRKAG2* gene, which encodes the γ2 regulatory subunit of AMP-activated protein kinase (AMPK), but in the sporadic form of the disease this gene is rarely implicated. Other genetic associations include mitochondrial DNA mutations and, in association with hypertrophic cardiomyopathy, *TNNI3* and *MYBPC3* gene variants.[84,85] WPWS manifests as supraventricular arrhythmias associated with palpitations, and pre-excitation and syncope. WPWS is caused by an abnormal accessory electrical circuit that is present at birth (known as "the bundle of Kent"), and surgical ablation of this pathway is almost always successful in eliminating the cause and symptoms of WPWS. However, the marginally less-effective but much less invasive measure of radiofrequency catheter ablation is now typically employed in WPWS.[86,87]

CPVT is observed clinically as exercise- or emotional stress-induced syncope and sudden cardiac death, and on the body-surface ECG as bidirectional or polymorphic ventricular tachycardia. Two genes involved in excitation-contraction coupling have been linked to CPVT: *RyR2* (which encodes the cardiac ryanodine receptor, a sarcoplasmic reticulum Ca^{2+} release channel) and *CASQ2* (encoding calsequestrin, which stores releasable Ca^{2+} within the sarcoplasmic reticulum). Increased RyR2 activity or decreased calsequestrin expression generates spontaneous Ca^{2+} transients and DADs. CPVT is treated with β blockers, ICD, and/or other antiarrhythmic medications.

Sinus rhythm is dictated by hyperpolarization-activated, cyclic-nucleotide gated monovalent cation channels known as HCN or pacemaker channels (and to a greater or lesser extent, Ca^{2+} oscillations, a matter of current debate). Hence, HCN4 mutation is associated with sinus-mediated pathologic slowing of the heart rate (sinus bradycardia). *SCN5A* sodium channel gene mutations have been linked to sick sinus syndrome, and atrial standstill—which is also associated with a loss-of-function sequence variant in the gene encoding connexin 43 (Cx43), a transmembrane protein that forms gap junctions important to intercellular coupling.

hERG Drug Interactions

I_{Kr} is the dominant phase 3 repolarization current (see Figure 24-1, *A*), and by an evolutionary quirk, the hERG α subunit has a propensity for inhibition by a wide range of otherwise potentially clinically useful drugs (see Figure 24-4). This unfortunate situation has led drug regulatory agencies including the FDA to mandate that all potential new medications, and current medications linked to increased sudden death or QT prolongation, are subjected to time-consuming and expensive testing for potential hERG antagonism and QT prolongation in experimental preparations including canine Purkinje fibers, which are part of the specialized conduction system of the heart that rapidly conducts signals from the atrial-ventricular node (AV node) to the ventricles. Indeed, hERG safety concerns have spawned an industry in their own right, with companies being formed the major directive of which is to facilitate hERG safety testing via product development or outsourcing of cellular electrophysiology.[88] QT prolongation and TdP thought to result from block of cardiac hERG channels has resulted in withdrawal of drugs for a variety of indications. Between 1997 and 2001, ten prescription drugs were withdrawn from the U.S. market, four because of links to increased incidence of TdP: the antihistamines Seldane (terfenadine) and Hismanal (astemizole), the heartburn medication Propulsid (cisapride monohydrate), and the antibiotic grepafloxacin.

Interestingly, some medications (e.g., Trisenox [arsenic trioxide], a last-resort treatment for acute promyelocytic leukemia), and the majority of LQTS-linked *KCNH2* mutations, are now known to reduce I_{Kr} because of hERG misfolding and/or mistrafficking, rather than impaired conduction or gating of channels at the plasma membrane as was first thought. It remains to be seen whether this holds for other cardiac ion channels, but it is clinically relevant because it will influence the therapeutic strategies used to repair I_{Kr} in these cases: Small molecules have been identified that fix LQTS-associated mutant hERG channels, probably by creating nucleation points to aid channel folding.[89-92] Future antiarrhythmics could even be targeted toward enhancing "normal" hERG trafficking to overcome other repolarization deficiencies.

Gene Therapy Guided by Molecular Genetics of Inherited Arrhythmias

An interesting experimental approach to treatment of arrhythmias is to introduce genes that regulate cardiac rhythm based on their ability to regulate specific ion channels. Three examples stand out in the literature; it should be noted that gene therapy is currently only in experimental and trial phases owing to an array of side effects, not specific to the introduced gene but rather to the delivery method, often a virus.

In the first example, researchers have exploited the ability of the KCNE3 K^+ channel β subunit to accelerate ventricular repolarization by increasing current through the KCNQ1 K_v α subunit. In the heart, KCNQ1-KCNE1 normally generates the slowly activating I_{Ks} repolarizing current. However, in the colon, KCNQ1 complexes with KCNE3, a subunit that locks the KCNQ1 voltage sensor (and thus pore) open, producing a constitutively active yet K^+-selective channel that regulates cAMP-stimulated chloride secretion in vivo.[93,94] When KCNE3 was introduced into guinea-pig ventricular cavity by injection of adenovirus containing the *KCNE3* gene, the result was a shortening of the action potential and a reduction in QT interval, stemming from the resultant increase in KCNQ1 current (which would have been especially marked at negative voltages, where KCNQ1-KCNE1 is typically closed).[95]

Second, introduction of HCN channel genes into quiescent ventricular myocytes shows promise for converting them into pacemaker cells. HCN expression endows them with automaticity, the ability to fire spontaneously, because HCN channels open in response to hyperpolarization and initiate depolarization.[96,97]

Third, a natural polymorphism (Q9E) in the KCNE2 ancillary subunit that regulates the hERG K_v α subunit, increases the sensitivity of hERG-KCNE2 channels to block by the macrolide antibiotic clarithromycin. The polymorphism was discovered in an African-American woman with ventricular fibrillation precipitated by clarithromycin, and was later found to be present in 3% of African Americans but absent in Caucasian Americans. This finding was exciting because it uncovered a pharmacogenomic mechanism for increased susceptibility to adverse effects for a significant fraction of a specific ethnic group. However, it was also utilized ingeniously to engineer experimentally chamber-specificity to erythromycin susceptibility with therapeutic goals in mind. Thus, viral introduction of Q9E-KCNE2 into porcine atrium rendered hERG channels within the atrium several-fold more susceptible to block by clarithromycin than their ventricular, wild-type hERG-KCNE2 counterparts. Clarithromycin was found to selectively prolong the atrial refractory period in these pigs without significantly affecting ventricular action potentials, exploiting the increased sensitivity of the mutant KCNE2-containing atrial channels.[25,98-100]

Future work will build upon all these discoveries to create bench-to-bedside medicine that utilizes each patient's own molecular lesion to tailor highly patient- and target-specific, bespoke gene- and stem-cell-related therapies.

KEY POINTS

- Antiarrhythmic drugs are organized into the Singh-Vaughan Williams classification, which is a useful framework for categorizing by primary mode of action.
- Most antiarrhythmics can be classified into more than one of the four categories. Amiodarone, one of the most efficacious, falls into all four classes.
- Class I antiarrhythmics block voltage-gated Na^+ channels and are subcategorized into Ia, Ib, and Ic depending on their binding kinetics, which dictate their effects on cardiac myocyte action potentials. They are used for ventricular arrhythmias, but are currently less commonly used because of potential proarrhythmic effects.
- Class II antiarrhythmics block β adrenergic signaling and slow heart rate. Sinus tachycardia and ventricular tachycardia are treated with β blockers.
- Class III antiarrhythmics block K^+ channels, prolonging the cardiac myocyte action potential and refractory period. They are used for conversion and prevention of atrial fibrillation/flutter, and in the case of amiodarone in the treatment of ventricular tachycardia/fibrillation.
- Class IV antiarrhythmics block Ca^{2+} channels, slowing nodal conduction and reducing intracellular $[Ca^{2+}]$, without eliminating sympathetic regulation. Ca^{2+} channel blockers are used for treatment of idiopathic rhythms, ectopic atrial tachycardias, and atrioventricular nodal reentrant supraventricular tachycardias.
- Atrial fibrillation is most commonly treated with Na^+ channel blockers (Class 1a) or K^+ channel blockers (class III).
- A number of drugs from a variety of drug classes often used in anesthesia, as well as certain channel mutations, can predispose to torsades de pointes by blocking specific K^+ channels and prolonging the QT interval. This is usually treated with intravenous magnesium.

Key References

Abbott GW, Sesti F, Splawski I, et al. MiRP1 forms I_{Kr} potassium channels with HERG and is associated with cardiac arrhythmia. *Cell.* 1999;97:175-187. Reported the discovery of a secondary molecular component to I_{Kr}, and also the first description of an ion channel polymorphism increasing susceptibility to drug-induced arrhythmia. (Ref. 25)

Anderson CL, Delisle BP, Anson BD, et al. Most LQT2 mutations reduce Kv11.1 (hERG) current by a class 2 (trafficking-deficient) mechanism. *Circulation.* 2006;113:365-373. A groundbreaking paper indicating a major shift in our understanding of the mechanism of hERG-linked arrhythmias. (Ref. 91)

Baker JG, Hill SJ, Summers RJ. Evolution of beta blockers: from antianginal drugs to ligand-directed signalling. *Trends Pharmacol Sci.* 2011;32:227-234. An up-to-the-minute summary of the class II antiarrhythmics. (Ref. 7)

Catterall WA. Molecular mechanisms of gating and drug block of sodium channels. *Novartis Foundation Symposium.* 2002;241:206-232. In-depth review and discussion from one of the leaders in the mechanisms of sodium channel function and pharmacology. (Ref. 10)

Keating MT, Sanguinetti MC. Molecular and cellular mechanisms of cardiac arrhythmias. *Cell.* 2001;104:569-580. A clear, concise review of cardiac arrhythmia mechanisms. (Ref. 27)

Roden DM. Antiarrhythmic drugs: past, present and future. *J Cardiovasc Electrophysiol.* 2003;14:1389-1396. A summary of antiarrhythmic agents and their mechanisms of action. (Ref. 16)

Sanguinetti MC, Jiang C, Curran ME, et al. A mechanistic link between an inherited and an acquired cardiac arrhythmia: hERG encodes the I_{Kr} potassium channel. *Cell.* 1995;81:299-307. The article that defined the primary molecular basis for I_{Kr} and drug-induced arrhythmias. (Ref. 24)

Sanguinetti MC, Chen J, Fernandez D, et al. Physicochemical basis for binding and voltage-dependent block of hERG channels by structurally diverse drugs. *Novartis Foundation Symposium.* 2005;266:159-170. (Ref. 28)

Singh BN. Antiarrhythmic actions of amiodarone: a profile of a paradoxical agent. *Am J Cardiol.* 1996;78:41-53. A useful description of the complex mechanisms of amiodarone mode of action. (Ref. 54)

Westfall TC, Westfall DP. Adrenergic agonists and antagonists. In: Brunton LL, Chabner BA, Knollmann BC, eds. *Goodman & Gilman's The Pharmacological Basis of Therapeutics.* New York: McGraw Hill; 2011. Current knowledge of β blockers and their mechanisms of action. (Ref. 53)

References

1. Roden DM, George Jr AL. The cardiac ion channels: relevance to management of arrhythmias. *Annu Rev Med.* 1996;47:135-148.
2. Chaudhry GM, Haffajee CI. Antiarrhythmic agents and proarrhythmia. *Criti Care Med.* 2000;28:N158-164.
3. Boylan M. Galen: on blood, the pulse, and the arteries. *J History Biol.* 2007;40:207-230.
4. McMullen ET. Anatomy of a physiological discovery: William Harvey and the circulation of the blood. *J R Soc Med.* 1995;88:491-498.
5. Besterman E, Creese R. Waller—pioneer of electrocardiography. *Br Heart J.* 1979;42:61-64.
6. Snellen HA. Willem Einthoven Memorial Symposium on Developments in Electrocardiography 1927-1977, Leiden, The Netherlands, 28 October 1977. Introduction. *Eur J Cardiol.* 1978;8:201-203.
7. Baker JG, Hill SJ, Summers RJ. Evolution of beta blockers: from antianginal drugs to ligand-directed signalling. *Trend Pharmacol Sci.* 2011;32:227-234.
8. Singh BN. Comparative mechanisms of antiarrhythmic agents. *Am J Cardiol.* 1971;28:240-242.
9. Cobbe SM. Clinical usefulness of the Vaughan Williams classification system. *Eur Heart J.* 1987;8(Suppl A):65-69.
10. Catterall WA. Cellular and molecular biology of voltage-gated sodium channels. *Physiol Rev.* 1992;72:S15-S48.
11. Catterall WA. Molecular mechanisms of gating and drug block of sodium channels. *Novartis Foundation Symposium.* Chichester: Wiley; 2002;241:206-218; discussion 218-232.
12. Ragsdale DS, McPhee JC, Scheuer T, et al. Common molecular determinants of local anesthetic, antiarrhythmic, and anticonvulsant block of voltage-gated Na+ channels. *Proc Natl Acad Sci U S A.* 1996;93:9270-9275.
13. Lee CH, Ruben PC. Interaction between voltage-gated sodium channels and the neurotoxin, tetrodotoxin. *Channels (Austin).* 2008;2:407-412.
14. Desai SP, Marsh JD, Allen PD. Contractility effects of local anesthetics in the presence of sodium channel blockade. *Reg Anesth.* 1989;14:58-62.
15. Payandeh J, Scheuer T, Zheng N, et al. The crystal structure of a voltage-gated sodium channel. *Nature.* 2011;475:353-358.
16. Roden DM. Antiarrhythmic drugs: past, present and future. *J Cardiovasc Electrophysiol.* 2003;14:1389-1396.
17. Zicha S, Tsuji Y, Shiroshita-Takeshita A, et al. Beta blockers as antiarrhythmic agents. *Hndbk Exp Pharmacol.* 2006;235-266.
18. Bristow MR. Beta-adrenergic receptor blockade in chronic heart failure. *Circulation.* 2000;101:558-569.
19. Deal KK, England SK, Tamkun MM. Molecular physiology of cardiac potassium channels. *Physiol Rev.* 1996;76:49-67.
20. Wulff H, Castle NA, Pardo LA. Voltage-gated potassium channels as therapeutic targets. *Nat Rev Drug Disc.* 2009;8:982-1001.
21. Doyle DA, Morais Cabral J, Pfuetzner RA, et al. The structure of the potassium channel: molecular basis of K+ conduction and selectivity. *Science.* 1998;280:69-77.

22. Long SB, Campbell EB, Mackinnon R. Crystal structure of a mammalian voltage-dependent Shaker family K+ channel. *Science.* 2005; 309:897-903.

23. Sanguinetti MC, Curran ME, Zou A, et al. Coassembly of K(V) LQT1 and minK (IsK) proteins to form cardiac I(Ks) potassium channel. *Nature.* 1996;384:80-83.

24. Sanguinetti MC, Jiang C, Curran ME, et al. A mechanistic link between an inherited and an acquired cardiac arrhythmia: hERG encodes the IKr potassium channel. *Cell.* 1995;81:299-307.

25. Abbott GW, Sesti F, Splawski I, et al. MiRP1 forms IKr potassium channels with HERG and is associated with cardiac arrhythmia. *Cell.* 1999;97:175-187.

26. McCrossan ZA, Abbott GW. The MinK-related peptides. *Neuropharmacology.* 2004;47:787-821.

27. Keating MT, Sanguinetti MC. Molecular and cellular mechanisms of cardiac arrhythmias. *Cell.* 2001;104:569-580.

28. Sanguinetti MC, Chen J, Fernandez D, et al. Physicochemical basis for binding and voltage-dependent block of hERG channels by structurally diverse drugs. *Novartis Foundation Symposium.* 2005;266: 159-166; discussion 166-170.

29. Swartz KJ, MacKinnon R. Mapping the receptor site for hanatoxin, a gating modifier of voltage-dependent K+ channels. *Neuron.* 1997; 18:675-682.

30. Abbott GW, Xu X, Roepke TK. Impact of ancillary subunits on ventricular repolarization. *J Electrocardiol.* 2007;40:S42-S46.

31. Roepke TK, Kontogeorgis A, Ovanez C, et al. Targeted deletion of kcne2 impairs ventricular repolarization via disruption of I(K,slow1) and I(to,f). *FASEB J.* 2008;22:3648-3660.

32. Zhang M, Jiang M, Tseng GN. MinK-related peptide 1 associates with Kv4.2 and modulates its gating function: potential role as beta subunit of cardiac transient outward channel? *Circ Res.* 2001; 88:1012-1019.

33. Panaghie G, Abbott GW. The impact of ancillary subunits on small-molecule interactions with voltage-gated potassium channels. *Curr Pharmaceut Design.* 2006;12:2285-2302.

34. Bosch RF, Li GR, Gaspo R, et al. Electrophysiologic effects of chronic amiodarone therapy and hypothyroidism, alone and in combination, on guinea pig ventricular myocytes. *J Pharmacol Exp Ther.* 1999;289:156-165.

35. Kiehn J, Wible B, Lacerda AE, et al. Mapping the block of a cloned human inward rectifier potassium channel by dofetilide. *Mol Pharmacol.* 1996;50:380-387.

36. Proenza C, O'Brien J, Nakai J, et al. Identification of a region of RyR1 that participates in allosteric coupling with the alpha(1S) (Ca(V)1.1) II-III loop. *J Biological Chemistry.* 2002;277:6530-6535.

37. Catterall WA, Perez-Reyes E, Snutch TP, Striessnig J. International Union of Pharmacology. XLVIII. Nomenclature and structure-function relationships of voltage-gated calcium channels. *Pharmacol Rev.* 2005;57:411-425.

38. Rowland E. Antiarrhythmic drugs—class IV. *Eur Heart J.* 1987; 8(Suppl A):61-63.

39. Hockerman GH, Dilmac N, Scheuer T, Catterall WA. Molecular determinants of diltiazem block in domains IIIS6 and IVS6 of L-type Ca(2+) channels. *Mol Pharmacol.* 2000;58:1264-1270.

40. Hockerman GH, Johnson BD, Scheuer T, Catterall WA. Molecular determinants of high affinity phenylalkylamine block of L-type calcium channels. *J Biol Chem.* 1995;270:22119-22122.

41. Kraus R, Reichl B, Kimball SD, et al. Identification of benz(othi)azepine-binding regions within L-type calcium channel alpha1 subunits. *J Biol Chem.* 1996;271:20113-20118.

42. Cabo C, Wit AL. Cellular electrophysiologic mechanisms of cardiac arrhythmias. *Cardiol Clin.* 1997;15:517-538.

43. Wit AL. Electrophysiological basis for antiarrhythmic drug action. *Clin Physiol Biochem.* 1985;3:127-134.

44. Lazzara R, Scherlag BJ. Electrophysiologic basis for arrhythmias in ischemic heart disease. *Am Journal Cardiol.* 1984;53:1B-7B.

45. Zipes DP, Foster PR, Troup PJ, Pedersen DH. Atrial induction of ventricular tachycardia: reentry versus triggered automaticity. *Am J Cardiol* .1979;44:1-8.

46. Ashley EA, Niebauer J. *Cardiology Explained.* London: Remedica; 2004.

47. Singh BN. Acute management of ventricular arrhythmias: role of antiarrhythmic agents. *Pharmacotherapy.* 1997;17:56S-64S; discussion 89S-91S.

48. Trujillo TC, Nolan PE. Antiarrhythmic agents: drug interactions of clinical significance. *Drug Safety.* 2000;23:509-532.

49. Anderson JL. Clinical implications of new studies in the treatment of benign, potentially malignant and malignant ventricular arrhythmias. *Am J Cardiol.* 1990;65:36B-42B.

50. Campbell TJ. Subclassification of class I antiarrhythmic drugs: enhanced relevance after CAST. *Cardiovasc Drugs Ther.* 1992;6: 519-528.

51. Watanabe H, et al. Flecainide prevents catecholaminergic polymorphic ventricular tachycardia in mice and humans. *Nat Med.* 2009; 15:380-383.

52. Boriani G, Diemberger I, Biffi M, Martignani C, Branzi A. Pharmacological cardioversion of atrial fibrillation: current management and treatment options. *Drugs.* 2004;64:2741-2762.

53. Westfall TC, Westfall DP. Adrenergic agonists and antagonists. In: Brunton LL, Chabner BA, Knollmann BC, eds. *Goodman & Gilman's The Pharmacological Basis of Therapeutics.* New York: McGraw Hill; 2011.

54. Singh BN. Antiarrhythmic actions of amiodarone: a profile of a paradoxical agent. *Am Journal Cardiol.* 1996;78:41-53.

55. Karam R, Marcello S, Brooks RR, Corey AE, Moore A. Azimilide dihydrochloride, a novel antiarrhythmic agent. *Am J Cardiol.* 1998; 81:40D-46D.

56. Nair LA, Grant AO. Emerging class III antiarrhythmic agents: mechanism of action and proarrhythmic potential. *Cardiovasc Drugs Ther.* 1997;11:149-167.

57. Nattel S. The molecular and ionic specificity of antiarrhythmic drug actions. *J Cardiovasc Electrophysiol.* 1999;10:272-282.

58. Jost N, et al. Effect of the antifibrillatory compound tedisamil (KC-8857) on transmembrane currents in mammalian ventricular myocytes. Curr Med *Chemistry.* 2004;11:3219-3228.

59. Barrett TD, et al. Tedisamil and dofetilide-induced torsades de pointes, rate and potassium dependence. *Br J Pharmacol.* 2001; 32:1493-1500.

60. Chen YH, et al. KCNQ1 gain-of-function mutation in familial atrial fibrillation. *Science.* 2003;299:251-254.

61. Ellinor PT, et al. Mutations in the long QT gene, KCNQ1, are an uncommon cause of atrial fibrillation. *Heart.* 2004;90: 1487-1488.

62. Zhang DF, et al. [KCNE3 R53H substitution in familial atrial fibrillation]. *Chin Med J.* 2005;118:1735-1738.

63. Yang T, Yang P, Roden DM, Darbar D. Novel KCNA5 mutation implicates tyrosine kinase signaling in human atrial fibrillation. *Heart Rhythm.* 2010;7:1246-1252.

64. Abraham RL, Yang T, Blair M, Roden DM, Darbar D. Augmented potassium current is a shared phenotype for two genetic defects associated with familial atrial fibrillation. *J Mol Cell Cardiol.* 2010; 48:181-190.

65. Anantharam A, Markowitz SM, Abbott GW. Pharmacogenetic considerations in diseases of cardiac ion channels. *J Pharmacol Exp Ther.* 2003;307:831-838.

66. Du YM, et al. Molecular determinants of Kv1.5 channel block by diphenyl phosphine oxide-1. *J Mol Cell Cardiol.* 2010;48:1111-1120.

67. Fedida D, et al. The mechanism of atrial antiarrhythmic action of RSD1235. *J Cardiovasc Electrophys.* 2005;16:1227-1238.

68. Fedida D, Orth PM, Hesketh JC, Ezrin AM. The role of late I and antiarrhythmic drugs in EAD formation and termination in Purkinje fibers. *J Cardiovasc Electrophysiol.* 2006;17(Suppl 1): S71-S78.

69. Voigt N, et al. Inhibition of IK,ACh current may contribute to clinical efficacy of class I and class III antiarrhythmic drugs in patients with atrial fibrillation. *NaunynSchmiedebergs Arch Pharmacol.* 2010;381:251-259.

70. Nademanee K, Singh BN. Control of cardiac arrhythmias by calcium antagonism. *Ann N Y Acad Sci.* 1988;522:536-552.

71. Singh BN, Nademanee K, Feld G. Antiarrhythmic effects of verapamil. *Angiology.* 1983;34:572-590.

72. Weiner B. Hemodynamic effects of antidysrhythmic drugs. *J Cardiovasc Nurs.* 1991;5:39-48.

73. Singh BN, Nademanee K. Use of calcium antagonists for cardiac arrhythmias. *Am J Cardiol.* 1987;59:153B-162B.

74. Fodor JG, et al. The role of diltiazem in treating hypertension and coronary artery disease: new approaches to preventing first events. *Can J Cardiol.* 1997;13:495-503.

443

75. Abbott GW. Molecular mechanisms of cardiac voltage-gated potassium channelopathies. *Curr Pharmaceut Des*. 2006;12:3631-3644.

76. Wang Q, et al. SCN5A mutations associated with an inherited cardiac arrhythmia, long QT syndrome. *Cell*. 1995;80:805-811.

77. Wang Q, Bowles NE, Towbin JA. The molecular basis of long QT syndrome and prospects for therapy. *Mol Med Today*. 1998;4:382-388.

78. Brugada R, et al. Sudden death associated with short-QT syndrome linked to mutations in hERG. *Circulation*. 2004;109:30-35.

79. Borggrefe M, et al. Short QT syndrome. Genotype-phenotype correlations. *J Electrocardiol*. 2005;38:75-80.

80. Grunnet M. Repolarization of the cardiac action potential. Does an increase in repolarization capacity constitute a new antiarrhythmic principle? *Acta Physiol (Oxf)*. 2010;198(Suppl 676):1-48.

81. Benito B, Brugada J, Brugada R, Brugada P. Brugada syndrome. *Rev Esp Cardiol*. 2009;62:1297-1315.

82. Shimizu W, Horie M. Phenotypic manifestations of mutations in genes encoding subunits of cardiac potassium channels. *Circ Res*. 2011;109:97-109.

83. Roepke TK, Abbott GW. Pharmacogenetics and cardiac ion channels. *Vasc Pharmacol*. 2006;44:90-106.

84. Ehtisham J, Watkins H. Is Wolff-Parkinson-White syndrome a genetic disease? *J Cardiovasc Electrophysiol*. 2005;16:1258-1262.

85. Gollob MH, Green MS, Tang AS, Roberts R. PRKAG2 cardiac syndrome: familial ventricular preexcitation, conduction system disease, and cardiac hypertrophy. *Curr Opin Cardiol*. 2002;17:229-234.

86. Akhtar M, Tchou PJ, Jazayeri M. Mechanisms of clinical tachycardias. *Am J Cardiol*. 1988;61:9A-19A.

87. Tischenko A, et al. When should we recommend catheter ablation for patients with the Wolff-Parkinson-White syndrome? *Curr Opinion Cardiol*. 2008;23:32-37.

88. Hanton G, Tilbury L. Cardiac safety strategies. 25-26 October 2005, the Radisson SAS Hotel, Nice, France. *Exp Opin Drug Safety*. 2006;5:329-333.

89. Delisle BP, et al. Thapsigargin selectively rescues the trafficking defective LQT2 channels G601S and F805C. *J Biol Chem*. 2003;278:35749-35754.

90. Delisle BP, et al. Intragenic suppression of trafficking-defective KCNH2 channels associated with long QT syndrome. *Mol Pharmacol*. 2005;68:233-240.

91. Anderson CL, Delisle BP, Anson BD, et al. Most LQT2 mutations reduce Kv11.1 (hERG) current by a class 2 (trafficking-deficient) mechanism. *Circulation*. 2006;113:365-373.

92. Gong Q, Anderson CL, January CT, Zhou Z. Pharmacological rescue of trafficking defective hERG channels formed by coassembly of wild-type and long QT mutant N470D subunits. *Am J Physiol*. 2004;287:H652-H658.

93. Panaghie G, Abbott GW. The role of S4 charges in voltage-dependent and voltage-independent KCNQ1 potassium channel complexes. *J Gen Physiol*. 2007;129:121-133.

94. Schroeder BC, et al. A constitutively open potassium channel formed by KCNQ1 and KCNE3. *Nature*. 2000;403:196-199.

95. Mazhari R, Nuss HB, Armoundas AA, Winslow RL, Marban E. Ectopic expression of KCNE3 accelerates cardiac repolarization and abbreviates the QT interval. *The Journal of Clinical Investigation*. 2002;109:1083-1090.

96. Satin J, et al. Mechanism of spontaneous excitability in human embryonic stem cell derived cardiomyocytes. *J Physiol*. 2004;559:479-496.

97. Siu CW, Lieu DK, Li RA. HCN-encoded pacemaker channels: from physiology and biophysics to bioengineering. *J Membrane Biol*. 2006;214:115-122.

98. Burton DY, et al. The incorporation of an ion channel gene mutation associated with the long QT syndrome (Q9E-hMiRP1) in a plasmid vector for site-specific arrhythmia gene therapy: in vitro and in vivo feasibility studies. *Hum Gene Ther*. 2003;14:907-922.

99. Perlstein I, et al. Posttranslational control of a cardiac ion channel transgene in vivo: clarithromycin-hMiRP1-Q9E interactions. *Hum Gene Ther*. 2005;16:906-910.

100. Tester DJ, Will ML, Haglund CM, Ackerman MJ. Compendium of cardiac channel mutations in 541 consecutive unrelated patients referred for long QT syndrome genetic testing. *Heart Rhythm*. 2005;2:507-517.

101. Vandenberg JI, Walker BD, Campbell TJ. hERG K+ channels: friend and foe. *Trends Pharmacol Sci*. 2001;22:240-246.

Chapter 25

PULMONARY PHYSIOLOGY

Andrew B. Lumb and Deborah Horner

This chapter provides an outline of the physiology of the respiratory system by describing the control systems and mechanisms of air movement into and out of the lungs to allow oxygen and carbon dioxide to exchange with blood. Emphasis is placed on those systems where the molecular physiology is understood as these systems constitute targets for the actions of drugs on the respiratory system, both beneficial and harmful.

PULMONARY VENTILATION

Ventilation is the process by which air is drawn into and out of the lungs and delivered to the alveoli for gas exchange. It can be divided into an active inspiratory phase and most often a passive expiratory phase. Contraction of the inspiratory muscles increases the volume of the chest cavity, so reducing intrathoracic pressure and causing air to move down its pressure gradient from the mouth. To achieve this, the respiratory muscles must overcome the inherent elasticity of the respiratory system as well as resistance to gas flow in the airways. This resistance comprises elastic resistance of lung tissue and chest wall, resistance from surface forces at the alveolar gas/liquid interface, frictional resistance to gas flow through the airways, resistance to deformation of thoracic tissues, and finally inertia associated with movement of gas and tissue.

Expiration is usually a passive process during which the respiratory muscles relax, allowing the elastic tissues of the chest wall to return to their resting position. The point at which the tendency for the lung to contract equals the tendency of the chest wall to expand is the resting position of the respiratory system, the functional residual capacity (FRC).

Muscles of Ventilation

During inspiration, a subatmospheric pressure occurs throughout the airway. Collapse of large airways is prevented by their cartilaginous structure and of small airways by the elasticity of surrounding lung tissue, but in the pharynx collapse can easily occur. In conscious individuals, upper airway collapse is prevented by a combination of both tonic muscle activity and phasic inspiratory contraction of the pharyngeal dilator muscles. This muscle activity is controlled via reflex stimulation of mechanoreceptors in the larynx and pharynx that respond to subatmospheric pressure by rapidly (<50 ms) activating the pharyngeal dilators. Similar responses in the laryngeal muscles result in abduction of the vocal cords during inspiration and adduction in expiration. Adduction of the cords in early expiration is believed to act to slow expiratory flow rate and thus help prevent alveolar collapse.[1]

The diaphragm is the principal muscle for inspiration and is responsible for around three quarters of the tidal volume during resting inspiration in the supine posture. Intercostal muscles also contribute to inspiration, particularly when in an upright position and when there is increased ventilation, for example with exercise or with dyspnea from lung pathology. The external intercostal and parasternal portion of the internal intercostal muscles are normally active during inspiration, but changes in posture and other activities involving movement of the trunk affect which muscles are active in each phase of respiration. Other muscles such as the scalenes and sternocleidomastoids can also contribute to inspiration.

When the patient is supine, the weight of the abdominal contents assists in passive expiration by pushing the diaphragm cephalad. When the patient is upright or while hyperventilating however, the internal intercostals and abdominal wall muscles contract to assist expiration. Many of the respiratory muscles have additional functions including maintenance of posture, coughing, sneezing, and speech. Each of these functions must be integrated with the muscles' primary role in breathing.

The sensitivity of different muscles to neuromuscular blocking (NMB) agents is variable (Chapter 19). The diaphragm is considered to be the most resistant to neuromuscular blockade, which means that when compared to other muscles, for example the adductor pollicis, it requires a larger dose of relaxant to achieve full paralysis and is often the first muscle to recover function.[2,3] This resistance to NMB drugs can be explained by increased acetylcholine receptor density and acetylcholine release as well as lower acetylcholine esterase activity leading to greater synaptic acetylcholine concentrations in the diaphragm. Onset of diaphragmatic block is relatively fast, however, due to its high blood flow.

CONTROL OF AIRWAY DIAMETER

Gas flow within the airways is predominantly turbulent in the pharynx, larynx, and large airways, becoming more laminar in smaller airways as gas velocity decreases. For laminar flow, the flow rate is related to the fourth power of the radius (r^4) of a straight tube as described by the Poiseuille equation.[4] Lung volume has a large effect on airway diameter, so the relationship between lung volume and airway resistance is hyperbolic. Airway resistance is low at FRC, and increasing lung volume further has little effect. In contrast, a small reduction in lung volume results in a large increase in resistance. The main sites of resistance within the airway are the nose and major bronchi. Speed of airflow rapidly decreases as air passes from large to small airways, the aggregate cross sectional area increasing to very large values after the eighth generation of airway (small bronchi, 1-2 mm diameter).

Airway disease causes bronchospasm, increased airway lining fluid, and mucosal edema, all of which reduce the diameter of the airways. This reduction in diameter in turn causes increased airway resistance and decreased gas flow. A large proportion of current pharmacotherapy for airway disease targets airway smooth muscle in an attempt to increase airway diameter and gas flow.

Cellular Physiology

Most bronchial smooth muscle is found in the 12th to 16th generations of airway, which are bronchioles typically with a diameter of less than 1 mm. They have no cartilaginous support and their walls contain a high proportion of smooth muscle relative to luminal diameter.

Four mechanisms are involved in controlling muscle tone in small airways: neural pathways, humoral (via blood) control, direct physical and chemical effects, and local cellular mechanisms. Neural control is the most important in normal lung, with direct stimulation and humoral control contributing under some circumstances. Cellular mechanisms, particularly mast cells, have little influence under normal conditions but are important in airway disease.

NEURAL CONTROL

The parasympathetic nervous system is the most important determinant of bronchomotor tone and when activated can completely obliterate the lumen of small airways.[5] Both afferent and efferent nerve fibers travel via the vagus nerve (X) with efferent ganglia in the bronchial walls. Afferent nerves arise from receptors under the tight junctions of the bronchial epithelium and respond either to noxious stimuli acting directly on the receptors or to cytokines released by cellular mechanisms such as mast cell degranulation. Efferent nerves release acetylcholine, which acts at M_3 muscarinic receptors to cause contraction of airway smooth muscle, while also stimulating M_2 prejunctional muscarinic receptors to exert negative feedback on acetylcholine release. Stimulation of any part of the reflex arc results in bronchoconstriction. Some degree of resting tone is normally present and therefore permits a small degree of bronchodilation when vagal tone is reduced in a similar fashion to vagal control of heart rate.[6]

In contrast to the parasympathetic system, the sympathetic system is poorly represented in the lung and not yet proven to be of major importance in humans. Indeed it appears unlikely that there is any direct sympathetic innervation of airway smooth muscle.

The airways are provided with a third autonomic control system, the nerves of which are neither adrenergic nor cholinergic, and are referred to as noncholinergic parasympathetic nerves (Figure 25-1).[6,7] This is the only potential bronchodilator nervous pathway in humans, though the exact role of these nerves remains uncertain. The efferent fibers run in the vagus nerve and pass to the smooth muscle of the airways where they cause slow (minutes) and prolonged relaxation of bronchi. The major neurotransmitter is vasoactive intestinal peptide (VIP), which produces airway smooth muscle relaxation by promoting production of nitric oxide (NO). How NO relaxes airway smooth muscle is not as fully understood as its effect on vascular smooth muscle. It is likely that NO activates guanylyl cyclase to produce cyclic guanosine monophosphate (cGMP) and muscle relaxation. Resting airway tone does involve NO mediated bronchodilation, but whether this is from local cellular production of NO or noncholinergic parasympathetic nerves and VIP-mediated release of NO is unknown.[5]

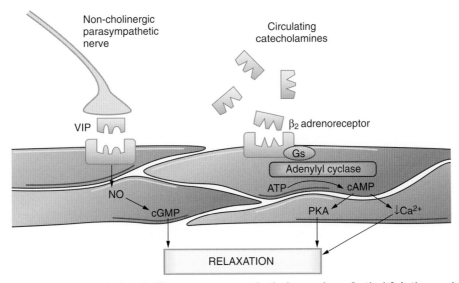

Figure 25-1 Schematic diagram of the two major bronchodilator systems present in the human airway. On the left is the neural bronchodilator pathway, involving fibers of the vagus nerve that release vasoactive intestinal peptide (VIP), which in turn increases nitric oxide (NO) production to stimulate the formation of cyclic guanosine monophosphate (cGMP) and bring about relaxation of airway smooth muscle cells. On the right is the G protein (Gs)-coupled β_2 adrenoreceptor, which responds to circulating epinephrine to cause relaxation of the airway via production of cyclic adenosine monophosphate (cAMP) and activation of protein kinase A (PKA).

HUMORAL CONTROL[8]

Despite the minimal significance of sympathetic innervation, airway smooth muscle has plentiful β_2-adrenergic receptors that are highly sensitive to circulating epinephrine and act via complex second messenger systems (see Figure 25-1 and described later).[9] Basal levels of epinephrine probably do not contribute to airway muscle tone, but this mechanism is brought into play during exercise or during the sympathetic "stress response." There are a few α-adrenergic receptors that cause bronchoconstriction, but these are not thought to be of physiologic significance.

Physical and Chemical Effects

Direct stimulation of the respiratory epithelium activates the parasympathetic reflex described above causing bronchoconstriction. This is a protective reflex that evolved to prevent inhaled particles gaining access to the lower respiratory tract by effectively reducing airway size and air flow to distal lung units. This type of protection is necessary because the thin alveolar capillary membrane (to facilitate gas transfer) is a vulnerable interface between the internal milieu and the outside world. Physical factors known to produce bronchoconstriction include mechanical stimulation of the upper airway, for example by laryngoscopy, and the presence of a foreign body in the airway. Inhalation of particulate matter, an aerosol of water or just cold air can also cause bronchoconstriction, particularly in patients with asthma. Many chemical stimuli also result in bronchoconstriction including liquids with low pH such as gastric acid and gases such as sulfur dioxide, ammonia, ozone, and nitrogen dioxide.

Local Cellular Mechanisms

Inflammatory cells found in the lung include mast cells, eosinophils, neutrophils, macrophages, and lymphocytes. These inflammatory cells are stimulated by a variety of pathogens, but some can also be activated by the direct physical factors described above. Once activated, cytokine production causes

amplification of the response, and a variety of mediators are released that can cause bronchoconstriction (Table 25-1). These mediators are produced in normal individuals, but patients with airway disease are usually "hyperresponsive" and so develop bronchospasm more easily.

Molecular Physiology

There are two opposing systems that control bronchial smooth muscle tone: signaling pathways resulting in increased intracellular cyclic adenosine monophosphate (cAMP), reduced intracellular Ca^{2+}, and bronchodilation, and pathways resulting in increased inositol triphosphate (IP_3), increased Ca^{2+}, and bronchoconstriction.

BRONCHODILATOR PATHWAY

These pathways are summarized in Figure 25-1. The molecular basis for the function of the β_2-adrenoreceptor is now clearly elucidated.[10] This G protein–coupled receptor contains 413 amino acids and has seven transmembrane helices. The agonist binding site is deep within the hydrophobic core of the protein, which sits within the lipid bilayer of the cell membrane. This affects the interaction of drugs at the binding site. Lipophilic drugs form a depot in the lipid bilayer from which they can repeatedly interact with the binding site of the receptor, producing a longer duration of action than hydrophilic drugs. Receptors exist in either activated or inactivated form, the former state occurring when the third intracellular loop is bound to the α-subunit of the Gs-protein. Agonists of the β_2 receptor probably do not induce a significant conformational change in the protein structure but rather stabilize the activated conformation, allowing this to predominate.

β_2-adrenoreceptor stimulation results in activation of Gs, a GTP-binding regulatory protein, which in turn activates adenylyl cyclase. This enzyme catalyzes the conversion of adenosine triphosphate (ATP) to cAMP.[10] cAMP inhibits the

Table 25-1. Mediators Involved in Control of Bronchial Smooth Muscle Activity in Inflamed Airways

SOURCE	Bronchoconstriction MEDIATOR	RECEPTOR	Bronchodilatation MEDIATOR	RECEPTOR
Mast cells, other proinflammatory cells	Histamine	H_1	Prostaglandin E_2	EP
	Prostaglandin D_2	TP	Prostacyclin (PGI_2)	EP
	Prostaglandin $F_{2\alpha}$	TP		
	Leukotrienes C_4, D_4, E_4	$CysLT_1$		
	PAF	PAF		
	Bradykinin	B_2		
C-fibers	Substance P	NK_2		
	Neurokinin A	NK_2		
	CGRP	CGRP		
Endothelial, epithelial cells	Endothelin	ET_B		

From Barnes PJ. Pharmacology of airway smooth muscle. *Am J Respir Crit Care Med*. 1998;158:S123-S132; and Thirstrup S. Control of airway smooth muscle tone.
I—Electrophysiology and contractile mediators. *Respir Med*. 2000;94:328-336.

B, Bradykinin; *CGRP*, calcitonin gene-related peptide; *EP*, prostaglandin E-specific prostanoid receptor; *ET*, endothelin; *H*, histamine; *LT*, leukotriene; *PAF*, platelet activating factor; *PG*, prostaglandin; *NK*, neurokinin; *TP*, thromboxane-specific prostanoid receptor.

release of Ca^{2+} from intracellular stores as well as activating protein kinase A, which in turn phosphorylates proteins regulating the interaction of actin and myosin. As a result of these actions, smooth muscle cells relax, leading to bronchodilatation (see Figure 25-1).

Intracellular cAMP is rapidly hydrolyzed by phosphodiesterase (PDE). Seven subtypes of PDE have been identified with subtypes 3 and 4 predominating in the airways. Several phosphodiesterase inhibitors are available (e.g., theophylline), which function by prolonging smooth muscle relaxation resulting from β_2 receptor stimulation. However, they are nonspecific inhibitors and as a result, their use in the treatment of bronchoconstriction is limited by side effects.[11]

Two β_2 receptor genes are present in humans, with a total of 18 polymorphisms described, giving rise to a large number of possible phenotypic variants.[12] Some clinical differences are observed between variants, but the contribution that different β_2 receptor phenotypes make to the overall prevalence of asthma appears to be minimal.[12,13]

BRONCHOCONSTRICTOR PATHWAY

Stimulation of M_3 acetylcholine receptors (Figure 25-2) results in the activation of a different G-protein (Gq) that in turn activates phospholipase C, stimulating the formation of IP_3. IP_3 binds to receptors on the sarcoplasmic reticulum promoting the release of Ca^{2+} from intracellular stores. Myosin light chain kinase is activated by Ca^{2+} and in turn phosphorylates myosin chains and activates myosin ATPase. As a result, crossbridges are formed between actin and myosin and contraction of smooth muscle occurs.[11] IP_3 is then converted to inactive inositol diphosphate (IP_2) by IP_3 phosphatase. Other mediators of bronchoconstriction, for example tachykinin and histamine, exert their effects via similar mechanisms resulting in an increase in IP_3 production (see Table 25-1).[14]

There are many interactions between the IP_3 and cAMP signalling pathways. Activation of Gq also results in synthesis of diacylglycerol from phosphatidylinositol bisphosphate by phospholipase C. Diacylglycerol in turn activates protein kinase C (PKC), which phosphorylates many downstream proteins including G proteins and the intracellular domain of the β_2 adrenoreceptor itself. This causes the β_2 adrenoreceptor

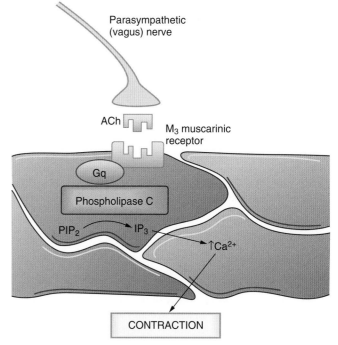

Parasympathetic (vagus) nerve

ACh

M_3 muscarinic receptor

Gq

Phospholipase C

PIP_2 IP_3

↑Ca^{2+}

CONTRACTION

Figure 25-2 Schematic diagram of the parasympathetic bronchoconstrictor system in human airways. Reflex activation of parasympathetic nerves by a variety of stimuli (see text for details) results in acetylcholine (ACh) release. Acting via M_3 muscarinic cholinergic receptors, a Gq protein activates phospholipase C, which converts phosphatidylinositol biphosphate (PIP_2) into inositol trisphosphate (IP_3), which promotes release of Ca^{2+} from intracellular stores in the stimulated cells. The increase in Ca^{2+} then activates the contractile machinery.

to become uncoupled from its G protein, resulting in downregulation of the transduction pathway.[10,11] Frequent stimulation of the receptor results in desensitization to its agonist via a similar mechanism.[15]

BRONCHOCONSTRICTION IN AIRWAY DISEASE

Bronchoconstriction as part of airway disease occurs as a result of complex interactions between proinflammatory cells and mediators. Mast cells are ubiquitous in airway epithelium and can be activated physically, for example by coughing, as well as by allergens and infection. Both allergens and infection exert their effects via IgE, complement, and cytokines. The latter cause chemotaxis and activation of other inflammatory cells including neutrophils, macrophages, eosinophils, and lymphocytes, which in turn lead to augmentation of the inflammatory response.

Another key pathway in the generation of bronchoconstriction is modulated by the noncholinergic parasympathetic system described earlier. C fiber nerve endings release inflammatory mediators, including tachykinins, which are thought to play an important part in the genesis of bronchial hyper-responsiveness.[14]

The physiologic complexity of bronchoconstriction presents many potential therapeutic targets for the treatment of asthma (see Chapter 26). Currently, steroids are the mainstay of treatment. Their antiinflammatory action reduces mucosal edema and swelling as well as smooth muscle tone, vascular permeability, and pulmonary vascular resistance. Glucocorticoids exert their effects by downregulating synthesis of certain proteins leading to a reduction in inflammatory cytokines such as interleukin(IL)-β, IL-6, IL-11, prostaglandins, bronchoconstrictor receptors such as neurokinin receptors, and inflammatory enzymes such as cyclooxygenase 2. In addition, glucocorticoids increase antiinflammatory cytokines and the numbers of bronchodilator receptors such as β_2 adrenoreceptors.[16]

Cytoplasmic glucocorticoid receptors consist of a single protein with two centrally bound zinc atoms. Agonists bind to the receptor within the cytoplasm resulting in a conformational change that allows the receptor to enter the nucleus. The receptor then regulates DNA transcription by directly binding to specific regulatory DNA sequences and interacting with other transcription factors to modify gene expression. Steroid responsiveness varies between individuals and this might be due to the variable requirement for other transcription factors to interact with the glucocorticoid receptor.[17]

OXYGENATION

The PO_2 of dry air at sea level is 159 mmHg (21.2 kPa). Oxygen is diluted by water vapor and expired carbon dioxide as it passes through the respiratory tract and then moves down its partial pressure gradient across the alveolar capillary barrier into the blood, then from arterial capillary blood into tissues and cells. PO_2 finally reaches its lowest level in the mitochondria where it is consumed in oxidative phosphorylation. At this point, the PO_2 is probably within the range 3.8 to 22.5 mmHg (0.5-3 kPa), varying within different tissues and cell types. This stepwise reduction in PO_2 from air to mitochondria is known as the oxygen cascade, and any step in the cascade can be affected under pathologic circumstances to result in tissue hypoxia (see Chapter 2).

There are about 300 million alveoli in the human lung. These thin-walled air sacs form the basic unit of gas exchange and are approximately 0.3 mm in diameter. Alveoli begin to appear in the lung at the level of the respiratory bronchioles, the level at which gas movement ceases to be tidal and moves instead by diffusion. The walls of alveoli are very thin, approximately 0.5 µm, to allow easy diffusion of respiratory gases. In order for gas to enter pulmonary capillaries it must

first traverse the alveolar-capillary barrier. This consists of the alveolar fluid, alveolar epithelial cell, interstitial tissue, basement membranes, and finally the pulmonary capillary endothelium. To minimize the distance between capillary endothelium and red blood cells (RBCs), the diameter of the pulmonary capillaries is small so that the RBCs must flatten in order to pass, bringing the RBC membrane into close contact with the capillary wall. This might explain why drugs such as salicylates, which increase the deformability of RBCs, can increase diffusing capacity.[18] Diffusion occurs quickly across the blood-gas barrier so that RBCs become fully saturated with oxygen within 0.25 second of entering the pulmonary capillary. This is only a third of the time the cell spends in the capillary in a resting subject and means that a diffusion barrier is rarely a cause of poor oxygen uptake, the only examples in humans being extreme hypoxia at altitude or extreme exercise in elite athletes.

Surfactant, a phospholipid-based fluid produced by type II alveolar cells lining the alveoli, has several important functions. Alveoli within the lung differ in size and shape. Without surfactant, small alveoli are significantly more difficult to expand than those with larger resting volumes because smaller alveoli are intrinsically less compliant. Small alveoli are prevented from collapsing by surfactant. Surface tension tends to collapse a bubble and a similar situation occurs within the alveolus. As the size of alveoli decreases their tendency to collapse increases, and surfactant reduces this tendency. Surfactant also has a role in the prevention of pulmonary edema. The negative interstitial pressure created by surface tension tends to draw fluid into the alveolus from the surrounding pulmonary capillaries. By reducing surface tension, surfactant minimizes this effect. In neonates, a lack of surfactant leads to respiratory distress syndrome. The mainstay of management is replacement with exogenous surfactant.

Ventilation and Perfusion Relationships

Matching ventilation and perfusion is critical to optimize oxygen transfer. Gas exchange is optimal when ventilation and perfusion are evenly distributed throughout the lung. In a contrasting and extreme example, if 100% of perfusion is to one lung and 100% of ventilation is to the other lung, no gas exchange occurs even though total ventilation and perfusion might be normal.

DISTRIBUTION OF VENTILATION
Ventilation to different regions of lung is influenced by several factors. The right lung is bigger than the left and therefore receives a greater proportion of total ventilation in the upright and supine positions. The effect of gravity is also important. Lung tissue can be considered as semifluid or gel-like within the chest cavity. The weight of tissue above compresses tissues below making the density of tissues at the bases greater than at the apices. The dependent bases are therefore less expanded and so more compliant, which in turn means they are better ventilated. With the body in the lateral position, the lower, dependent lung is better ventilated than the upper, nondependent lung, and similarly, in the supine position, the posterior part of the lung is better ventilated than the anterior part. Gravity is not the only influence, and airway distribution also affects ventilation. Scanning techniques with the ability to measure ventilation in areas of lung only a few microliters

in volume show increased ventilation in central compared with peripheral lung regions.[19] This observation probably results from unequal branching patterns of the airways.

DISTRIBUTION OF PERFUSION

The flow of blood through the pulmonary circulation equals the flow through the systemic circulation, from about 6 L/min[-1] under resting conditions, to as much as 25 L/min[-1] during exercise. It is remarkable that such a range of flow can normally be achieved with minimal increase in pulmonary vascular pressures, due to the considerably lower pulmonary vascular resistance (PVR) compared with that in the systemic circulation. PVR determines total blood flow to the lungs but the regional distribution of blood flow is not uniform. Flow progressively increases down the lung in an upright subject with flow per unit of lung volume increasing by 11% per centimeter of descent.[20] The relative contribution of gravity to regional pulmonary blood flow remains controversial, in that gravity is not the only determinant.[19,21,22]

Total PVR is influenced by a variety of both passive and active factors. Passive factors include:

1. *Transmural pressure.* If extravascular pressure is greater than intravascular hydrostatic pressure, the vessel will collapse, obstructing blood flow. This situation occurs in some lung regions during positive pressure ventilation and can increase regional PVR and reduce perfusion.
2. *Lung volume.* PVR is at its lowest at FRC. As lung volume increases, some pulmonary capillaries become narrowed and stretched, while a reduction in lung volume makes some capillaries more tortuous or kinked, both of which increase PVR.
3. *Vascular architecture.* The branching pattern of the pulmonary vasculature might be responsible for gravity-independent variation in blood flow, known as the *fractal hypothesis.* Two aspects of vascular structure contribute to variations in flow. Because of the exponential relationship between flow and radius, bifurcations of pulmonary arteries into two slightly different size vessels has a large effect on the flow rates in each.[19] In addition, pulmonary arteries are more numerous than pulmonary airways as a result of

small extra branches, often given off at right angles, throughout the pulmonary arterial tree. Mathematical modeling indicates that these "supernumerary" branches contribute significantly to the heterogeneity of regional perfusion.[23]

VENTILATION IN RELATION TO PERFUSION

Ventilation can be related to perfusion using the ventilation/perfusion ratio ($\dot{V}/\dot{Q}$). If alveolar ventilation is 4 L/min[-1] and pulmonary blood flow 5 L/min[-1], then the $\dot{V}/\dot{Q}$ ratio equals 0.8. If ventilation and perfusion of all alveoli were the same, then $\dot{V}/\dot{Q}$ would be 0.8 throughout the lung. But ventilation and perfusion are not uniform for all the reasons described, and alveoli range from unventilated to unperfused with all possible combinations in between. Alveoli with no ventilation ($\dot{V}/\dot{Q}$ ratio of 0) have Po_2 and Pco_2 values that are the same as those of mixed venous blood because the trapped air in the unventilated alveoli equilibrates with mixed venous blood. Alveoli with no perfusion ($\dot{V}/\dot{Q}$ ratio of ∞) have Po_2 and Pco_2 values that are the same as humidified inspired gas because there is no gas exchange to alter the composition of the alveolar gas. All other alveoli have Po_2 and Pco_2 values in between those of mixed venous blood and inspired gas depending on their $\dot{V}/\dot{Q}$ ratio (Figure 25-3).

SHUNT

Admixture of arterial blood with poorly oxygenated or mixed venous blood is an important cause of arterial hypoxemia. Venous admixture refers to the degree of admixture of mixed venous blood with pulmonary end-capillary blood that would be required to produce the observed difference between the Po_2 of arterial and pulmonary end-capillary blood. There are several sources of venous admixture. Physiologic sources include the venae cordis minimae (Thebesian veins) that drain blood from the myocardium directly into the chambers of the left heart and the bronchial veins that drain into the pulmonary veins. Pathologic causes include right-to-left shunting in congenital heart disease, particularly conditions involving obstruction of the right ventricular outflow tract (e.g., Fallot's tetralogy). More commonly, pulmonary pathology causes

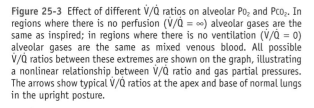

Figure 25-3 Effect of different $\dot{V}/\dot{Q}$ ratios on alveolar Po_2 and Pco_2. In regions where there is no perfusion ($\dot{V}/\dot{Q}$ = ∞) alveolar gases are the same as inspired; in regions where there is no ventilation ($\dot{V}/\dot{Q}$ = 0) alveolar gases are the same as mixed venous blood. All possible $\dot{V}/\dot{Q}$ ratios between these extremes are shown on the graph, illustrating a nonlinear relationship between $\dot{V}/\dot{Q}$ ratio and gas partial pressures. The arrows show typical $\dot{V}/\dot{Q}$ ratios at the apex and base of normal lungs in the upright posture.

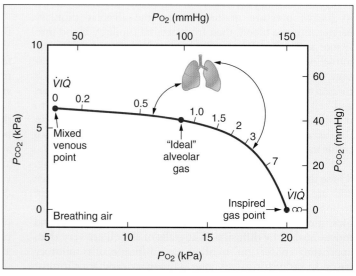

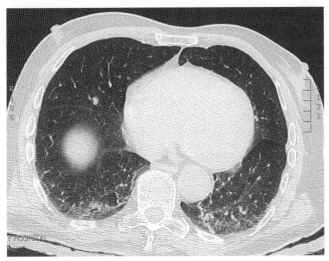

Figure 25-4 Computed tomography scan of the chest during general anesthesia with muscle relaxation. The slice shown is at the level of the dome of the right diaphragm, which is visible in the center of the right hemithorax. Patches of atelectasis in this supine patient can be seen throughout the dependent regions of both lungs.

increased venous admixture, usually resulting from pulmonary blood flow past nonventilated or poorly ventilated alveoli in conditions such as pneumonia, atelectasis, and acute lung injury.

EFFECTS OF GENERAL ANESTHESIA

General anesthesia has a marked effect on $\dot{V}/\dot{Q}$ relationships. Following induction of anesthesia, changes in the dimensions of the thoracic cavity due to muscle relaxation, in particular loss of tonic activity in the diaphragm, lead to a 10% to 20% reduction in FRC. As FRC approaches closing capacity, atelectasis occurs in the dependent parts of the lung (Figure 25-4) resulting in areas of lung that are perfused but not ventilated ($\dot{V}/\dot{Q} = 0$), increasing shunt and therefore impairing oxygenation. Even in dependent areas without atelectasis, the $\dot{V}/\dot{Q}$ ratio is less than 1 and oxygenation poor. Atelectasis and areas with a low $\dot{V}/\dot{Q}$ ratio are more likely in patients whose closing capacity is already equal to or greater than FRC prior to anesthesia, for example in older patients, infants, and the obese, in whom severe impairment of oxygenation can occur during anesthesia.

In nondependent areas of lung the converse problem occurs. These areas are, relative to dependent regions, well ventilated. General anesthesia commonly leads to low cardiac output and pulmonary hypotension, resulting in reduced perfusion to nondependent regions. As a result of these two effects, $\dot{V}/\dot{Q}$ ratios in nondependent regions are normally greater than 1, and there are some areas with ventilation but no perfusion ($\dot{V}/\dot{Q} = \infty$) which constitutes the alveolar dead space. Without compensatory increases in ventilation, these regions of lung lead to reduced carbon dioxide elimination and give rise to the large difference between end-expiratory and arterial P_{CO_2} commonly seen during general anesthesia. Although $\dot{V}/\dot{Q}$ ratios throughout the lung as a whole remain normal during general anesthesia, there is increased scatter of $\dot{V}/\dot{Q}$ ratios in different lung regions leading to impairment of both oxygenation and carbon dioxide elimination.

Pulmonary Vascular Resistance

In addition to the passive changes in PVR already described, pulmonary blood vessels are also under active control. The pulmonary vasculature is normally kept in a state of active vasodilatation.[24] There are many mechanisms involved in the active control of PVR. Some vasodilators, for example prostaglandins and VIP, act directly on smooth muscle cells via the cAMP second messenger system. In contrast, vasoconstrictors activate G protein–coupled receptors leading to increased IP3. Nitric oxide plays an important role in pulmonary blood vessels, and it is likely that NO acts as a final common pathway for relaxation of pulmonary vascular smooth muscle from a variety of different stimuli.[24] Nitric oxide synthase (NOS) produces NO by converting L-arginine to L-citrulline. Pulmonary NOS exists in two forms: constitutive and inducible NOS. The inducible form (iNOS or NOS2) is produced by many cells in response to activation by inflammatory mediators. Constitutive NOS (cNOS or NOS3) is always present in some cells, including pulmonary endothelium, producing short bursts of NO in response to changes in Ca^{2+} levels. Nitric oxide diffuses from the site of production to the smooth muscle cell where it activates guanylyl cyclase to produce cGMP, which in turn activates protein kinase G. This system is similar to the cAMP pathway and causes relaxation by a combination of effects on cytosolic Ca^{2+} levels and the activity of enzymes controlling myosin activity.

Hypoxic Pulmonary Vasoconstriction

Vasoconstriction in response to hypoxia represents the fundamental difference of pulmonary blood vessels compared to systemic vessels. Hypoxic pulmonary vasoconstriction (HPV) is mediated both by mixed venous (pulmonary arterial) and alveolar P_{O_2}, the greater influence being from the alveolus. In addition, bronchial arterial P_{O_2} influences tone in the larger pulmonary arteries via the vasa vasorum.

Regional HPV is beneficial as a means of diverting pulmonary blood flow away from areas of lung with a low oxygen partial pressure and is an important mechanism for optimizing $\dot{V}/\dot{Q}$ relationships. It is also important in the fetus to minimize perfusion of the unventilated lungs. However, long-term HPV, either continuous or intermittent, can lead to remodeling of the pulmonary vasculature and irreversible pulmonary hypertension.

The pressor response to hypoxia results from constriction of small arterioles of 30 to 200 μm in diameter and begins within a few seconds of P_{O_2} reduction. In humans, hypoxia in a single lobe of the lung results in a rapid decline in perfusion of the lobe such that within 5 minutes regional blood flow is half that during normoxia.[25] With prolonged hypoxia, HPV is biphasic: the initial rapid response reaches a plateau after about 5 minutes, with the second phase occurring after around 40 minutes and reaching a maximal response 2 to 4 hours after the onset of hypoxia (Figure 25-5).[26,27]

CELLULAR PHYSIOLOGY OF HYPOXIC PULMONARY VASOCONSTRICTION

Neural connections to the lung are not required as HPV occurs in isolated lung preparations and in humans following lung transplantation. Attempts to elucidate the mechanisms of HPV have been hampered by species differences, the

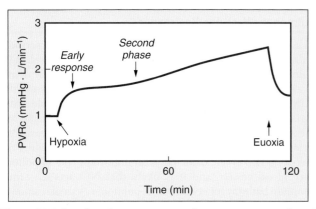

Figure 25-5 Hypoxic pulmonary vasoconstrictor response to prolonged hypoxia (end-tidal Po_2 50 mmHg). The early response is complete within a few minutes, then a more potent second phase begins after about 40 minutes. Note that when euoxia is restored, pulmonary vascular resistance corrected for cardiac output (PVRc) does not immediately return to baseline. *(Modified from Talbot NP, Balanos GM, Dorrington KL, et al. Two temporal components within the human pulmonary vascular response to ~2 h of iso-capnic hypoxia. J Appl Physiol. 2005;98:1125-1139.)*

multitude of systems affecting pulmonary vascular tone, and a lack of appreciation of the biphasic nature of the response. Uncertainties remain regarding the exact cellular mechanisms of HPV, but there is now agreement that contraction of pulmonary artery smooth muscle cells (PASMC) in response to hypoxia is an inherent property of these cells and that pulmonary endothelial cells only act to modulate the PASMC response.[28]

MOLECULAR PHYSIOLOGY

Hypoxia leads to a small increase in intracellular Ca^{2+} concentration within the PASMC, and also a rho kinase-mediated increase in the Ca^{2+} sensitivity of the smooth muscle contractile proteins.[29] The change in Ca^{2+} results from opening of L-type voltage-gated Ca^{2+} channels (Ca_v1), stimulated by hypoxia-induced inhibition of voltage-gated K^+ (Kv) channels. The molecular oxygen sensor that affects Kv channels remains controversial and might be an inherent property of the Kv channels, although mitochondria, nicotinamide adenine dinucleotide phosphate oxidases, and reactive oxygen species are also involved.[30-32]

Modulation by the endothelial cell of the PASMC response to hypoxia can either enhance or inhibit HPV.[28] Inhibitors of HPV include prostacyclin (PGI_2) and NO, both of which maintain some perfusion of hypoxic lung regions, although their role in normal lung is uncertain. For example, prostacyclin is a potent pulmonary vasodilator, but cyclooxygenase, which is required for its production, is inhibited by hypoxia and might therefore diminish its vasodilator effects.[27] Similarly, basal NO secretion by endothelial cells might act to moderate HPV, but hypoxia also inhibits endothelial NO production and so enhances HPV. Molecules that enhance HPV include thromboxane A_2 and endothelin, the latter being released by endothelial cells in response to hypoxia.[33] It is a potent vasoconstrictor peptide, and has a prolonged effect on pulmonary vascular tone such that this mechanism is probably involved in the second slow phase of HPV (see Figure 25-5). Endothelin is believed to be involved in producing the pulmonary hypertension associated with altitude hypoxia,

even though attempts to enhance HPV with endothelin infusions have not been successful.[27] Two groups of endothelin receptors are described, ET_A and ET_B, and their relative expression varies between the central and peripheral pulmonary vasculature. Apart from its vasoconstrictor effects, endothelin also stimulates cellular proliferation of vascular endothelial cells and pulmonary fibroblasts, and so has an important role in the pulmonary vascular remodeling that accompanies long-term hypoxia.

HPV is therefore a complex and poorly elucidated reflex. In normal subjects, HPV within the lung is inhomogeneous, with intense vasoconstriction in some areas and relative over-perfusion elsewhere.[34] The degree of this inhomogeneity varies between individuals, and this has important implications when travelling to high altitude. Subjects susceptible to high-altitude pulmonary edema have a more intense and inhomogenous HPV response.[34] Although this has never been studied, this raises the possibility that the same subgroup of patients would tolerate hypoxia due to lung disease poorly.

CONTROL OF BREATHING

Early in fetal development the respiratory center forms within the brainstem and is responsible for subconscious rhythmic breathing throughout life. Breathing is controlled by a complex network of physical and chemical reflexes that can be overridden by voluntary control and interrupted by acts such as swallowing, sneezing, vomiting, hiccupping, and coughing. The control system can also be fine-tuned to accommodate for posture, speech, voluntary movement, and exercise. The respiratory pattern is generated within the medulla and coordinates the voluntary and involuntary demands of respiratory activity via multiple neuronal connections.

Respiratory Center

There are two main groups of respiratory neurons: the dorsal and ventral respiratory groups.

The dorsal respiratory group lies close to the nucleus tractus solitarius, which is the area of the brain where visceral afferents from cranial nerves IX and X terminate. This group comprises mainly inspiratory neurons and is responsible for timing of the respiratory cycle.

The ventral respiratory group is a column of respiratory neurons divided into four subgroups.[35] The caudal group has both inspiratory and expiratory functions as well as controlling the force of contraction of the contralateral inspiratory muscles. The rostral subgroup is mainly composed of the nucleus ambiguous and controls the airway dilator functions of the larynx, pharynx, and tongue. The pre-Bötzinger complex is believed to be the anatomic location of the central pattern generator (CPG), while the Bötzinger complex is within the nucleus retrofacialis and has widespread expiratory functions (Figure 25-6).

CENTRAL PATTERN GENERATION

Unlike the heart, where inherent rhythm is initiated by a single pacemaker cell, respiratory rhythm begins with associated groups of neurons generating regular bursts of activity.[36] This activity can be recorded throughout the medulla but is concentrated in the pre-Bötzinger complex. Respiratory

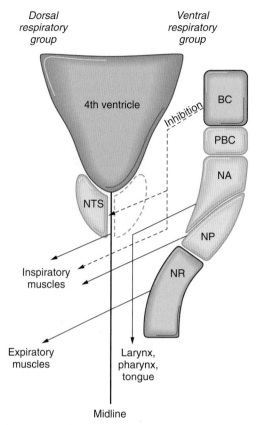

Dorsal respiratory group

Ventral respiratory group

4th ventricle

BC

Inhibition

PBC

NA

NTS

NP

NR

Inspiratory muscles

Expiratory muscles

Larynx, pharynx, tongue

Midline

Figure 25-6 Location of respiratory neurons in the medulla. For clarity, the dorsal respiratory group (nucleus tractus solitarius, NTS) is shown only on the left and the ventral respiratory group (VRG) is shown only on the right. The VRG consists of the Bötzinger (BC) and pre-Bötzinger (PBC) complexes, the rostral VRG area including the nucleus ambiguous (NA), and the caudal VRG area including the nucleus para-ambigualis (NP) and nucleus retroambigualis (NR). Areas with predominantly expiratory activity are shaded purple, and those with inspiratory activity shaded yellow. The dotted lines are expiratory pathways that inhibit inspiratory neurons.

neuron networks that exhibit spontaneous activity achieve this by a combination of intrinsic membrane properties and excitatory and inhibitory feedback mechanisms. In practice, both inhibitory and excitatory neurotransmitters have a dual effect to: (1) recruit other cells by direct activation and (2) modulate the spontaneous activity of a single cell by effects on its own membrane ion channels, for example, by slowing the rate at which an action potential travels along a dendrite.

CONNECTIONS TO THE RESPIRATORY CENTER

The pontine respiratory group, previously known as the pneumotaxic center, was believed to be important in controlling the timing of the respiratory cycle. It is no longer considered essential for generation of the respiratory rhythm but exerts fine control over medullary neurons, for example, setting the lung volume at which inspiration is terminated. The pons also coordinates input from other centers, for example, the hypothalamus, cortex, and nucleus tractus solitarius, integrating cortical and peripheral sensory information, such as odors, temperature, and visceral and cardiovascular inputs with the respiratory rhythm. Voluntary interruption of breathing is possible within limits determined by arterial blood gas tensions. This is necessary for conscious activities such as speech. It is possible that cortical signals bypass the

respiratory center, overriding it by acting directly on the lower motor neurons supplying respiratory muscles.[37]

A number of different peripheral receptors also provide input to the respiratory center. Chemical and irritant receptors are found in the nasopharynx, larynx, and trachea. When stimulated by irritants such as smoke and gastric acid, a reflex is initiated that protects the lungs from inhalational injury, resulting in laryngeal closure, apnea and bronchoconstriction, coughing, and sneezing.[38] Paintal's juxtapulmonary capillary receptors (J receptors) are small C fiber endings in alveolar walls close to pulmonary capillaries. Stimulation can occur in response to pulmonary vascular congestion, pulmonary embolus, or exercise; and results in rapid, shallow breathing; apnea; and mucus secretion.[38,39]

Pulmonary stretch receptors can be divided into two groups. *Slowly adapting stretch receptors* are situated in bronchial smooth muscle and are stimulated by lung inflation, maintaining firing rate when lung inflation is maintained and thus acting as a lung volume sensor. *Rapidly adapting stretch receptors* are located in the superficial mucosal layer of the airways and are stimulated by a change in tidal volume, respiratory frequency, or lung compliance.[40] Stimulation of pulmonary stretch receptors leads to inhibition of inspiration in response to lung distension and a reduction in respiratory rate by increasing expiratory time. This reflex was first described in 1868 by Hering and Breuer who noted that lightly anesthetized, spontaneously breathing animals ceased or decreased ventilation effort during sustained lung distention. Although this weak reflex has little clinical significance in adult humans, it is more pronounced in neonates and infants.[41]

Baroreceptors located in the carotid sinus and aortic arch are primarily concerned with regulation of the circulation, but can promote hyperventilation in response to a large decrease in arterial pressure.

MOLECULAR PHYSIOLOGY

There are a variety of different neurotransmitters involved in the CPG and respiratory control.[42] Excitatory transmitters include glutamate which activates both N-methyl-D-aspartate (NMDA) and non-NMDA type receptors. Inhibitory transmitters such as glycine and γ-aminobutyric acid (GABA) act via glycine and $GABA_A$ receptors to hyperpolarize and inhibit respiratory neurons.

Neuromodulators influence CPG output but are not involved in rhythm generation. The exact role of neuromodulators is unclear but they are important for both normal and abnormal breathing. For example, opioids have a profound effect on breathing, suggesting the presence of opioid receptors in the respiratory center. However, the opioid antagonist naloxone has no effect on respiration in resting normal subjects.[42] Other neuromodulators include acetylcholine, serotonin, and substance P. They exert their effects via a final common intracellular signaling pathways within CPG neurons involving protein kinase A and protein kinase C, modulating the activity of GABA, glycine, and glutamate-regulated K^+ and Cl^- channels.[43]

Chemical Control of Ventilation

For many years it was believed that the respiratory center itself was sensitive to carbon dioxide. However, it is now known that both peripheral and central chemoreceptors are responsible for the effect of carbon dioxide on breathing, the latter accounting for about 80% of the total ventilatory response.[44] Because of their reliance on extracellular pH (see later), the central chemoreceptors are regarded as monitors of steady-state arterial Pco_2 and tissue perfusion in the brain, while the peripheral chemoreceptors respond more to short-term and rapid changes in arterial Pco_2.[45]

CENTRAL CHEMORECEPTORS

Central chemoreceptors are located 0.2 mm below the ventrolateral surface of the medulla in the retrotrapezoid nucleus (RTN) inside the blood-brain barrier (BBB). As arterial Pco_2 rises, so does the CO_2 content of cerebrospinal fluid. This occurs because the BBB is permeable to CO_2 but not to hydrogen ions. CO_2 diffuses across the BBB into the cerebrospinal fluid (CSF) where it is hydrated to carbonic acid, which quickly ionizes to increase CSF hydrogen ion concentration and hence reduce pH. The mechanism by which a change in pH causes stimulation of chemoreceptor neurons remains controversial: the RTN might contain pH-sensitive K^+ channels, and release of ATP has been proposed.[44] Increases in arterial Pco_2 lead to an increase in respiratory rate and depth of breathing until steady-state hyperventilation is achieved after a few minutes. The response is linear over the range that is usually studied, with alveolar ventilation increasing by around 2 L/min^{-1} for each 1 mmHg increase in arterial Pco_2 (Figure 25-7). As Pco_2 continues to rise, the point of maximal ventilatory stimulation is reached, probably in the range of 100 to 200 mmHg (13.3 to 26.7 kPa). Beyond this point, respiratory fatigue and CO_2 narcosis occur.

Decreasing Pco_2 produces a fall in alveolar ventilation, but once arterial Pco_2 is less than about 30 mmHg (4 kPa), there are two possible physiologic responses. Some individuals reduce ventilation further, becoming apneic if Pco_2 continues to fall, while others continue to breathe regardless of the reduction in Pco_2.[46] This variable ventilatory response to low

Pco_2 almost certainly arises from cortical control of respiration, maintaining breathing despite a lack of chemical drive, particularly when awake (see Figure 25-7).

The Pco_2/ventilation response curve is the response of the entire respiratory system to the challenge of raised Pco_2. Apart from reduced sensitivity of the central chemoreceptors, the overall response can be blunted by partial neuromuscular blockade or by obstructive or restrictive lung disease. These factors must be taken into account when drawing conclusions from a reduced response; for example, severe airway obstruction will cause a blunted response to Pco_2 even when the central response is normal. Nevertheless, the slope of the Pco_2/ventilation response curve remains one of the most valuable parameters in the assessment of the responsiveness of the respiratory system to CO_2 and its depression by drugs. The response to raised Pco_2 is greatest over the first few hours and then begins to decline over the next 48 hours. This is partly due to redistribution of bicarbonate out of the CSF and increased renal excretion of bicarbonate, which reduces cerebral hydrogen ion concentration, in turn reducing stimulation of central chemoreceptors.

PERIPHERAL CHEMORECEPTORS

The peripheral chemoreceptors are the fast-responding monitors of arterial blood located in the carotid bodies close to the bifurcation of the common carotid artery.[47] The carotid bodies contain large sinusoids with a very high rate of perfusion, about 10 times that predicted by their metabolic rate, which is itself very high. This results in a small arterial/venous Po_2 difference, which allows for rapid (1- to 3-second) response to changes in arterial blood Po_2. Increased ventilation in response to activation of peripheral chemoreceptors occurs in response to various stimuli:

1. *Reduced arterial Po_2.* Glomus (type I) cells within the carotid body are in synaptic contact with neurons of the glossopharyngeal nerve. Discharge rate in the afferent nerves from the carotid body increases exponentially in response to falling arterial Po_2.
2. *Acidemia.* Elevated arterial Pco_2 or H^+ concentration both stimulate ventilation; the magnitude of the stimulus is the same whether the change in pH is due to a respiratory or metabolic cause. Quantitatively, the change produced by elevated Pco_2 on the peripheral chemoreceptors is only about one-sixth of that caused by the action on the central chemosensitive areas. This response does, however, occur very rapidly, and only develops when a "threshold" value of arterial Pco_2 is exceeded.[45,48,49]
3. *Hypoperfusion.* Stimulation of peripheral chemoreceptors by hypoperfusion can occur as a result of severe systemic hypotension, possibly by causing a "stagnant hypoxia" of the chemoreceptor cells.
4. *Hyperthermia.* An increase in body temperature increases the rate of firing from peripheral chemoreceptor neurons.

   Chemical stimulation by a wide range of substances causes increased ventilation via the peripheral chemoreceptors. These substances fall into two groups. The first comprises agents such as nicotine and acetylcholine that stimulate sympathetic ganglia. The second group of chemical stimulants comprises substances such as cyanide and carbon monoxide that block the cytochrome system and so prevent oxidative metabolism. Some drugs also stimulate respiration via the peripheral chemoreceptors, for example, doxapram.

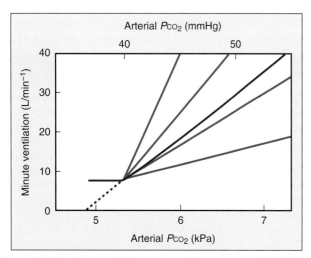

Figure 25-7 The Pco_2 ventilation response. The response to CO_2 is highly variable between individuals as shown by the four *blue* response lines. The population average is shown in purple, and is hockey stick shaped because when Pco_2 falls below the normal value, an awake subject continues to breathe despite the lack of respiratory drive from CO_2. In an anesthetized subject, when this voluntary drive for respiration is lost, the dotted line shows the continuation of the slope to the point where it meets the x-axis and apnea occurs.

MOLECULAR PHYSIOLOGY

There is now general agreement that oxygen-sensitive K^+ channels are responsible for the hypoxic response of the peripheral chemoreceptor type I cells.[28,47] Hypoxia inhibits the activity of K^+ channels, altering the membrane potential of the cell and stimulating Ca^{2+} channels to open, allowing an influx of extracellular Ca^{2+} that stimulates transmitter release. Stimulation of the chemoreceptors by increased arterial P_{CO_2} is dependent on carbonic anhydrase, present in the type I cell, and there is therefore the possibility of both raised P_{CO_2} and decreased arterial pH acting through an increase in intracellular H^+ concentration, as in the central chemoreceptors.

Various neurotransmitters have been identified within the carotid body with dopamine, acetylcholine, and ATP being the most prominent. Norepinephrine, angiotensin II, substance P, and enkephalins have also been described, although the specific role of each is uncertain. Acetylcholine and ATP are the most likely neurotransmitters involved in signaling between type I cells and afferent nerves.[50] The other transmitters seem to have autocrine rather than neurotransmitter roles, in that their release into the carotid body tissues modulates the response of the cells to various stimuli.[50] For example, dopamine is abundant in type I cells and released in response to hypoxia; its presence causes inhibition of Ca^{2+} channels so effectively 'damping' the acute response. Similarly, the α_2 adrenoceptor agonist clonidine reduces the ventilatory response to acute hypoxia indicating that norepinephrine also has an inhibitory effect.[51] Angiotensin II increases the sensitivity of the K^+ channels to hypoxia, and can be produced locally within the carotid body in response to long-term hypoxia or poor carotid body perfusion, as seen in heart failure.[52]

The gain of the carotid bodies is under nervous system control. There is an efferent pathway in the carotid sinus nerve, which, on excitation, decreases chemoreceptor activity. Excitation of the sympathetic innervation to the carotid body causes an increase in activity.

Ventilatory Response to Sustained Hypoxia

Moderate degrees of sustained hypoxia, with arterial oxyhemoglobin saturation (SO_2) of about 80%, result in a triphasic physiologic response. The initial acute hypoxic response is an immediate and rapid increase in ventilation. Sudden imposition of hypoxia results in stimulation of ventilation within the lung-to-carotid body circulation time (about 6 seconds). Ventilation continues to increase for 5 to 10 minutes, rapidly reaching high levels. Shortly after the acute hypoxic response reaches a peak, there is a period of hypoxic ventilatory decline (HVD) where the minute ventilation falls, reaching a plateau level, still above the resting ventilation, after 20 to 30 minutes (Figure 25-8). The individual degree of HVD correlates with the acute hypoxic response: the greater the initial increase in ventilation, the greater the subsequent decline. Although not completely elucidated, the mechanism of HVD appears to have a significant central component, and HVD represents a change in ventilatory drive rather than a decline in the sensitivity of receptors to hypoxia.[53,54] Once HVD is complete, continued isocapnic hypoxia results in a second, slower rise in ventilation over several hours (see Figure 25-8). Ventilation continues to increase for at least 8 hours and reaches a plateau by 24 hours.[53] The most likely explanation for this is a direct

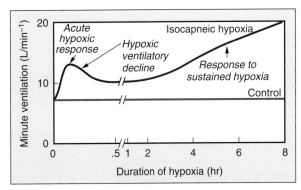

Figure 25-8 Time course of the ventilatory response to sustained hypoxia (arterial $SO_2 \approx 80\%$). When arterial P_{CO_2} is maintained at normal levels despite the changes in minute ventilation (isocapnia), the response is triphasic. The acute hypoxic response occurs within seconds, but lasts only for a few minutes, before hypoxic ventilatory decline returns the minute ventilation towards normal. Over several hours, a further and more pronounced ventilatory response occurs that reaches a plateau after 24 hours.

effect of hypoxia on the carotid bodies, possibly mediated by angiotensin II.

EMERGING DEVELOPMENTS

Remodeling of Airways

Repeated inflammation in small airways results in morphologic changes to both airway smooth muscle and epithelial cells. Hyperplasia of smooth muscle cells thickens the airway wall, even when the muscle is relaxed, and increases the degree of airway narrowing that occurs with small amounts of muscle contraction. In the long term, there is thickening of the epithelial cell basement membrane and changes to the extracellular matrix, eventually resulting in collagen deposition and long-term loss of lung function. The role of airway remodeling in asthma is unknown, but remodeling does lead to long-term lung damage in chronic obstructive pulmonary disease. Airway remodeling can begin before asthma becomes severe, or is even diagnosed at all, and even though reducing airway inflammation with steroids can delay remodeling, drugs to reverse the structural changes are yet to be discovered.[55]

Iron and Hypoxic Pulmonary Vasoconstriction

A fascinating recent finding relates iron metabolism to the intensity of individual HPV response. Increased iron availability (achieved by intravenous infusion) attenuates HPV, while reducing iron availability by administration of desferrioxamine enhances the response.[56] This finding indicates that HPV in humans is at least partially mediated via hypoxia-inducible factor (HIF), a ubiquitous transcription factor that is activated by hypoxia to initiate a range of responses to protect the cell from damage. One of the crucial oxygen-dependent steps in this reaction requires iron as a cofactor, explaining why iron status influences HPV. These observations might be highly significant for patients given that normal subjects have widely varying iron status, depending on such factors as sex, diet, and chronic illness, and also open up the possibility of therapeutic interventions for hypoxic critically ill patients.[57]

CO_2 Oscillations and Control of Ventilation

For decades the traditional teaching on the roles of CO_2 and O_2 in respiratory control has remained unchanged despite certain anomalies. For example, ventilation increases massively during exercise with no measurable change in arterial blood gas partial pressures. With resting ventilation, gas movement in and out of an alveolus is by diffusion, but as tidal volume increases, gas movement becomes cyclical. As a result, the P_{CO_2} of alveolar gas, and later arterial blood, begins to oscillate in phase with respiration, while the mean values remain unchanged. These oscillations of P_{CO_2} are sensed by the peripheral chemoreceptors and enhance respiratory drive, in effect providing positive feedback to breathing to maintain normal mean arterial P_{CO_2} even when metabolic production of CO_2 is very high. This system is believed to contribute to the ventilatory response to exercise and is particularly important if the subject is also hypoxic, for example, at high altitude.[58]

KEY POINTS

- The diaphragm is the principal muscle for inspiration and is responsible for 75% of tidal volume during resting inspiration in the supine posture. It is among the most resistant muscles to neuromuscular blockade, and compared to other muscles, for example, the adductor pollicis, requires a larger dose of relaxant to achieve full paralysis and is often the first muscle to recover function.
- Most bronchial smooth muscle is found in the 12th to 16th generation of the airway. Four mechanisms are involved in controlling muscle tone in small airways: neural, humoral (via blood), direct physical and chemical, and local cellular. Neural control is the most important in normal lung.
- Overall ventilation and perfusion are well matched and approximately equal, but in smaller regions of lung there are discrepancies between the two that can adversely affect gas exchange. For example, during general anesthesia there is a wider than normal spread of $\dot{V}/\dot{Q}$ ratios throughout the lung that impairs both oxygenation and carbon dioxide elimination.
- Regional HPV is beneficial as a means of diverting pulmonary blood flow away from areas of lung with low P_{O_2} and is an important mechanism for optimizing $\dot{V}/\dot{Q}$ relationships. Long-term HPV, either continuous or intermittent, leads to remodeling of the pulmonary vasculature and irreversible pulmonary hypertension.
- Uncertainties remain regarding the exact cellular mechanism of HPV, but there is now agreement that contraction of pulmonary artery smooth muscle cells in response to hypoxia is involved.
- Breathing is controlled by a complex network of physical and chemical reflexes that can be overridden by voluntary control and interrupted by acts such as swallowing, sneezing, vomiting, hiccupping, and coughing. The respiratory pattern is generated within the medulla, which coordinates the voluntary and involuntary demands of respiratory activity via multiple neuronal connections.
- Reflex control of breathing occurs in response to both CO_2 and O_2. Minute volume of ventilation increases in a linear fashion in response to increasing P_{CO_2}, a response that is highly variable between individuals. The response to hypoxia is exponential in nature such that below a P_{O_2} of approximately 60 mmHg (8 kPa), the ventilatory response curve is very steep.

Key References

Dehnert C, Risse F, Ley S, et al. Magnetic resonance imaging of uneven pulmonary perfusion in hypoxia in humans. *Am J Respir Crit Care Med.* 2006;174:1132-1138. This study used contrast-enhanced magnetic resonance imaging to demonstrate that individuals who previously had high altitude pulmonary edema had a more intense and patchy pulmonary vascular response to 2 hours of hypoxia (FiO2 = 0.12). These were otherwise healthy subjects, but the prospect that patients who develop hypoxia are also likely to have such a variable pulmonary vascular response is likely to lead to therapeutic interventions in the future. (Ref. 34)

Del Negro CA, Hayes JA. A 'group pacemaker' mechanism for respiratory rhythm generation. *J Physiol.* 2008;586:2245-2246. The concept of neuronal groups generating rhythmic activity (a 'group pacemaker') is quite a recent one and a departure from the conceptually simpler single 'pacemaker neuron.' This review considers the evidence that central pattern generation of respiratory rhythm is an example of a group pacemaker. (Ref. 36)

Galvin I, Drummond GB, Nirmalan M. Distribution of blood flow and ventilation in the lung: gravity is not the only factor. *Br J Anaesth.* 2007;98:420-428. For decades, physiologists have taught students that gravity is the main influence on both regional ventilation and perfusion in the lung, despite microgravity experiments in space clearly demonstrating that inhomogeneity of both still exists. This review comprehensively addresses the history of these studies and the various mechanisms underlying the current view that gravity, and the weight of the lung, is not the major determinant of regional $\dot{V}/\dot{Q}$ matching. (Ref. 19)

Talbot NP, Balanos GM, Dorrington KL, et al. Two temporal components within the human pulmonary vascular response to approximately 2 hours of isocapnic hypoxia. *J Appl Physiol.* 2005;98:1125-1139. This study of human volunteers provides the first clear demonstration of the biphasic nature of hypoxic pulmonary vasoconstriction (see Figure 25-6). This finding allowed the very different mechanisms of the two phases to be elucidated (oxygen-sensitive Kv channels for phase 1 and endothelin release for phase 2), and has significant implications for patients whose lungs are hypoxic, either through disease or anesthesia manipulations (e.g., during one-lung ventilation). (Ref. 26)

Weir K, López-Barneo J, Buckler KJ, et al. Acute oxygen-sensing mechanisms. *N Engl J Med.* 2005;353:2042-2055. In 1775, Joseph Priestley was the first to recognize that both oxygen deficiency and excess were harmful to animals, but more than 300 years later we remain mostly ignorant of how tissues detect and respond to extremes of P_{O_2}. This review considers how many different tissues respond to varying oxygen levels, including the common cellular mechanisms shared by tissues as diverse as the pulmonary vasculature and the placenta. (Ref. 28)

References

1. Kuna ST, Insalaco G, Woodson GE. Thyroarytenoid muscle activity during wakefulness and sleep in normal adults. *J Appl Physiol.* 1988;65:1332-1339.
2. Hemmerling TM, Donati F. Neuromuscular blockade at the larynx, the diaphragm and the corrugator supercilii muscle: a review. *Can J Anaesth.* 2003;50:779-794.

3. Donati F. Onset of action of relaxants. *Can J Anaesth.* 1988;35:S52–S58.
4. Lumb AB. *Nunn's Applied Respiratory Physiology.* 7th ed. Edinburgh: Churchill Livingstone; 2010.
5. Canning BJ, Fischer A. Neural regulation of airway smooth muscle tone. *Respir Physiol.* 2001;125:113-127.
6. Canning BJ. Reflex regulation of airway smooth muscle tone. *J Appl Physiol.* 2006;101:971-985.
7. Widdicombe JG. Autonomic regulation: i-NANC/e-NANC. *Am J Respir Crit Care Med.* 1998;158:S171-S175.
8. Thomson NC, Dagg KD, Ramsay SG. Humoral control of airway tone. *Thorax.* 1996;51:461-464.
9. Hakonarson H, Grunstein MM. Regulation of second messengers associated with airway smooth muscle contraction and relaxation. *Am J Respir Crit Care Med.* 1998;158:S115-S122.
10. Johnson M. The β-adrenoceptor. *Am J Respir Crit Care Med.* 1998;158:S146-S153.
11. Barnes PJ. Pharmacology of airway smooth muscle. *Am J Respir Crit Care Med.* 1998;158:S123-S132.
12. Hall IP, Sayers I. Pharmacogenetics and asthma: false hope or new dawn? *Eur Respir J.* 2007;29:1239-1245.
13. Wjst M. β₂-adrenoreceptor polymorphisms and asthma. *Lancet.* 2006;368:710-711.
14. Reynolds PN, Holmes MD, Scicchitano R. Role of tachykinins in bronchial hyper-responsiveness. *Clin Exp Pharmacol Physiol.* 1997;24: 273-280.
15. Johnson M. The β-adrenoceptor. *Am J Respir Crit Care Med.* 1998; 158:S146-S153.
16. van der Velden VHJ. Glucocorticoids: mechanisms of action and anti-inflammatory potential in asthma. *Mediat Inflam.* 1998;7:229-237.
17. Barnes PJ. Molecular mechanisms of glucocorticoid action in asthma. *Pulm Pharmacol Therap.* 1997;10:3-19.
18. Betticher DC, Reinhart WH, Geiser J. Effect of RBC shape and deformability on pulmonary O_2 diffusing capacity and resistance to flow in rabbit lungs. *J Appl Physiol.* 1995;78:778-783.
19. Galvin I, Drummond GB, Nirmalan M. Distribution of blood flow and ventilation in the lung: gravity is not the only factor. *Br J Anaesth.* 2007;98:420-428.
20. Brudin LH, Rhodes CG, Valind SO, Jones T, Hughes JB. Interrelationship between regional blood flow, blood volume, and ventilation in supine humans. *J Appl Physiol.* 1994;76:1205-1210.
21. Hughes M, West JB. Gravity is the major factor determining the distribution of blood flow in the human lung. *J Appl Physiol.* 2008; 104:1531-1533.
22. Glenny R. Gravity is not the major factor determining the distribution of blood flow in the healthy human lung. *J Appl Physiol.* 2008; 104:1533-1536.
23. Burrowes KS, Hunter PJ, Tawhai MH. Anatomically based finite element models of the human pulmonary arterial and venous trees including supernumerary vessels. *J Appl Physiol.* 2005;99:731-738.
24. Cooper CJ, Landzberg MJ, Anderson TJ, et al. Role of nitric oxide in the local regulation of pulmonary vascular resistance in humans. *Circulation.* 1996;93:266-271.
25. Morrell NW, Nijran KS, Biggs T, Seed WA. Magnitude and time course of acute hypoxic pulmonary vasoconstriction in man. *Respir Physiol.* 1995;100:271-281.
26. Talbot NP, Balanos GM, Dorrington KL, et al. Two temporal components within the human pulmonary vascular response to ~2 h of isocapnic hypoxia. *J Appl Physiol.* 2005;98:1125-1139.
27. Aaronson PI, Robertson TP, Ward JPT. Endothelium-derived mediators and hypoxic pulmonary vasoconstriction. *Respir Physiol Neurobiol.* 2002;132:107-120.
28. Weir K, López-Barneo J, Buckler KJ, et al. Acute oxygen-sensing mechanisms. *N Engl J Med.* 2005;353:2042-2055.
29. Aaronson PI, Robertson TP, Knock GA, et al. Hypoxic pulmonary vasoconstriction: mechanisms and controversies. *J Physiol.* 2006;570: 53-58.
30. Coppock EA, Martens JR, Tamkun MM. Molecular basis of hypoxia-induced pulmonary vasoconstriction: role of voltage-gated K^+ channels. *Am J Physiol.* 2001;281:L1-L12.

31. Sommer N, Dietrich A, Schermuly RT, et al. Regulation of hypoxic pulmonary vasoconstriction: basic mechanisms. *Eur Respir J.* 2008; 32:1639-1651.
32. Waypa GB, Schumacker PT. Hypoxic pulmonary vasoconstriction: redox events in oxygen sensing. *J Appl Physiol.* 2005;98:404-414.
33. Dupuis J, Hoeper MM. Endothelin receptor antagonists in pulmonary arterial hypertension. *Eur Respir J.* 2008;31:407-415.
34. Dehnert C, Risse F, Ley S, et al. Magnetic resonance imaging of uneven pulmonary perfusion in hypoxia in humans. *Am J Respir Crit Care Med.* 2006;174:1132-1138.
35. Rekling JC, Feldman JL. Pre-Bötzinger complex and pacemaker neurones: hypothesized site and kernel for respiratory rhythm generation. *Annu Rev Physiol.* 1998;60:385-405.
36. Del Negro CA, Hayes JA. A 'group pacemaker' mechanism for respiratory rhythm generation. *J Physiol.* 2008;586:2245–2246.
37. Horn EM, Waldrop TG. Suprapontine control of respiration. *Respir Physiol.* 1998;114:201-211.
38. Widdicombe JG. Afferent receptors in the airways and cough. *Respir Physiol.* 1998;114:5-15.
39. Kubin L, Alheid GF, Zuperku EJ, McCrimmon DR. Central pathways of pulmonary and lower airway vagal afferents. *J Appl Physiol.* 2006;101:618-627.
40. Widdicombe J. Airway receptors. *Respir Physiol.* 2001;125:3-15.
41. Rabbette PS, Fletcher ME, Dezateux CA, Soriano-Brucher H, Stocks J. Hering-Breuer reflex and respiratory system compliance in the first year of life: a longitudinal study. *J Appl Physiol.* 1994;76:650-656.
42. Ramirez JM, Telgkamp P, Elsen FP, Quellmalz UJA, Richter DW. Respiratory rhythm generation in mammals: synaptic and membrane properties. *Respir Physiol.* 1997;110:71-85.
43. Richter DW, Lalley PM, Pierrefiche O, et al. Intracellular signal pathways controlling respiratory neurons. *Respir Physiol.* 1997;110: 113-123.
44. Gourine AV. On the peripheral and central chemoreception and control of breathing: an emerging role of ATP. *J Physiol.* 2005;568: 715-724.
45. Nattie E. Why do we have both peripheral and central chemoreceptors? *J Appl Physiol.* 2006;100:9-10.
46. Lumb AB, Nunn JF. Ribcage contributions to CO_2 response during rebreathing and steady state methods. *Respir Physiol.* 1991;85:97-110.
47. López-Barneo J, Ortega-Sáenz P, Pardal R, Pascual A, Piruat JI. Carotid body oxygen sensing. *Eur Respir J.* 2008;32:1386-1398.
48. Tansley JG, Pedersen MEF, Clar C, Robbins PA. Human ventilatory response to 8 h of euoxic hypercapnia. *J Appl Physiol.* 1998;84:431-434.
49. Mohan R, Duffin J. The effect of hypoxia on the ventilatory response to carbon dioxide in man. *Respir Physiol.* 1997;108:101-115.
50. Nurse CA. Neurotransmission and neuromodulation in the chemosensory carotid body. *Auton Neurosci.* 2005;120:1–99.
51. Foo IT, Warren PM, Drummond GB. Influence of oral clonidine on the ventilatory response to acute and sustained isocapnic hypoxia in human males. *Br J Anaesth.* 1996;76:214-220.
52. Leung PS. Novel roles of a local angiotensin-generating system in the carotid body. *J Physiol.* 2006;575:4.
53. Robbins PA. Hypoxic ventilatory decline: site of action. *J Appl Physiol.* 1995;78:373-374.
54. Garcia N, Hopkins SR, Elliott AR, Aaron EA, Weinger MB, Powell FL. Ventilatory response to 2-h sustained hypoxia in humans. *Respir Physiol.* 2000;124:11-22.
55. Fixman ED, Stewart A, Martin JG. Basic mechanisms of development of airway structural changes in asthma. *Eur Respir J.* 2007;29: 379-389.
56. Smith TG, Balanos GM, Croft QP, et al. The increase in pulmonary arterial pressure caused by hypoxia depends on iron status. *J Physiol.* 2008;586:5999-6005.
57. Joyner MJ, Johnson BD. Iron lung? New ideas about hypoxic pulmonary vasoconstriction. *J Physiol.* 2008;586:5837-5838.
58. Collier DJ, Nickol AH, Milledge JS, et al. Alveolar P_{CO_2} oscillations and ventilation at sea level and at high altitude. *J Appl Physiol.* 2008; 104:404-415.

PULMONARY PHARMACOLOGY

Charles W. Emala, Sr.

The most widely used medications in pulmonary medicine are those delivered via inhalation for small airway diseases such as asthma, chronic obstructive pulmonary disease (COPD), and cystic fibrosis. Using the lung as a vehicle for drug delivery is well known to anesthesiologists who routinely deliver volatile anesthetics to the lungs for systemic distribution (see Chapter 3).

Three classes of medication are inhaled for therapeutic treatment of chronic lung diseases including β₂-adrenoceptor agonists, anticholinergic drugs (muscarinic receptor antagonists), and glucocorticoid steroids. Although combinations of β₂-adrenoceptor agonists and steroids are now the most widely used therapies in bronchoconstrictive diseases, this was not always so. In 1896, medical textbooks advocated the smoking of "asthma cigarettes" made from the dried leaf or fruiting tops of the *Datura stramonium* plant, commonly known as jimson weed, devil's trumpet, or thornapple. These plants contain tropane alkaloids such as atropine, hyoscyamine, and scopolamine that function as anticholinergics and relieve reflex-induced bronchoconstriction. Modern use of anticholinergics has evolved with the introduction of inhaled ipratropium bromide in the 1980s.

Methylxanthines were first recognized as having therapeutic effects for asthma when coffee was recommended as early as the 1860s and again in Osler's 1914 text.[1,2] By the 1940s, intravenous aminophylline was recognized as effective for asthma even though today the mechanisms for this beneficial effect are not clearly established. The likely mechanisms involve elevations of cyclic adenosine monophosphate (cAMP) in airway smooth muscle due to phosphodiesterase inhibition, antagonism of adenosine receptors, and/or systemic release of catecholamines. Nonetheless, the low therapeutic benefit to toxicity ratio led to its elimination from first-line asthma therapies.

The β-adrenoceptor agonists (see Chapters 13 and 22) have been the mainstay of asthma maintenance and rescue therapy since the development of metered dose inhalers in the 1950s. However, in 1910, Melland described dramatic relief of acute asthmatic symptoms by subcutaneous administration of epinephrine.[3] Inhaled epinephrine and isoproterenol were the initial therapeutics directed at β₂ adrenoceptors, but due to increased asthma death rates, agents more selective for the β₂ adrenoceptor were introduced in the 1960s.[4,5]

By the 1970s, it was recognized that systemic steroids dramatically improve asthma maintenance therapy. But the devastating complications of long-term systemic steroid use led to the search for alternative therapies in mild asthmatics and alternative routes of delivery of steroids for severe asthmatics. With the development of inhaled steroids, combination inhalers that combine selective β_2-adrenoceptor agonists with steroids became the mainstay of asthma therapy and ultimately culminated in the combination of long-acting β_2-adrenoceptor agonists (LABAs) with steroids. However, by the early 2000s it was recognized that LABAs alone are associated with increased asthma deaths. In 2009 this led to a warning from the U.S. Food and Drug Administration (FDA) that LABAs should not be used alone in the treatment of asthma, but should be used in combination with inhaled steroids. Studies continue to examine whether LABAs added to inhaled steroids are indeed superior to inhaled steroids alone, and whether the continued use of LABAs is warranted given safety concerns.[6]

β_2-ADRENOCEPTOR AGONISTS

Structure-Activity

All short acting β_2-adrenoceptor agonists (Table 26-1) are small molecules with a molecular structure very similar to the endogenous nonselective agonist epinephrine (Figure 26-1). The LABAs salmeterol and formoterol have modified long side chains with additional aromatic moieties to increase lipophilicity, which prolongs their duration at the site of action.

Mechanism and Metabolism

Among the hundreds of types of G protein–coupled receptors (GPCRs), the biochemical understanding of β-adrenoceptor ligand binding, G protein interactions, and mechanisms of receptor phosphorylation, desensitization, and internalization have served as the prototypical model for GPCR function. The effectiveness of β_2-adrenoceptors in asthma and COPD results from their combined effect at reducing inflammatory cell activation and directly relaxing airway smooth muscle. The potency of β_2-adrenoceptors as bronchodilators is largely due to the multiple signaling mechanisms activated within airway smooth muscle cells that all favor smooth muscle relaxation. Classically, β_2-adrenoceptors couple the Gs stimulatory G protein that activates membrane-associated adenylyl cyclase to synthesize the second messenger cAMP. cAMP activates a number of targets, including protein kinase A, that ultimately result in the opening of Ca^{2+}-activated K^+ channels and subsequent plasma membrane hyperpolarization, decreased intracellular entry of Ca^{2+}, and a decrease in the sensitivity of the contractile proteins to Ca^{2+}.

The long-lasting effects of LABAs, such as salmeterol and formoterol are thought to result from binding to two sites within the β_2-adrenoceptor: the classic ligand binding site and an exo-site on the receptor to which the hydrophobic tail binds irreversibly.[7] A second mechanism proposed to contribute to the prolonged duration of drug effect is high lipophilicity that allows the LABAs to dissolve within the lipid bilayer of the airway smooth muscle cell and serve as an agonist depot.[8]

The majority (80%-100%) of albuterol is excreted in the urine; its primary metabolic route is sulfate conjugation by sulfotransferase 1A3. Salmeterol is extensively metabolized to

Table 26-1. β_2-Adrenoceptor Agonists and Anticholinergic Drugs Used for Treatment of Bronchospasm

	FORMULATION	DELIVERY METHOD
Short-acting Inhaled β_2-adrenoceptor Agonists		
Albuterol	Generic	Nebulization
	Proair HFA	MDI
	Proventil HFA	MDI
	Ventolin HFA	MDI
Levalbuterol	Xopenex	MDI and Nebulization
Metaproterenol	Generic	Nebulization
Pirbuterol	Maxair	MDI
Short-acting Inhaled β_2-adrenoceptor Agonists-anticholinergic Combinations		
Albuterol + ipratropium bromide	Generic	Nebulization
	Duoneb	Nebulization
	Combivent	MDI
Long-acting Inhaled β_2-adrenoceptor Agonists (LABA)		
Formoterol	Foradil Aerolizer	DPI
	Perforomist	Nebulization
Salmeterol	Serevent Diskus	DPI
Arformoterol	Brovana	Nebulization
LABA-corticosteroid Combinations		
Salmeterol/fluticasone	Advair Diskus	DPI
	Advair HFA	MDI
Formoterol/mometasone	Dulera	MDI
Formoterol/budesonide	Symbicort	MDI
Short-acting Oral β_2-adrenoceptor Agonists		
Albuterol	Generic	Oral
	VoSpire ER	Oral
Metaproterenol	Generic	Oral
Terbutaline	Generic	Oral
Inhaled Anticholinergics		
Ipratropium bromide	Generic	Nebulization
	Atrovent HFA	MDI
Tiotropium bromide	Spiriva	DPI

DPI, Dry powder inhaler; *HFA,* hydrofluoroalkane propellant; *MDI,* metered dose inhaler.

α-hydroxysalmeterol (aliphatic oxidation) by CYP 3A4 with 25% eliminated in the urine and the majority in the feces. The xinafoate moiety of salmeterol xinafoate has no pharmacologic activity and is highly protein bound (>99%) with an elimination half-life of 11 days. Formoterol is metabolized by glucuronidation and *O*-demethylation by CYP 2D6 and CYP 2C. About 60% of oral or intravenous formoterol is excreted in the urine and the remainder in the feces.

Clinical Pharmacology

PHARMACOKINETICS, PHARMACODYNAMICS, AND THERAPEUTIC EFFECTS

Inhaled β_2-adrenoceptor agonists are rapidly absorbed through the respiratory epithelium, reaching the airway smooth muscle within a few minutes. The therapeutic effect of inhaled β_2 agonists depends on local tissue concentrations that are not reflected in plasma drug concentrations.[9] Regardless of the delivery device used, only about 10% of the inhaled dose actually reaches the peripheral airways to mediate bronchodilation.[10] The mean time for a 15% increase in forced expiratory volume in 1 second (FEV_1) was 6 minutes following two albuterol inhalations with a peak effect occurring at 55 minutes and a mean duration of effect of 2.6 hours.[11] A comparison of the racemic formulation to the levo (R-)

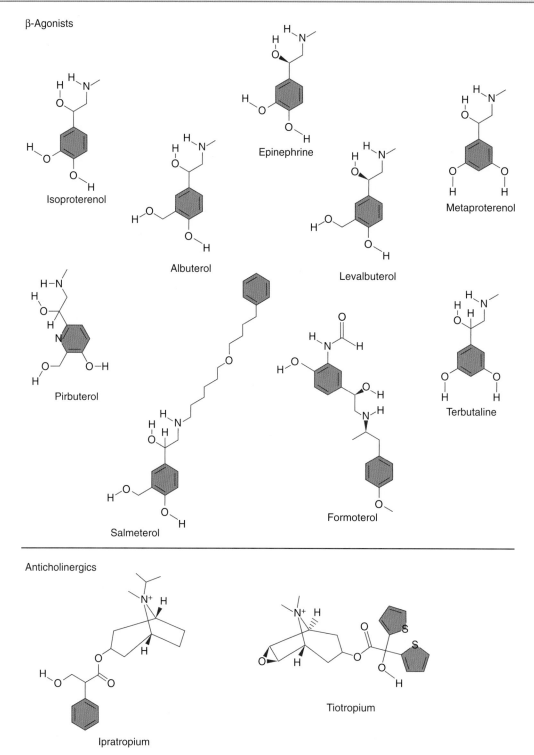

Figure 26-1 Structures of β-receptor agonists and anticholinergic drugs used as bronchodilators.

enantiomer of albuterol given by nebulization to healthy volunteers demonstrated a shorter time to maximum plasma concentrations for the R-enantiomer (0.2 hour for R-, 0.3 hour for RS-) but a longer half-life (1.5 hours for RS-, 3.4 hours for R-).[12] Limited pharmacokinetic data are available for salmeterol because plasma concentrations often cannot be detected even 30 minutes after a therapeutic dose of 50 μg. Salmeterol-induced airway relaxation is slow in onset,

prolonged in duration, and resistant to washout. After inhalation of 400 μg of salmeterol, plasma concentrations of 0.2 and 2 μg/L were achieved at 5 and 15 minutes in healthy volunteers.[13] In a separate study, a second peak plasma concentration occurred 45 to 90 minutes after inhalation, likely reflecting gastrointestinal absorption of swallowed drug.[14] LABAs can require up to 30 minutes to first achieve bronchodilator effects with a duration of 12 hours.

ADVERSE EFFECTS

The β agonists can produce dose-related cardiovascular effects (arrhythmias, tachycardia), hypokalemia, and elevations of blood glucose. Acute adverse effects are more common with oral than inhaled β_2 agonists, and most commonly include tachycardia, nervousness, irritability, and tremor. Changes in plasma concentrations of K^+ and glucose are seen at doses far exceeding those used clinically.[15] Paradoxical bronchospasm has been reported with β agonists. An initial concern regarding an increased death rate in asthmatics using salmeterol was raised in 1993 when 12 of 16,787 patients using salmeterol died, but this outcome was attributed to the severity of the patients' illnesses at the time of study entry.[16] The Salmeterol Multicenter Asthma study Research Trial (SMART), conducted at more than 6000 sites and enrolling more than 26,000 patients, was stopped after an interim data analysis revealed a small but significant increase in respiratory-related morbidity and mortality.[16] A meta-analysis of 19 trials involving more than 33,000 patients also revealed an increased risk of hospitalization for asthma exacerbations, life-threatening asthma attack, or asthma-related death.[17] Although the mechanism for these increased risks are unknown, speculations include the lack of anti-inflammatory effect, downregulation of β_2 adrenoceptors, or incorrect use of these LABAs as rescue inhalers. These findings led to a "black box" by the FDA warning that LABAs should not be used as monotherapy and should only be used in patients in whom asthma symptoms are not adequately controlled by low- to medium-dose inhaled steroids or whose disease severity warrants two maintenance therapies. Subsequently the FDA initiated a clinical trial protocol in cooperation with academic experts and manufacturers of LABAs that consists of five clinical trials, four in adults and one in children. The trials will be multinational, randomized, and double-blind, occurring from 2011 to 2017 and recruiting 11,700 adults.[6]

Drug Interactions

The β agonists can potentiate the hypokalemic effect of non–potassium-sparing diuretics. Serum levels of digoxin are reduced after the oral or intravenous administration of albuterol. The vascular effects of β agonists can be exacerbated by patients currently or recently taking monoamine oxidase inhibitors or tricyclic antidepressants. An increased risk of cardiovascular side effects can occur when salmeterol is used along with strong cytochrome P450 3A4 (CYP 3A4) inhibitors.

Clinical Application

COMMON APPLICATIONS

The use of long-acting β_2 agonists in combination with inhaled steroids is an option for patients whose bronchospasm is not adequately controlled using monotherapy with low to medium doses of inhaled corticosteroids as recommended by the Global Initiative for Asthma (GINA) and an expert report from the U.S. National Institutes of Health.[18,19] Conversely, the use of inhaled LABAs without steroids is not approved by the FDA due to an increased rate of asthma deaths with this therapy. Short-acting β agonists are recommended as rescue therapy for breakthrough episodes of bronchospasm and the frequency of use of rescue therapy is often used as an indicator of the adequacy of asthma maintenance therapy. Inhaled short-acting β agonists can be given to treat active wheezing in the preoperative or intraoperative period. They can also be administered prophylactically in patients at risk for bronchospasm, especially in those patients in whom intubation of the trachea is planned.

RATIONALE FOR DRUG SELECTION AND ADMINISTRATION

The anesthesiologist most commonly administers short-acting β_2-adrenoceptor agonists (e.g., albuterol) by inhalation via nebulization or metered dose inhalers either preoperatively or intraoperatively. Either modality can be connected to the inspiratory circuit of the anesthesia machine, but effective drug delivery to the airway smooth muscle is variable. This is affected by timing of drug administration relative to inspiration and the volume of dead space (endotracheal tube dimensions and anatomic dead space of the upper trachea/bronchi). Many studies have addressed the efficacy of delivering inhaled β_2-agonists in mechanically ventilated patients. Nebulization is more effective than metered dose inhalers.[20] A location 15 cm upstream from the endotracheal tube on the inspiratory side of an anesthesia circuit was optimal in an in vitro model.[21] The mode of mechanical ventilation and the humidity of the circuit are also important factors in delivery; a dry circuit and spontaneous breaths under continuous positive airway pressure (CPAP) enhance delivery compared to continuous mandatory volume, assist control, or pressure control ventilator settings.[22] It is also possible to administer selective β_2-adrenoceptor agonists parenterally (e.g., terbutaline). Emergency treatment of bronchospasm in the emergency department utilizes inhaled short-acting β_2 agonists and systemic corticosteroids.[23] Rescue therapy from intractable bronchospasm can require intravenous epinephrine, but systemic administration of these therapies is associated with significant cardiovascular effects.

The propellants in most inhalers were chlorofluorocarbons (CFCs) until an international agreement entitled "The Montreal Protocol on Substances That Deplete the Ozone Layer" led to the banning of this propellant and its replacement with hydrofluoroalkanes (HFAs). Substantial new technology was involved to make HFAs suitable for metered-dose inhalers.[24] This provided the opportunity to improve the performance of inhaled β_2-agonist formulations and enhanced the ability of inhaled steroids to reach smaller peripheral airways.[25] Ultra-long acting β_2-adrenoceptor agonists (olodaterol and sibenadet) that achieve effective bronchodilation for 24 hours are in development.[26,27] Clinical trials continue to determine whether the risk of LABAs are mitigated by the concurrent use of inhaled corticosteroids.[6]

ANTICHOLINERGICS

Structure-Activity

Inhaled anticholinergic drugs (Table 26-1) are a mainstay in the long-term management of COPD and are a component of some asthma regimens.[28] Ipratropium bromide (nebulization or metered dose inhaler) and tiotropium bromide (dry powder inhaler) (Figure 26-1) antagonize the effects of acetylcholine released from airway parasympathetic nerves on M_3 muscarinic receptors on airway smooth muscle (Figure 26-2).

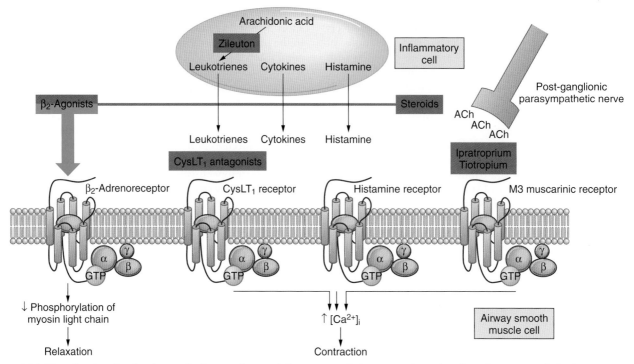

Figure 26-2 Sites of action of major classes of pulmonary drugs on inflammatory and airway smooth muscle cells. Inflammatory cells in the airway release a wide variety of mediators that affect signal transduction of several types of cells in the airway (epithelium, smooth muscle, and nerves). 5-Lipoxygenase inhibitors (e.g., zileuton) block the synthesis of leukotrienes while CysLT$_1$ antagonists block the effect of leukotrienes on airway cells. Steroids nonspecifically block activation of many inflammatory cells in the airway responsible for cytokine production that alter signaling pathways of airway cells favoring edema, mucus secretion, and airway smooth muscle contraction. β_2-adrenoceptor agonists both directly relax airway smooth muscle and block activation of inflammatory cells. Muscarinic receptor antagonists block M$_3$ muscarinic receptors on airway smooth muscle as well as muscarinic receptors on epithelium and nerves. The determinants of airway smooth muscle contraction are an increase in intracellular Ca^{2+} concentration ([Ca^{2+}]$_i$) as well as the sensitivity of the contractile proteins to a given concentration of Ca^{2+} (dictated by phosphorylation of the myosin light chain [MLC$_{20}$] and termed *calcium sensitization*).

Mechanism and Metabolism

Parasympathetic nerves traveling within the vagus nerve release acetylcholine to act upon M$_2$ and M$_3$ muscarinic receptors on airway smooth muscle. The nerve terminals also express autoinhibitory M$_2$ muscarinic receptors that respond to released acetylcholine to inhibit further neurotransmitter release. The M$_3$ muscarinic receptor on airway smooth muscle is a G protein–coupled receptor (Gq) that activates phospholipase C to generate diacylglycerol and inositol phosphates from membrane phospholipids. Diacylglycerol activates a number of targets, primarily protein kinase C isoforms. Inositol phosphates elevate intracellular Ca^{2+} primarily via release from the sarcoplasmic reticulum. This entire signaling cascade is blocked upstream by ipratropium or tiotropium's antagonism of cell surface airway smooth muscle muscarinic receptors (see Figure 26-1).

Inhaled ipratropium is metabolized to eight metabolites that have little to no anticholinergic activity, and are excreted in approximately equal proportions in feces and urine.

Clinical Pharmacology

PHARMACOKINETICS, PHARMACODYNAMICS, AND THERAPEUTIC EFFECTS

Inhaled ipratropium has an initial onset of 15 minutes with a peak effect at 1 to 2 hours and a duration of 3 to 6 hours. Tiotropium bromide has an onset of 30 minutes, a peak effect

at 3 hours, and a duration of 24 hours. Only 7% of inhaled ipratropium is bioavailable; the elimination half-life is 3.5 hours by all routes of administration.

Inhaled anticholinergics are indicated for the relief of bronchoconstriction in COPD and asthma by blockade of M$_3$ muscarinic receptor on airway smooth muscle. They can be used both prophylactically and as maintenance therapy. Their slower onset of action compared to inhaled β_2 agonists make them unacceptable as rescue therapy for acute exacerbations.

ADVERSE EFFECTS

Anticholinergics inhibit mucosal secretions and thus dry mouth is common (antisialagogue effect). As with β agonists, paradoxical bronchospasm has been reported with ipratropium. COPD patients using ipratropium bromide have an increased risk of adverse cardiac events that occur less commonly with tiotropium.[29-31] Inhaled anticholinergics increase the risk of acute urinary retention over fourfold in men with benign prostatic hypertrophy due to effects on parasympathetic innervation to the detrusor muscles of the bladder. Inhaled ipratropium can also worsen acute narrow angle glaucoma due to its parasympathetic effects.

Clinical Application

Anticholinergics have been used to treat obstructive airway disease since the early use of deadly nightshade genus

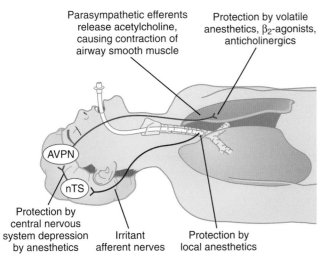

Figure 26-3 Sites of action of major classes of anesthetics on reflex-induced bronchoconstriction. Irritation of the upper airway by foreign bodies, including endotracheal tubes or suction catheters initiates an afferent irritant reflex arc resulting in the release of acetylcholine from parasympathetic nerves onto muscarinic receptors on airway smooth muscle resulting in bronchoconstriction. Anesthetics and other agents work at different levels of this irritant reflex to block bronchoconstriction. Local anesthetics can attenuate the initial afferent stimulus while multiple classes of anesthetics (general, intravenous, local) can attenuate the glutamatergic and GABAergic relay at the nucleus of the solitary tract (nTS) to the airway vagal preganglionic neurons (AVPN). Direct effects of volatile anesthetics, β2-adrenoceptor agonists, or muscarinic receptor antagonists attenuate the effects of acetylcholine on airway smooth muscle.

Table 26-2. Inhaled and Systemic Steroids for Treatment of Bronchospasm

	FORMULATION	DELIVERY METHOD
Inhaled		
Ciclesonide	Alvesco HFA	MDI
Mometasone	Asmanes Twisthaler	DPI
Budesonide	Generic	Nebulization
	Pulmicort Flexhaler	DPI
	Pulmicort Respules	Nebulization
Fluticasone	Flovent Diskus	DPI
	Flovent HFA	MDI
Beclomethasone	Qvar HFA	MDI
Systemic		
Methylprednisolone	Generic	Oral
	Medrol	Oral
Methylprednisolone sodium succinate	Generic	Parenteral
	Solu-Medrol	Parenteral
Prednisolone	Generic	Oral
	Orapred	Oral
	Pediapred	Oral
	Prelone	Oral
	Veripred 20	Oral
Prednisone	Generic	Oral
	Sterapred	Oral
Hydrocortisone sodium succinate	Solu-Cortef	Parenteral

DPI, Dry powder inhaler; *HFA,* hydrofluoroalkane propellant; *MDI,* metered dose inhaler.

(*Atropa*) plants and asthma cigarettes.[32] Although inhaled β2-adrenoceptor agonists with steroids are often the initial therapy for the bronchoconstrictive diseases asthma and COPD, there is evidence of equivalence or even superiority of inhaled anticholinergics in the treatment of COPD.[33] In the perioperative setting, the choice of anticholinergic is mechanistically sound because bronchoconstriction following airway irritation involves parasympathetic nerve release of acetylcholine onto M3 muscarinic receptors on airway smooth muscle.

Instrumentation of the upper airway with an endotracheal tube or suction catheter is a potent stimulus for reflex-induced bronchoconstriction (see Figure 26-3). This reflex originates in the airway wall where irritant nerve fibers travel in the vagal nerve complex to the nucleus of the solitary tract (nTS) which synapses via GABAA and glutamate receptors on the airway-related vagal preganglionic neurons (AVPNs).[34] The efferent outflow from this brainstem nucleus travels back down the vagus to release acetylcholine onto M3 muscarinic receptors on airway smooth muscle. The M3 muscarinic receptor via Gq-coupling increases intracellular Ca2+, resulting in smooth muscle contraction and airway narrowing. Thus anticholinergic blockade of M3 muscarinic receptors are an ideal target to attenuate reflex-induced bronchoconstriction.

Two inhaled antimuscarinics are available: the relatively quick onset and short duration ipratropium bromide and the longer duration tiotropium bromide.[35] Ipratropium bromide is available in either nebulized or metered dose inhaler formulations making this an ideal preoperative or intraoperative treatment for the anesthesiologist faced with a patient with bronchoconstriction induced by airway irritation. A new

inhaled anticholinergic drug, aclidinium, demonstrates bronchodilation for a similar duration as tiotropium with preclinical evidence of a reduced risk of anticholinergic heart rate effects.[36-38]

INHALED STEROIDS

Structure-Activity

The specific structures of the inhaled corticosteroids on a steroidal backbone are illustrated in Figure 26-4. Their formulations and delivery methods are summarized in Table 26-2, along with formulations of systemic steroids that are used in moderate to severe cases, particularly during initial presentation and acute exacerbations. For a more detailed discussion of systemic corticosteroid pharmacology, see Chapter 31.

Mechanism and Metabolism

Corticosteroids interact with intracellular steroid receptors that translocate to the nucleus and interact with transcription factor complexes to regulate inflammatory protein synthesis. The stimulation of gene transcription (transactivation) correlates with negative side effects of corticosteroids, while repression of transcription factors (e.g., NF-κB and AP-1) is responsible for antiinflammatory effects.[39] Although steroids affect the inflammatory response of lymphocytes, eosinophils, neutrophils, macrophages, monocytes, mast cells, and basophils, particular attention has focused on the role of a subset of interleukin (IL), producing T lymphocytes in asthma. CD+ Th2 cells that produce IL-4, IL-5, and IL-13 are particularly

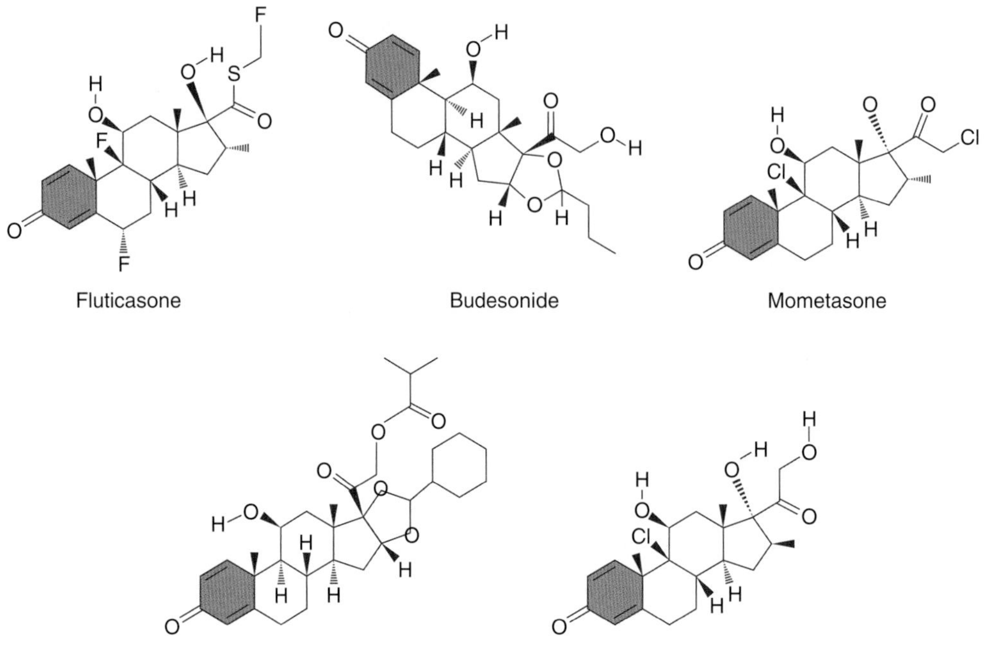

Fluticasone

Budesonide

Mometasone

Ciclesonide

Beclomethasone

Figure 26-4 Structures of inhaled corticosteroids.

important in orchestrating the complex inflammatory events in asthmatic lungs and are inhibited by inhaled steroids. Mast cell and basophil numbers are increased in asthma, and release of mediators (histamine, leukotrienes) in asthmatic airways is enhanced. Although inhaled steroids also suppress these cells, more specific therapy with oral leukotriene antagonists has allowed reduction in inhaled steroid use in some patients.

Corticosteroids exhibit high first-pass metabolism by the liver by CYP 3A4.

Clinical Pharmacology

PHARMACOKINETICS, PHARMACODYNAMICS, AND THERAPEUTIC EFFECTS

Beclomethasone dipropionate is a prodrug that is rapidly activated by hydrolysis to the active monoester 17-beclomethasone monopropionate, which has an affinity for the glucocorticoid receptor that is 25 times that of the parent compound. Ciclesonide is an inactive prodrug that is converted to the active metabolite desisobutyrylciclesonide in the lung. Forty percent to 90% of an inhaled corticosteroid is swallowed and therefore available for systemic absorption (and potential systemic side effects). Thus a low oral bioavailability of inhaled corticosteroids is desirable; it ranges from 1% for fluticasone propionate to 26% for 17-beclomethasone monopropionate.

In contrast to oral absorption, most of the drug deposited in the lung will be absorbed systemically and is not subjected to first-pass hepatic metabolism. Deposition and thus absorption from the lung is more a function of the efficiency of the delivery device than the properties of the drug itself. Fluticasone has only 1% oral bioavailability due to first pass metabolism but when delivered to the lung by dry powder or metered dose inhalers total systemic bioavailability is 17% and 25%,

respectively.[40] The transition from CFC- to HFA-powered metered dose inhalers has resulted in unanticipated improvement in the delivery of smaller particles deposited deeper in the lung with less oropharyngeal deposition and thus less systemic absorption. Most of the inhaled corticosteroids (approximately 70%) are bound to plasma proteins, and exhibit half-lives of 3 to 8 hours due to high extraction and metabolism by the liver.

The efficacy of inhaled corticosteroids in asthma has been shown in many studies usually with comparable benefits to systemic steroids with fewer side effects. Asthma patients discharged from the emergency department with 40-mg oral prednisone daily versus 600 µg inhaled budesonide four times a day exhibited similar rates of asthma relapse and similar improvements in FEV_1, asthma symptoms, and peak expiratory flow.[41] Personalized medicine may be able to predict respondents to specific therapies, including inhaled corticosteroids.[42]

ADVERSE EFFECTS

Many studies report no or minimal side effects on adrenal function, bone density or subcapsular cataracts, while some studies contend a dose-dependent effect of all inhaled steroids on these parameters.[43,44] A year-long study in adults receiving inhaled fluticasone or beclomethasone and a 12-week study in children receiving inhaled fluticasone showed no effect on bone density.[45,46]

Drug Interactions

Numerous reports exist of clinically significant Cushing's syndrome and adrenal insufficiency in both children and adults secondary to the combination of fluticasone propionate or budesonide with a CYP 3A4 inhibitor (e.g., ketoconazole, itraconazole, ritonavir).[47] Most patients were on high doses of inhaled corticosteroids. Plasma concentrations of mometasone furoate and a metabolite of ciclesonide increased with ketoconazole administration.

Clinical Application

Inhaled corticosteroids are commonly recommended as initial therapy for asthma. The introduction of inhaled steroids in the 1970s revolutionized therapy for bronchospastic diseases by allowing the delivery of steroids directly to the airway with a reduction in the systemic toxicity of chronic oral steroid ingestion. Although the precise mechanisms of asthma remain undefined, a significant component of asthma involves a complex interplay between inflammatory and structural cells of the airway on which steroids are efficacious. Inhaled glucocorticoids are the most effective anti-inflammatory medications for the treatment of asthma. Inhaled corticosteroids reduce the symptoms, frequency of exacerbations, airway hyperresponsiveness, airway inflammation, and asthma mortality.[48-50] A review of clinical studies suggests that inhaled fluticasone is more efficacious than inhaled budesonide as a monotherapy, and that either a combination of fluticasone/salmeterol or budesonide/formoterol was more effective than corresponding monotherapies with inhaled corticosteroids or inhaled long-acting β_2 agonists.[51] However, an ongoing controversy regarding the uncertain risk/benefit of adding inhaled long-acting β_2 agonists to inhaled glucocorticoids for asthma therapy led to an unprecedented series of clinical trials coordinated between the FDA and drug manufacturers of long-acting β_2 agonists to be completed in 2017.[6] Combination inhaled corticosteroids and long-acting β_2 agonists are also useful in COPD.[52,53]

METHYLXANTHINES AND PHOSPHODIESTERASE INHIBITORS

Structure-Activity

Theophylline is a close structural analogue of caffeine on a purine backbone. Aminophylline is two theophylline molecules with a 1,2 ethanediamine moiety. Roflumilast is a halide-modified benzamide molecule synthesized from 3-(cyclopropylmethoxy)-4-hydroxybenzaldehyde. The X-ray crystal structure of roflumilast docked within the catalytic sites of phosphodiesterase 4 has been determined, showing with unprecedented mechanistic molecular detail the target site of a medication newly added to clinical medicine.[54]

Mechanism and Metabolism

Methylxanthines have anti-inflammatory and bronchodilating effects. Although these drugs are phosphodiesterase (PDE) inhibitors in vitro, this is not likely to occur at the therapeutic levels achieved.[55] The methylxanthines release catecholamines from the adrenal gland, which might contribute to their beneficial activity in asthma, and also function as nonselective antagonists of four known subtypes of adenosine receptors (A_1, A_{2a}, A_{2b}, and A_3).[56,57] Additional mechanisms that have been proposed for the beneficial effects of methylxanthines in bronchoconstrictive diseases include modulation of

intracellular Ca^{2+} flux through ryanodine receptors, modulation of histone deacetylase activity, and increased peroxisome-proliferator-activated receptor γ expression.[58]

A new class of oral medication was introduced in 2011 for severe COPD. Roflumilast, a type 4 PDE inhibitor, inhibits degradation of cAMP in cells of the airway (airway smooth muscle, epithelium, and inflammatory cells) and elsewhere that express the type 4 PDE isoenzyme. Roflumilast and its active metabolite N-oxide roflumilast are highly selective inhibitors of PDE4 (which in turn is highly selective for cAMP) and are inactive against PDE isoforms 1, 2, 3, 5, and 7. The selectivity of roflumilast is distinct from that of the PDE inhibitors used in heart failure (milrinone, inamrinone, and cilostazol) that target cAMP-selective PDE3 and from the inhibitors used for erectile dysfunction (sildenafil and tadalafil) that target the cGMP-selective PDE5 isoforms. The selectivity of roflumilast for type 4 phosphodiesterase is suggested to produce fewer side effects than the nonselective (PDE types 3, 4, and 5) inhibition by theophylline.

Theophylline is extensively (>70%) metabolized in the liver by N-demethylation by CYP 1A2 primarily to 3-methylxanthine. Theophylline is also 8-hydroxylated to 1,3 dimethyluric acid, which is subsequently N-demethylated to 1-methyluric acid. In neonates it is directly 7-methylated to caffeine. About 10% is excreted in the urine unchanged. Many drug classes affect its metabolism and thus serum concentrations (see later).

Roflumilast is metabolized in liver by CYP 3A4 and 1A2 to roflumilast N-oxide (also a potent PDE4 inhibitor) and then O-deacylated and glucuronidated for urinary excretion.

Clinical Pharmacology

PHARMACOKINETICS, PHARMACODYNAMICS, AND THERAPEUTIC EFFECTS

Theophylline is 40% protein bound with a volume of distribution of 0.5 L/kg. Oral theophylline is well absorbed from the gastrointestinal tract, resulting in 90% to 100% bioavailability, with peak serum levels occurring within 1 to 2 hours of ingestion. Sustained release formulations are available due to the relatively short half-life of 8 hours in healthy adults. The elimination half-life varies widely: from 30 hours in premature neonates to 3.5 hours in children, 8 hours in nonsmoking adults, 5 hours in smoking adults, and 24 hours in those with NYHA class III-IV congestive heart failure. The intravenous dose required to achieve a therapeutic concentration of 10 to 20 µg/mL varies fourfold in an otherwise healthy adult population. For rapid treatment of acute bronchospasm, a loading dose followed by maintenance infusion is frequently employed. In children, the rate of clearance of theophylline is 40% greater than in adults.

Following oral administration of roflumilast, the time to peak plasma concentrations is 1 hour, with nearly 99% being protein bound. With daily dosing, steady-state levels are achieved in 4 days with a mean plasma half-life of 17 hours.

The role of methylxanthines as anti-inflammatory and the role of bronchodilators in asthma and COPD are well established. However, methylxanthines are also respiratory stimulants and have been evaluated in central apnea, obstructive sleep apnea, and periodic breathing (Cheyne-Stokes respiration).[59] Clinical trials have shown a benefit in central sleep apnea but not obstructive sleep apnea.[60] In animal studies, roflumilast did not protect against leukotriene D4 or serotonin-induced bronchoconstriction, and there is no evidence that roflumilast is bronchodilatory in humans with COPD. This suggests that its primary therapeutic benefit is due to its anti-inflammatory effects via PDE4 inhibition in airway inflammatory cells.

ADVERSE EFFECTS

Adverse reactions are uncommon at serum theophylline levels below 20 μg/mL. Adverse reactions at serum concentrations between 20 and 25 μg/mL include nausea, vomiting, diarrhea, headache, and insomnia. Symptoms of overdosage at concentrations over 30 μg/mL include seizures, tachyarrhythmias, congestive heart failure, tachypnea, hematemesis, and reflex hyperexcitability. Methylxanthine use during anesthesia was also problematic due to the release of catecholamines in combination with volatile anesthetics that sensitized the myocardium to their arrhythmogenic effects (e.g., halothane).[61] Moreover, aminophylline does not add additional bronchodilatory effect to the bronchodilation achieved by maintenance levels of volatile anesthetics.[62]

Drug Interactions

Many medications can increase the serum concentrations of theophylline enhancing their potential for toxicity including cimetidine, mexiletine, ticlopidine, propranolol, ciprofloxacin, alcohol, allopurinol, disulfiram, erythromycin, and estrogens. Cigarette and marijuana smoking and medications that induce liver metabolism (e.g., carbamazepine, phenytoin, thiabendazole) reduce theophylline serum concentrations.

SPECIAL POPULATIONS

Theophylline should be used with caution in patients with active peptic ulcer disease, seizure disorders, cardiac arrhythmias, compromised cardiac function, angina, hypertension, hyperthyroidism, or liver disease.

Clinical Application

Theophylline is among the most widely prescribed medication for the treatment of asthma worldwide, but is recommended as second- or third-line therapy behind inhaled corticosteroids and inhaled β-agonists due to theophylline's potential for systemic toxicity. By the 1980s, several studies reported that inhaled β2-agonists were superior to aminophylline or theophylline in acute asthmatic exacerbations.[63] Aminophylline and theophylline formulations are less commonly used as maintenance therapy in the United States due to their low therapeutic index.

LEUKOTRIENE RECEPTOR INHIBITORS AND 5-LIPOXYGENASE INHIBITORS

Structure-Activity

Leukotrienes are synthesized from arachidonic acid by 5-lipoxygnase. They are so named due to their source from leukocytes and the presence of three conjugated double bonds in their structure. The discovery that the slow reacting substance of anaphylaxis (SRS-A) was a mixture of leukotrienes

Table 26-3. Targeted Anti-inflammatory Therapies for Bronchospasm

	FORMULATION	MODE OF ACTION
Leukotriene Receptor Antagonists		
Zafirukast	Accolate	Leukotriene D4 and E4 receptor antagonist
Montelukast	Singulair	Cysteinyl leukotriene receptor antagonist
5-Lipoxygenase Inhibitor		
Zileuton	Zyflo	Inhibits leukotriene synthesis
Cell Release Inhibitors		
Omalizumab	Xolair	Inhibits IgE binding to mast cells and basophils

released from mast cells and basophils sparked the search for antagonists of leukotriene receptors. Independent medicinal chemistry strategies were employed to identify both of the antagonists in clinical use (Table 26-3). Montelukast was discovered by modifying a quinoline with leukotriene structural elements. Zafirlukast was based on a compound incorporating components from both FPL 55712 and the natural leukotrienes.[64]

Mechanism

The cysteinyl leukotrienes LTC_4, LTD_4, LTE_4 and LTB_4 are products of plasma membrane phospholipids that increase smooth muscle contraction, microvascular permeability, and airway mucus secretion. These leukotrienes mediate their airway effects primarily through the $CysLT_1$ receptor subtype, which is widely expressed on cells including mast cells, monocytes, macrophages, eosinophils, basophils, neutrophils, T and B lymphocytes, airway smooth muscle cells, microvascular endothelial cells, bronchial fibroblasts, and pluripotent hemopoietic stem cells.[65,66] The enzyme 5-lipoxygenase converts arachidonic acid to LTA_4, an upstream precursor to the active cysteinyl leukotrienes. This enzyme is inhibited by the only 5-lipoxygenase inhibitor approved for asthma, zileuton. Montelukast and zafirlukast are antagonists of the $CysLT_1$ receptor that directly block the effect of LTC_4, LTD_4, and LTE_4 on this receptor.

Clinical Pharmacology

PHARMACOKINETICS, PHARMACODYNAMICS, METABOLISM

The leukotriene receptor antagonists montelukast and zafirlukast are rapidly absorbed after oral administration and are more than 99% bound to albumin. They achieve peak plasma concentrations within 3 to 5 hours and undergo extensive metabolism by cytochrome P450 subtypes in the liver. Zileuton causes an increase in liver enzymes in 2% of patients and should be avoided in patients with active liver disease or persistent elevation of liver enzymes.

Drug Interactions

Certain anticonvulsants (phenytoin, carbamazepine, oxcarbazepine, phenobarbital) and rifamycin antibiotics can decrease plasma concentrations of montelukast. Coadministration of zafirlukast with warfarin increases prothrombin times by 35%. Coadministration of zafirlukast with oral theophylline reduces zafirlukast plasma concentrations by 30%, and coadministration of zafirlukast with aspirin decreases zafirlukast concentrations. Zileuton is a weak inhibitor of CYP 1A2 and has been shown to increase theophylline and propranolol concentrations. It can increase prothrombin times in patients coadministered warfarin.

Clinical Application

Leukotriene receptor antagonists and 5-lipoxygenase inhibitors are commonly used as adjuvant therapy in asthma.[67-69] The potential for toxicity from this therapy appears less than that of inhaled steroids, and leukotriene receptor antagonists can allow a reduction in the amount of steroid use. They are effective as additional therapy for acute asthma. An investigational intravenous formulation of montelukast has an onset within 10 minutes and improves airway obstruction for at least 2 hours.[70]

MONOCLONAL ANTIBODIES

Structure-Activity

Omalizumab is a recombinant human IgG$_1$κ monoclonal antibody (150 kDa) that selectively binds to human IgE and is effective as an adjuvant therapy in adults with moderate to severe asthma. This antibody binds to the constant region of circulating IgE molecules preventing their binding to the high (FceRI) and low (FceRII) affinity IgE receptors on mast cells, basophils, B lymphocytes, dendritic cells, and macrophages, impairing mediator release from these cells. One IgE molecule has two antigenic binding sites for omalizumab and omalizumab in turn has two antigen binding sites, thus IgE/anti-IgE complexes are formed with molecular masses of 500 to 1000 kDa.

Mechanism and Metabolism

As an anti-IgE antibody, omalizumab binds to circulating IgE molecules interrupting the allergic cascade. It is effective at treating patients with allergic asthma that exhibit a high concentration of IgE molecules. Neutralizing IgE molecules prevents the activation of degranulation of many IgE-presenting cells including mast cells and basophils and thus prevents release of histamine, leukotrienes, and cytokines involved in the inflammatory component of reactive airway disease.

The IgE/anti-IgE small immune complexes do not precipitate in the kidney and are easily cleared by the liver reticuloendothelial system (RES) and endothelial cells. Intact IgG is also excreted in the bile with serum elimination half-life of 26 days.

Clinical Pharmacology

PHARMACOKINETICS, PHARMACODYNAMICS, AND THERAPEUTIC EFFECTS

Omalizumab is administered subcutaneously every 2 to 4 weeks based on serum IgE levels and body weight. Absorption is slow after subcutaneous injection with peak serum concentrations achieved at 7 to 8 days with 62% bioavailability. Serum free IgE levels are reduced within 1 hour of the initial dose of omalizumab. In addition to a reduction in serum free IgE levels, omalizumab reduces expression of high affinity IgE receptors on inflammatory cells and reduces circulating numbers of eosinophils. The beneficial effects of omalizumab in severe persistent asthmatics include improvements in respiratory systems and quality of life, a reduction in emergency room visits, and reduction in steroid use and rescue asthma medications.[71-73]

ADVERSE EFFECTS

Anaphylaxis has been reported in 0.2% of patients receiving omalizumab occurring as early as the first dose and as late as 1 year after the initiation of therapy. Although concerns were raised about a small increase in malignant neoplasms and a case of lymphoma in early studies with omalizumab, subsequent review by independent oncologists reported no causal relationship between omalizumab and cancer development.[73] Fever, arthralgia, and rash sometimes accompanied by lymphadenopathy occur in some patients 1 to 5 days after omalizumab injections. Parasitic infections are more common in patients receiving omalizumab than in controls.[74]

Clinical Application

Omalizumab is used as adjuvant therapy in severe persistent asthmatics older than 6 years who have elevated serum IgE levels and who demonstrate positive skin tests or in vitro reactivity to a seasonal aeroallergen when symptoms are not adequately controlled with an inhaled corticosteroid.

ANESTHETIC AGENTS AS BRONCHODILATORS

Most volatile anesthetics are potent bronchodilators yet the mechanism by which this occurs is unknown.[75] With the exception of desflurane, volatile anesthetics dose-dependently bronchodilate airways and protect against reflex-induced bronchoconstriction during intubation in both asthmatics and patients with COPD.[76-78] The mechanisms of direct airway smooth muscle relaxation by inhaled anesthetics include reduction in Ca^{2+} sensitivity of contractile proteins and interruption of G protein coupling of procontractile receptor agonists (e.g., acetylcholine).[79,80]

The intravenous anesthetics vary in their ability to blunt bronchoconstriction induced by intubation. Historically, ketamine was the induction drug of choice for asthmatics due to its release of catecholamines with their effect on airway smooth muscle β$_2$-adrenoceptors. In the mid-1990s it was recognized that propofol is very protective against bronchoconstriction during intubation in both asthmatics and patients with COPD compared to thiobarbiturates or etomidate.[81,82] A direct clinical comparison between propofol and ketamine for bronchoprotective effects has not been done. The mechanism of bronchoprotection afforded by intravenous anesthetics is incompletely understood but might include direct interaction of anesthetics with GABA$_A$ receptors expressed on airway smooth muscle.[83] Intravenous, epidural, and inhaled local anesthetics have all been shown to inhibit histamine-induced bronchoconstriction.[84-86]

Table 26-4. Mucolytics, Surfactants, and α_1 Proteinase Inhibitors

	FORMULATION	MODE OF ACTION
Mucolytics		
Acetylcysteine	Mucomyst	Reduced viscosity of mucus by cleavage of disulfide bonds
Dornase alfa	Pulmozyme	Reduced viscosity of mucus by cleavage of leukocyte DNA
Surfactant Substitutes		
Poractant alfa	Curosurf	Reduced surface tension in alveolus
Calfactant	Infasurf	
Beractant	Survanta	
α_1 proteinase inhibitors	Aralast Glassia Prolastin-C Zemaira	Inhibit neutrophil elastase in α_1-proteinase inhibitor genetic deficiency, protecting protein components of alveolar wall

MUCOLYTIC THERAPIES

Structure-Activity

Inhaled mucolytics allow direct deposition of drugs to reduce mucus viscosity in pulmonary diseases, primarily cystic fibrosis (Table 26-4). Acetylcysteine by inhalation serves as a sulfhydryl donor to cleave disulfide bounds in mucus resulting in lower viscosity. Acetylcysteine is also used orally as an antidote for acetaminophen overdose. Dornase alfa is a recombinant human deoxyribonuclease I enzyme produced in cultured Chinese hamster ovary cells. The 37 kDa native human enzyme cleaves DNA from injured and dead leukocytes reducing the overall viscosity of pulmonary secretions.

Mechanism and Metabolism

Respiratory mucins contain disulfide bonds that contribute to the structure of mature mucins and are the target of sulfhydryl donors such as acetylcysteine. Tenacious airway secretions of cystic fibrosis arise in part from dying and dead leukocytes responding to airway infection and inflammation. The DNA of these dying cells contributes to the viscosity of secretions and is the substrate for dornase alfa degradation.

Acetylcysteine is rapidly deacetylated or oxidized in vivo to form cysteine or diacetylcystine, respectively.

Clinical Pharmacology

PHARMACOKINETICS, PHARMACODYNAMICS, AND THERAPEUTIC AND ADVERSE EFFECTS

Inhalation of dornase alfa in cystic fibrosis patients results in measurable DNAse activity in sputum within 15 minutes. Inhalation of 10 mg of dornase alfa three times a day for 6 days did not raise serum DNAse levels above endogenous levels.[87] Inhaled acetylcysteine has been associated with stomatitis, bronchoconstriction, nausea, vomiting, fever, rhinorrhea, and drowsiness. Bronchoconstriction responds to bronchodilators but gas exchange can initially worsen due to thin secretions traveling to more distal airways.[88,89] Thus acetylcysteine delivery through a bronchoscope or endotracheal tube should be followed by suctioning to prevent deterioration in gas exchange.[90]

Clinical Application

Inhaled acetylcysteine (by nebulization or direct tracheal instillation) is indicated in patients with viscous, increased or inspissated secretions with chronic COPD, tuberculosis, primary amyloidosis of the lung, or cystic fibrosis. Dornase alfa is effective in lowering the viscosity of pulmonary secretions with high DNA content from injured and dead leukocytes such as in cystic fibrosis. Twice daily use of dornase alfa reduces the incidence of pulmonary infections requiring parenteral antibiotics by 29%.

EMERGING DEVELOPMENTS

Smoking

Although the topic is not traditionally a part of pulmonary pharmacology, perioperative smoking cessation therapy is an emerging part of anesthesia practice.[91] As part of a multidisciplinary team, anesthesiologists are increasingly participating in individualized efforts to promote smoking cessation in perioperative patients.[92] Often regarded as the single most preventable cause of premature death in industrialized societies, smoking is also a major underlying factor in excess postoperative morbidity and mortality.[93] Studies suggest that a coordinated smoking cessation program instituted perioperatively when patients are motivated about personal health can be effective in helping smokers to quit the habit.[94,95] Some advocate that anesthesiologists should play a lead role in this process.[96,97] This mandates that anesthesiologists must be conversant with drug and nondrug therapies applied to assist patients in smoking cessation. The anesthesiologist, as a perioperative physician, has the opportunity to participate in interventions that have long-term impacts on pulmonary health. The stress of the perioperative period has been recognized as a "teachable moment," a time in the patient's life when he or she may be most receptive to advice regarding smoking cessation.[98]

Novel Therapeutic Approaches

It has long been recognized that clinical asthma is a mixture of disease phenotypes such that a variety of mechanisms can lead to airway hyperresponsiveness.[99] Future pharmacologic therapy will undoubtedly make use of better phenotypic and genotypic characterization in individual patients. This may allow more directed therapy particularly in the area of anti-inflammatory therapies where nonspecific steroid approaches might be replaced by targeting specific immunomodulatory mediators such as elevated IgE (e.g., omalizumab) or specific interleukins (e.g., IL-13).[100,101]

A nonpharmacologic therapy directed at airway smooth muscle hyperresponsiveness is bronchial thermoplasty. The belief is that eliminating airway smooth muscle from mid-sized airways by heat destruction will improve asthma symptoms. This invasive procedure, which requires repeated bronchoscopies, resulted in some short-term pulmonary complications but long-term improvements in the use of rescue medications, prebronchodilator FEV_1, and quality of life measurements.[102] A blinded randomized trial reported an improvement in scores on an asthma quality of life questionnaire but no statistical change in several secondary effectiveness end-points including FEV_1 (before or after bronchodilator), symptom-free days, or rescue medication use.[103] Thus the mechanism, efficacy, and future of this therapy currently are unresolved.[104,105]

KEY POINTS

- Inhaled corticosteroids are the preferred initial therapy for the management of asthma.
- The use of LABAs has been associated with increased risk of asthma-related death.
- Anticholinergics block acetylcholine, released from parasympathetic nerves, acting upon muscarinic receptors on airway smooth muscle. Anticholinergics are more often efficacious in chronic obstructive lung disease than in asthma.
- Intubation or suctioning can induce reflex-induced bronchoconstriction via a reflex arc that can be blocked at different levels by local anesthetics, intravenous anesthetics, or volatile anesthetics.
- Propofol is the preferred intravenous anesthetic for induction in patients with asthma or chronic obstructive lung disease.
- Volatile anesthetics, with the exception of desflurane, are potent bronchodilators.
- Personalized therapy for asthma is evolving with the introduction of monoclonal antibodies directed against IgE or IL-13.

Key References

Brown RH, Mitzner W, Zerhouni E, et al. Direct in vivo visualization of bronchodilation induced by inhalational anesthesia using high-resolution computed tomography. *Anesthesiology*. 1993;78:295-300. Direct visualization and quantification of airway bronchodilation during inhalation of volatile anesthetics. (Ref. 75)

Castro M, Musani AI, Mayse ML, et al. Bronchial thermoplasty: a novel technique in the treatment of severe asthma. *Ther Adv Respir Dis*. 2010;4:101-116. The first randomized and blinded clinical trial of bronchial thermoplasty for control of asthma. (Ref. 103)

Chowdhury BA, Seymour SM, Levenson MS. Assessing the safety of adding LABAs to inhaled corticosteroids for treating asthma. *N Engl J Med*. 2011;364:2473-2475. Summarizes the ongoing controversy and planned clinical trials to assess the safety of using long-acting β_2-adrenoceptor agonists as combined therapy with inhaled corticosteroids. (Ref. 6)

Chu EK, Drazen JM. Asthma: one hundred years of treatment and onward. *Am J Respir Crit Care Med*. 2005;171:1202-1208. This historical review summarizes the origins of pharmacologic therapy for hyperreactive airway disease. (Ref. 32)

Haxhiu MA, Kc P, Moore CT, et al. Brain stem excitatory and inhibitory signaling pathways regulating bronchoconstrictive responses. *J Appl Physiol*. 2005;98:1961-1982. Defines the neural signaling pathways that mediate reflex-induced bronchoconstriction induced by airway irritation. (Ref. 34)

Lazarus SC. Clinical practice. Emergency treatment of asthma. *N Engl J Med*. 2010;363:755-764. Current recommended therapy for treating acute bronchospasm in the emergency department, which is applicable to other acute care settings such as the operating room and intensive care unit. (Ref. 23)

Pizov R, Brown RH, Weiss YS, et al. Wheezing during induction of general anesthesia in patients with and without asthma: a randomized blinded trial. *Anesthesiology*. 1995;82:1111-1116. Established propofol as the preferred intravenous anesthetic for anesthetic induction in asthmatics. (Ref. 81)

References

1. Salter H. *Asthma, Its Pathology and Treatment*. London: John Churchill; 1860.
2. Osler W, McCrae T. *Bronchial Asthma. The Principles and Practice of Medicine*. 8th ed. New York, London: D. Appleton and Co; 1914:627-631.
3. Melland B. The treatment of spasmodic asthma by the hypodermic injection of adrenalin. *Lancet*. 1910;i:1407-1411.
4. Fraser PM, Speizer FE, Waters SD, Doll R, Mann NM. The circumstances preceding death from asthma in young people in 1968 to 1969. *Br J Dis Chest*. 1971;65:71-84.
5. Inman WH, Adelstein AM. Rise and fall of asthma mortality in England and Wales in relation to use of pressurised aerosols. *Lancet*. 1969;2:279-285.
6. Chowdhury BA, Seymour SM, Levenson MS. Assessing the safety of adding LABAs to inhaled corticosteroids for treating asthma. *N Engl J Med*. 2011;364:2473-2475.
7. Cazzola M, Testi R, Matera MG. Clinical pharmacokinetics of salmeterol. *Clin Pharmacokinet*. 2002;41:19-30.
8. Anderson GP, Linden A, Rabe KF. Why are long-acting beta-adrenoceptor agonists long-acting? *Eur Respir J*. 1994;7:569-578.
9. Hochhaus G, Schmidt EW, Rominger KL, Mollmann H. Pharmacokinetic/dynamic correlation of pulmonary and cardiac effects of fenoterol in asthmatic patients after different routes of administration. *Pharm Res*. 1992;9:291-297.
10. Taburet AM, Schmit B. Pharmacokinetic optimisation of asthma treatment. *Clin Pharmacokinet*. 1994;26:396-418.
11. Bleecker ER, Tinkelman DG, Ramsdell J, et al. Proventil HFA provides bronchodilation comparable to Ventolin over 12 weeks of regular use in asthmatics. *Chest*. 1998;113:283-289.
12. Gumbhir-Shah K, Kellerman DJ, DeGraw S, Koch P, Jusko WJ. Pharmacokinetic and pharmacodynamic characteristics and safety of inhaled albuterol enantiomers in healthy volunteers. *J Clin Pharmacol*. 1998;38:1096-1106.
13. Brogden RN, Faulds D. Salmeterol xinafoate. A review of its pharmacological properties and therapeutic potential in reversible obstructive airways disease. *Drugs*. 1991;42:895-912.
14. Barnhart ER. *Salmeterol xinofoate. Physician's Desk Reference*. Oradell, NJ: Medical Economics Co; 1998:108-111.
15. Bennett JA, Tattersfield AE. Time course and relative dose potency of systemic effects from salmeterol and salbutamol in healthy subjects. *Thorax*. 1997;52:458-464.
16. Castle W, Fuller R, Hall J, Palmer J. Serevent nationwide surveillance study: comparison of salmeterol with salbutamol in asthmatic patients who require regular bronchodilator treatment. *Br Med J*. 1993;306:1034-1037.
17. Salpeter SR, Buckley NS, Ormiston TM, Salpeter EE. Meta-analysis: effect of long-acting beta-agonists on severe asthma exacerbations and asthma-related deaths. *Ann Intern Med*. 2006;144:904-912.
18. Global Initiative for Asthma (GINA). GINA At-a-Glance Asthma Management Reference. Available at: http://www.ginasthma.org/uploads/users/files/GINA_AtAGlance_2011.pdf. Accessed August 17, 2011.
19. Expert Panel Report 3 (EPR3): Guidelines for the Diagnosis and Management of Asthma. Available at: http://www.nhlbi.nih.gov/guidelines/asthma/index.htm. Accessed August 17, 2011.
20. Manthous CA, Hall JB, Schmidt GA, Wood LD. Metered-dose inhaler versus nebulized albuterol in mechanically ventilated patients. *Am Rev Respir Dis*. 1993;148:1567-1570.
21. Ari A, Areabi H, Fink JB. Evaluation of aerosol generator devices at 3 locations in humidified and non-humidified circuits during adult mechanical ventilation. *Respir Care*. 2010;55:837-844.
22. Fink JB, Dhand R, Duarte AG, Jenne JW, Tobin MJ. Aerosol delivery from a metered-dose inhaler during mechanical ventilation. An in vitro model. *Am J Respir Crit Care Med*. 1996;154:382-387.
23. Lazarus SC. Clinical practice. Emergency treatment of asthma. *N Engl J Med*. 2010;363:755-764.
24. Leach CL. The CFC to HFA transition and its impact on pulmonary drug development. *Respir Care*. 2005;50:1201-1208.
25. Gentile DA, Skoner DP. New asthma drugs: small molecule inhaled corticosteroids. *Curr Opin Pharmacol*. 2010;10:260-265.
26. Casarosa P, Kollak I, Kiechle T, et al. Functional and biochemical rationales for the 24-hour-long duration of action of olodaterol. *J Pharmacol Exp Ther*. 2011;337:600-609.

27. Connolly S, Alcaraz L, Bailey A, et al. Design-driven LO: the discovery of new ultra long acting dibasic beta(2)-adrenoceptor agonists. *Bioorg Med Chem Lett.* 2011;21:4612-4616.
28. Anzueto A, Miravitlles M. Efficacy of tiotropium in the prevention of exacerbations of COPD. *Ther Adv Respir Dis.* 2009;3:103-111.
29. Anthonisen NR, Connett JE, Enright PL, Manfreda J. Hospitalizations and mortality in the Lung Health Study. *Am J Respir Crit Care Med.* 2002;166:333-339.
30. Singh S, Loke YK, Furberg CD. Inhaled anticholinergics and risk of major adverse cardiovascular events in patients with chronic obstructive pulmonary disease: a systematic review and meta-analysis. *JAMA.* 2008;300:1439-1450.
31. Wood-Baker R, Cochrane B, Naughton MT. Cardiovascular mortality and morbidity in chronic obstructive pulmonary disease: the impact of bronchodilator treatment. *Intern Med J.* 2010;40: 94-101.
32. Chu EK, Drazen JM. Asthma: one hundred years of treatment and onward. *Am J Respir Crit Care Med.* 2005;171:1202-1208.
33. Scullion JE. The development of anticholinergics in the management of COPD. *Int J Chron Obstruct Pulmon Dis.* 2007;2: 33-40.
34. Haxhiu MA, Kc P, Moore CT, et al. Brain stem excitatory and inhibitory signaling pathways regulating bronchoconstrictive responses. *J Appl Physiol.* 2005;98:1961-1982.
35. Yohannes AM, Willgoss TG, Vestbo J. Tiotropium for treatment of stable COPD: a meta-analysis of clinically relevant outcomes. *Respir Care.* 2011;56:477-487.
36. Joos GF, Schelfhout VJ, Pauwels RA, et al. Bronchodilatory effects of aclidinium bromide, a long-acting muscarinic antagonist, in COPD patients. *Respir Med.* 2010;104:865-872.
37. Alagha K, Bourdin A, Tummino C, Chanez P. An update on the efficacy and safety of aclidinium bromide in patients with COPD. *Ther Adv Respir Dis.* 2011;5:19-28.
38. Gavalda A, Miralpeix M, Ramos I, et al. Characterization of aclidinium bromide, a novel inhaled muscarinic antagonist, with long duration of action and a favorable pharmacological profile. *J Pharmacol Exp Ther.* 2009;331:740-751.
39. Schacke H, Schottelius A, Docke WD, et al. Dissociation of transactivation from transrepression by a selective glucocorticoid receptor agonist leads to separation of therapeutic effects from side effects. *Proc Natl Acad Sci U S A.* 2004;101:227-232.
40. Winkler J, Hochhaus G, Derendorf H. How the lung handles drugs: pharmacokinetics and pharmacodynamics of inhaled corticosteroids. *Proc Am Thorac Soc.* 2004;1:356-363.
41. Fitzgerald JM, Shragge D, Haddon J, et al. A randomized, controlled trial of high dose, inhaled budesonide versus oral prednisone in patients discharged from the emergency department following an acute asthma exacerbation. *Can Respir J.* 2000;7:61-67.
42. Tantisira KG, Lasky-Su J, Harada M, et al. Genomewide association between GLCCI1 and response to glucocorticoid therapy in asthma. *N Engl J Med.* 2011;365:1173-1183.
43. Li JT, Ford LB, Chervinsky P, et al. Fluticasone propionate powder and lack of clinically significant effects on hypothalamic-pituitary-adrenal axis and bone mineral density over 2 years in adults with mild asthma. *J Allergy Clin Immunol.* 1999;103:1062-1068.
44. Lipworth BJ. Systemic adverse effects of inhaled corticosteroid therapy: a systematic review and meta-analysis. *Arch Intern Med.* 1999;159:941-955.
45. Medici TC, Grebski E, Hacki M, Ruegsegger P, Maden C, Efthimiou J. Effect of one year treatment with inhaled fluticasone propionate or beclomethasone dipropionate on bone density and bone metabolism: a randomised parallel group study in adult asthmatic subjects. *Thorax.* 2000;55:375-382.
46. Ljustina-Pribic R, Stojanovic V, Petrovic S. The influence of inhaled fluticasone on bone metabolism and calciuria in asthmatic children. *J Aerosol Med Pulm Drug Deliv.* 2011;24:201-204.
47. De WE, Malfroot A, De S I, Vanbesien J, De SJ. Inhaled budesonide induced Cushing's syndrome in cystic fibrosis patients, due to drug inhibition of cytochrome P450. *J Cyst Fibros.* 2003;2:72-75.
48. Juniper EF, Kline PA, Vanzieghem MA, Ramsdale EH, O'Byrne PM, Hargreave FE. Effect of long-term treatment with an inhaled corticosteroid (budesonide) on airway hyperresponsiveness and clinical asthma in nonsteroid-dependent asthmatics. *Am Rev Respir Dis.* 1990;142:832-836.
49. The Childhood Asthma Management Program Research Group. Long-term effects of budesonide or nedocromil in children with asthma. *N Engl J Med.* 2000;343:1054-1063.
50. Suissa S, Ernst P, Benayoun S, Baltzan M, Cai B. Low-dose inhaled corticosteroids and the prevention of death from asthma. *N Engl J Med.* 2000;343:332-336.
51. Frois C, Wu EQ, Ray S, Colice GL. Inhaled corticosteroids or long-acting beta-agonists alone or in fixed-dose combinations in asthma treatment: a systematic review of fluticasone/budesonide and formoterol/salmeterol. *Clin Ther.* 2009;31:2779-2803.
52. Yawn BP, Raphiou I, Hurley JS, Dalal AA. The role of fluticasone propionate/salmeterol combination therapy in preventing exacerbations of COPD. *Int J Chron Obstruct Pulmon Dis.* 2010;5:165-178.
53. Sharafkhaneh A, Mattewal AS, Abraham VM, Dronavalli G, Hanania NA. Budesonide/formoterol combination in COPD: a US perspective. *Int J Chron Obstruct Pulmon Dis.* 2010;5:357-366.
54. Card GL, England BP, Suzuki Y, et al. Structural basis for the activity of drugs that inhibit phosphodiesterases. *Structure.* 2004;12:2233-2247.
55. Polson JB, Krzanowski JJ, Fitzpatrick DF, Szentivanyi A. Studies on the inhibition of phosphodiesterase-catalyzed cyclic AMP and cyclic GMP breakdown and relaxation of canine tracheal smooth muscle. *Biochem Pharmacol.* 1978;27:254-256.
56. Peach MJ. Stimulation of release of adrenal catecholamine by adenosine 3′:5′-cyclic monophosphate and theophylline in the absence of extracellular Ca2+. *Proc Natl Acad Sci U S A.* 1972;69:834-836.
57. Fredholm BB, Brodin K, Strandberg K. On the mechanism of relaxation of tracheal muscle by theophylline and other cyclic nucleotide phosphodiesterase inhibitors. *Acta Pharmacol Toxicol (Copenh).* 1979;45:336-344.
58. Kong H, Jones PP, Koop A, Zhang L, Duff HJ, Chen SR. Caffeine induces Ca2+ release by reducing the threshold for luminal Ca2+ activation of the ryanodine receptor. *Biochem J.* 2008;414:441-452.
59. Tilley SL. Methylxanthines in asthma. *Handb Exp Pharmacol.* 2011;439-456.
60. Javaheri S, Parker TJ, Wexler L, Liming JD, Lindower P, Roselle GA. Effect of theophylline on sleep-disordered breathing in heart failure. *N Engl J Med.* 1996;335:562-567.
61. Roizen MF, Stevens WC. Multiform ventricular tachycardia due to the interaction of aminophylline and halothane. *Anesth Analg.* 1978;57:738-741.
62. Tobias JD, Kubos KL, Hirshman CA. Aminophylline does not attenuate histamine-induced airway constriction during halothane anesthesia. *Anesthesiology.* 1989;71:723-729.
63. Siegel D, Sheppard D, Gelb A, Weinberg PF. Aminophylline increases the toxicity but not the efficacy of an inhaled beta-adrenergic agonist in the treatment of acute exacerbations of asthma. *Am Rev Respir Dis.* 1985;132:283-286.
64. Bernstein PR. Chemistry and structure-activity relationships of leukotriene receptor antagonists. *Am J Respir Crit Care Med.* 1998;157: S220-S226.
65. Austen KF. The mast cell and the cysteinyl leukotrienes. *Novartis Found Symp.* 2005;271:166-175.
66. Singh RK, Gupta S, Dastidar S, Ray A. Cysteinyl leukotrienes and their receptors: molecular and functional characteristics. *Pharmacology.* 2010;85:336-349.
67. Liu MC, Dube LM, Lancaster J. Acute and chronic effects of a 5-lipoxygenase inhibitor in asthma: a 6-month randomized multicenter trial. Zileuton Study Group. *J Allergy Clin Immunol.* 1996; 98:859-871.
68. Berger W, De Chandt MT, Cairns CB. Zileuton: clinical implications of 5-Lipoxygenase inhibition in severe airway disease. *Int J Clin Pract.* 2007;61:663-676.
69. Amlani S, Nadarajah T, McIvor RA. Montelukast for the treatment of asthma in the adult population. *Expert Opin Pharmacother.* 2011; 12:2119-2128.
70. Camargo CA Jr, Gurner DM, Smithline HA, et al. A randomized placebo-controlled study of intravenous montelukast for the treatment of acute asthma. *J Allergy Clin Immunol.* 2010;125:374-380.
71. Busse WW, Massanari M, Kianifard F, Geba GP. Effect of omalizumab on the need for rescue systemic corticosteroid treatment in patients with moderate-to-severe persistent IgE-mediated allergic asthma: a pooled analysis. *Curr Med Res Opin.* 2007;23:2379-2386.
72. Corren J, Casale T, Deniz Y, Ashby M. Omalizumab, a recombinant humanized anti-IgE antibody, reduces asthma-related emergency

room visits and hospitalizations in patients with allergic asthma. *J Allergy Clin Immunol*. 2003;111:87-90.

73. Rodrigo GJ, Neffen H, Castro-Rodriguez JA. Efficacy and safety of subcutaneous omalizumab vs placebo as add-on therapy to corticosteroids for children and adults with asthma: a systematic review. *Chest*. 2011;139:28-35.

74. Cruz AA, Lima F, Sarinho E, et al. Safety of anti-immunoglobulin E therapy with omalizumab in allergic patients at risk of geohelminth infection. *Clin Exp Allergy*. 2007;37:197-207.

75. Brown RH, Mitzner W, Zerhouni E, Hirshman CA. Direct in vivo visualization of bronchodilation induced by inhalational anesthesia using high-resolution computed tomography. *Anesthesiology*. 1993;78:295-300.

76. Goff MJ, Arain SR, Ficke DJ, Uhrich TD, Ebert TJ. Absence of bronchodilation during desflurane anesthesia: a comparison to sevoflurane and thiopental. *Anesthesiology*. 2000;93:404-408.

77. Klock PA Jr., Czeslick EG, Klafta JM, Ovassapian A, Moss J. The effect of sevoflurane and desflurane on upper airway reactivity. *Anesthesiology*. 2001;94:963-967.

78. Rooke GA, Choi JH, Bishop MJ. The effect of isoflurane, halothane, sevoflurane, and thiopental/nitrous oxide on respiratory system resistance after tracheal intubation. *Anesthesiology*. 1997;86:1294-1299.

79. Jones KA, Wong GY, Lorenz RR, Warner DO, Sieck GC. Effects of halothane on the relationship between cytosolic calcium and force in airway smooth muscle. *Am J Physiol (Lung Cell Mol Physiol)*. 1994;266:L199-L204.

80. Nakayama T, Penheiter AR, Penheiter SG, et al. Differential effects of volatile anesthetics on M3 muscarinic receptor coupling to the Galphaq heterotrimeric G protein. *Anesthesiology*. 2006;105:313-324.

81. Pizov R, Brown RH, Weiss YS, et al. Wheezing during induction of general anesthesia in patients with and without asthma: a randomized blinded trial. *Anesthesiology*. 1995;82:1111-1116.

82. Eames WO, Rooke GA, Wu RS, Bishop MJ. Comparison of the effects of etomidate, propofol, and thiopental on respiratory resistance after tracheal intubation. *Anesthesiology*. 1996;84:1307-1311.

83. Gallos G, Gleason NR, Virag L, et al. Endogenous gamma-aminobutyric acid modulates tonic guinea pig airway tone and propofol-induced airway smooth muscle relaxation. *Anesthesiology*. 2009;110:748-758.

84. Groeben H, Foster WM, Brown RH. Intravenous lidocaine and oral mexiletine block reflex bronchoconstriction in asthmatic subjects. *Am J Respir Crit Care Med*. 1996;154:885-888.

85. Groeben H, Schwalen A, Irsfeld S, Tarnow J, Lipfert P, Hopf HB. High thoracic epidural anesthesia does not alter airway resistance and attenuates the response to an inhalational provocation test in patients with bronchial hyperreactivity. *Anesthesiology*. 1994;81:868-874.

86. Groeben H, Irsfeld S, Stieglitz S, Lipfert P, Hopf HB. Lidocaine and bupivacaine, both dose dependently attenuate the response to

inhalational challenge in awake volunteers with bronchial hyperreactivity. *Anesthesiology*. 1994;81:A1470.

87. Aitken ML, Burke W, McDonald G, Shak S, Montgomery AB, Smith A. Recombinant human DNase inhalation in normal subjects and patients with cystic fibrosis. A phase 1 study. *JAMA*. 1992;267:1947-1951.

88. Kory RC, Hirsch SR, Giraldo J. Nebulization of N-acetylcysteine combined with a bronchodilator in patients with chronic bronchitis. A controlled study. *Dis Chest*. 1968;54:504-509.

89. Lourenco RV, Cotromanes E. Clinical aerosols II. Therapeutic aerosols. *Arch Intern Med*. 1982;142:2299-2308.

90. Lieberman J. The appropriate use of mucolytic agents. *Am J Med*. 1970;49:1-4.

91. Quraishi SA, Orkin FK, Roizen MF. The anesthesia preoperative assessment: an opportunity for smoking cessation intervention. *J Clin Anesth*. 2006;18:635-640.

92. Warner DO. Helping surgical patients quit smoking: why, when, and how. *Anesth Analg*. 2005;101:481-487.

93. Turan A, Mascha EJ, Roberman D, et al. Smoking and perioperative outcomes. *Anesthesiology*. 2011;114:837-846.

94. Sadr AO, Lindstrom D, Adami J, et al. The efficacy of a smoking cessation programme in patients undergoing elective surgery: a randomised clinical trial. *Anaesthesia*. 2009;64:259-265.

95. Moller A, Villebro N, Pedersen T. Interventions for preoperative smoking cessation. *Cochrane Database Syst Rev*. 2001;CD002294.

96. Warner DO. Feasibility of tobacco interventions in anesthesiology practices: a pilot study. *Anesthesiology*. 2009;110:1223-1228.

97. Warner DO. Surgery as a teachable moment: lost opportunities to improve public health. *Arch Surg*. 2009;144:1106-1107.

98. Shi Y, Warner DO. Surgery as a teachable moment for smoking cessation. *Anesthesiology*. 2010;112:102-107.

99. Handoyo S, Rosenwasser LJ. Asthma phenotypes. *Curr Allergy Asthma Rep*. 2009;9:439-445.

100. Kraft M. Asthma phenotypes and interleukin-13–moving closer to personalized medicine. *N Engl J Med*. 2011;365:1141-1144.

101. Corren J, Lemanske RF, Hanania NA, et al. Lebrikizumab treatment in adults with asthma. *N Engl J Med*. 2011;365:1088-1098.

102. Pavord ID, Cox G, Thomson NC, et al. Safety and efficacy of bronchial thermoplasty in symptomatic, severe asthma. *Am J Respir Crit Care Med*. 2007;176:1185-1191.

103. Castro M, Musani AI, Mayse ML, Shargill NS. Bronchial thermoplasty: a novel technique in the treatment of severe asthma. *Ther Adv Respir Dis*. 2010;4:101-116.

104. Shifren A, Chen A, Castro M. Point: efficacy of bronchial thermoplasty for patients with severe asthma. Is there sufficient evidence? Yes. *Chest*. 2011;140:573-575.

105. Michaud G, Ernst A. Counterpoint: efficacy of bronchial thermoplasty for patients with severe asthma. Is there sufficient evidence? Not yet. *Chest*. 2011;140:576-577.

GASTROINTESTINAL AND ENDOCRINE SYSTEMS

Chapter 27

LIVER AND GASTROINTESTINAL PHYSIOLOGY

Randolph H. Steadman, Michelle Braunfeld, and Hahnnah Park

During perioperative management, the gastrointestinal (GI) tract usually receives consideration after the cardiovascular and respiratory systems. However, potential perioperative problems such as aspiration, ileus, and nausea and vomiting are common and significant. Additionally, end-stage liver disease—often associated with multisystem organ failure—can be life threatening. It is incumbent on the anesthesiologist to understand the physiologic basis of these conditions to minimize associated complications and optimize patient outcomes.

LIVER

The liver weighs approximately 1.5 kg, or about 2% of total body weight in an adult. Functionally, the liver metabolizes carbohydrates, proteins, fats, hormones, and foreign substances. In addition, it filters and stores blood; stores vitamins, glycogen and iron; and produces bile and coagulation factors.

Anatomy

The functional unit of the liver is the lobule, or liver acinus, a structure roughly 1×2 mm that consists of plates of hepatocytes located in a radial distribution about a central vein (Figure 27-1). Bile canaliculi are located between the plates and collect bile formed in the hepatocytes. The canaliculi drain into bile ducts that are located at the periphery of the lobule next to portal venules and hepatic arterioles. The bile ducts join to form the common hepatic duct. The cystic duct from the gallbladder and the pancreatic duct join the common hepatic duct before entering the duodenum. The sphincter of Oddi controls the flow of bile into the small intestine.[1,2]

Portal venules empty blood from the GI tract into the hepatic sinusoids, the space between the plates of hepatocytes that serve as the capillaries of the liver. Hepatic arterioles supply well-oxygenated blood to the septa located between the plates of hepatocytes and the sinusoids. The liver typically contains between 50,000 and 100,000 lobules.

The large pores of endothelium lining the sinusoids allow plasma and its proteins to move readily into the tissue spaces surrounding hepatocytes, an area known as the spaces of Disse, or perisinusoidal spaces. This fluid drains into the lymphatic system. The liver is responsible for generating about half of the lymph.

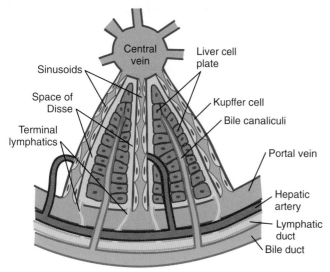

Figure 27-1 The structure of the liver lobule, or acinus. Hepatocytes radiate outward from the central vein. Blood enters the lobule from the periphery via the portal vein and hepatic artery and then flows by the plates of hepatocytes before entering the central vein. Bile flows in the opposite direction.

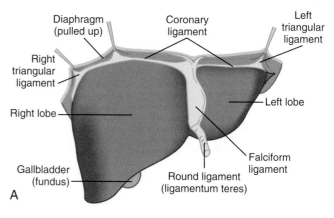

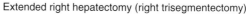

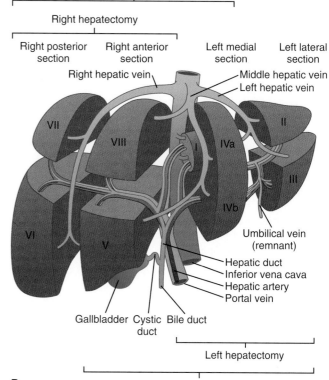

Figure 27-2 Liver anatomy. **A,** Surface anatomy of the liver depicting the right and left lobes, separated by the falciform ligament. **B,** The Couinaud segments of the liver and the accompanying vascular structures. The segments resected during various partial hepatectomies are illustrated.

Macroscopically the liver is divided unequally into right and left lobes by the falciform ligament (Figure 27-2, *A*). More recently a segmental, or surgical, anatomy has been described, known as Couinaud's classification. The liver is divided into eight segments based on the anatomy of the portal and hepatic veins (see Figure 27-2, *B*).

Blood Supply

The liver receives almost 25% of cardiac output via a dual supply. The portal venules conduct blood from the portal vein that drains the GI tract. The portal vein supplies 75% of liver flow, about 1 L/min. The hepatic arterioles supply 25% of blood flow. Each system contributes about 50% of the hepatic oxygen supply (Figure 27-3).

The high hepatic blood flow is due to low vascular resistance in the portal vein. The average portal vein pressure is 9 mmHg while hepatic venous pressure averages 0 mmHg, for a 9 mmHg pressure gradient. However, when hepatocytes are injured and replaced by fibrous tissues, blood flow is impeded, resulting in portal hypertension, the hallmark of cirrhosis. Sinusoidal pressures greater than 5 mmHg are abnormal and define portal hypertension (see later).[3] Sympathetic innervation from T3 to T11 controls resistance in the hepatic venules. Changes in compliance in the hepatic venous system help regulate cardiac output and blood volume. In the presence of reduced portal venous flow, the hepatic artery can increase flow by as much as 100% to maintain hepatic oxygen delivery. The reciprocal relationship between flow in the two afferent vessels is termed the *hepatic arterial buffer response*.[4]

The microcirculation of the liver lobule is divided into three zones that receive varying oxygen content.[5] Zone 1 receives oxygen-rich blood from the adjacent portal vein and hepatic artery. As blood moves through the sinusoid it passes from the intermediate zone 2 into zone 3, which surrounds the central vein. Zone 3 receives blood that has passed through zones 1 and 2, reducing the oxygen content. Pericentral hepatocytes have a greater quantity of cytochrome P450 (CYP)

enzymes and are the site of anaerobic metabolism. Hypoxia and reactive metabolic intermediates from biotransformation affect this zone more prominently than other zones.

Volatile anesthetics decrease hepatic blood flow; however, newer agents (isoflurane, desflurane, and sevoflurane) reduce flow less than older agents such as halothane.[6,7]

Liver Function

STORAGE

Due to its ability to distend, the liver is capable of storing up to 1 L of blood. Thus the liver serves as a reservoir capable of accepting blood, as in the presence of heart failure, or

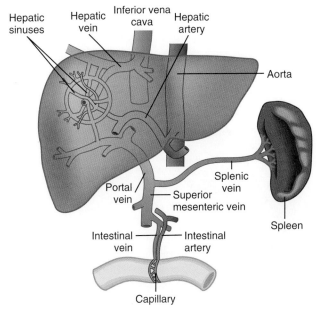

Hepatic sinuses
Hepatic vein
Inferior vena cava
Hepatic artery
Aorta
Portal vein
Splenic vein
Superior mesenteric vein
Spleen
Intestinal vein
Intestinal artery
Capillary

Figure 27-3 The splanchnic circulation.

releasing blood at times of low blood volume. The liver also stores vitamins, particularly vitamins B_{12} (1-year supply), D (3-month supply), and A (10-month supply). Excess body iron is transported via apoferritin to the liver for storage as ferritin, which is released when circulating iron levels are low. Thus the liver apoferritin system serves for iron storage and as a blood iron buffer.

FILTERING AND CLEANSING
Kupffer cells, a type of reticuloendothelial cell, line the venous sinusoids. Kupffer cells are macrophages that phagocytize bacteria that enter the sinusoids from the intestines. Less than 1% of bacteria that enter the liver pass through to the systemic circulation.

METABOLISM OF NUTRIENTS
The liver is involved in energy production and storage from nutrients absorbed from the intestines. The liver helps regulate blood glucose concentrations through its glucose buffer function. This is accomplished by storing glucose as glycogen, converting other carbohydrates (principally fructose and galactose) to glucose, and synthesizing glucose from amino acids and triglycerides (gluconeogenesis).[8] In patients with altered liver function, glucose loads are poorly tolerated, and blood glucose concentration can rise several-fold higher than the postprandial levels found in patients with normal hepatic function.

The liver synthesizes fat, cholesterol, phospholipids, and lipoproteins. It also metabolizes fat efficiently, converting fatty acids to acetyl coenzyme A (CoA), an excellent energy source. Some of the acetyl-CoA enters the citric acid cycle to liberate energy for the liver. The liver generates more acetyl-CoA than it consumes, so it packages the excess as acetoacetic acid for use by the rest of the body via the citric acid cycle. The majority of cholesterol synthesized in the liver is converted to bile salts and secreted in the bile. The remainder is distributed to the rest of the body where it is used to

form cellular membranes. Fat synthesis from protein and carbohydrates occurs almost exclusively in the liver, and the liver is responsible for most fat metabolism.

The liver also plays a key role in protein metabolism. The liver synthesizes all of the plasma proteins with the exception of gamma globulins, which are formed in plasma cells. The liver is capable of forming 15 to 50 g of protein per day, an amount sufficient to replace the body's entire supply of proteins in several weeks. Albumin is the major protein synthesized by the liver, and is the primary determinant of plasma oncotic pressure. The liver also synthesizes the nonessential amino acids from ketoacids, which it also synthesizes.

The liver can deaminate amino acids, a process that is required before their use for energy production or conversion to carbohydrates or fats. Deamination results in the formation of ammonia, which is toxic. Intestinal bacteria are an additional source of ammonia. The liver is responsible for the removal of ammonia through the formation of urea.

SYNTHESIS OF COAGULATION FACTORS
Blood clotting factors, except factors III (tissue thromboplastin), IV (calcium), and VIII (von Willebrand factor), are synthesized in the liver. Vitamin K is required for the synthesis of the Ca^{2+}-binding proteins prothrombin (factor II) and factors VII, IX, and X.

BILE SECRETION
Hepatocytes produce roughly 500 mL of bile daily. Between meals, the high pressure in the sphincter of Oddi diverts bile to the gallbladder for storage (Figure 27-4). The gallbladder holds 35 to 50 mL of bile in concentrated form. The presence of fat in the duodenum causes release of the hormone cholecystokinin from duodenal mucosa, which reaches the gallbladder via the circulation and stimulates gallbladder contraction. Bile contains bile salts, bilirubin, and cholesterol. Bile salts serve as a detergent, solubilizing fat into complexes called micelles, which are absorbed. Bile salts are returned to the liver via the portal vein, completing the enterohepatic circulation. Bile salts are needed for fat absorption, and cholestasis can result in steatorrhea and vitamin K deficiency.

Bilirubin and Jaundice

Bilirubin is the major end product of hemoglobin breakdown, which occurs when red blood cells reach the end of their 120-day life span. After phagocytosis by reticuloendothelial cells, hemoglobin is split into globin and heme. The heme releases iron and a four pyrrole nucleus that forms biliverdin, which is converted to free, or unconjugated, bilirubin. Unconjugated bilirubin is conjugated in the liver, primarily with glucuronic acid, before it is secreted into bile for transport to the intestines. In the intestines, a portion of conjugated bilirubin is converted to urobilinogen by bacteria. Some urobilinogen is reabsorbed from the intestines into the blood, but most is excreted back into the intestines. A small amount is excreted into urine as urobilin. Urobilinogen that remains in the intestines is oxidized to stercobilin and excreted in feces.

Jaundice is the yellow-green tint of body tissues that results from bilirubin accumulation in extracellular fluid. Skin discoloration is usually visible when plasma bilirubin reaches three times normal values. Bilirubin accumulation can occur due to increased breakdown of hemoglobin (hemolysis) or

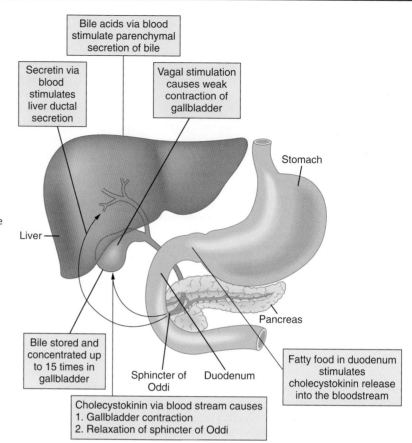

Figure 27-4 Neural and hormonal factors that regulate bile secretion.

obstruction of bile ducts. Hemolytic jaundice is associated with an increase in unconjugated (indirect) bilirubin, while obstructive jaundice is associated with increases in conjugated (direct) bilirubin.[9]

Liver Regeneration

The liver has the unique ability to restore itself after injury or partial hepatectomy. As much as two thirds of the liver can be removed with regeneration of the remaining liver in a matter of weeks.[10] Control over this process is not completely understood, but hepatocyte growth factor, produced by mesenchymal cells in the liver, is involved. Other growth factors, such as epidermal growth factor (EGF) and cytokines, tumor necrosis factor (TNF), and interleukin-6 can also stimulate regeneration. The mechanism responsible for returning the liver to a quiescent state might involve transforming growth factor-β, a known inhibitor of hepatocyte proliferation. The signal for cessation of regeneration appears to be related to the ratio of liver to body weight.[10,11] In the presence of inflammation, as with viral hepatitis, regeneration is significantly impaired.

Portal Hypertension

Ongoing inflammation results in fibrosis that constricts blood flow in the sinusoids. An increase in pressure of 5 to 7 mmHg can result in transudation of lymph from the surface of the liver into the peritoneal cavity. Larger pressure increases, to 15 mmHg, can increase lymphatic flow as much as 20-fold,

which overwhelms the ability to reabsorb this protein-rich fluid, causing formation of ascites.[12]

Resistance to portal blood flow causes collateral vessels to develop between portal and systemic veins. With increased pressure in the splenic vein, collateral vessels to esophageal veins develop. These enlarge and protrude into the esophageal lumen, producing esophageal varicies. Variceal size predicts the likelihood of rupture. Within 2 years of diagnosis of portal hypertension, approximately 30% of patients suffer variceal hemorrhage.[13] The 6-week mortality after variceal hemorrhage is 30%, which increases to 50% with a second episode of bleeding. Prophylaxis to prevent bleeding includes nonselective β blockers, long-acting nitrates, and endoscopic ligation.[14]

Portal hypertension results in portosystemic shunting. Shunted blood circumvents the filtering system of the liver. This results in the entry of drugs, ammonia, and other toxins normally handled by the liver into the systemic circulation; hepatic encephalopathy often ensues.[15] Splanchnic vasodilatation reduces renal perfusion, resulting in renal failure (hepatorenal syndrome). During the early stages of acute renal injury the kidneys can be functionally normal and the changes reversible. In the absence of improvement in liver function, renal injury can become permanent.[16]

Systemic vasodilatation leads to hyperdynamic circulation characterized by low normal blood pressure, low systemic vascular resistance and high cardiac output. Response to vasoconstrictors is often attenuated due to endogenous vasodilators, an ineffective splanchnic reservoir, and increased sympathetic tone.[17]

Hepatic Drug Metabolism and Excretion

The liver metabolizes and excretes many drugs into the bile. The liver is also responsible for metabolism of a number of hormones, including thyroxine and the steroids estrogen, cortisol, and aldosterone.

Intrinsic hepatic clearance of a compound divided by the hepatic blood flow determines the extraction ratio. The extraction ratio indicates the efficiency with which various drugs are cleared. Efficiently extracted drugs include opioids, β blockers (except atenolol), calcium channel blockers, and tricyclic antidepressants. Poorly extracted drugs include warfarin, aspirin, ethanol, and phenobarbital. Elimination of poorly extracted drugs is limited by intrinsic clearance and/or protein binding rather than hepatic blood flow, while elimination of highly extracted drugs is dependent on blood flow (see Chapter 4).

Anesthetic Pharmacology and the Liver

Volatile anesthetic agents decrease hepatic blood flow. Agents currently in use—isoflurane, sevoflurane, and desflurane—affect hepatic blood flow less than older agents. Despite reductions in hepatic blood flow, liver function testing fails to show alterations of hepatic function after administration of current inhaled anesthetics.[18,19] Fewer data exist on the effects of inhaled anesthetics on patients with chronic liver disease. Central neuraxial blockade decreases hepatic blood flow proportionally to the decrease in systemic blood pressure. Hepatic blood flow can be restored by administration of vasopressors.

Hepatic dysfunction affects the pharmacokinetics of intravenous anesthetics through alterations in protein binding (due to reduced plasma proteins), increases in the volume of distribution, and reductions in hepatic metabolism.[20] The pharmacodynamic effects of opioids and sedatives can be enhanced in end-stage liver failure patients with encephalopathy. Although opioids have been used successfully to treat biliary colic, they can also produce spasm of the sphincter of Oddi.[21] Glucagon, opioid antagonists, nitroglycerin, and atropine reverse this effect. Intermediate duration neuromuscular blocking agents that undergo hepatic elimination have a prolonged duration of action in the presence of liver disease. Atracurium and cisatracurium are not dependent on hepatic elimination, so dosing alterations are not required in patients with hepatic disease.

Etiology and Severity of Liver Disease

The most common causes of liver failure are hepatitis C and alcoholic liver disease. Other causes include biliary cirrhosis, autoimmune disease, drug-induced liver disease, metabolic disorders, and hepatocellular cancer.[22] Biliary cirrhosis includes several forms of cholestatic disease including primary biliary cirrhosis, sclerosing cholangitis, and biliary atresia. Nonalcoholic steatohepatitis (also called fatty liver disease), an increasingly recognized cause, is associated with obesity and type 2 diabetes mellitus. The severity of liver disease can be graded using the Child-Turcotte-Pugh (CTP) scoring system (Table 27-1).[23] Patients with the most severe disease have a CTP score of 10 points or more (class C). These patients have exceedingly high perioperative mortality

Table 27-1. Modified Child-Turcotte-Pugh Scoring System*

PARAMETERS	1 POINT	2 POINTS	3 POINTS
Albumin (g/dL)	>3.5	2.8-3.5	<2.8
Prothrombin time			
Seconds prolonged	<4	4-6	>6
International normalized ratio	<1.7	1.7-2.3	>2.3
Bilirubin (mg/dL)†	<2	2-3	>3
Ascites	Absent	Slight-moderate	Tense
Encephalopathy	None	Grade I-II	Grade III-IV

*Class A = 5.6 points, B = 7 to 9 points, and C = 10 to 15 points.
†For cholestatic diseases (e.g., primarily biliary cirrhosis), the bilirubin level is disproportionate to the impairment in hepatic function and an allowance should be made. For these conditions, assign 1 point for a bilirubin level less than 4 mg/dL, 2 points for a bilirubin level of 4 to 10 mg/dL, and 3 points for a bilirubin level over 10 mg/dL.
Modified from Pugh RN, Murray-Lyon IM, Dawson JL, et al. Transection of the oesophagus for bleeding oesophageal varices. *Br J Surg.* 1973;60:646-649.

(up to 75%).[24] Class B (7-9 points) patients also have significant perioperative mortality (30%). Preoperative risk modification, through treatment of encephalopathy and ascites, appears to reduce risk.[25]

An alternative mortality risk stratification for patients with liver disease undergoing nonhepatic surgery is the Model for End-Stage Liver Disease (MELD) score. The MELD score was developed to predict 90-day mortality in patients undergoing transjugular intrahepatic portosystemic shunt procedures.[26] It has since been validated for risk stratification of patients with liver disease in a number of different settings, including patients awaiting liver transplantation. The MELD score is used to allocate donor grafts to liver transplant candidates with the greatest urgency (highest predicted 90-day mortality).[27] It is calculated as follows: MELD = $3.78 \times \ln$ bilirubin (mg/dL) + $11.2 \times \ln$ INR + $9.57 \times \ln$ creatinine (mg/dL) + 6.43. A pioneering study included 140 peripheral, intraabdominal, and intrathoracic procedures in 131 patients whose MELD scores ranged from 6 to 43. Overall mortality was 16%, which correlated with MELD score and was confined to nonperipheral procedures.[28] Abdominal surgery carries more risk than nonabdominal surgery due to significant reductions in hepatic blood flow.[28,29] Laparoscopic surgery, which is controversial because of the requirement for pneumoperitoneum, appears to reduce perioperative risk.[30]

Hepatic Surgery

Hepatic resection surgery, most commonly for hepatocellular carcinoma and metastatic cancer, has become safer over the last several decades. In a single center series, the overall mortality was 4%, although subgroups with cirrhosis and biliary obstruction had higher mortality (9% and 21%, respectively).[31] This improvement in survival after hepatic resection is attributed to a number of factors, including improved patient selection, volumetric studies designed to assess predicted remnant liver mass, portal vein embolization (to decrease the mass of resected tissue and stimulate regeneration of the liver remnant), and use of intraoperative ultrasound to delineate vascular anatomy and the extent of pathology. Additionally, the success of liver transplantation, with a 5-year patient survival of 74%, has given rise to a generation of hepatobiliary surgeons skilled in liver resection.[32]

Liver transplantation is recognized as definitive management for patients with acute and chronic liver failure. The liver is the second most commonly transplanted organ, after the kidney. Anesthetic management for patients undergoing liver transplantation is challenging due to unpredictable, sometimes massive, blood loss, coagulation abnormalities, electrolyte and acid-base disturbances, and hemodynamic, pulmonary, renal, neurologic, and infectious derangements.[33]

GASTROINTESTINAL TRACT

The GI, or alimentary, tract provides the body with substrates for energy needs and essential nutrients through food digestion and absorption. Water, electrolytes, vitamins, and nutrients are supplied to the body via the exclusive function of the GI tract. Control of the process requires local, nervous system, and hormonal input.

Anatomy

The anatomy of the digestive tract consists of one continuous tube connected with the external environment. It is separated into distinct sections, each adapted to specialized functions (Figure 27-5).

A typical cross section of the gut consists of multiple layers (Figure 27-6). Moving from the outside to within, the gut is made up of the serosa, a longitudinal muscle layer, a circular muscle layer, submucosa, and mucosa. The enteric nervous system plexuses lie within the gut layers. As a barrier to the external environment, an epithelial layer lines the innermost portion of the gut.

Properties of the Gastrointestinal Tract

Food moves forward in the alimentary tract by peristalsis. This movement consists of a contractile ring that circles the gut, moving solids and liquids in front of the contractile ring forward. Peristalsis is stimulated by distention of the gut, chemical, or physical irritation of the epithelial lining in the gut, and strong parasympathetic nerve signals.[34]

Chyme is a semifluid mixture consisting of a mixture of food and stomach secretions. In the stomach and when initially expelled from the stomach, chyme is highly acidic with a pH of around 2. In the duodenum, pancreatic secretions of bicarbonate help to raise its pH (see later).

Respiration and Pharyngeal Swallowing

Swallowing occurs as a negligible interruption of about six seconds to the respiratory cycle. Even while talking, the act of swallowing is so rapid that it poses no threat to respiration.

Lower Esophageal Sphincter

Located between the esophagus and stomach, the smooth muscle of the lower esophageal sphincter, also known as the *gastroesophageal sphincter* or *cardiac sphincter*, remains constricted with an intraluminal pressure of about 30 mmHg while the higher portions of the esophagus remain normally relaxed.[35] Tonic constriction prevents the reflux of acidic stomach contents. Initiated by swallowing, a peristaltic wave helps coordinate the passage of food into the stomach, causing a "receptive relaxation" of the lower esophageal sphincter. Esophageal reflux is prevented by the valvelike mechanism of the distal end of the esophagus, which resists reflux of stomach contents as a result of high intraabdominal pressure.

Achalasia is a disorder in which the lower esophageal sphincter loses the ability to relax in response to swallowing. The esophagus distends, which can lead to chronic regurgitation and aspiration. Another disorder that can lead to reflux is Zenker's diverticulum, a weakness at the junction of

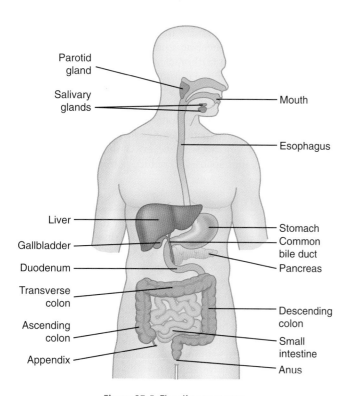

Figure 27-5 The alimentary tract.

Parotid gland
Salivary glands
Mouth
Esophagus
Liver
Stomach
Gallbladder
Common bile duct
Duodenum
Pancreas
Transverse colon
Descending colon
Ascending colon
Small intestine
Appendix
Anus

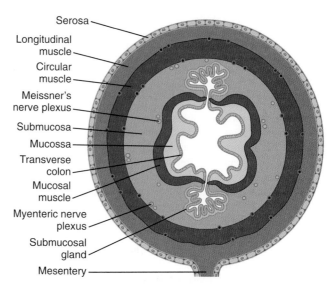

Figure 27-6 A cross section of the intestines.

Serosa
Longitudinal muscle
Circular muscle
Meissner's nerve plexus
Submucosa
Mucossa
Transverse colon
Mucosal muscle
Myenteric nerve plexus
Submucosal gland
Mesentery

the thyropharyngeus and cricopharyngeus muscles in the hypopharynx.

Neural Control

ENTERIC NERVOUS SYSTEM

Important in controlling GI movement and secretion, the enteric nervous system is composed of an outer plexus (myenteric or Auerbach's plexus) and an inner submucosal plexus (Meissner's plexus). The outer plexus lies between the longitudinal and circular muscle layers of the gut and exerts main control over GI movements (see Figure 27-6). The inner plexus is the main control for GI secretion and local blood flow.

The myenteric plexus extends throughout the entire length of the gut as a linear chain of interconnected neurons. Lying within intestinal smooth muscle, the myenteric plexus focuses on muscle control. Upon stimulation, the plexus causes an increase in gut wall tone and in intensity of rhythmical contractions. While mostly associated with excitatory muscle activity, there is also an inhibitory function of the myenteric plexus. Possibly through secretion of vasoactive intestinal polypeptide (or some other inhibitory peptide), the myenteric plexus can inhibit intestinal sphincter muscles such as the pyloric sphincter and the ileocecal valve, which normally impede the movement of gut contents.[36] As a part of the inner wall, the submucosal plexus focuses on controlling local muscle intestinal secretion, local absorption, and local contraction.

PARASYMPATHETIC STIMULATION

The cranial and sacral division of the parasympathetic system stimulates activity of the enteric nervous system. The cranial parasympathetic nerves originate almost entirely in the vagus nerves; however, some also exist at the mouth and pharyngeal regions of the tract. These nerves innervate the esophagus, stomach, pancreas, and a part of the intestines.[35]

The sacral parasympathetic nerves run from the second through fourth sacral segments of the spinal cord (S2 to S4) and pass through to the distal half of the large intestine to end in the anus. Concerned mainly with defecation reflexes, these fibers supply the sigmoidal, rectal, and anal regions of the GI tract.[37,38]

SYMPATHETIC STIMULATION

The sympathetic innervation of the GI tract originates in segments T5 to L2 of the spinal cord. Preganglionic fibers pass from the spinal column to the sympathetic chains. From the chains, sympathetic nerve fibers enter various outlying sympathetic ganglia such as the celiac ganglia and other mesenteric ganglia. These ganglia relay sympathetic stimulation via postganglionic fibers to all parts of the gut by releasing mainly norepinephrine and a smaller amount of epinephrine (see Chapter 12).

In contrast to the parasympathetic system, the sympathetic nervous system primarily inhibits GI tract activity. The strength of stimulation is proportional to the amount of secreted norepinephrine causing a range of inhibition from slight to very strong inhibition capable of causing a cessation of movement.[37,38] Hence, patients undergoing emergency surgery should be considered at risk for aspiration of stomach contents.

Hormonal Control

GI hormones are important for the physiologic control of GI motility. Key hormones, along with their stimuli, site of secretion, and actions are listed in Table 27-2.

Splanchnic Circulation

The blood supply of the GI system is a part of an extensive system called the *splanchnic circulation*. This system supplies and drains multiple organs including the gut, spleen, pancreas, and liver. The arterial supply includes the celiac, superior mesenteric, and inferior mesenteric arteries. Venous drainage of the visceral organs occurs via the splenic, superior mesenteric, and inferior mesenteric veins. Splanchnic blood reaches the liver via the portal vein, which is a confluence of the splenic and superior mesenteric veins. (For more on the splanchnic circulation see the liver section earlier.)

Stomach Emptying

The rate of stomach emptying varies depending upon the signals from the stomach and the duodenum. The duodenum is the primary regulator of the rate at which chyme enters the small intestine.

ENTEROGASTRIC NERVOUS REFLEX

The enterogastric nervous reflex of the duodenum inhibits stomach emptying. Food entering the duodenum elicits various nervous reflexes that regulate the rate of stomach emptying. Factors initiating this reflex include (1) duodenal distention, (2) irritation of duodenal mucosa, (3) acidity of chyme, (4) osmolality of chyme, and (5) presence of certain breakdown products in chyme.[35]

Three parallel nerve circuits control stomach emptying: the gut enteric nervous system from the duodenum to the stomach; extrinsic nerves that travel to the prevertebral sympathetic ganglia and return to the stomach by the inhibitory sympathetic nerve fibers; and the vagus nerves to the brain that inhibit excitatory signals sent to the stomach. Altogether, these affect stomach emptying by inhibiting the propulsive contractions of the pyloric pump and by increasing the tone of the pyloric sphincter.[39]

The association between abdominal mesenteric manipulation and cardiovascular perturbances is well established.[40,41] The proposed mechanism is afferent sympathetic stimulation from mesenteric traction, resulting in systemic vasodilation which provokes a compensatory increase in cardiac output.[41] Although bradycardia is frequently invoked as part of this response, the change in heart rate is variable. The existence of a reflex arc has been suggested in which stimulation of the celiac plexus results in inhibition of sympathetic activity, leading to increased vagal tone and bradycardia. However, bradycardia in response to mesenteric traction has not been consistently demonstrated in controlled studies.

Secretory Functions

The secretory function of the digestive glands is highly specialized to correspond with the food type and amount of food present in the gut. Secretions consist of digestive enzymes for

Table 27-2. Key Gastrointestinal Hormones

HORMONE	STIMULI FOR SECRETION	SITE OF SECRETION	ACTION

Gastrin	Protein
	Distention
	Nerve
	(Acid inhibits release)
		G cells of the antrum, duodenum, and jejunum	Stimulates
			  Gastric acid secretion
			  Mucosal growth

Cholecystokinin	Protein
	Fat
	Acid
		I cells of the duodenum, jejunum, and ileum	Stimulates
			  Pancreatic enzyme secretion
			  Pancreatic bicarbonate secretion
			  Gallbladder contraction
			  Growth of exocrine pancreas
			Inhibits
			  Gastric emptying (stomach contraction)
			  Appetite

Secretin	Acid
	Fat
		S cells of the duodenum, jejunum, and ileum	Stimulates
			  Pepsin secretion
			  Pancreatic bicarbonate secretion
			  Biliary bicarbonate secretion
			  Growth of exocrine pancreas
			Inhibits
			  Gastric acid secretion

Gastric inhibitory peptide	Protein
	Fat
	Carbohydrates
		K cells of the duodenum and jejunum	Stimulates
			  Insulin release
			Inhibits
			  Gastric acids secretion
			  Gastric motility

Motilin	Fat
	Acid
	Nerve
		M cells of the duodenum and jejunum	Stimulates
			  Gastric motility
			  Intestinal motility

Modified from Hall JE. *Guyton and Hall textbook of medical physiology.* 12th ed. Philadelphia: Saunders Elsevier; 2011.

the breakdown of food, and mucus for the protection and lubrication of the GI tract. Estimated amounts and pH of daily secretions are listed in Table 27-3.

AUTONOMIC STIMULATION

The parasympathetic nervous system stimulates an increase in alimentary glandular secretion. The glossopharyngeal and vagus parasympathetic nerves innervate glands of the upper tract; these include the salivary glands, esophageal glands, gastric glands, pancreas, and Brunner's glands in the duodenum. Glands in the large intestine also receive parasympathetic innervation. Other glands of the gut secrete in response to local neural and hormonal stimuli rather than as a result of nerve innervation.

Sympathetic stimulation to alimentary tract glandular secretion is less straightforward than parasympathetic stimulation. Sympathetic stimulation has a dual effect causing a slight increase in glandular secretion if stimulated alone, but with preexisting parasympathetic or hormonal stimulation, sympathetic stimulation reduces secretions. This results from vasoconstriction of blood vessels that supply the glands.[42]

GASTRIC SECRETIONS

The stomach mucosa contains oxyntic or gastric glands and pyloric glands. Oxyntic glands secrete hydrochloric acid, pepsinogen, intrinsic factor and mucus; and pyloric glands secrete mucus and the hormone gastrin.[35]

The pyloric glands contain G cells (or gastrin cells) that secrete gastrin in a large form (G-34) and a smaller form (G-17) when stimulated by protein-containing foods in the antrum of the stomach. Gastrin is released into the blood and rapidly transported to the enterochromaffin-like cells (ECL

Table 27-3. Daily Secretion of Intestinal Juices

	DAILY VOLUME (ML)	pH
Saliva	1000	6.0-7.0
Gastric secretion	1500	1.0-3.5
Pancreatic secretion	1000	8.0-8.3
Bile	1000	7.8
Small intestine secretion	1800	7.5-8.0
Brunner's gland secretion	200	8.0-8.9
Large intestinal secretion	200	7.5-8.0
Total	6700	

Modified from Hall JE. *Guyton and Hall textbook of medical physiology.* 12th ed. Philadelphia: Saunders Elsevier; 2011.

cells) of the stomach. This rapid transport is a result of the rapid mixing of gastric juices in the stomach. Histamine is also rapidly released into the deep oxyntic glands stimulating gastric hydrochloric acid secretion (Figure 27-7).[43, 44]

PANCREATIC DIGESTIVE ENZYMES

The pancreas secretes enzymes that are important for the digestion of proteins, carbohydrates, and fats. For the digestion of proteins, the pancreas releases the proteases trypsin, chymotrypsin, and carboxypolypeptidase. Carboxypolypeptidase is capable of breaking down some proteins entirely to their constituent amino acids. Trypsin and chymotrypsin split proteins into smaller, various sized peptides. Fats are digested by pancreatic lipase, cholesterol esterase, and phospholipase.

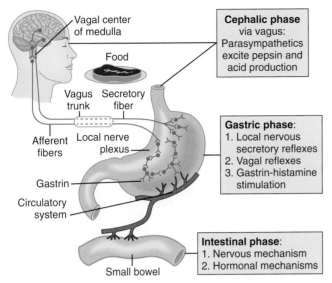

Figure 27-7 Phases of gastric secretion and their regulation.

Pancreatic lipase breaks down triglycerides to fatty acids and glycerol. Cholesterol esterase and phospholipase hydrolyze cholesterol esters and phospholipids, respectively. Pancreatic amylase breaks down carbohydrates (including starch and glycogen), randomly cleaving carbohydrate chains into disaccharides and trisaccharides.

The proteolytic digestive enzymes released by the pancreas are inactive forms (proenzymes) when synthesized (to prevent autodigestion of the pancreas). Release into the intestinal tract and interaction with various components of the intestinal fluid activates the enzymes by proteolytic processing. Trypsinogen can be activated by the enzyme enterokinase, which is released by the intestinal mucosa when contacted by chyme, or by previously secreted and activated trypsin (autoactivation).

BICARBONATE IONS
In addition to digestive enzymes, the pancreas releases large amounts of bicarbonate that neutralize the acidity of chyme as it enters the duodenum. Pancreatic secretions also contain digestive enzymes and water. Pancreatic enzymes are secreted from the acini of the pancreatic glands, whereas bicarbonate ions and water are secreted from the epithelial cells of the ducts that lead from the acini. Concentrations of bicarbonate can reach 145 mM, allowing neutralization of the hydrochloric acid released from the stomach.[45]

Absorption of Nutrients

Most nutrient absorption occurs in the small intestinal mucosa in the valvulae conniventes (folds of Kerckring). The stomach lacks such a highly increased surface area, only allowing absorption of highly lipid-soluble substances, such as alcohol and aspirin, through its epithelium. Villi and the brush border of microvilli contribute to the high absorptive properties of the small intestine by adding to the total absorptive area. Daily absorption from the small intestine consists of several hundred grams of carbohydrates, 100 or more grams of fat, 50 to 100 g of amino acids, 50 to 100 g of salt ions, and 7 to 8 L of water.[35]

GLUCOSE
Glucose is mostly absorbed by an Na^+-dependent glucose cotransporter mediated by a coupled secondary active transport process. These cotransporter proteins use an electrochemical potential difference instead of ATP to function. The movement of Na^+ by ATP through the basolateral membrane into the extracellular compartment by the Na^+/K^+ ATPase reduces Na^+ within the cell. The cotransporter allows Na^+ to move down its concentration gradient into the cell from the intestinal lumen, along with a glucose molecule. After glucose enters cells, it is transported by facilitated diffusion into the bloodstream. The initial active transport of Na^+ out of the epithelial cell provides the electrochemical motive force for moving glucose from the intestinal lumen to the bloodstream.[35]

FATS
Digestion of fats yields monoglycerides and fatty acids. These hydrophobic molecules travel through the alimentary tract in the form of bile micelles, which are soluble in chyme. When they reach the microvilli of the intestinal cell brush border, monoglycerides and fatty acids diffuse through the membrane into epithelial cells. Within epithelial cells, fatty acids and monoglycerides are used to synthesize new triglycerides. These triglycerides are released as chylomicrons and travel through the thoracic lymph duct to be released into the bloodstream.[46]

Gastrointestinal Disorders

Table 27-4 lists GI and neurologic disorders, many of which have anesthetic implications. Risks from these conditions include aspiration, diabetes mellitus, malabsorption with malnutrition, and nausea/vomiting.

Aspiration is a concern in patients who have eaten recently, have acid reflux disease, or disorders of GI motility. Cricoid pressure, or the Sellick maneuver, is the posterior displacement of the cricoid cartilage, intended to close the esophagus and decrease the risk of aspiration. However, cricoid pressure lowers resting lower esophageal sphincter pressure, so the benefit is confined to the physical barrier created. Questions exist about the efficacy of the mechanical effect due to lateral displacement of the esophagus, which is exacerbated by posterior pressure on the cricoid cartilage. Despite little evidence supporting benefit, the use of cricoid pressure is well entrenched. Because it can worsen the view with laryngoscopy, it should be abandoned if difficulties with intubation or ventilation are encountered.[47,48]

Nausea and vomiting are the most common postoperative patient complaints, after pain. The neural pathways involved are both peripheral and central. Vagal and sympathetic afferent nerves can activate the chemoreceptor trigger zone and vomiting center, located in the medulla close to the area postrema and fourth ventricle. Neurotransmitters involved include acetylcholine, dopamine, histamine, substance P, and serotonin. The vestibular apparatus, toxic substances in the GI tract, and opioids can also provide a stimulatory effect. Clinical risk factors for postoperative nausea and vomiting (PONV) include female gender, nonsmoking status, history of motion sickness, perioperative opioid use, and use of inhaled anesthetics, particularly nitrous oxide (see Chapter 29).

Table 27-4. Gastrointestinal Disorders

GI DISORDER	TYPE OF DISORDER	DESCRIPTION	CAUSE	ABNORMALITIES	CLINICAL RELATION
Disorders of swallowing and of the esophagus	Myasthenia gravis or botulism	Prevents normal swallowing	Paralysis of swallowing muscles Failure of neuromuscular transmission Deep anesthesia	Complete abrogation of swallowing action Failure of glottis to close Failure of soft palate and uvula to close the posterior nares → food reflux into nose	Patients under deep anesthesia may aspirate due to blocked reflex mechanism of swallowing
	Achalasia	Failure of lower esophageal sphincter to relax during swallowing	Damage in neural network of myenteric plexus in lower two thirds of esophagus	Lower esophagus remains spastically contracted Food fails to pass from esophagus to stomach Prolonged constriction can cause ulceration of esophageal mucosa	Balloon inflated on the end of a swallowed esophageal tube to stretch the blocked esophagus Antispasmodic drugs to relax smooth muscle
Disorders of the stomach	Achlorhydria (and hypochlorhydria, diminished acid secretion)	When pH of gastric secretions fail to decrease below 6.5 after maximal stimulation	Failure of stomach to secrete hydrochloric acid	Pepsin also fails to be secreted, which requires acid medium for activity	
Disorders of small intestine	Pancreatitis	Inflammation of pancreas; comes in form of acute pancreatitis or chronic pancreatitis	Drinking excess alcohol Blockage of the papilla of Vater by a gallstone	With gallstone blockage: accumulation of trypsinogen within pancreas activates trypsin and other proteolytic enzymes, causing rapid digestion and destruction of pancreas	
	Sprue	Inadequate absorption of nutrients from small intestine mucosa	Nontropical sprue: (idiopathic sprue, celiac disease, gluten enteropathy) result of toxic effects of gluten	Destruction of intestinal enterocytes thus decreasing absorptive surface area	Removal of wheat and rye flour from diet results in cure within weeks
			Tropical sprue: often occurs in tropics	Possibly by inflammation of intestinal mucosa from unidentified infectious agents	Treat with antibacterial agents
Disorders of large intestine	Megacolon (Hirschsprung's disease)	Severe constipation	Lack or deficiency of ganglion cells in myenteric plexus in a segment of the sigmoid colon	Tremendous accumulation of fecal matter within colon Failure of defecation reflexes and/or strong peristaltic motility	Requires surgical removal of involved bowel. May present with toxic megacolon
	Diarrhea	Rapid movement of fecal matter through large intestine	Enteritis: inflammation of intestinal tract caused by either virus or bacteria (e.g., cholera)	Increased motility of intestinal wall Increased quantity of fluid	Intravenous fluid to replace fluid and electrolytes as rapidly as lost
			Psychogenic diarrhea: excessive stimulation of the parasympathetic nervous system	Increased motility Excess secretion of mucus in distal colon	
			Ulcerative colitis: extensive areas of walls of large intestine become inflamed and ulcerated; cause is unknown	Repeated diarrheal bowel movements	Ileostomy to heal ulcers or Surgical removal of entire colon
Gastrointestinal tract	Chemoreceptor trigger zone	Initiation of vomiting by drugs or by motion sickness	Nervous signals arising in chemoreceptor trigger zone for vomiting		
			Drugs (amorphine, morphine, some digitalis derivatives)		
			Rapid change of direction or rhythm of motion of body		

Anesthetic Pharmacology and the Gastrointestinal Tract

Anesthetic drugs that affect the GI tract in clinically significant ways include the depolarizing neuromuscular blocker succinylcholine, anticholinergic drugs, cholinesterase inhibitors, and opioids.

Succinylcholine mimics the effect of acetylcholine at the neuromuscular junction, producing an initial muscle contraction that is clinically evident as fasciculation (see Chapter 19). Fasciculation is associated with increased intragastric pressure, potentially sufficient to overcome the lower esophageal sphincter and result in reflux of gastric contents with possible aspiration. Prevention of fasciculation with the use of a "de-fasciculating" or subparalytic dose of a nondepolarizing neuromuscular blocking agent might prevent or reduce the increase in intragastric pressure.[49] However that intervention is not entirely benign, being itself associated with partial paralysis, aspiration, and patient complaints of difficulty breathing.[50]

Commonly used anticholinergic drugs include atropine, glycopyrrolate, and scopolamine. Scopolamine is used primarily for its central effects, while atropine and glycopyrrolate are more commonly used for their peripheral effects. Some of these uses are as antisialagogues and as antagonists of the muscarinic effects of neuromuscular blocker reversal agents (cholinesterase inhibitors), which include bradycardia, nausea, increased gastric fluid secretion, and increased GI motility (see Chapter 19). Cholinesterase inhibitors also have potentially salutary effects on the GI tract, such as increasing lower esophageal tone, or treating ileus.[2]

Opioids are strongly associated with nausea and vomiting due to stimulation of the chemoreceptor trigger zone. They also produce constipation by reducing peristaltic activity throughout the small and large intestines and increasing tone in the pyloric sphincter, ileocecal valve, and anal sphincter.[2] Opioid-induced biliary spasm can confound diagnosis of cardiac disease, and might also be misinterpreted as a biliary stone or stricture on cholangiogram. Opioids also cause pancreatic duct contraction, releasing pancreatic amylase and lipase and also potentially confounding a diagnosis of pancreatitis; however, the clinical significance of these effects has been challenged.[51]

Studies have documented the salutary effects of regional anesthesia and analgesia on GI motility as compared to general anesthesia for abdominal surgery.[52] It is believed that a contributing factor to postoperative ileus is sympathetic stimulation caused by the surgical stress response and pain. Neuraxial regional anesthesia, which blocks afferent pain signals and efferent sympathetic outflow, can potentially minimize the depressive effects of surgery on postoperative GI motility.

KEY POINTS

- The liver has a dual afferent blood supply consisting of systemic blood from the hepatic artery and portal venous blood from the splanchnic circulation.
- The liver plays a key role in provision of energy requirements through the synthesis and metabolism of carbohydrates, proteins, and fats.
- The liver detoxifies and transforms exogenous and endogenous compounds, including anesthetics. Altered liver function can lead to encephalopathy and alter the metabolism, volume of distribution, and protein binding of drugs.
- Bile production by the liver is important in the absorption of fats. Biliary obstruction results in steatorrhea and vitamin K deficiency.
- End-stage liver disease is associated with multisystem organ failure. In addition to encephalopathy, hyperdynamic changes occur in the cardiovascular system; pleural effusions and ascites reflect decreased oncotic pressure and elevated portal pressure; varices and coagulopathy lead to GI bleeding; infections occur due to decreased reticuloendothelial function; and renal failure can result from alterations in renal blood flow.
- The GI tract is functionally divided into sections that systematically break down food to its discrete components that are absorbed and presented to the liver for storage or use.
- Surgical trauma affects GI function, particularly if surgery is intraabdominal.
- Anesthetic agents can affect the function of the GI tract.
- While GI dysfunction might not present a problem in the operating room, it is a contributor to perioperative morbidity in the forms of aspiration, postoperative nausea and vomiting, postoperative ileus, and delayed feeding.
- Considered selection of anesthetic agents and technique can mitigate the untoward effects of anesthesia and surgery on GI function.

Key References

Friedman LS. Surgery in the patient with liver disease. *Trans Am Clin Climatol Assoc.* 2010;121:192-205. A recent review describing liver disease-related contraindications to elective surgery. (Ref. 24)

Hall JE. *Guyton and Hall textbook of medical physiology.* 12th ed. Philadelphia: Saunders Elsevier; 2011. A definitive physiology text with excellent explanations of liver and gastrointestinal physiology. (Ref. 35)

Mushlin PS, Gelman S. Hepatic physiology and pathophysiology. In: Miller RD, ed. *Miller's Anesthesia.* 7th ed. Philadelphia: Churchill Livingstone Elsevier; 2009:411-440. The definitive anesthesia text with an excellent chapter on the implications of liver and gastrointestinal pathophysiology on perioperative care. (Ref. 20)

Northup PG, Wanamaker RC, Lee VD, et al. Model for End-Stage Liver Disease (MELD) predicts nontransplant surgical mortality in patients with cirrhosis. *Ann Surg.* 2005;242:244-251. Because of its ability to predict wait list mortality, the MELD score was adopted to allocate organs for liver transplant candidates. The authors examine the MELD score's ability to predict survival after nontransplant surgery in patients with cirrhosis. (Ref. 28)

Schubert ML, Peura DA. Control of gastric acid secretion in health and disease. *Gastroenterology.* 2008;134:1842-1860. An in-depth review of gastric acid secretion. (Ref. 43)

Teh SH, Nagorney DM, Stevens SR, et al. Risk factors for mortality after surgery in patients with cirrhosis. *Gastroenterology.* 2007;132:1261-1269. Examines the ability of the MELD score to predict perioperative mortality in 772 cirrhotics. (Ref. 29)

Ziser A, Plevak D, Wiesner R. Morbidity and mortality in cirrhotic patients undergoing anesthesia and surgery. *Anesthesiology.* 1999;90:42-53. Reports the effects of a number of risk factors on short- and long-term perioperative mortality of 733 cirrhotic patients. (Ref. 25)

References

1. Bell G, Emslie-Smith D, Paterson C. *Textbook of Physiology and Biochemistry*. 9th ed. New York: Churchill Livingstone; 1976.
2. Stoelting RK, Hillier SC. *Pharmacology & Physiology in Anesthetic Practice*. 4th ed. Philadelphia: Lippincott Williams & Wilkins; 2006.
3. Shah VH, Kamath PS. Portal hypertension and gastrointestinal bleeding. In: Mark Feldman M, Lawrence S, Friedman M, Lawrence J, Brandt M, eds. *Sleisinger and Fordtran's Gastrointestinal and Liver Disease*. 9th ed. Philadelphia: Saunders Elsevier; 2010.
4. Lautt WW. Mechanism and role of intrinsic regulation of hepatic arterial blood flow: hepatic arterial buffer response. *Am J Physiol*. 1985;249(5 Pt 1):G549-G556.
5. Jones A. Anatomy of the normal liver. In: Zakim D, Boyer TD, eds. *Hepatology: A Textbook of Liver Disease*. 3rd ed. Philadelphia: WB Saunders; 1996.
6. Gelman S, Fowler KC, Smith LR. Liver circulation and function during isoflurane and halothane anesthesia. *Anesthesiology*. 1984;61(6):726-730.
7. Crawford MW, Lerman J, Saldivia V, Carmichael FJ. Hemodynamic and organ blood flow responses to halothane and sevoflurane anesthesia during spontaneous ventilation. *Anesth Analg*. 1992;75(6):1000-1006.
8. Nordlie RC, Foster JD, Lange AJ. Regulation of glucose production by the liver. *Annu Rev Nutr*. 1999;19:379-406.
9. O'Leary JG, Pratt DS. Cholestasis and cholestatic syndromes. *Curr Opin Gastroenterol*. 2007;23(3):232-236.
10. Olthoff KM. Hepatic regeneration in living donor liver transplantation. *Liver Transpl*. 2003;9(10 Suppl 2):S35-S41.
11. Viebahn CS, Yeoh GC. What fires Prometheus? The link between inflammation and regeneration following chronic liver injury. *Int J Biochem Cell Biol*. 2008;40(5):855-873.
12. Heneghan MA, Harrison PM. Pathogenesis of ascites in cirrhosis and portal hypertension. *Med Sci Monit*. 2000;6(4):807-816.
13. de Franchis R, Primignani M. Natural history of portal hypertension in patients with cirrhosis. *Clin Liver Dis*. 2001;5(3):645-663.
14. Garcia-Tsao G, Bosch J. Management of varices and variceal hemorrhage in cirrhosis. *N Engl J Med*. 2010;362(9):823-832.
15. Jalan R, Hayes PC. Hepatic encephalopathy and ascites. *Lancet*. 1997;350(9087):1309-1315.
16. Chung RT, Jaffe DL, Friedman LS. Complications of chronic liver disease. *Crit Care Clin*. 1995;11(2):431-463.
17. Rakela J, Krowka M. Cardiovascular and pulmonary complications of liver disease. In: Zakim D, Boyer TD, eds. *Hepatology: A Textbook of Liver Disease*. 3rd ed. Philadelphia: WB Saunders; 1996.
18. Kharasch ED, Frink EJ Jr, Artru A, Michalowski P, Rooke GA, Nogami W. Long-duration low-flow sevoflurane and isoflurane effects on postoperative renal and hepatic function. *Anesth Analg*. 2001;93(6):1511-1520.
19. Weiskopf RB, Eger EI 2nd, Ionescu P, et al. Desflurane does not produce hepatic or renal injury in human volunteers. *Anesth Analg*. 1992;74(4):570-574.
20. Mushlin PS, Gelman S. Hepatic physiology and pathophysiology. In: Miller RD, ed. *Miller's Anesthesia*. 7th ed. Philadelphia: Churchill Livingstone Elsevier; 2009:411-440.
21. Radnay PA, Duncalf D, Novakovic M, Lesser ML. Common bile duct pressure changes after fentanyl, morphine, meperidine, butorphanol, and naloxone. *Anesth Analg*. 1984;63(4):441-444.
22. Quinn PG, Johnston DE. Detection of chronic liver disease: costs and benefits. *Gastroenterologist*. 1997;5(1):58-77.
23. Pugh RN, Murray-Lyon IM, Dawson JL, Pietroni MC, Williams R. Transection of the oesophagus for bleeding oesophageal varices. *Br J Surg*. 1973;60(8):646-649.
24. Friedman LS. Surgery in the patient with liver disease. *Trans Am Clin Climatol Assoc*. 2010;121:192-205.
25. Ziser A, Plevak D, Wiesner R. Morbidity and mortality in cirrhotic patients undergoing anesthesia and surgery. *Anesthesiology*. 1999;90(1):42-53.
26. Malinchoc M, Kamath PS, Gordon FD, Peine CJ, Rank J, ter Borg PC. A model to predict poor survival in patients undergoing transjugular intrahepatic portosystemic shunts. *Hepatology*. 2000;31(4):864-871.
27. Freeman RB Jr, Wiesner RH, Harper A, et al. The new liver allocation system: moving toward evidence-based transplantation policy. *Liver Transpl*. 2002;8(9):851-858.
28. Northup PG, Wanamaker RC, Lee VD, Adams RB, Berg CL. Model for End-Stage Liver Disease (MELD) predicts nontransplant surgical mortality in patients with cirrhosis. *Ann Surg*. 2005;242(2):244-251.
29. Teh SH, Nagorney DM, Stevens SR, et al. Risk factors for mortality after surgery in patients with cirrhosis. *Gastroenterology*. 2007;132(4):1261-1269.
30. D'Albuquerque LA, de Miranda MP, Genzini T, Copstein JL, de Oliveira e Silva A. Laparoscopic cholecystectomy in cirrhotic patients. *Surg Laparosc Endosc*. 1995;5(4):272-276.
31. Belghiti J, Hiramatsu K, Benoist S, Massault P, Sauvanet A, Farges O. Seven hundred forty-seven hepatectomies in the 1990s: an update to evaluate the actual risk of liver resection. *J Am Coll Surg*. 2000;191(1):38-46.
32. 2009 Annual Report of the U.S. Organ Procurement and Transplantation Network and the Scientific Registry of Transplant Recipients: Transplant Data 1999-2008. U.S. Department of Health and Human Services, Health Resources and Services Administration, Healthcare Systems Bureau, Division of Transplantation, Rockville, MD. Available at: http://optn.transplant.hrsa.gov/ar2009/default.htm.
33. Steadman RH. Anesthesia for liver transplant surgery. *Anesthesiol Clin North Am*. 2004;22(4):687-711.
34. Huizinga JD, Lammers WJ. Gut peristalsis is governed by a multitude of cooperating mechanisms. *Am J Physiol Gastrointest Liver Physiol*. 2009;296(1):G1-G8.
35. Hall JE. *Guyton and Hall textbook of medical physiology*. 12th ed. Philadelphia: Saunders Elsevier; 2011.
36. Adelson DW, Million M. Tracking the moveable feast: sonomicrometry and gastrointestinal motility. *News Physiol Sci*. 2004;19:27-32.
37. Furness JB. Types of neurons in the enteric nervous system. *J Auton Nerv Syst*. 2000;81(1-3):87-96.
38. Gonella J, Bouvier M, Blanquet F. Extrinsic nervous control of motility of small and large intestines and related sphincters. *Physiol Rev*. 1987;67(3):902-961.
39. Read NW, Houghton LA. Physiology of gastric emptying and pathophysiology of gastroparesis. *Gastroenterol Clin North Am*. 1989;18(2):359-373.
40. Doyle DJ, Mark PW. Reflex bradycardia during surgery. *Can J Anaesth*. 1990;37(2):219-222.
41. Seltzer JL, Ritter DE, Starsnic MA, Marr AT. The hemodynamic response to traction on the abdominal mesentery. *Anesthesiology*. 1985;63(1):96-99.
42. Xue J, Askwith C, Javed NH, Cooke HJ. Autonomic nervous system and secretion across the intestinal mucosal surface. *Auton Neurosci*. 2007;133(1):55-63.
43. Schubert ML, Peura DA. Control of gastric acid secretion in health and disease. *Gastroenterology*. 2008;134(7):1842-1860.
44. Dockray GJ, Varro A, Dimaline R, Wang T. The gastrins: their production and biological activities. *Annu Rev Physiol*. 2001;63:119-139.
45. Allen A, Flemstrom G. Gastroduodenal mucus bicarbonate barrier: protection against acid and pepsin. *Am J Physiol Cell Physiol*. 2005;288(1):C1-19.
46. Iqbal J, Hussain MM. Intestinal lipid absorption. *Am J Physiol Endocrinol Metab*. 2009;296(6):E1183-1194.
47. Garrard A, Campbell AE, Turley A, Hall JE. The effect of mechanically-induced cricoid force on lower oesophageal sphincter pressure in anaesthetised patients. *Anaesthesia*. 2004;59(5):435-439.
48. Ellis DY, Harris T, Zideman D. Cricoid pressure in emergency department rapid sequence tracheal intubations: a risk-benefit analysis. *Ann Emerg Med*. 2007;50(6):653-665.
49. Miller RD, Way WL. Inhibition of succinylcholine-induced increased intragastric pressure by nondepolarizing muscle relaxants and lidocaine. *Anesthesiology*. 1971;34(2):185-188.
50. El-Orbany M, Connolly LA. Rapid sequence induction and intubation: current controversy. *Anesth Analg*. 2010;110(5):1318-1325.
51. Thompson DR. Narcotic analgesic effects on the sphincter of Oddi: A review of the data and therapeutic implications in treating pancreatitis. *Am J Gastroenterol*. 2001;96(4):1266-1272.
52. Moraca RJ, Sheldon DG, Thirlby RC. The role of epidural anesthesia and analgesia in surgical practice. *Ann Surg*. 2003;238(5):663-673.

Chapter 28

NUTRITIONAL AND METABOLIC THERAPY

Robert G. Martindale, T. Miko Enomoto, and Mary McCarthy

Macronutrients have traditionally been regarded as a means to provide basic energy for cellular homeostasis while amino acids are considered necessary for protein synthesis. However, surgical, traumatically injured, and critically ill patients are in a dynamic state between systemic inflammation, immune suppression, and persistent chronic inflammatory states.[1] It often takes weeks or months for the inflammatory states resulting from major surgical intervention or intensive care unit (ICU) admission to resolve. Multiple factors including timing of insult, anesthesia and sedation provided, and prestress comorbidities influence the duration of the hyperdynamic inflammatory state.

As a result of recent elucidation of metabolic pathways using tracer technology, gene regulation, proteomics, and genomics, research supporting the benefits of supplemental specific nutrients has increased exponentially.[2-6] Although it has long been realized that preoperative malnutrition is a risk factor for poor wound healing, perioperative complications, and even mortality, the most commonly considered anesthetic implication of a patient's nutritional state is fasting status.[7-9] While the gastric volume and pH at the time of induction of anesthesia affect the risk of aspiration of stomach contents, other aspects of nutritional state significantly influence ability to tolerate procedures and heal in the setting of disease and surgical insult, and should be of concern to all perioperative physicians.

FASTING IN THE PERIOPERATIVE PERIOD

Time elapsed from last oral intake is perhaps the most immediate and relevant issue regarding how nutrition affects perioperative anesthesia care. The risk of aspiration on induction presents a severe, potentially modifiable risk such that the American Society of Anesthesiology issues fasting guidelines for patients undergoing elective procedures requiring anesthesia. The 2011 updated guidelines recommend fasting times for clear liquids of 2 or more hours, 4 or more hours for breast milk, 6 or more hours for a light meal, and 8 or more hours for a fatty meal prior to undergoing general or regional anesthesia or sedation.[10]

If not for the risk of aspiration, might it be optimal to continue nutrition through the surgical period? Currently only a few reports exist on feeding up to the time of surgery and even feeding during non-intraabdominal surgery. This is mainly in burn and orthopedic procedures, but has recently been extended to other surgical groups.[11] The standard of routinely continuing nutritional therapy during procedures is only established for parenteral nutrition (PN), in that there is no increased risk for aspiration due to increased gastric volume. However, there are data to suggest that continuing postpyloric tube feeding in the critically ill, mechanically ventilated patient presenting for nonabdominal surgery does not increase the incidence of aspiration, suggesting that enteral nutrition can be safely continued in the perioperative period.[12]

BENEFITS OF EARLY ENTERAL FEEDING

Early enteral nutrition (EN) in the ICU has a myriad of reports explaining the diverse mechanisms to support the observed benefits (Table 28-1). The gastrointestinal tract comprises the largest immune organ in the body and is responsible for the production of more than 80% of the immunoglobulin (Ig) transported to extraintestinal sites. The ability of the gut to function appropriately to this end is dependent upon the maintenance of both structural and functional integrity. The integrity of the gut, in turn, is greatly dependent upon continued exposure to luminal nutrient substrates. Both adaptive and innate immune defenses are active in this process. Innate mechanisms depend on epithelial tight junctions and secretory capabilities of the mucosa. Secretory IgA is an important component of the adaptive immune system, in that antigens are tagged and presented to dendritic cells within Peyer patches, which are in highest concentration in the distal small bowel. Gut disuse over a period of as little as 5 days can result in a dramatic decrease in the mass of gut-associated lymphoid tissue (GALT) and reduced production of secretory intestinal IgA.[3,5,13] These changes are completely reversed with reinstitution of enteral nutrition therapy.[4] Increases in intestinal permeability have been shown to correlate with the development and severity of multiple organ dysfunction syndrome (MODS).[6,14]

Goals of nutrition support therapy now focus on the attenuation of metabolic and oxidative stress by downregulating the severity of systemic inflammatory responses, accentuating the compensatory antiinflammatory adaptive immune response, and promoting an earlier return to a homeostatic baseline. It has become increasingly apparent

that the nonutilized gut can contribute significantly to the proinflammatory state of critically ill patients, further emphasizing the role for early EN therapy in appropriate patients.[15]

TIMING OF NUTRIENT DELIVERY

The optimal time to start nutrition support is influenced by a host of factors including age, premorbid conditions, route of nutrient delivery, metabolic state, organ perfusion, and function.[16,17] Although literature evaluating nutritional support for critically ill patients has analyzed heterogeneous populations, these diverse studies provide a foundation to guide nutritional therapy in a wide range of ICU patient types (e.g., burn, trauma, abdominal surgery, oncologic surgery).[18,19]

The reported benefits of early EN are, among others, prevention of adverse structural and functional alterations to the mucosal barrier, augmentation of visceral blood flow, and enhancement of local and systemic immune response.[20,21] The clinical benefits of early EN have been the focus of three recent metaanalyses, which report benefits of reducing infections, length of hospital stay, and in some reports improved mortality with minimal risk.[20,22-24] Despite these acknowledged benefits, nutrition delivery remains suboptimal in a significant percentage of critically ill patients.[25,26]

Acknowledging that the early initiation of nutrition support constitutes best practice, a multidisciplinary approach to determining appropriate timing in the individual patient cannot be overemphasized. Enteral feeding should not proceed until appropriate resuscitation has been undertaken (Table 28-2). Early resuscitation remains a cornerstone of ICU therapy. Early and aggressive resuscitation, or "early goal-directed therapy" involves the placement of invasive lines including central venous and arterial catheters with continuous venous oxygen saturation, blood pressure, and/or cardiac output monitoring, and more recently noninvasive cardiac output monitors, to evaluate overall intravascular volume status. Volume resuscitation is continued with appropriate arterial and central pressure, cardiac output, and/or tissue perfusion goals; if unable to reach these goals, vasopressor medications are added in the hypotensive (mean arterial pressures <65 mm Hg) vasodilated patient (see Chapters 22 & 33).[27] Any single laboratory or hemodynamic parameter

Table 28-1. Metabolic Benefits of Early Enteral Feeding

Attenuates inflammatory response to stress/critical illness
Prevents mucosal atrophy, loss of gut barrier
Luminal delivery maintains GALT and MALT
Supports systemic immune response
Helps maintain normal gut bacterial flora (microbiome)
Decreases insulin resistance, better glycemic control
Maintains vagal mediated antiinflammatory reflex
Luminal (portal) nutrient delivery allows for hepatic first-pass metabolic effects
More balanced nutrient delivery possible when compared to parenteral nutrition

GALT, Gut-associated lymphoid tissue; *MALT,* mucosal associated lymphoid tissue.

Table 28-2. Considerations Before Any Nutritional Intervention, Either Enteral or Parenteral, in Intensive Care Unit Settings

Optimize Timing and Intensity of Resuscitation
Correct volume deficits, electrolytes, acid-base disorders
Obtain infection source control if it is in question
Appropriate Antibiotics
Early, aggressive broad-spectrum antibiotics, then deescalate as cultures become available
Attempt to Maximize Visceral Perfusion
Prevents loss of gut mucosal integrity
Consider Specific Organ Support as Indicated
Examples: pulmonary, renal, cardiac, hepatic
Glycemic Control
Intravenous insulin drips (protocols) to maintain glycemic control in range of 140-80 mg/dL

signaling the successful resuscitation of the critically ill patient in shock remains elusive. Generally, trends in hemodynamic parameters including mean arterial pressures, central venous pressures, cardiac output, and pressor requirements in conjunction with urine output, arterial blood base deficit, serum lactate, and venous oxygen saturation are used to determine the relative adequacy of resuscitation.

Splanchnic circulation can increase by as much as 40% to 60% in the setting of enteral feeding. The specific actions of digestion and absorption increase the metabolic demand and oxygen utilization by the gastrointestinal tract.[28] If supply falls short of demand, rare but devastating complications can ensue (Figure 28-1). Fortunately, nonocclusive mesenteric ischemia (NMI) remains an uncommon complication in inadequately resuscitated patients in which early enteral feeding is used. NMI most commonly affects the distribution of the superior mesenteric artery, which can result in ischemia and possibly necrosis of portions of the affected small and large bowel. Hypovolemia and underresuscitation can exaggerate the already hypoperfused and dysregulated splanchnic circulation in the ICU setting. Enteral feeding in the hemodynamically unstable patient should be undertaken with extreme caution.[19]

Treatment of NMI is usually supportive. Hemodynamic performance is optimized and intraarterial vasodilators can be used as an adjunct. Patients who go on to require laparotomy and resection of nonviable bowel have very poor outcomes with mortality as high as 80%.[29] Following adequate resuscitation and assuming no other absolute contraindication to enteral feeding exist (i.e., bowel obstruction), enteral support should be initiated as soon as possible.

Numerous reports continue to support the concept that bowel sounds and evidence of bowel function, that is, passing flatus or stool, is not required for EN.[30] The approach of waiting for these signs can contribute to unnecessary delays in feeding. In a randomized trial, oral feeding initiated within 48 hours of gastrectomy, without waiting for traditional predictors of feeding tolerance (i.e., passing flatus) demonstrated the safety of the approach.[31] There was no increase in morbidity and a reduction in hospital stay. A recent metaanalysis examining 15 studies and 1240 patients with gastrointestinal anastomoses demonstrated reduced postoperative complications when feeding was initiated within 24 hours of operation.[24] Other meta-analysis, specifically in ICU and trauma patients, report significant decrease in mortality, as well as infectious complications.[14,32]

Although the benefits of early EN have been confirmed in many populations, feeding immediately after the diagnosis of sepsis is associated with an entirely different set of problems. Gastrointestinal dysfunction in the ICU ranges from 30% to 70%, depending on the diagnosis, premorbid condition, ventilation mode, medications, and metabolic state.[17,33]

GASTROINTESTINAL DYSFUNCTION

Proposed mechanisms of ICU and postoperative gastrointestinal dysfunction can be divided into three general categories: mucosal barrier disruption, altered motility, and atrophy of the mucosa and GALT. Barrier disruption seems to most commonly be associated with splanchnic hypoperfusion, which is precipitated by numerous factors in the critical care setting and immediate perioperative period, including hypovolemia, increased catecholamines, increased proinflammatory cytokines, and decreased cardiac output. All ultimately lead to reduced mucosal blood flow, barrier disruption, altered gastrointestinal motility, and changes in the bacterial flora and virulence of the host gut microbiome.[34-37] Membrane toll-like receptors (TLR) been implicated in altered motility with resultant changes in intestinal bacterial flora and the potential for translocation. Lipopolysaccharide (LPS), or endotoxin, has been demonstrated to stimulate TLR-4 resulting in impaired smooth muscle function in the gastrointestinal tract, which contributes to dysmotility.[38]

The proposed mechanisms inducing postoperative ileus following bowel manipulation have recently been described (Figure 28-2).[34,39] Following visceral manipulation, activation of transcription factors is noted, with upregulation of ICAM-1 (intracellular adhesion molecule-1) on the endothelium of the muscularis vessels. Leukocyte extravasation into the muscularis occurs, with resultant upregulation of iNOS (inducible nitric oxide synthase), COX-2 (cyclooxygenase-2), IL-6 (interleukin-6), and STAT-3 (signal transducer and activator of transcription-3) phosphorylation. This, combined with the T-cell changes, underlies the inflammatory process leading to decreased contractile response and altered electrical activity, resulting in ileus.[34,39]

As previously stated, recent approaches to maximize gut function in the postoperative and critical care settings include maintenance of visceral perfusion, glycemic control, electrolyte correction, early EN, and minimization of medications that alter gastrointestinal function, such as anticholinergic agents, narcotics, and high-dose vasopressors.[30] Gastrointestinal intolerance should be continually reassessed

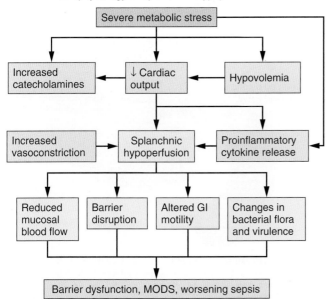

Figure 28-1 Pathophysiology of splanchnic hypo-perfusion often associated with critical illness. *GI*, Gastrointestinal; *MODS*, multiple organ dysfunction syndrome. *(Modified from Schmidt H, Martindale R. The gastrointestinal tract in critical illness: nutritional implications. Curr Opin Clin Nutr Metab Care. 2003;6:587-591; Mutlu GM, et al. GI complications in patients receiving mechanical ventilation. Chest. 2001;119:1222-1241.)*

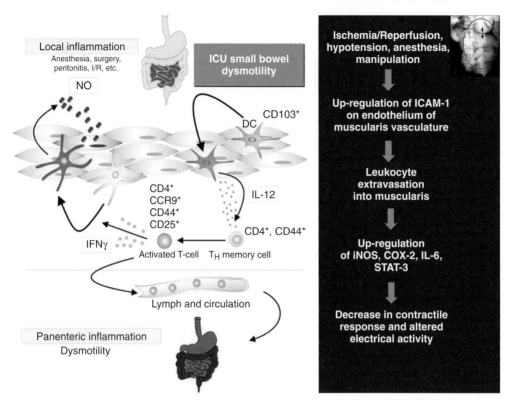

Figure 28-2 Current theories on the mechanism of intensive care unit and postoperative ileus. *(Left panel, Modified from Wehner S, Vilz TO, Stoffels B, et al. Immune mediators of postoperative ileus.* Langenbecks Arch Surg. *2012;397:591-601. Right panel, Modified from Kalff JC, Turler A, Schwarz NT, et al. Intra-abdominal activation of a local inflammatory response within the human muscularis externa during laparotomy.* Ann Surg. *2003;237:301-315.)* See text for more detailed explanation and definition of abbreviations.

and can manifest clinically in a variety of forms, including acidosis, abdominal distention, increased gastric residual volumes or nasogastric output, abdominal pain, or diarrhea. The segmental contractility of the gastrointestinal tract should be considered because dysmotility can be focal (affecting predominately either the proximal or distal bowel) or diffuse. Impaired gastric and proximal GI motility (Figure 28-3) can be addressed and overcome rather efficiently through the placement of postpyloric feeding tubes. Postpyloric tubes can be placed successfully at the bedside in more than 80% of patients.[40]

Prokinetic agents can be used early and are helpful in some patients. Erythromycin acts on motilin receptors, resulting in increased motility, and can be used on a short-term basis but is limited due to tachyphylaxis. The concern of potentially inducing antibiotic class resistance must be considered. Metoclopramide, a $5HT_4$ receptor agonist, works via cholinergic stimulation and is primarily efficacious in the proximal gut. When using metoclopramide, one must also consider the potential for extrapyramidal side effects, especially in patients with altered mental status from traumatic head injury of cerebral vascular events. Alvimopan, a peripherally acting mu-opioid antagonist, has demonstrated some success in the setting of dysmotility associated with opioid administration in the postoperative setting.[41] No single prokinetic agent will have uniform success in the ICU; the factors contributing to gastrointestinal dysmotility in each individual patient must be considered. Caution should be used when using prokinetic agents on patients at high risk for bowel necrosis or obstruction.

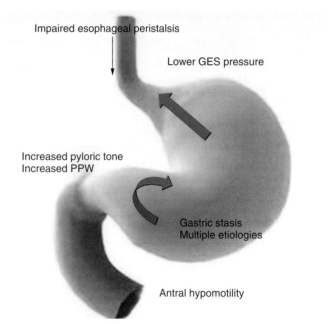

Figure 28-3 Mechanisms involved in gastric dysmotility in the intensive care unit population. *GES,* Gastroesophageal sphincter; *PPW,* pyloric pressure wave. *(Modified from Caddell KA, Martindale R, McClave SA, et al. Can the intestinal dysmotility of critical illness be differentiated from postoperative ileus?* Curr Gastroenterol Rep. *2011;13:358-367.)*

NUTRITION AND METABOLISM IN THE CRITICALLY ILL

Early EN can be accomplished in the ICU and postoperative settings using standardized protocols, with little morbidity and a gastrointestinal tolerance rate in the 70% to 85% range.[21,42] A recent study in which investigators implemented a standardized, evidence-based enteral feeding protocol, reported shortened duration of mechanical ventilation and a reduced mortality.[43]

Several reports have now shown that using specific nutrients such as fish oils, selected amino acids (i.e., arginine, glutamine, leucine), antioxidants, and nucleic acids in quantities greater than necessary for "normal" metabolism, has multiple outcome benefits including shortened length of ICU and hospital stay, decreased incidence of infections, and reduced mortality in some cases.[44-46] A wide range of select specific nutrients has been reported to benefit the critically ill patient when delivered at pharmacologic quantities. Many of these compounds are now considered to be therapeutic agents in the management of complex, catabolically stressed patients (Table 28-3). The recent collaboration between the Society of Critical Care Medicine (SCCM) and the American Society of Parenteral and Enteral Nutrition (ASPEN) resulted in Guidelines for the Provision and Assessment of Nutrition Support Therapy in the Adult Critically Ill Patient. These guidelines describe the rationale for the use of immunonutrients, based on the available evidence that the use of metabolic and immune modulating formulations should receive the highest recommendation based on large randomized trials with clear-cut results.[44] Similar recommendations for the use of immune-modulating nutrients in the surgical patient are endorsed by the European Society of Enteral and Parenteral Nutrition (ESPEN).[47] Since the publication of both the SCCM/ASPEN and ESPEN guidelines in 2009, an additional study supporting these pharmaconutrient concepts have been published.[48,49]

In 1794, John Hunter described in his book, *A Treatise on Blood, Inflammation and Gunshot Wounds, A Mechanism of Inflammation*, an observation that "many types of injury produce a similar inflammation.[50] Along that same concept in

1904, Sir William Osler stated "except on few occasions the patient appears to die from the body's response to infection rather than from it." These two extremely insightful and prophetic comments were both made more than 100 years ago. The current strategy in the ICU of using nutrition therapy to modulate inflammation and immune response in the surgical, traumatically injured, and critically ill populations is now widely accepted. Efforts are made to attenuate or control the metabolic response to stress and trauma rather than allowing the extremes of the immediate systemic inflammatory response syndrome (SIRS) and the more prolonged persistent inflammation, immunosuppression, and catabolism syndrome (PICS).[1] Until just recently, the concept of a compensatory antiinflammatory response (CARS) was used as a framework to understand the postinsult metabolic and immunologic response, accounting for the progression to MODS. With new metabolic studies taking advantage of genomic and proteomic expression, CARS has evolved to PICS, which better describes the metabolic response to stress.

The metabolic response to stress includes a hyperdynamic cardiac and pulmonary state, insulin resistance, hyperglycemia, accelerated protein catabolism from muscle, poor adaptation to starvation, and increased oxidative stress.[51] Unabated, the metabolic response to stress can culminate in immune suppression.[52] During this hyperdynamic phase of critical illness, surgery, or trauma, the loss of lean body mass continues despite delivery of seemingly adequate enteral or parenteral protein and calories. In effect, administration of standard "calories and protein" to the hyperdynamic patient will not reverse the adverse effects of ongoing loss of lean body tissue. The hyperdynamic state-induced loss of lean body tissue is made worse by "muscle unloading" (Figure 28-4). Pharmaconutrition or immunonutrition is defined as the provision of key nutrients that modulate the inflammatory and/or the catabolic response associated with critical illness. This concept is distinctly separate from the delivery of adequate enteral or parenteral nutrition to meet the needs of the organism for normal cell metabolism and growth. The use of select nutrients for their therapeutic effects has received greater attention as part of current surgical, trauma, and ICU care throughout the world.

Several immune and/or metabolic modulating enteral formulas are now available globally. These products contain

Table 28-3. Nutrients/Compounds Reported to Have Immune and/or Metabolic Activity

Arginine	Ginger	**Selenium**
Boswellia	Glucosamine	Shark cartilage
Caffeine	**Glutamine**	Taurine
Capsaicin	Glutathione	Threonine
Carnitine	**Leucine**	Tumeric
Chamomile	Licorice	**Vitamin C**
Creatine	Probiotics	**Vitamin E**
Curry paste	**Omega-3 FA (EPA/DHA)**	Willow bark
Cysteine	Resveratrol	**Zinc**
Echinacea	Saffron	
Garlic		

The above compounds have all been reported to alter metabolic or immune function in human models. The majority of data is with the vitamins E and C, trace mineral zinc and selenium, the amino acids, glutamine, arginine, and leucine, in addition to the fish oils (shown in bold).

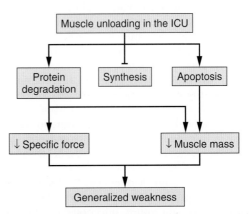

Figure 28-4 Explanation for muscle loss during unloading of muscle in the intensive care unit. These effects culminate in prolonged, generalized muscle weakness. Weakness lasts for weeks to months; up to 50% of survivors do not return to preICU function at 1 year.

various nutrients identified and reported as beneficial during critical illness. Well over 100 prospective randomized human trials have been conducted with various combinations of these immune and metabolic modulating nutrients in various ICU, surgical, and medical populations. A wide range of methodologic quality is observed in these studies from relatively small, poorly designed studies to large prospective, randomized clinical trials with intention to treat analysis. The majority of these studies report a clear benefit of reduced intensive care and hospital length of stay, decreased antibiotic use, and reduced rates of infection.[44,49] These nutrients, including glutamine, fish oils, and arginine, have been credited with a reduction in infections and length of stay in surgical patients, as well as a similar favorable, although less dramatic, impact on these outcomes in other ICU populations.

SPECIFIC NUTRIENTS

For decades amino acids were believed to modulate intermediary metabolism, but the clinical outcome benefits of specific amino acids have only been reported in recent years. Dietary supplementation with the amino acids glutamine, arginine, and leucine has been the focus of the majority of clinical trials, but other amino acids, specifically glycine, taurine, citrulline, and glutamate, have received interest recently.[53]

Glutamine

Since the early 1980s, glutamine has gained popularity in the critical care and surgical arena following reports of its metabolic and outcome benefits, ranging from decreasing mortality in critical care and trauma to enhancing mood in psychiatry.[54] Although little controversy exists over the potential benefits of glutamine in the surgical setting, some doubt still exists about the need for routine supplementation in all ICU populations.[55]

Glutamine is a nonessential amino acid that can be synthesized in most tissues of the body.[56] Skeletal muscle, by virtue of its mass, produces the majority of endogenous glutamine. During major catabolic insults, demand for glutamine outstrips the endogenous supply, resulting in its designation as a conditionally essential amino acid. Glutamine serves as the primary oxidative fuel for rapidly dividing tissues, such as the small bowel mucosa, proliferating lymphocytes, and macrophages.[57] Glutamine has numerous roles in intermediary metabolism, including maintenance of acid-base status, as a precursor of urinary ammonia, and in interorgan nitrogen transfer for the biosynthesis of nucleotides, amino sugars, arginine, glutathione, and glucosamine.[58,59] During periods of stress, glutamine can provide the carbon skeleton for gluconeogenesis and is the primary substrate for renal gluconeogenesis.[60] In addition to the proposed benefits described, glutamine supplementation has recently been shown to be effective in decreasing peripheral insulin resistance in stressed human and other mammalian models.[61-63] In addition, glutamine supports optimal gut growth and repair, as well as decreasing sepsis and other infectious conditions, while enhancing nitrogen balance and supporting endogenous antioxidant functions via nuclear factor kappa B (NFκB) and glutathione.[64]

There is a growing volume of human data regarding the use of parenteral and enteral glutamine supplementation.[65] There is little dispute that administration by the parenteral route as a dipeptide currently yields a better clinical outcome than the enteral route in the ICU population.[66] The majority of enterally delivered glutamine, estimated at 70%-80%, is metabolized in the viscera, with only a fraction reaching the systemic circulation. Even so, outcome benefits have been reported with the delivery of enteral glutamine.[65,67] As a result of the constraints by the U.S. Food and Drug Administration, parenteral glutamine is not readily available in the United States. Intravenous glutamine is widely used by much of the world in the form of glutamine dipeptide.[68]

In animal models and limited human experience, supplemental glutamine has been shown to enhance intestinal adaptation after massive small bowel resection and to attenuate intestinal and pancreatic atrophy.[59,69] Glutamine appears to maintain gastrointestinal tract mucosal thickness, stabilize DNA and protein content, and reduce bacteremia and mortality after chemotherapy, and following sepsis or endotoxemia.[63,65] Glutamine has also been reported to enhance glutathione synthesis, the primary endogenously produced antioxidant in mammalian species.[62]

An additional mechanism explaining some of the benefits observed with glutamine supplementation is the induction of heat shock proteins (HSP-70, -32, -27), which are critical to the cell's ability to survive injury and attenuate the proinflammatory SIRS during critical illness.[70-73] HSPs are a family of highly conserved cytosolic chaperone proteins involved in cell protection during various metabolic stresses.[74] They assist in cellular recovery following injury and partially protect the cell and involved organ from subsequent failure.[73]

CLINICAL OUTCOME STUDIES USING GLUTAMINE

In humans undergoing surgical stress, use of glutamine-supplemented parenteral nutrition appears to help maintain nitrogen balance and the intracellular glutamine pool in skeletal muscle tissue.[75] In trauma patients, a reduction in pneumonia by more than 50% has been demonstrated with glutamine supplementation compared to an isonitrogenous, isocaloric control.[67] In critically ill patients, glutamine supplementation attenuates villous atrophy and the increased intestinal mucosal permeability associated with parenteral nutrition.[76,77] In a randomized blinded trial of 84 critically ill patients, of which 71% were septic on admission, parenteral glutamine supplementation showed significant improvement in mortality at 6 months.[78] Parenteral nutrition supplemented with glutamine has also resulted in fewer infections, improved nitrogen balance, and significantly shorter mean hospital length of stay in bone marrow transplantation patients.[79] Oral glutamine supplementation reduced severity and decreased duration of stomatitis that occurred during chemotherapy in patients receiving bone marrow.[80] Glutamine supplementation at the level of 30 g/day in esophageal cancer patients undergoing radiation was associated with preserved lymphocyte response and decreased gut permeability.[81] In a multicenter, prospective, blinded trial involving 114 ICU patients with multiple trauma, complicated surgery, or pancreatitis, total parenteral nutrition supplemented with the dipeptide L-alanyl-L-glutamine was compared to L-alanine + L-proline control. The glutamine supplemented group had significantly fewer infections, decreased incidence of pneumonia, and better glycemic control.[68]

In 2002, a meta-analysis evaluating the use of glutamine in the ICU population concluded that, in surgical patients, glutamine supplementation may be associated with a reduction in infectious complication rates and shorter hospital stay.[82] Large multicenter trials using glutamine have recently been published with mixed results depending on dosing, concentrations, patient heterogeneity, and route of delivery.[66,83] A large multicenter trial in the United Kingdom in which patients received 20 g/day resulted in no benefit in reducing infections, length of hospital stay, or modified Sequential Organ Failure Assessment (SOFA) score.[83] In the Scandinavian glutamine trial in which glutamine dipeptide was delivered at a dose of 0.283 g/kg/24 hours, there was a reduced mortality benefit in those patients who received glutamine for more than 3 days.[66]

DELIVERY OF GLUTAMINE

While the balance of animal and human data provides evidence that glutamine is beneficial in a variety of experimental and clinical models, the recommendation for routine enteral glutamine supplementation in critically ill patients remains somewhat equivocal as illustrated by the recent Scottish and Scandinavian multicenter trials.[83,84] Although it seems clear that glutamine is a contributor to restoring homeostasis in the critically ill surgical and trauma populations, well-designed clinical trials with clearly defined endpoints, relatively homogenous populations, and adequate statistical power are still needed. Currently, adequate clinical studies are available to support the use of glutamine supplementation in most surgical settings. There is no disputing that glutamine stores are rapidly depleted in critical illness or injury and providing supplemental glutamine as a metabolic fuel for enterocytes and immune cells supports barrier and immune function. The data currently available favor the parenteral route over the enteral route for glutamine supplementation although benefit has been reported for both. Glutamine supplementation receives a strong recommendation (grade A) to reduce mortality in critically ill patients receiving parenteral nutrition but glutamine supplemented enteral formulation receives a somewhat weaker recommendation (grade B), and only in burn and trauma patients. For its role in protecting cells against injury and preventing complications, such as infection and mortality in surgical, trauma, and critical care settings, glutamine has earned its reputation as an important pharmaconutrient.

Arginine

Arginine is considered a nonessential amino acid under normal physiologic conditions of cell growth and development. Arginine becomes conditionally essential in the stressed mammalian host and plays a significant role in the intermediary metabolism of the critically ill patient.[85] Key contributions of arginine include it being a secretagogue for the release of growth hormone, prolactin, and insulin, and it stimulates the proliferation and activation of T cells.[86,87] L-Arginine is available to the host from endogenous synthesis as part of the urea cycle (via citrulline conversion in the kidney), from endogenous protein breakdown, and from dietary protein sources (current Western diet only contributes about 20% to 25% of total arginine).

Arginine is a prominent intermediate in polyamine synthesis (one of the primary regulators of cell growth and proliferation) and proline synthesis (wound healing and collagen synthesis), and is the only biosynthetic substrate for nitric oxide (NO) production from the three isoforms of nitric oxide synthase (eNOS, iNOS, nNOS). Nitric oxide is a potent intracellular signaling molecule influencing virtually every mammalian cell type. Arginine also serves as a potent modulator of immune function via its effects on lymphocyte proliferation and differentiation, as well as its benefits in improved bactericidal action via the arginine nitric oxide pathway (Figure 28-5).[56,86]

As mentioned earlier, the de novo synthesis and dietary intake is reduced in acute surgical and major metabolic insults. Following these insults, immature cells of myeloid origin are present in the circulation and lymph tissue; these cells express high levels of arginase-1, an enzyme that degrades arginine to ornithine. While exogenous and endogenous supply of arginine is decreased, the cellular demand for arginine is increased. This accelerated demand for arginine in the settings of trauma, surgery, sepsis, and critical care is driven mainly by the upregulation of arginase in several tissues (arginase I and arginase II), yielding urea and ornithine, and of iNOS, yielding NO and citrulline.[56,88] This state of relative arginine deficiency is manifested in the suppression of T-lymphocyte function and proliferation. Other signs of T-cell dysfunction after surgery or trauma include a decrease in the number of circulating CD4 cells, increased production of IL-2 and interferon-γ, as well as loss of the zeta chain peptide, which is essential in the T-cell receptor complex. These changes in arginase activity result in impaired immune function at multiple levels of the immune response.[89] This defect in immune competence can contribute to increased risk of infection for critically ill patients.

Making generalized statements about amino acid metabolism in critical care is extremely difficult because the ICU population is such a heterogeneous group. Without strong scientific evidence validating the toxicity or benefits of most popular dietary supplements, let alone an amino acid with the metabolic complexity of arginine, making global recommendations is naive. Both animal and human data are available to support arguments for and against the use of supplemental arginine in ICU populations. These results will strongly depend on dose given, model chosen to study, and duration of therapy. Trends are beginning to show the majority of the literature supporting use of arginine supplementation in both medical and surgical populations.[90,91]

CLINICAL OUTCOME STUDIES USING ARGININE

Of all the pharmaconutrients, arginine has prompted the most controversy. The theoretical concept that arginine may pose a threat to the surgical or critically ill patient is mainly based on the perception that postoperative or septic surgical patients are often hemodynamically unstable, with upregulated iNOS enzyme activity. Consequently, by delivering supplemental arginine in metabolic states of upregulated iNOS, an increase in nitric oxide will result in vasodilation and hypotension leading to even greater hemodynamic instability and organ dysfunction.[92] This hypothesis has not held up in clinical practice; a nonselective nitric oxide synthase inhibitor was administered in high doses to counteract vasodilation and hypotension in patients with severe sepsis in septic shock and

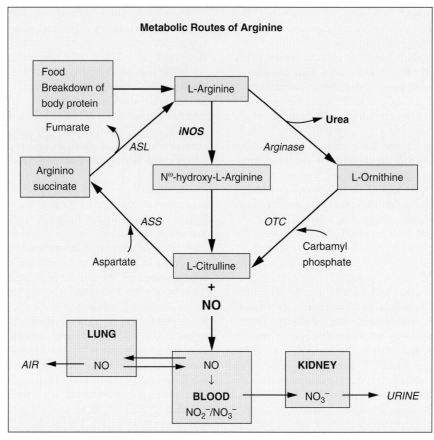

Figure 28-5 Metabolic pathways for arginine. In critical illness, the exogenous supply of L-arginine is reduced, and endogenous demand is increased by increases in arginase and iNOS activity. Reduced levels of L-arginine lead to T-cell dysfunction and impaired immune responses resulting in infection. *ASL,* Arginosuccinate lyase; *ASS,* arginosuccinate synthase; *NO,* nitric oxide; *NO_2^-,* nitrate; *NO_3^-,* nitrate; *iNOS,* inducible nitric oxide synthase; *OTC,* ornithine transcarbamylase.

28-day mortality was significantly increased when compared to patients receiving placebo.[93] In fact, in this study, the highest mortality occurred within 72 hours in the treatment group. An alternate, equally valid hypothesis would be that controlled vasodilation would be beneficial in critical illness and sepsis. Shock, by definition, is inadequate delivery of oxygen and nutrients to maintain normal tissue and cellular function.[92] Vasodilation resulting from supplemental arginine is a cellular adaptive mechanism that could increase delivery of oxygen to the cell. This concept was illustrated in a study in which investigators attempted to modulate asymmetric-dimethylarginine (ADMA) in septic patients by tight glycemic control, but was unsuccessful in altering the course of sepsis. As with other studies, the investigators were left to question whether the effect of an endogenous inhibitor of nitric oxide synthases is preferable to potentially beneficial effects of arginine.[94,95]

ADMA has been shown to increase in states of inflammation in acute infections and other stress models.[95] It has been suggested that an imbalance of arginine and ADMA is associated with altered endothelial cell function and cardiac dysfunction. Some investigators reported that elevated arginine and lower ADMA resulted in reduced mortality in septic patients.[96] A lower ratio of arginine to ADMA resulted in poor organ perfusion and decreased cardiac output. Until recently, few studies had evaluated supplemental arginine

as a single agent in the critically ill and septic patient population. An elaborate series of tracer studies in a clinical trial dealing with citrulline and arginine metabolism in septic patients has shed light on this controversy.[97] The complex metabolic alterations noted in sepsis that contribute to reduced citrulline and arginine availability suggest that supplemental arginine might in fact be beneficial in the septic population. In another study using tracer technology, investigators evaluated arginine in sepsis and also concluded that arginine might be deficient in sepsis because of inadequate de novo synthesis.[98]

These recent findings relating to arginine were published after the release of the Society of Critical Care Medicine and American Society for Parenteral and Enteral Nutrition Guidelines (2009) but will certainly be incorporated into future versions of the guidelines. Arginine is perhaps the most controversial of the immune-modulating nutrients, but it is important to reiterate that investigations examining the physiologic impact of arginine, and its related enzymes the nitric oxide synthases, have been conducted in different critically ill populations (e.g., medical vs. surgical, severely septic vs. nonseptic) using variable dosing, thereby making generalizations to all ICU populations difficult. There may be subgroups of patients whose vascular function is improved by L-arginine supplementation, and there may be other subgroups who simply do not benefit from L-arginine dietary supplementation. Arginine dose and patient selection are likely important factors affecting any nutrition study outcome.[99]

Arginine is available to the host from numerous sources. "Normal" arginine intake for a western diet is 5 to 7 g/day, while endogenous production of arginine is estimated at 15 to 20 g/day. Studies using different doses of arginine, from 5 to 30 g/day in the normal host, have shown varying results. It appears that orally delivered arginine supplementation up to 30 g/day is safe with few gastrointestinal side effects.[53,88] The current routinely used critical care enteral formulas deliver 0 to 18.7 g of supplemental arginine per liter of formula. It is estimated that on average, an ICU patient receiving arginine-supplemented enteral feeding at prescribed rates would receive 15 to 30 g/day of supplemental arginine.

Several factors must be considered when deciding whether arginine fits into the therapeutic plan of the critically ill patient. One must evaluate organ systems involved, timing of nutrient delivery, and location and route of delivery. The appropriate and safe level in the critically ill or hypermetabolic patient in which a proinflammatory state exists is much more difficult to determine. Arginine is very tightly regulated within the cell by multiple mechanisms including regulation of arginine transporters, as well as arginase and NOS enzymatic activity, and the colocalization of enzymes in the membrane leads to variable concentration within the intracellular space.[88] Arginine appears safe and beneficial in the levels delivered by commercially available supplemental formulations.

As with other studies on pharmaconutrients, in those reporting results with arginine supplementation, the arginine is given with other so-called immune or metabolically active agents, that is, fish oils or nucleic acids. The potential interactions between arginine and other delivered nutrients must also be considered. In very different models, several studies have both shown that delivery of an omega-3 fatty acid with arginine significantly alters the arginine metabolism via arginase and iNOS and possibly yields more available arginine.[100,101] Ornithine alpha-ketoglutarate (OKG) and citrulline are other nutrients that have been reported to have potential interaction with arginine. Citrulline is poorly metabolized by the liver and essentially bypasses first-pass hepatic nutrient metabolism, making it highly bioavailable via the oral route. Citrulline is then converted to arginine in the kidney, making citrulline a key component in arginine homeostasis, especially in the critical ill population.[88] It is clear that additional research is needed on the influence of arginine in specific populations, specific disease conditions, and the gene-nutrient interactions.

DELIVERY OF ARGININE
Arginine is safe and beneficial at doses delivered in immune and metabolic modulating formulas for most all hemodynamically stable ICU populations able to tolerate enteral feeding. This would include medical and surgical ICU patients, trauma patients, major surgical patients, and post-myocardial infarction or pulmonary hypertension patients. Elective major surgical patients across multiple surgical specialties can be expected to benefit from a reduction of surgical infections when arginine containing formulations are applied in the perioperative setting.[49] The optimal dose of arginine to

be delivered is yet to be determined. Arginine plasma levels fall rapidly in critical illness, trauma, and sepsis.[102] This decline in plasma levels is multifactorial and results from decreased dietary intake, increased uptake in tissues, and increased metabolism, mainly from the upregulation of arginase and iNOS (see Figure 28-5). Arginine transport in catabolic states is accelerated in several tissues including liver, intestine, lymphocytes, and endothelium.[103]

Omega-3 Fatty Acids
Although lipids are a mainstay in nutritional therapy for the critically ill and surgical populations, controversy exists regarding their digestion, absorption, and utilization in hyperdynamic surgical settings.[104,105] The heterogeneous nature of the ICU population makes lipid administration in these groups somewhat challenging. Although uncertainty exists regarding which lipid formulation to deliver, there is no debate regarding the need to meet the essential fatty acid and cellular oxidation requirements. The use of lipids in this manner replaces malabsorbed lipid nutrients and serves as a daily source of calories shown to be equally nitrogen-sparing with glucose when administered continuously for 4 days.[106] The beneficial antiinflammatory effects of omega-3 fatty acids, primarily eicosapentaenoic acid and docohexanoic acid (EPA and DHA), have been well documented in several chronic inflammatory diseases, including rheumatoid arthritis, Crohn's disease, ulcerative colitis, lupus erythematosus, multiple sclerosis, and asthma (Table 28-4).[107-110]

In addition to the use of antiinflammatory lipids in the setting of chronic illness, the use of specific antiinflammatory lipid substrates in the acute hyperdynamic setting to maintain vital organ function and to modulate key processes such as immunity, inflammation, and antioxidant defenses has now become routine in many surgical and ICU settings.[111] In numerous randomized clinical trials, appropriate use of the omega-3 fatty acids EPA/DHA can partially attenuate the

Table 28-4. Lipid Choices in Intensive Care Unit Stress States

Lipid absorption and utilization is very dependent on source, route, and metabolic state of the patient.
Enteral vs. Parenteral Lipids
Enteral superior to parenteral: significantly more lipid options enterally
Lipid Substrate
SCFA (requires colonic fermentation of soluble fibers)
  Acetate, butyrate, propionate
  Increase utilization in stress models
MCFA
  6-12 carbons
  Dual absorption via portal and lymphatics
  No carnitine required to enter inner mitochondria membrane for β oxidation
  Increase utilization
LCFA
  Omega-6
  Omega-3
  Utilization variable depending on carnitine, oxygenation, for example

LCFA, Long chain fatty acids; *MCFA,* medium chain fatty acids; *SCFA,* short chain fatty acids.

metabolic response, reverse or minimize loss of lean body tissue, prevent oxidative injury in a variety of tissues, and improve outcome by modulating synthesis of proinflammatory and antiinflammatory mediators.[104,111-113] The mechanisms of these effects are multiple and include changes in cell membrane phospholipids, alterations in gene expression, and modifications to endothelial expression of intracellular adhesion molecule 1 (ICAM-1), E-selectin, and other endothelial receptors regulating vascular integrity and function. Additionally, EPA and DHA derivatives, including resolvins, docosatrienes, and neuroprotectins, are potent effectors of the resolution of inflammation.[104,114] Resolvins regulate polymorphonuclear neutrophil transmigration. Neuroprotectins decrease neutrophil infiltration, proinflammatory gene signaling, and NFκB binding. These protective mediators are found to be highly conserved among species, from primitive fish to mammals.[115] Data also support the potential beneficial influence of EPA on preventing loss of diaphragm function in sepsis, and resistance to gram-negative pathogens such as *Pseudomonas* (Figure 28-6).[116,117]

EPA and DHA can be thought of as not just *passively* modulating the inflammatory process but as *actively* involved in the resolution of inflammation.[118,119] Use of enteral and parenteral formulations containing antiinflammatory lipids, primarily EPA and DHA, can be used as pharmacologic agents to modulate the hyperdynamic response and outcomes in surgical and critically ill patients.

CLINICAL OUTCOME STUDIES USING 20 AND 22 CARBON OMEGA-3 FATTY ACIDS

When evaluating the literature regarding the use of omega-3 fatty acids, it is important to take into account the species evaluated, experimental model, as well as total quantity of

macronutrient delivered, carbon structure, and lipid ratios. Variable and occasionally contradictory results exist for cell cultures, animal models, or in human clinical trials depending on these factors. Other significant factors include the route of delivery, timing of delivery in relation to the specified event, and the percent of lipid calories delivered. If the omega-3 fat is delivered as the 18 carbon α-linolenic acid form (canola oil or flaxseed oil), it often has little effect in humans.[120] However, if it is given as EPA or DHA, rapid and dramatic effects have been reported.[121] Other issues to evaluate include the amount of antioxidant vitamins and micronutrients delivered simultaneously. This is especially important for vitamin E, in that the amount of polyunsaturated fatty acid delivered can alter vitamin E requirements.[122]

DELIVERY OF OMEGA-3 FATTY ACIDS

As with the other pharmaconutrients previously discussed, the optimal dose, timing, and formulation of omega-3 fatty acids is unknown. Guided by a recent metaanalysis that aggregated the results of three randomized clinical trials conducted in patients with acute respiratory distress syndrome (ARDS), an enteral formula enriched with fish oils appears to significantly reduce mortality by as much as 49%, ventilator days, and ICU length of stay by up to 6 days.[123] More recent prospective, randomized trials of fish oils and borage oil in ARDS have shown no benefit.[124,125] Several issues should be resolved before abandoning the use of fish oils in ARDS, such as the method of feeding, background nutrition, and the patient's absorptive capacity with bolus delivery of the pharmacologic agents. While there is variability in outcome benefit seen in results from clinical trials using omega-3 antiinflammatory therapy in critically ill patients, doses greater than 5 g/day have consistently shown significant benefit in this population, specifically those with ALI/ARDS or sepsis/septic shock.[126] Numerous other studies in ICU populations continue to support the use of fish oils.[127]

TIMING OF DELIVERY OF NUTRIENTS AS PHARMACOLOGIC AGENTS

The timing for optimal delivery of pharmaconutrients appears to be before the stressful or traumatic event. A now classic study demonstrated that when arginine, fish oils, and nucleic acids were given as oral supplements 5 to 7 days before major gastrointestinal surgery there was a lower infection rate and a lower overall complication rate.[128] Most recently, a metaanalysis of 35 studies concluded that when arginine is given preoperatively, benefits include a significant decrease in infectious complications.[49]

As opposed to the surgical setting when the planned metabolic stress is known, to date there is inadequate supportive literature to yield the optimal time to deliver immune and metabolically active nutrients once the stressful event has taken place. Timing will depend on several factors such as the route of delivery, dosing, and method of delivery (e.g., bolus as a single agent, infusion with other nutrients). Growing evidence from mammalian models of sepsis and shock suggest that once the oxidative stress has damaged the cell's energy production potential via inducing mitochondrial damage, the detrimental changes are irreversible.[129,130] Once the patient has been adequately resuscitated and able to receive enteral

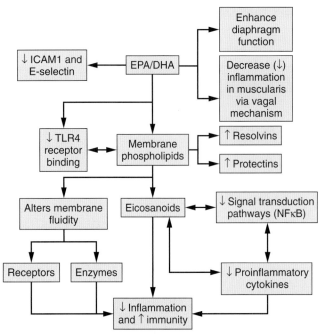

Figure 28-6 Multiple beneficial effects of eicosapentanoic acid and docosa hexaenoic acid in the critical care setting. *DHA,* Docosahexaenoic acid; *EPA,* eicosapentaenoic acid; *ICAM-1,* intracellular adhesion molecule-1; *NFκB,* nuclear factor kappa B; *TLR-4,* toll-like receptor-4.

New Definition of Malnutrition
Three Distinct Forms of Malnutrition

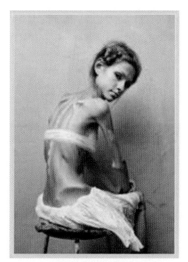

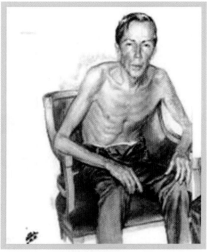

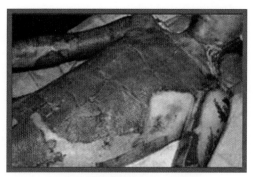

Starvation-related	Chronic disease-related	Acute disease or injury-related
No inflammation	Mild-mod inflammation	Severe inflammation
Example: Anorexia nervosa	Example: COPD, pancreatic cancer, sarcopenic obesity	Example: Burn, trauma, major infection, surgery

Figure 28-7 Refined definitions for malnutrition. *COPD,* Chronic obstructive pulmonary disease. *(Modified from Jensen GL, Mirtallo J, Compher C, et al. Adult starvation and disease-related malnutrition: a proposal for etiology-based diagnosis in the clinical practice setting from the international consensus guideline committee.* J Parenter Enteral Nutr. *2010;34:156-159.)*

feeding, these agents should be safe. One study specifically evaluated delivery of glutamine during shock resuscitation in the emergency department and found it to be safe and associated with enhanced intestinal tolerance to subsequent enteral feeding.[131]

Regarding route of delivery of metabolically active nutrients, no prospective randomized trials have evaluated or compared enteral with parenteral route. The optimal route of delivery for the majority of active nutrients remains uncertain, although it appears that the parenteral route is favorable for glutamine.[44] Parenteral EPA and DHA are reported to have beneficial influences within 1 to 24 hours, while enteral delivery might need 12 to 72 hours for beneficial or antiinflammatory effects.[132,133]

EMERGING DEVELOPMENTS

NEW PROTOCOLS AND MALNUTRITION DEFINITIONS

Protocols to deliver early nutrition effectively and safely either parenterally or enterally have been widely published.[42,43,134-138] These protocols have reported advantages in decreasing ventilator days, length of ICU stay, and even mortality.[21,134] The "CAN WE FEED" protocol links resuscitation with clinical assessment and nutrient delivery.[42] This protocol has rapidly gained widespread acceptance in ICUs across the globe.

Recently developed definitions for malnutrition (Figure 28-7) will aid in the ability to better define the various populations and allow specific therapies to improve outcomes.[139] Despite the controversies in critical care nutrition (Table 28-5), most major nutrition societies agree on the majority of issues (Table 28-6).

Table 28-5. Current Issues and Problems with Intensive Care Unit Nutrition

Failure to predict who will need support?
  Lack of adequate assessment markers
  Surrogate markers albumin, prealbumin, CRP, IGF-1 not currently useful
Controversy regarding what is the best formula to feed?
  Lack of understanding of "neutraceutical" approach
  Glutamine, arginine, fish oils (DHA, EPA), carnitine
Overreliance and inappropriate use of parenteral nutrition (PN)
  Starting PN for "one or two" days
  Nonphysiologic lipid and amino acid solutions (in United States)
The morbidly obese critically ill patient
  How many calories, IBW, ABW, BMI remain in question
Failure to maximize use of early enteral feeding
Failure to get adequate safe early enteral access
Unfounded indications for stopping and holding enteral feeding
Diagnostic tests, NPO for OR, "road trips", bathing

ABW, Actual body weight; *BMI,* body mass index (formula: weight (kg)/ [height(m)]²; *CRP,* C-reactive protein; *IBW,* ideal body weight; *IGF-1,* insulin-like growth factor-1.

Additional Metabolically Active Nutrients

Several other specific nutrients have been reported to be beneficial in the surgical population. Antioxidants such as vitamins C and E, and trace minerals like selenium and zinc, which function as cofactors for several potent endogenous antioxidant enzymes (superoxide dismutase and glutathione peroxidase), have received attention for their ability to improve outcomes in surgical and trauma patients.[140]

Other amino acids, including citrulline, taurine, leucine, and creatine, have also had variable success in improving metabolic outcomes or surrogate markers following major

Table 28-6. Critical Care Guidelines

Areas of common agreement: ADA, ASPEN, CPG, ESPEN, SCCM
All agree with:
  Early enteral feeding
  Enteral superior to parenteral nutrition
  Fish oils beneficial (except ADA)
  Postpyloric feeding preferable if possible
  Supplemental antioxidants
  Use of glutamine (except ADA)
  Use of arginine in surgery patients
    Preop in addition to postop when possible

ADA, American Dietetic Association; *ASPEN*, American Society of Parenteral and Enteral Nutrition; *CPG*, Canadian Clinical Practice Guidelines; *ESPEN*, European Society of Parenteral and Enteral Nutrition; *SCCM*, Society of Critical Care Medicine.

surgery or major trauma.[53] As with glutamine and arginine, these amino acids alter gene expression and intracellular protein turnover, and regulate metabolic pathways.[113,141]

Several studies show probiotics can decrease the inflammatory response, stabilize and support the mucosal surface, improve immune function, and decrease infectious complications in a wide range of surgical populations.[142,143] Probiotics are defined as "live microbial organisms which beneficially affect human health through the prevention of specific disease states."[144] Recent large prospective studies have reported significant decreases in ventilator-associated pneumonia (VAP) in several ICU settings. Studies suggest that probiotics reduce the incidence of VAP locally by promoting selective colonization and perhaps systematically by immunomodulation.[145]

A recent prospective randomized double-blinded placebo-controlled trial of mechanically ventilated patients at high risk of developing VAP examined the influence of probiotic therapy.[146] The probiotic group not only had about 50% lower incidence of VAP, but also had reduced total antibiotic use and *Clostridium difficile* diarrhea compared to placebo-treated patients. An earlier metaanalysis concluded that the incidence of VAP was significantly lower in patients treated with probiotics.[147] A recent literature review on the prevention of VAP concludes that probiotic therapy may be associated with a reduction in VAP but does not appear to reduce mortality.[145] The majority of studies report trends suggesting a treatment effect of probiotics in terms of reducing the incidence of VAP, but which probiotic to use, the optimal timing, duration of therapy, route, and methods of delivery are controversial.

Future Studies

The use of protocols to enhance the safe, early delivery of enteral nutrients is now well established. A large number of new or ongoing randomized controlled trials will soon advance our understanding of the mechanisms that drive the benefits, harms, toxicities, or null effects of pharmaconutrients. Future studies must focus on evidence-based therapies that impact clinically relevant surgical endpoints such as length of stay, infectious morbidity, and mortality, as well as more subtle clues of successful modulation of the stress response, wound healing, time to tracheal extubation, hemodynamic stability, and early mobility. The translation from human trials, mammalian models, and basic science studies has resulted in better understanding of immune and metabolic nutrients. Focused nutrition therapy has now reached a point where early aggressive enteral feeding via protocols and the use of pharmaconutrients should be incorporated into standard surgical and ICU practice. Novel therapies such as probiotics and specific amino acid therapy, combined with exercise in the ICU setting (even with ongoing mechanical ventilation), will undoubtedly change practice in the future. The questions of optimal doses, timing, and routes of these nutrients remain to be determined.

KEY POINTS

- Preoperative malnutrition is a risk factor for poor wound healing, perioperative complications, and mortality.
- The metabolic response to stress includes a hyperdynamic cardiac and pulmonary state, insulin resistance, hyperglycemia, and accelerated protein catabolism from muscle; unabated, this can culminate in PICS, MODS, and death.
- Early enteral feeding in critically ill patients is associated with numerous benefits, including attenuation of the inflammatory response to stress, prevention of loss of gut barrier function, maintenance of GALT, maintenance of normal gut bacteria, and support of the systemic immune response, among others.
- Enteral feeding should not begin until relative hemodynamic stability and other acute resuscitation issues have been accomplished. Institution of enteral feeding prematurely can result in NMI, a devastating complication with a high mortality rate.
- Pharmaconutrition or immunonutrition is defined as the provision of key nutrients that may modulate the inflammatory and/or the catabolic response associated with critical illness. Pharmaconutrition is distinct from the delivery of balanced macronutrient energy supply to support normal cell metabolism and division.
- Glutamine, arginine, and fish oils are the most prominent pharmaconutrients in contemporary nutritional therapy. The optimal dosage and timing of delivery of these pharmaconutrients are not yet well established.
- Nutritional therapy in the ICU is best accomplished on a multidisciplinary basis according to evidence-based protocols and multifaceted assessments.

Key References

Doig GS, Heighes PT, Simpson F, et al. Early enteral nutrition reduces mortality in trauma patients requiring intensive care: a meta-analysis of randomised controlled trials. *Injury.* 2011;42:50-56. An important meta-analysis suggesting that early enteral nutrition improves survival. The study acknowledges the need for larger, confirmatory clinical trials. (Ref. 14)

Gentile LF, Cuenca AG, Efron PA, et al. Persistent inflammation and immunosuppression: a common syndrome and new horizon for surgical intensive care. *J Trauma Acute Care Surg.* 2012;72:1491-1501. An important paper clarifying the evolving epidemiologic terms and concepts relating to persistent inflammation and immunosuppression in the ICU (i.e., SIRS, CARS, MODS, PICS). (Ref. 1)

Martindale RG, McClave SA, Vanek VW, et al. Guidelines for the provision and assessment of nutrition support therapy in the adult critically ill patient: Society of Critical Care Medicine and American Society for Parenteral and Enteral Nutrition: executive summary. *Crit Care Med.* 2009;37:1757-1761. A summary of current evidence-based practice guidelines for the provision of nutritional support in critically ill patients. (Ref. 44)

Moncure M, Samaha E, Moncure K, et al. Jejunostomy tube feedings should not be stopped in the perioperative patient. *J Parenter Enteral Nutr.* 1999;23:356-359. A prospective study suggesting that postpylorus tube feedings need not be stopped in the perioperative period. (Ref. 12)

References

1. Gentile LF, Cuenca AG, Efron PA, et al. Persistent inflammation and immunosuppression: a common syndrome and new horizon for surgical intensive care. *J Trauma Acute Care Surg.* 2012;72(6):1491-1501.
2. Hall MJ, Williams SN, DeFrances CJ, Golosinskiy A. Inpatient care for septicemia or sepsis: a challenge for patients and hospitals. *NCHS Data Brief.* 2011;(62):1-8.
3. Kochanek KD, Xu J, Murphy SL, et al. Deaths: preliminary data for 2009. *National Vital Statistics Reports.* 2011;59(4):1-51.
4. Sands KE, Bates DW, Lanken PN, et al. Epidemiology of sepsis syndrome in 8 academic medical centers. *J Am Med Assoc.* 1997;278(3):234-240.
5. Manship L, McMillin RD, Brown JJ. The influence of sepsis and multisystem and organ failure on mortality in the surgical intensive care unit. *Am Surg.* 1984;50(2):94-101.
6. Hotchkiss RS, Karl IE. The pathophysiology and treatment of sepsis. *N Engl J Med.* 2003;348(2):138-150.
7. Cruse PJ, Foord R. A five-year prospective study of 23,649 surgical wounds. *Arch Surg.* 1973;107(2):206-210.
8. Studley HO. Percentage of weight loss: a basic indicator of surgical risk in patients with chronic peptic ulcer. 1936. *Nutr Hosp.* 2001;16(4):140-143.
9. Reinhardt GF, Myscofski JW, Wilkens DB, Dobrin PB, Mangan Jr JE, Stannard RT. Incidence and mortality of hypoalbuminemic patients in hospitalized veterans. *J Parenter Enteral Nutr.* 1980;4(4):357-359.
10. Practice guidelines for preoperative fasting and the use of pharmacologic agents to reduce the risk of pulmonary aspiration: application to healthy patients undergoing elective procedures: a report by the American Society of Anesthesiologist Task Force on Preoperative Fasting. *Anesthesiology.* 1999;90(3):896-905.
11. Schricker T, Wykes L, Meterissian S, et al. The anabolic effect of perioperative nutrition depends on the patient's catabolic state before surgery. *Ann Surg.* August 9, 2012 [Epub ahead of print].
12. Moncure M, Samaha E, Moncure K, et al. Jejunostomy tube feedings should not be stopped in the perioperative patient. *J Parenter Enteral Nutr.* 1999;23(6):356-359.
13. Buchman AL, Moukarzel AA, Bhuta S, et al. Parenteral nutrition is associated with intestinal morphologic and functional changes in humans. *J Parenter Enteral Nutr.* 1995;19(6):453-460.
14. Doig GS, Heighes PT, Simpson F, Sweetman EA. Early enteral nutrition reduces mortality in trauma patients requiring intensive care: a meta-analysis of randomised controlled trials. *Injury.* 2011;42(1):50-56.
15. Petrov MS, Loveday BP, Pylypchuk RD, McIlroy K, Phillips AR, Windsor JA. Systematic review and meta-analysis of enteral nutrition formulations in acute pancreatitis. *Br J Surg.* 2009;96(11):1243-1252.
16. Lewis SJ, Egger M, Sylvester PA, Thomas S. Early enteral feeding versus "nil by mouth" after gastrointestinal surgery: systematic review and meta-analysis of controlled trials. *Br Med J.* 2001;323(7316):773-776.
17. Mutlu GM, Mutlu EA, Factor P. Prevention and treatment of gastrointestinal complications in patients on mechanical ventilation. *Am J Respir Med.* 2003;2(5):395-411.
18. Martindale RG, Shikora SA, Nishikawa R, Siepler JK. The metabolic response to stress and alterations in nutrient metabolism. In: Shikora SA, Martindale RG, Schwaitzberg SD, eds. Nutritional considerations in the intensive care unit: science, rationale, and practice. Kendall/Hunt Publishing Co. Dubuque, IA, 2002: 11-19.
19. Martindale RG, McClave SA, Vanek VW, et al. Guidelines for the provision and assessment of nutrition support therapy in the adult critically ill patient: Society of Critical Care Medicine and American Society for Parenteral and Enteral Nutrition: executive summary. *Crit Care Med.* 2009;37(5):1757-1761.
20. Marik PE, Zaloga GP. Early enteral nutrition in acutely ill patients: a systematic review. *Crit Care Med.* 2001;29(12):2264-2270.
21. Heyland DK, Cahill NE, Dhaliwal R, Sun X, Day AG, McClave SA. Impact of enteral feeding protocols on enteral nutrition delivery: results of a multicenter observational study. *J Parenter Enteral Nutr.* 2010;34(6):675-684.
22. Zaloga GP, Roberts PR, Marik P. Feeding the hemodynamically unstable patient: a critical evaluation of the evidence. *Nutr Clin Pract.* 2003;18(4):285-293.
23. Heyland DK, Dhaliwal R. Early enteral nutrition vs. early parenteral nutrition: an irrelevant question for the critically ill? *Crit Care Med.* 2005;33(1):260-261.
24. Osland E, Yunus RM, Khan S, Memon MA. Early versus traditional postoperative feeding in patients undergoing resectional gastrointestinal surgery: a meta-analysis. *J Parenter Enteral Nutr.* 2011;35(4):473-487.
25. Martins JR, Shiroma GM, Horie LM, Logullo L, Silva Mde L, Waitzberg DL. Factors leading to discrepancies between prescription and intake of enteral nutrition therapy in hospitalized patients. *Nutrition.* 2012;28(9):864-867.
26. McClave SA, Sexton LK, Spain DA, et al. Enteral tube feeding in the intensive care unit: factors impeding adequate delivery. *Crit Care Med.* 1999;27(7):1252-1256.
27. Rivers E, Nguyen B, Havstad S, et al. Early goal-directed therapy in the treatment of severe sepsis and septic shock. *N Engl J Med.* 2001;345(19):1368-1377.
28. Revelly JP, Tappy L, Berger MM, Gersbach P, Cayeux C, Chiolero R. Early metabolic and splanchnic responses to enteral nutrition in postoperative cardiac surgery patients with circulatory compromise. *Intensive Care Med.* 2001;27(3):540-547.
29. Park WM, Gloviczki P, Cherry Jr KJ, et al. Contemporary management of acute mesenteric ischemia: factors associated with survival. *J Vasc Surg.* 2002;35(3):445-452.
30. Caddell KA, Martindale R, McClave SA, Miller K. Can the intestinal dysmotility of critical illness be differentiated from postoperative ileus? *Curr Gastroenterol Rep.* 2011;13(4):358-367.
31. Suehiro T, Matsumata T, Shikada Y, Sugimachi K. Accelerated rehabilitation with early postoperative oral feeding following gastrectomy. *Hepatogastroenterology.* 2004;51(60):1852-1855.
32. Doig GS, Heighes PT, Simpson F, Sweetman EA, Davies AR. Early enteral nutrition, provided within 24 h of injury or intensive care unit admission, significantly reduces mortality in critically ill patients: a meta-analysis of randomised controlled trials. *Intensive Care Med.* 2009;35(12):2018-2027.
33. Schmidt H, Martindale R. The gastrointestinal tract in critical illness: nutritional implications. *Curr Opin Clin Nutr Metab Care.* 2003;6(5):587-591.
34. Kalff JC, Turler A, Schwarz NT, et al. Intra-abdominal activation of a local inflammatory response within the human muscularis externa during laparotomy. *Ann Surg.* 2003;237(3):301-315.
35. Ritz MA, Fraser R, Tam W, Dent J. Impacts and patterns of disturbed gastrointestinal function in critically ill patients. *Am J Gastroenterol.* 2000;95(11):3044-3052.
36. Alverdy J, Zaborina O, Wu L. The impact of stress and nutrition on bacterial-host interactions at the intestinal epithelial surface. *Curr Opin Clin Nutr Metab Care.* 2005;8(2):205-209.
37. Ayala A, Chung CS, Grutkoski PS, Song GY. Mechanisms of immune resolution. *Crit Care Med.* 2003;31(8 Suppl):S558-S571.
38. Scirocco A, Matarrese P, Petitta C, et al. Exposure of toll-like receptors 4 to bacterial lipopolysaccharide (LPS) impairs human colonic smooth muscle cell function. *J Cell Physiol.* 2010;223(2):442-450.
39. Wehner S, Vilz TO, Stoffels B, Kalff JC. Immune mediators of postoperative ileus. *Langenbecks Arch Surg.* 2012;397(4):591-601.
40. Gatt M, MacFie J. Bedside postpyloric feeding tube placement: a pilot series to validate this novel technique. *Crit Care Med.* 2009;37(2):523-527.
41. Wolff BG, Michelassi F, Gerkin TM, et al. Alvimopan, a novel, peripherally acting mu opioid antagonist: results of a multicenter,

randomized, double-blind, placebo-controlled, phase III trial of major abdominal surgery and postoperative ileus. *Ann Surg.* 2004;240(4):728-735.

42. Miller KR, Kiraly LN, Lowen CC, Martindale RG, McClave SA. "CAN WE FEED?" A mnemonic to merge nutrition and intensive care assessment of the critically ill patient. *J Parenter Enteral Nutr.* 2011;35(5):643-659.

43. Kozar RA, McQuiggan MM, Moore EE, Kudsk KA, Jurkovich GJ, Moore FA. Postinjury enteral tolerance is reliably achieved by a standardized protocol. *J Surg Res.* 2002;104(1):70-75.

44. Martindale RG, McClave SA, Vanek VW, et al. Guidelines for the provision and assessment of nutrition support therapy in the adult critically ill patient: Society of Critical Care Medicine and American Society for Parenteral and Enteral Nutrition: executive summary. *Crit Care Med.* 2009;37(5):1757-1761.

45. Hardy G, Manzanares W. Pharmaconutrition: how has this concept evolved in the last two decades? *Nutrition.* 2011;27(10):1090-1092.

46. Cerantola Y, Hubner M, Grass F, Demartines N, Schafer M. Immunonutrition in gastrointestinal surgery. *Br J Surg.* 2011;98(1):37-48.

47. Weimann A, Braga M, Harsanyi L, et al. ESPEN guidelines on enteral nutrition: surgery including organ transplantation. *Clin Nutr.* 2006;25(2):224-244.

48. Marimuthu K, Varadhan KK, Ljungqvist O, Lobo DN. A meta-analysis of the effect of combinations of immune modulating nutrients on outcome in patients undergoing major open gastrointestinal surgery. *Ann Surg.* 2012;255(6):1060-1068.

49. Drover JW, Dhaliwal R, Weitzel L, Wischmeyer PE, Ochoa JB, Heyland DK. Perioperative use of arginine-supplemented diets: a systematic review of the evidence. *J Am Coll Surg.* 2011;212(3):385-399, 399.e1.

50. Hunter J. *A Treatise on the Blood, Inflammation and Gunshot Wounds.* London: Nicol; 1794.

51. Cuthbertson D, Tilstone WJ. Metabolism during the postinjury period. *Advances in Clinical Chemistry.* 1969;12:1-55.

52. Atiyeh BS, Gunn SW, Dibo SA. Metabolic implications of severe burn injuries and their management: a systematic review of the literature. *World J Surg.* 2008;32(8):1857-1869.

53. Wu G. Amino acids: metabolism, functions, and nutrition. *Amino Acids.* 2009;37(1):1-17.

54. Wischmeyer PE. Glutamine: role in gut protection in critical illness. *Curr Opin Clin Nutr Metab Care.* 2006;9(5):607-612.

55. Alpers DH. Glutamine: do the data support the cause for glutamine supplementation in humans? *Gastroenterology.* 2006;130(2 Suppl 1):S106-S116.

56. Santora R, Kozar RA. Molecular mechanisms of pharmaconutrients. *J Surg Res.* 2010;161(2):288-294.

57. Curi R, Newsholme P, Procopio J, Lagranha C, Gorjao R, Pithon-Curi TC. Glutamine, gene expression, and cell function. *Front Biosci.* 2007;12:344-357.

58. Sacks GS. Effect of glutamine-supplemented parenteral nutrition on mortality in critically ill patients. *Nutr Clin Pract.* 2011;26(1):44-47.

59. Ziegler TR, Bazargan N, Leader LM, Martindale RG. Glutamine and the gastrointestinal tract. *Curr Opin Clin Nutr Metab Care.* 2000;3(5):355-362.

60. Griffiths RD. Glutamine: establishing clinical indications. *Curr Opin Clin Nutr Metab Care.* 1999;2(2):177-182.

61. Roth E. Nonnutritive effects of glutamine. *J Nutr.* 2008;138(10):2025S-2031S.

62. Weitzel LR, Wischmeyer PE. Glutamine in critical illness: the time has come, the time is now. *Crit Care Clin.* 2010;26(3):515-525.

63. Grau T, Bonet A, Minambres E, et al. The effect of L-alanyl-L-glutamine dipeptide supplemented total parenteral nutrition on infectious morbidity and insulin sensitivity in critically ill patients. *Crit Care Med.* 2011;39(6):1263-1268.

64. Rodas PC, Rooyackers O, Hebert C, Norberg A, Wernerman J. Glutamine and glutathione at ICU admission in relation to outcome. *Clin Sci (Lond).* 2012;122(12):591-597.

65. Wernerman J. Glutamine supplementation. *Ann Intensive Care.* 2011;1(1):25.

66. Wernerman J, Kirketeig T, Andersson B, et al. Scandinavian glutamine trial: a pragmatic multi-centre randomised clinical trial of intensive care unit patients. *Acta Anaesthesiol Scand.* 2011;55(7):812-818.

67. Houdijk AP, Rijnsburger ER, Jansen J, et al. Randomised trial of glutamine-enriched enteral nutrition on infectious morbidity in patients with multiple trauma. *Lancet.* 1998;352(9130):772-776.

68. Dechelotte P, Hasselmann M, Cynober L, et al. L-alanyl-L-glutamine dipeptide-supplemented total parenteral nutrition reduces infectious complications and glucose intolerance in critically ill patients: the French controlled, randomized, double-blind, multicenter study. *Crit Care Med.* 2006;34(3):598-604.

69. Byrne TA, Wilmore DW, Iyer K, et al. Growth hormone, glutamine, and an optimal diet reduces parenteral nutrition in patients with short bowel syndrome: a prospective, randomized, placebo-controlled, double-blind clinical trial. *Ann Surg.* 2005;242(5):655-661.

70. Singleton KD, Serkova N, Beckey VE, Wischmeyer PE. Glutamine attenuates lung injury and improves survival after sepsis: role of enhanced heat shock protein expression. *Crit Care Med.* 2005;33(6):1206-1213.

71. Ziegler TR, Ogden LG, Singleton KD, et al. Parenteral glutamine increases serum heat shock protein 70 in critically ill patients. *Intensive Care Med.* 2005;31(8):1079-1086.

72. Hamiel CR, Pinto S, Hau A, Wischmeyer PE. Glutamine enhances heat shock protein 70 expression via increased hexosamine biosynthetic pathway activity. *Am J Physiol Cell Physiol.* 2009;297(6):C1509-C1519.

73. Wischmeyer PE, Heyland DK. The future of critical care nutrition therapy. *Crit Care Clin.* 2010;26(3):433-441.

74. Macario AJ, Conway de Macario E. Sick chaperones, cellular stress, and disease. *N Engl J Med.* 2005;353(14):1489-1501.

75. Wischmeyer PE. Glutamine: role in critical illness and ongoing clinical trials. *Curr Opin Gastroenterol.* 2008;24(2):190-197.

76. Nose K, Yang H, Sun X, et al. Glutamine prevents total parenteral nutrition-associated changes to intraepithelial lymphocyte phenotype and function: a potential mechanism for the preservation of epithelial barrier function. *J Interferon Cytokine Res.* 2010;30(2):67-80.

77. Ren ZG, Liu H, Jiang JW, et al. Protective effect of probiotics on intestinal barrier function in malnourished rats after liver transplantation. *Hepatobiliary Pancreat Dis Int.* 2011;10(5):489-496.

78. Griffiths RD. Outcome of critically ill patients after supplementation with glutamine. *Nutrition.* 1997;13(7-8):752-754.

79. Ziegler TR, Young LS, Benfell K, et al. Clinical and metabolic efficacy of glutamine-supplemented parenteral nutrition after bone marrow transplantation. A randomized, double-blind, controlled study. *Ann Intern Med.* 1992;116(10):821-828.

80. Anderson PM, Schroeder G, Skubitz KM. Oral glutamine reduces the duration and severity of stomatitis after cytotoxic cancer chemotherapy. *Cancer.* 1998;83(7):1433-1439.

81. Yoshida S, Matsui M, Shirouzu Y, Fujita H, Yamana H, Shirouzu K. Effects of glutamine supplements and radiochemotherapy on systemic immune and gut barrier function in patients with advanced esophageal cancer. *Ann Surg.* 1998;227(4):485-491.

82. Novak F, Heyland DK, Avenell A, Drover JW, Su X. Glutamine supplementation in serious illness: a systematic review of the evidence. *Crit Care Med.* 2002;30(9):2022-2029.

83. Andrews PJ, Avenell A, Noble DW, et al. Randomised trial of glutamine, selenium, or both, to supplement parenteral nutrition for critically ill patients. *Br Med J.* 2011;342:d1542.

84. Wernerman J, Kirketeig T, Andersson B, et al. Scandinavian glutamine trial: a pragmatic multi-centre randomised clinical trial of intensive care unit patients. *Acta Anaesthesiol Scand.* 2011;55(7):812-818.

85. Zhu X, Herrera G, Ochoa JB. Immunosuppression and infection after major surgery: a nutritional deficiency. *Crit Care Clin.* 2010;26(3):491-500.

86. Popovic PJ, Zeh 3rd HJ, Ochoa JB. Arginine and immunity. *J Nutr.* 2007;137(6 Suppl 2):1681S-1686S.

87. Zhou M, Martindale RG. Arginine in the critical care setting. *J Nutr.* 2007;137(6 Suppl 2):1687S-1692S.

88. Morris Jr SM. Arginine: master and commander in innate immune responses. *Sci Signal.* 2010;3(135):pe27.

89. Bansal V, Ochoa JB. Arginine availability, arginase, and the immune response. *Curr Opin Clin Nutr Metab Care.* 2003;6(2):223-228.

90. Luiking YC, Poeze M, Dejong CH, Ramsay G, Deutz NE. Sepsis: an arginine deficiency state? *Crit Care Med.* 2004;32(10):2135-2145.

91. Marik PE. Arginine: too much of a good thing may be bad! *Crit Care Med.* 2006;34(11):2844-2847.

92. Martindale RG, McCarthy MS, McClave SA. Guidelines for nutrition therapy in critical illness: are not they all the same? *Minerva Anestesiol.* 2011;77(4):463-467.

93. Lopez A, Lorente JA, Steingrub J, et al. Multiple-center, randomized, placebo-controlled, double-blind study of the nitric oxide synthase inhibitor 546C88: effect on survival in patients with septic shock. *Crit Care Med.* 2004;32(1):21-30.

94. Iapichino G, Albicini M, Umbrello M, et al. Tight glycemic control does not affect asymmetric-dimethylarginine in septic patients. *Intensive Care Med.* 2008;34(10):1843-1850.

95. Zoccali C, Maas R, Cutrupi S, et al. Asymmetric dimethyl-arginine (ADMA) response to inflammation in acute infections. *Nephrol Dial Transplant.* 2007;22(3):801-806.

96. Visser M, Vermeulen MA, Richir MC, et al. Imbalance of arginine and asymmetric dimethylarginine is associated with markers of circulatory failure, organ failure and mortality in shock patients. *Br J Nutr.* 2012;107(10):1458-1465.

97. Luiking YC, Poeze M, Ramsay G, Deutz NE. Reduced citrulline production in sepsis is related to diminished de novo arginine and nitric oxide production. *Am J Clin Nutr.* 2009;89(1):142-152.

98. Kao CC, Bandi V, Guntupalli KK, Wu M, Castillo L, Jahoor F. Arginine, citrulline and nitric oxide metabolism in sepsis. *Clin Sci (Lond).* 2009;117(1):23-30.

99. Boger RH. The pharmacodynamics of L-arginine. *J Nutr.* 2007;137(6 Suppl 2):1650S-1655S.

100. Bansal V, Syres KM, Makarenkova V, et al. Interactions between fatty acids and arginine metabolism: implications for the design of immune-enhancing diets. *J Parenter Enteral Nutr.* 2005;29(1 Suppl):S75-S80.

101. Alexander JW, Metze TJ, McIntosh MJ, et al. The influence of immunomodulatory diets on transplant success and complications. *Transplantation.* 2005;79(4):460-465.

102. Chiarla C, Giovannini I, Siegel JH. Plasma arginine correlations in trauma and sepsis. *Amino Acids.* 2006;30(1):81-86.

103. Pan M, Choudry HA, Epler MJ, et al. Arginine transport in catabolic disease states. *J Nutr.* 2004;134(Suppl 10):2826S-2829S; discussion 2853S.

104. Calder PC. Rationale and use of omega-3 fatty acids in artificial nutrition. *Proc Nutr Soc.* 2010;69(4):565-573.

105. Calder PC, Yaqoob P. Understanding omega-3 polyunsaturated fatty acids. *Postgrad Med.* 2009;121(6):148-157.

106. Jeejeebhoy K, Anderson G, Nakhooda A. Metabolic studies in total parenteral nutrition in man. *J Clin Invest.* 1975;57:125-136.

107. Bhangle S, Kolasinski SL. Fish oil in rheumatic diseases. *Rheum Dis Clin North Am.* 2011;37(1):77-84.

108. Weitz D, Weintraub H, Fisher E, Schwartzbard AZ. Fish oil for the treatment of cardiovascular disease. *Cardiol Rev.* 2010;18(5):258-263.

109. Wilczynska-Kwiatek A, Bargiel-Matusiewicz K, Lapinski L. Asthma, allergy, mood disorders, and nutrition. *Eur J Med Res.* 2009;14(Suppl 4):248-254.

110. Turner D, Shah PS, Steinhart AH, Zlotkin S, Griffiths AM. Maintenance of remission in inflammatory bowel disease using omega-3 fatty acids (fish oil): a systematic review and meta-analyses. *Inflamm Bowel Dis.* 2011;17(1):336-345.

111. Singer P, Shapiro H, Theilla M, Anbar R, Singer J, Cohen J. Anti-inflammatory properties of omega-3 fatty acids in critical illness: novel mechanisms and an integrative perspective. *Intensive Care Med.* 2008;34(9):1580-1592.

112. Pittet YK, Berger MM, Pluess TT, et al. Blunting the response to endotoxin in healthy subjects: effects of various doses of intravenous fish oil. *Intensive Care Med.* 2010;36(2):289-295.

113. Wischmeyer P. Nutritional pharmacology in surgery and critical care: 'you must unlearn what you have learned.' *Curr Opin Anaesthesiol.* 2011;24(4):381-388.

114. Massaro M, Scoditti E, Carluccio MA, Campana MC, De Caterina R. Omega-3 fatty acids, inflammation and angiogenesis: basic mechanisms behind the cardioprotective effects of fish and fish oils. *Cell Mol Biol (Noisy-le-grand).* 2010;56(1):59-82.

115. Serhan CN, Krishnamoorthy S, Recchiuti A, Chiang N. Novel anti-inflammatory—pro-resolving mediators and their receptors. *Curr Top Med Chem.* 2011;11(6):629-647.

116. Supinski GS, Vanags J, Callahan LA. Eicosapentaenoic acid preserves diaphragm force generation following endotoxin administration. *Crit Care.* 2010;14(2):R35.

117. Tiesset H, Bernard H, Bartke N, et al. (Omega-3) long-chain PUFA differentially affect resistance to *Pseudomonas aeruginosa* infection of male and female cftr-/- mice. *J Nutr.* 2011;141(6):1101-1107.

118. Serhan CN, Yacoubian S, Yang R. Anti-inflammatory and proresolving lipid mediators. *Annu Rev Pathol.* 2008;3:279.

119. Bannenberg G, Serhan CN. Specialized pro-resolving lipid mediators in the inflammatory response: an update. *Biochim Biophys Acta.* 2010;1801(12):1260-1273.

120. Calder PC. Omega-3 polyunsaturated fatty acids and inflammatory processes: nutrition or pharmacology? *Br J Clin Pharmacol.* July 6, 2012 [Epub ahead of print].

121. Pluess TT, Hayoz D, Berger MM, et al. Intravenous fish oil blunts the physiological response to endotoxin in healthy subjects. *Intensive Care Med.* 2007;33(5):789-797.

122. Atkinson J, Harroun T, Wassall SR, Stillwell W, Katsaras J. The location and behavior of alpha-tocopherol in membranes. *Mol Nutr Food Res.* 2010;54(5):641-651.

123. Jones NE, Heyland DK. Pharmaconutrition: a new emerging paradigm. *Curr Opin Gastroenterol.* 2008;24(2):215-222.

124. Rice TW, Wheeler AP, Thompson BT, et al. Enteral omega-3 fatty acid, gamma-linolenic acid, and antioxidant supplementation in acute lung injury. *J Am Med Assoc* 2011;306(14):1574-1581.

125. Stapleton RD, Martin TR, Weiss NS, et al. A phase II randomized placebo-controlled trial of omega-3 fatty acids for the treatment of acute lung injury. *Crit Care Med.* 2011;39(7):1655-1662.

126. Todd SR, Gonzalez EA, Turner K, Kozar RA. Update on postinjury nutrition. *Curr Opin Crit Care.* 2008;14(6):690-695.

127. van der Meij BS, van Bokhorst-de van der Schueren MA, Langius JA, Brouwer IA, van Leeuwen PA. Omega-3 PUFAs in cancer, surgery, and critical care: a systematic review on clinical effects, incorporation, and washout of oral or enteral compared with parenteral supplementation. *Am J Clin Nutr.* 2011;94(5):1248-1265.

128. Braga M, Gianotti L, Nespoli L, Radaelli G, Di Carlo V. Nutritional approach in malnourished surgical patients: a prospective randomized study. *Arch Surg.* 2002;137(2):174-180.

129. Garrabou G, Moren C, Lopez S, et al. The effects of sepsis on mitochondria. *J Infect Dis.* 2012;205(3):392-400.

130. Galley HF. Oxidative stress and mitochondrial dysfunction in sepsis. *Br J Anaesth.* 2011;107(1):57-64.

131. McQuiggan M, Kozar R, Sailors RM, Ahn C, McKinley B, Moore F. Enteral glutamine during active shock resuscitation is safe and enhances tolerance of enteral feeding. *J Parenter Enteral Nutr.* 2008;32(1):28-35.

132. Calder PC. Fatty acids and inflammation: the cutting edge between food and pharma. *Eur J Pharmacol.* 2011;668(Suppl 1):S50-S58.

133. van der Meij BS, van Bokhorst-de van der Schueren MA, Langius JA, Brouwer IA, van Leeuwen PA. Omega-3 PUFAs in cancer, surgery, and critical care: a systematic review on clinical effects, incorporation, and washout of oral or enteral compared with parenteral supplementation. *Am J Clin Nutr.* 2011;94(5):1248-1265.

134. Martin CM, Doig GS, Heyland DK, Morrison T, Sibbald WJ, Southwestern Ontario Critical Care Research Network. Multicentre, cluster-randomized clinical trial of algorithms for critical-care enteral and parenteral therapy (ACCEPT). *Can Med Assoc J.* 2004;170(2):197-204.

135. Davies AR, Morrison SS, Bailey MJ, et al. A multicenter, randomized controlled trial comparing early nasojejunal with nasogastric nutrition in critical illness. *Crit Care Med.* 2012;40(8):2342-2348.

136. Marshall AP, Cahill NE, Gramlich L, MacDonald G, Alberda C, Heyland DK. Optimizing nutrition in intensive care units: empowering critical care nurses to be effective agents of change. *Am J Crit Care.* 2012;21(3):186-194.

137. Heyland DK, Dhaliwal R, Jiang X, Day AG. Identifying critically ill patients who benefit the most from nutrition therapy: the development and initial validation of a novel risk assessment tool. *Crit Care.* 2011;15(6):R268.

138. Marr AB, McQuiggan MM, Kozar R, Moore FA. Gastric feeding as an extension of an established enteral nutrition protocol. *Nutr Clin Pract.* 2004;19(5):504-510.

139. Jensen GL, Mirtallo J, Compher C, et al. Adult starvation and disease-related malnutrition: a proposal for etiology-based

diagnosis in the clinical practice setting from the international consensus guideline committee. *J Parenter Enteral Nutr*. 2010;34(2): 156-159.

140. Heyland DK, Dhaliwal R, Suchner U, Berger MM. Antioxidant nutrients: a systematic review of trace elements and vitamins in the critically ill patient. *Intensive Care Med*. 2005;31(3):327-337.

141. Jayarajan S, Daly JM. The relationships of nutrients, routes of delivery, and immunocompetence. *Surg Clin North Am*. 2011;91(4): 737-753.

142. Jeppsson B, Mangell P, Thorlacius H. Use of probiotics as prophylaxis for postoperative infections. *Nutrients*. 2011;3(5):604-612.

143. Lundell L. Use of probiotics in abdominal surgery. *Dig Dis*. 2011;29(6):570-573.

144. Fuller R. Probiotics in human medicine. *Ann Med*. 1990;22: 37-41.

145. Heineman J, Bubenik S, McClave S, Martindale R. Fighting fire with fire: is it time to use probiotics to manage pathogenic bacterial diseases? *Curr Gastroenterol Rep*. 2012;14(4):343-348.

146. Morrow LE, Kollef MH, Casale TB. Probiotic prophylaxis of ventilator-associated pneumonia. A blinded, randomized, controlled trial. *Am J Respir Crit Care Med*. 2010;182:1058-1064.

147. Siempos II, Ntaidou TK, Falagas ME. Impact of the administration of probiotics on the incidence of ventilator-associated pneumonia: a meta-analysis of randomized controlled trials. *Crit Care Med*. 2010;38(3):954-962.

Chapter 29

PHARMACOLOGY OF POSTOPERATIVE NAUSEA AND VOMITING

Rachel Whelan and Christian C. Apfel

HISTORICAL PERSPECTIVE

In the first half of the 20th century, one of the most feared complications of general anesthesia was postoperative vomiting, primarily because aspiration of gastric contents into the lungs could lead to death. Early prophylaxis sometimes consisted of advising patients to consume olive oil before general anesthesia to shield the intestinal wall from emetogenic gases. Prevention of postoperative vomiting was one of the primary motivations for developing local/regional anesthesia blocks, first with cocaine and procaine, then with lidocaine. Postoperative nausea, on the other hand, was considered too minor a complication to measure—until the development in the 1950s and 1960s of anesthetic drugs that could be cleared more rapidly (e.g., halothane, barbiturates, and novel opioids), which meant that patients spent more of the immediate postoperative period awake.[1]

While the antiemetic effect of some drugs, like anticholinergics, were first described more than a century ago, modern understanding of the specific receptor pathways and intracellular processes involved in postoperative nausea and vomiting (PONV) is relatively recent. It was not until the 1950s that interest in antiemetic drugs took off, with the identification of histamine and dopamine receptors in the nausea and vomiting pathway, and hence the clinical utility of H_1 and D_2 receptor antagonists like cyclizine, chlorpromazine, and promethazine. This surge in research on antiemetics was largely driven by advances in chemotherapy and a focus on chemotherapy-related outcomes. For example, neuro-oncologists first noticed the antiemetic effect of corticosteroids before the same observation was made for PONV in the 1990s.[1]

The development of 5-hydroxytryptamine type 3 (5-HT$_3$) receptor antagonists marks the greatest shift in antiemetic drug research. Early 5-HT$_3$ receptor antagonists were not more effective than other available antiemetics, but they were the first to be specifically designed by the pharmaceutical industry to target chemotherapy-induced nausea and vomiting (CINV) and PONV. This led to an increase in large, well-designed PONV studies, marketing of antiemetic agents, and a focus on PONV as a significant postoperative outcome.[1] The first-generation 5-HT$_3$ receptor antagonists are associated with QTc prolongation, but the newest 5-HT$_3$ receptor antagonists, palonosetron, appears to have improved efficacy, duration of action, and side-effect profile compared to its predecessors. Neurokinin-1 (NK1) receptor antagonists, such as aprepitant, are the newest class of antiemetic drugs, and they too benefit from a long duration of action and favorable side-effect profile. As current understanding of the nausea and vomiting pathway, pharmacokinetics and pharmacodynamics, and genetics continues to improve, antiemetic drugs are likely to become safer and easier to tailor to individual patients.

MECHANISMS OF NAUSEA AND VOMITING

Despite thousands of studies, new insights into target receptor function, and the successful development of novel antiemetic agents, the actual mechanisms of nausea and vomiting remain unknown. Most antiemetic drugs act upon one of several putative neurotransmitter pathways. 5-HT$_3$ receptor antagonists are the most commonly used antiemetic class of drugs (Table 29-1). Other classes include dopamine (D$_2$), histamine (H$_1$), NK1, GABA$_A$, opioid, and muscarinic cholinergic receptor antagonists.

The receptors upon which antiemetics act certainly play a role in nausea and vomiting. However, given that only 20% to 30% of patients respond to any one agent, nausea and vomiting cannot be solely attributed to activity of one—or several—of these receptor classes. It is also likely that individual variability plays a larger role than previously acknowledged. While it is essential to understand and investigate the drug-receptor relationship, the therapeutic potential of targeting specific receptor classes is limited.

Nausea and vomiting can be triggered by a variety of stimuli, including toxins, anxiety, adverse drug reactions, pregnancy, radiation, chemotherapy, and motion. These stimuli are integrated by the vomiting center in the nucleus tractus solitarius (NTS), located primarily in the medulla as well as in the lower pons. The vomiting center receives input from the adjacent chemoreceptor trigger zone (CTZ), the gastrointestinal (GI) tract, the vestibular system, and the cerebral cortex (Figure 29-1).

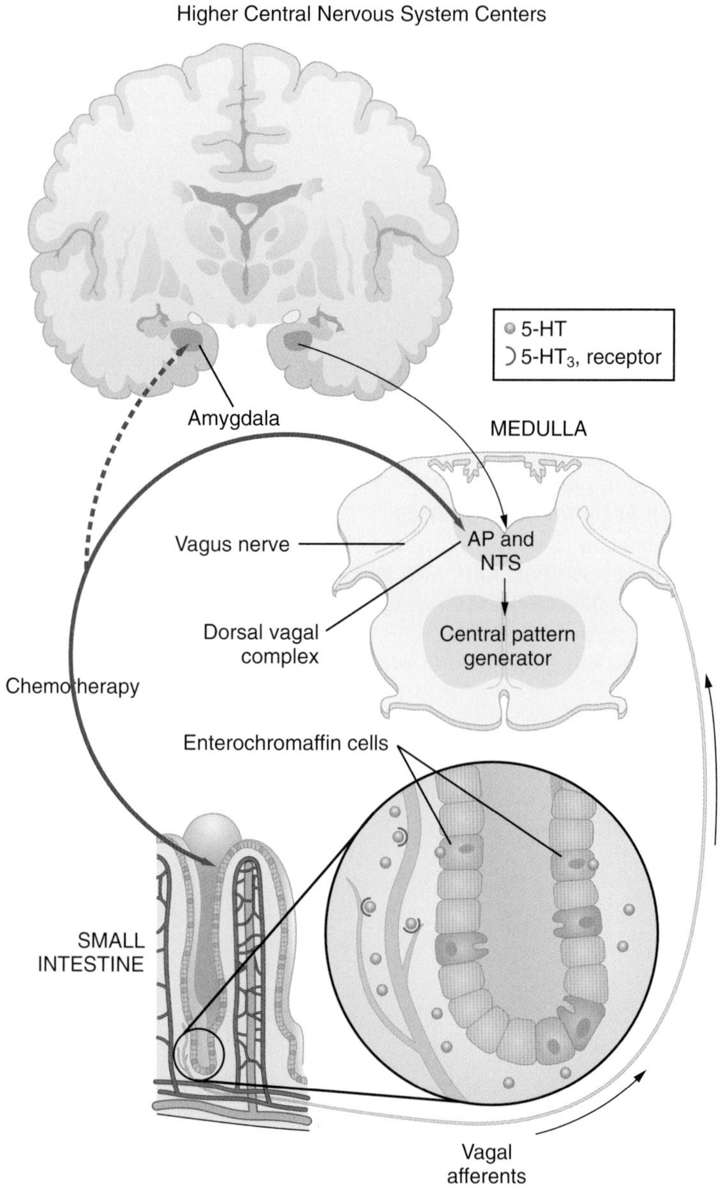

Figure 29-1 Schematic of pathways involved in postoperative nausea and vomiting. *5-HT,* 5-hydroxytryptamine; *5-HT₃,* 5-hydroxytryptamine type 3 receptor; *AP,* area postrema; *NTS,* nucleus tractus solitarius.

The CTZ is located at the caudal end of the fourth ventricle in the area postrema, a highly vascularized structure that lacks a true blood-brain barrier. Therefore chemosensitive receptors in the CTZ can be directly stimulated by toxins, metabolites, and drugs that circulate in the blood and cerebrospinal fluid. The CTZ communicates with the vomiting center primarily via D_2 receptors as well as $5\text{-}HT_3$ receptors. Enterochromaffin cells in the GI tract release serotonin, which stimulates vagal afferents that terminate in the CTZ and communicate information regarding intestinal luminal compounds and gastric tone. The vestibular system, located in the bony labyrinth of the temporal lobe, detects changes in equilibrium, which can cause motion sickness. Histamine (histamine-1 receptor, H_1) and acetylcholine (muscarinic acetylcholine receptors, mACh) are the neurotransmitters that communicate between the vestibular system and the vomiting center. Anticipatory or anxiety-induced nausea and vomiting probably originates in the cerebral cortex. The cortex has direct input to the vomiting center (VC) via several types of neuroreceptors.

SEROTONIN RECEPTOR ANTAGONISTS

Serotonin ($5\text{-}HT_3$) receptors are ligand-gated Na^+ and K^+ channels found throughout the central and peripheral nervous systems, notably in the CTZ and afferent fibers of the vagus nerve in both the gut and central nervous system (Figure 29-1). Serotonin activation of the CTZ and vagal afferents can both trigger the vomiting reflex. Serotonin plays an important role in anesthesia-, chemotherapy-, and radiation-induced nausea and vomiting. Serotonin receptor antagonists can be used as antiemetic treatment because they inhibit both central and peripheral stimulation of $5\text{-}HT_3$ receptors, and they are effective, nonsedative, and generally well tolerated. Thus $5\text{-}HT_3$ receptor antagonists are currently the most commonly used antiemetic agents for PONV, CINV, and rescue treatment.

Ondansetron

Ondansetron was the first $5\text{-}HT_3$ receptor antagonist approved by the U.S. Food and Drug Administration (FDA), and at the time of its development, was the safest and most effective treatment for early CINV.[2] Its reputation for superior CINV prophylaxis carried over to PONV, but a factorial trial in more than 5000 patients showed that 4 mg ondansetron was only as effective as 4 mg dexamethasone and 1.25 mg droperidol for PONV.[3] Contrary to the common clinical impression that ondansetron is less effective against nausea than against vomiting, the relative risk reduction (risk ratio) of ondansetron is the same for nausea and for vomiting.[4] However, ondansetron's plasma half-life is only about 4 hours, which is probably why several studies found it to be more efficacious when administered toward the end rather than at the beginning of anesthesia.[5] Like other $5\text{-}HT_3$ receptor antagonists, ondansetron's side effects are generally mild to moderate and include constipation and headache, the latter of which is increased by about 3%.[6] First-generation $5\text{-}HT_3$ receptor antagonists like ondansetron have also been associated with QTc prolongation, which potentially increases the risk of cardiac arrhythmia and cardiac arrest.[7] The QTc

prolongation associated with ondansetron use is similar to that caused by droperidol.[8]

Even though $5\text{-}HT_3$ receptor antagonists are among the most effective antiemetic treatments for CINV, 20% to 30% of patients do not respond to $5\text{-}HT_3$ receptor antagonism in the early phase of CINV.[9] Furthermore, 50% to 60% of high-risk patients do not respond to these drugs in the late phase of CINV.[10,11] Several studies have shown that responsiveness to ondansetron appears to be modulated by variations in cytochrome P450 enzyme 2D6 (CYP 2D6) activity and the *ABCB1* gene. The ability to predict patient responsiveness to $5\text{-}HT_3$ receptor antagonists based on genetic testing for known polymorphisms could prove to be an important breakthrough in individualizing antiemetic therapy.

Ondansetron is partially metabolized by hepatic CYP 2D6. There are numerous CYP 2D6 polymorphisms, each associated with one of four metabolic phenotypes: poor (no functional alleles), intermediate (less activity than one functional allele), extensive (two functional alleles, and the most common phenotype), and ultrarapid (three functional alleles). Ultrarapid metabolizers can degrade ondansetron more quickly and are therefore less likely to benefit from prophylaxis with the drug. In fact, several studies have shown that patients with three CYP 2D6 alleles, especially those with three functional alleles, are significantly more likely to experience PONV after prophylaxis with ondansetron than patients with fewer alleles (Figure 29-2).[9,12] Ultrarapid metabolism by CYP 2D6 is believed to be responsible for prophylactic ondansetron failures in individuals with an ultrarapid metabolic genotype, whereas other enzymes that metabolize ondansetron, namely CYP 3A4, CYP 2E1, and CYP 1A2, are thought to play a larger role in drug clearance in individuals with poor, intermediate, and extensive metabolism genotypes.[12]

Ondansetron pharmacokinetics also appear to be modulated by polymorphisms of the gene that codes for the drug efflux transporter adenosine triphosphate-binding cassette subfamily B member 1 (*ABCB1*). The *ABCB1* pump transports at least three $5\text{-}HT_3$ receptor antagonists, including ondansetron, across the blood-brain barrier, thereby limiting accumulation of these drugs in the central nervous system.[13] Polymorphisms of *ABCB1* that reduce its activity increase the concentration of $5\text{-}HT_3$ receptor antagonists in the brain, which enhances efficacy. Indeed, cancer patients with a 3435C>T genetic polymorphism were less likely to experience chemotherapy-induced vomiting (CIV) in the first 24 hours after prophylaxis with ondansetron.[13] Similarly, 3435C>T and/or 2677G>T/A polymorphisms are associated with a lower incidence of PONV in surgery patients, but only within the first 2 postoperative hours.[14]

Granisetron and Dolasetron

Other first-generation $5\text{-}HT_3$ receptor antagonists include granisetron and dolasetron. Both drugs have a plasma half-life about twice as long as ondansetron. In general, $5\text{-}HT_3$ receptor antagonists are considered to be equally effective at equipotent doses. Compared to 4 mg ondansetron, 12.5 mg dolasetron and 1 mg granisetron appear to be the minimal effective dose for the prevention of PONV.[15] Both drugs are associated with similar side effects to ondansetron, including QTc prolongation. CYP 2D6, the enzyme responsible for partial metabolism of ondansetron, is the primary enzyme for

Table 29-1. Properties of Individual Antiemetic Drugs

	CHEMICAL NAME	EMPIRICAL FORMULA	ADMINI-STRATION	PONV	*Daily Dosage (mg)* CINV	C_{MAX} (NG/ML)
5-HT₃ Receptor Antagonists						
Ondansetron (Zofran)	1, 2, 3, 9-tetrahydro-9-methyl-3-[(2-methyl-1H-imidazol-1-yl)methyl]-4H-carbazol-4-one, monohydrochloride, dihydrate	$C_{18}H_{19}N_3O$	IV IM Oral Sup	4 4 16 16	32 (0.15 mg/kg × 3) 8 8 × 2 16	
Granisetron (Kytril)	endo-N-(9-methyl-9-azabicyclo [3.3.1] non-3-yl)-1-methyl-1H-indazole-3-carboxamide hydrochloride	$C_{18}H_{24}N_4O$	IV Oral TD	1 1 3.1	10 mcg/kg 2 3.1	64
Dolasetron (Anzemet)	(2α,6α,8α,9αβ)-octahydro-3-oxo-2,6-methano-2H-quinolizin-8-yl-1H- indole-3-carboxylate monomethanesulfonate, monohydrate	$C_{19}H_{20}N_2O_3$	IV Oral	12.5 100	100	
Tropisetron (Navoban)	1αH,5αH-Tropan-3α-yl indole-3-carboxylate	$C_{17}H_{20}N_2O_2$	IV Oral	2 5	5 5	15.1 3.46
Palonosetron (Aloxi)	(3aS)-2-[(S)-1-Azabicyclo [2.2.2]oct-3-yl]-2,3,3α,4,5,6-hexahydro-1- oxo-1Hbenz[de] isoquinoline hydrochloride	$C_{19}H_{24}N_2O$	IV Oral	0.075 0.075	0.25 0.5	5.6
D₂ Receptor Antagonists						
Droperidol	1-[1-[3-(p-Fluorobenzoyl) propyl]-1,2,3,6-tetrahydro-4-pyridyl]-2-benzimidazolinone	$C_{22}H_{22}FN_3O_2$	IV IM	0.625-1.25 × 6-8 0.625-1.25 × 6-8	25	3.2
Haloperidol (Haldol)	4-[4-(p-chloro-phenyl)-4-hydroxypiperidino]-4'—fluorobutyrophenone	$C_{21}H_{23}ClFNO_2$	IV IM Oral	1-2		
Metoclopramide (Reglan)	4-amino-5-chloro-N-[2-(diethylamino) ethyl]-2-methoxybenzamide monohydrochloride monohydrate	$C_{14}H_{22}ClN_3O_2$	IV IM Oral	25-50 25-50	100 (1-2 mg/kg) × 8-12	
Corticosteroids						
Dexamethasone	9-fluoro-11β, 17,21-trihydroxy-16α-methylpregna-1,4-diene-3,20-dione	$C_{22}H_{29}FO_5$	IV IM SC Oral	4	4 × 4 4 × 4 4 × 4	
NK1 Receptor Antagonists						
Aprepitant (Emend)	5-([(2R,3S)-2-((R)-1-[3,5-bis(trifluoromethyl) phenyl]ethoxy)-3-(4-fluorophenyl)morpholino] methyl)-1H-1,2,4-triazol-3(2H)-one	$C_{23}H_{21}F_7N_4O_3$	Oral	40	125 D1/80 D2-3	0.7 (40 mg); 1.6 (125 mg); 1.4 (80 mg)
Anticholinergics						
Transdermal Scopolamine (Transderm-Scop)	α-(hydroxymethyl) benzeneacetic acid 9-methyl-3-oxa-9-azatricyclo [3.3.1.0²,⁴] non-7-yl ester	$C_{17}H_{21}NO_4$	TD	0.5		
Opioid Receptor Antagonists						
Alvimopan (Entereg)	[[2(S)-[[4(R)-(3-hydroxyphenyl)-3(R),4-dimethyl-1-piperidinyl]methyl]-1-oxo-3-phenylpropyl] amino]acetic acid dihydrate	$C_{25}H_{32}N_2O_4$	Oral			
GABA Agonists						
Diazepam (Diastat, Valium)	7-chloro-1,3-dihydro-1-methyl-5-phenyl-2H-1,4-benzodiazepin-2-one	$C_{16}H_{13}ClN_2O$	IV IM Oral Sup			
Lorazepam (Ativan)	7-chloro-5-(o-chlorophenyl)-1,3-dihydro-3-hydroxy-2H-1,4-benzodiazepin-2-one	$C_{15}H_{10}Cl_2N_2O_2$	IV IM Oral TD		1.5 mg/m² 2.5 × 2	20
Midazolam	8-chloro-6-(2-fluorophenyl)-1-methyl-4H-imidazo [1,5-a][1,4]benzodiazepine hydrochloride	$C_{18}H_{13}ClFN_3$	IV IM Oral			90
H₁ Receptor Antagonists						
Dimenhydrinate (Dramamine)	2- (diphenylmethoxy)-N,N -dimethylethylamine hydrochloride	$C_{17}H_{21}NO$	IV IM Oral Sup	50-100 × 4-6 50-100 × 4-6 50-100 × 4-6		80-110
Promethazine (Phenergan)	10-[2- (Dimethylamino)propyl] phenothiazine monohydrochloride	$C_{17}H_{20}N_2S$	IV IM Oral Sup	12.5-25 × 4-6 12.5-25 × 4-6 25 × 2 25 × 2		

CINV, Chemotherapy-induced nausea and vomiting; *D,* day; *D₂,* dopamine 2; *EPS,* extrapyramidal symptoms; *5-HT₃,* 5-hydroxytryptamine type 3 (serotonin); *GABA,* γ-aminobutyric acid-A; *H₁,* histamine 1; *IM,* intramuscular; *IV,* intravenous; *NK1,* neurokinin-1; *PONV,* postoperative nausea and vomiting; *QTc,* heart-rate corrected *QT* interval; *Sup,* suppository; * indicates duration of action; *C_max,* maximum plasma concentration; *AUC,* area under the curve; *T_max,* time to maximum plasma concentration; *VD,* volume of distribution.

AUC (NG•H/ML)	T_MAX (H)	BIOAVAILABILITY	VD (L/KG)	PROTEIN BOUND	METABOLISM	PLASMA HALF-LIFE (H)	ADVERSE EFFECTS	OTHER
							Constipation, headache, QTc prolongation	No sedation
	0.4 0.7 1.5-2.2	56%		70%-76%	CYP3A4, CYP1A2, CYP2D6	4		
		60%	3	65%	CYP3A	3-14		
527	48							
	0.6 1	75%	5.8	69%-77%	CYP2D6, CYP3A, flavin monooxygenase	8		HPB black box warning (Canada)
20.7 32.9	2.6	60%-80%		71%	CYP3A4, CYP1A2, CYP2D6	6-8		
35.8		97%	8.3	62%	CYP2D6, CYP3A, CYP1A2	40		No QTc prolongation
							EPS, QTc prolongation	
69	17.8		1.5	>90%		2-3		FDA black box warning
	0.2-0.3 3-6	50%-60%	18	92%		12-36		
	1-2	80%	3.5	30%		5-6	Cumulative CINV doses associated with significant EPS	10 mg PONV dose insufficient EPS <1% at 25-50 mg
		80%-90%		70%	CYP3A4	36-54*	Hyperglycemia	Most dose response studies suggest that 4 mg is sufficient
								No sedation
7.8 (40 mg); 19.6 (125 mg); 21.2 (80 mg)	3 (40 mg); 4 (80-125 mg)	60%-65% (80-125 mg)		>95%	CYP3A4, CYP1A2, CYP2C19	9-13		
	<24	10%-50%				72*		
	2	6%		80%-90%	Intestinal flora		Sedation	Limited evidence
	0.5-2 1-1.5	90%-100%	0.8-1.0	95%-98%	CYP2C19, CYP3A4	20		
	2	90%		85%		9-16		
	0.5	>90%	1-3.1	97%	CYP3A4	2-6		
	2-3	61%		78%	CYP2D6	2-9		
		25%		93%		16-19	Necrosis that may require amputation	FDA black box warning

dolasetron metabolism.[12] In contrast, granisetron is primarily metabolized by CYP 3A4 and not at all by CYP 2D6.[12] Therefore the efficacy of dolasetron might be modulated by the CYP 2D6 polymorphisms mentioned earlier, while *ABCB1* polymorphisms might play a larger role in enhancing the efficacy of granisetron.

Palonosetron

Palonosetron is the newest and most effective 5-HT₃ receptor antagonist for preventing acute and delayed emesis associated with chemotherapy and for reducing nausea severity (Figure 29-3).[16,17] Palonosetron is characterized by 2500-fold greater affinity than serotonin and 100-fold greater affinity than other 5-HT₃ receptor antagonists.[18] Palonosetron also has a long half-life of 40 hours. However, palonosetron's high binding affinity and long half-life cannot explain its superiority to other 5-HT₃ receptor antagonists. High binding affinity does not account for palonosetron's superiority against higher doses of dolasetron or ondansetron (i.e., higher doses of less potent drugs do not overcome the potency difference). Simi-

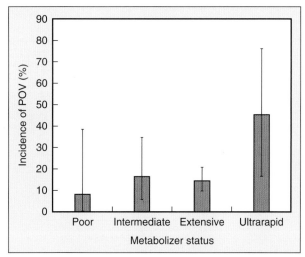

Figure 29-2 Patients with a genotype associated with ultrarapid metabolism (i.e., three functional copies of CYP 2D6) are at increased risk for postoperative vomiting (POV) after prophylaxis with ondansetron in the first 24 postoperative hours. (*Adapted from Candiotti KA, Birnbach DJ, Lubarsky DA, et al. The impact of pharmacogenomics on postoperative nausea and vomiting: do CYP2D6 allele copy number and polymorphisms affect the success or failure of ondansetron prophylaxis? Anesthesiology. 2005;102:543-549.*)

larly, a long half-life cannot account for palonosetron's superiority against more frequent redosing of ondansetron.[17]

Instead, recent research suggests that palonosetron's high efficacy can be attributed to the manner in which it binds to 5-HT₃ receptors.[17] While other 5-HT₃ receptor antagonists bind only to the agonist binding site, palonosetron also binds at an allosteric site that increases receptor affinity for the receptor antagonist at the agonist binding site.[16] Given that granisetron and ondansetron induce little to no receptor internalization, this allosteric binding might also be responsible for palonosetron's relatively high rate (50%-60%) of receptor internalization and low receptor exocytosis. Internalized receptor-antagonist complexes are less likely to be dissociated, and, in turn, bound receptors are less likely to be exocytosed and subsequently reactivated by agonists at the cell surface. The low receptor density at the cell surface due to palonosetron results in prolonged inhibition of receptor function, that is, protection against delayed emesis. Indeed, studies have shown that prophylaxis with palonosetron decreases CIV in a significant proportion of patients in the 5 days following chemotherapy treatment.[19]

Another mechanism that contributes to palonosetron's high efficacy is its inhibition of cross-talk between 5-HT₃ and NK1 receptor signaling pathways.[20] Palonosetron and the NK1 agonist substance P (SP) cannot bind to each other's respective target receptors. However, serotonin and SP enhance each other's potency, and 5-HT₃ receptor antagonists and NK1 receptor antagonists block activation of vagal afferents by the other agonist.[20] Palonosetron is associated with a sixfold reduction in serotonin enhancement of SP potency in vitro (Figure 29-4). Granisetron and ondansetron, on the other hand, had no effect on SP potency in vitro. In an in vivo study in rat nodose ganglia, palonosetron reduced cisplatin-induced SP activation for hours after cisplatin administration.[20] Palonosetron thus appears to have a prolonged downstream effect upon SP function in vitro and in vivo, that might be due to palonosetron's ability to cause 5-HT₃ receptor internalization and reduce receptor density at the cell surface.

Studies have shown that 0.25 mg and 0.075 mg palonosetron are effective doses for preventing CINV and PONV, respectively, and with a half-life of 40 hours, palonosetron provides therapeutic effect for a 72-hour period.[19,21] Unlike other 5-HT₃ receptor antagonists, palonosetron is not associated with QTc prolongation. Palonosetron's long half-life

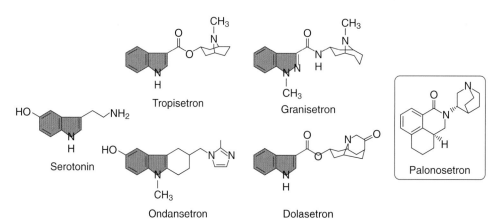

Figure 29-3 Palonosetron and other 5-HT₃ receptor antagonists. The structure of the serotonin is shown on the left.

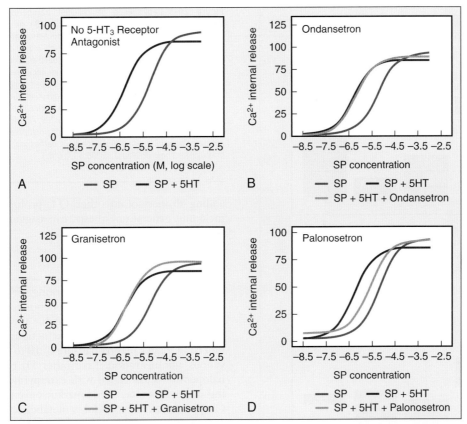

Figure 29-4 The effect of 5-HT$_3$ receptor antagonists on serotonin enhancement of substance P (SP)-induced intracellular Ca^{2+} release. NG108-15 neuroblastoma cells were incubated with SP and subsequently exposed to serotonin. **A,** Serotonin (5HT) enhancement of the SP response. Ondansetron **(B),** granisetron **(C),** and palonosetron **(D)** were preincubated with NG108-15 cells for 2 hours, then removed, after which serotonin was added and the SP response was measured. Unlike ondansetron and granisetron, palonosetron can partially reduce serotonin enhancement of SP activity. *(From Rojas C, Li Y, Zhang J, et al. The antiemetic 5-HT$_3$ receptor antagonist palonosetron inhibits substance P-mediated responses in vitro and in vivo. J Pharmacol Exp Ther. 2010;335:362-368.)*

makes it a potentially important treatment for postdischarge nausea and vomiting (PDNV), although its relative efficacy in this setting has yet to be demonstrated.

DOPAMINE RECEPTOR ANTAGONISTS

Droperidol

Low dose (0.625-1.25 mg IV) droperidol is an effective antiemetic for treatment of PONV and opioid-induced nausea and vomiting (OINV), with similar efficacy against nausea (RR [relative risk] = 0.65) and vomiting (RR = 0.65).[3,22] Droperidol has a short half-life of 3 hours, and, if used for the prevention of PONV, should be administered toward the end of anesthesia. At low doses, droperidol is an α-adrenergic receptor blocker that causes increased sedation (RR = 1.32).[23] Therefore, for PONV prophylaxis droperidol should be administered at the minimum effective dose of 0.625 mg IV to reduce the risk of adverse effects. For OINV prophylaxis, although 50 µg of morphine is the most effective dose to add to a morphine or piritramide patient-controlled analgesia (PCA) infusion pump, 25 µg of morphine is the safer, recommended dose.[24]

In 2001, reports of arrhythmia and death associated with use of droperidol led the FDA to attach a "black box" warning to the drug's label, after which droperidol use decreased 10-fold in the United States. According to the new label, droperidol is contraindicated in patients with known or suspected QT prolongation. Therefore absence of QT prolongation must be confirmed by electrocardiogram (ECG) before droperidol administration, and ECG monitoring must be continued for 2 to 3 hours after drug administration. Many hospitals have removed droperidol from their formularies or placed restrictions upon its use, so that droperidol usage is less than 2% of cases in the United States, even though more than 90% of anesthesiologists believe that the FDA black box warning is unwarranted.[25]

Those who argue against the black box warning question the clinical relevance of droperidol-induced QT prolongation, particularly because QT prolongation is associated with general anesthesia itself. QTc prolongation after placebo, 0.625 mg droperidol, and 1.25 mg droperidol were 12, 15, and 22 msec, respectively.[26] Similarly, 0.75 mg droperidol and 4 mg ondansetron were associated with 17- and 20-msec QT prolongation, respectively.[8] It is possible, however, that these studies were inadequately powered to include patients with a rare but clinically significant predisposition to QT prolongation.[8,26] Of note, there are polymorphisms in the hERG receptor that occur in about 0.5% to 2% of the population, and it is possible that these are the patients who are at high risk when exposed to droperidol (see Chapter 24). Thus it is not possible to exclude the possibility that

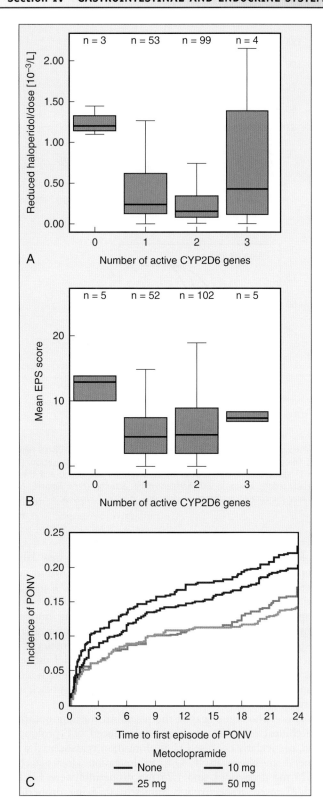

Figure 29-5 Dependence of reduced haloperidol serum trough levels (**A**) and extrapyramidal symptoms (EPS) (**B**) on CYP 2D6 genotype after haloperidol doses of 2 to 24 mg. 0 = no active alleles. 1 = 1 active allele. 2 = 2 active alleles. 3 = 1 active and 1 or 2 duplication alleles. Black lines show medians, blue boxes show interquartile ranges, and error bars show ranges of measured data. **C,** Cumulative incidence of PONV in treatment groups receiving placebo or 10, 25, and 50 mg metoclopramide. *(A and B, From Brockmoller J, Kirchheiner J, Schmider J, et al. The impact of the CYP2D6 polymorphism on haloperidol pharmacokinetics and on the outcome of haloperidol treatment. Clin Pharmacol Ther. 2002;72:438-552; C, From Wallenborn J, Gelbrich G, Bulst D, et al. Prevention of postoperative nausea and vomiting by metoclopramide combined with dexamethasone: randomised double blind multicentre trial. Br Med J. 2006;333:324.)*

adding droperidol to other QT prolonging interventions, including general anesthesia, can trigger QT prolongations that leads to cardiac arrhythmia.[27]

Haloperidol

As a result of the black box warning for droperidol, interest in haloperidol, an older butyrophenone, was renewed. Haloperidol is an effective treatment for psychiatric disorders at high doses and is an effective antiemetic at low doses. Haloperidol has a longer plasma half-life of 10 to 20 hours after intravenous administration. Like other D_2 receptor antagonists, haloperidol is associated with extrapyramidal effects, including acute dystonia, pseudoparkinsonism, and akathisia (see Chapter 11).[28] Haloperidol is metabolized in the liver, where 23% of haloperidol is reduced by a carbonyl reductase into a functional metabolite with high binding affinity to σ opioid and D_2, and D_3 receptors.[28] However, there is significant interindividual variation in haloperidol pharmacokinetics.[28]

Plasma concentrations of haloperidol correlate with dosage, drug efficacy, and incidence of adverse effects.[28] Although CYP 3A4 is the primary enzyme responsible for haloperidol metabolism, with CYP 2D6 appearing to play only a minor role, several studies have shown that certain CYP 2D6 genotypes are associated with poor metabolism and are correlated with higher haloperidol plasma concentrations and lower drug clearance than genotypes associated with extensive metabolism (Figure 29-5, *A* and *B*). Specifically, individuals with 0, 1, 2, and greater than two active CYP 2D6 alleles are considered poor, intermediate, extensive (most common), and ultrafast metabolizers, respectively. Thus poor metabolizers are at higher risk for adverse effects than are intermediate and extensive metabolizers.[28]

Reports of QT prolongation, torsades de pointes, and sudden death associated with use of haloperidol similar to those associated with droperidol led the FDA to issue an FDA alert for haloperidol in 2007. It has not received a black box label because these severe adverse effects occurred in patients who had received off-label IV administration of haloperidol at doses greater 35 mg/day, whereas only intramuscular administration has been approved by the FDA.

Metoclopramide

Metoclopramide, a procainamide derivative and a benzamide prokinetic agent, is the most commonly used D_2 receptor antagonist for antiemetic prophylaxis, primarily for PONV and chemotherapy associated with low emetogenic risk. It is assumed that both the central D_2 receptor antagonist activity at the CTZ and vomiting center and peripheral activity in the GI tract contribute to the antiemetic effect. Metoclopramide acts upon peripheral D_2, muscarinic, and 5-HT$_4$ receptors to induce prokinetic activity. Opioids can cause delayed gastric emptying, but metoclopramide enhances gastric motility and increases intestinal peristalsis, which reduces reflux of stomach contents and the urge to vomit. Because of its short half-life of 5 to 6 hours, metoclopramide is likely to have greatest efficacy if administered at the end of surgery.

Metoclopramide was first prescribed for CINV in high doses (e.g., 200 mg every 4-6 hours), which cause extrapyramidal symptoms in more than 10% of patients.[29] To reduce the incidence of adverse effects, metoclopramide is available in vials of just 10 mg. However, extensive studies and a meta-analysis have demonstrated that 10 mg metoclopramide has no clinically relevant antiemetic effect.[30] In fact, a large and well-designed dose-response study in more than 3000 patients demonstrated that doses of 25 and 50 mg metoclopramide are effective by reducing PONV by about 37% (RR = 0.63, a similar efficacy as other commonly used antiemetics), while the rate for extrapyramidal symptoms was less than 1% (see Figure 29-5, C).[31]

Like haloperidol, metoclopramide is metabolized primarily by CYP 2D6. Although several studies have shown CYP 2D6 polymorphisms that result in reduced CYP 2D6 activity are associated with a higher incidence of metoclopramide adverse effects, no studies have investigated yet whether CYP 2D6 polymorphisms influence the antiemetic efficacy of the drug. Given that nearly 25% of metoclopramide is excreted unchanged, however, the effect of CYP 2D6 polymorphisms might be relatively small, at least in patients with normal renal function.

Like other D_2 receptor antagonists, metoclopramide is associated with severe cardiac adverse effects.[32] High doses are associated with a high incidence of extrapyramidal symptoms, but lower doses (25-50 mg) are associated with less than 1% incidence of dyskinetic and/or extrapyramidal symptoms.[31] It is important to note that the FDA issued a black box warning for metoclopramide, given the high risk of developing tardive dyskinesia if metoclopramide use extends beyond 12 weeks. However, this concern likely does not apply to a short-term course of metoclopramide in the perioperative setting.

Other D_2 receptor antagonists such as alizapride, perphenazine, and prochlorperazine might be as effective as other commonly used antiemetics, but they are rarely used, and their side-effect profiles are unclear compared with that of other antiemetics.[22]

CORTICOSTEROIDS

Dexamethasone is a synthetic glucocorticoid with antiinflammatory and immunosuppressant properties. With 20 to 30 times the binding affinity for glucocorticoid receptors of endogenous cortisol, dexamethasone is a potent treatment for PONV and CINV. Even though dexamethasone is one of the most commonly used antiemetics, its mechanism of action remains unclear. Studies in animal models suggest that dexamethasone acts on the glucocorticoid receptor-rich bilateral nucleus tractus solitarius (i.e., the vomiting center), but not the area postrema.[33]

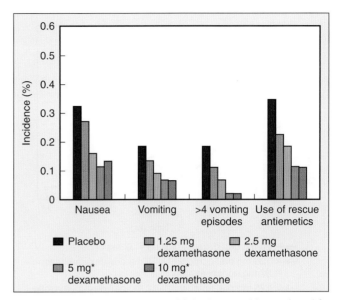

Figure 29-6 Incidence of nausea, vomiting, severe vomiting, and need for rescue antiemetics 0 to 24 hours after dexamethasone prophylaxis in a dose-ranging study. *P < .05 compared to placebo. (From Wang JJ, Ho ST, Lee SC, et al. The use of dexamethasone for preventing postoperative nausea and vomiting in females undergoing thyroidectomy: a dose-ranging study. Anesth Analg. 2000;91:1404-1407.)

Although 8 mg is the most commonly used dose for prevention of PONV, dose-response studies suggest that 5 mg is the minimum effective dose for PONV prophylaxis (Figure 29-6).[34] Furthermore, a large factorial trial in more than 5000 patients found that 4 mg dexamethasone has similar efficacy to 4 mg ondansetron or 1.25 mg droperidol.[35] Thus ambulatory surgery guidelines recommend 4 to 5 mg dexamethasone.[36] Dexamethasone is more effective when given at the beginning rather at the end of surgery, which suggests that there is a delay in onset of action by about 2 hours.[37] Furthermore, a single intraoperative dose of dexamethasone has not been associated with adverse effects.[36] However, like other intravenous drugs containing phosphate esters, dexamethasone has been associated with perineal burning and itching when injected in awake patients.[38] In addition, doses of 12 to 20 mg can be given for CINV.[39]

Dexamethasone is an effective and well-tolerated component of antiemetic combination therapy.[35] Adding aprepitant to the typical treatment regimen for CINV—a 5-HT$_3$ receptor antagonist (ondansetron) and a corticosteroid (dexamethasone)—further reduces the incidence of CINV. The doses of aprepitant recommended for CINV (125 mg day 1, 80 mg days 2-3) moderately inhibits CYP 3A4, the enzyme responsible for dexamethasone metabolism. In fact, aprepitant's inhibition of CYP 3A4 activity approximately doubles the plasma concentration of dexamethasone (Figure 29-7). Given that dexamethasone has high (80%) oral bioavailability, and that aprepitant also increases the peak plasma concentration and half-life of dexamethasone, aprepitant's inhibition of CYP 3A4 activity probably plays a larger role in systemic rather than first-pass clearance of dexamethasone.[40] Therefore doses of dexamethasone that are coadministered with aprepitant should be reduced by half to maintain dexamethasone plasma concentrations that are similar to regimens without aprepitant. The pharmacokinetics of ondansetron, which is partially metabolized by CYP 3A4, are not affected by aprepitant.[40]

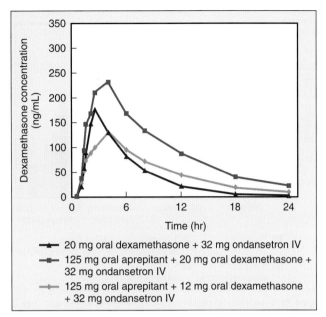

Figure 29-7 Mean plasma concentration profiles of dexamethasone when combined with other antiemetics. Aprepitant markedly increased the plasma concentration of dexamethasone. *(From McCrea JB, Majumdar AK, Goldberg MR, et al. Effects of the NK1 receptor antagonist aprepitant on the pharmacokinetics of dexamethasone and methylprednisolone.* Clin Pharmacol Ther. *2003;74:17-24.)*

NK1 RECEPTOR ANTAGONISTS

NK1 receptors are G protein–coupled receptors found in both the central and peripheral nervous system. NK1 receptors are found in the GI tract and in high concentrations in regions responsible for regulating the vomiting reflex, including the brainstem nuclei, nucleus tractus solitarius, and area postrema. Substance P (SP), a member of the tachykinin family of neuropeptides, is the dominant ligand of NK1 receptors. In animal models, SP activation of NK1 receptors in the area postrema induces retching, and NK1 receptor antagonists reduce emesis associated with a range of stimuli, including cisplatin, cyclophosphamide, irradiation, ipecacuanha, copper sulfate, opioids, and motion.[41] NK1 receptor antagonists competitively inhibit SP binding to central NK1 receptors, effectively preventing neurotransmission within the central pattern generator for vomiting.[42] Because cisplatin increases plasma levels of SP, NK1 receptor antagonists are particularly important for the prevention and treatment of CINV.[43]

Aprepitant

Currently, aprepitant is the only FDA-approved NK1 receptor antagonist. Aprepitant has greater efficacy for preventing vomiting than any other single intervention, with relative risk reductions of more than 50%.[41,44] Furthermore, aprepitant has greater efficacy against both acute and delayed postoperative vomiting (POV) and chemotherapy-induced vomiting (CIV).[43,45,46] Aprepitant is available as an oral capsule that is easy to coadminister with other surgical premedication for PONV prophylaxis. Whereas aprepitant is highly effective on its own, it reaches its optimal efficacy against early emesis when combined with other antiemetics, such as 5-HT$_3$

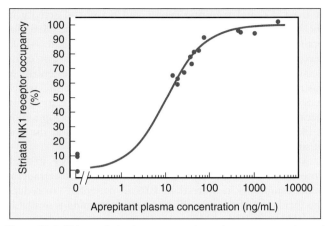

Figure 29-8 High correlation between aprepitant plasma concentration and NK1 receptor occupancy [0.97 (*P* < 0.001; 95% CI = 0.94-1.00)]. *(From Bergstrom M, Hargreaves RJ, Burns HD, et al. Human positron emission tomography studies of brain neurokinin 1 receptor occupancy by aprepitant.* Biol Psychiatry. *2004;55:1007-1012.)*

receptor antagonists and/or dexamethasone.[43,45,46] Its efficacy against nausea, however, appears to be comparable to other treatment options.[41] Like 5-HT$_3$ receptor antagonists, aprepitant is nonsedative; it has a long half-life of 9 to 13 hours. Furthermore, aprepitant is not associated with QTc prolongation.[41] Aprepitant is primarily metabolized by CYP 3A4; CYP 1A2 and CYP 2C19 also contribute to its metabolism.

Positron emission tomography studies have shown that aprepitant can penetrate the blood-brain barrier to bind to NK1 receptors in the area postrema.[47] The FDA-approved dose of aprepitant for PONV prophylaxis is 40 mg, which is associated with only 75% receptor occupancy (Figure 29-8). Doses of 100 mg or more, such as the FDA-approved 125 mg for CINV prophylaxis, are sufficient to achieve greater than 90% NK1 receptor occupancy. Cancer patients typically receive 125 mg aprepitant the day of chemotherapy, followed by 2 days of 80 mg aprepitant.[48] Aprepitant doses as high as 375 mg are associated with the same level of receptor occupancy as 125 mg and thus have no clinical advantage.

ANTICHOLINERGIC DRUGS

The neurotransmitter acetylcholine acts on cholinergic receptors in the CTZ, vestibular system, and cerebellum. According to the current model of motion sickness, an orientation disparity comparator in the cerebellum compares expected sensory input from memory with actual sensory input, and any significant discrepancy between the two triggers symptoms of motion sickness. Acetylcholine might be involved in integrating sensory stimuli in the vestibular nuclei, as well as transmitting information regarding expected sensory input to the cerebellum. Therefore anticholinergic agents like scopolamine might facilitate habituation to motion by preventing acetylcholine from relaying signals to the comparator, and instead allowing a new sensory pattern to develop that reflects the actual environment.[49] Acetylcholine released from the gut wall also appears to increase gut motility and secretion. Anticholinergic agents thus play an important role in the prevention of motion sickness and PONV.

Scopolamine

Scopolamine is a competitive antagonist of acetylcholine at muscarinic receptors, and the most effective single agent for preventing motion sickness.[49] Scopolamine is available in oral, parenteral, and transdermal formulations. The 0.3- to 0.6-mg oral and 0.2-mg parenteral doses are associated with a short duration of action of 5 to 6 hours and some adverse effects, most commonly dry mouth, drowsiness, and blurred vision.[50] Redosing with oral or parenteral doses can result in variable drug plasma concentrations, which if too high are associated with severe autonomic and central nervous system effects and if too low are associated with inadequate antiemetic efficacy.

A transdermal formulation of scopolamine was developed to overcome the limited half-life and clinical efficacy of the oral and parenteral formulations. A transdermal delivery system is also an advantage when oral doses are intolerable. Transdermal scopolamine (TDS) is available in a thin (0.2 mm) patch made up of four layers: an outer membrane, a drug reservoir mixed with mineral oil and polyisobutylene, a rate-limiting microporous membrane, and an adhesive layer closest to the skin. In vitro studies using human cadavers show wide variation in skin permeability between both application sites and individuals. Therefore the patch is recommended for use at the postauricular site, a highly permeable area, and the rate-limiting microporous membrane has been designed to deliver scopolamine at a slower rate than that achieved in the least porous postauricular skin sample tested.[49] In addition, the adhesive layer contains a 140-μg priming dose of scopolamine to overcome the skin as the primary compartment before a more constant scopolamine delivery leads to steady-state plasma concentrations.

The drug reservoir contains 1.5 mg scopolamine that is released at a constant rate of about 5 μg/hr for 3 days. The controlled drug delivery decreases the incidence of adverse side effects compared to oral and parenteral formulations.[51,52] This delivery rate maintains therapeutic plasma concentrations, estimated to be greater than 50 pg/mL. Plasma concentrations greater than 50 pg/mL and antiemetic efficacy are both observed 6 hours after patch application (Figure 29-9, *A*).[53,54] Drug efficacy peaks at plasma concentrations greater than 100 pg/mL, observed 8 to 12 hours after application. Therefore TDS should be administered ideally 4 to 6 hours before an antiemetic effect is required. However, supplementing TDS with 0.3 to 0.6 mg oral scopolamine results in therapeutic plasma concentrations after only 1 hour (see Figure 29-9, *B* and *C*).[55]

TDS is an effective antiemetic intervention, associated with a risk reduction of 0.56 and 0.54 for PON and POV, respectively, if applied the night before surgery, and with a risk reduction of 0.61 and 0.74 for PON and POV, respectively, if applied the day of surgery.[56] Interestingly, despite wide variation between individual plasma concentrations, correlation of plasma concentrations 8 hours after TDS application in the same individual on different occasions is still 0.52 ($P < 0.05$).[57]

TDS is generally well-tolerated; adverse effects are similar to those associated with oral and parenteral scopolamine. The most common adverse effects are dry mouth, allergic contact dermatitis, and drowsiness. The drowsiness appears to be associated with PONV more than motion

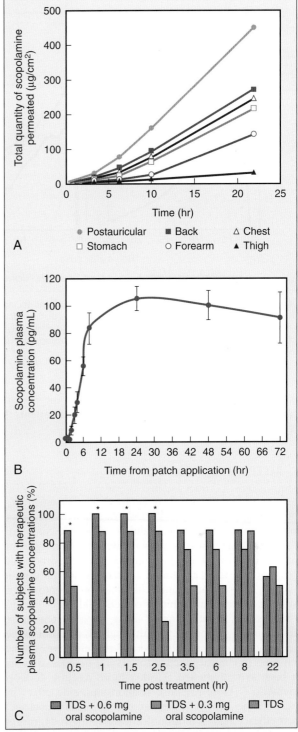

Figure 29-9 A, In vitro permeation of scopolamine at 30°C from various patch locations. **B,** Transdermal scopolamine (TDS) effects on plasma concentrations. Plasma concentrations of scopolamine persist up to 72 hours after TDS application (n = 15). **C,** Percentage of subjects with plasma scopolamine concentration greater than 50 pg/mL, 0 to 22 hours after treatment in three experimental groups. *$P < 0.05$ for oral scopolamine groups compared to TDS alone. *(From Nachum Z, Shupak A, Gordon CR. Transdermal scopolamine for prevention of motion sickness: clinical pharmacokinetics and therapeutic applications. Clin Pharmacokinet. 2006;45:543-566.)*

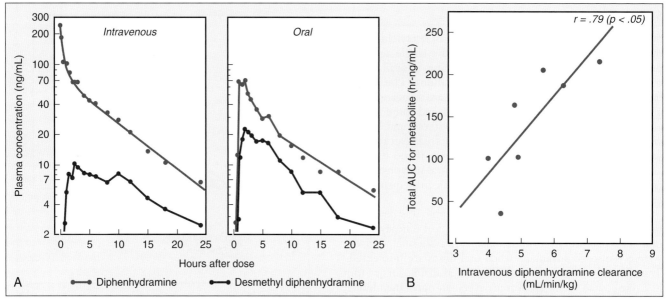

Figure 29-10 A, Plasma concentrations of diphenhydramine and its metabolite desmethyl diphenhydramine following intravenous and oral administration of diphenhydramine. **B,** Relation of clearance of intravenous diphenhydramine to total area under the plasma concentration-time curve (AUC) for the metabolite desmethyl diphenhydramine, as determined by linear regression analysis. Appearance of the metabolite thus mirrors the disappearance of diphenhydramine. *(From Blyden GT, Greenblatt DJ, Scavone JM, et al. Pharmacokinetics of diphenhydramine and a demethylated metabolite following intravenous and oral administration.* J Clin Pharmacol. *1986;26:529-533.)*

sickness.[49] Scopolamine is not recommended for pediatric patients and should be used with caution in older patients due to the sedative effects and the risk of delirium.

H₁ RECEPTOR ANTAGONISTS

H₁ receptor antagonists can be used for management of motion sickness, PONV, and OINV. Agents like diphenhydramine, promethazine, and cyclizine are reversible competitive H₁ receptor antagonists with moderate anticholinergic (antimuscarinic) and weak antidopaminergic activity. Although the mechanism of their antiemetic efficacy is not fully understood, H₁ receptor antagonists likely act on receptors in the vestibular system and vomiting center.[23] Side effects include drowsiness, dry mouth, blurred vision, urinary retention, and extrapyramidal symptoms.[22,58] Although H₁ receptor antagonists are generally well tolerated and cost effective, and have been used in clinical practice for several decades, they have not been as well studied as other more recently developed antiemetics.[59] Dose-response relationships, side effect profiles, and the benefit of repeat dosing remain unclear.[58,60] Their efficacy against motion sickness might give H₁ receptor antagonists an important role in antiemetic prophylaxis for ambulatory patients.[61]

Dimenhydrinate and Diphenhydramine

Dimenhydrinate is a theoclate salt composed of diphenhydramine, an ethanolamine derivative, and 8-chlorotheophylline, a chlorinated theophylline derivative, in a 1:1 ratio. Dimenhydrinate must be metabolized into its active ingredient diphenhydramine to attain antiemetic efficacy. Therefore dimenhydrinate has a slower onset of action, and is administered as a 60-mg dose to match the potency of 30-mg

diphenhydramine.[59] Diphenhydramine itself undergoes N-demethylation to its principal metabolite monodesmethyl-diphenhydramine (DMDP) in the liver.[62] Oral diphenhydramine bioavailability ranges from 43% to 72%, probably due to first-pass metabolism, with peak plasma concentrations of approximately 64 ng/mL after approximately 2.5 hours.[62,63] Plasma concentration of diphenhydramine covaries with that of DMDP (Figure 29-10, *A*). The observed plasma half-life of oral dimenhydrinate is 3 to 9.3 hours, and the elimination half-lives after intravenous and oral administration are 8.4 and 9.2 hours, respectively, for diphenhydramine, and 9.3 and 7.3 hours, respectively, for DMDP (see Figure 29-10, *B*).[64] The observed metabolite area under the curve (AUC) after oral administration (218 hr-ng/mL) is significantly larger than after intravenous administration (145 hr-ng/mL).[64] Sedative and performance-impairing side effects are typically associated with diphenhydramine doses greater than or equal to 50 mg, and differ from placebo only within the first 3 hours.[62,65] While there is a positive correlation between plasma concentration and sedative effects, there is also wide variation between individuals in the severity and persistence of these effects.[65]

A systematic review incorporating 18 clinical trials and 3045 patients demonstrated that diphenhydramine is associated with decreased POV and PONV, although its impact upon PON was not significant.[58] In addition, 50 mg IV dimenhydrinate is similarly effective to 4 mg IV ondansetron for the prevention of PONV in patients undergoing elective laparoscopic cholecystectomy.[66] For management of motion sickness, 100 mg oral dimenhydrinate is superior to TDS, while 50 mg is similarly effective as TDS.[49]

For OINV management, diphenhydramine can be safely and effectively coadministered with morphine via a PCA pump, especially given the two drugs' similar pharmacokinetic profiles. Administering 30 mg diphenhydramine at

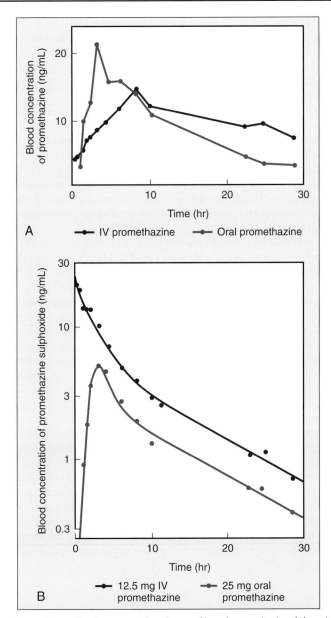

Figure 29-11 Blood concentration-time profiles of promethazine **(A)** and promethazine sulphoxide **(B)** in a human volunteer following administration of 12.5 mg IV (purple) or 25 mg oral (blue) promethazine. *(From Taylor G, Houston JB, Shaffer J, et al. Pharmacokinetics of promethazine and its sulphoxide metabolite after intravenous and oral administration to man. Br J Clin Pharmacol. 1983;15:287-293.)*

induction, followed by a 4.8:1 diphenhydramine-morphine solution via a PCA pump, reduced emesis without morphine-sparing or sedative effects.[59] The initial intraoperative dose serves to establish a therapeutic plasma concentration before the infusion, thereby minimizing the risk of sedative side effects associated with larger diphenhydramine doses during the postoperative period.

Promethazine

Promethazine is a phenothiazine derivative and a potent antihistamine with moderate antimuscarinic activity. Although more than 80% is absorbed, promethazine undergoes extensive first-pass hepatic glucuronidation and sulphoxidation, resulting in low absolute bioavailability of approximately 25%.[67] Peak plasma concentrations of promethazine (2.4-18.0 ng/mL) are observed between 1.5 and 3 hours after administration (Figure 29-11, *A*). Like other drugs that undergo extensive hepatic first-pass metabolism, plasma concentrations of its metabolite, promethazine sulphoxide (PMZSO), peak earlier and higher following oral administration compared to intravenous administration (see Figure 29-11, *B*).[67] Overall, however, PMZSO plasma AUCs are not significantly different following oral or intravenous administration. Time to effect after intravenous and intramuscular injection is 5 and 20 minutes, respectively.[68] With a plasma half-life after intravenous and intramuscular injection of 9 to 16 hours and 6 to 13 hours, respectively, promethazine's duration of effect is typically 4 to 6 hours, up to 12 hours.[68]

Promethazine is also effective for rescue treatment of established PONV and has been combined with 5-HT₃ receptor antagonists and TDS to reduce both the frequency and severity of PONV.[69-72] For PONV management, 12.5 to 25 mg is administered toward the end of surgery and every 4 hours, as needed, with doses of coadministered analgesics and/or barbiturates reduced accordingly.[68] Studies investigating a 6.25-mg promethazine dose to reduce the incidence of sedative side effects have produced conflicting results on antiemetic efficacy.[71] Because H_1 receptors are involved in the development of inflammatory pain and hyperalgesia, administering antihistamines like promethazine can also reduce pain levels in addition to incidence of emesis. In one study, preoperative administration of 0.1 mg/kg IV promethazine reduced postoperative morphine consumption by approximately 30% in the first 24 postoperative hours.[73]

Promethazine received a black box warning from the FDA in 2004 indicating that the drug should not be used in children younger than 2 years of age due to potential fatal respiratory depression. The warning label also recommends that promethazine should be administered with caution and at the lowest effective dose in children 2 years of age and older. The promethazine hydrochloride injection also received a black box warning from the FDA in 2009 indicating that severe tissue injuries, including gangrene, can rarely be associated with intravenous administration of promethazine. In anesthesia practice it is important to inject promethazine only through a well-established and secure IV line.

GABA RECEPTOR AGONISTS

Propofol

Propofol has several mechanisms of action, including potentiation of γ-aminobutyric acid-A (GABA$_A$) receptors. Administration of propofol-based total intravenous anesthesia (TIVA) instead of volatile anesthetics can reduce the incidence of PONV by about 20%.[35] That propofol has antiemetic effects is supported by the finding that repeat doses of 20 mg propofol via a patient-controlled delivery device in the postanesthesia care unit (PACU) significantly reduced PONV.[74] However, this effect could not be reproduced in a similar study, and another study found that both propofol and midazolam had antiemetic properties only under clinical sedation.[75,76] Therefore it is likely that the reduced incidence of PONV after TIVA with propofol compared to general anesthesia with inhaled gas is at least in part a result of not administering volatile anesthetics rather than the potential antiemetic effects of propofol.

Some patients experience anticipatory nausea and vomiting before chemotherapy begins or earlier in the treatment regimen than expected. As a learned response to chemotherapy, anticipatory nausea and vomiting can affect up to 25% of patients by the fourth treatment cycle.[77,78] However, much about its pathogenesis and management remains unclear.

Benzodiazepines

Benzodiazepines are currently the most commonly used anxiolytics. These agents act as positive modulators of $GABA_A$ receptors. Increased $GABA_A$ receptor activity results in varying levels of central nervous system depression including sedative, hypnotic, anxiolytic, anticonvulsant, muscle relaxant, and amnesic effects. In addition to decreased anxiety, the mechanism of action of benzodiazepines is believed to involve $GABA_A$ receptor-mediated reduction of dopamine and $5\text{-}HT_3$ receptor activity in the CTZ.[79] Another specific pathway that has been suggested is that benzodiazepines decrease adenosine reuptake, thereby leading to decreased synthesis, release, and postsynaptic activity of dopamine in the CTZ.[80,81]

$GABA_A$ receptor activation is also associated with reduced opioid analgesia.[82] Opioids are believed to produce an analgesic effect by inhibiting GABA-receptor pain modulation in the periaqueductal gray matter and the rostral ventral medulla. In one study, 0.75 mg IV flumazenil, a benzodiazepine antagonist, enhanced postoperative morphine analgesia in patients who received IV diazepam preoperatively, compared to patients who did not receive flumazenil.[82] Therefore opioid analgesia can be improved by using benzodiazepines of short duration of action, and/or by coadministering flumazenil with morphine in the immediate postoperative period.

Diazepam is typically administered as a 5- to 10-mg dose 2 hours before surgery. The agent appears to be effective against both nausea (RR = 0.50, 95% CI: 0.25-0.99) and vomiting (RR = 0.85, 95% CI: 0.58-1.24).[22] Due to a long half-life of more than 24 hours, other benzodiazepines with shorter durations of action, such as lorazepam and midazolam, can be used instead.

Lorazepam is the preferred agent for anticipatory nausea and vomiting. It can also be used for the prophylaxis and treatment of PONV and CINV.[83] Like diazepam, lorazepam appears to have a greater effect on nausea (RR = 0.55, 95% CI 0.33-0.93) than vomiting (RR = 0.61, 95% CI 0.33-1.13) compared to placebo.[22] For PONV prophylaxis, patients receive 0.05 mg/kg (up to 4 mg maximum) 1 to 2 hours before surgery. For anticipatory nausea and vomiting, guidelines recommend 0.5 to 2 mg lorazepam on the night before and morning of surgery, and for CINV management, 0.5 to 2 mg every 4 to 6 hours on days 1 to 4 post-treatment.[84] Lorazepam might be insufficient as an antiemetic on its own, but can be safely combined with other antiemetic agents to manage CINV.[85] A randomized controlled trial found lorazepam effective in managing anticipatory, acute, and delayed CINV, especially when co-administered with 2 mg/kg metoclopramide IV.[86] Mild sedation (lethargy but arousable without any disorientation) and amnesia (no memory of chemotherapy treatment) were more common in patients treated with lorazepam.

Lorazepam is readily absorbed into the bloodstream with an absolute bioavailability of 90%. Peak plasma concentrations of 20 ng/mL after a 2-mg dose are reached approximately 2 hours after administration. The plasma half-life of lorazepam is approximately 12 hours, and 18 hours for its primary metabolite, lorazepam glucuronide.

Intravenous midazolam is the most commonly used premedication in ambulatory surgery for induction of general anesthesia and preoperative sedation due to its rapid onset of action, relatively short half-life, low cost, and low incidence of side effects.[87] For PONV prophylaxis, a 2-mg dose of midazolam can be given before or after induction or postoperatively as a continuous infusion. Several studies have shown that midazolam is similarly effective to ondansetron without an increased incidence of sedative side effects.[88-90]

Midazolam is rapidly metabolized to 1′-hydroxymidazolam by both hepatic and intestinal CYP 3A4. Therefore drugs like aprepitant that inhibit CYP 3A4 activity could lead to prolonged sedation due to increased exposure to midazolam. In a study in which healthy volunteers received a 2-mg dose of oral midazolam during the week preceding the study, a second dose on day 1, and a third on day 5, participants were randomized to receive an aprepitant dosing regimen similar to CINV (125 mg day 1 and 80 mg days 2-5) or PONV prophylaxis (40 mg day 1 and 25 mg days 2-5).[91] CINV doses of aprepitant led to a 2.3-fold increase in midazolam plasma AUC on day 1 and a 3.3-fold increase on day 5 (Figure 29-12, A, upper panel), as well as increased maximum observed plasma concentrations and half-life of midazolam. The latter can be explained by inhibition of both first-pass metabolism and systemic clearance of midazolam by aprepitant. PONV doses of aprepitant had no significant effect on oral midazolam metabolism (Figure 29-12, A, lower panel). Because aprepitant cannot inhibit first-pass metabolism of CYP 3A4 substrates when they are given intravenously, it is not surprising that both CINV and PONV doses of aprepitant have no significant effect on intravenous midazolam metabolism (see Figure 29-12, B).[90,92,93]

OPIOID RECEPTOR ANTAGONISTS

Although the FDA has not specifically approved the use of $5\text{-}HT_3$ and D_2 receptor antagonists for OINV, these agents significantly reduce the incidence of nausea and vomiting after opioid administration.[94-98] Antiemetic agents that specifically target opioid receptors might also have efficacy against OINV, which has the advantage of simultaneously targeting multiple other opioid-induced adverse effects, such as, postoperative ileus.[99]

Alvimopan

Alvimopan, a trans-3,4-dimethyl-4-(3-hydroxyphenyl) piperidine, is approved by the FDA to reverse postoperative ileus after colectomy. Although opioids do have some peripherally mediated analgesic effects, opioid analgesia primarily involves central μ, κ, and δ receptors in the rostral anterior cingulate cortex , the brainstem, and the dorsal horn of the spinal cord (see Chapter 15).[100] Opioid agonist activity at peripheral receptors in the gut, on the other hand, inhibits the release of acetylcholine from the mesenteric plexus and stimulates

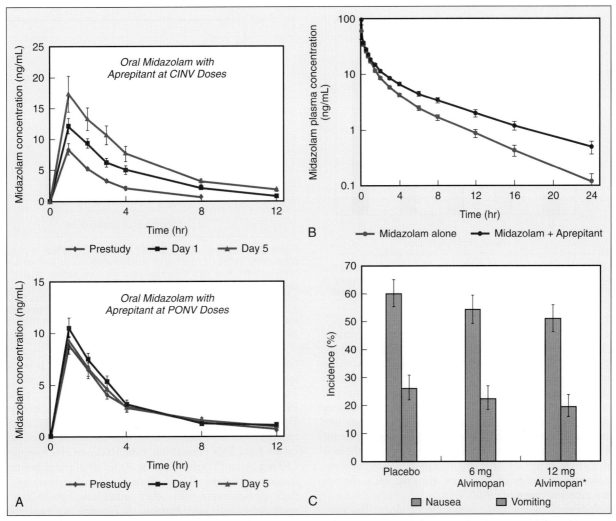

Figure 29-12 Interaction between midazolam and aprepitant. **A,** Plasma concentration-time profiles of 2 mg oral midazolam prestudy, day 1, and day 5 when coadministered with 125 mg aprepitant day 1 and 80 mg days 2 to 5 in eight healthy male subjects *(upper panel)*. Plasma concentration-time profiles of 2 mg oral midazolam prestudy, day 1, and day 5 when coadministered with 40 mg aprepitant day 1 and 25 mg days 2 to 5 *(lower panel)*. **B,** Plasma concentrations of midazolam when administered intravenously, alone, and with 125 mg oral aprepitant in 12 healthy subjects. **C,** Incidence of opioid-induced nausea and vomiting after prophylaxis with 6 and 12 mg alvimopan. *(**A,** From Majumdar AK, McCrea JB, Panebianco DL, et al. Effects of aprepitant on cyto-chrome P450 3A4 activity using midazolam as a probe. Clin Pharmacol Ther. 2003;74:150-156; **B,** From Majumdar AK, Yan KX, Selverian DV, et al. Effect of aprepitant on the pharmacokinetics of intravenous midazolam. J Clin Pharmacol. 2007;47:744-750; **C,** From Adolor Corporation. Entereg (alvimopan) Capsules for postoperative ileus FDA Advisory Panel briefing document. http://www.fda.gov/ohrms/dockets/ac/08/briefing/2008-4336b1-02-Adolor.pdf.)*

μ receptors, thereby reducing muscle tone and peristaltic activity. The resulting delayed gastric emptying and gastric distention stimulate visceral mechanoreceptors and chemo-receptors, which trigger nausea and vomiting via a seroto-nergic signaling pathway. Alvimopan's high polarity and large zwitterionic structure prevent penetration of the blood-brain barrier, such that potency at binding peripheral μ receptors is 200 times that of central μ receptors.[99,101] By selectively targeting peripheral μ receptors, alvimopan prevents periph-eral opioid emetogenic effects without affecting their central analgesic effects.[102,103]

Because of its high binding affinity (K_i = 0.4 nM) and low dissociation rate ($t_{1/2}$ = 30-44 min), alvimopan has low bio-availability (6%).[104] Alvimopan is quickly absorbed, with a time to maximum plasma concentration of 2 hours after administration. Alvimopan also has a long half-life of 10 to 17 hours.[104] Plasma clearance averages at 400 mL/min and is primarily mediated by biliary secretion. Alvimopan is metabolized by intestinal flora, with an active but clinically

irrelevant amide hydrolysis metabolite (ADL 08-0011) that has lower binding affinity than alvimopan itself.

Alvimopan is only available as a 12 mg oral capsule. Patients can be given 12 mg 30 minutes to 5 hours before surgery, followed by 12 mg twice a day for up to 7 days after surgery (max of 15 doses).[104] Furthermore, 12 mg alvimopan has been shown to reduce OINV and to be well-tolerated by ambula-tory patients in the postdischarge period (Figure 29-12, *C*).[103]

RISK-BASED PROPHYLAXIS AND MULTIMODAL THERAPY

Although all FDA-approved antiemetics have been proven to be safe in multiple clinical trials, no agent is without side effects. Therefore only patients at moderate to high risk for PONV should receive prophylaxis. A simplified risk score, such as the Apfel score, can be useful for predicting PONV in adult patients undergoing inhalational anesthesia and thus

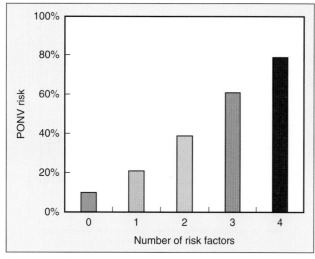

Figure 29-13 The Apfel simplified risk score for postoperative nausea and vomiting based on the number of risk factors (female gender, history of motion sickness and/or PONV, non-smoking, use of postoperative opioids).

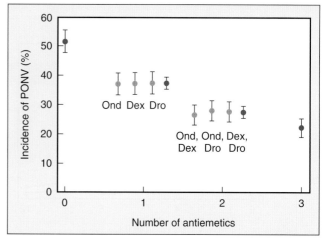

Figure 29-14 Results of the IMPACT trial showing effect of multimodal prophylactic antiemetic therapy on postoperative nausea and vomiting. N = 5161 patients. Blue dots = average value for each number of prophylactic antiemetics. Orange dots = incidence for each antiemetic or combination of antiemetics. *Ond,* Ondansetron; *Dex,* dexamethasone; *Dro,* droperidol. *(From Apfel CC, Korttila K, Abdalla M, et al. A factorial trial of six interventions for the prevention of postoperative nausea and vomiting. N Engl J Med. 2004;350:2441-2451.)*

for identifying which patients should be targeted for prophylaxis. The positive predictors included in the Apfel score are female gender, history of motion sickness or PONV, non-smoking, and use of postoperative opioids.[105] The incidence of PONV associated with one, two, three, and four risk factors is 10%, 21%, 39%, 61%, and 79%, respectively (Figure 29-14). An easy-to-remember guideline is that one antiemetic intervention is recommended for each risk factor present. It is also important to note that multimodal therapy should include drugs of different receptor classes, because repeat dosing of drugs of the same receptor class do not improve protection against PONV.[106]

No antiemetic agent can completely eliminate the incidence of PONV. A Cochrane review found the overall relative risk for antiemetics to be 0.60 to 0.80, that is, a relative risk reduction (RRR) of 20% to 40%.[22] However, the treatment effect might be slightly optimistic given that there is evidence of publication bias toward small studies with more positive results.

The *International Multicenter Protocol to quantify the relative impact of single and combined Antiemetics in a randomized Controlled Trial of factorial design* (IMPACT) found that the RRs for 4 mg ondansetron, 4 mg dexamethasone, and 1.25 mg droperidol all equal approximately 0.75 (i.e., a RRR of 25% for each intervention; see Figure 29-14).[35] The study also demonstrated that each antiemetic intervention acted independently, which means that the efficacy of combination therapy can be estimated by multiplying the RR associated with each intervention. This independence of action implies that each additional antiemetic intervention is associated with less effectiveness than the previous one due to an already decreased baseline risk of PONV.

EMERGING DEVELOPMENTS

Novel Antiemetic Drugs

With the success of novel antiemetics like aprepitant and palonosetron, there is great promise for other new agents currently under investigation. These include newer NK1

receptor antagonists like the intravenous prodrug of aprepitant known as fosaprepitant, as well as the phase 3–ready rolapitant (rolapitant hydrochloride, Schering-Plough SCH619734), both developed for CINV prevention. Upon injection, fosaprepitant is rapidly converted to aprepitant and therefore has the same mechanism of action as aprepitant. For CINV prevention, patients can receive fosaprepitant 150 mg as an IV infusion over 20 to 30 minutes before chemotherapy on the day of chemotherapy, followed by 2 to 3 days of treatment with other antiemetic agents like dexamethasone and ondansetron. Rolapitant appears to have several advantages to aprepitant, including a long half-life of 180 hours. It is more rapidly absorbed and does not inhibit CYP 2C9, 2C19, 2D6, and 3A4 or P-glycoprotein in vitro, suggesting that rolapitant has a low risk of interacting with concomitant medications.[107] Oral doses of rolapitant appear to be rapidly absorbed and well tolerated without significant side effects. A dose-response study reported that rolapitant reduced POV up to 120 hours after surgery in high-risk patients, and that 70 mg and 200 mg were the most effective doses in terms of complete response.[107] However, the optimal rolapitant dose has yet to be determined. In addition, rolapitant is currently available only in an oral formulation and therefore must be administered preoperatively.

Postdischarge Nausea and Vomiting

As the number of surgeries performed on an outpatient basis continues to grow, there is increasing interest in using antiemetic agents to prevent and treat postdischarge nausea and vomiting (PDNV). Because outpatient procedures are typically less invasive and shorter in duration than inpatient procedures, the relatively lower exposure to emetogenic inhalational anesthetics and opioids predicts a relatively lower incidence of PONV in the PACU. However, a study in 2170 ambulatory patients in the United States found that the incidence of nausea and vomiting after discharge from the hospital was 37%, even after intraoperative prophylaxis with ondansetron or dexamethasone.[108] PDNV is particularly a concern because it occurs when patients no longer have access to fast-acting intravenous rescue treatment, and PDNV limits their ability to tolerate oral antiemetics. Ideal antiemetics for PDNV should have a long duration of action with a safe side effect profile, such as palonosetron, TDS, aprepitant, and rolapitant. However, further studies are required to investigate the absolute and relative value of these and other antiemetics in the postdischarge setting.

KEY POINTS

- Despite new insights into relevant target receptor function and the successful development of novel antiemetic agents, the actual mechanisms of PONV remain unknown.
- Ondansetron is the most commonly used serotonin type 3 (5-HT$_3$) receptor antagonist for prevention and treatment of PONV and CINV, probably because it is not associated with sedation that might slow recovery from anesthesia.
- Low-dose droperidol (0.625 to 1.25 mg), a dopamine type 2 (D$_2$) receptor antagonist, used to be the most commonly used antiemetic for the prevention of PONV; however, potential for torsades de pointes and cardiac arrest led to an FDA black box warning that has significantly reduced its usage in the United States.
- Metoclopramide is an alternative D$_2$ receptor blocker; 25 mg is the minimally effective dose for preventing PONV. Extrapyramidal symptoms associated with the 25-mg dose affect less than 1% of patients, but like other D$_2$ antagonists, arrhythmias have been described.
- The antiemetic effect of glucocorticoids such as dexamethasone is well established although poorly understood. Most dose-response studies suggest that 4 mg is the minimally effective dose with equal efficacy as 4 mg ondansetron and 1.25 mg droperidol.
- Aprepitant is the first FDA-approved NK1 receptor antagonist. An oral dose of 40 mg aprepitant reduces nausea by about 30% and vomiting by more than 50%. It is thus particularly useful for surgeries wherein postoperative vomiting might impact the success of the surgery.
- Transdermal scopolamine is the only approved anticholinergic for prevention of PONV. Relative risk reduction is comparable to other antiemetics; its long duration of action makes transdermal scopolamine a suitable antiemetic for preventing PDNV in ambulatory patients.
- H$_1$ antagonists such as dimenhydrinate, cyclizine, and promethazine are less popular, mainly because of their sedative and psychotropic side effects and the potential for vein irritation and tissue damage.
- Alvimopan is a peripheral opioid receptor antagonist that is indicated for the prevention of ileus after colectomies. Secondary data analyses suggest that it might reduce OINV.
- The effectiveness of antiemetics when given prophylactically is critically dependent on the patient's risk for PONV. This can be easily assessed using a simplified risk score for PONV consisting of four risk factors: female sex, history of motion sickness and/or PONV, nonsmoking status, and anticipated use of postoperative opioids.

Key References

Apfel CC, Korttila K, Abdalla M, et al. A factorial trial of six interventions for the prevention of postoperative nausea and vomiting. *N Engl J Med.* 2004;350:2441-2451. A large multicenter trial in more than 5000 patients demonstrating that the relative risk reduction for three commonly used antiemetic interventions are all in the range of 25%, that efficacy is independent of patient risk, and that antiemetic drugs of different classes act independently of each other. (Ref. 35)

Apfel CC, Laara E, Koivuranta M, et al. A simplified risk score for predicting postoperative nausea and vomiting: conclusions from cross-validations between two centers. *Anesthesiology.* 1999;91:693-700. According to the simplified PONV risk score reported in this study, patients are likely to benefit from receiving antiemetic prophylaxis if they have at least two of the following four risk factors: female gender, history of PONV and/or motion sickness, nonsmoking status, and use of postoperative opioids. (Ref. 105)

Candiotti KA, Birnbach DJ, Lubarsky DA, et al. The impact of pharmacogenomics on postoperative nausea and vomiting: do CYP2D6 allele copy number and polymorphisms affect the success or failure of ondansetron prophylaxis? *Anesthesiology.* 2005;102:543-549. The CYP2D6 gene is responsible for metabolism of several antiemetic drugs, including ondansetron. Patients with three functional copies of the CYP2D6 gene were more likely to require rescue treatment for vomiting after prophylaxis with ondansetron. Some interindividual differences in response to prophylaxis might therefore be due to genetic variations between patients. (Ref. 12)

Carlisle J, Stevenson C. Drugs for preventing postoperative nausea and vomiting. *Cochrane Database Syst Rev.* 2006;3:CD004125. A systematic review of more than 730 trials that assessed the efficacy of all antiemetic agents as well as their associated side effects. The individual relative risk versus placebo for all effective antiemetics ranged between 0.60 and 0.80. (Ref. 22)

Cubeddu LX, Hoffmann IS, Fuenmayor NT, et al. Efficacy of ondansetron (GR 38032F) and the role of serotonin in cisplatin-induced nausea and vomiting. *N Engl J Med.* 1990;322:810-816. One of the first papers to show that ondansetron safely and effectively reduced the incidence of CINV in cancer patients undergoing chemotherapy. The results also suggested that cisplatin treatment triggered enterochromaffin cells to release serotonin and that ondansetron worked by blocking 5-HT$_3$ receptors. (Ref. 2)

Hvarfner A, Hammas B, Thorn SE, et al. The influence of propofol on vomiting induced by apomorphine. *Anesth Anal.* 1995;80:967-969. This study reported that propofol did not protect against nausea and vomiting at nonsedative doses, but that at sedative doses, propofol did have an antiemetic effect similar to that of midazolam. Therefore the antiemetic effect often attributed to propofol is more likely an effect of sedation. (Ref. 76)

Kovac AL, O'Connor TA, Pearman MH, et al. Efficacy of repeat intravenous dosing of ondansetron in controlling postoperative nausea and vomiting: a randomized, double-blind, placebo-controlled multicenter trial. *J Clin Anesth.* 1999;11:453-459. Patients who received 4 mg IV ondansetron for prophylaxis against PONV did not benefit from additional doses of ondansetron in the PACU. This study highlights the importance of administering antiemetics of different receptor classes for prophylaxis and/or rescue treatment to increase protection against PONV. (Ref. 106)

Rojas C, Stathis M, Thomas AG, et al. Palonosetron exhibits unique molecular interactions with the 5-HT$_3$ receptor. *Anesth Analg.* 2008;107:469-478. The first molecular-level study to differentiate between palonosetron and first generation 5-HT$_3$ receptor antagonists. Only palonosetron binds allosterically and cooperatively to the 5-HT$_3$ receptor, and its effect on receptor function persists longer than its binding to the receptor at the cell surface, suggesting that palonosetron induces receptor internalization. These unique mechanisms might account for palonosetron's superior efficacy against delayed PONV. (Ref. 16)

Wallenborn J, Gelbrich G, Bulst D, et al. Prevention of postoperative nausea and vomiting by metoclopramide combined with dexamethasone: randomised double blind multicentre trial. *Br Med J.* 2006;333:324. A dose-response trial in 3140 patients that determined that 25 mg was the minimum effective dose of metoclopramide for PONV prophylaxis, and that the commonly used dose of 10 mg was insufficient. Extrapyramidal symptoms associated with the 25-mg dose affected less than 1% of patients. (Ref. 31)

References

1. Raeder J. History of postoperative nausea and vomiting. *Int Anesth Clin.* 2003;41:1-12.
2. Cubeddu LX, Hoffmann IS, Fuenmayor NT, Finn AL. Efficacy of ondansetron (GR 38032F) and the role of serotonin in cisplatin-induced nausea and vomiting. *N Engl J Med.* 1990;322:810-816.
3. Apfel CC, Korttila K, Abdalla M, et al. An international multicenter protocol to assess the single and combined benefits of antiemetic interventions in a controlled clinical trial of a 2x2x2x2x2x2 factorial design (IMPACT). *Control Clin Trials.* 2003;24:736-751.
4. Jokela RM, Cakmakkaya OS, Danzeisen O, et al. Ondansetron has similar clinical efficacy against both nausea and vomiting. *Anaesthesia.* 2009;64:147-151.
5. Tang J, Wang B, White PF, Watcha MF, Qi J, Wender RH. The effect of timing of ondansetron administration on its efficacy, cost-effectiveness, and cost-benefit as a prophylactic antiemetic in the ambulatory setting. *Anesth Analg.* 1998;86:274-282.
6. Tramer MR, Reynolds DJ, Moore RA, McQuay HJ. Efficacy, dose-response, and safety of ondansetron in prevention of postoperative nausea and vomiting: a quantitative systematic review of randomized placebo-controlled trials. *Anesthesiology.* 1997;87:1277-1289.
7. Benedict CR, Arbogast R, Martin L, Patton L, Morrill B, Hahne W. Single-blind study of the effects of intravenous dolasetron mesylate versus ondansetron on electrocardiographic parameters in normal volunteers. *J Cardiovasc Pharmacol.* 1996;28:53-59.
8. Charbit B, Albaladejo P, Funck-Brentano C, Legrand M, Samain E, Marty J. Prolongation of QTc interval after postoperative nausea and vomiting treatment by droperidol or ondansetron. *Anesthesiology.* 2005;102:1094-1100.
9. Kaiser R, Sezer O, Papies A, et al. Patient-tailored antiemetic treatment with 5-hydroxytryptamine type 3 receptor antagonists according to cytochrome P-450 2D6 genotypes. *J Clin Oncol.* 2002;20:2805-2811.
10. Gregory RE, Ettinger DS. 5-HT$_3$ receptor antagonists for the prevention of chemotherapy-induced nausea and vomiting. A comparison of their pharmacology and clinical efficacy. *Drugs.* 1998;55:173-189.
11. Hickok JT, Roscoe JA, Morrow GR, King DK, Atkins JN, Fitch TR. Nausea and emesis remain significant problems of chemotherapy despite prophylaxis with 5-hydroxytryptamine-3 antiemetics: a University of Rochester James P. Wilmot Cancer Center Community Clinical Oncology Program Study of 360 cancer patients treated in the community. *Cancer.* 2003;97:2880-2886.
12. Candiotti KA, Birnbach DJ, Lubarsky DA, et al. The impact of pharmacogenomics on postoperative nausea and vomiting: do CYP2D6 allele copy number and polymorphisms affect the success or failure of ondansetron prophylaxis? *Anesthesiology.* 2005;102:543-549.
13. Babaoglu MO, Bayar B, Aynacioglu AS, et al. Association of the ABCB1 3435C>T polymorphism with antiemetic efficacy of 5-hydroxytryptamine type 3 antagonists. *Clin Pharmacol Ther.* 2005;78:619-626.
14. Choi EM, Lee MG, Lee SH, Choi KW, Choi SH. Association of ABCB1 polymorphisms with the efficacy of ondansetron for postoperative nausea and vomiting. *Anaesthesia.* 2010;65:996-1000.
15. Philip BK, McLeskey CH, Chelly JE, et al. Pooled analysis of three large clinical trials to determine the optimal dose of dolasetron mesylate needed to prevent postoperative nausea and vomiting. The Dolasetron Prophylaxis Study Group. *J Clin Anesth.* 2000;12:1-8.
16. Rojas C, Stathis M, Thomas AG, et al. Palonosetron exhibits unique molecular interactions with the 5-HT$_3$ receptor. *Anesth Analg.* 2008;107:469-478.
17. Rojas C, Thomas AG, Alt J, et al. Palonosetron triggers 5-HT(3) receptor internalization and causes prolonged inhibition of receptor function. *Eur J Pharmacol.* 2010;626:193-199.
18. Wong EH, Clark R, Leung E, et al. The interaction of RS 25259-197, a potent and selective antagonist, with 5-HT$_3$ receptors, in vitro. *Br J Pharmacol.* 1995;114:851-859.
19. Gralla R, Lichinitser M, Van Der Vegt S, et al. Palonosetron improves prevention of chemotherapy-induced nausea and vomiting following moderately emetogenic chemotherapy: results of a double-blind randomized phase III trial comparing single doses of palonosetron with ondansetron. *Ann Oncol.* 2003;14:1570-1577.
20. Rojas C, Li Y, Zhang J, et al. The antiemetic 5-HT$_3$ receptor antagonist palonosetron inhibits substance P-mediated responses in vitro and in vivo. *J Pharmacol Exp Ther.* 2010;335:362-368.
21. Kovac AL, Eberhart L, Kotarski J, Clerici G, Apfel C. A randomized, double-blind study to evaluate the efficacy and safety of three different doses of palonosetron versus placebo in preventing postoperative nausea and vomiting over a 72-hour period. *Anesth Analg.* 2008;107:439-444.
22. Carlisle J, Stevenson C. Drugs for preventing postoperative nausea and vomiting. *Cochrane Database Syst Rev.* 2006;3:CD004125.
23. Kovac AL. Prevention and treatment of postoperative nausea and vomiting. *Drugs.* 2000;59:213-243.
24. Culebras X, Corpataux J-B, Gaggero G, Tramer MR. The antiemetic efficacy of droperidol added to morphine patient-controlled analgesia: a randomized, controlled, multicenter dose-finding study. *Anesth Analg.* 2003;97:816-821.
25. Habib AS, Gan TJ. The use of droperidol before and after the Food and Drug Administration black box warning: a survey of the members of the Society of Ambulatory Anesthesia. *J Clin Anesth.* 2008;20:35-39.
26. White PF, Song D, Abrao J, Klein KW, Navarette B. Effect of low-dose droperidol on the QT interval during and after general anesthesia: a placebo-controlled study. *Anesthesiology.* 2005;102:1101-1105.
27. Scuderi PE. You (still) can't disprove the existence of dragons. *Anesthesiology.* 2005;102:1081-1082.
28. Brockmoller J, Kirchheiner J, Schmider J, et al. The impact of the CYP2D6 polymorphism on haloperidol pharmacokinetics and on the outcome of haloperidol treatment. *Clin Pharmacol Ther.* 2002;72:438-452.
29. Parlak I, Erdur B, Parlak M, et al. Midazolam vs. diphenhydramine for the treatment of metoclopramide-induced akathisia: a randomized controlled trial. *Acad Emerg Med.* 2007;14:715-721.
30. Henzi I, Walder B, Tramer MR. Metoclopramide in the prevention of postoperative nausea and vomiting: a quantitative systematic review of randomized, placebo-controlled studies. *Br J Anaesth.* 1999;83:761-771.
31. Wallenborn J, Gelbrich G, Bulst D, et al. Prevention of postoperative nausea and vomiting by metoclopramide combined with dexamethasone: randomised double blind multicentre trial. *Br Med J.* 2006;333:324.
32. Bentsen G, Stubhaug A. Cardiac arrest after intravenous metoclopramide—a case of five repeated injections of metoclopramide causing five episodes of cardiac arrest. *Acta Anaesthesiol Scand.* 2002;46:908-910.
33. Ho CM, Ho ST, Wang JJ, Tsai SK, Chai CY. Dexamethasone has a central antiemetic mechanism in decerebrated cats. *Anesth Analg.* 2004;99:734-739.
34. Wang JJ, Ho ST, Lee SC, Liu YC, Ho CM. The use of dexamethasone for preventing postoperative nausea and vomiting in females undergoing thyroidectomy: a dose-ranging study. *Anesth Analg.* 2000;91:1404-1407.
35. Apfel CC, Korttila K, Abdalla M, et al. A factorial trial of six interventions for the prevention of postoperative nausea and vomiting. *N Engl J Med.* 2004;350:2441-2451.
36. Gan TJ, Meyer TA, Apfel CC, et al. Society for ambulatory anesthesia guidelines for the management of postoperative nausea and vomiting. *Anesth Analg.* 2007;105:1615-1628.
37. Wang JJ, Ho ST, Tzeng JI, Tang CS. The effect of timing of dexamethasone administration on its efficacy as a prophylactic antiemetic for postoperative nausea and vomiting. *Anesth Analg.* 2000;91:136-139.
38. Perron G, Dolbec P, Germain J, Bechard P. Perineal pruritus after I.V. dexamethasone administration. *Can J Anaesth.* 2003;50:749-750.
39. Jordan K, Sippel C, Schmoll HJ. Guidelines for antiemetic treatment of chemotherapy-induced nausea and vomiting: past, present, and future recommendations. *Oncologist.* 2007;12:1143-1150.

40. McCrea JB, Majumdar AK, Goldberg MR, et al. Effects of the neurokinin1 receptor antagonist aprepitant on the pharmacokinetics of dexamethasone and methylprednisolone. *Clin Pharmacol Ther.* 2003;74:17-24.

41. Apfel CC, Malhotra A, Leslie JB. The role of neurokinin-1 receptor antagonists for the management of postoperative nausea and vomiting. *Curr Opin Anaesthesiol.* 2008;21:427-432.

42. Saito R, Takano Y, Kamiya H. Roles of substance P and NK1 receptor in the brainstem in the development of emesis. *J Pharmacol Sci.* 2003;91:87-94.

43. Van Belle S, Lichinitser MR, Navari RM, et al. Prevention of cisplatin-induced acute and delayed emesis by the selective neurokinin-1 antagonists, L-758,298 and MK-869. *Cancer.* 2002;94: 3032-3041.

44. Gan TJ, Apfel CC, Kovac A, et al. A randomized, double-blind comparison of the NK1 antagonist, aprepitant, versus ondansetron for the prevention of postoperative nausea and vomiting. *Anesth Analg.* 2007;104:1082-1089.

45. Navari RM, Reinhardt RR, Gralla RJ, et al. Reduction of cisplatin-induced emesis by a selective neurokinin-1-receptor antagonist. L-754,030 Antiemetic Trials Group. *N Engl J Med.* 1999;340:190-195.

46. Hesketh PJ, Grunberg SM, Gralla RJ, et al. The oral neurokinin-1 antagonist aprepitant for the prevention of chemotherapy-induced nausea and vomiting: a multinational, randomized, double-blind, placebo-controlled trial in patients receiving high-dose cisplatin—the Aprepitant Protocol 052 Study Group. *J Clin Oncol.* 2003;21: 4112-4119.

47. Bergstrom M, Hargreaves RJ, Burns HD, et al. Human positron emission tomography studies of brain neurokinin 1 receptor occupancy by aprepitant. *Biol Psychiatry.* 2004;55:1007-1012.

48. Chawla SP, Grunberg SM, Gralla RJ, et al. Establishing the dose of the oral NK1 antagonist aprepitant for the prevention of chemotherapy-induced nausea and vomiting. *Cancer.* 2003;97:2290-2300.

49. Nachum Z, Shupak A, Gordon CR. Transdermal scopolamine for prevention of motion sickness: clinical pharmacokinetics and therapeutic applications. *Clin Pharmacokinet.* 2006;45:543-566.

50. Parrott AC. The effects of transdermal scopolamine and four dose levels of oral scopolamine (0.15, 0.3, 0.6, and 1.2 mg) upon psychological performance. *Psychopharmacology.* 1986;89: 347-354.

51. Price NM, Schmitt LG, McGuire J, Shaw JE, Trobough G. Transdermal scopolamine in the prevention of motion sickness at sea. *Clin Pharmacol Ther.* 1981;29:414-419.

52. Graybiel A, Knepton J, Shaw J. Prevention of experimental motion sickness by scopolamine absorbed through the skin. *Aviat Space Environ Med.* 1976;47:1096-1100.

53. Parrott AC. Transdermal scopolamine: a review of its effects upon motion sickness, psychological performance, and physiological functioning. *Aviat Space Environ Med.* 1989;60:1-9.

54. Clissold SP, Heel RC. Transdermal hyoscine (Scopolamine). A preliminary review of its pharmacodynamic properties and therapeutic efficacy. *Drugs.* 1985;29:189-207.

55. Nachum Z, Shahal B, Shupak A, et al. Scopolamine bioavailability in combined oral and transdermal delivery. *J Pharmacol Exp Ther.* 2001;296:121-123.

56. Apfel CC, Zhang K, George E, et al. Transdermal scopolamine for the prevention of postoperative nausea and vomiting: a systematic review and meta-analysis. *Clin Ther.* 2010;32:1987-2002.

57. Gil A, Nachum Z, Dachir S, et al. Scopolamine patch to prevent seasickness: clinical response vs. plasma concentration in sailors. *Aviation, space, and environmental medicine.* 2005;76:766-770.

58. Kranke P, Morin AM, Roewer N, Eberhart LH. Dimenhydrinate for prophylaxis of postoperative nausea and vomiting: a meta-analysis of randomized controlled trials. *Acta Anaesthesiol Scand.* 2002;46:238-244.

59. Lin TF, Yeh YC, Yen YH, Wang YP, Lin CJ, Sun WZ. Antiemetic and analgesic-sparing effects of diphenhydramine added to morphine intravenous patient-controlled analgesia. *Br J Anaesth.* 2005; 94:835-839.

60. Eberhart LHJ, Seeling W, Ulrich B, Morin AM, Georgieff M. Dimenhydrinate and metoclopramide alone or in combination for prophylaxis of PONV. *Can J Anaesth.* 2000;47:780-785.

61. Turner KE, Parlow JL, Avery ND, Tod DA, Day AG. Prophylaxis of postoperative nausea and vomiting with oral, long-acting dimenhydrinate in gynecologic outpatient laparoscopy. *Anesth Analg.* 2004:1660-1664.

62. Scavone JM, Greenblatt DJ, Harmatz JS, Engelhardt N, Shader RI. Pharmacokinetics and pharmacodynamics of diphenhydramine 25 mg in young and elderly volunteers. *J Clin Pharmacol.* 1998;38: 603-609.

63. Luna BG, Scavone JM, Greenblatt DJ. Doxylamine and diphenhydramine pharmacokinetics in women on low-dose estrogen oral contraceptives. *J Clin Pharmacol.* 1989;29:257-260.

64. Blyden GT, Greenblatt DJ, Scavone JM, Shader RI. Pharmacokinetics of diphenhydramine and a demethylated metabolite following intravenous and oral administration. *J Clin Pharmacol.* 1986;26: 529-533.

65. Carruthers SG, Shoeman DW, Hignite CE, Azarnoff DL. Correlation between plasma diphenhydramine level and sedative and antihistamine effects. *Clinical Pharmacol Ther.* 1978;23:375-382.

66. Kothari SN, Boyd WC, Bottcher ML, Lambert PJ. Antiemetic efficacy of prophylactic dimenhydrate (Dramamine) vs ondansetron (Zofran): a randomized, prospective trial inpatients undergoing laparoscopic cholecystectomy. *Surg Endosc.* 2000;14:926-929.

67. Taylor G, Houston JB, Shaffer J, Mawer G. Pharmacokinetics of promethazine and its sulphoxide metabolite after intravenous and oral administration to man. *Br J Clin Pharmacol.* 1983;15:287-293.

68. Phenergan (promethazine hydrochloride) Injection, Solution [package insert]. Deerfield, IL: Baxter Healthcare Corporation; 1997.

69. Kreisler NS, Spiekermann BF, Ascari CM, et al. Small-dose droperidol effectively reduces nausea in a general surgical adult patient population. *Anesth Analg.* 2000;91:1256-1261.

70. Khalil S, Philbrook L, Rabb M, et al. Ondansetron/promethazine combination or promethazine alone reduces nausea and vomiting after middle ear surgery. *J Clin Anesth.* 1999;11:596-600.

71. Gan TJ, Candiotti KA, Klein SM, et al. Double-blind comparison of granisetron, promethazine, or a combination of both for the prevention of postoperative nausea and vomiting in females undergoing outpatient laparoscopies. *Can J Anaesth.* 2009;56:829-836.

72. Tarkkila P, Torn K, Tuominen M, Lindgren L. Premedication with promethazine and transdermal scopolamine reduces the incidence of nausea and vomiting after intrathecal morphine. *Acta Anaesthesiol Scand.* 1995;39:983-986.

73. Chia YY, Lo Y, Liu K, Tan PH, Chung NC, Ko NH. The effect of promethazine on postoperative pain: a comparison of preoperative, postoperative, and placebo administration in patients following total abdominal hysterectomy. *Acta Anaesthesiol Scand.* 2004;48:625-630.

74. Gan TJ, El-Molem H, Ray J, Glass PS. Patient-controlled Antiemesis: A Randomized, Double-Blind Comparison of Two Doses of Propofol versus Placebo. *Anesthesiol.* 1999;90:1564-1570.

75. Scuderi PE, D'Angelo R, Harris L, Mims GR, Weeks DB, James RL. Small-dose propofol by continuous infusion does not prevent postoperative vomiting in females undergoing outpatient laparoscopy. *Anesth Analg.* 1997;84:71-75.

76. Hvarfner A, Hammas B, Thorn SE, Wattwil M. The influence of propofol on vomiting induced by apomorphine. *Anesth Analg.* 1995;80:967-969.

77. Morrow GR, Rosenthal SN. Models, mechanisms and management of anticipatory nausea and emesis. *Oncology.* 1996;53(Suppl 1): 4-7.

78. Morrow GR, Roscoe JA, Kirshner JJ, Hynes HE, Rosenbluth RJ. Anticipatory nausea and vomiting in the era of 5-HT₃ antiemetics. *Support Care Cancer.* 1998;6:244-247.

79. Takada K, Murai T, Kanayama T, Koshikawa N. Effects of midazolam and flunitrazepam on the release of dopamine from rat striatum measured by in vivo microdialysis. *Br J Anaesthesia.* 1993;70: 181-185.

80. Phillis JW, Bender AS, Wu PH. Benzodiazepines inhibit adenosine uptake into rat brain synaptosomes. *Brain Res.* 1980;195:494-498.

81. Di Florio T. The use of midazolam for persistent postoperative nausea and vomiting. *Anaesth Intens Care.* 1992;20:383-386.

82. Gear RW, Miaskowski C, Heller PH, Paul SM, Gordon NC, Levine JD. Benzodiazepine mediated antagonism of opioid analgesia. *Pain.* 1997;71:25-29.

83. Jordan K, Kasper C, Schmoll HJ. Chemotherapy-induced nausea and vomiting: current and new standards in the antiemetic prophylaxis and treatment. *Eur J Cancer.* 2005;41:199-205.

84. Effective interventions for CINV: NCCN Antiemesis Clinical Practice Guidelines in Oncology. *ONS News*. 2004;19:17-18.

85. Kris MG, Hesketh PJ, Somerfield MR, et al. American Society of Clinical Oncology guideline for antiemetics in oncology: update 2006. *J Clin Oncol*. 2006;24:2932-2947.

86. Malik IA, Khan WA, Qazilbash M, Ata E, Butt A, Khan MA. Clinical efficacy of lorazepam in prophylaxis of anticipatory, acute, and delayed nausea and vomiting induced by high doses of cisplatin. A prospective randomized trial. *Am J Clin Oncol*. 1995;18:170-175.

87. Bauer KP, Dom PM, Ramirez AM, O'Flaherty JE. Preoperative intravenous midazolam: benefits beyond anxiolysis. *J Clin Anesth*. 2004;16:177-183.

88. Unlugenc H, Guler T, Gunes Y, Isik G. Comparative study of the antiemetic efficacy of ondansetron, propofol and midazolam in the early postoperative period. *Eur J Anaesthesiol*. 2003;20:668-673.

89. Sanjay OP, Tauro DI. Midazolam: an effective antiemetic after cardiac surgery—a clinical trial. *Anesth Analg*. 2004;99:339-343.

90. Lee Y, Wang JJ, Yang YL, Chen A, Lai HY. Midazolam vs ondansetron for preventing postoperative nausea and vomiting: a randomised controlled trial. *Anaesthesia*. 2007;62:18-22.

91. Majumdar AK, McCrea JB, Panebianco DL, et al. Effects of aprepitant on cytochrome P450 3A4 activity using midazolam as a probe. *Clin Pharmacol Ther*. 2003;74:150-156.

92. Emend (aprepitant) [package insert]. Whitehouse Station, NJ: Merck & Co., Inc.; 2006. http://www.emend.com/emend/shared/documents/pi.pdf.

93. Majumdar AK, Yan KX, Selverian DV, et al. Effect of aprepitant on the pharmacokinetics of intravenous midazolam. *Journal of Clinical Pharmacology*. 2007;47:744-750.

94. Rung GW, Claybon L, Hord A, et al. Intravenous ondansetron for postsurgical opioid-induced nausea and vomiting. *Anesth Analg*. 1997;84:832-838.

95. Chung F, Lane R, Spraggs C, et al. Ondansetron is more effective than metoclopramide for the treatment of opioid-induced emesis in post-surgical adult patients. *Eur J Anaesthesiol*. 1999;16:669-677.

96. Sussman G, Shurman J, Creed MR, et al. Intravenous ondansetron for the control of opioid-induced nausea and vomiting. International S3AA3013 Study Group. *Clinical therapeutics*. 1999;21:1216-1227.

97. Herndon CM, Jackson KC, 2nd, Hallin PA. Management of opioid-induced gastrointestinal effects in patients receiving palliative care. *Pharmacotherapy*. 2002;22:240-250.

98. Aldrete JA. Reduction of nausea and vomiting from epidural opioids by adding droperidol to the infusate in home-bound patients. *J Pain Symptom Manage*. 1995;10:544-547.

99. Bates JJ, Foss JF, Murphy DB. Are peripheral opioid antagonists the solution to opioid side effects? *Anesth Aanalgesia*. 2004;98:116-122.

100. Machelska H, Stein C. Immune mechanisms in pain control. *Anesth Analg*. 2002;95:1002-1008.

101. Schmidt W. Alvimopan*(ADL 8-2698) is a novel peripheral opioid antagonist. *Am J Surg*. 2001;182:S27-S38.

102. Paulson DM, Kennedy DT, Donovick RA, et al. Alvimopan: an oral, peripherally acting, mu-opioid receptor antagonist for the treatment of opioid-induced bowel dysfunction—-a 21-day treatment-randomized clinical trial. *J Pain*. 2005;6:184-192.

103. Herzog T, Coleman R, Guerrieri J. A double-blind, randomized, placebo-controlled phase III study of the safety of alvimopan in patients who undergo simple total abdominal hysterectomy. *Am J Obstet Gynecol*. 2006;195:445-453.

104. Adolor Corporation. Entereg (alvimopan) Capsules for postoperative ileus FDA Advisory Panel briefing document. http://www.fda.gov/ohrms/dockets/ac/08/briefing/2008-4336b1-02-Adolor.pdf.

105. Apfel CC, Laara E, Koivuranta M, Greim CA, Roewer N. A simplified risk score for predicting postoperative nausea and vomiting: conclusions from cross-validations between two centers. *Anesthesiology*. 1999;91:693-700.

106. Kovac AL, O'Connor TA, Pearman MH, et al. Efficacy of repeat intravenous dosing of ondansetron in controlling postoperative nausea and vomiting: a randomized, double-blind, placebo-controlled multicenter trial. *J Clin Anesth*. 1999;11:453-459.

107. Gan TJ, Gu J, Singla N, et al. Rolapitant for the prevention of postoperative nausea and vomiting: a prospective, double-blinded, placebo-controlled randomized trial. *Anesth Analg*. 2011;112:804-812.

108. Apfel CC, Philip BK, Cakmakkaya OS, et al. Who is at risk for post-discharge nausea and vomiting after ambulatory surgery? *Anesthesiology*. 2012;117(3):475-486.

Chapter 30

ENDOCRINE PHYSIOLOGY

Julie L. Huffmyer and Edward C. Nemergut

Endocrine physiology encompasses processes that range from master regulation by the incredibly small, but critically important organ, the pituitary gland that, in effect, communicates with all other endocrine organs via hormones, to the much larger pancreas that controls energy utilization processes of the body. This chapter reviews normal endocrine physiology and pathophysiology, as well as the basic anesthetic implications associated with the five major endocrine organs relevant to anesthesiologists: the pituitary gland, the parathyroid glands, the thyroid gland, the adrenal glands, and the pancreas.

PITUITARY PHYSIOLOGY

The pituitary gland controls the function of many other endocrine glands, often being referred to as the "master gland." Despite its central role in the endocrine system, the pituitary is extremely small—about the size of a pea—and weighs only about 0.5 g. It is attached to the hypothalamus by the pituitary stalk (or infundibulum) and rests in the sella turcica, a small bony cavity in the sphenoid bone at the base of the brain. The pituitary secretes at least eight hormones that regulate organ function and are critical to survival.

Both functionally and anatomically, the pituitary can be divided into the anterior lobe (or adenohypophysis) and the posterior lobe (or neurohypophysis). The lobes are different enough from one another that they can almost be considered as entirely different glands. In fact, consistent with their distinct structure and function, the embryonic origin of each lobe is entirely different: the anterior pituitary arises from oral ectoderm whereas the posterior pituitary arises from neuroectoderm.

Anterior Pituitary

The anterior pituitary is a glandular secretory organ. The most important hormones produced by the anterior pituitary include adrenocorticotropic hormone (ACTH), thyroid-stimulating hormone (TSH), growth hormone (GH), prolactin (PRL), and the two gonadotropins, luteinizing hormone (LH) and follicle-stimulating hormone (FSH). Melanocyte-stimulating hormone (MSH) is also produced by the anterior pituitary but is not required for homeostasis.

The anterior pituitary is composed of three cell types as identified with traditional aniline dye stains: acidophils, basophils (often collectively referred to as chromophils), and chromophobes. The chromophils are the principal secretory cell types whereas the chromophobes are not thought to have secretory function. Today, five cell types producing the six major hormones are best differentiated using immunohistochemical staining. These are:

- Somatotrophs, which produce GH (acidophilic)
- Mammotrophs, which produce PRL (acidophilic)
- Corticotrophs, which produce ACTH, MSH, and various endorphins (basophilic)
- Thyrotrophs, which produce TSH (basophilic)
- Gonadotrophs, which produce FSH and LH (basophilic)

In general, the balance of releasing factors secreted by the hypothalamus and inhibiting factors secreted by each hormone's target organ control the secretion of each hormone produced by the anterior pituitary. For example, TSH stimulates the thyroid to produce triiodothyronine (T_3) and tetraiodothyronine (T_4). The secretion of TSH by the anterior pituitary is stimulated by the secretion of thyrotropin-releasing hormone by the hypothalamus, but inhibited by both thyroid hormones (T_3 and T_4), creating a feedback loop. The releasing and inhibiting factors for each hormone are summarized in Table 30-1. The exception to this principle is prolactin, which is under tonic-inhibition by dopamine secreted by the hypothalamus.

The action of releasing factors secreted by the hypothalamus is facilitated by the presence of a portal blood supply to the anterior pituitary. The hypothalamus secretes releasing factors into a primary capillary plexus from which they travel to a secondary capillary plexus in the anterior pituitary.

HYPERPITUITARISM AND ANTERIOR LOBE TUMORS

Essentially all cases of hyperpituitarism occur secondary to pituitary adenoma. These tumors are commonly encountered in clinical practice. They represent approximately 10% of diagnosed brain neoplasms, and as many as 20% of people have a pituitary tumor on postmortem examination, suggesting that most pituitary adenomas are asymptomatic.[1]

Although the majority of pituitary adenomas are asymptomatic, most tumors present in three discrete ways:

(1) hormonal hypersecretion, (2) local mass effects (including pituitary hypofunction due to compression of the normal gland), or (3) incidental discovery during cranial imaging for an unrelated condition. Approximately 75% of pituitary tumors are "functioning" and produce a single predominant hormone; these patients typically present with the signs and symptoms of hormone excess. For example, patients with a TSH-secreting adenoma have pituitary hyperthyroidism and present with the signs and symptoms of hyperthyroidism. Patients with Cushing disease (secondary to an ACTH-secreting adenoma) and acromegaly (secondary to a growth hormone-secreting adenoma) merit special attention and are discussed below. The perioperative management of patients with pituitary tumors undergoing surgery has been extensively reviewed.[2] Pituitary adenomas are often classified based upon their size at the time of discovery. Tumors larger than 10 mm in any dimension are classified as "macroadenomas"; tumors smaller than 10 mm are classified as "microadenomas."

The mass effects produced by pituitary tumors can be extensive and problematic given the location of the pituitary gland within the brain. Patients can present with varying degrees of hypopituitarism secondary to compression of normal anterior pituitary tissue by the expanding intrasellar mass. Seventy percent to 90% of patients with nonfunctioning pituitary macroadenomas exhibit deficiencies in at least one pituitary hormone with formal testing.[3] Thus, while it is easy to focus on the signs and symptoms of glucocorticoid excess in a patient with Cushing disease, for example, the patient with Cushing disease might also suffer from pituitary hypothyroidism. Furthermore, prolactin is frequently elevated in patients with all varieties of pituitary tumors secondary to disruption in normal inhibitory tone from the hypothalamus. Regardless, posterior pituitary dysfunction is unusual, even among patients with very large tumors.

Gigantism and Acromegaly

The unregulated hypersecretion of growth hormone by the anterior pituitary leads to increased production of insulin-like growth factor 1 (IGF-1) by the liver. Children in whom the epiphyses have not closed experience gigantism. In contrast, acromegaly develops in adults. Cardiac disease, hypertension, and ventricular hypertrophy are the most important causes of

Table 30-1. Major Hormones of the Anterior Pituitary

HORMONE	SYMBOL	PROTEIN STRUCTURE	RELEASING FACTOR (FROM HYPOTHALAMUS)	INHIBITING FACTORS	ANATOMIC TARGET	EFFECTS
Adrenocorticotropic hormone	ACTH	Polypeptide	Corticotropin-releasing hormone	Glucocorticoids	Adrenal gland	Secretion of glucocorticoids
Thyroid-stimulating hormone	TSH	Glycoprotein	Thyrotropin-releasing hormone	T_3 and T_4	Thyroid gland	Secretion of thyroid hormones
Growth hormone	GH	Polypeptide	Growth hormone-releasing hormone	Growth hormone, insulin-like growth factor 1 (IGF-1), somatostatin	Liver, adipose tissue	Growth, anabolic, promotes lipid and carbohydrate metabolism
Prolactin	PRL	Polypeptide	(See text)	Dopamine	Ovaries, mammary glands	Milk production, lipid and carbohydrate metabolism
Luteinizing hormone	LH	Glycoprotein	Gonadotropin-releasing hormone	Estrogen, testosterone	Gonads	Sex hormone production
Follicle-stimulating hormone	FSH	Glycoprotein	Gonadotropin-releasing hormone	Estrogen, testosterone	Gonads	Sex hormone production

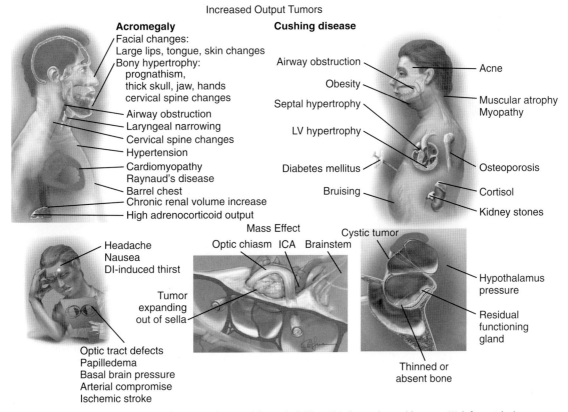

Increased Output Tumors

Acromegaly
Facial changes:
Large lips, tongue, skin changes
Bony hypertrophy:
prognathism,
thick skull, jaw, hands
cervical spine changes
Airway obstruction
Laryngeal narrowing
Cervical spine changes
Hypertension
Cardiomyopathy
Raynaud's disease
Barrel chest
Chronic renal volume increase
High adrenocorticoid output

Cushing disease
Airway obstruction
Obesity
Septal hypertrophy
LV hypertrophy
Diabetes mellitus
Bruising
Acne
Muscular atrophy
Myopathy
Osteoporosis
Cortisol
Kidney stones

Mass Effect
Optic chiasm ICA Brainstem
Cystic tumor
Headache
Nausea
DI-induced thirst
Tumor
expanding
out of sella
Hypothalamus
pressure
Residual
functioning
gland
Optic tract defects
Papilledema
Basal brain pressure
Arterial compromise
Ischemic stroke
Thinned or
absent bone

Figure 30-1 Manifestations of acromegaly. *DI,* Diabetes insipidus; *ICA,* internal carotid artery; *LV,* left ventricular.

morbidity and mortality in acromegalic patients. Patients with acromegaly have a characteristic facies as the soft tissues of the nose, mouth, tongue, and lips become thicker and contribute to the acromegalic appearance. Airway obstruction and obstructive sleep apnea (OSA) can affect up to 70% of acromegalic patients.[4] A high risk of perioperative airway compromise has been well documented in acromegalic patients.[5] Other manifestations of acromegaly are summarized in Figure 30-1.

Cushing Disease
Cushing disease specifically results from the unregulated hypersecretion of ACTH by a pituitary adenoma and consequent hypercortisolism. Systemic hypertension is among the most common manifestations.[2] Increased endogenous corticosteroids have been shown to cause systemic hypertension by a variety of mechanisms. Secondary to hypertension, a high prevalence of left ventricular hypertrophy and concentric remodeling has been reported. Glucose intolerance occurs in at least 60% of patients, with overt diabetes mellitus (DM) present in up to one third of all patients. Patients are typically obese with characteristic "moon facies." Although not as common as in acromegaly, patients frequently have OSA. Despite the association with OSA, endotracheal intubation is not usually more difficult.[5] Other manifestations of acromegaly are summarized in Figure 30-1.

Prolactinomas
Prolactinomas are the most frequently observed type of hyperfunctioning pituitary adenoma, representing 20% to 30% of all clinically recognized pituitary tumors and half of all functioning tumors. Despite their frequency,

prolactinoma is not associated with significant mortality. In women, hyperprolactinemia causes amenorrhea, galactorrhea, loss of libido, and infertility. In men, symptoms of hyperprolactinemia are relatively nonspecific and include decreased libido, impotence, premature ejaculation, erectile dysfunction, and oligospermia.

Posterior Pituitary
Unlike the anterior pituitary, the posterior pituitary gland (neurohypophysis) is not really a secretory gland, but rather a collection of axon terminals arising from the supraoptic and paraventricular nuclei of the hypothalamus. The posterior pituitary is principally responsible for the secretion of oxytocin and vasopressin, also known as antidiuretic hormone (ADH).

ADH is synthesized in the supraoptic and paraventricular nuclei of the hypothalamus. After initial synthesis, the precursor hormone is transported down the axon into the posterior lobe of the pituitary where ADH undergoes final maturation to active hormone and is stored in vesicles for future release. Plasma osmolarity is the primarily stimulus for ADH secretion; however, other factors such as left atrial distention, circulating blood volume, exercise, and certain emotional states can also alter ADH release. ADH is considerably more sensitive to small changes in osmolarity than to similar changes in blood volume. A 1% to 2% increase in osmolarity is sufficient to increase ADH secretion. ADH binds to vasopressin 2 (V_2) receptors on the renal collecting ducts, which increases their permeability to water. This results in a significant increase in water reabsorption. Additionally, ADH increases blood pressure by increasing systemic vascular resistance through

Table 30-2. Syndrome of Inappropriate Antidiuretic Hormone (SIADH) and Diabetes Insipidus (DI)

	SIADH	DI
Associated conditions	1. Neurologic disease (SAH, TBI) 2. Neoplasia (especially non–small cell lung cancer) 3. Nonneoplastic lung disease 4. Drugs (carbamazepine)	1. Pituitary surgery 2. TBI 3. SAH (especially secondary to anterior communicating artery aneurysm)
Presentation	Hyponatremia	Polyuria
Plasma volume (awake patients)	Euvolemic (or slightly hypervolemic)	Euvolemic (practically speaking) Hypovolemic if not allowed access to fluids or unconscious
Serum osmolarity	Hypotonic (<275 mOsm/L)	Hypertonic (>310 mOsm/L)
Serum Na$^+$	Falling (<135 mEq/L)	Rising (>145 mEq/L)
Urine volume	Low (but not normally absent)	Voluminous (4 to 18 L/day)
Urine osmolarity	Relatively high (>100 mOsm/L)	Relatively low (<200 mOsm/L)
Urinary Na$^+$	>30 mEq/L	Normal (or variable)
Treatment	Fluid restriction If Na$^+$ < 120 mEq/L consider hypertonic saline to correct sodium (but no faster than 1 mEq/L/h) Intravenous urea Demeclocycline Lithium (rarely used)	Supportive DDAVP

DDAVP, Desmopressin (1-desamino-8-D-arginine vasopressin); *DI*, diabetes insipidus; *SAH*, subarachnoid hemorrhage; *SIADH*, syndrome of inappropriate diuretic hormone; *TBI*, traumatic brain injury.

interaction with V_{1a} receptors on blood vessels. The effect of ADH on blood pressure is mild in health, but becomes much more important in hypovolemic shock. It is used therapeutically as a vasopressor (see Chapter 22).

Diabetes Insipidus and Syndrome of Inappropriate Antidiuretic Hormone

The absence of ADH secretion results in pituitary diabetes insipidus (DI), whereas oversecretion or "inappropriately high" levels of ADH (or ADH-like hormones) results in the syndrome of inappropriate ADH (SIADH). DI is most commonly associated with pituitary surgery and is most often transient. Whereas 18% of 881 patients undergoing transsphenoidal surgery experienced early postoperative DI, only 2% had persistent DI 1 week after surgery.[6] Its onset is heralded by the abrupt onset of polyuria, accompanied by thirst and polydipsia. SIADH is most commonly associated with central nervous system injury or trauma as well as certain cancers, especially lung cancer. Unlike DI, which typically presents with polyuria, SIADH typically presents with the signs and symptoms of hyponatremia. Characteristics of DI and SIADH are summarized in Table 30-2.

Like ADH, oxytocin is also synthesized in the supraoptic and paraventricular nuclei of the hypothalamus and transported down long axons into the posterior pituitary for release. The principal physiologic functions of oxytocin are to stimulate cervical dilation and uterine contraction during labor and to allow milk to be let down into the subareolar sinuses during lactation. Oxytocin is one of the few hormones involved in a positive feedback loop. For example, uterine contractions stimulate oxytocin release from the posterior pituitary, which in turn increases uterine contractions.

PARATHYROID PHYSIOLOGY

The parathyroid glands, of which there are usually four, are small, bilateral, pea-sized glands located posterior to the thyroid gland in the neck. The glands possess a rich vascular supply via the inferior thyroid artery and consist mainly of chief cells primarily responsible for secreting parathyroid hormone (PTH) in response to hypocalcemia.

PTH plays a chief role in bone remodeling and Ca^{2+} homeostasis. PTH stimulates bone resorption and consequently release of Ca^{2+} into the bloodstream. In addition, PTH causes Ca^{2+} reabsorption into the circulation and phosphate excretion via the kidney. PTH facilitates vitamin D conversion to its activated form such that it facilitates intestinal and renal absorption of Ca^{2+}. Activated vitamin D also acts on bone to increase resorption, thus leading to further Ca^{2+} release into the bloodstream. Primary control of the release of PTH comes via negative feedback inhibition once elevated vitamin D and plasma Ca^{2+} levels are detected by a parathyroid Ca^{2+}-sensing receptor.[7] Other mechanisms also affect the release of PTH: (1) increased phosphate levels lead to increases in production and release of PTH; (2) hypomagnesemia, like hypocalcemia, causes release of PTH; (3) adrenergic agonists such as epinephrine increase PTH release through β-adrenergic receptors on parathyroid cells.[8] Indeed, this effect of adrenergic agonists is transient and very mild during hypercalcemia but more pronounced at lower Ca^{2+} levels.[8] In addition, β-adrenergic antagonists such as propranolol decrease PTH in normal patients, but seem to have less effect of secondary hyperparathyroidism.[8] Calcitonin counteracts the effects of PTH as it inhibits bone resorption and increases excretion of Ca^{2+} through the kidneys.

The net result of the interactions of PTH, Ca^{2+}, vitamin D, and calcitonin is maintenance of normal plasma Ca^{2+} concentration, which in turn helps maintain normal cellular function, nerve transmission, membrane stability, bone integrity, coagulation, and intracellular signaling. Normal plasma Ca^{2+} levels are 8.5 to 10.5 mg/dL (2.1-2.6 mM). The majority of Ca^{2+} is stored in the bones and teeth. Only 1% is found in plasma in three portions: ionized or unbound Ca^{2+} (50%; this form is sensed by the Ca^{2+} receptors in the parathyroid gland), protein-bound Ca^{2+} (40%), and Ca^{2+} bound to citrate and phosphate (10%). Protein-bound Ca^{2+} is primarily bound to albumin with implications for changes in blood pH. Acidosis causes a decrease in protein binding, thus leading to higher ionized Ca^{2+} (normally 1.0-1.2 mM), whereas alkalosis results in higher protein binding, thus reducing the free Ca^{2+} fraction in blood.[9]

Primary Hyperparathyroidism

Primary hyperparathyroidism is excess PTH production and release most often due to parathyroid gland hyperplasia or tumor. The elevated PTH increases bone resorption and extracellular Ca^{2+}. It occurs most commonly in patients aged 30 to 50 years and is more common in women than men.[10] Clinically, patients exhibit increased intact PTH levels, hypercalcemia, hypercalciuria, hypophosphatemia, nephrolithiasis, osteoporosis, and neuromuscular changes such as fatigue, weakness, and difficulties with cognition. Nausea, vomiting, constipation, and anorexia are common symptoms of hypercalcemia and patients may also complain of depression, confusion, and psychosis. Despite these manifestations, primary hyperparathyroidism is most often asymptomatic and detected incidentally on routine laboratory analysis as isolated hypercalcemia. Treatment of primary hyperparathyroidism centers on surgical excision of the parathyroid glands or tumor because there is increased risk of morbidity and cardiovascular mortality with long-standing hypercalcemia and untreated hyperparathyroidism.[8]

Multiple Endocrine Neoplasia

Two familial syndromes that include hyperparathyroidism as a component are multiple endocrine neoplasia (MEN) type 1 and type 2 syndromes. MEN1 is a rare, autosomal dominant syndrome in which tumors develop in the parathyroid glands, pancreas, and anterior pituitary gland of affected individuals. Most patients present with hyperparathyroidism. MEN2 is also an autosomal dominant syndrome but has incomplete penetrance and variable expression. MEN2A represents the combination of medullary thyroid carcinoma, pheochromocytoma, and hyperparathyroidism. Generally in MEN2B there is lack of parathyroid involvement. MEN2 syndromes have hyperparathyroidism as a feature in 10% to 25% of patients with mild hypercalcemia.[8] (Topic is reviewed elsewhere.[11,12])

Secondary Hyperparathyroidism

Secondary hyperparathyroidism is a complication most commonly due to chronic renal failure, but can result from any disease that causes chronic hypocalcemia. Early in the course of renal failure decreased vitamin D and ionized Ca^{2+} levels cause increased production and release of PTH. The kidneys are also unable to excrete the phosphate load, which contributes to low serum Ca^{2+}. Over time, the parathyroid glands become more resistant to the negative feedback mechanism of vitamin D and Ca^{2+} on PTH release, such that an increase in Ca^{2+} results in less efficient inhibition of PTH release. Hyperphosphatemia also further results in uremia-induced parathyroid gland hyperplasia, and PTH production and release. Goals of treatment of secondary hyperparathyroidism include maintaining Ca^{2+} and phosphate levels close to normal, reducing PTH secretion, and treating preexisting bone disease. These treatments focus on dietary phosphate restriction, maintaining daily Ca^{2+} intake greater than or equal to

1500 mg, administration of phosphate binder agents, and vitamin D replacement.

Anesthetic considerations for patients with hyperparathyroidism (whether primary or secondary) focus on the effects of hypercalcemia. Preoperative evaluation should focus on eliciting the cause of the hyperparathyroidism and the degree of hypercalcemia. If hypercalcemia is mild to moderate and patients are without severe cardiovascular or renal complications, most surgery can proceed without further evaluation. Patients can have polydipsia and polyuria, and can present for surgery to remove renal calculi because nephrolithiasis is common. The electrocardiogram (ECG) can show shortened PR and QT intervals as well as cardiac arrhythmias.[8] Patients can be hypertensive, and severe hypercalcemia can cause significant hypovolemia such that volume resuscitation is required. Severe hypercalcemia should be treated preoperatively. Aggressive volume resuscitation with diuretic administration once volume status has been repleted can be used to acutely lower serum Ca^{2+} levels. Loop diuretics such as furosemide decrease the reabsorption of Ca^{2+} from the proximal tubules. For patients with renal dysfunction or failure, hemodialysis is immediately effective to reduce Ca^{2+} levels. Medications such as mithramycin and calcitonin can also be used but have significant side-effect profiles and should be administered with caution.

Induction and maintenance of anesthesia should proceed carefully but are without specific requirements as to choice of agent. Most anesthetic concerns for parathyroid surgery focus on emergence and postoperative care. After surgery in the area of the thyroid and parathyroid glands, recurrent laryngeal nerve damage, airway swelling, and hematoma formation are real potential complications. The recurrent laryngeal nerves innervate all muscles of the larynx with the exception of the cricothyroid, which is supplied by the external laryngeal nerve. If the recurrent laryngeal nerve is completely paralyzed, the vocal cord will be abducted and will vibrate and cause stridor and hoarseness.[8] If the recurrent laryngeal nerve is partially paralyzed the vocal cord will be adducted. Thus a partial lesion is more concerning for airway obstruction and a complete lesion more concerning for possible aspiration risk.[8] Hypocalcemia can occur quickly after parathyroid removal and thus patients should be monitored with serial Ca^{2+}, Mg^{2+}, phosphate, and PTH levels. Hypocalcemia can also present with rapid onset of weakness and airway compromise.

Hypoparathyroidism

Hypoparathyroidism is associated with other endocrine disorders and neoplasias and as a result of surgical removal of the parathyroid glands. Hypocalcemia is the major acute result of inadvertent removal of the parathyroid glands. Hypocalcemic tetany can manifest as painful spasms of the facial muscles and extremities and laryngeal muscle spasm with upper airway obstruction. ECG changes associated with hypocalcemia include prolonged QT interval and possible heart block. Pseudohypoparathyroidism is not due to reduced PTH levels, but instead to reduced target sensitivity to PTH due to a receptor defect. Patients exhibit low plasma Ca^{2+} levels, high phosphate levels, and high PTH levels. Patients with pseudohypoparathyroidism appear either normal and have renal resistance to PTH or are short in stature with skeletal abnormalities as a result of generalized hormone resistance.

There are few anesthetic considerations for the patient with a history of hypoparathyroidism presenting for surgery. The patient should have baseline Ca^{2+}, phosphate, and Mg^{2+} levels and an ECG to determine QT interval. Hypocalcemia can be treated with calcium gluconate bolus and infusion in order to maintain serum Ca^{2+} levels.

THYROID PHYSIOLOGY

The thyroid gland is an acinar gland positioned in the neck, just anterior to the trachea with a rich vascular supply from the superior and inferior thyroid arteries. Weighing up to 25 g, the thyroid gland has a right and left lobe connected by the thyroid isthmus. Several cell types make up the thyroid gland including follicular cells (involved in thyroid hormone synthesis), endothelial cells (line the capillaries and provide blood supply to follicles), parafollicular or C cells (produce calcitonin), and fibroblasts, lymphocytes, and adipocytes (structural support for the thyroid). Other structures close to the thyroid gland include the trachea and esophagus as well as the recurrent laryngeal nerves and superior laryngeal nerve.

Thyrotropin-releasing hormone (TRH) is produced in the hypothalamus and released in response to decreased free circulating thyroid hormone. TRH binds to a G protein–coupled receptor in the anterior pituitary causing an increase in intracellular Ca^{2+}. Increased intracellular Ca^{2+} then causes release of TSH into the bloodstream, which stimulates the thyroid gland to increase the synthesis and release of T_4 and T_3 into the systemic circulation. T_4 and T_3 inhibit further secretion of TSH by inhibiting secretion of TRH. Thus thyroid hormone production and secretion are regulated via negative feedback by the hypothalamic-pituitary-thyroid (HPA) axis. Other mediators that inhibit TSH release include dopamine, somatostatin, and glucocorticoids.

Iodide is required for thyroid hormone synthesis and the body readily absorbs the necessary iodine from dietary sources.[13] Iodine is then converted to iodide before it is absorbed by the thyroid gland.[13] In the follicle of the thyroid, thyroglobulin, a glycoprotein possessing several tyrosine residues, is iodinated, yielding monoiodinated tyrosine (MIT) and diiodinated tyrosine (DIT) residues. MIT and DIT ultimately are synthesized to T_3 and T_4 via thyroid peroxidase. The thyroid gland releases more T_4 than T_3, and mainly in the liver T_4 is converted to T_3 as a result of the deiodination of T_4. T_4 is less active than T_3 in that it has decreased affinity for the thyroid hormone receptor but both T_3 and T_4 are able to be stored in the thyroid gland for a 2- to 3-month supply. Thyroid hormones circulate in the bloodstream bound to proteins, mainly to the thyroid binding globulin but also to albumin. A small amount of each hormone circulates in an unbound, free form ready to enter the cell and bind to the thyroid hormone receptor. T_4 binds more avidly to proteins and thus has a longer half-life of 7 days compared to T_3, which has a half-life of 1 day. Thyroid hormone metabolism involves the sequential removal of iodine. Thus T_4, a relatively inactive thyroid hormone, is deiodinated to T_3, the active thyroid hormone. Removal of one more iodine to T_2 yields a completely inactive product. In addition, thyroid hormones can be conjugated in the liver to increase solubility and allow biliary excretion.

Thyroid hormone receptors are found in virtually all tissues. Thyroid hormones play a chief role in cellular energy metabolism and are involved in the following[14]:

- Transcription of cell membrane sodium-potassium adenosine triphosphate (ATP)-ase, leading to increase in oxygen consumption
- Transcription of uncoupling protein
- Fatty acid oxidation and heat generation with production of ATP
- Protein synthesis and breakdown
- Epinephrine-induced glycogenolysis and gluconeogenesis with effects on insulin-induced glycogen synthesis and glucose utilization
- Cholesterol synthesis and lipoprotein receptor regulation

Thyroid hormones play a major role in normal growth and development. Specific systems to note include the skeletal system in which thyroid hormone is essential for bone growth, and the cardiovascular system in which thyroid hormone has inotropic and chronotropic effects as evidenced by increased cardiac output, and effects on blood volume and systemic vascular resistance. Thyroid hormone differentiates adipose tissue and regulates triglyceride and cholesterol metabolism in the liver. Thyroid hormone also controls production of pituitary hormones and expression of genes involved in central nervous system myelination, cell differentiation, migration, and signaling.

Thyroid disease and dysfunction occurs as a result of alterations in levels of thyroid hormones, impaired metabolism of thyroid hormones, or resistance to effects of thyroid hormones. The thyroid gland can undergo changes that contribute to altered thyroid function. Thyroid hyperplasia or enlargement occurs in Graves disease and thyroid destruction occurs in Hashimoto thyroiditis. Table 30-3 differentiates hypothyroidism from hyperthyroidism based on laboratory values and clinical manifestations.

Table 30-3. Disorders of Thyroid Function

	HYPOTHYROIDISM	HYPERTHYROIDISM
Laboratory values	Low free T_4 Low or normal T_3 High TSH	High T_4 High T_3 Low TSH
Clinical manifestations	Fatigue, lethargy Constipation Decreased appetite Cold intolerance Abnormal menses Hair loss Hoarse voice Brittle nails, dry skin Myxedema Delayed reflexes Reduced stroke volume Decreased heart rate Decreased cardiac output Decreased mental function Impaired memory	Palpitations Widened pulse pressure Tachycardia Increased blood volume Ophthalmopathy Nervousness Irritability Hyperactivity Heat intolerance Weight loss Decreased or absent menses Increased gastric motility and bowel function Warm moist skin Fine tremor Excessive sweating

TSH, Thyroid-stimulating hormone.

Hypothyroidism

Hypothyroidism is divided into primary and secondary hypothyroidism. Primary hypothyroidism refers to disease at the level of the thyroid gland itself. In adults this is most often due to autoimmune disease causing destruction of thyroid tissue. Surgical excision or radioactive iodine therapy are iatrogenic causes for hypothyroidism and require thyroid hormone replacement. Secondary hypothyroidism implies dysfunction outside of the thyroid gland, most likely in the hypothalamus or pituitary gland, characterized by decreased TSH secretion from the pituitary gland and decreased thyroid hormone release from the thyroid gland. Medications such as lithium, amiodarone, iron, and cholestyramine can be iatrogenic causes of hypothyroidism.[15] Symptoms of hypothyroidism are vague and nonspecific including fatigue, lethargy, painful joints and muscles, cold intolerance, constipation, change in voice quality (rough or gravely), bradycardia, low voltage of ECG, and heart failure symptoms.

Myxedema coma refers to severe hypothyroidism characterized by decreased mental status and coma, hypothermia, bradycardia, hyponatremia, heart failure, and respiratory failure. Myxedema coma is rare, and most commonly presents in the postoperative period after a trigger such as infection, exposure to cold temperatures, and excessive sedation and analgesic medications.[15] A patient with myxedema coma should be treated in the intensive care unit with supportive therapy and urgent administration of intravenous levothyroxine and glucocorticoids for likely concomitant adrenal insufficiency, as well as aggressive volume replacement.[15-17]

Hyperthyroidism

Hyperthyroidism refers to excessive thyroid gland function such that excess thyroid hormone is produced and released. Patients most commonly experience increased metabolism and autonomic nervous system disturbances. For adults, the most common cause of hyperthyroidism is Graves disease or diffuse toxic goiter, an autoimmune disease in which thyroid hormone is produced in an autonomous fashion due to TSH receptor stimulation by antibodies. Patients with Graves disease often have thyroid eye disease as well evidenced by exophthalmos or protruding eyes due to lymphocyte and fibroblast infiltration of the extraocular tissues and eye muscles. Other conditions leading to hyperthyroidism include toxic nodular goiter, toxic adenomatous disease of the thyroid, administration of excessive thyroid hormone, excess iodine intake, thyroiditis, follicular carcinoma, and TSH-producing tumor of the pituitary gland. Clinical features of hyperthyroidism or thyrotoxicosis include weight loss, tremor, heat intolerance, sweating, tachycardia, cardiac arrhythmias such as atrial fibrillation, heart failure, dyspnea, diarrhea, nausea, vomiting, anxiety, irritability, insomnia, and depression.

Thyroid storm presenting in the perioperative period can mimic malignant hyperthermia (MH) and as such anesthesiologists need to be aware and vigilant for this concerning complication of undiagnosed or undertreated hyperthyroidism. Symptoms are nonspecific and similar to those of MH: hyperpyrexia (up to 41°C), tachycardia, weakness, and delirium. Treatment requires intensive care and is supportive, with β blockers being helpful to reduce the adrenergic surge, antithyroid medications and iodine to reduce thyroid gland

output, and cooling measures such as antipyretics, cool fluids and blankets as well as control of respiratory status and minute ventilation to treat increased carbon dioxide production.[18] Antithyroid medications (e.g., propylthiouracil) must be given before iodine, which also blocks the release of thyroid hormone.[18,19]

Sick euthyroid syndrome affects patients with chronic nonthyroid medical conditions and diseases as patients appear euthyroid clinically but have evidence of thyroid dysfunction on laboratory testing. Usually patients have decreased T_3 and T_4, decreased T_4 binding to thyroid binding globulin but normal TSH and otherwise normal imaging of the thyroid gland itself.[14] Factors known to precipitate sick euthyroid syndrome include stress, starvation, malnutrition, surgical trauma, myocardial infarction, chronic renal failure, diabetic ketoacidosis, cirrhosis, sepsis, and hyperthermia. Medications such as propranolol and amiodarone can also induce sick euthyroid syndrome as they impair conversion of T_4 to T_3.[15]

THYROIDITIS

Thyroiditis, or inflammation of the thyroid gland, can be acute or chronic and can lead to abnormalities of thyroid function. Acute thyroiditis is rare and infectious. Patients present with a painful thyroid gland, chills, and fever and appear hyperthyroid. Chronic thyroiditis (otherwise known as Hashimoto thyroiditis, chronic lymphocytic thyroiditis, or autoimmune thyroiditis) represents an autoimmune condition of the thyroid gland in which there is lymphocytic infiltration of the thyroid gland and circulating autoimmune antibodies. The antibodies prevent iodide uptake and thyroid hormone synthesis. Autoimmune thyroiditis is the most common cause of adult hypothyroidism.[15] Early in the course of the disease patients can have variable levels of T_3, T_4, and TSH but usually have antibodies to thyroid peroxidase and thyroglobulin. Once chronic hypothyroidism develops, patients manifest low T_3 and T_4 and high TSH levels although the increased TSH usually dissipates over time.

Hypothyroid patients presenting for surgery can be more sensitive to the effects of anesthetic agents and can have a prolonged recovery from anesthesia. Patients with mild to moderate hypothyroidism are at low risk for complications when undergoing surgery and anesthesia.[10,20] If possible, patients should be rendered euthyroid before surgery and patients should receive their thyroid supplementation medication on the day of surgery. It is important to maintain body temperature in hypothyroid patients because hypothermia puts patients at risk for increased complications related to recovery from anesthesia, wound healing, and coagulation.

The major anesthetic consideration for a patient with a history of hyperthyroidism before surgery is their current thyroid status and medication history. It is helpful to obtain the most recent thyroid function tests and attempt to elicit symptoms of hyperthyroidism such as tachycardia, atrial fibrillation, diarrhea, and weight loss. In the case of the patient presenting for thyroid surgery, it is vital to consider the size of the thyroid gland, any compressive symptoms the patient is experiencing due to an enlarged gland or goiter such as dysphagia, respiratory symptoms such as dyspnea, stridor, and respiratory distress. Imaging of the neck may be helpful to reveal tracheal compression or deviation as well as retrosternal extension of the thyroid gland.[18] Such patients can require awake, fiberoptic intubation with maintenance of spontaneous ventilation due to compression of the trachea. Thyroid surgery for patients with retrosternal extension may require sternal splitting and partial sternotomy. In patients having emergency surgery with a concern for possible untreated or inadequately treated hyperthyroidism, a short-acting β blocker such as esmolol can be used to control tachycardia. During surgery in the neck, manipulation of the carotid sinus and bodies can induce hemodynamic instability that may not be well tolerated by patients who have coexistent cardiovascular disease. Other anesthetic considerations for the intraoperative and postoperative period, especially with regard to vocal cord dysfunction, are reviewed in the anesthetic considerations section above in parathyroid disease.

Postoperative complications related to thyroid surgery are critical for every anesthesiologist to be vigilant of and understand how to treat quickly. Airway obstruction due to hemorrhage in the neck, recurrent laryngeal nerve injury and tracheal compression must be treated immediately. Hemorrhage in the neck after thyroid surgery causes early airway compression and the neck wound must be opened and allowed to drain. Stitch and staple removers should be present at the bedside of every patient after thyroid surgery.[18] After release of the airway compression, the neck wound can be explored and the hemorrhage treated surgically.

ADRENAL GLAND PHYSIOLOGY

The adrenal glands are small (3-5 cm in length) and are located just superior to each kidney. There are two parts to each adrenal gland: the outer adrenal cortex derives from mesodermal tissue and the inner medulla derives from neural crest cells. The cortex makes up 90% of the adrenal mass and produces the steroid hormones glucocorticoids, mineralocorticoids, and androgens (cortisol, aldosterone, and dehydroepiandrosterone) as a result of hypothalamic-pituitary-adrenal (HPA) stimulation. The medulla makes up the remaining 10% of adrenal mass and synthesizes and releases the catecholamines epinephrine and norepinephrine as a result of sympathetic stimulation. Blood supply of the adrenal glands comes from branches of the suprarenal arteries. The venous drainage includes a renal vein for each adrenal gland. Steroid hormones are all synthesized from the same initial first step,

the conversion of cholesterol to pregnenolone by cytochrome P450 enzymes.

Adrenal Cortex Physiology

Cortisol is released from the adrenal gland in a pulsatile fashion, following a circadian rhythm sensitive to light, sleep, stress, and disease, due to stimulation by ACTH from the anterior pituitary gland. Cortisol is mainly bound to a carrier called *transcortin;* some cortisol is also bound to albumin and a minimal amount of cortisol circulates unbound, which is the biologically active portion. Glucocorticoids such as cortisol have a multitude of actions such as protein breakdown and gluconeogenesis, fatty acid mobilization, and prevention of muscle protein synthesis (Table 30-4). The main effect of glucocorticoids is to increase serum glucose concentration. At high circulating levels, glucocorticoids cause catabolism and breakdown of lean body mass, including bone and muscle. They also affect the immune response by exerting an antiinflammatory effect.

Aldosterone is synthesized and released from the adrenal cortex zona glomerulosa, regulated not by the HPA axis but instead as a result of the renin-angiotensin-aldosterone system, which is responsible for maintaining salt and water homeostasis. When intravascular volume and renal perfusion are decreased, renin is released and through the angiotensin-converting enzyme (ACE), angiotensin II is released, which binds to a G protein–coupled receptor and stimulates aldosterone release. Aldosterone increases Na^+ and water absorption through the kidneys and K^+ is excreted. The other main stimulant for aldosterone release is K^+. Aldosterone helps maintain K^+ homeostasis and is responsible for preventing hyperkalemia by increasing K^+ excretion via the kidneys, gastrointestinal tract, diaphoresis, and salivation.

CUSHING SYNDROME

Glucocorticoid excess (Cushing syndrome) can occur for a number of reasons, including overproduction of cortisol by an adrenal mass, excessive stimulation of a normal adrenal gland to produce cortisol due to excessive ACTH production by the pituitary gland, or iatrogenic administration of glucocorticoids. Cushing syndrome manifests initially by a large increase in weight, usually central in the abdominal region.

Table 30-4. Glucocorticoid Effects

METABOLISM	HEMODYNAMIC	IMMUNE FUNCTION	CENTRAL NERVOUS SYSTEM
Muscle protein breakdown	Maintains vascular integrity	Increases antiinflammatory cytokines	Regulates perception and emotion
Increases nitrogen excretion	Maintains vascular reactivity	Decreases proinflammatory cytokines	Decreases corticotropin-releasing hormone
Increases gluconeogenesis	Maintains responsiveness to catecholamines	Decreases inflammation	Decreases adrenocorticotropic hormone release
Increases plasma glucose	Maintains fluid volume	Inhibits prostaglandin and leukotriene production	
Increases hepatic glycogen synthesis		Inhibits bradykinin and serotonin inflammatory effects	
Decreases glucose utilization		Decreases eosinophil, basophil, and lymphocyte counts	
Decreases amino acid utilization		Impairs cell-mediated immunity	
Increases fat mobilization		Increases neutrophil, platelet, and red blood cell counts	
Redistributes fat			

Patients also can appear to have moon facies and a buffalo hump of adipose tissue at the posterior cervical region. Other characteristics of Cushing syndrome include hypertension, glucose intolerance, change in menses for women (usually decreased or absent), decreased libido, spontaneous ecchymoses, muscle wasting and weakness, thin friable skin, and osteoporosis due to bone resorption.

Anesthetic considerations for patients with Cushing syndrome entail supporting the patient with the effects of glucocorticoid excess during the perioperative period. Some patients are obese with the attendant risks for difficult airway management and positioning. Osteoporosis presents risks during positioning of inadvertent bony fractures. Patients can have preexisting muscle weakness and be sensitive to the effects of neuromuscular blocking agents. Patients with Cushing syndrome tend to be hypervolemic with hypokalemic metabolic alkalosis. Many patients are on chronic diuretic therapy with potassium replacement.

GLUCOCORTICOID DEFICIENCY

Glucocorticoid deficiency (Addison disease) is less common and results from dysfunction of the adrenal gland (primary deficiency) or from lack of ACTH stimulation of adrenal glucocorticoid production (secondary deficiency). Clinical manifestations include weakness, fatigue, hypoglycemia, hypotension, and weight loss. Exogenous administration of glucocorticoids in the treatment of chronic medical conditions results in downregulation of corticotropin-releasing hormone and ACTH. Thus sudden withdrawal of exogenous glucocorticoids during a stressful period or critical illness can precipitate a medical emergency and addisonian crisis. Patients can experience circulatory collapse, fever, hypoglycemia, and mental obtundation as a result of the acute decrease in cortisol and the inability to secrete cortisol as a result of stress.

Anesthetic considerations for patients with glucocorticoid deficiency (whether chronic or acute) include steroid replacement therapy during the perioperative period, which represents a time of acute physiologic stress. If a patient has taken the equivalent dose of prednisone 20 mg for 5 days, their HPA axis can be suppressed and their adrenal glands might not be able to respond to physiologic stress by production of cortisol.[21,22] Exogenous glucocorticoid therapy for a 1-month period places patients at risk for HPA axis suppression for a year after the treatment is discontinued.[21,22] Thus "stress dose" steroids should be considered for these patients during the perioperative period. Historically, stress dose steroid therapy consisted of hydrocortisone 100 mg every 8 hours. This can precipitate hyperglycemia and decreased wound healing in some patients, thus a lower dose regimen might be considered: hydrocortisone 25 mg at induction of anesthesia, followed by a total of 100 mg of hydrocortisone over the next 24 hours.[15] This lower dose regimen decreases the risks of excessive steroid replacement and allows for plasma cortisol levels equal to that of healthy patients undergoing elective surgery. The initial bolus dose of hydrocortisone can be increased based on the urgency and complexity of the surgical procedure.[23]

HYPERALDOSTERONISM

Aldosterone excess can take several forms based on the pathophysiology. Primary hyperaldosteronism or Conn syndrome is due to adrenal oversecretion of aldosterone by benign adrenal tumors. Patients have hypertension due to Na^+ and water retention and hypokalemia due to K^+ excretion as well as muscle weakness and metabolic alkalosis. Secondary hyperaldosteronism usually results from another pathologic state, which reduces the effective circulating blood volume such as cirrhosis with ascites or congestive heart failure. This decrease in the effective circulating volume causes continuous stimulation of the renin-angiotensin-aldosterone system with overproduction of aldosterone.[24] Tertiary hyperaldosteronism, or Bartter syndrome, is a renal disorder that leads to increased renin release in order to compensate for excessive Na^+ loss. The excess renin causes excess production of angiotensin II and aldosterone. Anesthetic considerations include correction of fluid and electrolyte abnormalities preoperatively. Patients might be on a potassium-sparing diuretic such as spironolactone, which helps manage the hypokalemia and hypervolemia, and helps control hypertension.

HYPOALDOSTERONISM

Aldosterone deficiency also can take several forms. Primary hypoaldosteronism, or Addison disease, occurs as a result of destruction of the adrenal gland due to infection, injury, autoimmune problems, or genetic disorders. In Addison disease, renin activity is increased, which helps differentiate primary hypoaldosteronism from the other forms of deficiency. Clinical manifestations include hyponatremia, hypovolemia, hypotension, hyperkalemia, and metabolic acidosis. Secondary hypoaldosteronism results from decreased renin stimulation, usually from renal insufficiency, but the adrenal glands are normal. Anesthetic considerations include preoperative preparation with mineralocorticoid therapy such as fludrocortisone, which helps correct the hypovolemia and hyperkalemia.

ADRENAL MEDULLA PHYSIOLOGY

The adrenal medulla is the inner part of the adrenal gland and is highly vascular, made up of two types of chromaffin cells: those that produce epinephrine and those that produce norepinephrine. Catecholamines such as epinephrine and norepinephrine are made from the amino acid tyrosine through multiple enzymatic conversions: Tyrosine $\Rightarrow$ L-DOPA (L-3,4-dihydroxyphenylalanine) $\Rightarrow$ dopamine $\Rightarrow$ norepinephrine $\Rightarrow$ epinephrine.

The synthesis of catecholamines can be regulated by changes in the first enzymatic reaction of the pathway (tyrosine hydroxylase) such that the enzyme is inhibited acutely by increase in catecholamine production and chronically by an increase in tyrosine hydroxylase synthesis. Catecholamines are released in direct response to sympathetic nervous stimulation of the adrenal medulla. Acetylcholine released from the preganglionic sympathetic nerve terminals binds to nicotinic receptors in the chromaffin cells of the adrenal medulla. Depolarization of these cells leads to activation of Ca^{2+} channels. The influx of Ca^{2+} causes the vesicles containing the catecholamines to release their contents, including the catecholamines and other molecules such as chromogranins, ATP, and various peptides. Catecholamines have a very short half-life, on the order of just 10 seconds up to about 2 minutes, and undergo uptake at extraneuronal sites and degradation by catechol-O-methyltransferase (COMT) or monoamine

Table 30-5. Physiologic Effects of Adrenergic Stimulation

α-ADRENERGIC RECEPTOR STIMULATION	β-ADRENERGIC RECEPTOR STIMULATION
Vasoconstriction	Vasodilation
Intestinal relaxation	Intestinal relaxation
Bladder and intestinal sphincter contraction	Bladder wall relaxation
Pilomotor contraction	
Bronchoconstriction	Bronchodilation
Uterine smooth muscle contraction	Uterine relaxation
Increased cardiac contractility	Cardioacceleration, increased contractility
Hepatic glucose production	Glycogenolysis, lipolysis
Iris dilation	

oxidase (MAO). The degradation by COMT and MAO of norepinephrine and epinephrine, mostly in the liver, produces the metabolite vanillylmandelic acid (VMA), which is excreted in the urine and can be measured as an index of cumulative catecholamine secretion.

The physiologic effects of the catecholamines epinephrine and norepinephrine are mediated by G protein–coupled receptors found in many tissues (Table 30-5). α Adrenoreceptor activation causes activation of phospholipase C, which then activates protein kinase C via diacylglycerol. This causes an increase in intracellular Ca^{2+} and corresponding increase in smooth muscle contraction. β Adrenoceptor stimulation leads to increase in cyclic adenosine monophosphate (cAMP) and depending on which subtype of β receptor is stimulated, effects vary from increasing myocardial contractility, vasodilation, bronchial smooth muscle relaxation, and lipolysis. Catecholamines are secreted due to sympathetic stimulation and play a chief role in the stress response to perceived or real physical or psychologic injury, including hemorrhage, severe hypoglycemia, trauma, surgical trauma, and fear. The basic physiologic effects attributed to catecholamine secretion are mental arousal and alertness, pupillary dilation, diaphoresis, bronchial smooth muscle dilation, tachycardia, reduced activity of gastrointestinal tract, sphincter constriction, and uterine muscle relaxation. Catecholamines allow for the expenditure of energy in order to provide substrate for the stress. As such, glucose is mobilized from the liver through glycogen breakdown and fat breakdown.

Pheochromocytoma

Pheochromocytoma represents the most significant disease associated with adrenal medullary tissue. This tumor causes overproduction of catecholamines. Patients present with signs of excess catecholamine effects such as severe sustained or paroxysmal hypertension, headache, sweating, and palpitations. Most pheochromocytomas are benign and located unilaterally in an adrenal gland, but approximately 10% can be malignant and 10% can be bilateral/extraadrenal in origin.[25] Unrecognized pheochromocytoma can present intraoperatively due to sympathetic stimulation or surgical stimulation in the area of the undiagnosed tumor. Under general anesthesia the signs of undiagnosed pheochromocytoma include tachycardia and hypertension.

Preoperative evaluation and assessment should concentrate on treatment with α-adrenergic blockers and volume replacement. Arterial blood pressure, orthostatic blood pressure measurements, heart rate, and ECG are critical and might warrant further cardiovascular evaluation including echocardiography. At the time of diagnosis, patients with pheochromocytoma are usually hypovolemic with a normal to elevated hematocrit. Preoperative α-adrenergic blocker therapy with phenoxybenzamine or phentolamine helps correct the hypertension and vasoconstriction as well as reducing the intravascular volume deficit. A drop in hematocrit usually signals an appropriate level of α-blocking therapy. β-blocker therapy can be started after the α-blocker therapy has been started in order to help control heart rate and blood pressure.[26] There is a theoretical risk of unopposed α agonism and massive vasoconstriction if β-blocker therapy is starting before α antagonists.[15]

Management of resection of a pheochromocytoma mandates intraarterial blood pressure monitoring for immediate evaluation of rapid changes in blood pressure as well as targeting therapeutic interventions and laboratory analysis associated with hemorrhage and volume resuscitation. Central venous access may be helpful to allow infusion of vasoactive substances and large volumes of fluid and blood products if required. Induction should proceed in a careful, smooth fashion, with strict blood pressure control and a deep, adequate plane of anesthesia should be achieved before laryngoscopy and intubation in order to prevent the sympathetic activation due to inadequate anesthesia and intubation. Intraoperative hypertension can be treated with phentolamine, nitroprusside, or nicardipine. Phentolamine blocks α receptors, is relatively short acting, and prevents effects of catecholamines. Nitroprusside is easily titratable, with rapid onset and offset, but can result in cyanide accumulation with high doses. Potential anesthetic drugs to avoid include those that stimulate sympathetic nervous system activity or block parasympathetic activity such as ketamine, ephedrine, and pancuronium. After the tumor is resected with a decrease in the levels of catecholamines and residual antihypertensive therapies, hypotension can complicate the intraoperative and postoperative course, but in some patients hypertension continues to be problematic and requires treatment.[27] The hypotension is usually responsive to fluid resuscitation and adrenergic agonist therapy if necessary. Persistent hypertension is treated with antihypertensive medications as well as serial surveillance for recurrence of the pheochromocytoma.[27]

PANCREAS PHYSIOLOGY

The pancreas plays a key role in digestion, metabolism, utilization, and storage of energy substrate with exocrine and endocrine capacities. The pancreas is located in the retroperitoneal space, near the duodenum. Most of the mass of the pancreas is made up of exocrine cells, which secrete an alkaline digestive fluid into the pancreatic duct and duodenum. Making up 1% to 2% of the mass of the pancreas and within the pancreatic lobules there are small clusters of endocrine cells, the islets of Langerhans, which include α, β, and δ cells. The β cells make up about 75% of the total mass of the islets and secrete insulin. Eighteen percent to 20% of endocrine cells are α cells, which secrete glucagon, and the remaining

5% are δ cells, which secrete somatostatin. The arterial blood supply to the pancreas consists of branches from the splenic artery and the superior and inferior pancreaticoduodenal arteries. The islets receive 10% to 15% of the pancreatic blood flow, thus their rich vascularization allows easy access for the hormones to be secreted by the islet cells into the bloodstream. Venous drainage is directly to the portal vein of the liver, thus the liver performs first-pass metabolism on the pancreatic hormones before their release into the systemic circulation.

Insulin synthesis begins with an inactive protein, preproinsulin, which undergoes cleavage to proinsulin and then to insulin by cleavage of the C-peptide linkage structure. Insulin is thus made up of two amino acid peptides, α and β linked by a disulfide bond. The insulin and C peptide make up secretory granules that are stored in β cells and released in response to increased blood glucose. Glucose enters β cells via the GLUT-2 receptor, where it is used to generate ATP. ATP causes closure of the ATP-sensitive K^+ channels, membrane depolarization, and Ca^+ influx, which then triggers exocytosis of insulin secretory granules into the circulation. Overall, insulin has an anabolic effect on target organs and increases the synthesis of carbohydrates, fats, and proteins (Table 30-6).

Glucose transporters play a key role in the utilization of glucose mediated by insulin. There are several glucose transporters with variable tissue distributions and functions.[28] GLUT-1 transporters are found in most tissues but with high concentrations in human red blood cells and in the blood vessels of the brain; GLUT-1 assists with glucose uptake by skeletal muscle and fat under basal conditions. GLUT-2 transporters are low-affinity transporters, found in pancreatic β cells, the liver, intestine, and kidney; GLUT-2 assures that glucose uptake by β cells and hepatic cells occurs only when circulating glucose concentrations are elevated. GLUT-3 transporters are found in neurons; GLUT-1 and GLUT-3 allow glucose to cross the blood-brain barrier and gain access to the brain. GLUT-4 transporters are found in striated muscle and fat, and within storage vesicles inside the cell; GLUT-4 mediates insulin-stimulated glucose transport into fat and muscle cells. GLUT-5 transporters are found in spermatozoa and the small intestine, and primarily transport fructose.

Glucagon is an amino acid polypeptide hormone secreted by the α-cells of the islets of Langerhans and plays a vital role in glucose homeostasis by antagonizing the effects of insulin. Glucagon release is inhibited by increased blood glucose levels and somatostatin and stimulated by hypoglycemia, high amino acid levels after amino acid–rich food intake, epinephrine, and vagal stimulation. The primary target tissues for the effects of glucagon are the liver and adipose tissue sites. The main effect of glucagon is to increase serum glucose concentration by causing hepatic gluconeogenesis and glycogen breakdown. The effects of glucagon on adipose tissue primarily occur during periods of stress and food deprivation.

Diabetes Mellitus

DM results from impaired secretion of insulin from the pancreas and/or reduced tissue sensitivity. Type 1 DM has been referred to as insulin-dependent DM due to the destruction of the β cells in the pancreas, thus necessitating administration of exogenous insulin to avoid diabetic ketoacidosis. It is associated with onset in younger age patients and makes up 2% to 5% of cases of DM. Type 2 DM is more frequent and results from loss of normal regulation of insulin secretion from the pancreas and insulin sensitivity. It is associated with adult onset, obesity, mild levels of hyperglycemia, and insulin resistance. The mean normal blood glucose is about 72 mg/dL (4 mM). The diagnosis of diabetes is made when fasting serum glucose is greater than 126 mg/dL (7 mM) or at random glucose levels greater than 200 mg/dL (11 mM) with associated symptoms of DM such as polyuria, polydipsia, and polyphagia. With DM there is impaired insulin released such that glucose cannot be taken up by the cells as energy substrate and thus glucose levels are elevated. Increased glucose concentrations cause elevated plasma osmolarity and glycosuria, accompanied by water and Na^+ loss in the urine (polyuria). Patients become very dehydrated and thirst (polydipsia) as well as hunger (polyphagia) are compensatory mechanisms in that the cells are starving because they are unable to utilize glucose.

Diabetic ketoacidosis (DKA) can occur perioperatively; it is an acute event that anesthesiologists must understand and for which they must be vigilant. DKA is characterized by elevated blood glucose, ketone body formation (in the forms of acetoacetate and β-hydroxybutyrate), and anion gap metabolic acidosis that result from decreased availability of insulin and elevated levels of the counterregulatory hormones glucagon, catecholamines, cortisol, and growth hormone. Lactic acidosis can coexist with the anion gap metabolic acidosis with DKA. DKA can be precipitated by infection, stress, surgery, inadequate doses of exogenous insulin, and untreated DM. Patients manifest tachypnea, severe abdominal pain, nausea, and vomiting as well as altered mental status. Treatment of DKA involves aggressive fluid volume resuscitation, insulin to treat the hyperglycemia, and replacement of K^+ deficit. Patients with DKA require intensive care and frequent laboratory analysis for glucose, K^+, serum ketones, and acid-base status.

There are three main defects involved in type 2 DM. First, there is inadequate response of the β cells of the pancreas to

Table 30-6. Effects of Insulin

	GLUCOSE TRANSPORT INTO FAT AND MUSCLE	GLYCOGEN BREAKDOWN IN MUSCLE AND LIVER
Carbohydrate metabolism	Glycolysis in fat and muscle	Glycogenolysis and gluconeogenesis in liver
	Glycogen synthesis in fat, muscle, and liver	
Lipid metabolism	Fatty acid synthesis	Lipolysis in fat (causes decreased plasma fatty acids)
	Uptake of triglycerides from circulation into fat and muscle	Fatty acid oxidation in muscle and liver
	Cholesterol synthesis in liver	Ketogenesis
Protein metabolism	Amino acid transport into tissues	Protein breakdown in muscle
	Protein synthesis in muscle, fat, and liver	Urea formation

glucose loads, such that at basal conditions patients produce and secrete insulin but with meals or serum glucose elevation there is much less secretion of insulin than in normal patients. Second, type 2 DM patients also have a decreased response of peripheral tissues to the actions of insulin. Third, patients with type 2 DM have increased hepatic glucose production.[29] These impairments contribute to an overall higher fasting glucose level. Approximately 80% of patients with type 2 DM are considered obese and have a sedentary lifestyle, both of which are well-known risk factors.[30,31]

Anesthetic considerations for patients with diabetes include a thorough preoperative evaluation to determine whether the patient requires insulin and to determine end organ damage. Hemoglobin A_{1C} levels are helpful in preoperative evaluation for identifying patients at risk for perioperative hyperglycemia and further complications. Hemoglobin A_{1C} levels less than 6% are considered normal (with good glycemic control); those patients with levels greater than 8% are considered to have poorly controlled DM and often have postoperative complications.[32,33] Patients with diabetes are at high risk for cardiovascular complications including myocardial ischemia and infarction, thus a preoperative ECG should be obtained. Diabetic autonomic dysfunction has many implications for the patient undergoing surgery and anesthesia. It limits the ability of the myocardium to compensate for changes in volume status such as reduced preload as well as predisposing patients to cardiovascular instability, hypotension, and sudden cardiac death. Delayed gastric emptying and risk for aspiration can also be attributed to autonomic dysfunction and the attendant gastroparesis. Longstanding DM also places patients at risk for renal dysfunction and failure, so evidence of these end-organ complications should be sought. Patients with DM have decreased immune system function and microvascular disease, and are thus at risk for infections and delayed or impaired wound healing.

The intraoperative care of the patient with diabetes focuses on control of blood glucose. There has been much controversy surrounding what level of glucose should be targeted for patients with diabetes undergoing surgery. Hyperglycemia in surgical patients is a common problem in the perioperative period for patients with and without known DM. There are many reasons postulated for this hyperglycemia including poorly controlled DM preoperatively, insulin resistance, increased inflammatory response associated with surgical trauma, increased stress response characterized by increased secretion of counterregulatory hormones, and requirement for catecholamine-based vasopressors such as epinephrine.[15,34,35] The effects of these changes lead to increased gluconeogenesis, glycogenolysis, and insulin resistance in the periphery.

Multiple studies have illustrated the importance of good glycemic control in surgical patients. The Portland Diabetes Project demonstrated the connection between hyperglycemia in the perioperative period and increased morbidity in the form of increased infections and deep sternal wound infections as well as increased mortality.[36,37] In addition, intensive insulin therapy to control serum glucose to levels less than 110 mg/dL (6.1 mM) in the intensive care unit population was shown to significantly reduce morbidity and mortality.[38] However, concerns over tight glycemic control have surfaced as a result of studies showing that intensive glucose control intraoperatively led to an increased incidence of stroke and death.[39]

Thus there is no one generalizable glucose goal that one can point to for patients with DM having surgery and anesthesia. One approach is to learn as much about each patient's glycemic control before surgery. If a patient has a hemoglobin A_{1C} of 9%, there is likely very poor control and as such rapidly controlling that patient's blood glucose to a narrow strict or "low" target range could lead to complications such as severe hypoglycemia and even stroke or death. Instead a patient whose DM is poorly controlled can be treated in a moderate fashion, aiming to reduce the blood glucose slowly over time to less than 200 mg/dL (11 mM) intraoperatively via an insulin infusion. Insulin infusions are more physiologic, rapidly titratable, and easier to control than intravenous insulin boluses.[40] Currently, there is a paucity of evidence-based data to demonstrate that strict glucose control is superior to more moderate control intraoperatively. Refer to several other sources on blood glucose management.[15,16,41]

KEY POINTS

- The most important hormones produced by the anterior pituitary include ACTH, TSH, GH, PRL, and the two gonadotropins, LH and FSH.
- The balance of releasing factors secreted by hypothalamus and inhibiting factors secreted by each hormone's target organ control the secretion of each hormone produced by the anterior pituitary.
- Cardiac disease, hypertension, and ventricular hypertrophy are the most important causes of morbidity and mortality in acromegalic patients.
- ADH, produced by the posterior pituitary gland in response to a very mild increase in osmolarity, binds to vasopressin receptors on the renal collecting ducts and causes an increase in water reabsorption.
- The end result of the interactions PTH, calcium, vitamin D, and calcitonin is to maintain normal plasma calcium concentration, which in turn helps maintain normal cellular function, nerve transmission, membrane stability, bone integrity, coagulation, and intracellular signaling.
- Thyroid hormones play a major role in normal growth and development, controlling the rate of metabolism and many body functions.
- Glucocorticoids such as cortisol have a multitude of actions such as protein breakdown and gluconeogenesis, fatty acid mobilization, and prevention of muscle protein synthesis.
- Catecholamines, such as epinephrine and norepinephrine, are produced by the adrenal medulla and secreted due to sympathetic stimulation and play a chief role in the stress response to perceived or real physical or psychologic injury, including hemorrhage, severe hypoglycemia, trauma, surgical trauma, and fear.
- Insulin, secreted by the β cells of the pancreas, has an anabolic effect on target organs and causes the synthesis of carbohydrates, fats, and proteins.
- Type 2 diabetes mellitus involves three main defects in glucose and insulin metabolism: inadequate response of the pancreatic β cells to glucose, decreased response of the peripheral tissues to effects of insulin, and increased hepatic glucose production.

Key References

Gandhi GY, Nuttall GA, Abel MD, et al. Intensive intraoperative insulin therapy versus conventional glucose management during cardiac surgery. *Ann Intern Med.* 2007;146:233-243. This study called into question the safety of the adoption of strict glucose control for all patients, in that it showed an increased incidence of death and stroke in patients having cardiac surgery managed with intensive glucose control (serum glucose <110 mg/dL). (Ref. 39)

Henzen C, Suter A, Lerch E, et al. Suppression and recovery of adrenal response after short-term, high-dose glucocorticoid treatment. *Lancet.* 2000;355:542-545. Acute and chronic treatment with glucocorticoid therapy and adrenal gland suppression often become concerns for anesthesiologists in the perioperative period. This study reported the recovery of adrenal function after short-term high-dose glucocorticoid treatment and use of the low-dose corticotropin test for evaluation of adrenal recovery. (Ref. 21)

Mihai R, Farndon JR. Parathyroid disease and calcium metabolism. *Br J Anaesth.* 2000;85:29-43. This well-written manuscript provides a thorough review of parathyroid anatomy, calcium homeostasis, and parathyroid hormone regulation, as well as the various classifications of hyperparathyroidism including treatment options and anesthetic considerations for parathyroid surgery. (Ref. 8)

Nemergut EC, Dumont AS, Barry UT, et al. Perioperative management of patients undergoing transsphenoidal pituitary surgery. *Anesth Analg.* 2005;101:1170-1181. This review gives attention to a variety of conditions including Cushing disease, acromegaly, and hyperthyroidism and the implications of transsphenoidal surgery to resect pituitary masses. (Ref. 2)

Van Den Berghe G, Wouters P, Weekers F, et al. Intensive insulin therapy in critically ill patients. *N Engl J Med.* 2001;345:1359-1367. This landmark study in 2000 showed a significant reduction in morbidity and mortality with strict glucose control (blood glucose <110 mg/dL) in surgical intensive care unit patients. (Ref. 38)

References

1. Burrow GN, Wortzman G, Rewcastle NB, et al. Microadenomas of the pituitary and abnormal sellar tomograms in an unselected autopsy series. *N Engl J Med.* 1981;304:156-158.
2. Nemergut EC, Dumont AS, Barry UT, et al. Perioperative management of patients undergoing transsphenoidal pituitary surgery. *Anesth Analg.* 2005;101:1170-1181.
3. Singer PA, Sevilla LJ. Postoperative endocrine management of pituitary tumors. *Neurosurg Clin N Am.* 2003;14:123-138.
4. Guilleminault C, van den Hoed J. Acromegaly and narcolepsy. *Lancet.* 1979;2:750-751.
5. Nemergut EC, Zuo Z. Airway management in pituitary disease: a review of 746 patients. *J Neurosurg Anesth.* 2006;18:73-77.
6. Nemergut EC, Zuo Z, Jane JA Jr, et al. Predictors of diabetes insipidus after transphenoidal surgery: a review of 881 patients. *J Neurosurg.* 2005;103:448-454.
7. Bringhurst FB, Demay MB, Kronenberg HM. Hormones and disorders of mineral metabolism. In: Kronenberg HM, ed. *Williams Textbook of Endocrinology.* 11th ed. Philadelphia: Saunders; 2008:1203-1268.
8. Mihai R, Farndon, JR. Parathyroid disease and calcium metabolism. *Br J Anaesth.* 2000;85:29-43.
9. Molina PE: Parathyroid gland & Ca^{2+} & PO_4^- regulation. In: Molina PE, ed. *Endocrine Physiology.* 3rd ed. Available at: http://www.accessmedicine.com/content.aspx?aID=6169587.
10. Edwards R. Thyroid and parathyroid disease. *Int Anesthesiol Clin.* 1997;35:63-83.
11. Thakker RV. Mutliple endocrine neoplasia type 1. *Best Pract Res Clin Endocrinol Metab.* 2010;24:355-370.
12. Wohllk N, Schweizer H, Erlic Z, et al. Multiple endocrine neoplasia type 2. *Best Pract Res Clin Endocrinol Metab.* 2010;24:371-387.
13. Leung AM, Pearce EN, Braverman LE. Perchlorate, iodine, and the thyroid. *Best Pract Res Clin Endocrinol Metab.* 2010;24:133-141.
14. Molina PE. Thyroid gland. In: Molina PE, ed. *Endocrine Physiology.* 3rd ed. http://www.accessmedicine.com/content.aspx?aID=6169456.
15. Kohl BA, Schwartz S. How to manage perioperative endocrine insufficiency. *Anesthesiol Clin.* 2010;28:139-155.
16. Mercado DL, Petty BG. Perioperative medication management. *Med Clin N Am.* 2003;87:41-57.
17. Bennett-Guerrero E, Kramer DC, Schwinn DA. Effect of chronic and acute thyroid hormone reduction on perioperative outcome. *Anesth Analg.* 1997;85:30-36.
18. Farling PA. Thyroid disease. *Br J Anaesth.* 2000;85:15-28.
19. Graham GW, Unger BP, Coursin DB. Perioperative management of selected endocrine disorders. *Int Anesthesiol Clin.* 2000;38:31-67.
20. Weinberg AD, Brennan MD, Gorman CA, et al. Outcome of anesthesia and surgery in hypothyroid patients. *Arch Int Med.* 1983;143:893-897.
21. Henzen C, Suter A, Lerch E, et al. Suppression and recovery of adrenal response after short-term, high-dose glucocorticoid treatment. *Lancet.* 2000;355:542-545.
22. Hopkins RL, Leinung MC. Exogenous Cushing's syndrome and glucocorticoid withdrawal. *Endocrinol Met Clin N Am.* 2005;34:371-384.
23. Kohl BA, Schwartz S. Surgery in the patient with endocrine dysfunction. *Anesthesiol Clin.* 2009;27:687-703.
24. Molina PE. Adrenal gland. In: Molina PE, ed. *Endocrine Physiology.* 3rd ed. Available at: http://www.accessmedicine.com/content.aspx?aID=6169718.
25. Lenders JW, Eisenhofer G, Mannelli M, et al. Phaeochromocytoma. *Lancet.* 2005;366:665-675.
26. Roizen MF, Schreider BD, Hassan SZ. Anesthesia for patients with pheochromocytoma. *Anesthesiol Clin N Am.* 1987;5:269-275.
27. Plouin P-F, Amar L, Lepoutre C. Phaeochromocytomas and functional paragangliomas: clinical management. *Best Pract Res Clin Endocrinol Met.* 2010;24:933-941.
28. Shepherd PR, Kahn BB. Glucose transporters and insulin action—implications for insulin resistance and diabetes mellitus. *N Engl J Med.* 1999;341:248-257.
29. Lin Y, Sun Z. Current views on type 2 diabetes. *J Endocrinol.* 2010;204:1-11.
30. Venables MC, Jeukendrup AE. Physical inactivity and obesity: links with insulin resistance and type 2 diabetes mellitus. *Int J Exp Diabetes Res.* 2009;25:S18-S23.
31. Weinstein AR, Sesso HD, Lee IM, et al. Relationship of physical activity vs body mass index with type 2 diabetes in women. *J Am Med Assoc.* 2004;292:1188-1194.
32. Nathan DM, Singer DE, Hurxthal K, et al. The clinical information value of the glycosylated hemoglobin assay. *N Engl J Med.* 1984;310:341-346.
33. Umpierrez GE, Isaacs SD, Bazargan N, et al. Hyperglycemia: an independent marker of in-hospital mortality in patients with undiagnosed diabetes. *J Clin Endocrinol Metab.* 2002;87:978-982.
34. Friedberg SJ, Lam YW, Blum JJ, et al. Insulin absorption: a major factor in apparent insulin resistance and the control of type 2 diabetes mellitus. *Metab Clin Exp.* 2006;55(5):614-619.
35. Furnary AP. Clinical benefits of tight glycaemic control: focus on the perioperative setting. *Best Pract Res Clin Anaesthesiol.* 2009;23(4):411-420.
36. Zerr KJ, Furnary AP, Grunkemeier GL, et al. Glucose control lowers the risk of wound infection in diabetics after open heart operations. *Ann Thorac Surg.* 1997;63(2):356-361.
37. Furnary AP, Zerr KJ, Grunkmeier GL, et al. Continuous intravenous insulin infusion reduces the incidence of deep sternal wound infection in diabetic patients after cardiac surgical procedures. *Ann Thorac Surg.* 1999;67(2):352-360.
38. Van Den Berghe G, Wouters P, Weekers F, et al. Intensive insulin therapy in critically ill patients. *N Engl J Med.* 2001, 345(19):1359-1367.
39. Gandhi GY, Nuttall GA, Abel MD, et al. Intensive intraoperative insulin therapy versus conventional glucose management during cardiac surgery. *Ann Int Med.* 2007, 146:233-243.
40. Fleisher, LA, Beckman JA, Brown KA, et al. ACC/AHA 2007 guidelines on perioperative cardiovascular evaluation and care for noncardiac surgery: a report of the American College of Cardiology/American Heart Association Task Force on Practice Guidelines. *Circulation.* 2007;116:e418-499.
41. Garber AJ, Moghissi ES, Bransome ED Jr, et al. American College of Endocrinology position statement on inpatient diabetes and metabolic control. *Endocrinol Pract.* 2004;10(Suppl 2):4-9.

ENDOCRINE PHARMACOLOGY

Mark T. Keegan

Dysfunction of the complex physiologic processes of the endocrine systems can lead to significant and potentially life-threatening problems. Administration of exogenous hormones or drugs that mimic or antagonize hormonal effects to manipulate the metabolic milieu is important in many therapies. Endocrine pharmacotherapeutics range from simple supplementation of a missing hormone, such as insulin in the case of patients with type 1 diabetes mellitus (DM), to careful manipulation of physiologic processes with advanced pharmaceuticals in the case of assisted reproduction techniques. Many of these agents have implications for the practice of anesthesia, critical care, and pain. Historical perspectives are highlighted below with the discussion of individual drug classes.

DRUGS TO TREAT DISORDERS OF THE ENDOCRINE PANCREAS

Insulin

The discovery of insulin by Banting and Best represents a major milestone in modern medicine.[1] Within a few years of its discovery insulin had been purified and crystallized. Its amino acid sequence was established by Sanger in 1960. The protein was synthesized in 1963 and its three-dimensional structure elucidated in 1972. The first biosynthetic human insulin was approved by the U.S. Food and Drug Administration (FDA) in 1982.[2]

BASIC PHARMACOLOGY
Insulin is synthesized in β cells of the pancreatic islets of Langerhans. Pre-proinsulin (a single-chain 110 amino acid precursor) is initially formed. Subsequently the N-terminal 24 amino acid peptide is cleaved to form proinsulin. Removal of four basic amino acids and a connecting (C) peptide gives rise to insulin itself. The insulin molecule contains A and B peptide chains, usually composed of 21 and 30 amino acid residues, respectively. In most species a single insulin gene gives rise to a single protein product.

When pancreatic β cells are stimulated, insulin and C-peptide are released into the circulation in equimolar amounts. Therefore functional activity of pancreatic β cells is reflected by plasma C-peptide concentrations. It is also possible to differentiate endogenous from exogenous insulin by evaluating plasma C-peptide content. Human insulin, made by recombinant DNA techniques, is used exclusively in the United States. "Purified" insulin contains less than 10 ppm of proinsulin. Refrigeration is recommended but is not crucial.

Insulin is a member of a family of peptides known as *insulin-like growth factors* (IGFs). IGFs are produced in many tissues and regulate cellular growth and metabolism. Specific insulin receptors in the plasma membrane are similar to IGF receptors. The insulin receptor is a large transmembrane glycoprotein that mediates its actions through intracellular tyrosine kinase activity. Insulin binding leads to autophosphorylation of intracellular insulin receptor sites causing recruitment of numerous enzymes and mediating molecules that are activated or inactivated, leading to a myriad of intracellular events. Importantly, GLUT-4 transporters are translocated to the plasma membrane where they facilitate diffusion of glucose into cells. Other signals activate glycogen synthase, stimulate uptake of amino acids and protein synthesis, and regulate gene expression (see Chapter 30 for more information on the physiology of insulin). Insulin's hypoglycemic actions on liver, muscle, and adipose tissue are most important (Table 31-1).

When injected intravenously, insulin has a plasma half-life of 5 to 6 minutes. It is degraded in liver, kidney, and muscle. When renal function is severely impaired, insulin requirements decrease because of reduced breakdown. Liver metabolism of insulin operates at near maximal capacity and cannot compensate for loss of renal function. Although insulin is cleared relatively quickly from the circulation, its biologic effects persist for 30 to 60 minutes because it binds tightly to insulin receptors. Subcutaneous injection of insulin leads to slow release into the circulation and a sustained pharmacologic effect.

CLINICAL PHARMACOLOGY

Insulin is most commonly administered subcutaneously, but it can also be administered intravenously. In contrast to physiologic secretion of insulin, subcutaneous administration delivers insulin to the peripheral tissues rather than the portal system and the pharmacokinetics do not reproduce a normal rise and fall associated with ingestion of nutrients. Nonetheless, insulin treatment is lifesaving for patients with DM.

Insulin preparations are characterized by their duration of action or their species of origin. This latter classification is less relevant now due to the wide availability of synthetic human preparations. For historical reasons, doses and concentrations of insulin are expressed in units. In the past, preparations of the hormone were impure and were standardized by bioassay. One unit of insulin is equal to the amount of insulin required to reduce blood glucose concentration in a fasting rabbit to 45 mg/dL (2.5 mM). Insulin is supplied in solution or suspension at a concentration of 100 units/mL. Typically, a patient with type 1 DM requires between 20 and 60 units of exogenously administered insulin per day. Higher concentration insulin preparations are available for patients who are resistant to insulin. Table 31-2 details currently available insulin preparations and Figure 31-1 shows typical pharmacokinetic profiles of insulin and insulin analogues following subcutaneous administration.

Table 31-1. Hypoglycemic Actions of Insulin

LIVER	MUSCLE	ADIPOSE TISSUE
Inhibits hepatic glucose production (decreases gluconeogenesis and glycogenolysis)	Stimulates glucose uptake	Stimulates glucose uptake (amount is small compared to muscle)
Stimulates hepatic glucose uptake	Inhibits flow of gluconeogenic precursors to the liver (e.g., alanine, lactate, pyruvate)	Inhibits flow of gluconeogenic precursors to liver (glycerol) and reduces energy substrate for hepatic gluconeogenesis (nonesterified fatty acids)

Modified from Table 60.2 of Brunton LL, ed. *Goodman and Gilman's The Pharmacologic Basis of Therapeutics.* 11th ed. New York, NY: McGraw Hill; 2006.

Table 31-2. Insulin Preparations

PREPARATION		ONSET (HOURS)	PEAK (HOURS)	EFFECTIVE DURATION (HOURS)
Short-acting				
	Aspart	<0.25	0.5-1.5	3-4
	Glulisine	<0.25	0.5-1.5	3-4
	Lispro	<0.25	0.5-1.5	3-4
	Regular	0.5-1.0	2-3	4-6
Intermediate-acting				
	NPH	1-4	6-10	10-16
Long-acting				
	Detemir	1-4	—*	20-24
	Glargine	1-4	—*	20-24
Insulin combinations				
	75/25-75% protamine lispro, 25% lispro	<0.25	1.5	Up to 10-16
	70/30-70% protamine aspart, 30% aspart	<0.25	1.5	Up to 10-16
	50/50-50% protamine lispro, 50% lispro	<0.25	1.5	Up to 10-16
	70/30-70% NPH, 30% regular	0.5-1	Dual†	10-16

*Glargine and detemir have minimal peak activity.
†Dual: two peaks, one at 2 to 3 hours; the second one several hours later.
Copyright 2004 American Diabetes Association. Adapted with permission from Skyler JS. Insulin treatment. In: Lebovitz HE, ed. *Therapy for Diabetes Mellitus.* Alexandria, Va: American Diabetes Association; 2004.

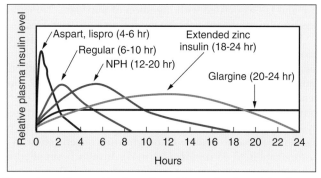

Figure 31-1 Pharmacokinetic profiles of human insulin and insulin analogues. The approximate relative duration of action of the various forms of insulin is shown. Duration varies widely both between and within individuals. *(From Hirsch IB. Insulin analogues. N Engl J Med. 2005;352:174-183.)*

Insulin is among the drugs that the Institute for Safe Medication Practices has highlighted as having an increased risk for patient harm when used in error. The administration of insulin is prone to error because of the variety of preparations used and the difficulty associated with administration of a small number of units.

Hypoglycemia is the most common adverse reaction associated with insulin administration. It can occur due to administration of an inappropriately large dose of insulin, when peak insulin effect does not coincide with carbohydrate intake, or due to superimposed factors such as exercise. Patients in the perioperative period are especially vulnerable to the development of hypoglycemia because of interruption of oral intake and alterations in insulin dosing regimens. The incidence of hypoglycemia increases when "tighter" glycemic control goals are adopted. Symptoms and signs of hypoglycemia include tachycardia, diaphoresis, tremor, palpitations, anxiety, and hunger. These can be absent during anesthesia. Neuroglycopenia can cause dizziness, blurred vision, and loss of consciousness, potentially progressing to coma, seizures, and even death. Lipodystrophy can occur at the sites of subcutaneous insulin injection, leading to alterations in subcutaneous fat. Lipoatrophy is probably secondary to an immune response to insulin. Enlargement of subcutaneous fat deposits (lipohypertrophy) can also occur and is thought to be due to the lipogenic action of insulin. Allergic reactions to insulin were more common before the use of recombinant human insulin or highly purified insulin preparations, although such reactions still occur. Local reactions cause erythema and induration, and are usually IgE mediated. Systemic reactions are less frequent and are usually IgG antibody mediated. Prolonged use of NPH (neutral protamine Hagedorn) insulin can lead to protamine sensitization that can manifest when a large dose of protamine is administered, as in the setting of cardiopulmonary bypass. Doses of subcutaneous insulin of more than 100 units per day can indicate insulin resistance, which can be due to antiinsulin antibodies or target cell receptor dysfunction. As with allergic reactions, the incidence of insulin resistance due to antibodies is decreasing with use of recombinant and highly purified preparations.

As detailed in Chapters 13 and 30, a number of hormones antagonize the effects of insulin. These include epinephrine, which inhibits the secretion of insulin and stimulates glycogenolysis, and adrenocorticotrophic hormone (ACTH), glucagon, and estrogens, which tend to cause hyperglycemia. Certain drugs (e.g., tetracycline, salicylates) can increase the duration of action of insulin.

INDIVIDUAL INSULIN PREPARATIONS

Regular Insulin
Regular insulin is a crystalline zinc insulin preparation, the effect of which appears within 30 minutes of subcutaneous injection. Regular insulin should be injected subcutaneously 30 to 45 minutes before meals. This causes the blood glucose to fall rapidly, reaching a nadir in 20 to 30 minutes.

Rapidly Acting Insulin Analogues
Regular insulin monomers form hexamers in currently available insulin preparations. The hexameric form delays absorption and onset of action. Insulin analogues have been developed that maintain a monomeric or dimeric configuration, increasing their speed of absorption and reducing time to onset to 5 to 15 minutes. They are identical to human insulin except for substitutions of amino acids at one or two positions. Such rapidly acting insulin preparations include insulin lispro, insulin aspart, and insulin glulisine. The use of insulin lispro rather than regular insulin can decrease the incidence of hypoglycemia and improve glycemic control. In clinical trials, insulin aspart has similar effects to insulin lispro on hypoglycemia frequency and glycemic control and causes less nocturnal hypoglycemia than regular insulin.[3] Insulin glulisine has similar properties.

Intermediate-Acting Insulin
Intermediate-acting insulins are designed to dissolve gradually when administered subcutaneously. NPH (or isophane) insulin is a soluble crystalline zinc insulin combined with protamine zinc insulin. Lente insulin is a mixture of crystallized (ultralente) and amorphous (semilente) insulins in an acetate buffer. Their onset of action is delayed to 2 to 4 hours with a peak response at 8 to 10 hours; duration of action is less than 24 hours.

Long-Acting Insulins
Ultralente insulin (an extended insulin zinc suspension) has a slower onset of action and a prolonged peak effect. It provides a low basal concentration of insulin throughout the day and is often used in combination with other insulin preparations. The desire for insulin preparations without peak effects prompted the development of long-acting insulin analogues including insulin glargine and insulin detemir. They lack a peak effect and have durations of action of 17 to 24 hours. Insulin glargine is produced by the addition of two arginine residues to the C-terminus of the insulin B chain and replacement of a single asparagine residue with a glycine in the A chain. The resulting insulin forms a solution with a pH of 4. The low pH stabilizes the hexamer and delays absorption but also means that glargine cannot be mixed with short-acting insulin preparations that are at neutral pH. Another long-acting preparation, insulin detemir, is synthesized by the addition of a saturated fatty acid to the lysine at position B29 in human insulin.

Inhaled Insulin
Inhaled insulin is a rapidly acting preparation that can be useful for patients with needle phobias and significant

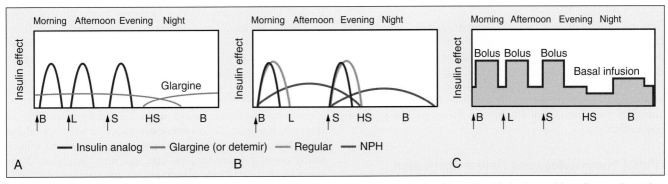

Figure 31-2 Commonly used insulin regimens. **A,** Administration of a long-acting insulin-like glargine (detemir could also be used but often requires twice-daily administration) to provide basal insulin and a short-acting insulin analogue before meals. **B,** A less intensive insulin regimen with twice-daily injection of NPH insulin providing basal insulin and regular insulin or an insulin analogue providing mealtime insulin coverage. Only one type of shorting-acting insulin would be used. **C,** The insulin level attained following subcutaneous insulin (short-acting insulin analogue) by an insulin pump programmed to deliver different basal rates. At each meal, an insulin bolus is delivered. *B,* Breakfast; *HS,* bedtime; *S,* supper. Upward arrow shows insulin administration at meal-time. *(Copyright 2008 American Diabetes Association. From Kaufman FR, ed.* Medical Management of Type 1 Diabetes. *5th ed. Modified with permission from the American Diabetes Association.)*

lipodystrophy.[4] It was approved by the FDA for preprandial, but not basal, use. Inhaled insulin is contraindicated in smokers because of the theoretical risk of promoting lung cancer formation by the growth stimulating effects of insulin.

CLINICAL APPLICATION

Subcutaneously administered insulin is the primary therapy for patients with type 1 DM and for many patients with type 2 DM. The American Diabetes Association recommends the following goals of therapy[5]:

- HbA1c (hemoglobin A1c) < 7%
- Preprandial capillary glucose 70 to 130 mg/dL (3.9-7.2 mM)
- Peak postprandial plasma glucose <180 mg/dL (10 mM)

A variety of insulin dosing regimens can be used to achieve these glycemic targets depending on multiple factors including age, compliance, frequency of significant hypoglycemia and hyperglycemia, and associated medical conditions. Figure 31-2 illustrates three potential regimens. Although the route is not FDA approved, regular insulin is often administered intravenously during the perioperative period, during labor and delivery, for the treatment of diabetic ketoacidosis, and as an infusion in the intensive care unit (ICU). The rapidly acting insulin analogues can be injected immediately before or after a meal, allowing for smoother glycemic control because the insulin dose can be titrated to the amount of food actually consumed. In addition, the rapidly acting insulin preparations are commonly used in insulin pumps. Intermediate-acting insulins are usually given once daily (often before breakfast) or twice daily. Long-acting insulin glargine can be administered at any time during the day, has a sustained absorption profile without a peak, and provides better once-daily glycemic control with less hypoglycemia than NPH or ultralente. It is sometimes combined with oral hypoglycemic agents (see later) in patients with type 2 DM. Insulin detemir is administered subcutaneously once or twice daily, and delivers glycemic control that is smoother and safer than NPH insulin.

ORAL HYPOGLYCEMIC AGENTS: SULFONYLUREAS, BIGUANIDES, THIAZOLIDINEDIONES

In the 1940s it was discovered that some sulfonamide antibiotics cause hypoglycemia. Subsequently, more than 20 members of the related sulfonylureas have been developed and used as oral hypoglycemic agents (OHAs). Other major classes of OHAs include the biguanides, the thiazolidinediones, the α-glucosidase inhibitors, and the meglitinides. OHAs are used in patients with type 2 DM.

Basic Pharmacology

SULFONYLUREAS

There are two generations of sulfonylurea drugs based on an arylsulfonylurea backbone, to which substitutions at the para position on the benzene ring and at a nitrogen residue in the urea moiety are made. First-generation agents include tolbutamide, chlorpropamide, tolazamide, and acetohexamide. Second-generation sulfonylureas are more potent and include glyburide, gliclazide, glipizide, and glimepiride. They act by increasing insulin secretion by stimulating pancreatic β cells. Sulfonylureas inhibit adenosine triphosphate (ATP)-dependent K$^+$ (K$_{ATP}$) channels in the β cells, causing Ca^{2+} entry and release of insulin storage granules. They can also decrease hepatic clearance of insulin and have other minor extrapancreatic effects.

BIGUANIDES

The biguanides reduce serum glucose by decreasing hepatic glucose output (presumably by decreasing gluconeogenesis) and by sensitizing peripheral tissues such as muscle and fat to the effects of insulin. They do not stimulate insulin release from the pancreas and so are very unlikely to cause hypoglycemia. As such, they are considered to be antihyperglycemic rather than hypoglycemic agents.

THIAZOLIDINEDIONES

The thiazolidinediones act at extrapancreatic sites to increase insulin sensitivity. They selectively stimulate nuclear peroxisome-proliferator-activated receptor-γ (PPARγ), thus activating insulin-responsive genes that regulate carbohydrate and lipid metabolism. The drugs also decrease hepatic glucose production. They are especially effective in obese patients, although the thiazolidinediones can cause weight gain as edema fluid.

Clinical Pharmacology and Clinical Application

SULFONYLUREAS

Sulfonylurea drugs are used in patients with type 2 DM in whom diet alone is insufficient to achieve glycemic control. They are absorbed from the gastrointestinal tract where food can interfere with their absorption, so sulfonylureas with short half-lives should be taken 30 minutes before eating. They are weakly acidic and highly protein bound, especially to albumin. Because they are metabolized by the liver with urinary excretion of metabolites, they should be used cautiously in the presence of renal or hepatic dysfunction; if used in such patients, second generation agents are typically chosen. Specific drugs have considerable variation in their duration of action and metabolism. Glyburide has significant fecal excretion. The metabolism of chlorpropamide is incomplete, with 20% excreted unchanged in the urine. Second generation sulfonylureas are approximately 100 times more potent than the first generation agents. Despite their relatively short half lives of 3 to 5 hours, they have hypoglycemic effects for 12 to 24 hours, and once daily dosing is possible for some.

The sulfonylureas can cause hypoglycemia, potentially leading to coma, especially in elderly patients who have renal or hepatic dysfunction. For first generation sulfonylureas, the risk of hypoglycemia is greatest for drugs that have a longer duration of action (e.g., chlorpropamide). This is not true of the second generation agents, however. For example, glimepiride causes hypoglycemia in 2% to 4% of patients, whereas glyburide causes hypoglycemia in 20% to 30% of patients, even though the drugs have similar durations of action. It appears that during hypoglycemia, protective mechanisms (inhibition of insulin secretion and promotion of glucagon secretion) are preserved in the presence of glimepiride but not in the presence of glyburide. Drugs that interfere with metabolism or excretion of sulfonylureas and drugs that displace them from plasma proteins can increase the risk of hypoglycemia. Sulfonylurea drugs can also cause cholestatic jaundice, aplastic and hemolytic anemias, agranulocytosis, hypersensitivity reactions, rashes, and nausea and vomiting. Chlorpropamide can cause flushing in association with alcohol ingestion. The sulfonylureas can also cause hyponatremia by potentiating the renal effects of antidiuretic hormone (ADH). They are not typically used in pregnant or lactating women.

The degree of cardiovascular risk associated with long-term use of sulfonylureas is controversial. The University Group Diabetes Program demonstrated a slightly higher incidence of cardiovascular events in patients with type 2 DM treated with tolbutamide compared with insulin or placebo. However, multiple other studies, including the large

United Kingdom Prospective Diabetes Study Group, demonstrated the absence of increased cardiovascular mortality in sulfonylurea users.[6] Indeed, glimepiride might decrease cardiovascular morbidity, in that it has beneficial effects on ischemic preconditioning.

BIGUANIDES

Metformin, approved for use in the United States in 1995, is the only biguanide in common use today. It is indicated for patients with type 2 DM in whom it was shown to reduce macrovascular complications in the United Kingdom Prospective Diabetes Study Group.[7] It is administered orally and is subsequently absorbed from the small intestine. Metformin is excreted unchanged in the urine, and is relatively contraindicated in patients with renal impairment. It is not bound to plasma proteins. Its half-life in plasma is 2 to 4 hours, and it is administered two to three times daily. The drug is sometimes administered in combination with other oral hypoglycemic agents. Metformin leads to a mild weight reduction in obese patients and has beneficial effects on lipid profiles (decreasing plasma triglycerides and cholesterol). The drug is also used in polycystic ovary syndrome.[8]

Phenformin, a similar compound to metformin, was withdrawn from the market because of its predisposition to cause lactic acidosis. Metformin is also associated with lactic acidosis but the incidence (<1 per 10,000 patient-years) is 10 to 20 times lower than that associated with phenformin. The mechanism is thought to be related to interaction with mitochondria that leads to decreased intracellular ATP, causing glucose to be metabolized anaerobically to lactate. In addition to cautions associated with renal impairment, a history of lactic acidosis, significant liver disease, cardiac failure, chronic hypoxic lung disease, and administration of radiographic iodinated contrast agents are relative or absolute contraindications. Metformin should be stopped if the patient develops sepsis or myocardial infarction because of the risk of lactic acidosis. It should also be stopped if plasma lactate is greater than 3 mM. It has been recommended that metformin should not be given on the day of surgery, because of concern for the development of lactic acidosis. Some advocate that it be held for 48 hours before surgery. However, in a study comparing a cohort of 443 patients who took metformin preoperatively and a group of 443 patients who did not, there was no difference between groups in hospital mortality, cardiac, renal, or neurologic morbidities.[9] Metformin is also associated with nausea, taste disturbances, abdominal discomfort, diarrhea, and anorexia, although fewer than 5% of patients have side effects severe enough to warrant cessation of the drug.

THIAZOLIDINEDIONES

Thiazolidinediones include pioglitazone, rosiglitazone, and troglitazone. They are used in patients with type 2 DM, either alone or in combination with insulin or other oral hypoglycemic agents. Maximum clinical effect does not occur for 6 to 12 weeks after initiation of therapy. They are taken orally, usually once daily, and are metabolized in the liver via the cytochrome P450 system. Drugs that interfere with cytochrome P450 enzymes alter their rate of metabolism.

Hepatic transaminase levels should be measured regularly in patients taking thiazolidinediones because these drugs can induce liver dysfunction, and hepatic disease is a contraindication to their use. In fact, troglitazone was withdrawn because of associated severe hepatic dysfunction. If elevations of transaminases or other signs of hepatic dysfunction occur during therapy, treatment should be stopped. The cardiovascular effects of the thiazolidinediones have also come under scrutiny. Some patients have developed significant peripheral edema and even overt heart failure. Patients who have hypertension and/or diastolic dysfunction are especially at risk. In 2010, rosiglitazone was the subject of FDA restrictions because of adverse cardiovascular effects, including myocardial infarction and stroke.

OTHER ORAL HYPOGLYCEMIC AGENTS

Both the meglitinide analogue repaglinide and the D-phenylalanine derivative nateglinide inhibit K_{ATP} channels in pancreatic β cells to stimulate insulin production. Compared to the sulfonylureas, these drugs have faster onset and shorter duration of action. Repaglinide is administered orally, peak blood levels are obtained within 1 hour, and the half-life is about 1 hour. It can be given multiple times per day before meals. It should be used with caution in patients with liver dysfunction because it is hepatically excreted, although a small portion is renally metabolized. Nateglinide is used to reduce postprandial hyperglycemia in patients with type 2 DM. It is given 1 to 10 minutes before meals. The drug is metabolized by the liver, with a smaller portion excreted unchanged in the urine. Nateglinide is less likely to cause hypoglycemia than repaglinide. Neither drug should be administered when fasting.

The α-glucosidase inhibitors (e.g., miglitol and acarbose) decrease gastrointestinal digestion of carbohydrates and absorption of disaccharides through their action at the intestinal brush border. They are usually administered in combination with insulin or other oral hypoglycemic agents, although they can be used as single-agent therapy in patients with predominantly postprandial hyperglycemia or in older adults. They do not cause hypoglycemia unless administered in combination with other glucose-lowering agents. α-Glucosidase inhibitors should be administered at the start of a meal. The drugs can be very effective in patients with type 2 DM who are severely hyperglycemic, although they have more modest effects in those with mild to moderate hyperglycemia. Gastrointestinal side effects can be problematic, although a slow up-titration of the dose lessens these symptoms.

Incretins are gastrointestinal hormones that augment glucose-dependent insulin secretion. They include glucose-dependent insulinotropic polypeptide (GIP) and glucagon-like peptide (GLP-1). Both are rapidly broken down by dipeptidyl peptidase IV. Exenatide is a GLP-1 receptor agonist with a clinically useful duration of action, and sitagliptin is a dipeptidyl peptidase IV inhibitor that prolongs the effect of the incretins. Both are potentially useful in patients with type 2 DM to amplify glucose-induced insulin release. Amylin is co-secreted with insulin from pancreatic β cells. This 37 amino acid peptide decreases gastric emptying, glucagon secretion, and appetite. Pramlintide, an injectable analogue of amylin, has been approved for the treatment of patients whose type 1 or type 2 DM is inadequately controlled despite insulin

therapy. Drugs that interact with gastrointestinal hormones can predispose patients to increased postoperative nausea and vomiting, their effects on gastric emptying can increase the likelihood of aspiration, and their hypoglycemic effects can lead to dangerously low plasma glucose in the perioperative period.[10] It is recommended that they be held on the day of surgery if possible.

Table 31-3 compares agents used for the treatment of DM.

Glucagon

BASIC PHARMACOLOGY

Glucagon is a 29 amino acid single-chain polypeptide secreted, like insulin, by the islets of Langerhans, but by the α cells rather than β cells.[2,11] Glucagon is important in the regulation of glucose and ketone body metabolism. Like insulin, glucagon is synthesized as a pro-hormone. Pre-proglucagon is a 180 amino acid polypeptide that gives rise to glucagon, GLP-1 and GLP-2, and glicentin-related pancreatic peptide. Pre-proglucagon is processed differently according to the tissue in which the hormone is secreted, and a variety of glucagon analogues of varying potency can be produced. Glucagon acts on a glycoprotein receptor on target cells that mediates its action through a G protein cyclic adenosine monophosphate (cAMP)/protein kinase A (PKA)-mediated mechanism. Glucagon activates glycogen phosphorylase, the rate-limiting step in glycogenolysis, leading to increased glucose concentrations. Glycolysis is also inhibited. Glucagon is active in the liver (to regulate glucose levels), adipose tissue (where it increases lipolysis), heart (where it acts as an inotrope), and the gastrointestinal tract (where it causes relaxation). Glucagon secretion is influenced by diet and by insulin. Both glucagon and insulin release are stimulated by ingestion of amino acids, presumably to minimize hypoglycemia if a pure protein meal is taken. In normal individuals, glucagon release is stimulated by hypoglycemia, a defense mechanism to maintain serum glucose concentration homeostasis. This response is attenuated in the presence of type 1 DM.

CLINICAL PHARMACOLOGY AND CLINICAL APPLICATION

Clinical preparations of glucagon are extracted from bovine and porcine pancreas because there is no structural difference between these preparations and human glucagon. The half-life of glucagon in plasma is 3 to 6 min, because it is broken down quickly in liver, kidney, plasma, and other sites.

Glucagon is used to treat severe hypoglycemia, especially in patients with DM when oral or intravenous (IV) administration of glucose is not possible. Intramuscular (IM), subcutaneous, or IV glucagon can be administered at a dose of 1 mg, with clinical improvement within 10 minutes. The antihypoglycemic effects of glucagon depend on the presence of adequate hepatic glycogen stores. The effect of glucagon is transient and steps should be taken to prevent recurrence of hypoglycemia after the initial effect has waned. Side effects include nausea and vomiting. Glucagon is also used to relax the gastrointestinal tract to improve imaging procedures and to treat biliary spasm and intussusception. It has also been used for its cardiac inotropic effects in instances of β blocker overdose. It is contraindicated in patients with pheochromocytoma in that it can stimulate release of catecholamines from the tumor.

Table 31-3. Therapeutic Agents for Diabetes Mellitus

	MECHANISM OF ACTION	EXAMPLES	HBA₁c REDUCTION (%) *	AGENT-SPECIFIC ADVANTAGES	AGENT-SPECIFIC DISADVANTAGES	CONTRAINDICATIONS
Oral						
Biguanides[‡]	↓ Hepatic glucose absorption	Metformin	1–2	Weight neutral, do not cause hypoglycemia, inexpensive	Diarrhea, nausea, lactic acidosis	CFR < 50 mL/min, congestive heart failure, radiographic contrast studies, seriously ill patients, acidosis
α-Glucosidase inhibitors[‡]	↓ GI glucose absorption	Acarbose, miglitol	0.5–0.8	Reduce postprandial glycemia	Flatulence, liver function tests	Renal/liver disease
Dipeptidyl peptidase-4 inhibitors[‡]	Prolong endogenous GLP-1 action	Sexagliptin, sitagliptin, vildagliptin	0.5–1.0	Do not cause hypoglycemia		Reduce dose with renal disease
Insulin secretagogues – sulfonylureas[‡]	↑ Insulin secretion	See text	1–2	Inexpensive	Hypoglycemia, weight gain	Renal/liver disease
Insulin secretagogues – nonsulfonylureas[‡]	↑ Insulin secretion	Repaglinide, nateglinide	1–2	Short onset of action, lower postprandial glucose	Hypoglycemia	Renal/liver disease
Thiazolidinediones[‡]	↓ Insulin resistance, ↑ glucose utilization	Rosiglitazone, pioglitazone	0.5–1.4	Lower insulin requirements	Peripheral edema, CHF, weight gain, fractures, macular edema Rosiglitazone may increase risk of CV disease	Congestive heart failure, liver disease
Bile acid sequestrants[‡]	Bind bile acids; mechanism of glucose-lowering not known	Colesevelam	0.5		Constipation, dyspepsia, abdominal pain, nausea, ↑ triglycerides, interfere with absorption of other drugs, intestinal obstruction	
Parenteral						
Insulin	↑ Glucose utilization, ↓ hepatic glucose production, and other anabolic actions	See text	Not limited	Known safety profile	Injection, weight gain, hypoglycemia	
GLP-1 agonists[‡]	↑ Insulin, ↓ glucagon, slow gastric emptying, satiety	Exenatide, liraglutide	0.5–1.0	Weight loss	Injection, nausea, ↑ risk of hypoglycemia with insulin secretagogues, pancreatitis	Renal disease, agents that also slow gastrointestinal motility, pancreatitis
Amylin agonists[†,‡]	Slow gastric emptying, ↓ glucagon	Pramlintide	0.25–0.5	Reduce postprandial glycemia; weight loss	Injection, nausea, ↑ risk of hypoglycemia with insulin	Agents that also slow gastrointestinal motility
Medical nutrition therapy and physical activity[‡]	↓ Insulin, resistance, ↑ insulin secretion	Low-calorie, low-fat diet, exercise	1–3	Other health benefits	Compliance difficult, long-term success low?	

Adapted with permission from Fauci AS, Braunwald E, Kasper DL, et al, eds. *Harrison's Principles of Internal Medicine.* 17th ed. New York: McGraw-Hill; 2008. Copyright © 2008 by The McGraw-Hill Companies, Inc. All rights reserved.

*A₁c reduction (absolute) depends partly on starting A₁c value.
[†]Used in conjunction with insulin for treatment of type 1 diabetes mellitus.
[‡]Used for treatment of type 2 diabetes mellitus.

Somatostatin Analogues

BASIC AND CLINICAL PHARMACOLOGY

The somatostatins are actually a group of related peptides and include the original 14 amino acid peptide somatostatin, a 28 amino acid peptide, and a 12 amino acid peptide. They are released by pancreatic islets (delta cells), in the central nervous system, and in the gastrointestinal tract. The somatostatins act as inhibitors of the release of thyroid-stimulating hormone (TSH) and growth hormone (GH) from the pituitary, of insulin and glucagon from the pancreas, and of a number of vasoactive peptides from the gastrointestinal tract. Somatostatin has a half-life of less than 6 minutes, but longer acting analogues such as octreotide and lanreotide have been developed.

CLINICAL APPLICATION

Somatostatin analogues are used to block hormone release in endocrine tumors. Octreotide and lanreotide are used for the treatment of carcinoid tumors, glucagonomas, VIPomas, and growth hormone–secreting tumors. Octreotide, which has been available for longer in the United States, can be given intravenously or subcutaneously and is useful in the perioperative period. The drug is administered in 50- or 100-μg aliquots, either prophylactically or in response to hemodynamic instability, bronchospasm, or other manifestations thought to be secondary to release of vasoactive mediators. Long-term somatostatin analogue use can lead to biliary abnormalities and gastrointestinal symptoms.

DRUGS TO TREAT DISORDERS OF THE HYPOTHALAMIC-PITUITARY-END-ORGAN AXIS

Thyroid Hormones

The physiology of the thyroid gland and of the hypothalamic-pituitary-thyroid axis is discussed in Chapter 30.

BASIC PHARMACOLOGY

The endogenous thyroid hormones thyroxine (T_4) and triiodothyronine (T_3) can be used as pharmacologic agents. T_4 is the pro-hormone product of the thyroid gland.[12] The thyroid secretes 80 to 100 μg of T_4 daily; its half life in the circulation is 6 to 7 days. Thus missing a morning dose of replacement T_4 on the morning of surgery has minimal impact. T_4 is metabolized to biologically active T_3 or biologically inactive reverse T_3. T_3 (3,5,3-triiodothyronine) is formed by extrathyroidal deiodination of T_4 (80%) and by direct thyroid secretion (20%). It is more potent and less protein bound than T_4; its half-life in the circulation is 24 to 30 hours. T_3 mediates most of the effects of thyroid hormones.

CLINICAL PHARMACOLOGY

Thyroxine (levothyroxine sodium) (T_4) is the hormone of choice for thyroid hormone replacement due to its consistent potency and its duration of action. Usually given orally, 50% to 80% of the administered dose of thyroxine is absorbed in the small intestine. Absorption is increased by fasting and decreased by administration of a number of drugs including sucralfate, cholestyramine, and mineral supplements. Levothyroxine supplementation is monitored by assay of serum TSH levels, with a goal of achieving a normal TSH concentration. Most patients require 75 to 150 μg per day. Dose adjustments take approximately 5 weeks to induce a new serum steady-state. In older patients and patients with cardiac disease, low-dose thyroxine supplementation should be started initially, with subsequent slow titration upward to avoid myocardial ischemia or arrhythmias. If enteral access is not possible, thyroxine can be prepared from a lyophilized powder and administered intravenously at 50% of the enteral dose.

Liothyronine sodium (T_3) is the salt of triiodothyronine. It is available in tablet and injectable forms. The average daily dose is 50 to 75 μg. Liothyronine is usually not used as primary replacement therapy because of its relatively short half-life.

Thyrotropin alfa is recombinant TSH and is administered intramuscularly. It is used as an adjunctive diagnostic tool for testing of serum thyroglobulin and in association with radio-iodine for ablation of remnants of thyroid tissue in patients with thyroid cancer. Common adverse effects include nausea and headache, paresthesias, arrhythmias, and hypersensitivity reactions.

CLINICAL APPLICATION

Myxedema coma is a rare, extreme form of hypothyroidism. It usually occurs in older women with undiagnosed hypothyroidism, especially in the setting of intercurrent illness. It can present with mental status changes and severe metabolic derangements, including hyponatremia and hypoglycemia, and can lead to hypotension and hypoventilation. Myxedema coma is associated with relatively high mortality. Therapy includes mechanical ventilation and rewarming and administration of IV levothyroxine and hydrocortisone, the latter because 5% to 10% of patients also have adrenal insufficiency.

THIOUREYLENE ANTITHYROID DRUGS

Basic and Clinical Pharmacology

Clinically used antithyroid drugs belong to the thioureylene class and include propylthiouracil (PTU), methimazole, and carbimazole. Carbimazole, used in Europe, is a prodrug of methimazole.[12]

Thioureylenes interfere with the incorporation of iodine into tyrosyl residues of thyroglobulin and inhibit the coupling of tyrosyl residues to form iodotyrosines. Blockade of the peroxidase enzyme prevents oxidation of iodide or iodotyrosyl groups to the active state. The coupling reaction might be more sensitive to antithyroid drugs than the iodination reaction. Inhibition of thyroid hormone synthesis leads to depletion of thyroid hormone stores and subsequently to a decrease in serum concentrations. PTU, but not methimazole, also inhibits peripheral conversion of T_4 to T_3 and has theoretical advantages in thyroid storm wherein such blockade of peripheral T_3 production is useful.

Both drugs, but especially methimazole, can produce agranulocytosis, which seems to be dose related and which can develop rapidly. The development of fever or pharyngitis in patients taking antithyroid medication should prompt evaluation including a complete blood count. The most common adverse effect of these drugs, however, is a mild, urticarial rash. Joint pain, headache, paresthesias, nausea, alopecia, and rarely vasculitis can also occur. Both drugs cross the placenta and appear in breast milk, although transfer is lower with PTU, making PTU the preferred agent in parturients and breast-feeding mothers.

Clinical Application

Antithyroid drugs are used as definitive treatment for hyperthyroidism, in conjunction with radioiodine for the treatment of Graves disease, and to control hyperthyroidism in preparation for surgical treatment. PTU is started at a dose of 100 mg every 8 hours or 150 mg twice daily. Methimazole, because of its relatively long duration of action, is given as a single daily dose. Doses of greater than 300 to 400 mg of PTU or 30 to 40 mg of methimazole are usually not required. Thyrotoxicosis usually improves within 3 to 6 weeks. Pretreatment serum T_3 concentrations, size of the goiter, and dose of medication administered all impact the rate of resolution of symptoms. Once the patient is euthyroid, typically within 3 months, the dose of antithyroid medication can be reduced. The drugs are usually not stopped, however, to reduce risk of recurrence of hyperthyroidism. Hypothyroidism can develop and necessitates reduction in dosage or even the administration of thyroid hormone supplementation. Some have advocated use of a combination of levothyroxine and methimazole, but there is no evidence that this is beneficial. Both PTU and methimazole must be given enterally.

Thyroid storm is a rare life-threatening exacerbation of hyperthyroidism that can be precipitated by surgical stress or intercurrent illness. It is more likely to occur with undiagnosed or untreated hyperthyroidism. It manifests as hyperthermia, agitation, confusion, and tachycardia. Patients can develop arrhythmias, myocardial ischemia and congestive heart failure. The differential diagnosis includes pheochromocytoma and malignant hyperthermia, and light anesthesia can mimic some of the features. Treatment of thyroid storm often requires multiple antithyroid agents administered simultaneously.

OTHER ANTITHYROID DRUGS

β Blockers (see Chapters 13 and 23) can be used as adjunctive therapies to improve the signs and symptoms of hyperthyroidism. β Blockers blunt tachycardia, tremor, and anxiety associated with the condition but do not affect synthesis or secretion of T_3 or T_4. They should not be used as single-agent therapy except for brief periods before sodium iodide [^{131}I] administration or before surgery.

Iodide has been used for many years for the treatment of hyperthyroidism and was the only therapy available before the introduction of the antithyroid drugs. Administration of large doses of iodide acutely inhibits synthesis of iodotyrosines and thyroid hormones (known as the Wolff-Chaikoff effect). The mechanism of the acute Wolff-Chaikoff effect is unclear but might be due to antagonism of TSH and cAMP-stimulated thyroid hormone release or generation of organic iodocompounds within the thyroid.

Inorganic iodine (Lugol's solution, consisting of 5% iodine and 10% KI) is used in preparation for thyroidectomy in patients with thyrotoxicosis. Administered enterally, iodine is converted to iodide in the intestine. It can be given alone, but is usually given 7 to 10 days immediately preoperatively after thyrotoxicosis has been controlled with an antithyroid drug. Saturated solution of potassium iodide is an alternative form of inorganic iodine. Doses are determined empirically and range from 1 to 5 drops three times per day. Inorganic iodide decreases the uptake of radioactive iodine, with uptake being inversely proportional to serum iodine concentration. Iodide was administered to populations at risk after the Chernobyl nuclear accidents as protection against thyroid cancer.

Iodinated contrast agents (e.g., iopanoic acid, ipodate sodium) can be used as temporary treatment for hyperthyroidism of any cause. These agents block peripheral conversion of T_4 to T_3 and are useful for very symptomatic hyperthyroidism and thyroid storm. They are not currently available in the United States.

Of the radioisotopes of iodine, ^{131}I has been used most commonly as an antithyroid medication.[13] It has a half-life of 8 days, meaning that the vast majority of its radioactivity has decayed within 60 days. It emits both β particles and gamma rays. ^{131}I is administered orally in capsule or solution form, is taken up into the thyroid in the same manner as nonradioactive iodide, and is incorporated into monoiodotyrosine and diiodotyrosine and subsequently into thyroid hormones that are stored in the thyroid follicles. Radioactivity damages thyroid parenchymal cells. Carefully chosen doses of radioactive iodine cause destruction of the thyroid gland without damage to adjacent tissues. ^{131}I is used to treat hyperthyroidism and is often the therapy of choice for Graves disease, especially in older patients and those in whom the disease has been difficult to control. Complete ablation of the thyroid is often recommended, with subsequent supplementation with L-thyroxine. More than half of patients to whom ^{131}I is administered require only one dose, but in others second or subsequent doses are required. Even when complete ablation of the thyroid gland is not desired, many patients develop hypothyroidism. Administration of PTU, but not methimazole, reduces the effectiveness of ^{131}I, presumably by blocking incorporation into thyroid hormone. ^{131}I is contraindicated in pregnancy because of concern for damage to the fetal thyroid gland. Theoretically the drug can cause cancer, and so there are concerns about its administration to younger patients. However, extensive experience with ^{131}I, as documented in the Cooperative Thyrotoxicosis Therapy Follow-up Study Group, has not demonstrated an increase in cancer mortality following ^{131}I treatment for Graves disease.[14] Another radioisotope of iodine, ^{129}I, primarily emits gamma rays, has a shorter half-life than ^{131}I, and is used for imaging of the thyroid gland.

DRUGS USED IN THE TREATMENT OF PHEOCHROMOCYTOMA

Basic and Clinical Pharmacology

α ANTAGONISTS

Phenoxybenzamine is a nonselective α-adrenergic receptor antagonist used in patients with pheochromocytoma or paraganglionoma. The drug blunts the effects of catecholamines released from the tumor and is usually administered preoperatively in preparation for pheochromocytoma resection. Phenoxybenzamine can cause a reflex tachycardia by inhibition of presynaptic α_2 adrenoceptors at postganglionic neurons, resulting in increased release of norepinephrine. It also causes orthostatic hypotension. Despite the use of phenoxybenzamine, significant elevations of blood pressure can still occur, especially with intraoperative tumor manipulation. Once a pheochromocytoma has been isolated from the circulation and removed, hypotension is common, and the residual effects of phenoxybenzamine contribute to this hypotension as drug effects dissipate over about 36 hours. Phenoxybenzamine is usually administered in the outpatient setting at an initial dose of 10 mg orally twice daily, increased in 10-mg increments daily until arterial blood pressure has stabilized and symptoms have reduced. Average dose is 44 mg/day (range 10-240 mg/day), and most patients require 10-14 days of therapy.[15]

Selective α_1-receptor antagonists include terazosin and prazosin. They do not cause reflex tachycardia, decreasing the need for preoperative β-receptor antagonists. They have a shorter duration of action, allowing adjustment before surgery and a shorter duration of hypotension after pheochromocytoma resection. In addition to their use in the management of patients with pheochromocytoma, selective α_1 antagonists can also be used in the treatment of benign prostatic hyperplasia. Side effects include dizziness and muscle weakness.

Doxazosin is a long-acting α_1 blocker administered once daily. Use of doxazosin before pheochromocytoma resection provides hemodynamic control similar to phenoxybenzamine.[16]

Phentolamine is an α_1 antagonist that can be given intravenously or intramuscularly. It can be used for management of hypertension associated with pheochromocytoma, especially in the perioperative period, when it is given intravenously in 5-mg doses. It has also been used for pralidoxime-associated hypertension. Phentolamine can also be administered subcutaneously in diluted form to decrease the effects of extravasation of α-adrenergic agonists and to reverse the effects of subcutaneously administered local anesthetics. The drug is metabolized in the liver and excreted in the urine.

α-METHYL PARATYROSINE (METYROSINE)

α-Methyl paratyrosine is a competitive inhibitor of tyrosine hydroxylase, the rate-limiting enzyme in the production of catecholamines. Administration reduces tumor stores of catecholamines, and can be used in the long-term management of patients with pheochromocytoma when surgery is contraindicated or when long-term management of malignant pheochromocytoma is required. It can also be used in the preoperative preparation of patients with pheochromocytoma. Metyrosine can be especially useful for patients with congestive heart failure in whom α blockers cause tachycardia and β blockers worsen congestive heart failure. The dose is 0.5 to 4 mg/day.

Clinical Application

Two different preoperative preparatory regimens for pheochromocytoma resection have been described.[17] Combination therapy with phenoxybenzamine, α and β blockers, and perhaps α-methyl paratyrosine should be used in "high-risk" patients. In "low-risk" patients, α-methyl paratyrosine and calcium channel blockers might be sufficient. Comparison of two preoperative regimens (one using the nonselective α blocker phenoxybenzamine; the other using α_1 blockers prazosin, doxazosin, or terazosin) found differences

in the need for intraoperative pressors and volume administration, but no differences in surgical outcome or length of hospital stay.[18]

Achieving satisfactory hemodynamic and symptom control in patients with pheochromocytoma can also involve use of calcium channel antagonists and β blockers. Intraoperative blood pressure control often requires use of readily titratable, rapidly acting vasodilators such as sodium nitroprusside and nicardipine (see Chapter 23).

CORTICOSTEROIDS

In the 1940s, Kendall and Hench at Mayo Clinic used products of the adrenal gland, especially cortisol (hydrocortisone), to treat rheumatoid arthritis, opening the door to widespread use of "steroids" in medicine.[19] The physiology of the hypothalamic-pituitary-adrenal access is described in Chapter 30.

Basic Pharmacology

All steroids, both endogenous and synthetic, are based on the cyclopentanophenanthrene ring, to which side group substitutions can be added to alter the pharmacodynamic and pharmacokinetic profile. The adrenal cortex synthesizes two classes of steroids: the corticosteroids and the androgens. Corticosteroids have traditionally been divided into glucocorticoids and mineralocorticoids according to their relative effects on carbohydrate metabolism, Na^+ retention, and inflammation. Glucocorticoids have more effect on carbohydrate metabolism and more potent antiinflammatory effects, whereas mineralocorticoids more powerfully cause distal renal tubular absorption of Na^+. Many steroids have both properties. Hydrocortisone is synthetically produced cortisol, the primary glucocorticoid in humans, and is used as the reference steroid (Table 31-4).

Transport of the steroid into the cytoplasm allows binding to cytoplasmic receptors, which translocate to the nucleus where they interact with glucocorticoid response elements in genes. Glucocorticoids repress or activate specific genes, interact with other transcription factors, modulate messenger RNA, and alter protein production.[20]

Clinical Pharmacology

Corticosteroid effects include alterations in protein, carbohydrate and lipid metabolic processes, preservation of cardiovascular and metabolic homeostasis, and actions on the nervous, endocrine and immune systems.[21] Steroids increase blood glucose, promote hepatic glycogen synthesis, and decrease sensitivity to insulin. Muscle tissue can be degraded leading to negative nitrogen balance. Antiinflammatory effects are mediated by stabilization of lysozymes, diminishing leucocyte response to local inflammation, promoting the formation of inhibitor of nuclear factor κB ($I_\kappa B$), and inhibition of proliferation of activated T cells (Figure 31-3).

In plasma, glucocorticoids are bound to albumin and transcortin, the levels of which are altered by states such as liver disease or pregnancy. Free, unbound glucocorticoid exerts physiologic effects. Glucocorticoids are metabolized primarily in the liver where they undergo oxidation-reduction

Table 31-4. Pharmacokinetics and Pharmacodynamics of Commonly Used Steroids

STEROID	ANTI-INFLAMMATORY POTENCY	EQUIVALENT DOSE (MG)	ELIMINATION HALF-TIME (HR)	DURATION OF ACTION (HR)	SODIUM-RETAINING POTENCY	ROUTE OF ADMINISTRATION
Cortisol	1	20	1.5-3.0	8-12	1	O, T, IV, IM, IA
Cortisone	0.8	25	0.5	8-36	0.8	O, T, IV, IM, IA
Prednisolone	4	5	2-4	12-36	0.8	O, T, IV, IM, IA
Prednisone	4	5	2-4	12-36	0.8	O
Methylprednisolone	5	4	2-4	12-36	0.5	O, T, IV, IM, IA, E
Betamethasone	25	0.75	5	36-54	0	O, T, IV, IM, IA,
Dexamethasone	25	0.75	3.5-5.0	36-54	0	O, T, IV, IM, IA
Triamcinolone	5	4	3.5	12-36	0	O, T, IV, IM, E
Fludrocortisone	10	2		24	250	O, T, IV, IM
Aldosterone	0				3000	

From Elisha S, Ouellette RG, and Joyce J. *Pharmacology for Nurse Anesthesiology.* Sudbury, Mass: Jones and Bartlett Learning; 2011. Table 18.3.
E, Epidural; *IA,* intraarticular; *IM,* intramuscular; *IV,* intravenous; *O,* oral; *T,* topical.

reactions to form dihydrocortisol and tetrahydrocortisol. These metabolites are conjugated with glucuronide or sulfate to water-soluble metabolites that are excreted in the urine. A small proportion of the water-soluble metabolites are eliminated via the intestine.

The serum half-lives of the synthetic glucocorticoids vary considerably. Hydrocortisone has a half-life of 80 minutes, whereas dexamethasone has a half-life of 270 minutes. The duration of physiologic effects is determined by the effects on gene regulation, which usually last significantly longer than the half-life. Glucocorticoids can be administered orally, intravenously, and intramuscularly. Preparations are specifically designed for topical use, and steroids can also be administered into the epidural space, synovial spaces, conjunctiva, and respiratory tract. If the enteral route is not available, an equivalent dose can be administered intravenously. The intravenous route is used as first-line therapy for allergic reactions (including anaphylaxis), and in severely ill patients. Inhaled steroids are commonly used for reactive airways disease (usually by metered-dose inhaler), epidural steroids are a mainstay of therapy in certain pain disorders, and topical steroid preparations are used in dermatologic conditions.

Fludrocortisone is the mineralocorticoid most commonly used in clinical practice. It is administered in association with glucocorticoids for primary and secondary adrenocortical insufficiency and for treatment of salt-losing adrenogenital syndrome. It is administered orally, and absorption is rapid and complete. The dose is 0.05 to 0.2 mg/day, although there is considerable interpatient variability. Its half-life is 18 to 36 hours. Side effects include congestive heart failure, hypertension and edema.

ADVERSE EFFECTS

High-dose and/or long-term corticosteroid therapy can cause side effects in many organs (Table 31-5). Hypertension is caused by renal Na$^+$ retention and potentiation of vasopressor responses to angiotensin II and catecholamines. In children, corticosteroids interfere with the proliferation and longevity of chondrocytes, thus slowing longitudinal growth. In adults, osteoporosis and an increased risk of fracture occur due to adverse effects on osteoblast function. Corticosteroid induced immunosuppressant effects on lymphocytes predispose to infection, and interfere with wound healing. Although corticosteroids are used in the treatment of allergic reactions,

patients can have allergic reactions to synthetic steroids. An allergy to a specific steroid can mean that the patient has an allergy to other synthetic steroids.

Negative feedback effects of exogenous steroids can blunt the function of the hypothalamic-pituitary-adrenal axis (HPAA), leading to absolute or relative adrenal suppression. This can lead to problems in stressful situations, such as during illness or in the perioperative period (see later).

Clinical Application

ADRENAL INSUFFICIENCY

Corticosteroid therapy is vital in patients with Addison's disease. Hydrocortisone, a short-acting agent, is often used. Dosing recommendations include 5 mg/m^2 body surface area three times per day, 10 mg in the morning and 5 mg in the evening, and 15 to 25 mg per day administered in two or three doses. These dosing regimens attempt to mimic physiologic steroid secretion, but early morning relative adrenal insufficiency can still occur. Longer-acting steroid preparations (prednisone, dexamethasone) can also be used, especially in those who are noncompliant with multiple dose regimens. Mineralocorticoids might also need to be administered, usually in the form of fludrocortisone, as mentioned earlier.

REACTIVE AIRWAYS DISEASE

Asthma and chronic obstructive pulmonary disease are inflammatory conditions in which corticosteroids are often used. Inhaled glucocorticoids are the agents of choice in the treatment of persistent asthma according to the National Asthma Education and Prevention Program. Regular treatment with steroids reduces symptom frequency, improves quality of life, decreases risk of serious exacerbations, and modulates bronchial hyperresponsiveness. In randomized controlled trials, inhaled budesonide decreases the incidence of asthma exacerbations more than placebo and inhaled terbutaline.[22,23] Inhaled glucocorticoids can be administered by metered-dose inhaler, dry powder inhaler, or nebulizer. Oral and intravenous corticosteroids are also administered for exacerbations of asthma and chronic obstructive pulmonary disease, and oral agents can be used on a long-term basis for severe reactive airways disease.

CORTICOSTEROID THERAPY IN NEUROLOGIC CRITICAL CARE

Glucocorticoids (usually dexamethasone) are administered in relatively large doses for the treatment and prevention of

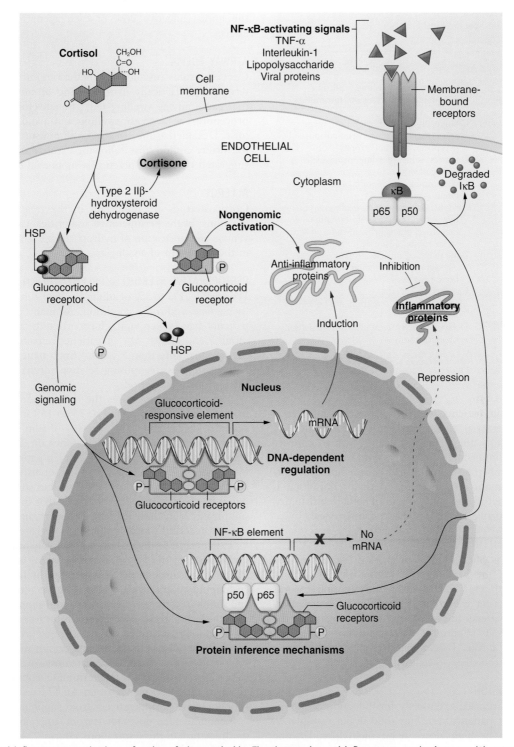

Figure 31-3 Anti-inflammatory mechanisms of action of glucocorticoids. The three major anti-inflammatory mechanisms are (1) nongenomic activation mediated by cytoplasmic glucocorticoid receptors, (2) genomic signaling involving DNA-dependent gene regulation via glucocorticoid receptor interaction with glucocorticoid response elements, and (3) protein interference mechanisms (e.g., NF-κB elements). Black arrows denote activation, the red line denotes inhibition, the red dashed arrows denote repression, and the red X denotes lack of product (i.e., no mRNA). *HSP,* Heat shock protein; *mRNA,* messenger RNA; *P,* phosphate; *TNF,* tumor necrosis factor α. *(From Rhen T, Cidlowski JA. Anti-inflammatory action of glucocorticoids—new mechanisms for old drugs.* N Engl J Med. *2005;353:1711-1723.)*

Table 31-5. Tissue-Specific Side Effects of High-Dose or Prolonged Glucocorticoid Therapy

TISSUE	SIDE EFFECTS
Adrenal gland	Adrenal atrophy, Cushing syndrome
Cardiovascular system	Dyslipidemia, hypertension, thrombosis, vasculitis
Central nervous system	Changes in behavior, cognition, memory, and mood (i.e., glucocorticoid-induced psychoses, cerebral atrophy)
Gastrointestinal tract	Gastrointestinal bleeding, pancreatitis, peptic ulcer
Immune system	Broad immunosuppression, activation of latent viruses
Integument	Atrophy, delayed wound healing, erythema, hypertrichosis, perioral dermatitis, petechiae, glucocorticoid-induced acne, striae rubrae distensae, telangiectasia
Musculoskeletal system	Bone necrosis, muscle atrophy, osteoporosis, retardation of longitudinal bone growth
Eyes	Cataracts, glaucoma
Kidney	Increased sodium retention and potassium excretion
Reproductive system	Delayed puberty, fetal growth retardation, hypogonadism

From Rhen T, Cidlowski JA. Antiinflammatory action of glucocorticoids—new mechanisms for old drugs. *N Engl J Med.* 2005;353:1711-1723.

cerebral edema in patients with brain tumors and certain patients with bacterial meningitis.[24] Despite encouraging experimental results, they have not been shown to improve outcome when administered to patients with ischemic stroke, intracerebral hemorrhage, aneurysmal subarachnoid hemorrhage, and traumatic brain injury. Methylprednisolone is often administered in the acute phase of spinal cord injury, although the evidence to support this is controversial.[25,26]

NAUSEA AND VOMITING

Dexamethasone is often used as prophylaxis against nausea and vomiting in the perioperative setting and in patients receiving chemotherapy. In the perioperative period it works best when administered early in the surgical procedure suggesting that its effects might be due to a decrease in the inflammatory effects of surgery.[27] Modulation of endorphins might also play a role. Dexamethasone might also have a central effect on the chemoreceptor trigger zone.

IMMUNOSUPPRESSION

Corticosteroids are used extensively for induction of immunosuppression in patients receiving solid organ transplants. They are given in high doses (e.g., methylprednisolone 500 mg) in the operating room and continued at lower doses for an indefinite period.

TREATMENT OF INFLAMMATORY CONDITIONS

Steroids are used to treat rheumatoid arthritis, connective tissue diseases (e.g., polyarteritis nodosa, Goodpasture syndrome, Wegener granulomatosis), ocular inflammation (e.g., iritis, uveitis), myasthenia gravis, inflammatory bowel disease, and cutaneous disorders. In addition to systemic therapy, steroids can be administered rectally and topically for bowel and cutaneous disorders, respectively. Steroids are usually used in conjunction with other immunosuppressants to allow use of the lowest effective dose of each agent to minimize side effects.

AIRWAY EDEMA

Corticosteroids (usually dexamethasone) are often administered prophylactically in the setting of surgical procedures that cause airway swelling (e.g., tonsillectomy, maxillofacial procedures) to decrease swelling and avoid airway compromise. Dexamethasone can also be administered as a treatment for airway compromise following extubation. A metaanalysis suggested that such a practice is supported by clinical data.[28]

ALLERGY

Corticosteroids are important in the treatment of allergic reactions. In the perioperative and critical care setting, intravenous administration of hydrocortisone is a key component in the treatment of anaphylaxis.

PERIOPERATIVE STEROID SUPPLEMENTATION

Worldwide, 1% to 3% of adults use long-term corticosteroids to manage a chronic condition. As many as 20% of these patients have taken oral glucocorticoids for more than 6 months and almost 5% of patients remain on oral steroid therapy for more than 5 years.[29] Such patients are at risk of adrenal suppression causing relative adrenal insufficiency in the perioperative period.

Major surgery increases the daily production of cortisol from the usual 15 to 20 mg to 75 to 150 mg. There is considerable debate about the necessity of administering perioperative "stress" doses of steroids. Since the 1950s, there have been reports of perioperative deaths in patients with adrenal insufficiency. The incidence of hypotensive crises due to adrenal insufficiency is low (1%-2%), but steroid supplementation has been justified on the basis that the risk of death is significant. Many have expressed concern, however, that perioperative steroid supplementation is overused.

Patients can be divided into those likely or unlikely to have suppression of the HPAA. Patients taking the equivalent of 20 mg of prednisone per day or more or those who have a cushingoid appearance are likely to have adrenal suppression and should receive perioperative steroid supplementation. On the other hand, those taking steroids for less than 3 weeks and those on long-term alternate-day therapy are unlikely to have suppression of the HPAA axis and do not need perioperative supplementation. For intermediate doses of steroids when the state of the HPAA axis is indeterminate, consideration can be given to the performance of an ACTH test or patients can simply receive perioperative steroid supplementation.

Recommended doses for steroid supplementation depend on the nature of the surgical procedure.[30,31] For minor procedures (e.g., hernia repair) the usual morning steroid dose should be taken and no additional supplementation is required. For patients undergoing a procedure associated with moderate surgical stress (e.g., joint replacement), hydrocortisone 50 mg can be given before the procedure, and hydrocortisone 25 mg given every 8 hours for 24 hours postoperatively. Subsequently the patient should receive the usual steroid dose. If a major surgical procedure is being performed (e.g., esophagectomy), 100 mg of hydrocortisone should be given before induction and hydrocortisone 50 mg IV administered every 8 hours for 24 hours. Subsequent steroid supplementation should be tapered relatively quickly to baseline levels.

ADRENOCORTICOTROPIC HORMONE AND STEROID ANTAGONISTS

Corticotropin or ACTH is used diagnostically in the ACTH test for adrenal insufficiency and therapeutically for a variety of conditions including acute exacerbations of multiple sclerosis, infantile spasms, and many rheumatologic and connective tissue diseases. Adverse effects are similar to those of the corticosteroids and include adrenal insufficiency after acute withdrawal.

Spironolactone is a potassium-sparing diuretic that acts to antagonize the actions of aldosterone on distal renal tubules.[32] It is used in the treatment of congestive heart failure, primary hyperaldosteronism, hypertension, and peripheral edema. Side effects include hyperkalemia, renal impairment, and gynecomastia. It is associated with tumor development in animals. Eplerenone is another aldosterone antagonist used to modify the renin-angiotensin-aldosterone system in patients with heart failure. It lacks the sexual side effects of spironolactone, but might be more likely to cause hyperkalemia.

Metyrapone and aminoglutethimide inhibit steroid synthesis. Metyrapone inhibits the 11-β-hydroxylation reaction, leading to a decrease in cortisol secretion and accumulation of 11-deoxycortisol. Mineralocorticoid deficiency does not occur because 11-deoxycorticosterone production (a mineralocorticoid) is increased. It can be used in situations of excess glucocorticoid production from adrenal or extraadrenal tumors. Aminoglutethimide inhibits cholesterol side-chain cleavage enzyme (a desmolase), leading to a decrease in both cortisol and aldosterone production. Like metyrapone it is used in the treatment of tumor-induced steroid excess. The commonly used induction agent etomidate blunts steroid production by inhibiting 11-β-hydroxylation, and there has been considerable controversy regarding the appropriateness of its use in patients with septic shock.[33]

POSTERIOR PITUITARY HORMONES, ANALOGUES, AND ANTAGONISTS

The posterior pituitary (neurohypophysis) secretes oxytocin and ADH. The latter is also known as arginine vasopressin (AVP) or vasopressin. These agents, their analogues, and their antagonists are used in clinical practice, especially in obstetrics and critical care.

Basic and Clinical Pharmacology

VASOPRESSIN AND DESMOPRESSIN

Arginine vasopressin, a 9–amino acid peptide with a 6 amino acid ring and 3 amino acid side chain, is a powerful vasoconstrictor that works by stimulating specific G protein–coupled receptors (V_1 receptors) in the vasculature. It also acts on the renal collecting ducts where it increases permeability to water and results in the production of more concentrated urine. This effect is mediated by V_2 receptors. V_3 receptors are found in the anterior pituitary and are coupled to various second messenger systems. They have a role in the secretion of ACTH.[34] Other vasopressin-like receptors regulate the release of factor VIII and von Willebrand factor. Desmopressin acetate (also known as DDAVP) is a long-acting synthetic analogue of vasopressin that has a much more pronounced antidiuretic effect and much fewer vasopressor properties than vasopressin. Compared with vasopressin, in desmopressin the first amino acid has been deaminated and the arginine at the eighth position is the *dextro* rather than *levo* form. Vasopressin can be administered intramuscularly or intravenously. It has a half-life in the circulation of about 15 minutes and is metabolized in the kidneys and the liver. Desmopressin can be given intravenously, subcutaneously, orally, or intranasally. It has a half-life of 1.5 to 2.5 hours. Oral bioavailability is less than 1%, but when given by the nasal route it is 3% to 4%. Adverse effects associated with use of vasopressin include headache and agitation. Abdominal pain and nausea can occur due to stimulation of abdominal smooth muscle and increased peristalsis. Allergic reactions, which include rashes, urticaria, and anaphylaxis, are rare. Hyponatremia with subsequent seizure activity can occur if an inappropriately high dose is administered. Thrombocytopenia can be caused by AVP-induced platelet aggregation mediated by V_1 receptors.[35] Extravasation can lead to skin necrosis and gangrene. Myocardial ischemia can occur at relatively high doses.

OXYTOCIN

Oxytocin is a cyclic nonapeptide structurally similar to AVP. The hormones differ by only two of their nine amino acids. An oxytocin precursor is produced by the paraventricular and supraoptic nuclei of the hypothalamus. After proteolysis, oxytocin is secreted by the posterior pituitary. There is also minor oxytocin release from regions of the hypothalamus, brainstem, and spinal cord. Oxytocin is synthesized to a significantly lesser extent in the ovary, uterus, and placenta. It is released in response to cervical dilation and suckling at the breast. Oxytocin plays an important role in pregnancy and labor where it stimulates the force and frequency of uterine contractions and milk ejection. It acts through G protein–coupled receptors that are closely related to vasopressin receptors (see Chapter 30). Oxytocin is used to induce or augment labor in selected pregnant women.[36]

Adverse effects of oxytocin include water retention and hyponatremia; when used at high doses in patients to whom hypotonic fluids are administered, this can lead to seizures and coma. Intravenous administration of oxytocin causes vasodilation with subsequent hypotension and reflex tachycardia. Hypotension can be severe in hypovolemic patients and in patients under anesthesia in whom compensatory reflexes are blunted. In contrast to the effects on the systemic vasculature, coronary vasoconstriction can occur.

Clinical Application

VASOPRESSIN AND DESMOPRESSIN

Both vasopressin and desmopressin can be used for treatment of pituitary diabetes insipidus (DI), which can occur due to disruption of the posterior pituitary after neurosurgery or trauma or in the setting of postpartum hemorrhage. Desmopressin is typically used in a dose of 10 to 40 µg per day in two or three divided doses delivered by intranasal spray. It can also be given orally or intravenously. In the ICU it can be given intravenously in a dose of 1 to 4 µg once or twice daily as needed to treat polyuria, polydipsia, and hypernatremia of pituitary origin.

Vasopressin has also been used in critically ill patients with bleeding esophageal varices or bleeding colonic diverticula. The doses required are relatively high and can cause coronary ischemia. Alternative therapies are more typically used now.

In doses larger than those used for the treatment of DI, vasopressin causes vasoconstriction and increases in both systemic and pulmonary blood pressure by direct effects on vascular smooth muscle. When vascular tone is low, the vasoconstrictive effects are more powerful. Studies of AVP serum concentrations in shock states have shown that there is relative AVP deficiency in patients with vasodilatory shock states such as sepsis. Administration of vasopressin in vasodilatory shock caused a dramatic increase in systemic blood pressure, even with acidemia in which the effectiveness of catecholamines is reduced.[37] Vasopressin use in critically ill patients has increased over the past 2 decades. It is used as an infusion at a dose of 0.03 to 0.04 units/min in septic shock. Its exact role has been debated; recommendations are that it be used as an adjunct to catecholamines rather than as a first-line single agent.[38] The results of a large prospective study (VASST) comparing low-dose vasopressin to norepinephrine in patients with septic shock failed to show a significant difference in 28-day mortality (Figure 31-4).[39] Vasopressin has also been introduced into algorithms for the treatment of cardiac arrest based on a prospective study that demonstrated effectiveness similar to that of epinephrine.[40] The American Heart Association recommendations for the treatment of ventricular fibrillation include the use of vasopressin 40 units via the intravenous or intraosseous route.

In addition to its role in the treatment of DI, desmopressin is also used in patients with uremia, liver disease, and some types of hemophilia to improve hemostatic function. It releases von Willebrand factor, prostaglandins, and tissue plasminogen activator from endothelial cells via V_2 receptors, increasing platelet adhesiveness. It can be used in the treatment of hemophilia A, mild to moderate von Willebrand disease type 1, and uremic platelet dysfunction. It is also used in the perioperative period, although the effectiveness of such therapy is debatable.[41]

OXYTOCIN

Oxytocin is administered by intravenous infusion. A starting dose of 0.5 to 2 mU/min can be titrated upward in increments of 1 to 2 mU/min until the desired contraction pattern is established, and decreased when a satisfactory contraction pattern and adequate cervical dilation are present. Infusion rates of 6 mU/min provide oxytocin levels similar to those of spontaneous labor; rates greater than 9 to 10 mU/min are rarely required, although high-dose oxytocin strategies have been employed using doses of more than 20 mU/min. As increased uterine contraction occurs, so too does an increase in the associated pain, and additional analgesia or adjustment of epidural analgesia might be required. Hyperstimulation leads to very frequent or sustained uterine contractions that can necessitate discontinuation of the infusion. Cessation of the infusion usually leads to rapid resolution of hyperstimulation because the plasma half-life of intravenous oxytocin is about 3 minutes. A low-dose oxytocin infusion administered as an "oxytocin challenge test" is performed in some pregnant women to assess fetal well-being.

Oxytocin is also used as a therapy for postpartum hemorrhage.[42] Ten units can be given intramuscularly, or 20 to 40 units diluted in a liter of crystalloid can be administered intravenously. If oxytocin fails to cause uterine contraction and postpartum hemorrhage is ongoing, administration of methylergonovine and/or prostaglandin F2 might be required.

OTHER AGENTS

Terlipressin is a vasopressin analogue, not currently available in the United States, with a longer duration of action than vasopressin. It is used with albumin administration for treatment of hepatorenal syndrome (HRS). Although it can improve short-term renal function and survival in patients with type 1 HRS, there is a paucity of evidence demonstrating an effect on overall mortality.[43]

Vaptans are relatively new drugs that antagonize the effects of AVP. Tolvaptan selectively antagonizes the effects of AVP at V_2 receptors in the renal collecting ducts, causing a marked, dose-dependent increase in solute-free water excretion.[44] In two multicenter trials, oral tolvaptan was effective in patients with euvolemic or hypervolemic hyponatremia, and is approved for the treatment of hyponatremia and heart failure.[45] Conivaptan antagonizes V_1a and V_2 receptors, which, in conditions associated with increased vasopressin levels, decreases renal water excretion. It is used to treat hyponatremia and has been used successfully to treat hyponatremia in

Figure 31-4 Kaplan-Meier survival curves for patients with septic shock randomized to receive vasopressin or norepinephrine. The dashed vertical line marks day 28. There was no significant difference in mortality rate calculated with the log-rank test. *(From Russell JA, Walley KR, Singer J, et al. Vasopressin versus norepinephrine infusion in patients with septic shock. N Engl J Med. 2008;358:877-887.)*

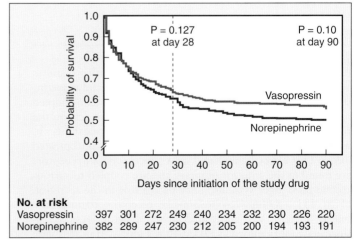

No. at risk										
Vasopressin	397	301	272	249	240	234	232	230	226	220
Norepinephrine	382	289	247	230	212	205	200	194	193	191

liver transplant candidates.[46] Use of vaptans for the treatment of hyponatremia allows avoidance of fluid restriction and continuation of natriuretic diuretics (for treatment of ascites) and prevents development of hepatic encephalopathy. Conivaptan is not approved for treatment of congestive heart failure. The most frequent side effect of the vaptans is thirst. They can also theoretically cause rapid hypernatremia and renal failure due to depletion of intravascular water.

Carbetocin is an analogue of oxytocin, still under investigation, that has a longer duration of action than oxytocin. Atosiban is a peptide agent that antagonizes the actions of oxytocin for the treatment of preterm labor. Its clinical utility is still under consideration and not currently available in the United States.[47]

GROWTH HORMONE, PROLACTIN, AND RELATED DRUGS

Growth Hormone

BASIC PHARMACOLOGY

GH is secreted from the anterior pituitary in a pulsatile manner. Secretion is high in childhood, maximal around the time of puberty, and decreases with age. Pituitary secretion is under the control of GH-releasing hormone (GHRH) and somatostatin from the hypothalamus, which increase and decrease GH secretion, respectively. Ghrelin (from the stomach) and IGF-1 (which mediates GH effects in the periphery) negatively feed back on GH release. GH is actually a mixture of peptides. A polypeptide of 191 amino acids is most prominent, and a 176 amino acid polypeptide makes up approximately 10% of secreted GH. These are bound to a number of GH-binding proteins. GH binds to specific cell surface receptors that are widely distributed. The hormone stimulates the longitudinal growth of bones, increases bone density when the epiphyses have closed, stimulates chondrocyte formation, and increases muscle mass. GH acts on the liver to stimulate gluconeogenesis and on fat cells to promote fat breakdown. It stimulates production of IGF-1 in liver and many tissues, and it is through IGF-1 that its anabolic action is mediated.

CLINICAL PHARMACOLOGY

Pharmaceutical GH is now produced by recombinant techniques, which has increased the safety of administration. Pharmacologic preparations include somatropin whose sequence matches that of native GH, and somatrem, a GH derivative. They have similar biologic activity but differ slightly in their method of preparation. The half-life of GH is less than 30 minutes, but its biologic half-life is up to 18 hours. GH is administered subcutaneously, once daily, or every second day, usually in the evening. Some preparations can also be given intramuscularly.

Adverse effects of GH administration include raised intracranial pressure manifesting as nausea, vomiting, headache, and visual changes. This is a rare complication but warrants periodic ophthalmoscopy to assess for the presence of papilledema. There could be an increased risk of cancers including leukemia, although the link is tenuous. GH is antagonistic to insulin and administration increases the risk of type 2 DM. Scoliosis and epiphyseal injuries have been associated with excessively rapid growth. In adults, arthralgias, myalgias, carpal tunnel syndrome, and peripheral edema can occur.

CLINICAL APPLICATION

GH is used as replacement therapy in children with short stature and severe GH deficiency. In addition, GH can be used in other conditions associated with short stature including Prader-Willi syndrome, Turner syndrome, and (somewhat controversially) in idiopathic short stature. It is also used in wasting associated with acquired immunodeficiency syndrome and for patients with short bowel syndrome.

Measurement of serum IGF-1 levels is used to monitor response in the initial phase of administration; later change in height is assessed. The duration of GH therapy must be individualized, although some children with GH deficiency require continuation of GH supplementation into adulthood.

Drugs Related to Growth Hormone

Sermorelin acetate is a synthetic analog of GHRH also available for treatment of GH deficiency. It is less effective than GH and not suitable for GH deficiency of pituitary origin. Recombinant human IGF-1 is also available for use in patients with GH resistance. Mecasermin is a complex of recombinant human IGF-1 and recombinant human IGF-binding protein-3 (rhIGFBP-3) used to treat children with severe IGF-1 deficiency unresponsive to GH. The rhIGFBP-3 is used to maintain an adequate half-life of the biologically active IGF-1. Subcutaneous administration can cause hypoglycemia and so should be given only around food ingestion. Elevations in intracranial pressure and liver blood tests can also occur. Pegvisomant is a GH receptor antagonist used in the treatment of acromegaly.[48] It is administered subcutaneously once daily with dosage adjusted to serum IGF-1 levels. It can cause liver dysfunction and, theoretically, loss of negative feedback of GH and IGF-1 can lead to increased growth of GH-secreting tumors.

Drugs Affecting Prolactin Physiology

Dopamine acts as an inhibitory transmitter for prolactin release. The release of prolactin from prolactin-secreting adenomas is also inhibited by dopamine and dopamine receptor agonists. Bromocriptine and cabergoline are ergot derivatives that act as dopamine-receptor agonists. Usually administered orally, they are useful in the treatment of hyperprolactinemia caused by prolactin-secreting pituitary tumors and in Parkinson disease, and can also be of use at higher doses in the suppression of GH release in acromegaly.[49] The half-life of bromocriptine (7 hours) is shorter than that of cabergoline (65 hours). Longer acting preparations of bromocriptine are available outside the United States. Side effects of dopamine agonists include headache, nausea and vomiting, postural hypotension, digital vasospasm, nasal congestion, nightmares, and insomnia. At high doses, pulmonary infiltrates and cardiac valvulopathies can develop. Bromocriptine was used for suppression of lactation and decrease of breast size when breast feeding was not desired, but this is no longer recommended because of the potential for coronary thrombosis and stroke. Pramipexole is a dopamine agonist used in the treatment of Parkinson disease and restless legs syndrome.[50]

SEX HORMONES AND RELATED DRUGS

Because many of these drugs are essentially identical to their endogenous hormone counterparts, their basic and clinical pharmacology behavior (i.e., structure-activity, mechanism, metabolism, pharmacokinetics, and clinical effects) mimic those of the endogenous hormones. Sex steroids include androgens, estrogens, and progestins. Their physiology is reviewed in Chapter 30.

Basic and Clinical Pharmacology

THE GONADOTROPINS

Gonadotropins include follicle stimulating hormone (FSH) and luteinizing hormone (LH). They are produced by the gonadotroph cells in the anterior pituitary. In women, both LH and FSH are involved in the production of ovarian steroids and in the regulation of the ovarian cycle. In men, FSH regulates spermatogenesis and supports developing sperm. LH stimulates testosterone production by Leydig cells. Human chorionic gonadotropin (hCG) controls estrogen and progesterone production during pregnancy. The three hormones have identical α chains and unique β chains, although the β chains of LH and hCG are very similar.

The gonadotropins are used in the treatment of infertility. They can stimulate spermatogenesis in men and induce ovulation in women. Preparations of FSH include urofollitropin or uFSH (a purified preparation of FSH extracted from the urine of postmenopausal women), and follitropin α and follitropin β (recombinant preparations). Lutropin α is recombinant human LH. It is used in association with follitropin α to stimulate follicle development in infertile women with LH deficiency. FSH and LH are also contained in human menopausal gonadotropins (hMG), which is another extract obtained from the urine of postmenopausal women. hCG is purified from the urine of pregnant women or made by recombinant techniques when it is known as choriogonadotropin α (rhCG). The former preparation is administered intramuscularly, the latter subcutaneously. It is typically used to cause final maturation of follicles and timed ovulation in assisted reproduction techniques.

Adverse effects of gonadotropin treatment include depression and emotional lability, headache, edema, and antibody production. Gynecomastia can be associated with gonadotropin treatment in men and is related to the level of treatment-associated testosterone production.

SEX STEROIDS

Androgens and Androgen Antagonists

Androgens include testosterone, dihydrotestosterone, and related compounds. They act through a specific androgen receptor. Hepatic metabolism limits the systemic availability of orally administered drug, so parenteral preparations are commonly used. Testosterone is used when there is a deficiency of endogenous testosterone, males with delayed puberty and hypogonadism, and inoperable breast cancer. A variety of compounds that activate the androgen receptor are also used in clinical practice. Therapeutic uses include catabolic and wasting states and, controversially, enhancement of athletic performance. Male contraception is a potential use for androgen administration but such therapy is still being refined. Administration of androgens is used to prevent attacks in both male and female patients with angioedema caused by C1-esterase inhibitor deficiency. Stanozolol and danazol, both of which are 17α-alkylated androgens, stimulate hepatic synthesis of the inhibitor. Danazol 200 mg is administered orally two to three times per day initially, with subsequent decrease in the long-term dose. If an attack occurs, dosage is increased by up to 200 mg/day. Side effects include hepatotoxicity and rarely benign intracranial hypertension. The drugs are also used to treat endometriosis and fibrocystic breast disease in women.

Nilutamide, bicalutamide, and flutamide are androgen receptor antagonists used in the treatment of metastatic prostate cancer. Nilutamide commonly causes visual changes and is associated with interstitial pneumonitis in 2% of recipients. All three drugs can cause hepatotoxicity and gynecomastia. Cyproterone is a weak antiandrogen used to reduce hirsutism. Finasteride and dutasteride antagonize the enzyme (5α-reductase) that converts testosterone to dihydrotestosterone. They are used in the treatment of benign prostatic hyperplasia and male-pattern baldness. Impotence and gynecomastia can occur as a result of their use.

Estrogens and Estrogen Antagonists

Estrogens and progestins are endogenous hormones that produce numerous physiologic actions, including developmental effects, control of ovulation and cyclical changes in the female reproductive tract, and actions on carbohydrate, protein, lipid, and mineral metabolism.[51]

Estrogens can be administered via oral, parenteral, transdermal, or topical routes. Oral drugs include estradiol, conjugated estrogens (including conjugated equine estrogens), esters of estrone and other estrogens, and ethinyl estradiol. The delivery of estrogens by transdermal patch allows a slow, sustained release of hormone to the systemic circulation. Preparations in oil are most suitable for intramuscular administration and have a prolonged duration of action. Estradiol and preparations of conjugated estrogen have been prepared for topical (vaginal) use. Systemic estrogens are bound to plasma proteins in varying degrees and metabolized in the liver. They also undergo enterohepatic circulation. Adverse effects of pharmacologic estrogen administration include nausea and vomiting, migraine headaches, breast tenderness, exacerbation of endometriosis, alterations in triglyceride and lipoprotein metabolism, increased risk of gynecologic malignancies, and increased risk of thromboembolic disease, especially in smokers.[52,53] In addition to thromboembolic disease, use of oral contraceptives is associated with hypertension, cholelithiasis, and the development of benign hepatomas.

Progestins and Progestin Antagonists

The progestins are compounds with actions similar to those of progesterone.[51] They include progesterone, a naturally occurring hormone, pregnanes (17α-acetoxyprogesterone derivatives), estranes (19-nortestosterone derivatives), and gonanes (norgestrel and related compounds). The progestins are used for contraception, either alone or in association with an estrogen, and are administered with estrogen as hormone replacement therapy in postmenopausal women. Progestins can be used in the diagnosis of secondary amenorrhea and can be employed to reduce endometrial hyperplasia induced by unopposed estrogens. Levonorgestrel is used as an emergency contraceptive measure. Mifepristone is an antiprogestin that can be used for termination of pregnancy. It is a derivative of the 19-norprogestin norethindrone and acts as a competitive antagonist at progesterone receptors. Mifepristone is orally active, has good bioavailability, and undergoes liver metabolism and enterohepatic circulation. Effects depend on the phase of the cycle in which it is administered. It can cause breakdown of the decidua, delay or prevent ovulation, and impair the development of a secretory endometrium. Ulipristal is another 19-norprogestin derivative that acts as a selective progesterone receptor modulator. It can be used as an emergency contraceptive for at least 72 hours after unprotected intercourse. Adverse effects include nausea, abdominal pain, and headache.

Clinical Application

GONADOTROPINS

In women with anovulation (e.g., those with polycystic ovarian syndrome or hypogonadotropic hypogonadism), gonadotropins are used to induce ovulation. They are also used for controlled ovarian hyperstimulation in assisted reproduction techniques. Careful monitoring of their effects using blood hormone concentrations and ultrasound visualization of the ovaries is required as they can cause ovarian hyperstimulation syndrome and multiple pregnancies. Ovarian hyperstimulation occurs in up to 4% of patients and, on occasion, a cycle might need to be abandoned because of the risk of hyperstimulation. Ovarian hyperstimulation results in painful ovarian enlargement, ascites, pleural effusions, and potentially intravascular volume depletion. Fever, ovarian cyst rupture, and thromboembolism can also occur. Treatment of infertility in men who have hypogonadism requires stimulation of FSH and LH by gonadotropins. hCG and hMG are administered for this purpose, although rFSH and rLH have been used more recently.

ESTROGENS

Estrogens are administered to decrease vasomotor symptoms, bone fractures, and urogenital atrophy in menopausal women. The long-term effects of estrogens on cardiovascular risk in postmenopausal women is a matter of debate.[54,55] In addition, estrogens are commonly administered as a component (with progestins) of combination oral contraceptive regimens. The combination of hormones inhibits ovulation by a negative feedback mechanism that prevents release of FSH and LH. A less frequent, but accepted, indication for estrogen treatment is in the setting of failure of ovarian development (e.g., Turner syndrome) in which estrogens are administered to induce puberty.

Selective estrogen receptor modulators (SERMs) are drugs that produce beneficial estrogen effects in some tissues (e.g., bone) and antagonize estrogen effects in others (e.g., breast), also with beneficial intent. Tamoxifen, administered orally, is the hormonal therapy of choice in women with early and advanced breast cancer and is used as palliative therapy in women with advanced breast cancer who have estrogen receptor positive tumors. Adverse effects include hot flashes and increased risk of thromboembolic disease and endometrial cancer. It is metabolized in the liver by cytochrome P450, and induces the activity of some isoforms. Metabolism to its more potent 4-hydroxy metabolite is influenced by genetic polymorphisms. Toremifene is similar to tamoxifen in structure and activity. Raloxifene is used to reduce the risk of breast cancer in postmenopausal women and in the prevention and treatment of osteoporosis. It inhibits proliferation of estrogen receptor-positive breast cancer cells and has an antiresorptive effect on bone that leads to a reduction in the incidence of vertebral fractures.

Clomiphene and fulvestrant antagonize the action of estrogen in all tissues. The former is used in the treatment of female infertility due to anovulation. Administered orally, it increases gonadotrophin levels and enhances follicular recruitment. Adverse effects of clomiphene include ovarian hyperstimulation, multiple births, ovarian cysts, hot flashes, and visual changes. Prolonged use might increase the risk of ovarian cancer. Fulvestrant is used in patients with advanced breast cancer.

HORMONAL CONTRACEPTIVES

Most oral contraceptives employ a combination of an estrogen and a progestin, with a theoretical efficacy of greater than 99.9%.[51] They are usually presented in 28-day packs, with pills for days 22 to 28 being inert. Preparations are monophasic, biphasic, or triphasic, depending on the relative amounts of estrogens and progestins, in an attempt to more closely mimic the natural menstrual cycle and limit the amount of hormone administered. Most preparations contain 30 to 35 μg of estrogen; those containing less than 35 μg are referred to as "low-dose." Preparations containing a combination of norelgestromin and ethinyl estradiol are available as patches and as an intravaginal ring. Combination contraceptives act by influencing the hypothalamic-pituitary-ovarian axis at multiple levels, but ultimately prevent ovulation, especially by suppressing FSH and LH.

Adverse effects of combination oral contraceptives are related to the dose of estrogen used and newer low-estrogen preparations have decreased risks.[56] Side effects include increased risk of venous thromboembolic disease, especially in women who smoke, myocardial infarction in smokers and those with other risk factors, hepatic adenomas and hepatocellular carcinoma, and cervical cancer in long-term oral contraceptive users who also have human papilloma virus infection. Combination oral contraceptives decrease the risk of endometrial and ovarian cancers. An association with breast cancer is controversial. Combination oral contraceptives are contraindicated in patients with active or previous thromboembolic disease, cerebrovascular disease, myocardial infarction, congenital hyperlipidemia, liver tumors or significant dysfunction, and certain cancers. The risk of cardiovascular side effects is significantly increased if combination oral contraceptives are administered to smokers older than 35 years.

Progestin-only preparations are also available. They block ovulation in only 60% to 80% of cycles but cause a thickening of cervical mucus that decreases sperm penetration and cause endometrial alterations that impair implantation. They have a slightly decreased theoretical efficacy (99%) compared to combination preparations. They are taken in pill form, administered intramuscularly, or placed subdermally or intravaginally. Side effects include breakthrough bleeding, headache, and alterations in lipid metabolism. The progestin-only preparations are contraindicated in liver disease, breast cancer, and undiagnosed vaginal bleeding.

PARATHYROID HORMONE AND DRUGS AFFECTING CALCIUM METABOLISM

Parathyroid hormone (PTH) helps regulate extracellular fluid Ca^{2+} concentration.[57] It influences bone osteoclast activity, renal distal tubular reabsorption of Ca^{2+}, and gastrointestinal Ca^{2+} absorption, the latter through its regulation of the synthesis of 1,25 dihydroxycholecalciferol (calcitriol). PTH also affects renal absorption of phosphate and bicarbonate. PTH secretion is regulated primarily by serum $[Ca^{2+}]$ and is influenced by phosphate, Mg^{2+}, and catecholamine levels.[58] The actions of PTH on metabolism are shown in Figure 31-5. See Chapter 30 for a more detailed discussion of PTH physiology. PTH is derived from pre-proparathyroid hormone, and subsequently from proparathyroid hormone, neither of which appears in plasma. During periods of hypocalcemia, PTH secretion is increased. The half-life of PTH in the plasma is 2 to 5 minutes. It is cleared mainly by the liver and kidneys. The physiologic effects of PTH on target tissues are mediated by PTH-specific G protein–coupled receptors.

With high levels of circulating PTH (e.g., in primary hyperparathyroidism), bone demineralization and osteopenia occur. PTH can be administered intermittently however, and this promotes bone growth. Teriparatide is recombinant human PTH 1-34 (a 34 amino acid terminal PTH fragment) used for the treatment of osteoporosis in postmenopausal women at high risk for fracture, as well as hypogonadal or primary osteoporosis in men and osteoporosis due to glucocorticoid administration.[59] Teriparatide reduces the risk of vertebral and nonvertebral fractures. Given via the subcutaneous route, it causes an increased serum Ca^{2+} that peaks at 4 to 6 hours. Adverse effects include transient hypercalcemia, orthostatic hypotension, chest pain, and syncope as well as gastrointestinal upset. It is also associated with the development of osteosarcoma in animals.

Vitamin D is used therapeutically for prevention and treatment of osteoporosis, prophylaxis against, and cure of, nutritional rickets, treatment of chronic renal failure metabolic rickets osteomalacia, and hypoparathyroidism. A number of preparations are available. Calcitriol (1,25-dihydroxy cholecalciferol) is administered orally or by injection. Doxercalciferol (1α- hydroxyvitamin D_2) is administered orally or

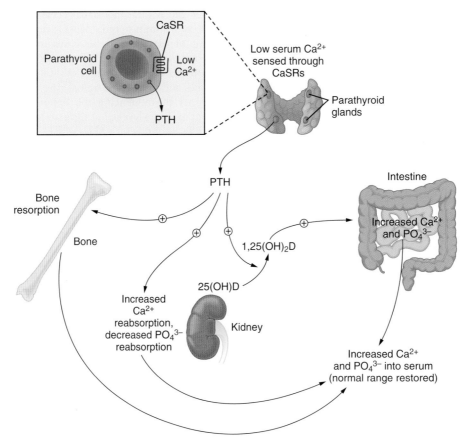

Figure 31-5 Control of mineral metabolism by parathyroid hormone. Levels of serum ionized calcium (Ca^{2+}) are tightly controlled through the action of parathyroid hormone (PTH) and 1,25-dihydroxyvitamin D (1,25[OH]$_2$D). Both the rate and magnitude of changes in serum ionized Ca^{2+} concentration are detected by extracellular Ca^{2+}-sensing receptors (CaSRs) expressed on parathyroid cells. When ionized Ca^{2+} decreases, release of PTH is triggered. Conversely, when ionized Ca^{2+} levels increase, PTH secretion is suppressed. PTH stimulates bone resorption, which delivers Ca^{2+} and phosphorus (PO_4^{3-}) into the circulation. In the kidney, PTH stimulates renal reabsorption of Ca^{2+} and promotes phosphate excretion. PTH also enhances the conversion of 25-hydroxyvitamin D (25[OH]D) to the active vitamin D metabolite 1,25(OH)2D, which increases transepithelial transport of Ca^{2+} and PO_4^{3-} through actions in intestinal cells. In concert, these steps restore ionized Ca^{2+} to the normal range, and through the actions of PTH and other factors (e.g., fibroblast-derived growth factor 23) in the kidney, reset the level of serum PO4 $^{3-}$ within the normal range. When the actions of PTH are reduced or lost, subsequent steps in the maintenance of homeostasis are impaired, resulting in hypocalcemia, hyperphosphatemia, and hypercalciuria. *(From Shoback D. Clinical practice. Hypoparathyroidism. N Engl J Med. 2008;359:391-403.)*

intravenously for the treatment of secondary hyperparathyroidism. It requires activation in the liver by 25-hydroxylation. Dihydrotachysterol is another form of vitamin D that requires activation in the liver. At high doses it mobilizes bone mineral and is used in the treatment of hypoparathyroidism. Ergocalciferol is used for prevention of vitamin D deficiency as well as therapeutically for the treatment of hypoparathyroidism, certain types of rickets and familial hypophosphatemia.

Calcitonin is a single chain peptide hormone secreted by the parafollicular C cells of the thyroid. It circulates in very low concentrations in plasma and causes hypocalcemia and hypophosphatemia by inhibition of osteoclastic bone resorption. The actions of calcitonin oppose those of PTH, although it does not appear essential for Ca^{2+} homeostasis. It is used pharmacologically to treat hypercalcemia (especially hypercalcemia related to malignancy), osteoporosis, and Paget disease. The therapeutic agent is derived from salmon or eel and administered subcutaneously, intramuscularly, or intranasally. Side effects are usually associated with the nasal route of administration and include rhinitis, flushing, back pain, and rare allergic reactions.

Cinacalcet mimics the effect of Ca^{2+} to inhibit PTH secretion (i.e., it is a calcimimetic) and lowers the concentration of Ca^{2+} at which PTH secretion is suppressed. It is used for the treatment of secondary hyperparathyroidism due to chronic renal disease and for patients with hypercalcemia associated with parathyroid carcinoma. Cinacalcet can cause hypocalcemia, which is especially problematic in patients prone to seizures.

Pyrophosphate analogues with two phosphate groups attached to a central carbon are known as bisphosphonates.[60] The bisphosphonates have a strong affinity for bone because their physical structure allows them to chelate Ca^{2+}. They inhibit bone resorption by concentrating at sites of active remodeling where they are absorbed into the bone matrix and subsequently inhibit osteoclasts. They also decrease osteoclast numbers. Members of this class include etidronate, zoledronate, pamidronate, alendronate, tiludronate, and risedronate. Bisphosphonates have limited bioavailability (1%-6%) when given orally because they are very poorly absorbed from the gastrointestinal tract and can be given intravenously to avoid this problem. Excretion is primarily renal, and poor renal function is a relative contraindication. Zoledronate can be nephrotoxic. The bisphosphonates can cause osteomalacia, especially the first generation bisphosphonate etidronate, and esophagitis. Although hypocalcemia associated with their use is unusual, it can occur especially in patients with malignancy. Intravenous administration can cause myalgias and fevers. Oral bisphosphonates increase phosphate retention in the tubules. The bisphosphonates are used in postmenopausal osteoporosis, Paget disease, corticosteroid-associated bone loss, and hypercalcemia due to malignancy.[61] They are also used for patients with multiple myeloma and metastatic breast cancer. They can be given as infrequently as weekly or monthly.

EMERGING DEVELOPMENTS

Glycemic Control in the Perioperative Period and in the Critically Ill

There is considerable controversy regarding optimal blood glucose concentration in the perioperative period and in critically ill patients.[62] Significant hyperglycemia is associated with multiple adverse effects including increased incidence of surgical site infections. Certain patient populations are adversely affected by hyperglycemia (e.g., patients with acute myocardial infarction, neurologic injury). In 2001, a single center study suggested that targeting "tight" glycemic control (80-110 mg/dL; 4.4-6.1 mM) in critically ill patients improved outcomes.[63] Over the course of the subsequent decade, glycemic control targets were lowered and the use of insulin infusions in the ICU became commonplace. Many practitioners extrapolated these data and targeted tighter glycemic control in the operating room. Quality initiatives also encouraged tighter glycemic control. However, the potential for hypoglycemia exists when intensive insulin therapy is employed. Hypoglycemia is associated with adverse neurologic outcomes and is a feared perioperative complication. Further data suggested that hypoglycemia in critically ill patients was independently associated with poor outcome. A number of studies and metaanalyses failed to demonstrate beneficial effects of "tight" glycemic control, and raised the question of whether the practice was, in fact, detrimental. The NICE SUGAR study, a prospective multicenter, multinational randomized controlled trial comparing tight glycemic control (target glucose 81-108 mg/dL; 4.5-6 mM) with conventional glycemic control (target glucose <180 mg/dL; 10 mM) failed to demonstrate a beneficial effect of intensive insulin therapy and, in fact, demonstrated increased mortality in the intensive insulin therapy group (Figure 31-6).[64] Current guidelines suggest that in-hospital glucose should be kept between 140 and 180 mg/dL (7.8-10 mM).[65]

Steroid Supplementation During Critical Illness

Steroid supplementation in the setting of severe sepsis and septic shock has also been a topic of debate over the past decade. Adrenal insufficiency can be a feature of the so-called endocrinopathy of critical illness.[66] Initial data suggested that supplementation with hydrocortisone and fludrocortisone in patients with septic shock improved outcomes.[67] The choice and dose of steroids, the need for performance of an ACTH test, the duration of steroid use, and the choice of patients in whom steroid supplementation is necessary are controversial. Recent multicenter studies, however, have failed to demonstrate any benefit to steroid administration in septic shock.[68,69]

High-dose corticosteroid administration in the early phase of the acute respiratory distress syndrome (ARDS) does not offer significant advantages. Low-dose steroids have been used in the fibroproliferative stage of ARDS to decrease the fibrosing alveolitis. A multicenter study demonstrated that in patients in whom ARDS had been present for 7 days, administration of a course of methylprednisolone allowed earlier liberation from mechanical ventilatory support, but ultimately no difference in outcome.[70]

Hormone Supplementation in Potential Organ Donors

A consensus conference on management of patients with brain death who are potential organ donors recommended that four-drug hormonal resuscitation (T_3, vasopressin, methylprednisolone, and insulin) be an integral component of donor management protocols.[71] Methylprednisolone 15/mg kg bolus, T_3 (4 µg bolus, then an infusion at 3 µg/hr),

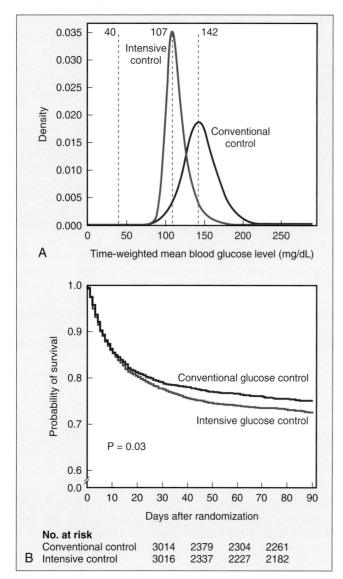

Figure 31-6. A, Density plot for the mean time-weighted blood glucose levels for individual patients in the NICE SUGAR study. Dashed lines indicate the modes in the intensive-control group *(blue)* and the conventional control group *(purple)*, as well as the upper threshold for severe hypoglycemia (40 mg/dl). **B,** Kaplan-Meier plots demonstrating improved survival with conventional glycemic control versus intensive glycemic control (*P* = 0.03) in the NICE SUGAR study. *(From Finfer S, Chittock DR, Su SY, et al. Intensive versus conventional glucose control in critically ill patients.* N Engl J Med. *2009;360:1283-1297.)*

arginine vasopressin (1 unit bolus, then 0.5-4 units/hr), and insulin (infused at a minimum of 1 unit/hr, titrating blood glucose to 120-180 mg/dL) are recommended. Hormonal supplementation is considered to increase the number of organs transplanted and to improve graft and recipient survival. The utility of thyroid hormone supplementation in the potential organ donor is supported by most clinical data, although conflicting data have also been published.[72] Corticosteroids are used to attenuate the effects of inflammatory cytokines generated as a result of brain death. In addition to potential advantages in lung donors, steroids have been demonstrated to improve graft survival after renal and cardiac

transplantation. Vasopressin is used to improve donor hemodynamics and insulin is used to optimize glycemic control that can result in improved graft function.

Key References

Banting FG, Best CH, Collip JB, et al. Pancreatic extracts in the treatment of diabetes mellitus. *Can Med Assoc J*. 1922;12:141-146. The original description of the use of insulin for the treatment of diabetes mellitus, work that resulted in a Nobel Prize. (Ref. 1)

Finfer S, Chittock DR, Su SY, et al. Intensive versus conventional glucose control in critically ill patients. *N Engl J Med*. 2009;360:1283-1297. An international prospective randomized control trial of more than 6000 critically ill adults comparing intensive glucose control with conventional glucose control. This landmark study demonstrated that, contrary to previous data, intensive glycemic control increased mortality. (Ref. 64)

Haahtela T, Jarvinen M, Kava T, et al. Comparison of a beta 2-agonist, terbutaline, with an inhaled corticosteroid, budesonide, in newly detected asthma. *N Engl J Med*. 1991;325:388-392. A prospective, randomized trial in patients with recently diagnosed, mild asthma, demonstrating the superiority of antiinflammatory therapy with inhaled budesonide over the use of inhaled terbutaline. (Ref. 23)

Hench PS, Kendall EC, Slocumb CH, et al. Effects of cortisone acetate and pituitary ACTH on rheumatoid arthritis, rheumatic fever, and certain other conditions. *Arch Intern Med (Chic)*. 1950;85:545-666. The original description of the use of corticosteroids for the treatment of rheumatoid arthritis and other inflammatory conditions, which resulted in a Nobel Prize. (Ref. 19)

Hulley S, Grady D, Bush T, et al. Randomized trial of estrogen plus progestin for secondary prevention of coronary heart disease in postmenopausal women. Heart and Estrogen/progestin Replacement Study (HERS) Research Group. *JAMA*. 1998;280:605-613.

In a study of more than 2700 postmenopausal women with established coronary disease, administration of estrogen and progesterone did not reduce the overall rate of cardiovascular events (Ref. 54)

Landry DW, Levin HR, Gallant EM, et al. Vasopressin deficiency contributes to the vasodilation of septic shock. *Circulation*. 1997;95:1122-1125. A small but important study demonstrating that vasopressin plasma levels are inappropriately low in vasodilatory shock, which led to a new therapeutic intervention. (Ref. 37)

Sprung CL, Annane D, Keh D, et al. Hydrocortisone therapy for patients with septic shock. *N Engl J Med*. 2008;358:111-124. A multicenter, randomized, double-blind, placebo-controlled trial that compared administration of intravenous hydrocortisone with placebo in patients with septic shock. Hydrocortisone did not improve survival or reversal of shock either overall or in patients who did not have a response to ACTH. (Ref. 68)

Steinberg KP, Hudson LD, Goodman RB, et al. Efficacy and safety of corticosteroids for persistent acute respiratory distress syndrome. *N Engl J Med*. 2006;354:1671-1684. A prospective, randomized trial from the Acute Respiratory Distress Syndrome Network (ARDSNet) in 180 patients with persistent ARDS that demonstrated lack of benefit and potential harm from the nonselective use of steroids. (Ref. 70)

Zaroff JG, Rosengard BR, Armstrong WF, et al. Consensus conference report: maximizing use of organs recovered from the cadaver donor: cardiac recommendations, March 28-29, 2001, Crystal City, Va. *Circulation*. 2002;106:836-841. A consensus conference involving members of the transplant community focusing on maximizing use of organs recovered from brain dead donors. Specific recommendations for hormonal supplementation have been incorporated into many management protocols. (Ref. 71)

References

1. Banting FG, Best CH, Collip JB, Campbell WR, Fletcher AA. Pancreatic extracts in the treatment of diabetes mellitus. *Can Med Assoc J*. 1922;12:141-146.
2. Powers A, D'Alessio D. Endocrine pancreas and pharmacotherapy of diabetes mellitus and hypoglycemia. In: Brunton L, Chabner B, Knollmann B, eds. *Goodman & Gilman's The Pharmacological Basis of Therapeutics*. 12th ed. New York: McGraw Hill; 2011.
3. Hirsch IB. Insulin analogues. *N Engl J*. 2005;352:174-183.
4. McMahon GT, Arky RA. Inhaled insulin for diabetes mellitus. *N Engl J Med*. 2007;356:497-502.
5. American Diabetes Association. Standards of medical care in diabetes. *Diabetes Care*. 2012;35(Suppl 1).
6. UK Prospective Diabetes Study (UKPDS) Group. A 6-year, randomized, controlled trial comparing sulfonylurea, insulin, and metformin therapy in patients with newly diagnosed type 2 diabetes that could not be controlled with diet therapy (UKPDS 24). *Ann Intern Med*. 1998;128:165-175.
7. UK Prospective Diabetes Study (UKPDS) Group. Intensive blood-glucose control with sulphonylureas or insulin compared with conventional treatment and risk of complications in patients with type 2 diabetes (UKPDS 33). *Lancet*. 1998;352:837-853.
8. Diamanti-Kandarakis E, Economou F, Palimeri S, Christakou C. Metformin in polycystic ovary syndrome. *Ann N Y Acad Sci*. 2010;1205:192-198.
9. Duncan AI, Koch CG, Xu M, et al. Recent metformin ingestion does not increase in-hospital morbidity or mortality after cardiac surgery. *Anesth Analg*. 2007;104:42-50.
10. Chen D, Lee SL, Peterfreund RA. New therapeutic agents for diabetes mellitus: implications for anesthetic management. *Anesth Analg*. 2009;108:1803-1810.
11. Habegger KM, Heppner KM, Geary N, Bartness TJ, DiMarchi R, Tschop MH. The metabolic actions of glucagon revisited. *Nat Rev Endocrinol*. 2010;6:689-697.
12. Brent G, Koenig R. Thyroid and anti-thyroid drugs. In: Brunton L, Chabner B, Knollmann B, eds. *Goodman & Gilman's The Pharmacological Basis of Therapeutics*. New York: McGraw Hill; 2011.
13. Ross DS. Radioiodine therapy for hyperthyroidism. *N Engl J Med*. 2011;364:542-550.
14. Ron E, Doody MM, Becker DV, et al. Cancer mortality following treatment for adult hyperthyroidism. Cooperative Thyrotoxicosis Therapy Follow-up Study Group. *JAMA*. 1998;280:347-355.
15. Kinney MA, Warner ME, vanHeerden JA, et al. Perianesthetic risks and outcomes of pheochromocytoma and paraganglioma resection. *Anesth Analg*. 2000;91:1118-1123.
16. Prys-Roberts C, Farndon JR. Efficacy and safety of doxazosin for perioperative management of patients with pheochromocytoma. *World J Surg*. 2002;26:1037-1042.
17. Pacak K. Preoperative management of the pheochromocytoma patient. *J Clin Endocrinol Metab*. 2007;92:4069-4079.
18. Weingarten TN, Cata JP, O'Hara JF, et al. Comparison of two preoperative medical management strategies for laparoscopic resection of pheochromocytoma. *Urology*. 2010;76:508 e6-11.
19. Hench PS, Kendall EC, Slocumb CH, Polley HF. Effects of cortisone acetate and pituitary ACTH on rheumatoid arthritis, rheumatic fever and certain other conditions. *Arch Intern Med (Chic)*. 1950;85:545-666.
20. Rhen T, Cidlowski JA. Antiinflammatory action of glucocorticoids—new mechanisms for old drugs. *N Engl J Med*. 2005;353:1711-1723.
21. Schimmer B, Funder J. ACTH, adrenal steroids, and pharmacology of the adrenal cortex. In: Brunton L, Chabner B, Knollmann B, eds. *Goodman & Gilman's The Pharmacological Basis of Therapeutics*. New York: McGraw Hill; 2011.
22. Pauwels RA, Pedersen S, Busse WW, et al. Early intervention with budesonide in mild persistent asthma: a randomised, double-blind trial. *Lancet*. 2003;361:1071-1076.
23. Haahtela T, Jarvinen M, Kava T, et al. Comparison of a beta 2-agonist, terbutaline, with an inhaled corticosteroid, budesonide, in newly detected asthma. *N Engl J Med*. 1991;325:388-392.
24. Gomes JA, Stevens RD, Lewin 3rd JJ, Mirski MA, Bhardwaj A. Glucocorticoid therapy in neurologic critical care. *Crit Care Med*. 2005;33:1214-1224.
25. Bracken MB, Collins WF, Freeman DF, et al. Efficacy of methylprednisolone in acute spinal cord injury. *JAMA*. 1984;251:45-52.
26. Bracken MB, Shepard MJ, Collins WF, et al. A randomized, controlled trial of methylprednisolone or naloxone in the treatment of acute spinal-cord injury. Results of the Second National Acute Spinal Cord Injury Study. *N Engl J Med*. 1990;322:1405-1411.
27. Wang JJ, Ho ST, Tzeng JI, Tang CS. The effect of timing of dexamethasone administration on its efficacy as a prophylactic antiemetic for postoperative nausea and vomiting. *Anesth Analg*. 2000;91:136-139.
28. McCaffrey J, Farrell C, Whiting P, Dan A, Bagshaw SM, Delaney AP. Corticosteroids to prevent extubation failure: a systematic review and meta-analysis. *Intensive Care Med*. 2009;35:977-986.
29. van Staa TP, Leufkens HG, Abenhaim L, Begaud B, Zhang B, Cooper C. Use of oral corticosteroids in the United Kingdom. *Q J Med*. 2000;93:105-111.
30. Coursin DB, Wood KE. Corticosteroid supplementation for adrenal insufficiency. *JAMA*. 2002;287:236-240.
31. Yong SL, Marik P, Esposito M, Coulthard P. Supplemental perioperative steroids for surgical patients with adrenal insufficiency. *Cochrane Database Syst Rev*. 2009;CD005367.
32. Jansen PM, Danser AH, Imholz BP, van den Meiracker AH. Aldosterone-receptor antagonism in hypertension. *J Hypertens*. 2009;27:680-691.
33. Albert SG, Ariyan S, Rather A. The effect of etomidate on adrenal function in critical illness: a systematic review. *Intensive Care Med*. 2011;37:901-910.
34. Barrett LK, Singer M, Clapp LH. Vasopressin: mechanisms of action on the vasculature in health and in septic shock. *Crit Care Med*. 2007;35:33-40.
35. Dunser MW, Fries DR, Schobersberger W, et al. Does arginine vasopressin influence the coagulation system in advanced vasodilatory shock with severe multiorgan dysfunction syndrome? *Anesth Analg*. 2004;99:201-206.
36. Smith JG, Merrill DC. Oxytocin for induction of labor. *Clin Obstet Gynecol*. 2006;49:594-608.
37. Landry DW, Levin HR, Gallant EM, et al. Vasopressin deficiency contributes to the vasodilation of septic shock. *Circulation*. 1997;95:1122-1125.
38. Kampmeier TG, Rehberg S, Westphal M, Lange M. Vasopressin in sepsis and septic shock. *Minerva Anesthesiol*. 2010;76:844-850.

39. Russell JA, Walley KR, Singer J, et al. Vasopressin versus norepinephrine infusion in patients with septic shock. *N Engl J Med.* 2008;358:877-887.

40. Wenzel V, Krismer AC, Arntz HR, Sitter H, Stadlbauer KH, Lindner KH. A comparison of vasopressin and epinephrine for out-of-hospital cardiopulmonary resuscitation. *N Engl J Med.* 2004; 350:105-113.

41. Levy JH. Pharmacologic methods to reduce perioperative bleeding. *Transfusion.* 2008;48:31S-38S.

42. Dyer RA, Butwick AJ, Carvalho B. Oxytocin for labour and caesarean delivery: implications for the anaesthesiologist. *Curr Opin Anaesthesiol.* 2011;24:255-261.

43. Gluud LL, Christensen K, Christensen E, Krag A. Systematic review of randomized trials on vasoconstrictor drugs for hepatorenal syndrome. *Hepatology.* 2010;51:576-584.

44. Gassanov N, Semmo N, Semmo M, Nia AM, Fuhr U, Er F. Arginine vasopressin (AVP) and treatment with arginine vasopressin receptor antagonists (vaptans) in congestive heart failure, liver cirrhosis and syndrome of inappropriate antidiuretic hormone secretion (SIADH). *Eur J Clin Pharmacol.* 2011;67:333-346.

45. Schrier RW, Gross P, Gheorghiade M, et al. Tolvaptan, a selective oral vasopressin V$_2$-receptor antagonist, for hyponatremia. *N Engl J Med.* 2006;355:2099-2112.

46. O'Leary JG, Davis GL. Conivaptan increases serum sodium in hyponatremic patients with end-stage liver disease. *Liver Transpl.* 2009; 15:1325-1329.

47. Usta IM, Khalil A, Nassar AH. Oxytocin antagonists for the management of preterm birth: a review. *Am J Perinatol.* 2010;28:449-460.

48. Melmed S. Medical progress: acromegaly. *N Engl J Med.* 2006;355: 2558-2573.

49. Sherlock M, Woods C, Sheppard MC. Medical therapy in acromegaly. *Nat Rev Endocrinol.* 2011;7:291-300.

50. Kushida CA. Pramipexole for the treatment of restless legs syndrome. *Expert Opin Pharmacother.* 2006;7:441-451.

51. Levin E, Hammes S. Estrogens and progestins. In: Brunton L, Chabner B, Knollmann B, eds. *Goodman & Gilman's The Pharmacological Basis of Therapeutics.* New York: McGraw Hill; 2011.

52. Grady D, Wenger NK, Herrington D, et al. Postmenopausal hormone therapy increases risk for venous thromboembolic disease. The Heart and Estrogen/Progestin Replacement Study. *Ann Intern Med.* 2000;132:689-696.

53. Rossouw JE, Anderson GL, Prentice RL, et al. Risks and benefits of estrogen plus progestin in healthy postmenopausal women: principal results from the Women's Health Initiative randomized controlled trial. *JAMA.* 2002;288:321-333.

54. Hulley S, Grady D, Bush T, et al. Randomized trial of estrogen plus progestin for secondary prevention of coronary heart disease in postmenopausal women. Heart and Estrogen/Progestin Replacement Study (HERS) Research Group. *JAMA.* 1998;280:605-613.

55. Grady D, Herrington D, Bittner V, et al. Cardiovascular disease outcomes during 6.8 years of hormone therapy: Heart and Estrogen/progestin Replacement Study follow-up (HERS II). *JAMA.* 2002;288:49-57.

56. Burkman R, Schlesselman JJ, Zieman M. Safety concerns and health benefits associated with oral contraception. *Am J Obstet Gynecol.* 2004;190:S5-S22.

57. Friedman P. Agents affecting mineral ion homeostasis and bone turnover. In: Brunton L, Chabner B, Knollmann B, eds. *Goodman & Gilman's The Pharmacological Basis of Therapeutics.* New York: McGraw Hill; 2011.

58. Shoback D. Clinical practice. Hypoparathyroidism. *N Engl J.* 2008; 359:391-403.

59. Reeve J. Recombinant human parathyroid hormone. *Br Med J.* 2002;324:435-436.

60. Licata AA. Discovery, clinical development, and therapeutic uses of bisphosphonates. *Ann Pharmacother.* 2005;39:668-677.

61. Favus MJ. Bisphosphonates for osteoporosis. *N Engl J Med.* 2010; 363:2027-2035.

62. Akhtar S, Barash PG, Inzucchi SE. Scientific principles and clinical implications of perioperative glucose regulation and control. *Anesth Analg.* 2010;110:478-497.

63. van den Berghe G, Wouters P, Weekers F, et al. Intensive insulin therapy in the critically ill patients. *N Engl J Med.* 2001;345:1359-1367.

64. Finfer S, Chittock DR, Su SY, et al. Intensive versus conventional glucose control in critically ill patients. *N Engl J Med.* 2009;360: 1283-1297.

65. Moghissi E, Korytkowski M, DiNardo M, et al. American Association of Clinical Endocrinologists and American Diabetes Association Consensus statement on inpatient glycemic control. *Endocrine Practice.* 2009;15:353-369.

66. Marik PE. Critical illness-related corticosteroid insufficiency. *Chest.* 2009;135:181-193.

67. Annane D, Sebille V, Charpentier C, et al. Effect of treatment with low doses of hydrocortisone and fludrocortisone on mortality in patients with septic shock. *JAMA.* 2002;288:862-871.

68. Sprung CL, Annane D, Keh D, et al. Hydrocortisone therapy for patients with septic shock. *N Engl J Med.* 2008;358:111-124.

69. Annane D, Cariou A, Maxime V, et al. Corticosteroid treatment and intensive insulin therapy for septic shock in adults: a randomized controlled trial. *JAMA.* 2010;303:341-348.

70. Steinberg KP, Hudson LD, Goodman RB, et al. Efficacy and safety of corticosteroids for persistent acute respiratory distress syndrome. *N Engl J Med.* 2006;354:1671-1684.

71. Zaroff JG, Rosengard BR, Armstrong WF, et al. Consensus conference report: maximizing use of organs recovered from the cadaver donor: cardiac recommendations, March 28-29, 2001, Crystal City, Va. *Circulation.* 2002;106:836-841.

72. Cooper DK, Novitzky D, Wicomb WN, Basker M, Rosendale JD, Myron Kauffman H. A review of studies relating to thyroid hormone therapy in brain-dead organ donors. *Front Biosci.* 2009;14:3750-3770.

Section V

FLUID, ELECTROLYTE, AND HEMATOLOGIC HOMEOSTASIS

RENAL PHYSIOLOGY

Joseph Meltzer

The kidney is a complex multifunctional organ that can be affected by anesthesia and the physiologic alterations of the perioperative period. The main functions of the kidney as related to anesthesia are (1) regulation of salt and water balance, (2) toxin and metabolite elimination (including drugs), (3) electrolyte homeostasis, (4) acid-base balance, and (5) hormone production. If these functions are not understood and recognized, significant problems can arise during and after surgery or intensive care. The anesthetist must understand the kidney's role in salt and water balance or else hypovolemia, volume overload, or acute renal failure can complicate surgery. The elimination of toxins and metabolites is important in the perioperative period; this function also includes the elimination of many anesthetic drugs, which can be viewed as exogenous toxins. Electrolyte balance is key for cardiovascular stability and prevention of dysrhythmias. Acid-base balance and maintenance of pH are vital for proper enzyme and cellular function. Hormones such as renin and erythropoietin play critical roles in blood pressure regulation and red blood cell production, critical concerns during the perioperative period. These many functions of the kidney help maintain homeostasis during periods of changing fluid and electrolyte intake and losses. Figure 32-1 shows the anatomic position and blood supply of the kidneys.

RENAL BLOOD FLOW AND GLOMERULAR FILTRATION RATE

Renal Blood Flow

The kidney is the most robustly perfused organ per gram of tissue in the human body, receiving 20% to 25% of cardiac output. Renal blood flow (RBF) is directly proportional to the "trans-renal gradient," the pressure difference between the renal artery and renal vein. RBF is inversely proportional to the resistance of the renal vasculature. Autoregulation of RBF is accomplished by changing renal vascular resistance as arterial pressure changes, thereby maintaining constant blood flow across a range of mean arterial pressure from 50 to 150 mmHg in normotensive people.[1]

While global RBF is relatively constant, its distribution within the kidney is quite heterogeneous. The renal cortex and renal cortical nephrons receive 90% of the RBF while the renal medulla and its juxtamedullary nephrons receive only

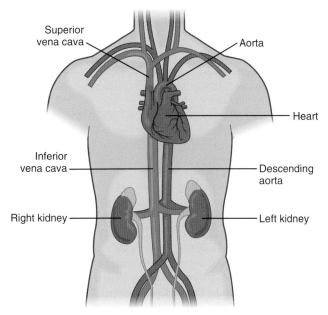

Figure 32-1 The anatomic position of the kidney. The kidneys are retro-peritoneal organs attached to the abdominal aorta and inferior vena cava by the renal arteries and veins, respectively. The right kidney most often lies caudal to the left kidney, inferior to the liver.

about 10%. This great disparity in regional blood flow makes the renal medulla sensitive to ischemic injury. RBF is calculated by determining both the clearance of a given substance from the plasma and the renal plasma flow (RPF).

Renal Clearance

The renal clearance of a substance is the volume of plasma completely cleared of a substance per unit time.

$$C = U \times V/P \qquad [1]$$

where C = clearance in mL/min or mL/24 hr; U = urine concentration in mg/min; V = urine volume/time in mL/min; P = plasma concentration in mg/mL.

Renal Plasma Flow

RPF is calculated by the clearance of para-aminohippuric acid (PAH), as at low concentrations this compound is completely cleared from the plasma by renal tubular filtration and secretion in a single pass.

$$RPF = C_{PAH} = U_{PAH} \times V/P_{PAH} \qquad [2]$$

where RPF = renal plasma flow in mL/min or mL/24 hr; C_{PAH} = clearance of PAH in mL/min or mL/24 hr; U_{PAH} = urine concentration of PAH in mg/mL; V = urine flow rate in mL/min or mL/24 hr; P_{PAH} = plasma concentration of PAH in mg/mL.

RBF (in mL/min) is determined via the following equation:

$$RBF = RPF/1 - \text{hematocrit} \qquad [3]$$

Glomerular Filtration Rate

Glomerular filtration rate (GFR) is measured by the clearance of inulin, a fructose polysaccharide that is readily filtered but not resorbed or secreted by the renal tubule.

$$GFR = U_{inulin} \times V/P_{inulin} = C_{inulin} \qquad [4]$$

where GFR = glomerular filtration rate in mL/min or mL/24 hr; U_{inulin} = urine concentration of inulin in mg/mL; V = urine flow rate in mL/min or mL/24 hr; P_{inulin} = plasma concentration of inulin in mg/mL; C_{inulin} = clearance of inulin in mL/min or mL/24 hr.

Normal GFR is about 120 mL/min in men and 100 mL/min in women. GFR can also be estimated with blood urea nitrogen (BUN) and plasma creatinine. BUN and plasma creatinine increase as GFR decreases. Notably, GFR decreases with age although plasma creatinine remains relatively constant due to a decrease in muscle mass. Creatinine clearance is less accurate than inulin clearance, but much more practical to measure.

$$GFR \approx U_{creatinine} \times V/P_{creatinine} = C_{creatinine} \qquad [5]$$

where GFR = glomerular filtration rate in mL/min or mL/24 hr; $U_{creatinine}$ = urine concentration of creatinine in mg/mL; V = urine flow rate in mL/min or mL/24 hr; $P_{creatinine}$ = plasma concentration of creatinine in mg/mL; $C_{creatinine}$ = clearance of creatinine in mL/min or mL/24 hr.

The filtration fraction (FF) is the fraction of RPF that is filtered across the glomerular capillaries and is normally about 0.20. Therefore 20% of the RPF is filtered, leaving 80% of the RPF to leave the glomerulus via the efferent arterioles, making up the peritubular capillary circulation.

$$FF = GFR/RPF \qquad [6]$$

where FF = filtration fraction; GFR = glomerular filtration rate; RPF = renal plasma flow.

Blood flow to the glomerulus is regulated by the afferent and efferent arteriolar sphincter tone, which adjusts glomerular filtration pressure. Afferent arteriolar dilation or efferent arteriolar constriction increase the FF and GFR. This auto-regulatory mechanism is capable of maintaining GFR across a wide range of blood pressures and is achieved, in part, via the juxtaglomerular apparatus (see later).

If blood pressure falls, there is a concomitant decrease in RBF and reduction in afferent arteriolar pressure as well as a decrease in filtered solute. This triggers release of renin by the macula densa in the juxtaglomerular apparatus. Renin, a selective protease, converts angiotensinogen to angiotensin I, which is subsequently converted to angiotensin II by angiotensin converting enzyme (ACE) in the lungs. Angiotensin II causes thirst (and water intake), vasoconstriction, and Na^+ and water retention (via aldosterone), all of which increase blood pressure, renal perfusion pressure, and thus RBF. Additionally, the kidney responds to low levels of catecholamines circulating when blood pressure drops by preferential efferent arteriolar vasoconstriction, which maintains GFR.[2]

AGE-RELATED RENAL CHANGES

RBF decreases by 10% per decade of life after age 50; parallel changes occur in the kidney's ability to handle acid and Na^+. Creatinine becomes increasingly unreliable as a marker of GFR in older adults due to loss of muscle and malnutrition. The National Kidney Foundation recommends using the Cockcroft-Gault formula for the calculation of GFR.[3]

$$GFR_{men} = 140 - age\ (years) \times weight\ (kg)/$$
$$serum\ creatinine\ (mg/dL) \times 72 \qquad [7]$$

$$GFR_{women} = 140\ age\ (years) \times weight\ (kg) \times 0.85/$$
$$serum\ creatinine\ (mg/dL) \times 72 \qquad [8]$$

In neonates, when adjusted for body surface area (BSA), RBF doubles during the first 2 weeks of postnatal life and continues to increase until it reaches adult values at about 2 years of age. This change is thought to be secondary to increasing cardiac output and dropping systemic vascular resistance. GFR parallels this rise in RBF.

GFR can be estimated in children based on the serum creatinine level and height as follows:

$$GFR = height\ (cm) \times k/serum\ creatinine\ (mg/dL) \qquad [9]$$

where k = 0.45 for infants; k = 0.55 for children; k = 0.70 for adolescents. Neonates are unable to excrete K^+ efficiently, therefore the normal range of serum potassium tends to be higher than in older children and adults. The normal serum potassium by age is summarized in Table 32-1.

THE NEPHRON

Each kidney contains 1.0 to 1.3 million nephrons, the functional unit of the kidney.[4] The glomerulus is made up of a tuftlike network of branching capillaries covered with epithelial cells that arc into Bowman's capsule, providing a large surface area for blood filtration (Figure 32-2).[5] Blood enters the glomerulus via an afferent arteriole and exits through an efferent arteriole. The basement membrane of the glomerulus acts as a filter. This membrane allows water, amino acids, and free ions to pass through it into Bowman's capsule; however, charged molecules, large proteins, and cellular elements including red blood cells cannot pass.

Fluid then flows from Bowman's capsule to the proximal tubule. The main function of the proximal tubule is to resorb Na^+ and water, but bicarbonate, Cl^-, glucose, amino acids, phosphate, and lactate are also transported. The loop of Henle leads from the proximal convoluted tubule to the distal

Table 32-1. Normal Values of Serum Potassium

AGE	SERUM POTASSIUM RANGE (mEq/L)
0-1 month	4.0-6.0
1 month to 2 years	4.0-5.5
2-17 years	3.8-5.0
>18 years	3.2-4.8

convoluted tubule. Its main function is to create and maintain a significantly increasing concentration gradient of osmolality within the renal medullary interstitium, thereby providing the downstream collecting ducts with the ability to concentrate urine by osmosis. The loop of Henle is also responsible for Ca^{2+} and Mg^{2+} resorption. The distal convoluted tubule carries hypotonic fluid from the loop of Henle to the collecting ducts and is responsible for subtle changes in Na^+, K^+, Ca^{2+}, phosphate, and acid-base homeostasis. The collecting ducts run down the steep concentration gradient created by the loop of Henle and allow significant water resorption and therefore the creation of concentrated, hypertonic urine.

The juxtaglomerular apparatus is a small structure made up of the macular densa (a portion of modified ascending limb of the loop of Henle), mesangial cells, and juxtaglomerular cells (Figure 32-3) that release renin in response to β-adrenergic stimulation, a decrease in afferent arteriolar perfusion pressure (sensed by a baroreceptor mechanism), and changes in Cl^- flow within the loop of Henle (sensed by chemoreceptors).[6] The role of each segment of the nephron is summarized in Table 32-2.

WATER AND THE KIDNEY

Regulation of plasma osmolarity is accomplished by varying the amount of water excreted by the kidney. Concentrated hyperosmotic urine is produced when circulating levels of antidiuretic hormone (ADH) are high. ADH is also known as *vasopressin* (see Chapter 30). With dehydration, ADH is released from the posterior pituitary in response to increased osmolality (sensed by magnocellular neurons in the hypothalamus), decreased circulating plasma volume and/or angiotensin II. ADH increases the number of aquaporin channels in the collecting ducts of the nephron, facilitating water reabsorption by osmosis. ADH secretion occurs in times of water deprivation or hemorrhage, or with syndrome of inappropriate ADH (SIADH). Without ADH, dilute urine is excreted due to reduced permeability of the distal tubules and collecting ducts to water, leading to little water reabsorption.

SALT AND THE KIDNEY

Sodium is resorbed all along the nephron, but the majority is resorbed isosmotically in the proximal convoluted tubule. Sodium regulation is controlled by two main mechanisms: (1) renin-angiotensin-aldosterone (Figure 32-4) and (2) atrial natriuretic peptide (ANP). Angiotensin II is the most powerful Na^+-retaining hormone. Its plasma levels increase with low blood pressure, hypovolemia, or salt and water loss. Angiotensin II stimulates aldosterone secretion, which increases Na^+ absorption. Additionally, angiotensin II constricts efferent arterioles, thus raising the filtration fraction, and directly stimulates Na^+ resorption in the proximal tubule. In times of salt and water overload and plasma volume expansion, the cardiac atria become distended and secrete the peptide ANP. ANP dilates the afferent arterioles in the glomerulus and constricts the efferent arterioles thus increasing GFR and increasing salt and water excretion. ANP also inhibits renin secretion, resulting in reduced angiotensin I, angiotensin II, and aldosterone production.[6]

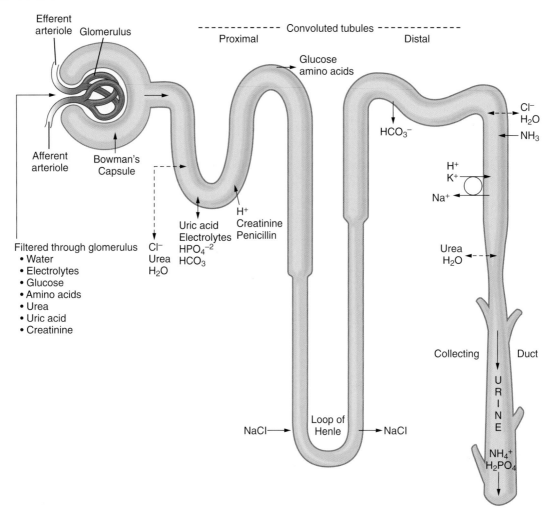

Figure 32-2 The structure of the nephron. The structure of the nephron, specialized tubular segments in particular, is uniquely suited to sodium, water, electrolyte and H+ ion handling. The afferent arteriole brings blood into the glomerulus while the efferent arteriole carries blood away from the glomerulus. Bowman's capsule (or glomerular capsule) is a cup-like sac that cradles the tuft-like glomerular capillaries at the beginning of the tubular component of the nephron that performs the first step in the filtration of blood to form urine. This leads to the proximal convoluted tubule, the most proximal segment of the renal tubule. It is responsible for the reabsorption of glucose, amino acids, and the majority of ions and water that is reabsorbed. The loop of Henle separates the proximal and distal convoluted tubules. Its main function is to create a concentration gradient in the renal medulla. By means of a counter-current multiplier, the loop of Henle creates an area of high urine concentration deep in the medulla, in the zone of the collecting duct establishing a concentration gradient. Water present in the filtrate in the collecting duct flows down this concentration gradient (via aquaporin channels) out of the collecting duct. This process reabsorbs water and creates concentrated urine for excretion. The distal convoluted tubule follows the loop of Henle and is involved in the secretion of ammonia and urea as well as the regulation of potassium, sodium, calcium, and pH. From the distal convoluted tubule, filtrate drains into collecting ducts. Each duct receives filtrate from the distal convoluted tubules of many nephrons. Inside these collecting ducts, water can be absorbed to regulate the final concentration of urine produced by the kidneys. On leaving the collecting ducts, urine enters the renal pelvis and flows into the ureters.

POTASSIUM AND THE KIDNEY

Potassium is filtered, resorbed, and secreted by the nephron. Potassium excretion can vary widely from 1% to 110% of the filtered load depending on dietary K+ intake, aldosterone levels, tubular flow rate, and acid-base balance. The proximal tubule reabsorbs 67% of the filtered K+ along with Na+ and water. The loop of Henle resorbs an additional 20% of filtered K+. The distal convoluted tubule and collecting duct reabsorb and secrete K+ and are responsible for regulation of K+ balance. Aldosterone stimulates K+ secretion by increasing Na+ entry into principal cells in the distal tubules.

Acidosis decreases K+ excretion and alkalosis increases K+ secretion. The primary mechanism by which increased hydrogen ion concentration inhibits K+ secretion is via the Na+, K+ ATPase pump.[7] Hydrogen ions and K+ effectively exchange for one another across the cell membrane via this pump. Urine flow rates also affect K+ secretion, and drugs that increase urine flow such as loop and thiazide diuretics cause dilution of luminal K+ concentration and increase the driving force for K+ secretion (see Chapter 34). The common causes of hyperkalemia and hypokalemia are summarized in Tables 32-3 and 32-4, respectively.

TOXIN AND METABOLITE EXCRETION

The kidney plays a major role in the excretion of drugs, hormones, and toxins. Uremic toxins and metabolites are cleared

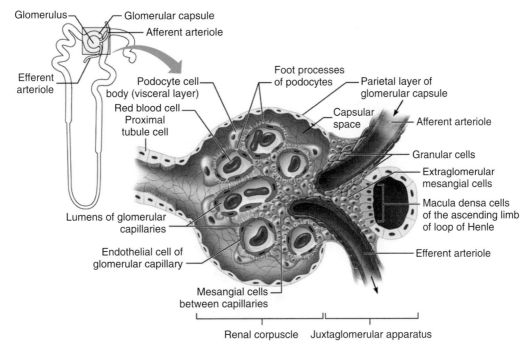

Figure 32-3 The structure of the glomerulus and macula densa (see text for a detailed explanation). The upper left shows the position of the glomerulus and justaglomerular apparatus relative to the entire nephron.

Table 32-2. Functional Divisions of the Nephron

SEGMENT	FUNCTION
Proximal tubule	Reabsorption: Na⁺, Cl⁻, water, bicarbonate, glucose, protein, amino acids, K⁺, Mg²⁺, Ca²⁺, phosphate, uric acid, urea Secretion: organic anions and cations Ammonia production
Loop of Henle	Reabsorption: Na⁺, Cl⁻, water, K⁺, Ca²⁺, Mg²⁺ Establishes concentration gradient within medulla
Distal tubule	Reabsorption: Na⁺, Cl⁻, water, K⁺, Ca²⁺, bicarbonate Secretion: H⁺, K⁺, Ca²⁺
Collecting duct	Reabsorption: Na⁺, Cl⁻, water, K⁺, bicarbonate Secretion: H⁺, K⁺ Ammonia production
Juxtaglomerular apparatus	Secretion of renin

Adapted from Rose BD, Post T. *Clinical Physiology of Acid-Base and Electrolyte Disorders.* 4th ed. New York: McGraw-Hill; 2001.

from the blood by filtration and secretion. The kidney freely filters water-soluble toxins such as creatinine and urea, which are excreted in the urine. Other toxins are removed from the blood and actively secreted. The kidney utilizes multiple pathways to metabolize drugs, including oxidation, dealkylation, reduction, hydrolysis, glucuronidation, sulfation, methylation, acetylation, and conjugation.[8]

ACID-BASE BALANCE

The main organs involved in acid-base balance are the lungs and the kidneys. The lungs excrete a volatile acid, carbon dioxide. The kidneys are responsible for handling nonvolatile

acids. The kidneys help regulate acid-base balance by excreting either acidic or basic urine. This is achieved via precise handling of the large amount of bicarbonate and acidic ions filtered continuously into the renal tubules. Volume depletion is associated with Na⁺ retention, which enhances bicarbonate reabsorption leading to alkalemia. Hypokalemia enhances bicarbonate reabsorption, also leading to alkalemia (contraction alkalosis).[9] There is ongoing controversy as to whether the kidney maintains acid-base homeostasis via ammonium (acid) excretion or chloride excretion. In any case, it is correct that the kidney reabsorbs bicarbonate and excretes acids to maintain acid-base balance.[10]

RENAL HORMONE PRODUCTION

The kidney secretes two hormones, erythropoietin (EPO) and calcitriol (1,25 [OH]₂ vitamin D₃), as well as the enzyme renin. EPO is a glycoprotein that acts on the bone marrow to increase red blood cell production in response to any condition that reduces the quantity of oxygen to the tissues. Most often EPO production is increased due to anemia, low blood volumes, or hypoxia such as experienced by people living at high altitudes, or with prolonged cardiac or pulmonary failure.

Calcitriol is the activated form of vitamin D. It acts in the intestine to increase the absorption of calcium from food, on the bone to mobilize stored calcium, and in the kidney itself to reabsorb phosphate. It is the downstream product of calciferol, which is synthesized from ingested vitamin D in skin exposed to ultraviolet light. Calciferol is subsequently converted by the liver to 25 [OH] vitamin D₃ and then carried to the kidney and converted to calcitriol in response to parathyroid hormone. The enzymatic function of renin, which is produced by the juxtaglomerular apparatus in response to hypotension, is described elsewhere in this chapter.

Renin-angiotensin-aldosterone system

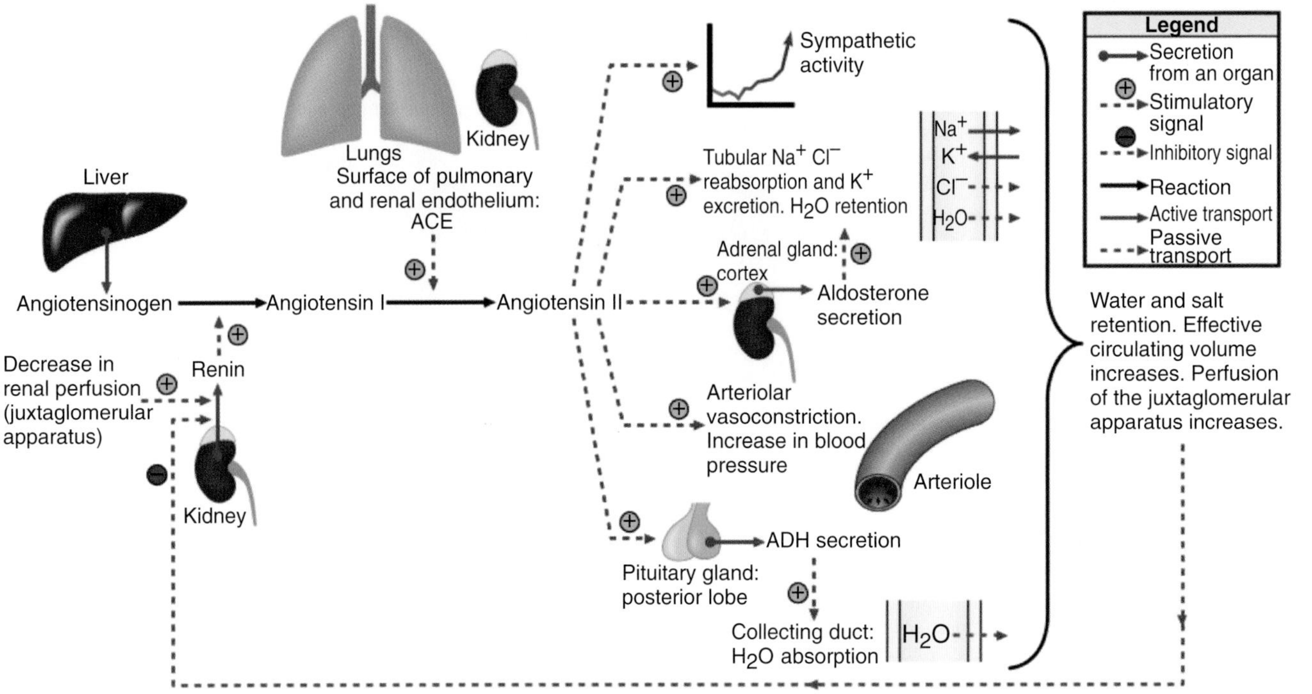

Figure 32-4 Renin-angiotensin-aldosterone system. The renin-angiotensin-aldosterone system regulates blood pressure and fluid balance. When blood volume is low, juxtaglomerular cells secrete renin into the circulation. Plasma renin then converts angiotensinogen released by the liver to angiotensin I. Angiotensin I is subsequently converted to angiotensin II by angiotensin converting enzyme (ACE) found in the lungs. Angiotensin II is a potent vasoactive peptide that causes blood vessels to constrict, resulting in increased blood pressure. Angiotensin II promotes ADH secretion by the posterior pituitary, increasing water reabsorption by the kidneys, resulting in decreased urinary output. Angiotensin II also stimulates the secretion of the hormone aldosterone from the adrenal cortex. Aldosterone causes the tubules of the kidneys to increase the reabsorption of sodium and water into the blood. This increases the volume of fluid in the body, which also increases blood pressure.

Table 32-3. Causes of Hyperkalemia

TRANSCELLULAR SHIFTS	DECREASED EXCRETION	INCREASED UPTAKE
Acidosis	Renal failure	K^+ supplements
β-Blockers	K^+-sparing diuretics	Blood transfusions
Insulin deficiency	Cyclosporin	K^+-containing
Burns	NSAIDs	medications
Tumor lysis	ACE-inhibitors	
syndrome	Mineralocorticoid	
Rhabdomyolysis	deficiency/resistance	

ACE, Angiotensin-converting enzyme; *NSAIDs,* nonsteroidal antiinflammatory drugs.

Table 32-4. Causes of Hypokalemia

TRANSCELLULAR SHIFTS	INCREASED EXCRETION	DECREASED UPTAKE
Insulin	Vomiting	Malnutrition
β-Agonists	Diarrhea	
	Nasogastric suction	
	Laxatives	
	Diuretics	
	Cisplatin	
	Amphotericin B	
	Renal tubular acidosis	
	Corticosteroids	

Defining Renal Failure

Acute kidney injury (AKI, formerly known as acute renal failure) is associated with increased perioperative morbidity, mortality, duration of hospital stay, and cost.[11,12] Arriving at a standardized definition of renal failure has been surprisingly difficult. Renal failure is usually divided into either AKI or chronic kidney disease (CKD) (previously termed chronic renal insufficiency or chronic renal failure).[13] More than 35 definitions have existed for renal failure.[14] The absence of a consensus definition has had a negative impact on basic science as well as clinical research in the field of AKI.

There is no consensus on the most effective way to assess renal function; either by defining which markers best gauge renal function or at what level any biomarker differentiates normal from abnormal renal function. Only recently has a unified standard for classifying and diagnosing AKI been accepted. The diagnosis of AKI requires both clinical history and relevant laboratory data. The Acute Kidney Injury Network (AKIN) introduced specific criteria for diagnosis of AKI including a rapid time course (less than 48 hours) and decrement of kidney function.[15] Reduction of kidney function was defined as either an absolute increase in serum creatinine of greater than 0.3 mg/dL, percentage increase in serum creatinine of more than 50%, or reduction in urine output to less than 0.5 mL/kg/hr for more than 6 hours. In addition to the AKIN, the Acute Dialysis Quality Initiative (ADQI) has attempted to uniformly define and stage AKI with the RIFLE

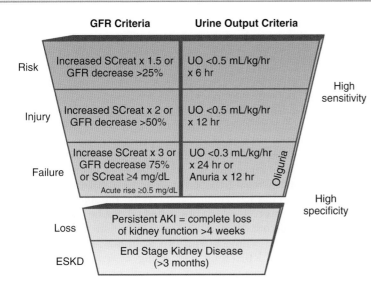

GFR Criteria | Urine Output Criteria

Risk — Increased SCreat x 1.5 or GFR decrease >25% | UO <0.5 mL/kg/hr x 6 hr

Injury — Increased SCreat x 2 or GFR decrease >50% | UO <0.5 mL/kg/hr x 12 hr

Failure — Increase SCreat x 3 or GFR decrease 75% or SCreat ≥4 mg/dL (Acute rise ≥0.5 mg/dL) | UO <0.3 mL/kg/hr x 24 hr or Anuria x 12 hr

High sensitivity

Oliguria

High specificity

Loss — Persistent AKI = complete loss of kidney function >4 weeks

ESKD — End Stage Kidney Disease (>3 months)

Figure 32-5 RIFLE criteria. *SCreat,* Serum creatinine; *GFR,* glomerular filtration rate; *UO,* urine output; *AKI,* acute kidney injury.

criteria (Risk, Injury, Failure, Loss, End-stage kidney disease).[16] These five categories represent three grades of increasing severity of AKI (risk, injury, and failure) and two outcome classes (loss, and end-stage kidney disease). Absolute increase of serum creatinine, percentage increase in creatinine, percentage reduction in GFR, and decrement in urine output over time define the categories. Figure 32-5 summarizes the RIFLE criteria. Rather than equating renal function and serum creatinine, the RIFLE criteria attempt to standardize the definition and severity of renal injury in order to facilitate evaluation, treatment, and communication amongst health care providers. A recent study demonstrated the utility of the RIFLE criteria as a predictor of mortality in patients admitted to the intensive care unit (ICU).[17]

RISK OF PERIOPERATIVE ACUTE KIDNEY INJURY

Predicting patients at risk for perioperative AKI would allow anesthesiologists to outline properly the perioperative risk to their patients as well as tailor management toward the prevention of AKI. Risks for perioperative AKI include advanced age, revised cardiac risk index score greater than 2, American Society of Anesthesiology Physical Status of IV or V, male sex, active congestive heart failure, hypertension, emergency surgery, high-risk surgery (intraperitoneal, intrathoracic, vascular), elevated preoperative creatinine, and diabetes mellitus.[18,19] Blood product transfusion, sepsis, as well as the possible exposure to hypovolemia and hypotension also probably place patients at risk for AKI.[20]

Certain surgical procedures carry a higher risk for AKI than others, in particular cardiac surgery, aortic surgery, and liver transplantation. Aortic clamping, employed in cardiac and aortic surgery, can significantly reduce renal perfusion and predispose the kidney to atheromatous emboli, possibly leading to AKI. Regardless of the position of the aortic cross-clamp in aortic surgery, RBF is reduced by about 50% during surgical preparation of the aorta.[2] Methods for renal protection during open thoracoabdominal aneurysm repair include maintaining distal aortic perfusion during aortic cross-clamping, infusing cold perfusate into the renal arteries during periods of ischemia, and the use of left heart bypass to maintain perfusion pressure during aortic cross-clamping.[21] The anatomic location and extent of the aortic aneurysm has profound implications on the ability to maintain kidney perfusion during surgery.

Patients undergoing liver transplantation are at significant risk for development of AKI. These patients can have preexisting renal dysfunction, and they can have intraoperative interruption of the inferior vena cava. There is significant risk of hemodynamic instability, bleeding, transfusion, and medication-induced nephrotoxicity.[22] Cardiac surgical patients are also at high-risk for AKI. Additionally, cardiopulmonary bypass induces hypotension, reduces aortic blood flow, and decreases RBF. Cardiopulmonary bypass not only induces an inflammatory cascade but also requires anticoagulation, both of which can lead to bleeding and worsening renal injury.

ACUTE KIDNEY INJURY IN SURGICAL PATIENTS

Acutely, renal function can deteriorate over a period of hours to days and is most often the result of multiple insults. AKI is a rapid loss of kidney function, which has multiple causes that have traditionally been categorized into three broad groups: *pre-renal, intrinsic-renal, and post-renal kidney injury.* Because reversible pre-renal azotemia and intrinsic-renal acute tubular necrosis from medullary ischemia are two ends of a continuum, the division is artificial. However, this division can be useful in guiding treatment options. The most common cause of perioperative renal injury is ischemia-reperfusion injury.[23] The traditional "pre-renal" causes of kidney injury include any mechanism that decreases effective blood flow to the kidney. Common causes of pre-renal kidney injury include dehydration, hypovolemia, hemorrhage, hypotension, and heart failure. Pre-renal injury is often rapidly reversible when the underlying mechanism is corrected, thus glomerular or tubular injury can be avoided.

"Intrinsic" causes of kidney injury can result from direct injury to the glomeruli, tubules, or interstitium. Common causes of intrinsic kidney injury include glomerulonephritis, acute interstitial nephritis, and acute tubular necrosis (ATN).[12] Infection and sepsis are common diagnoses leading to AKI. Chronically ill patients are at risk for toxin-mediated ATN from aminoglycoside antibiotics, intravenous contrast agents, or nonsteroidal antiinflammatory medications. Postrenal kidney injury involves obstruction at any point along the urinary outflow tract by malignancies, renal calculi, retroperitoneal fibrosis, a hypertrophied prostate, or an obstructed bladder catheter. Iatrogenic injury to the ureter can occur in lower abdominal surgery. Treatment of any type of kidney injury is centered on treating the underlying cause while providing supportive care and avoiding nephrotoxic substances and further renal insult.

ASSESSMENT AND MANAGEMENT OF ACUTE KIDNEY INJURY

Preoperative Approach

Managing patients with AKI depends on both the cause and the severity of injury. The most common and practical way to assess renal function is by factors included in the RIFLE criteria: serum creatinine, GFR, and urine output. Although commonly used and widely accepted, serum creatinine is unfortunately insensitive and not linearly related to GFR.[22] GFR, the gold standard of renal function, is impractical to measure. In patients of advanced age, serum creatinine is often an unreliable indicator of renal function due to decreased creatinine production secondary to reduced muscle mass. Therefore a normal or low serum creatinine is likely to overestimate GFR. Additionally, urine output may not be a reliable marker of renal function or injury for a number of reasons including diuretic therapy.

Patients presenting for surgery can have kidney injuries with a wide array of causes and severity. There is no proven preventive measure or treatment for AKI.[22] Therefore management of AKI centers on identifying and treating the underlying cause, supporting renal function by maintaining RBF and oxygen delivery, and avoiding nephrotoxic agents. Common pre-renal causes of AKI include hypovolemia secondary to bleeding, fluid losses, reduced oral intake, or diuretic administration. Bleeding, including gastrointestinal or posttraumatic, can lead to significant hypovolemia. Excessive fluid losses from the gastrointestinal tract (due to diarrhea or preoperative bowel preparation) or from the kidneys (excessive diuresis) can also cause pre-renal injury. Treatment of pre-renal injury can be simple, but requires quick recognition of the cause and appropriate treatment to avoid more permanent renal injury. Discontinuation of diuretics and optimization of fluid status and RBF by administration of isotonic crystalloid or colloid solutions can be necessary to prevent progression of the injury. There is little convincing evidence favoring colloids over crystalloids (see Chapter 33). In more acute situations, such as gastrointestinal bleeding, rapid administration of plasma expanders and/or blood products might be needed to reverse hemodynamic instability.

Sepsis should always be considered as a cause of renal injury in patients with signs of infection. Early and aggressive treatment should be initiated if sepsis is suspected including source control, appropriate antibiotics, early goal directed therapy, lung protective ventilation in the setting of acute lung injury (ALI) or acute respiratory distress syndrome (ARDS), avoidance of severe hyperglycemia, early enteral nutrition, and possible steroid therapy for adrenal insufficiency or refractory vasoplegia.[24-27] All bacterial infections should be treated quickly and appropriately with the initial empirical therapy often dictated by local and hospital antibiograms.[28]

"Renal-dose" dopamine remains in use probably because it is an effective diuretic and often increases urine output. It also is often effective in improving renal perfusion in patients with low cardiac output and/or bradycardia. Unfortunately, several studies showed no role for dopamine in the prophylaxis or treatment of AKI (see Chapter 22).[29-31]

Loop diuretics can be used in the setting of AKI but it is essential that euvolemia be restored before administration to avoid further renal hypoperfusion and exacerbation of AKI. Loop diuretics have multiple effects on the injured kidney. Loop diuretics can relieve obstructed tubules by mechanically clearing necrotic cells with increased urine flow. They increase prostaglandin synthesis with two main downstream effects: (1) increases RBF, thus augmenting oxygen delivery, and (2) decreases active tubular Na^+ reabsorption, decreasing metabolic demand.[22] Even so, most large studies have shown no direct positive effect of loop diuretics on prevention or treatment of AKI.[32]

INTRAOPERATIVE MANAGEMENT OF RENAL FUNCTION

There are no data supporting one particular anesthetic technique over another in regard to renal function. Supporting normal blood pressure, and therefore renal perfusion, maintaining euvolemia to ensure adequate perfusion and oxygen delivery to all tissues, and avoiding nephrotoxins are prudent.

Volatile anesthetics, used for maintenance of general anesthesia, can decrease GFR primarily as a result of decreased systemic vascular resistance and blood pressure.[22] This is worsened by hypovolemia and ADH secretion, commonly seen in the surgical stress response.[33] Sevoflurane can theoretically cause fluoride-induced renal injury via generation of the haloalkene compound A (see Chapter 3). This breakdown product is produced from sevoflurane when certain carbon dioxide absorbants are used. Compound A is nephrotoxic in laboratory animals but no studies have linked it to AKI in humans, despite low-flow anesthesia for many hours, and most consider this volatile agent safe for patients with renal dysfunction.[34]

After induction of general anesthesia, patients are placed on positive pressure ventilation with positive end-expiratory pressure (PEEP), which can reduce cardiac output, RBF, GFR, Na^+ excretion and urine flow rate.[35] The extent of this effect depends on mean airway pressures, the degree of reduction in venous return and cardiac output, and activation of the renin-angiotensin-aldosterone pathway.

Sodium bicarbonate can be administered to correct severe metabolic acidosis. Potential side effects such as hypercarbia, hypernatremia, rebound alkalosis, and worsening intracellular acidosis making administration of sodium bicarbonate of questionable efficacy in this setting.[36] Trishydroxymethylaminomethane (THAM) is a buffer that appears to control safely acidosis during surgery and should be considered as an alternative to sodium bicarbonate. However, THAM accumulates in patients with renal dysfunction, so its universal use is not recommended.

There is emerging evidence that blood transfusion, as well as anemia, is associated with development of AKI. However, significant bleeding during surgery often requires transfusion of blood products. Transfusion can lead to hyperkalemia, which is most often treated with loop diuretics. Preexisting kidney dysfunction or AKI might make the loop of Henle resistant or unresponsive to these diuretics.

Pressors are often required during surgery to reverse multifactorial hypotension and vasodilation. Norepinephrine and arginine vasopressin are two commonly used agents. Norepinephrine profoundly constricts the glomerular afferent arteriole, dropping filtration pressure, and thus can contribute to and prolong the course of AKI. In contrast, arginine vasopressin constricts the glomerular efferent arteriole and therefore can increase filtration pressure and consequently GFR.

To guide hemodynamic management during AKI, invasive monitors should be considered, including arterial line, central venous catheter, pulmonary arterial catheter, non-invasive cardiac output monitor, and/or transesophageal echocardiography. Because patients are anesthetized and paralyzed, pulse pressure variation and stroke volume variation can help guide hemodynamic management (see Chapter 21).[37,38] It appears that surgical patients receiving perioperative hemodynamic optimization with "goal-directed management" are at decreased risk for renal impairment.[39] Obviously, urine output must be closely monitored with a urinary catheter. Frequent point of care assessment of acid-base status and electrolyte balance aid in determining whether renal replacement therapy is needed.

ANESTHETIC DRUGS AND IMPAIRED RENAL FUNCTION

Anesthesiologists must be aware of medications that might accumulate or have adverse effects in patients with renal dysfunction. Barbiturates can be used safely in patients with renal dysfunction although these patients appear to have increased sensitivity possibly secondary to acidosis favoring a more rapid entry of drug into the brain. Most benzodiazepines undergo hepatic metabolism and conjugation before elimination in the urine so caution should be used when administering diazepam or midazolam to patients with renal impairment due to the presence of active metabolites. Lorazepam might be the benzodiazepine of choice due to the lack of active metabolites. Succinylcholine can be used safely in renal failure once the preadministration serum K^+ concentration has been determined and is at a safe level. If serum K^+ concentration is unknown or significantly elevated, a nondepolarizing neuromuscular blocker should be used. Some consider cisatracurium as the neuromuscular blocking agent of choice, in that it is broken down by Hoffman elimination, thereby having consistent duration of action in the face of AKI or renal failure. While the elimination of vecuronium is primarily hepatic, 15% to 25% is eliminated by the kidney. Similarly, rocuronium is primarily excreted by hepatic biotransformation and hepatobiliary excretion, but the duration of action seems to have greater variability in patients with renal failure and end-stage renal disease. This might be due to decreased clearance, increased potency, or changes in protein binding.[40] Sugammadex can be useful for patients with renal dysfunction who have received rocuronium. Morphine should be used with caution due to the accumulation of the active metabolite morphine-6-glucuronide. Similarly, meperidine should be avoided due to accumulation of the toxic metabolite normeperidine, which has been associated with seizures. Fentanyl, remifentanil, sufentanil, alfentanil, and hydromorphone are the opioids of choice for patients with, or at risk for, renal impairment because these drugs do not depend on renal clearance mechanisms.

COMMON PERIOPERATIVE MEDICATIONS THAT IMPAIR RENAL FUNCTION

Multiple medications used in the perioperative period can have adverse affects on renal function. Calcineurin inhibitors, such as tacrolimus and cyclosporine, are immunosuppressive medications used to prevent the rejection of transplanted organs such as lung, heart, kidney, and liver. Calcineurin inhibitors cause profound afferent arteriolar vasoconstriction and reduce GFR.[41] Antimicrobial drugs are often administered to patients undergoing surgery and can cause ATN (aminoglycosides) or tubulointerstitial nephritis (penicillins, cephalosporins, or fluoroquinolones). Nonsteroidal antiinflammatory drugs, including cyclooxygenase-2 inhibitors, inhibit prostaglandin synthesis and therefore prevent renal arteriolar vasodilation, potentially impairing renal autoregulation. Angiotensin-converting enzyme inhibitors and angiotensin receptor blocking drugs also inhibit autoregulation, but by a different mechanism (blockade of efferent arteriolar vasoconstriction).[42] Finally, radiographic contrast media can cause renal injury by two mechanisms. First, they can induce medullary vasoconstriction and reduce blood flow, resulting in ischemic injury. Second, they can have a direct cytotoxic effect in the vulnerable kidney.[43]

While most pharmacologic strategies to prevent AKI have proven unsuccessful, the prevention of contrast-induced nephropathy (CIN) is probably possible in many cases. Risk reduction involves judicious use of very low volumes of nonionic isosmolar contrast along with careful isotonic intravenous hydration with 0.9% normal saline or sodium bicarbonate to ensure adequate hydration prior to the administration of contrast agents.[44] Use of oral or intravenous N-acetylcysteine (NAC) is controversial. It was previously advocated to reduce the incidence of CIN; however, there is increasing evidence suggesting a lack of efficacy.[45] Despite the controversy, based on the ease of use and lack of side effects, oral NAC can be considered.

RENAL REPLACEMENT THERAPY DURING AND AFTER SURGERY

Although there are several renal replacement modalities, three major types exist: intermittent hemodialysis (iHD), peritoneal dialysis (PD), and continuous renal replacement therapies (CRRT). Intermittent hemodialysis, the standard treatment for severe renal failure for more than 4 decades, is most often used in patients without acute hemodynamic abnormalities. Peritoneal dialysis is often used in patients with CKD, but is contraindicated in patients with ascites. There are few data validating one method over another and there is debate over the timing and dosage of RRT in the perioperative period.[12] The RRT modality used is often determined by institutional experience and is quite variable. CRRT, particularly continuous venovenous hemodialysis (CVVHD), is the most widely used and safest modality for patients in the perioperative period with a tenuous hemodynamic status. Regardless of the method of RRT, complications such as bleeding, infection, and hypotension should be recognized.

RRT, either iHD or CRRT, might be required in the perioperative period. Sustained low-efficiency dialysis is a hybrid form of RRT that is essentially a slower version of iHD using the same machinery with slower blood blows, longer dialysis sessions (8-10 hours vs. 3-4 hours), and possibly a lower incidence of hypotension.[46] There are several forms of CRRT including, but not limited to, slow continuous ultrafiltration, continuous venovenous hemofiltration, CVVHD, and continuous venovenous hemodiafiltration. These forms of RRT use ultrafiltration, hemofiltration, and/or hemodialysis for solute and fluid removal. Despite development of these renal replacement therapies that can rapidly correct the metabolic and biochemical derangements of AKI, improvements in mortality have not materialized. The typical CVVHD circuit is represented in Figure 32-6.

HEPATORENAL SYNDROME

Patients with liver cirrhosis are at risk for all three types of AKI, but they can also develop a unique entity known as hepatorenal syndrome (HRS).[47] HRS is a form of pre-renal AKI thought to be the result of circulatory dysfunction secondary to an imbalance of circulating vasodilatory and vasoconstrictive factors. This dysfunction is likely the result of a decrease in systemic vascular resistance arising from splanchnic vasodilatation due to nitric oxide, prostaglandins, and other vasoactive substances released in patients with portal hypertension and advanced cirrhosis.[48] The vasodilatation triggers activation of the renin-angiotensin system, and along with sympathetic stimulation, results in intense renal vasoconstriction. In compensated cirrhosis, cardiac output and plasma volume both increase to restore effective arterial volume and thereby renal perfusion and function is preserved. However, in decompensated cirrhosis, cardiac output and heart rate are already maximal and cannot increase further to augment blood pressure, resulting in a further increase in circulating vasoconstrictors and renal vasoconstriction, Na^+ and water retention, and ascites formation.[49] This results in decreased renal perfusion pressure and reduced GFR.

Two types of HRS exist: type 1 HRS is characterized by a rapid decline in renal function, while type 2 HRS entails a more chronic deterioration in renal function that is associated with ascites formation. Differentiating HRS from ATN can be difficult because diagnosing the former involves excluding other causes of AKI and there is no single test that confirms HRS.[50] Although mortality is very high among patients with cirrhosis and renal failure, patients with type 1 HRS seem to have the worst prognosis—a 50% survival rate at 1 month and 20% survival rate at 6 months.[51]

Therapeutic options are limited for patients with HRS. Vasopressors are effective in AKI, primarily in the setting of type 1 HRS.[50,52] The mechanism seems to be reversal of splanchnic vasodilatation and the restoration of central blood volume and renal perfusion. Several vasoconstrictors have been studied, including terlipressin (a vasopressin analogue), octreotide, norepinephrine, and midodrine. The strongest evidence, including recent randomized controlled trials, seems to be in favor of vasopressin analogues, with possibly added benefit with coadministration of intravenous albumin.[52] Although they should be considered first-line therapy, this class of medications can be associated with cardiovascular and ischemic complications—greater than 10% in some studies. Overall, vasopressin analogues can be effective in 40% to 50% of patients with HRS, but 3- and 6-month mortality benefits in these studies are lacking.[50,52]

Despite maximum pharmacologic therapy, AKI and/or HRS can cause renal function to decline to the point of metabolic disarray, acidosis, severe electrolyte abnormalities, and/or volume overload. Once renal function has reached this level of severity, the patient should be treated with renal replacement therapy (RRT). While albumin combined with vasopressin (or its analogues) is of some benefit, optimal medical management should include evaluation for liver transplantation. Diagnostic criteria for HRS are summarized in Table 32-5.

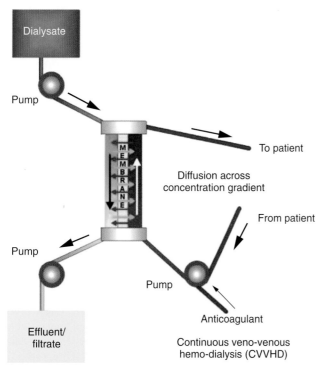

Figure 32-6 The continuous venovenous hemodialysis (CVVHD) circuit. CVVHD is similar to standard dialysis except that it is performed continuously over a longer period of time. Red tubing is the access line; it moves blood from the patient to the hemofilter. Blue tubing is the return line; it is used to convey blood from the hemofilter back to the patient. Green tubing is the dialysate line; it moves the dialysate from the source into the hemofilter. Yellow tubing is the effluent line; it removes the effluent from the dialyzer into a waste or effluent bag.

EMERGING DEVELOPMENTS

Prevention and Biomarkers for Acute Kidney Injury

Renal function and dysfunction is an important determinant and indicator of perioperative outcome. Anesthesiologists often give fluid in an attempt to increase renal perfusion and reduce perioperative AKI. There is very little evidence to

Table 32-5. Major Diagnostic Criteria of Hepatorenal Syndrome

Hepatic failure and ascites
Creatinine >1.5 mg/dL
No shock, ongoing bacterial infection, nephrotoxic agents, or fluid losses
No improvement after diuretic withdrawal and fluid resuscitation
Proteinuria <500 mg/day, normal renal sonography

Adapted from Meltzer J, Brentjens TE. Renal failure in patients with cirrhosis: hepatorenal syndrome and renal support strategies. *Curr Opin Anaesthesiol.* 2010;23:139-144.

suggest that a particular fluid should be used for the resuscitation of patients with or at risk of AKI; however, there is some evidence that 6% hydroxyethyl starch should be avoided in the setting of AKI because there is an emerging body of experiments and clinical studies that show that hydroxyethyl starch can induce and/or exacerbate renal injury.[53,54]

Detection and understanding of AKI is improving with time. Recently, there has been a promising search for biomarkers of renal function and injury. Serum cystatin C, a protein produced by all nucleated cells, is independent of age, sex, race, and muscle mass and is a better marker of GFR than creatinine[55]; further studies are needed for validation. Neutrophil gelatinase-associated lipocalin (NGAL) is a protein produced by renal tubular cells in the setting of renal injury.[56] It can be detected easily in the urine within minutes of induced injury and is highly sensitive and specific to AKI—levels are much less increased in chronic kidney disease. Although NGAL has been used in a variety of clinical scenarios, further research is necessary before it becomes widely accepted and used in clinical practice.

Many vasoactive drugs have been studied in hopes of finding a pharmacologic approach to prevention or treatment of renal injury. Renal vasoactive medications such as dopamine and prostaglandin infusions have not been effective. However, fenoldopam mesylate, a dopamine-1 receptor agonist originally approved for hypertensive emergencies, has shown some potential benefit (see Chapter 23). In a variety of surgical and ICU populations fenoldopam has been shown to reduce the risk of AKI, but only in small randomized trials or metaanalyses of these trials.[58-60]

KEY POINTS

- Main functions of the kidney are (1) regulation of salt and water balance, (2) toxin and metabolite elimination, (3) electrolyte homeostasis, (4) acid-base balance, and (5) hormone production.
- RBF is directly proportional to the "trans-renal gradient," the pressure difference between the renal artery and the renal vein. Autoregulation mechanisms maintain constant RBF over a range of blood pressures.
- Normal GFR is around 120 mL/min in men and 100 mL/min in women.
- RBF decreases by about 10% per decade of life after age 50; parallel changes occur in the kidney's ability to handle acid and sodium (Na^+).
- Regulation of plasma osmolarity is accomplished by varying the amount of water excreted by the kidney. Concentrated, hyperosmotic urine is produced when circulating levels of ADH are high.

- Na^+ regulation is controlled by two main mechanisms: (1) renin-angiotensin-aldosterone and (2) ANP.
- Potassium (K^+) excretion can vary widely from 1% to 110% of the filtered load depending on dietary K^+ intake, aldosterone levels, tubular flow rate, and acid-base balance.
- Risk factors for acute kidney injury include advanced age, revised cardiac risk index score greater than 2, American Society of Anesthesiologists Physical Status IV or V, male sex, active congestive heart failure, hypertension, emergency surgery, high-risk surgery, elevated preoperative creatinine, and diabetes mellitus.
- Procedures associated with the highest risk of acute kidney injury are cardiac surgery, aortic surgery, and liver transplantation.
- There is no evidence-based support for one anesthetic technique over another in regard to optimal renal function. Important goals include support of normal blood pressure and therefore renal perfusion; maintenance of euvolemia to ensure adequate perfusion and oxygen delivery to all tissues; and avoidance of nephrotoxins.
- Norepinephrine profoundly constricts the glomerular afferent arteriole, dropping filtration pressure, and can contribute to and prolong the course of AKI.
- Arginine vasopressin constricts the glomerular efferent arteriole and therefore can increase filtration pressure and GFR.

Key References

Bellomo R, Chapman M, Finfer S, et al. Low-dose dopamine in patients with early renal dysfunction: a placebo-controlled randomised trial. Australian and New Zealand Intensive Care Society (ANZICS) Clinical Trials Group. *Lancet.* 2000;356:2139-2143. The administration of low-dose dopamine by continuous infusion to critically ill patients at risk of renal failure does not confer clinically significant protection from renal dysfunction. (Ref. 29)

Bellomo R, Ronco C, Kellum JA, et al. Acute renal failure—definition, outcome measures, animal models, fluid therapy and information technology needs: the Second International Consensus Conference of the Acute Dialysis Quality Initiative (ADQI) Group. *Crit Care.* 2004;8:R204-R212. An introduction to the changing classification and nomenclature of acute kidney injury. (Ref. 16)

Borthwick E, Ferguson A. Perioperative acute kidney injury: risk factors, recognition, management, and outcomes. *Br Med J.* 2010;340:85-91. A good general look at which patients are at most risk of perioperative renal injury. (Ref. 20)

Finfer S, Bellomo R, Boyce N, et al. A comparison of albumin and saline for fluid resuscitation in the intensive care unit. *N Engl J Med.* 2004;350:2247-2256. A well-performed landmark trial of crystalloids versus colloids for fluid resuscitation in ICU patients revealing that the use of albumin or normal saline for fluid resuscitation results in similar outcomes at 28 days. Subgroup analysis supported albumin resuscitation for sepsis and saline resuscitation for brain injury. (Ref. 55)

Gines P, Schrier RW. Renal failure in cirrhosis. *N Engl J Med.* 2009;361:1279-1290. An outstanding review of the connection between renal failure and liver failure. (Ref. 49)

Kheterpal S, Tremper K, Heung M, et al. Development and validation of an acute kidney injury risk index for patients undergoing general surgery: results from a national data set. *Anesthesiology.* 2009;110:505-515. An investigation into the incidence and risk factors for postoperative acute kidney injury. (Ref. 18)

Rivers E, Nguyen B, Havstad S. Early goal-directed therapy in the treatment of severe sepsis and septic shock. *N Engl J Med.* 2001;345:1368-1377. A protocolized, goal-directed approach to the management of patients early in the course of severe, overwhelming infections improved survival significantly. The cornerstones of this early, goal-directed approach was monitoring, fluid resuscitation, and hemodynamic management. (Ref. 24)

References

1. Loutzenhiser R, Griffin K, Williamson G, et al. Renal autoregulation: new perspectives regarding the protective and regulatory roles of the underlying mechanisms. *Am J Physiol Regul Integr Comp Physiol.* 2006;290:R1153-1167.
2. Sladen RN. Renal physiology. In: Miller R, ed. *Miller's Anesthesia.* 6th ed. Philadelphia: Elsevier; 2005:77-182.
3. Stefan M, Iglesia LL, Fernandez G. Medical consultation and best practices for preoperative evaluation of elderly patients. *Hospital Practice.* 2011;39:41-51.
4. Rose BD, Post T. *Clinical Physiology of Acid-Base and Electrolyte Disorders.* 4th ed. New York: McGraw-Hill; 2001.
5. Guyton AC, Hall JE. Urine formation by the kidneys: I. Glomerular filtration, renal blood flow, and their control. In: Guyton AC, Hall JE, eds. *Textbook of Medical Physiology.* 9th ed. Philadelphia: WB Saunders; 1996:315-329.
6. Widmaier E, Ruff H, Strang K. *Vander's Human Physiology.* 12th ed. New York: McGraw-Hill; 2010.
7. Guyton AC and Hall JE. Integration of renal mechanisms for control of blood volume and extracellular fluid volume; and renal regulation of potassium, calcium, phosphate, and magnesium. In: Guyton AC, Hall JE, eds. *Textbook of Medical Physiology.* 9th ed. Philadelphia: WB Saunders; 1996:367-382.
8. Lohr JW, Willsky GR, Acara MA. Renal drug metabolism. *Pharmacol Rev.* 1998;50:107-142.
9. Brandis K. Acid-base physiology. Available at http://www.anaesthesiaMCQ.com.
10. Bellomo R, Ronco C. New paradigms in acid-base physiology. *Curr Opin Crit Care.* 1999;5:427.
11. Stewart J, Findlay G, Smith N, et al. Adding insult to injury. A review of patients who died in hospital with primary diagnosis of acute kidney injury. NCEPOD, 2009. Available at www.ncepod.org.
12. Bihorac, A, Yavas S, Subbiah S, et al. Long-term risk of mortality and acute kidney injury during hospitalization after major surgery. *Ann Surg.* 2009;249:851-858.
13. Thadhani R, Pascual M, Bonventre JV. Acute renal failure. *N Engl J Med.* 1996;334:1448-1460.
14. Kellum JA, Levin N, Bouman C, et al. Developing a consensus classification system for acute renal failure. *Curr Opin Crit Care.* 2002;8:509-514.
15. Mehta RL, Kellum JA, Shah SV. Acute Kidney Injury Network: report of an initiative to improve outcomes in acute kidney injury. *Crit Care.* 2007;11(2):R31.
16. Bellomo R, Ronco C, Kellum JA, et al. Acute renal failure—definition, outcome measures, animal models, fluid therapy and information technology needs: the Second International Consensus Conference of the Acute Dialysis Quality Initiative (ADQI) Group. *Crit Care.* 2004;8:R204-212.
17. Cholongitas E, Calvaruso V, Senzolo M, et al. RIFLE classification as predictive factor of mortality in patients with cirrhosis admitted to intensive care unit. *J Gastroenterol Hepatol.* 2009;24:1639-1647.
18. Kheterpal S, Tremper K, Heung M, et al. Development and validation of an acute kidney injury risk index for patients undergoing general surgery: results from a national data set. *Anesthesiology.* 2009;110:505-515.
19. Abelha FJ, Botelho M, Fernandez V, et al. Determinants of postoperative acute kidney injury. *Crit Care.* 2009;13:R79.
20. Borthwick E, Ferguson A. Perioperative acute kidney injury: risk factors, recognition, management, and outcomes. *Br Med J.* 2010;340:85-91.
21. Vaughn SB, LeMaire SA. Collard D. Case scenario: anesthetic considerations for thoracoabdominal aortic aneurysm repair. *Anesthesiology.* 2011;115:1093-1102.
22. Rymarz A, Serwacki M, Rutkowski M. Prevalence and predictors of acute renal injury in liver transplant recipients. *Transplant Proc.* 2009;15:475-483.
23. Wagener G, Brentjens TE. Anesthetic concerns in patients presenting with renal failure. *Anesth Clin.* 2010;28:39-54.
24. Rivers E, Nguyen B, Havstad S. Early goal-directed therapy in the treatment of severe sepsis and septic shock. *N Engl J Med.* 2001;345:1368-1377.
25. The Acute Respiratory Distress Syndrome Network Investigators. Ventilation with lower tidal volumes as compared with traditional tidal volumes for acute lung injury and the acute respiratory distress syndrome. *N Engl J Med.* 2000;342:1301-1308.
26. Finfer S, Chittock DR, Su SY. Intensive versus conventional glucose control in critically ill patients. *N Engl J Med.* 2009;360:1283-1297.
27. Sprung CL. Hydrocortisone therapy for patients with septic shock. *N Engl J Med.* 2008;358:111-124.
28. Dellinger RP, Levy MM, Carlet JM. Surviving Sepsis Campaign: international guidelines for management of severe sepsis and septic shock: 2008. *Crit Care Med.* 2008;36:296-327.
29. Bellomo R, Chapman M, Finfer S, et al. Low-dose dopamine in patients with early renal dysfunction: a placebo-controlled randomised trial. Australian and New Zealand Intensive Care Society (ANZICS) Clinical Trials Group. *Lancet.* 2000;356:2139-2143.
30. Friedrich JO, Adhikari N, Herridge MS, et al. Meta-analysis: low-dose dopamine increases urine output but does not prevent renal dysfunction or death. *Ann Intern Med.* 2005;142:510-524.
31. Lassnigg A, Donner E, Grubhofer G, et al. Lack of renoprotective effects of dopamine and furosemide during cardiac surgery. *J Am Soc Nephrol.* 2000;11:97-104.
32. Ho KM, Sheridan DJ. Meta-analysis of furosemide to prevent or treat acute renal failure. *Br Med J.* 2006;333:420-424.
33. Kusudo K, Ishii K, Rahman M. Blood flow-dependent changes in intrarenal nitric oxide levels during anesthesia with halothane or sevoflurane. *Eur J Pharmacol.* 2004;498:267-273.
34. Gentz BA, Malan TP. Renal toxicity with sevoflurane: a storm in a teacup? *Drugs.* 2001;61:2155-2162.
35. Doherty D, Sladen RN. Effects of positive airway pressure on renal function. In: Lumb PL, ed. *Postoperative Mechanical Ventilation.* Philadelphia: JB Lippincott; 1990:369-386.
36. Nahas GG, Sutin KM, Fermon C. Guidelines for the treatment of acidaemia with THAM. *Drugs.* 1998;55:191-224.
37. Solus-Biguenet H, Fleyfel M, Tavernier B. Non-invasive prediction of fluid responsiveness during major hepatic surgery. *Br J Anaesth.* 2006;97:808-816.
38. Biais M, Nouette-Gaulain K, Roullet S, et al. A comparison of stroke volume variation measured by Vigileo/FloTrac system and aortic Doppler echocardiography. *Anesth Analg.* 2009;109:466-469.
39. Brienza N, Giglio MT, Marucci M, et al. Does perioperative hemodynamic optimization protect renal function in surgical patients? A meta-analytic study. *Crit Care Med.* 2009;37:2079-2090.
40. Robertson EN, Driessen JJ, Booij LH. Pharmacokinetics and pharmacodynamics of rocuronium in patients with and without renal failure. *Eur J Anesth.* 2005;22:4-10.
41. Shihab FS. Cyclosporin nephropathy: pathology and clinical impact. *Semin Nephrol.* 1996;16:536-547.
42. Nolin TD, Himmelfarb J. Mechanisms of drug-induced nephrotoxicity. *Adverse Drug Reactions: Handbook of Experimental Pharmacology.* 2010;196:111-130.
43. Itoh Y, Yano T, Sendo T. Clinical and experimental evidence for prevention of acute renal failure induced by radiographic contrast media. *J Pharmacol Sci.* 2005;97:473-488.
44. Schweiger MJ. Prevention of contrast induced nephropathy: recommendations for the high risk patient undergoing cardiovascular procedures. *Cath Cardiovasc Interv.* 2007;69:135-160.
45. Thiele H, Hildbrand L, Schuler G. Impact of high-dose N-acetylcysteine versus placebo on contrast-induced nephropathy and myocardial reperfusion injury in unselected patients with ST-segment elevation myocardial infarction undergoing primary percutaneous coronary intervention: the LIPSIA-N-ACC Trial. *JACC.* 2010;55:2201-2209.
46. Petroni KC, Cohen NH. Continuous renal replacement therapy: anesthetic implications. *Anesth Analg.* 2002;94:1288-1297.
47. Meltzer J, Brentjens TE. Renal failure in patients with cirrhosis: hepatorenal syndrome and renal support strategies. *Curr Opin Anaesthesiol.* 2010;23:139-144.

48. Martin PY, Gines P, Schrier RW. Nitric oxide as a mediator of hemodynamic abnormalities and sodium and water retention in cirrhosis. *N Engl J Med*. 1998;339:533-541.

49. Gines P, Schrier RW. Renal failure in cirrhosis. *N Engl J Med*. 2009;361:1279-1290.

50. Salerno F, Gerbes A, Gines P, et al. Diagnosis, prevention and treatment of hepatorenal syndrome in cirrhosis. *Gut*. 2007;56:1310-1318.

51. Alessandria C, Ozdogan O, Guevara M. MELD score and clinical type predict prognosis in hepatorenal syndrome: relevance to liver transplantation. *Hepatology*. 2005;41:1282-1289.

52. Martin-Llahi M, Pepin MN, Guevara M. Terlipressin and albumin vs albumin in patients with cirrhosis and hepatorenal syndrome: a randomized study. *Gastroenterology*. 2008;134:1352-1359.

53. Schrier RW, Wang W. Acute renal failure and sepsis. *N Engl J Med*. 2004;351:159-169.

54. Schortgen F, Lacherade JC, Bruneel F. Effects of hydroxyethylstarch and gelatin on renal function in severe sepsis: a multicentre randomised study. *Lancet*. 2001;357:911-916.

55. Finfer S, Bellomo R, Boyce N, et al. A comparison of albumin and saline for fluid resuscitation in the intensive care unit. *N Engl J Med*. 2004;350:2247-2256.

56. Hojs R, Bevc S, Ekart R, et al. Serum cystatin C as an endogenous marker of renal function in patients with mild to moderate impairment of kidney function. *Nephrol Dial Transplant*. 2006;21:1855-1862.

57. Wagener G, Minhaz M, Mattis FA, et al. Urinary neutrophil gelatinase-associated lipocalin as a marker of acute kidney injury after orthotopic liver transplantation. *Nephrol Dial Transplant*. 2011;26:1717-1723.

58. Jones DT, Lee HT. Surgery in the patient with renal dysfunction. *Anesth Clin*. 2009;27:739-749.

59. Morelli A. Prophylactic fenoldopam for renal protection in sepsis: a randomized, double-blind, placebo controlled pilot trial. *Crit Care Med*. 2005;33:2681-2683.

60. Landoni G. Beneficial impact of fenoldopam in critically ill patients with or at risk for acute renal failure: a meta-analysis of randomized clinical trials. *Am J Kidney Dis*. 2007;1:56-68.

Chapter 33

INTRAVASCULAR VOLUME REPLACEMENT THERAPY

Christer Svensén and Peter Rodhe

HISTORICAL PERSPECTIVE

Plasma volume replacement is important in the perioperative period. The body and cardiovascular system are exposed to many challenges such as neurohumoral adaptations, evaporation, fluid redistribution, and blood loss that necessitate interventions. To achieve this, fluids are administered according to protocols based on tradition, expert recommendations, and often limited evidence. There is an ongoing debate concerning the ideal composition and amount of intravenous fluids necessary for perioperative management.[1-6] During the last century, recommendations varied from fluid restriction to giving liberal amounts for resuscitation.[7-12]

Surprisingly, intravenous fluids have been regarded as rather harmless, resulting in nothing worse than volume overload, which is often viewed as a minor problem.[13] However, intravenous fluids can be deleterious in large amounts if not timed according to patient needs.[3-5,14,15] In the late 1970s and early 1980s, acute lung injury due to increased filtration rate across pulmonary capillaries and subsequent pulmonary inflammation was suggested as a plausible consequence.[16] It has never been proven that large amounts of crystalloids cause acute respiratory distress syndrome (ARDS), however the link to abdominal compartment syndrome, which can be the result of large-volume crystalloid resuscitation, is compelling.[14] Traditionally, the rationale supporting liberal perioperative fluid administration included assumptions that preoperative fasting resulted in hypovolemia, that insensible losses increased considerably during surgery, and that some body fluid is distributed to a "third space."[11,17] Any resulting fluid overload was considered harmless because the kidneys had the capacity to eliminate the excess.[18]

The primary problem the clinician faces is that individual hydration and volume states are unknown before surgery. There is no simple test or physical maneuver to assess reliably either the level of hydration or the intravascular volume status. The clinician must rely on indirect nonspecific clinical signs to estimate the volume status of the cardiovascular system. Since the vascular system is highly reactive to neurohumoral changes and positioning, predicting the disposition of intravenous fluids is difficult.

Very few healthy stable surgical patients admitted for elective minor operations require significant amounts of fluid, and thus the perioperative fluid management of these

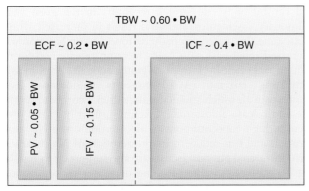

TBW ~ 0.60 • BW

ECF ~ 0.2 • BW   ICF ~ 0.4 • BW

PV ~ 0.05 • BW

IFV ~ 0.15 • BW

Figure 33-1 A static schematic of the distribution of body water. Water constitutes about 60% of body weight and is unequally distributed between extracellular and intracellular spaces. *BW,* Body weight in kg; *ECF,* extracellular fluid; *ICF,* intracellular fluid; *IFV,* interstitial fluid volume; *TBW,* total body water; *PV,* plasma volume.

patients is straightforward.[4,15,19] In contrast, for critically ill patients fluid management can be extremely demanding, and timing is very important.[20] These patients sometimes require large amounts of volume support, usually with monitoring by central venous pressure (CVPs), pulmonary artery occlusion pressure, invasive or non-invasive cardiac output monitoring, or transesophageal echocardiography to guide fluid resuscitation. However, evidence suggests that these monitors have limitations in measuring the adequacy of intravascular volume.[21,22]

CONVENTIONAL CONCEPTS

Body Water

With respect to traditional fluid therapy, the body is conceptualized as an interconnected group of anatomic spaces among which fluids distribute. However, this is a static concept that hardly reflects the complexity of how fluids dynamically distribute over time. Total body water (TBW) is the amount of sodium-free water in the whole body, commonly divided into the extracellular fluid (ECF) space and the intracellular fluid (ICF) space. Under normal conditions, ECF constitutes 20% of total body weight and ICF 40% of TBW for an adult.

The ECF consists of the plasma volume and the interstitial fluid volume (Figure 33-1). The plasma volume (PV) is relatively small, which is important to understand when boluses of fluids are given. The interstitial fluid volume (IFV) contains water but is mainly bound by a gel-like composition of proteoglycan filaments and collagen fibers (see later). Infused Na^+ distributes mainly within ECF, which contains equal Na^+ concentrations ([Na^+]) in PV and IFV(approximately 140 mM). The predominant intracellular cation, K^+, has an intracellular concentration ([K^+]) of approximately 150 mM.

MEASUREMENT OF BODY FLUID SPACES

There are several methods to measure the various fluid spaces. TBW can be estimated by anthropometric formulae, commonly validated from tracer dilution methods. Anthropometric predictions of various physiologic properties depend on height, weight, age, gender, and race; these population models

naturally result in various degrees of inaccuracy when applied to individuals. For example, TBW can be estimated by the formula: TBW (females) = −2.097 + 0.1069 • height (cm) + 0.2466 • body weight (kg).

Inaccuracy when applied to the individual can be substantial.[23] This equation does not take into account that TBW decreases with age.[24] The amount of body fat also influences TBW; fat varies inversely with water.[25] TBW can be measured by isotope dilution techniques, preferably with nonradioactive isotopes such as the stable water isotopes ^2H_2O and $H_2^{18}O$, and the precision can be as high as 1%.[26] However, these methods are not clinically feasible due to the complex experimental set-up and mixing time required for the tracer.[27] Another technique of estimating TBW is by bioelectrical impedance analysis. Although simple, quick, and cheap, there are many potential sources of error.[28]

ECF can also be estimated by tracer techniques. The most commonly used tracer is the bromide anion. Drawbacks of using bromide as a dilution tracer are that it requires a long mixing time and does not distribute equally through the ECF.[29] The blood volume is commonly predicted by anthropometric formulae but individual variation can be considerable.[30] Because the blood volume includes erythrocytes (in ICF) and the plasma volume (PV), the two components can be estimated individually. The volume of erythrocytes can be determined by isotope-labeling with ^{51}Cr and ^{99}Tc, for example, but there are other nonradioactive methods such as labeling erythrocytes with fluorescein.[29] A newer concept is to use a semiautomated blood volume analyzer that can provide rapid and fairly accurate information when assessing blood volume in blood loss situations and making critical transfusion decisions. It uses albumin-^{131}I and results are available in 20 minutes.[31]

MAINTENANCE REQUIREMENTS FOR WATER, SODIUM, AND POTASSIUM

TBW content is regulated by the intake and output of water. Water intake includes ingested liquids plus an average of 750 mL ingested in solid food and 350 mL generated metabolically. Perspiration losses are approximately 1000 mL • day^{-1} and gastrointestinal losses are about 200 mL • day^{-1} (Figure 33-2).

Thirst, the primary mechanism of controlling water intake, is triggered by an increase in plasma tonicity or by a decrease in ECV (see Chapters 31, 34). Reabsorption of filtered water and Na^+ is enhanced by changes mediated by the hormonal factors antidiuretic hormone (ADH), atrial natriuretic peptide (ANP), and aldosterone (see Chapters 32, 34). Renal water handling has three important components: (1) delivery of tubular fluid to the diluting segments of the nephron, (2) separation of solute and water in the diluting segment, and (3) variable reabsorption of water in the collecting ducts.[32] In the descending loop of Henle, water is reabsorbed while solute is retained to achieve a final osmolality of tubular fluid of ~1200 mOsm • kg^{-1}. This concentrated fluid is then diluted by active reabsorption of electrolytes in the ascending limb of the loop of Henle and distal tubule, both of which are relatively impermeable to water. As fluid exits the distal tubule and enters the collecting duct, osmolality is ~50 mOsm • kg^{-1}. Within the collecting duct water reabsorption is modulated by ADH (also called vasopressin). Vasopressin binds to V_2 receptors along the basolateral membrane of the

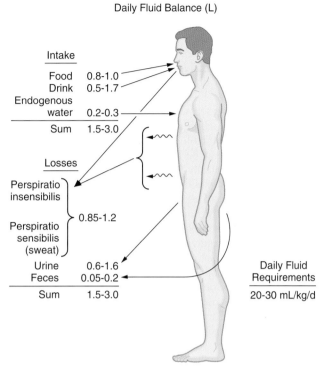

Daily Fluid Balance (L)

Intake
Food   0.8-1.0
Drink   0.5-1.7
Endogenous
water   0.2-0.3
Sum   1.5-3.0

Losses
Perspiratio
insensibilis   ⎫
               ⎬ 0.85-1.2
Perspiratio   ⎪
sensibilis   ⎭
(sweat)
Urine   0.6-1.6
Feces   0.05-0.2
Sum   1.5-3.0

Daily Fluid
Requirements

20-30 mL/kg/d

Figure 33-2 Schematic of daily fluids turnover. Arrow direction indicates intake or output. Water intake is required to offset gastrointestinal, urinary and insensible losses.

collecting duct cells and stimulates synthesis and insertion of aquaporin-2 water channels into the luminal membrane of collecting duct cells to facilitate water permeability.

Plasma hypotonicity suppresses ADH release, resulting in excretion of dilute urine. Hypertonicity stimulates ADH secretion, which increases the permeability of the collecting duct to water and enhances water reabsorption. In response to changing plasma [Na$^+$], differences in the secretion of ADH can vary urinary osmolality from 50 to 1200 mOsm • kg^{-1} and urinary volume from 0.4 to 20 L • day^{-1}. Other factors that stimulate ADH secretion, though none as powerfully as plasma tonicity, include hypotension, hypovolemia, and non-osmotic stimuli such as nausea, pain, and medications, including opioids.

Two powerful hormonal systems regulate total body Na$^+$. The natriuretic peptides, atrial natriuretic peptide (ANP), brain natriuretic peptide (BNP), and C-type natriuretic peptide, defend against Na$^+$ overload, and the renin-angiotensin-aldosterone axis defends against Na$^+$ depletion and hypovolemia.[33] ANP, released from the cardiac atria in response to increased atrial stretch, produces vasodilation and increases the renal excretion of Na$^+$ and water. ANP secretion is decreased during hypovolemia. Even in patients with chronic (nonoliguric) renal insufficiency, infusion of ANP in low doses (i.e., that do not produce hypotension) increases Na$^+$ excretion and augments urinary losses of retained solutes.[34] Aldosterone is the final common pathway in a complex response to decreased effective blood volume, whether decreased effective volume is true or relative (e.g., edematous states or hypoalbuminemia). In this pathway, decreased stretch in the baroreceptors of the aortic arch

and carotid body and stretch receptors in the great veins, pulmonary vasculature, and atria result in increased sympathetic tone. Increased sympathetic tone, in combination with decreased renal perfusion, leads to renin release and formation of angiotensin I from angiotensinogen. Angiotensin-converting enzyme (ACE) converts angiotensin I to angiotensin II, which stimulates the adrenal cortex to synthesize and release aldosterone.[35] Acting primarily in the distal tubules, high concentrations of aldosterone cause Na$^+$ reabsorption and can reduce urinary excretion of Na$^+$ nearly to zero. Intrarenal physical factors are also important in regulating Na$^+$ balance. Sodium loading decreases colloid osmotic pressure, thereby increasing the glomerular filtration rate (GFR), decreasing net Na$^+$ reabsorption, and increasing distal Na$^+$ delivery, which in turn suppresses renin secretion.

In healthy adults, sufficient water is required to offset gastrointestinal losses of 50 to 200 mL • day^{-1}, insensible losses of 850 to 1200 mL • day^{-1} (half of which is respiratory and half cutaneous), and urinary losses of about 1000 mL • day^{-1} (see Fig. 33-2). Urinary losses exceeding 1000 mL • day^{-1} can represent an appropriate physiologic response to extracellular volume (ECV) expansion or an inability to conserve salt or water.

Daily requirements for Na$^+$ and K$^+$ are approximately 75 mEq • day^{-1} and 40 mEq • day^{-1}, respectively, although wider ranges of Na$^+$ intake than K$^+$ intake are physiologically tolerated because conservation and excretion of Na$^+$ are more efficient than of K$^+$. Therefore healthy 70-kg adults require 2500 mL • day^{-1} of water containing a [Na$^+$] of 30 mM and a [K$^+$] of 15 to 20 mM. Intraoperatively, fluids containing Na$^+$-free water (i.e., [Na$^+$] <130 mM) are rarely used in adults because of the necessity for replacing isotonic losses and the risk of postoperative hyponatremia.

Interstitium

During surgery and trauma, extravasation of body fluid is enhanced. Capillary permeability increases and permits more fluid to escape to the interstitium. The ECV consists of the plasma (approximately in a 70-kg man, 3.5 L), the interstitial space (approximately 10.5 L), and small amounts of transcellular fluids such as gastrointestinal fluids, cerebrospinal fluid, and ocular fluid.[32] The interstitium is a mixture of fluid and fibrillar structures. The main nonfluid components are fibrils and the interstitial ground substance which can be subdivided into a colloid-rich and a water-rich phase. Fibrils are mainly collagenous, reticular, and elastic. The amorphous ground substance or gel-like matrix is produced by the same cell types as the fibrillar components. It contains several different glycosaminoglycans (mucopolysaccharides). It has been suggested that plasma proteins passing the capillary wall are mainly restricted to a random network of interstitial channels corresponding to colloid-poor, water-rich areas. Edema causes and increases hydration and depolymerization of the ground substance (Figure 33-3).[36]

Fluid distribution within the human body is related to the distribution of osmotically active substances. The physiologic distribution is maintained by biologic barriers and ATP-requiring pumps. The vascular wall is impermeable to larger molecules or proteins, with normal fluid distribution subject to an intact inner lining of the endothelial wall (glycocalyx).[37-39] When the outward and inward pressures are accounted

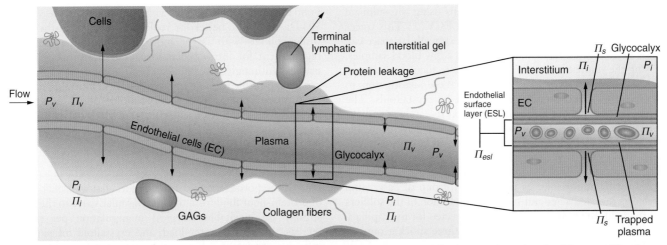

Figure 33-3 A capillary vessel with surrounding tissue. Endothelial cells permit leakage of water, small solutes, and proteins. Conditions can differ due to pathology. Abbreviations refer to the Starling formula, which is modified by the existence of the glycocalyx. The inner lining of the glycocalyx and trapped plasma together form the endothelial surface layer (ESL). A revised Starling formula would be as follows: $J_v = K_f ([P_v - P_i] - \sigma[\Pi_{esl} - \Pi_s])$. Within the ESL there is practically no circulation. J_v, Net filtration; K_f, filtration coefficient; P_i, interstitial hydrostatic pressure; P_v, capillary hydrostatic pressure; Π_i, interstitial oncotic pressure; Π_{esl}, oncotic pressure within the endothelial surface layer; Π_s, oncotic pressure beneath the endothelial surface layer; Π_v, venous vascular oncotic pressure; σ, reflection coefficient. *(Modified from Chappell D, Jacob M, Hofmann-Kiefer K, et al. A rational approach to perioperative fluid management.* Anesthesiology. *2008;109:723-740.)*

for, there is a small net filtration of fluid at all times. However, it seems that the deterioration of the glycocalyx, as seen in systemic inflammatory conditions, is of greater importance than the interstitial protein concentration for fluid escape over the endothelial wall.[40] The endothelial glycocalyx consists of a variety of transmembrane and membrane-bound molecules. These are mainly syndecans and membrane-bound glypicans, which contain heparan sulfate and chondroitin sulfate chains. The thickness of the glycocalyx is about 1 µm. Together with some plasma proteins that are membrane-bound, hyaluronan, and dissolved glycosaminoglycans, the inner endothelial surface layer is approximately tens of nanometers.[39] A degradation of the glycocalyx leads inevitably to increase of capillary leakage and interstitial edema, which is strongly correlated to a decrease in tissue oxygenation.[40] Reduction of the endothelial glycocalyx, such as in sepsis, major vascular surgery with global or regional ischemia, or diabetes mellitus can lead to changes such as increased permeability and release of proteases, tumor necrosis factor α, oxidized low-density lipoprotein, and atrial natriuretic peptide.[40,41]

Smaller molecules such as crystalloids are probably not much affected since they can escape through the barrier anyway.[42,43] Filtration normally leads to only a moderate shift and accumulation of fluid because both increased lymph flow and interstitial hydrostatic pressure, in combination with dilution of interstitial protein, limit excess accumulation of interstitial fluid. There is also normal transcapillary escape of albumin of about 5% of the intravascular albumin per hour, which is increased in a variety of diseases.[44] Transfer of albumin back to the intravascular space occurs via the lymph, but can be impeded by surgery and inflammation.[40]

THIRD SPACE

Clinicians frequently tend to replace losses to the third space during surgical procedures. The concept of the third space has been a topic of debate and controversy for decades.[29] Loss to the interstitial space is an inevitable phenomenon that consists mainly of small molecules leaving through an intact vascular barrier. When this loss due to trauma and surgery becomes pathologic it can be considered an accumulation within the interstitial space or the "functional" ECV.[15] This is normally removed by the lymphatic system as described earlier. However, when there is an overload, either by excessive fluid load or cessation of urinary production, the result is an even more pronounced accumulation of interstitial fluid. Fluid within the hypothetical third space is thought to be a "nonfunctional" body fluid separated from the interstitial space. Examples of the third space would be fluid in the peritoneal cavity, bowel, and traumatized tissues, with the key point being that losses to these spaces are no longer in rapid equilibrium with the ECF and thus are nonfunctional.[45]

A major problem is that the third space cannot be measured, and there is considerable controversy regarding its existence.[29] It is common belief that fluid spaces can be identified by applying a tracer intravenously. The tracer is assumed to equilibrate within the desired space and the dye or isotope enables identification of the distribution volume.[8] Unfortunately, interpretation of tracer kinetic trials is not simple. The volume measured is the volume-of-distribution of a tracer, and might not represent a volume of any clinical relevance. Furthermore, tracers are subject to differences in perfusion and equilibration time. For example, Na+ is rapidly transported to the intracellular compartment, bromide enters red blood cells, and is excreted in bile, and the sulphate tracer $^{35}SO_4$ is bound to plasma components and can accumulate in the liver and kidneys (and during shock in muscular tissue as well).[8,46] If the time for equilibration is too short, the concentration of any tracer in blood can be incorrectly high and the calculated volume-of-distribution will appear contracted.[46] To overcome this, tracer spaces should be calculated from multiple blood samples with continued sampling until equilibrium is demonstrated.

The theory behind the third space concept is mainly based on studies by Shires and coworkers in the early 1960s performed on both animals and humans using the sulphate tracer $^{35}SO_4^-$ to identify the functional ECV.[17,18] This tracer has a short equilibration time and the extracellular space can thus be calculated from a single or just a few blood samples. Using the sulphate tracer it was possible to identify an apparently contracted ECF space, which led these investigators to believe this space needed replacement by crystalloids. The Shires group had considerable impact on researchers and clinicians in the 1960s, but few other researchers have been able to replicate their findings. In a study of 50 young male war casualties, ECV was estimated by measuring the $^{35}SO_4^-$ concentration in multiple blood samples.[47] Comparison of one group with minor injuries to a control group of base camp subjects revealed a general state of dehydration of the soldiers in the field. In another study, when corrected for the capillary refill phenomenon, comparison of the three shock groups to the control group of combat subjects showed that the ECV changed in accordance with calculated fluid balance. Other investigators studied 10 healthy young male volunteers who were bled 11% to 14% of their blood volume with or without subsequent replacement with lactated Ringer's (LR) solution.[48] None of the subjects developed shock, and the ECV changed in accordance with the fluid balance.

Only trials using the sulphate tracer and short equilibration times have reported a "third space contraction." Other researchers using tracers such as Na^+ or bromide all report ECV expansion during surgical conditions. Trials calculating the ECV from multiple blood samples have found the ECV either unchanged or expanded following surgery.

The concept of a loss to third space needing replacement was introduced simultaneously with the conflict in Vietnam.[49] Liberal fluid administration together with improved evacuation and field surgical care (and improvement in other treatment modalities) might have saved many lives. Renal failure, which had been a major problem in World War II and the Korean conflict, was almost unheard of. On the other hand "the wet lung syndrome" (later diagnosed as ARDS) was reported in otherwise healthy soldiers resuscitated with large amounts of fluids after traumatic injury. However, the evidence for respiratory distress due to fluid overload is not compelling.[16]

Abdominal compartment syndrome is, on the other hand, linked to overzealous crystalloid administration. In a prospective randomized trial of patients undergoing colorectal surgery, a restricted intravenous fluid regimen omitting replacement of the "third space losses" significantly reduced postoperative complications compared with a standard regimen following traditional guidelines.[3] These results have been confirmed by another prospective randomized trials of more varied elective intraabdominal procedures.[5] Fluid kinetics studies indicate that the peripheral expandable fluid space during anesthesia and surgery is similar to that in awake volunteers.[50] The peripheral expandable space is in equilibrium with infused fluid, further contradicting the argument of an ECF contraction needing replacement during surgery.[51] Nevertheless there might be situations with low perfusion where cell membranes are altered and fluid does indeed shift to the intracellular space. These compartmental shifts might need replacement, but the use of aggressive fluid management in elective surgical procedures is not justified by evidence.

Numerous studies have argued that it should be beneficial to vary the choice of intravenous fluids in certain situations.

Fundamentally, crystalloids with molecules of less than 30 kDa should be better for replacing losses from the ECF, while colloids with larger molecules should be the ideal replacement for intravascular losses (apart from blood and plasma). Although these fluids show different properties, it has not been possible to show any differences in mortality in large randomized studies.[52-54] The crystalloid-colloid debate has recently focused more on side effects such as renal damage.[55]

Fluid Shifts and Losses During Surgery, and Their Replacement

Due to the porous nature of the endothelial wall, fluid shifts of protein-poor fluid from the intravascular space to the interstitium are inevitable. Surgical manipulation per se can increase interstitial water load, and crystalloid infusion can influence its extent.[56] Losses that consistently occur during surgical procedures include urinary output and insensible losses.[56] During trauma surgery and certain other major operations, blood loss constitutes a significant fluid loss. Urinary output and evaporation should affect the extracellular space (vascular system and interstitium) and should cause no net change in colloid osmotic pressure in the vascular system. On the contrary, intravascular loss (bleeding) contains blood components and thereby causes a change in colloid osmotic pressure.

To replace these losses it is logical to replace extracellular losses with crystalloid. The conventional perception of the distribution of crystalloids is that up to 80% are distributed to the interstitial space.[57] However, fluid shifts are context-sensitive. Sophisticated kinetic analysis (see section on body fluid dynamics later) demonstrates a central accumulation of fluid that eventually distributes to the periphery or is eliminated as urine.[51] In simple terms, this means that a crystalloid load initially exerts a substantial volume expansion effect (Figure 33-4), which is more pronounced during low pressure or bleeding, but the effect is transitory. This, however, has

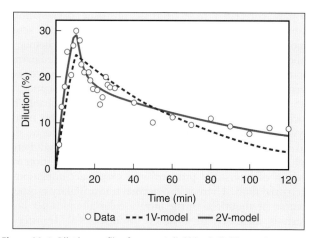

Figure 33-4 Dilution profiles for a crystalloid load. Fluid was given over 10 minutes, reflecting the time course of preload augmentation. Hemoglobin is used as an endogenous tracer to calculate plasma dilution, and the data fitted to nonlinear equations.[51] The broken *pink* curve is the kinetic profile of a one-compartment (one volume space) model, and the continuous *blue* curve shows the dilution profile of a two-compartment model (two volume spaces). The dilution is maximal when the infusion is turned off. The effect is transitory and the fluid is almost eliminated from the central space within 3 hours.

been challenged by those who advocate direct assessment of plasma and blood volume.[58] Colloids on the other hand have a more prolonged effect on intravascular volume.

To replace blood loss, it is plausible to replace intravascular loss either by giving blood or a colloid. Whole blood would be preferable but this is not usually possible due to logistical reasons and infectious and incompatibility risks (see Chapter 36).[59]

CLINICAL ASSESSMENT OF INTRAVASCULAR VOLUME IN CRITICALLY ILL PATIENTS

Visual estimation, the simplest technique for quantifying intraoperative blood loss, assesses the amount of blood absorbed by gauze sponges and laparotomy pads and adds an estimate of blood accumulation on the floor and surgical drapes and in suction containers. Assessment of the adequacy of intraoperative fluid resuscitation integrates multiple clinical variables, including heart rate, blood pressure, urinary output, arterial oxygenation, and pH. Tachycardia is an insensitive, nonspecific indicator of hypovolemia. In patients receiving potent inhalational agents, maintenance of satisfactory blood pressure implies adequate intravascular volume. During profound hypovolemia, indirect measurements of blood pressure can significantly underestimate true blood pressure. In patients undergoing extensive procedures, direct arterial pressure measurements are more accurate than indirect techniques. An additional advantage of direct arterial pressure monitoring can be recognition of increased systolic blood pressure variation accompanying positive pressure ventilation in the presence of hypovolemia.

Despite improvements in resuscitation and supportive care, there is a risk of organ dysfunction in patients with life-threatening conditions. Therefore it is important to evaluate the impact of fluid resuscitation on oxygen delivery often exacerbated by microcirculatory injury and increased tissue metabolic demands.[60] A key variable that has been associated with improved outcome in high-risk surgical patients and critically ill patients is systemic oxygen delivery (O_2) ≥ 600 mL $O_2 \cdot m^{-2} \cdot min^{-1}$ (equivalent to a CI of 3.0 L$\cdot m^{-2} \cdot min^{-1}$, a [Hb] of 14 g $\cdot dL^{-1}$, and 98% oxyhemoglobin saturation).[61] Boyd and colleagues randomized patients to conventional treatment or fluid plus dopexamine to maintain oxygen delivery ≥ 600 mL $O_2 \cdot m^{-2} \cdot min^{-1}$and demonstrated reduced mortality and complications in patients managed at the higher level of oxygen delivery.[62] Based on these results, the authors calculated that the cost of obtaining a survivor was 31% lower in the treatment group. In patients undergoing major elective surgery randomized into three groups (routine perioperative care; fluid and dopexamine perioperatively to maintain oxygen delivery ≥ 600 mL $O_2 \cdot m^{-2} \cdot min^{-1}$; and fluid plus epinephrine perioperatively to achieve the same endpoints), the two groups in which oxygen delivery was supported showed reduced mortality, and complications were significantly lower in the dopexamine group compared with the epinephrine group.[63] In patients randomized to conventional treatment or supplemented oxygen delivery ≥ 600 mL $O_2 \cdot m^{-2} \cdot min^{-1}$ using a combination of volume and dobutamine, an increase in mortality was observed in the treatment group, suggesting that aggressive elevations in DO_2 might be harmful.[64]

In summary, there is no apparent benefit of enhanced oxygen delivery for patients other than surgical patients and patients undergoing initial resuscitation from septic shock.[20] For surgical patients, early initiation of goal-directed resuscitation is associated with better outcome than delayed initiation.[65] Outcome can be strongly influenced by the choice of inotropic agents, and increased fluid given as part of goal-oriented resuscitation has been associated with an increased incidence of abdominal compartment syndrome in trauma patients.[14,66]

Conventional Indices of Resuscitation

Resuscitation of critically ill patients requires accurate assessment of intravascular volume status and the ability to predict the hemodynamic response to a fluid challenge. Indices of hemodynamic response such as blood pressure, cardiac output, heart rate, and oxygen delivery do not fully reflect the adequacy of tissue perfusion. Less than 50% of critical care patients given fluid boluses are volume responsive. Passive leg raising, however, represents an endogenous volume challenge that can be used to predict fluid responsiveness. This procedure rapidly returns 150 to 200 mL of blood from the veins in the lower extremities to the central circulation. As a result of increased ventricular preload, cardiac output is augmented according to the degree of preload reserve (see Chapter 21).[67]

Urinary Output and Clinical Signs of Hypovolemia

A reduction in renal perfusion normally results in dilatation of the afferent glomerular arteriole and constriction of the efferent arteriole so that glomerular filtration rate (GFR) is kept constant. However, if mean arterial pressure falls below 70 mm Hg (kidney autoregulatory threshold), renal perfusion pressure and glomerular filtration rate fall, leading to oliguria. However, the kidney is affected by many factors including cardiac function, osmotic load, intrathoracic pressure, intraabdominal pressure, and chronic renal insufficiency which make urine output an unreliable predictor of volume status.[32] Other signs of inadequate intravascular volume are peripheral cyanosis, skin mottling, tachycardia, hypotension, and cold extremities. All these signs are nonspecific and unreliable indicators of adequate resuscitation.

Response to Fluid Challenge

An important concept for guiding rational fluid administration is the use of the Frank-Starling curve for cardiac performance (Figure 33-5). In most clinical circumstances, a basic assumption is that the patient is on the ascending part of the Starling curve and has a submaximal cardiac output. When the subject reaches the flat part, more fluid administration has little effect on cardiac output/stroke volume and will only increase tissue edema. Although this concept applies to healthy volume-depleted patients, critically ill patients might also respond to a fluid challenge, and this concept can be applicable.[68]

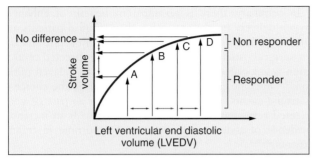

Figure 33-5 Relationship between preload and stroke volume. An incremental increase *(A-B)* in volume on the x-axis (left ventricular end-diastolic volume, LVEDV) increases stroke volume/cardiac output on the y-axis (responder). Eventually a deflection point is reached (between *C-D*), after which the heart will no longer perform increased work with increasing preload (nonresponder).

Static Measurements of Intravascular Volume

CENTRAL VENOUS PRESSURE

CVP is a common parameter used to guide fluid therapy.[69] However, the idea that CVP reflects intravascular volume is a common misconception.[70] CVP is usually measured in cm H_2O (1 cm H_2O is equivalent to 0.735 mm Hg or 10.2 kPa). The concept that fluids should be administered if the CVP falls more than 5 cm H_2O is still used today. The CVP, however, is influenced by many factors not related to actual fluid balance such as venous tone, intrathoracic pressure, and left and right ventricular compliance. Consequently there is poor correlation between CVP and the right ventricular end-diastolic volume, which it is intended to measure (see Chapter 21). Metaanalyses assessing the ability of CVP to predict fluid responsiveness show low predictability in that there is poor association between CVP and circulating blood volume.[71]

PULMONARY ARTERY OCCLUSION PRESSURE

The pulmonary artery catheter (PAC), is used to measure pulmonary artery occlusion pressure (PAOP) or pulmonary capillary wedge pressure (PCWP), which is intended to reflect left ventricular preload.[72] However, the PAOP is not a good indicator of preload.[73,74] The catheter measures pressure and not volume, the relationship is not direct but curvilinear, and clinical benefit is highly doubtful.[75,76] Left ventricular compliance is dependent on filling of the right ventricle, which means that the PAC suffers from the same limitations as the central venous catheter. Development of a PAC in which a rapid response thermistor and electrocardiogram facilitates measurement of right ventricular ejection allows calculation of right ventricular end systolic and end diastolic volumes. This should intuitively be a better measurement of preload but has not been convincingly validated.[73]

TRANSESOPHAGEAL ECHOCARDIOGRAPHY

Widely used in cardiothoracic surgery, transesophageal echocardiography has not proved a reliable predictor of fluid responsiveness in critically ill patients. There are conflicting results for use of left ventricular end-diastolic area (LVEDA) as a good predictor, because it is a static measurement.[77,78] Continuous measurements, such as positive pressure ventilation induced changes in vena-caval diameter and aortic flow velocity/stroke volume assessed by echocardiography all suffer limitations.

INTRATHORACIC BLOOD VOLUME INDEX AND GLOBAL END-DIASTOLIC VOLUME INDEX

Transpulmonary thermodilution is a method that uses a cold bolus as a single indicator for determination of the assessment of the largest volume of blood contained in the four heart chambers, called the global end-diastolic volume (GEDV). It requires the use of a specific thermodilution arterial catheter (Pulse Contour Cardiac Output Monitoring, PiCCO) that measures temperature changes following the injection of the bolus through a central vein catheter (normally the central vein catheter is placed in the neck, the arterial line in the femoral artery). It does not appear to be a good predictor of fluid responsiveness according to available studies.[22,79,80]

STROKE VOLUME VARIATION AND PULSE PRESSURE VARIATION

Intermittent positive pressure ventilation induces cyclic changes in cardiac loading conditions. Insufflation decreases preload and increases afterload of the right ventricle (RV). The increase in RV afterload is related to inspiratory increases in transpulmonary pressure. The RV preload reduction is due to the decrease in venous return pressure gradient which in turn is dependent of the inspiratory increase in pleural pressure. These simultaneous changes in RV preload and afterload lead to a decrease in RV stroke volume, which is at its minimum at the end of inspiration. The inspiratory reduction in RV stroke volume corresponds to a reduction of left ventricle (LV) filling delayed 2 or 3 heartbeats because of the filling of the lungs. Thus the LV preload reduction is at its minimum during inspiration. Changes in RV and LV stroke volume are greater when the ventricles work on the steep part of the Starling curve (see Figure 33-5). Thus change in LV stroke volume is an indicator of biventricular preload dependence.[81] According to a large systematic review, pulse pressure variation (PPV) and stroke volume variation (SVV) predict with a high degree of accuracy (ROC 0.94 and 0.84, respectively) patients who are likely to respond to a fluid challenge.[71] This suggests that currently PPV and SVV are the most accurate, dynamic tools for guidance of fluid management, but they are limited by arrhythmias and the requirement for mechanical ventilation. They are less reliable in critically ill patients under ventilatory support. Furthermore, PPV is a direct measurement while SVV is an indirect calculation from pulse contour analysis. PPV can be affected by the tidal volume, with the recommendation that tidal volume be at least 8 mL/kg.[21,22] Pleth variability index (PVI) is a measure of respiratory-induced variations in the plethysmographic waveform amplitude that like other dynamic indices has been shown to predict fluid responsiveness.[82] This is a rather new method provided by noninvasive hemoglobin measurement devices and some other monitors.[82]

ESOPHAGEAL DOPPLER CATHETER

This technique measures blood flow velocity in the descending aorta by means of a Doppler ultrasound device placed at the tip of a flexible probe. Patients need to be anesthetized or at least sedated in order to tolerate the probe; once in the esophagus, the catheter is rotated so that the transducer faces the aorta.[83] Because the width of the aorta is either measured or known, the cardiac output can be calculated when the heart rate is known. The flow time corrected for heartbeats (FTc) is considered an indicator for volume and afterload status. It appears to be a reliable predictor of fluid responsiveness, and has benefits for specific patient groups in reducing morbidity and hospital stay.[84-88] Performance depends on catheter positioning, but the required training for insertion is minimal.

NEAR INFRARED SPECTROSCOPY

New techniques such as near infrared spectroscopy are rapidly emerging and might allow monitoring of end organ markers of tissue perfusion and metabolism such as lactate and CO_2 and O_2 tensions.[89]

BODY FLUID DYNAMICS (MODELING FLUID THERAPY)

How do we analyze and quantify the volume and equilibrating process induced by infusing fluid into the human body? Is it possible to compare effects of different fluid therapies given in a variety of clinical situations?

A key problem in studying these phenomena is that infused fluid is added to a highly regulated system that attempts to maintain intravascular, interstitial, and intracellular volume through homeostatic adaptation. In order to describe these processes involved during equilibration of body fluids, we must use dynamic models to predict more accurately the time course of volume changes.[83,90] This modeling process is similar to pharmacokinetics for drugs. These analyses should permit estimation of peak volume expansion and rates of clearance of infused fluid and covariate analysis of other effects, such as changes in cardiac output or cardiac filling pressures.

As shown in Figure 33-6, the traditional clinical assumption of the distribution of infused crystalloids, one-third intravascular and two-thirds peripheral, is not always accurate due to large variations between individuals. The response to hypovolemia or hypervolemia depends highly on the starting hydration level, underlying pathology, and the general ability to eliminate and distribute fluid via homeostatic mechanisms.[91]

Computing Intravascular Expansion from an Endogenous Marker—Hemoglobin

If the intravascular volume V_b (mL) is defined as the distribution volume of hemoglobin (Hb), it is natural to use Hb as an endogenous tracer when analyzing volume expansion; assuming no loss of red cells, as plasma volume expands, Hb concentration decreases. Consider the relationship between the amount of Hb (X_{Hb}) and its concentration C_{Hb} (mmol/mL):

$$C_{Hb} = \frac{X_{Hb}}{V_b} \qquad [1]$$

If V_b is assumed to be a completely closed but expandable space (Figure 33-7), and fluid is infused by a constant rate R_i (mL/min), the concentration at any time point t can be computed:

$$C_{Hb}(t) = \frac{X_{Hb}}{V_b + R_i \cdot t} \qquad [2]$$

Since X_{Hb} is considered to be constant during infusion, Equations 1 and 2 can be combined:

$$V_b \cdot \left(\frac{C_{Hb}(0)}{C_{Hb}(t)} - 1\right) = R_i \cdot t \qquad [3]$$

Rewriting Equation 3 as:

$$\frac{1}{R_i} \cdot \left(\frac{C_{Hb}(0)}{C_{Hb}(t)} - 1\right) = Y = \frac{1}{V_b} \cdot t \cong \theta \cdot t + \varepsilon \qquad [4]$$

Equation 4 allows us to compute Y and ε (the residual error) by regression, to obtain an estimate of Y ($1/V_b$). The

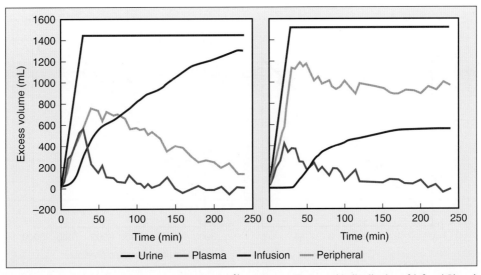

Figure 33-6 Mass balance computations for fluid infused over 30 minutes.[94] The figures illustrate the distribution of infused Ringer's solution in mL *(dark pink)* between plasma *(blue line)*, accumulated urine *(purple)*, and the peripheral fluid space *(yellow line)* for two subjects over time in minutes. The subject in the left panel responds quickly to the hypervolemia and has eliminated almost all the infused fluid during the observation time. The subject in the right panel has a less pronounced and slower elimination. *(Reprinted with permission from Rodhe P, Drobin D, Hahn RG, et al. Modelling of peripheral fluid accumulation after a crystalloid bolus in female volunteers—a mathematical study. Computat Math Method Med. 2010;25:1-11.)*

method is straightforward and only needs Hb data as an input. Figure 33-8 shows an example of experimental data obtained using the closed volume approach. In the right panel, the Hb-infusion estimation overestimates V_b by nearly 1 L. Although the predictions, based on gender, height, and weight, can differ considerably between individuals, the estimations based on the closed volume approach should be adjusted by an empirical correction term. This overestimation phenomenon might arise from two sources: (1) underestimating the rate of infusion or, more likely, (2) fluid is disappearing from the intravascular fluid space during infusion. Therefore the complexity of the fluid distribution model should be increased to understand intravascular volume changes.

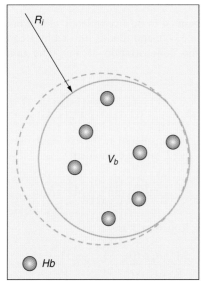

Figure 33-7 Closed volume approach. Fluid is infused at a rate of R_i which causes an expansion of the intravascular volume V_b. This in turn lowers the concentration of the endogenous marker hemoglobin *(Hb)*.

Plasma Volume Expansion

The plasma volume, at any time point t, can be computed from the hematocrit (HCT) as:

$$v_p(t) = v_b(t) \cdot (1 - HCT(t)) \qquad [5]$$

If the volume of erythrocytes is considered to be constant during observation time T (which is not true if bleeding is present), then the relation:

$$HCT(t) = \frac{HCT(0) \cdot V_b}{v_b(t)} \qquad [6]$$

holds for $0 \leq t \leq T$ where $V_b = v_b(0)$. Furthermore, the amount of Hb is constant and the relation:

$$v_b(t) = \frac{C_{Hb}(0) \cdot V_b}{C_{Hb}(t)} = \frac{C_{Hb}(0) \cdot V_p}{C_{Hb}(t) \cdot (1 - HCT(0))} \qquad [7]$$

also holds, $V_p = v_p(0)$. The *amount* of fluid a_p is now defined as $a_p(t) = v_p(t) - V_p$ and the relative change of plasma volume as:

$$D_p(t) = \frac{a_p(t)}{V_p} \qquad [8]$$

where D_p is dimensionless, referred to as the *dilution*. Then, using Equations 1, 5, 6, 7, and 8, a more compact formula can be derived:

$$D_p(t) = \frac{\dfrac{C_{Hb}(0)}{C_{Hb}(t)} - 1}{(1 - HCT(0))} \qquad [9]$$

Repeated measurements of Hb concentration can then be transformed into the dilution-time domain to describe plasma volume expansion (Figure 33-9). This constitutes a model for

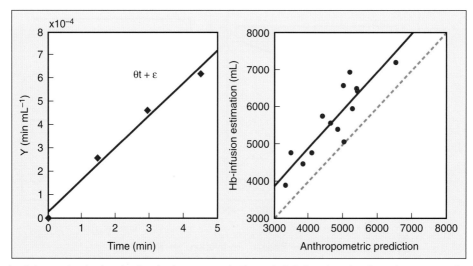

Figure 33-8 An example of data analyzed using the closed volume approach. The analysis is based on data from Figure 33-7. *Left,* Y is estimated by linear regression *(solid line)* from three consecutive time points (t = 1.5, 3, 4.5 min; *diamonds*) corresponding to three Hb values for one subject. V_b is then estimated by 1/y. *Right,* The distribution volume V_b was computed from 14 subjects *(circles)* receiving 1.5 mL/kg/min of lactated Ringer's solution.[95] Hb values were taken from arterial blood samples. Although there was a 1:1 relation between the anthropometric prediction and the Hb-infusion estimation, a bias of 770 mL was present.[30] The *dotted line* represents the line of identity, while the *solid line* represents the linear regression.

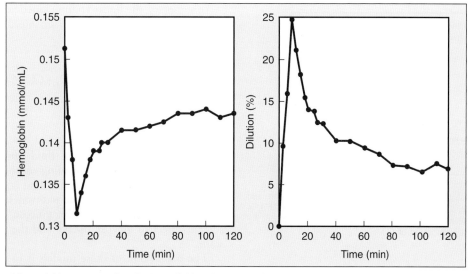

Figure 33-9 Example of hemoglobin concentration decrease *(left)* and corresponding dilution *(right)* following a crystalloid infusion over 10 minutes. *(Reprinted with permission from Svensen C, Olsson J, Rodhe P, et al. Arteriovenous differences in plasma dilution and the kinetics of lactated Ringer's solution. Anesth Analg. 2009;108:128-133.)*

Table 33-1. Basic Differences Between Traditional Pharmacokinetic Expressions and Their Similarities in Volume Kinetics

	PHARMACOKINETICS	VOLUME KINETICS
Observed agent	X (mg)	a (mL)
Concentration	C (mg/mL)	D (no unit)
Distribution volume	V (mL)	V (mL)
Mass at time t	$C(t) \cdot V$ (mg)	$D(t) \cdot V$ (mL)

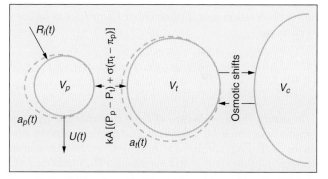

Figure 33-10 Basic volume kinetic model used to characterize the movement of fluid in the body. An infusion $R_i(t)$ of fluid causes an expansion by $a_p(t)$ in the central compartment V_p. This fluid is eliminated as $U(t)$ mL. There is also exchange of fluid with a peripheral compartment, here denoted by V_t, t for tissue. This exchange can be thought of as a whole body generalized effect of filtration mechanisms based on the Starling equation. If the administered fluid, given orally or intravenously, introduces osmotic imbalances, a third compartment representing the cellular fluid volume V_c is required.

intravascular fluid therapy that enables simulations to predict the effects of various fluids and dosing regimens.

The transformation of Hb concentration into dilution enables methods of analyzing infusion fluids using pharmacokinetic theories. This field is commonly referred as *volume kinetics for infusion fluids* or *fluid kinetics*. One conceptual problem with this approach is that we infuse fluid into fluid, where both fluids consist mainly of water. The term *concentration* becomes somewhat ambiguous from a unit perspective (Table 33-1).

Volume Kinetics for Infusion Fluids

Adaptation of pharmacokinetic/pharmacodynamic (PK/PD) nomenclature for infusion fluids has many advantages, not the least of which is treating infusion fluids as drugs, introducing concepts such as absorption, distribution, metabolism, and elimination. The process of *pharmacokinetic* modeling involves breaking down drug movement within the body into a finite number of compartments. Once the drug has reached its target area, the effect-site, the field of *pharmacodynamics* characterizes in quantitative terms the effects of the drug.[92] PK/PD modeling usually starts with some physiologic assumptions about the underlying process. From the closed volume approach, the following relation is derived:

$$v_b(t) = v_p(t) + VOE = a_p(t) - V_p + VOE = V_b + R_i(t) - U(t)$$
$$[10]$$

where $U(t)$ is a time-dependent loss of fluid due to the perturbation introduced by the infusion $R_i(t)$. Differentiating Equation 10 and considering *VOE* constant, the following relation is derived:

$$\frac{da_p}{dt} = \frac{dR_i}{dt} - \frac{dU}{dt}$$
$$[11]$$

Equation 11 forms the basis for volume kinetic modeling. Figure 33-10 shows the general pathways of fluid.

Fluid is largely eliminated by renal clearance. This clearance is mainly proportional to the volume expansion and therefore in its simplest form, renal clearance can be modeled by a first order approximation:

$$\frac{dU(t)}{dt} = Cl_1 \cdot D + Cl_0$$
$$[12]$$

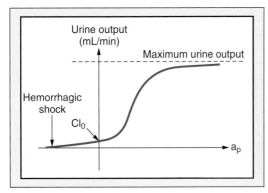

Figure 33-11 Relationship between intravascular volume expansion and urine output. The x-axis, a_p, denotes the plasma volume expansion. If a_p is zero, the plasma volume is considered to be at its optimal volume, or its baseline, having a basal elimination of Cl_0.

Cl_0 (mL/min) is often referred to as *basal elimination* and reflects ongoing losses of water due to respiration, sweating and basal renal filtration. For an adult, Cl_0 is about 0.5 to 1.5 mL/min, which is consistent with findings from volume kinetics computations.[93] If the total urine (U_{tot}) is known during observation time T, then either Cl_1 or Cl_0 can be computed from:

$$\int_0^T \frac{dU(t)}{dt}\,dt = U_{tot} = Cl_1 \cdot \int_0^T D \cdot dt + Cl_0 \cdot T \approx Cl_1 \cdot AUC(D) + Cl_0 \cdot T$$

[13]

In reality, the mechanisms of renal clearance are far more complex, governed by a feedback system that involves hormones including antidiuretic hormone, renin-angiotensin, atriopeptin, aldosterone, and angiotensin II. Specialized cell receptors are also involved including baroreceptors and osmoreceptors that regulate salt and water homeostasis. It is, however, possible to generalize fluid clearance from an intravascular expansion viewpoint, disregarding the turnover of Na^+ and other ions, within certain limits. The physiologic homeostatic mechanisms to maintain blood volume seem to be among the most highly developed.

Figure 33-11 displays a theoretical representation of intravascular volume expansion versus urine output. Normally, the human body is thought to oscillate around $a_p = 0$ depending on fluid intake and fluid and salt homeostasis. In a clinical setting, or for pathologic reasons, this relationship might be challenged. In this case, the linear relationship in Equation 12 will not hold, and a nonlinear model must be used, reflecting the shape of the relationship shown in Figure 33-11 for renal elimination.[94]

The exchange of fluid with the peripheral fluid space V_t can also be approximated in a linear relationship as:

$$\frac{dQ(t)}{dt} = Cl_d \cdot \left(\frac{a_p}{V_p} - \frac{a_t}{V_t} \right)$$

[14]

where Cl_d (mL/min) is the distribution clearance, reflecting a generalized impact on perfusion and permeability properties in various tissues.[95] During infusion, the initial intravascular volume expansion causes a flow into V_t when $Q > 0$. If $Q < 0$, the peripheral fluid space is thought to be saturated in relation to V_p, which results in a flow back to the intravascular space.[96]

In summary, the linear volume kinetic equations of an isoosmotic intravenous fluid, with no bleeding, can be represented by:

$$\frac{da_p}{dt} = \frac{dR_i(t)}{dt} - Cl_1 \cdot D_p - Cl_0 - Cl_t \cdot \left(D_p - D_t \right)$$

$$\frac{da_t}{dt} = Cl_t \cdot \left(D_p - D_t \right)$$

[15]

This model for infusion of fluid can be rewritten and extended in many ways, depending on the type of fluid and the clinical scenario in which the fluid is given.[94-100] If given orally, one needs to model the pathway before entering the central fluid space. If it contains glucose, one might have to add the effect of glucose uptake and the associated osmolar shifts.[99]

The main point of these models is to provide a platform to compare the effects of various fluids and dosing regimens on volume expansion, and the distribution and elimination of body fluids. Although clinicians are sometimes intimidated by the mathematics, it is only necessary to understand the models in conceptual terms.

The central fluid space, V_p, will presumably include tissues that quickly equilibrate with the intravascular volume. That is why V_p sometimes is referred as a functional distribution volume, rather than the plasma volume.[94,95] If the infused fluid is eliminated rapidly, there might be no exchange of fluid with the peripheral fluid space and no expansion in V_t. In this case, Cl_t will not be an identifiable parameter and Equation 15 will collapse into one equation:

$$\frac{da_p}{dt} = \frac{dR_i(t)}{dt} - Cl_1 \cdot D_p - Cl_0$$

[16]

Estimation of Volume Kinetic Parameters

Currently, there is no standardization for volume kinetic experiments regarding the ideal length of an infusion or the optimal rate. To evaluate the linear volume kinetic properties of a fluid, a brisk infusion for 10 to 30 minutes is recommended.[90] The empirical Hb values are then transformed into the dilution-time plane by Equation 9.

The volume kinetic model governed by the parameters Cl_0, Cl_1, Cl_d, V_p, and V_t (see Equation 15) is then fitted by nonlinear regression to the empirical values of Hb obtained. In this model, Cl_1 can be regarded as the *elimination efficacy*, that is, the ability to eliminate excess fluid. Cl_1 is typically reduced by hypovolemia, general and spinal anesthesia, and pregnancy (although it is increased during preeclampsia).[101-103] Cl_1 is also variably reduced by surgery.[104,105] In the linear form, Cl_1 can vary between individuals depending on hydration status (see Figure 33-11).[97]

V_p is often close to the expected plasma volume for crystalloid solutions but is reduced significantly for "volume potent" solutions such as 7.5% saline or Dextran 70 due to the simultaneous osmotic shifts into the vascular volume.[51] V_t is assumed to reflect the volume of interstitial fluid space, but volume kinetics findings indicate a smaller volume than expected.[102] The reason for this is that some parts of the interstitial space are not reachable during the time frame of volume kinetic evaluations and/or some parts are not expandable.[90] The parameter Cl_d reflects the rate and proportion that the peripheral fluid space accumulates fluid due to expansion of the intravascular volume. A high Cl_d indicates that fluid is transported readily into the peripheral fluid space, thus potentially forming edema if not given carefully.

Population Kinetics for Infusion Fluids

Volume kinetics for infusion fluids offers a tool for describing the dynamics of intravascular volume expansion with a set of a few parameters. However, these methods only give us an understanding of the *intrasubject* processes during fluid infusion. In order to develop dosing guidelines for different clinical situations and intravenous fluids, one needs to analyze how the effect of fluid administration varies across subjects and the volume effects of gender, age, weight, or type of anesthesia.

Population kinetic methodology is based on the statistical assumption of the presence of *mixed effects* to the basic model that arise from random effects and fixed effects. The fixed effects can be coupled to individual characteristics. V_p seems to have a strong correlation to predicted blood volume, which is in turn dependent on height and weight. Therefore it is reasonable to assume that weight might have a fixed effect on V_p.

The *random effect* is commonly modeled from two sources of variability: interindividual, which is the random variability between individuals, and the residual error, which can be due to noise in data. These effects, either random or fixed, are estimated along with the structural parameters to quantify variabilities. Population kinetic modeling of infusion fluids is a nascent area of study even though some analysis exists.[83]

Pharmacodynamics of Infusion Fluids

The concept of pharmacodynamics can be confusing for infusion fluids when one of the active ingredients is water. Where and what is the effect-compartment in volume kinetics? What is the endpoint of infused fluids (i.e., the targeted therapeutic effect)? In volume kinetics, the focus is mainly on the intravascular expansion effect of infused fluids. From this methodology one can create nomograms for different types of fluids to produce a certain level of dilution and therefore a targeted level of volume expansion.[106]

One of the most important endpoints of infusion fluids is to guarantee adequate perfusion of critical organs. This effect, or capillary filtration, depends heavily on hydrostatic pressure, the status of the endothelial glycocalyx, osmolar and oncotic content, and cardiac output. To fully evaluate the dynamics of an infused fluid with regard to the filtration effect, these quantities should be measured: capillary pressure, serum osmolarity, albumin concentration, among others. Therapeutic interventions to repair the glycocalyx have been suggested but this area needs further research.[38]

As the fluid dynamic model grows in complexity, it is often necessary to increase the resolution of the pharmacokinetic model in order to adequately describe arteriovenous differences due to net filtration effects, perfusion and flow through specific organs (especially the kidney), variability of vessel compliance, turnover of proteins, and even the adequacy of the lymphatic pump. This is beyond traditional PK/PD modeling and enters the physiologic domain, sometimes referred

to as *physiologic-based pharmacokinetics* (PBPK). Fluid dynamics is commonly modeled by the "lumped element method," which simplifies hydrodynamics, a complex field in physics, into a compartmental model with expandable volumes. Flows, fluidity, and resistance govern the flows between compartments.[107,108] They can also be referred to as their *electrical analogues*, in that they can be modeled by electrical circuits.[109] They can be further extended to take into account the dynamics of osmolar and oncotic content.[110] From these methodologies, full-body simulators have been developed, which in a more comprehensive way, quantify intravascular fluid expansion and fluid distribution due to infusion fluids.[110-112]

GUIDING PRINCIPLES AND CLINICAL RECOMMENDATIONS

Fluid distribution is guided by both *osmolality* and *tonicity*. Osmolality is the number of particles dissolved in water solution. The usual osmolality is 295 mOsm in body fluids. However, the tonicity also determines the distribution of fluids. Tonicity is the degree to which the solution moves fluid in or out of the ICF. Sodium chloride 0.9% for instance does not move fluid from the ICF and is thereby both iso-osmotic and isotonic. In comparison, ethanol raises the osmolality but does not redistribute water. Osmolality and tonicity are thus not equivalent.[93]

Hypotonic solutions are solutions with an osmolality lower than what is found in plasma. They are poor expanders and should be regarded as "water," which distributes to all compartments of the body.[93]

Isotonic solutions are solutions that have an osmolality close to the extracellular osmolality of the body. This includes solutions that contain Na^+ such as sodium chloride 0.9%, and acetated or lactated Ringer's. Both acetate and lactate are metabolized to bicarbonate that acts as a buffer. Isotonic solutions expand the whole of ECV.[93]

Hypertonic solutions have an osmolality higher than ECV. These include solutions such as hypertonic saline and mannitol. They rapidly expand ECV by mobilizing water from the ICV. If the hypertonic solutions do not contain colloids, the volume effect is transitory and after 60 to 120 minutes most of the plasma volume expansion is gone.

Crystalloids

Crystalloids are solutions that contain solutes with molecular weight less than 30 kDa, usually either salt or glucose; they are able to crystallize, hence the name. These solutes pass easily through the capillary membrane, a thin fenestrated endothelium that divides the plasma volume. Crystalloids can be hypotonic, isotonic, or hypertonic (Table 33-2).

NORMAL SALINE

Normal saline, sodium chloride 9 mg/mL (0.9%) in water, is a common solution for perioperative management in the United States. It is also widely used for mixing drugs for intravenous infusions. In parts of Europe it is mostly used for correcting metabolic alkalosis, particularly the hypochloremic alkalosis in connection with vomiting. There is a risk of hyperchloremic metabolic acidosis if normal saline is infused in large amounts.[113]

Table 33-2. Properties and Components of Selected Crystalloid Solutions Compared with Plasma

SOLUTION	OSMOLALITY mOsm	pH	Na⁺ (mM)	K⁺ (mM)	HCO₃⁻ (mM EQUIVALENT)	Cl⁻ (mM)	GLUCOSE % (mM)
Plasma	295	7.4	140	3.6-5.1	30	100	5
0.9% saline (9 mg/mL)	308	5.0	154	0	0	154	0
3% saline (30 mg/mL)	1026		513	0	0	513	0
7.5% saline (75 mg/mL)	2400	3.5-7	1250	0	0	1250	0
Ringer's lactate	273	6.5	130	4	28	109	0
Ringer's acetate	270	6	130	4	30	110	0
Ringer Fundinᵃ	309	5.1-5.9	140	4	24	127	5
Plasmalyte Aᵃ	294	7.4	140	5	50	98	0
Hartmann's solutionᵇ	280	6.5	131	5	29	111	0
Buffered glucose, 2.5%ᶜ and 5%	270 (2.5%)-440 (5%)	6-7	70	0	25	45	2.5-5
5% glucose in 0.9% saline (D5NS)	560	4	154	0	0	154	(278)
5% glucose in water (D5W)	253	4	0	0	0	0	(278)
5% glucose in 0.45% saline	505	4	77	0	0	77	(278)

ᵃBalanced—electrolyte content similar to plasma.
ᵇVery similar to lactated Ringer's.
ᶜSometimes called Rehydrex.

HYPERTONIC SALINE

These are solutions that are made hypertonic in order to move fluid from the ICF to the ECF. They were originally developed for prehospital use because quick restoration of the blood volume was desirable (the small size of bags were attractive). Large randomized trials have, however, cast doubt on the clinical benefit in these settings.[114,115] These solutions (3%) are currently mostly used to raise the level of sodium during hyponatremia and in the acute treatment of cerebral edema.

RINGER'S SOLUTIONS

Ringer's solutions are either called *lactated* or *acetated Ringer's solutions*, named for a British physiologist, or *Hartmann's solution*, named for a U.S. pediatrician who in the 1930s added lactate as a buffer to prevent acidosis in septic children.[114,116] In the United States and worldwide, mainly lactated Ringer's (LR), or Hartmann's solution as it is called in the United Kingdom, is used (see Table 33-2) as the initial crystalloid for resuscitation and for perioperative maintenance. The buffer ion in acetated Ringer's (AR) is acetate, which is mostly used in Scandinavia. While both ions are metabolized to bicarbonate, acetate is more quickly metabolized.[117] Lactate is metabolized in the liver and kidneys while acetate is metabolized in most tissues. Furthermore, lactate requires more oxygen for metabolism and causes a slight increase in plasma glucose, providing a theoretical advantage for the acetated Ringer's solution.[118]

Ringer's solutions are the fluids of choice for almost every situation. Although they are slightly hypotonic and low caloric, few side effects are observed. All Ringer's solutions are slightly vasodilatory and inflammatory. They distribute from the plasma to the interstitium in approximately 25 to 30 minutes with a distribution half-time of approximately 8 minutes.[98] However, this is a static concept of distribution. The fluid load is either readily eliminated or distributed to the interstitium. The volume effect of a crystalloid such as LR could be substantial depending on the effects of anesthesia, surgery, trauma, and hemorrhage.[83] However, the concept of calculating volume effects based on hemoglobin dilution (hematocrit dilution) is sometimes challenged by researchers

who claim the effects are overestimated.[58] If LR is used to compensate for blood loss, there is a conventional perception of giving three times the lost volume as replacement according to the static distribution profile mentioned earlier. These recommendations originate from studies in controlled hemorrhage models.[49] However, these studies suffer from difficulties with methodology and they do not fully emulate the clinical environment. Ringer's solutions should be used as initial fluids in major hemorrhage according to Advanced Trauma Life Support protocols but with some caution.[119] If there is ongoing bleeding, surgical hemostasis is necessary and if the patient does not improve, the fluid therapy strategy should be revised. For perioperative fluid management, Ringer's solutions are ideal for maintenance. Important guiding principles governing the use of maintenance fluids such as Ringer's solutions are:

- The extracellular deficit after fasting is low.[120]
- The basal fluid loss via insensible mechanisms is also low and approximately 0.5 mL/kg/hr, extending to 1 mL/kg/hr during more extensive surgery.[56]
- Evidence for a fluid consuming third space is not compelling.[29]
- Fluids are context-sensitive (there is momentarily a limited space in the plasma volume before a fluid load is eliminated), meaning that they should be infused and titrated according to needs and not too rapidly.[90,121]

Crystalloids in general have a tendency to accumulate peripherally during surgery due to neurohumoral protective mechanisms, such as increased levels of antidiuretic hormone, renin, and aldosterone. Caution must be used when crystalloids are infused for purposes other than pure replacement of extracellular losses because edema can result.

In summary, isotonic crystalloids are an inexpensive solution for initial resuscitation. They are also nearly ideal as a maintenance solution and for the replacement of basal fluid losses.

GLUCOSE SOLUTIONS

These solutions contain glucose and are thereby distributed to all body fluid compartments because glucose is eventually metabolized to carbon dioxide and water.[93] Elimination of glucose occurs by insulin-dependent uptake and metabolism by cells. In healthy volunteers, the half-time is 15 minutes but it is considerably longer during surgery.[99,122] Although glucose solutions initially have volume expanding efficacy similar to or even better than Ringer's solutions, they are seldom used for that purpose.[99] Solutions that contain 2.5% (hypotonic) and 5% glucose (isotonic) are readily distributed to the ICF because of the osmotic strength of the glucose.

The glucose-containing solutions are not administered commonly in the perioperative setting, in part due to the potential adverse effects of hyperglycemia. When they are administered perioperatively, they are never given plain but are usually part of a buffered mixture such as buffered glucose 2.5% (Rehydrex) (see Table 33-2). Establishing and maintaining a stable plasma glucose level in critically ill patients is an issue that has been of great recent interest.[123,124] Glucose solutions with ongoing insulin therapy

perioperatively might be necessary in some patients, but they require frequent serum glucose checks and careful standardization of care.

Colloids

Colloids are large molecular weight solutions that pass the endothelial wall with difficulty (Table 33-3). Plasma losses out of the circulation should ideally be replaced by iso-oncotic colloids, presuming the vascular barrier to be primarily intact and recognizing that colloidal volume effects are context-sensitive.[15] Colloids are mainly advocated because of superior volume efficacy and attractive rheologic and antiinflammatory properties. However, in large randomized studies, colloids have no superiority over crystalloids in terms of major outcome measures such as mortality.[53,54] They are more expensive than crystalloids and can have a more unfavorable profile of side effects.

Table 33-3. Properties and Components of Selected Intravenous Colloid Solutions

SOLUTION	OSMOLALITY (mOsm)	Na$^+$ (mM)	MOLECULAR WEIGHT (kDa)—MEAN VALUES/DEGREE OF SUBSTITUTION (DS)—C$_2$/C$_6$ RATIO	INITIAL VOLUME EXPANSION (%)	PLASMA HALF-LIFE (HR)/DOSAGE LIMIT	POSSIBLE SIDE EFFECTS
Plasma	295	140	Varying	Low		TRALI
Albumin 4%, 5%	300	130-160	69	70-100	16-24; No limit	Anaphylaxis (rare), fever, rash
Albumin 20%, 25%	1500	125	69	200-300	16-24; No limit	Anaphylaxis (rare), fever, rash, fluid overload
Hespan (hexastarch) 6% in 0.9% sodium chloride	309	154	600/0.75	100-160	20 mL/kg/d	Alteration of coagulation / Pruritus / Renal dysfunction
Hextend (hexastarch with added calcium) 6% in lactated electrolyte solution	307	143	670/0.75	100-160	1.4 hr/20 mL/kg/d	Alteration of coagulation / Pruritus / Renal dysfunction
Voluven (tetrastarch) 6% in 0.9% sodium chloride	296	140	130/0.40/9:1	1:1	50 mL/kg/d	Alteration of coagulation / Pruritus / Renal dysfunction
Venofundin	309	154	130/0.42/6:1	1:1	50 mL/kg/d	Alteration of coagulation / Pruritus / Renal dysfunction
Volulyte 6% in balanced salt solution	296	140	130/0.4/691	1:1	50 mL/kg/d	Alteration of coagulation / Pruritus / Renal dysfunction
Gelofusin 4% solution in 0.9% saline	274	154	30	1:1 initially but effect transient	No upper limit Hypervolemia is a concern	Anaphylaxis
10% dextran 40 (Rheomacrodex)* in 0.9% saline	350	154	40	175	1.5 g/kg/d	Anaphylaxis / Alteration of coagulation / Renal dysfunction
3% dextran 60 (Plasmodex)* in 0.9% saline	270	130	60	50	1.5 g/kg/d	Anaphylaxis / Alteration of coagulation / Renal dysfunction
6% dextran 70 (Macrodex)* in 0.9% saline	300	154	70	100	1.5 g/kg/d	Anaphylaxis / Alteration of coagulation / Renal dysfunction
HyperHES 7.2% NaCl with 6% starch	2464	1232	200	7-8 times NS	4 mL/kg BW 2-5 minutes Titrate to response	Anaphylaxis (rare) / Hypernatremia (transient)
Hypertonic saline-dextran (HSD), 7.5% NaCl with dextran 70, Rescueflow	2567	1283	70	7-8 times NS	4 mL/kg BW 2-5 minutes Titrate to response	Anaphylaxis (rare) / Hypernatremia (transient)

*Preinduce with Hapten (dextran-1) 20 mL 2 minutes before infusion.

ALBUMIN

Albumin is a natural colloid abundant in plasma (molecule weight 69 kDa). Commercially available strengths are 3.5%-5%. Hyperoncotic albumin, 20%-25%, is also available in some regions. There is normal translocation of albumin over the endothelium to the interstitium, and 60% of albumin is located extravascularly. Albumin is transported back to the circulation system via the lymphatic system. Albumin 5% expands plasma volume by 80% of the infused volume; infusion of 10 mL/kg albumin 5% increases serum albumin by 10% for 6 to 8 hours. In critically ill patients, there is increased leakage of albumin and supplementation of more albumin only contributes to peripheral edema (i.e., "albumin trapping"). Despite excellent volume-expanding efficacy of albumin, randomized clinical trials have found no superiority over crystalloids.[52]

DEXTRAN-CONTAINING SOLUTIONS

Dextran is a complex branched glucan (polysaccharide made of many glucose molecules). Dextran is synthetized from sucrose by certain lactic-acid bacteria, the best known are *Leuconostoc bacteroides* and *Streptococcus mutans*. When used as a component of colloid solutions, dextrans are mixed in normal saline as an isotonic solution. A hypertonic mixture, Rescueflow, is limited to prehospital use for treatment of hypotension during bleeding, but the benefit is doubtful.[114,115] Additionally, there is a similar solution combined with starch but studies are limited.

The isotonic versions of dextran solutions are either 6% or 10%. The molecular sizes of the dextran molecules are 40, 60, or 70 kDa. The most widely used plasma expander, 6% dextran 70 (Macrodex), expands plasma with the same volume as the infused amount, and the solution resides in the plasma for about 3 to 4 hours.[51] Dextrans have excellent rheologic properties and 10% dextran 40 (Rheomacrodex) is used for this purpose in vascular surgeries. It has larger plasma volume expanding efficacy but shorter half life than 6% dextran 70. Dextran molecules are excreted by the kidneys or metabolized by an endogenous hydrolase (dextranase) to carbon dioxide and water.

Dextrans are associated with anaphylactic reactions. This is, however, a rare occurrence and can be considerably reduced by infusing a low molecular weight dextran (dextran-1, Hapten) a few minutes before the infusion of the main solution.

HETASTARCH

Hetastarches are synthetic colloids consisting of polysaccharides prepared from either grain or corn. The most common concentration is 6%. Artificial starch–containing solutions for plasma volume expansion are characterized by their molar substitution and molecular weight. The molar substitution is an expression for how many hydroxyethyl groups there are for every 100 glucose units. This prevents the molecule from degradation by amylase. The average molecular weights range from 70 to 670 kDa, depending on the type of solution. Hydroxyethyl groups are attached by ether linkage primarily at C-2 of the glucose unit and to a lesser extent at C-3 and C-6. The polymer resembles glycogen, and the polymerized D-glucose units are joined primarily by α-1,4 linkages with occasional α-1,6 branching linkages.

Over the past decades there has been a trend to focus on the development of starch solutions with a molecular weight of around 130 kDa (tetrastarch). The older hetafractions and pentafractions have been associated with considerable side effects such as renal and coagulation problems.[55,125] The degree of substitution seems to be optimal, around 0.45 to 0.60 and a C2/C6 ratio less than eight seems advantageous (see Table 33-3).

Starches are mixed in normal saline (Hespan, Voluven) or balanced salt solution (Hextend, Volulyte). They all expand plasma volume by 1:1. Elimination of starch occurs mostly by renal elimination; larger molecules are cleaved by endogenous α-amylase in the plasma into smaller fragments and excreted or subjected to phagocytosis by the reticuloendothelial system. The expected plasma half time is 3 to 4 hours for a low molecular weight starch (130 kDa) before elimination occurs in a patient with intact endothelium.

Starches are used for plasma volume expansion with a substantial effect. Their use can be complicated by undesirable renal and coagulation effects. They are particularly popular during goal-directed therapy wherein cardiac output or stroke volume variation measurement methods show real-time effect of the therapy, although there is currently no clinical outcome difference between colloids and crystalloids in the perioperative setting.[54,84,85,126] There has been a long standing issue with renal compromise with high molecular starch (200/0.5) for critically ill patients.[55,127] A randomized clinical trial has shown that for low molecular starch (130/0.42) there was an increased mortality and need for renal replacement therapy for patients with severe sepsis and septic shock.[128] However, a randomized study with ICU patients in general given either HES 130/0.4 or saline showed no increased mortality within 90 days, but there was an issue with increased need for renal replacement therapy.[129]

GELATIN

Gelofusine is a 4% solution of succinylated gelatin mixed in normal saline. When the molecule is succinylated it becomes negatively charged and its volume expands. These solutions consist of polypeptides derived from bovine sources. They have a transient volume effect that lasts for 2 to 3 hours.

SUMMARY

In summary, colloids are intravenous solutions that contain osmotically active large molecules. Colloids expand plasma volume more significantly and for a longer period than crystalloid solutions. Disadvantages of colloid solutions include greater expense, variable anticoagulant effects, renal issues, and occasional anaphylactic reactions. Despite their popularity during goal-directed fluid therapy in critically ill patients, studies demonstrating clear outcome advantages for colloid solutions have not been forthcoming.

Clinical Fluid Therapy Guidelines

BASAL REQUIREMENTS AND REHYDRATION

Daily fluid requirements are 20 to 25 mL/kg in older adults and 25 to 30 mL/kg in middle-aged adults. This basal fluid requirement compensates for perspiration, urinary, and fecal losses.

Elective surgical patients should be normovolemic when they arrive; considering modern preoperative fasting rules, most patients present in a slightly dehydrated state that would, even for a minor surgery, benefit from a small amount of crystalloid solution (1-1.5 L) before and during surgery.[19] Larger deficits, such as during intestinal obstruction, have to be carefully scrutinized and more than 50% of the deficit needs to be replaced before surgery starts. If blood is lost, existing guidelines vary between 60 and 100 g/L in hemoglobin as trigger points for transfusion. Older patients will most likely benefit from a transfusion trigger of 80 to 100 g/L (see Chapter 36).

DAY SURGERY CASES: MINOR SURGERY

For most brief outpatient surgery cases, 1000 to 1500 mL of a crystalloid should be adequate to address the preoperative fluid deficit and ongoing maintenance needs. Treating mild hypotension with large volumes of resuscitation fluid is typically unnecessary.

SURGERY UNDER SPINAL OR EPIDURAL BLOCK

Recent evidence shows that preloading before spinal and epidural blocks has little impact on the hemodynamic stability after the block.[130] Crystalloids are minimally effective and then only when given as a rapid load (called *coload* in this perspective to differ it from *preload*) immediately after induction of the block. Most experts agree that treating hypotension with a vasopressor in this setting is more prudent.

GASTROINTESTINAL SURGERY

Most of the recent fluid therapy outcome studies are focused on gastrointestinal surgery. Optimal fluid therapy for open abdominal surgery has been a matter of controversy for decades. The Brandstrup study sparked the debate regarding liberal versus restrictive fluid therapy that continues today.[3] Restrictive fluid therapy aimed for a net balance in water intake and output as measured by body weight before and after surgery, Numerous studies have shown a lower rate of perioperative complications when more restrictive fluid therapy regimens are instituted.[5] The more liberal fluid therapies might be associated with more complications in part because evaporative fluid loss is often grossly overestimated (and replaced) as are losses to the presumed third space that might not exist.[29,131]

The following guidelines might apply:

- The current practice in many parts of Europe is to apply an ERAS concept (Enhanced Recovery After Surgery) to perioperative fluid management of gastrointestinal surgery patients.[132]
- Perioperative fluid management in this setting is guided by the use of semiinvasive devices such as the esophageal Doppler (Cardio Q) wherein small incremental boluses (150-200 mL) of colloids are given in addition to a low maintenance rate of crystalloids (2-3 mL/kg/hr). The concept is to incrementally give fluids to a deflection point on the Frank-Starling curve (see above and Chapter 21).

EMERGING DEVELOPMENTS

Historically, providers gave large amounts of fluids because fluids were regarded as rather harmless. In the last 20 years or so, there is increasing concern that intravenous fluid therapy needs to be more individualized. The long-lasting debate on the choice of fluids, crystalloids or colloids, has been replaced by a more fruitful one on the amount, rate, and timing for giving intravenous fluids. Colloids have been targeted as deleterious to the kidneys during serious conditions such as sepsis. Discussions are focused on the benefits of zero fluid balance and individualized protocols according to goal-directed guidance. Noninvasive monitoring devices seem promising to guide fluid therapy in the future.

KEY POINTS

- The body consists to a large extent of water. Crucial is an intake of approximately 2 L daily to maintain homeostasis.
- Fluid therapy has conventionally been recognized as harmless, but should be regarded as an individual therapy with considerable side effects.
- The so-called third space is not likely to be significant and should not be overzealously treated with crystalloid solutions.
- It is difficult to continuously measure the physiologic effects of fluid therapy. Static measurements such as central venous pressure or systemic blood pressure do not adequately show the efficacy of administered fluids. Instead, pulse pressure or stroke volume variation measured invasively or noninvasively better reflect the results of administered fluids.
- Fluid kinetics, similar to pharmacokinetics, is a recent tool to better understand the dynamics of fluid distribution.
- Fluid effects are context-sensitive: they distribute intravascularly if there is space for them (bleeding), otherwise they are eliminated, either renally or more likely interstitially during anesthesia and surgery.
- Crystalloids and colloids have different physiologic properties. However, in large randomized clinical studies there is no significant difference in outcomes.
- Restrictive fluid therapy is gaining popularity and is increasingly supported by evidence for specific procedures such as gastrointestinal surgeries.

Key References

Brandstrup B, Tønnesen H, Beier-Holgersen R, et al. Effects of intravenous fluid restriction on postoperative complications: comparison of two perioperative fluid regimens. *Ann Surg.* 2003;238:641-648. Initiated the debate on fluid therapy in the early 2000s by demonstrating the potential advantages of restrictive or zero balance fluid therapy for gastrointestinal surgery. (Ref. 3)

Chappell D, Jacob M, Hofmann-Kiefer K, et al. A rational approach to perioperative fluid management. *Anesthesiology.* 2008;109:723-740. An excellent review of evidence-based fluid therapy. (Ref. 15)

Connolly C, Kramer G, Hahn RG, et al. Isoflurane but not mechanical ventilation promotes third-space fluid losses during crystalloid volume loading. *Anesthesiology.* 2003;98:670-681. A kinetic paper that shows fluid distribution after anesthetic perturbations. Isoflurane anesthesia promoted interstitial fluid accumulation in this model. (Ref. 100)

Finfer S, Bellomo R, Boyce N, et al. A Comparison of Albumin and Saline for Fluid Resuscitation in the Intensive Care Unit (SAFE Study). *N Engl J Med.* 2004;350:2247-2256. Study showing that colloids were not superior to crystalloids in an ICU setting of nearly 7000 patients. (Ref. 52)

Rivers E, Nguyen B, Havstad SV, et al. Early goal directed therapy in the treatment of severe sepsis and septic. *N Engl J Med.* 2001;345:1368-1377. A randomized clinical study highlighting the importance of early management of septic patients. (Ref. 20)

Svensen C, Hahn RG. Volume kinetics of Ringer solution, dextran 70, and hypertonic saline in male volunteers. *Anesthesiology.* 1997;87:204-212. An early work on fluid kinetics, pharmacokinetics for fluids, that gives a plausible explanation to the distribution of fluids. (Ref. 51)

References

1. Healey MA, Davis RE, Liu FC, Loomis WH, Hoyt DB. Lactated ringer's is superior to normal saline in a model of massive hemorrhage and resuscitation. *J Trauma*. 1998;45:894-899.
2. Reid F, Lobo DN, Williams RN, Rowlands BJ, Allison SP. (Ab) normal saline and physiological Hartmann's solution: a randomized double-blind crossover study. *Clin Sci*. 2003;104:17-24.
3. Brandstrup B, Tønnesen H, Beier-Holgersen R, et al. Effects of intravenous fluid restriction on postoperative complications: comparison of two perioperative fluid regimens. *Ann Surg*. 2003;238: 641-648.
4. Holte K, Sharrock NE, Kehlet H. Pathophysiology and clinical implications of perioperative fluid excess. *Br J Anaesth*. 2002;89: 622-632.
5. Nisanevich V, Felsenstein I, Almogy G, et al. Effect of intraoperative fluid management on outcome after intraabdominal surgery. *Anesthesiology*. 2005;103:25-32.
6. Jacob M, Chappell D, Rehm M. Clinical update: perioperative fluid management. *Lancet*. 2007;369:1984-1986.
7. Cannon WB, Fraser J, Cowell E. The preventive treatment of wound shock. *JAMA*. 1918;70:618-621.
8. Shires T, Williams J, Brown FT. A method for the simultaneous measurement of plasma volume, red blood cell mass and extracellular fluid space in man using radioactive 131I, S35O, and Cr51. *Journal of Laboratory & Clinical Medicine*. 1960;55:776.
9. Shires GT, Williams J, Brown F. Acute changes in extracellular fluid associated with major surgical procedures. *Ann Surg*. 1961;154:803-810.
10. Shires GT, Coln D, Carrico J, Lightfoot S. Fluid therapy in hemorrhagic shock. *Archives of Surgery*. 1964;88:688-693.
11. Shires GT, Cunningham JN, Baker CR, et al. Alterations in cellular membrane function during hemorrhagic shock in primates. *Ann Surg*. 1972;176:288-295.
12. Roberts JP, Roberts JD, Jr., Skinner C, et al. Extracellular fluid deficit following operation and its correction with Ringer's lactate: a reassessment. *Ann Surg*. 1985;202:1-8.
13. Farstad M, Haugen O, Rynning SE, Onarheim H, Husby P. Fluid shift is moderate and short-lived during acute crystalloid hemodilution and normothermic cardiopulmonary bypass in piglets. *Acta Anaesthesiol Scand*. 2005;49:949-955.
14. Balogh Z, McKinley BA, Cocanour CS, et al. Supranormal trauma resuscitation causes more cases of abdominal compartment syndrome. *Arch Surg*. 2003;138:637-642.
15. Chappell D, Jacob M, Hofmann-Kiefer K, Conzen P, Rehm M. A rational approach to perioperative fluid management. *Anesthesiology*. 2008;109:723-740.
16. Ashbaugh DG, Bigelow DB, Petty TL, Levine BE. Acute respiratory distress in adults. *Lancet*. 1967;2:319-323.
17. Holte K, Kehlet H. Compensatory fluid administration for preoperative dehydration—does it improve outcome? *Acta Anaesthesiol Scand*. 2002;46:1089-1093.
18. Watenpaugh DE, Yancy CW, Buckey JC, et al. Role of atrial natriuretic peptide in systemic responses to acute isotonic volume expansion. *J Appl Physiol*. 1992;73:1218-1226.
19. Holte K, Klarskov B, Christensen D, et al. Liberal vs restrictive fluid administration to improve recovery after laparoscopic cholecystectomy: a randomised, double-blind study. *Ann Surg*. 2004; 240:892-899.
20. Rivers EP, Nguyen B, Havstad SV, et al. Early goal directed therapy in the treatment of severe sepsis and septic shock. *N Engl J Med*. 2001;345:1368-1377.
21. Marik PE. Techniques for assessment of intravascular volume in critically ill patients. *J Intensive Care Med*. 2009;24:329-337.
22. Hofer CK, Cannesson M. Monitoring fluid responsiveness. *Acta Anaesthesiol Taiwan*. 2011;49:59-65.
23. Watson PE, Watson ID, Batt RD. Total body water volumes for adult males and females estimated from simple anthropometric measurements. *Am J Clin Nutr*. 1980;33:27-39.
24. Morgenstern BZ, Wuhl E, Nair KS, Warady BA, Schaefer F. Anthropometric prediction of total body water in children who are on pediatric peritoneal dialysis. *J Am Soc Nephrol*. 2006;17:285-293.
25. Sheng HP, Huggins RA. A review of body composition studies with emphasis on total body water and fat. *Am J Clin Nutr*. 1979;32: 630-647.
26. Schoeller DA. Hydrometry. In: Roche AF, Heymsfield SB, Lohman TG, eds. *Human Body Composition*. Champaign, IL: Human Kinetics; 1996:25-44.
27. Hahn RG, Prough DS, Svensen C. *Perioperative Fluid Management*. New York: Informa Healthcare USA; 2007.
28. Bolton MP, Ward LC, Khan A, et al. Sources of error in bioimpedance spectroscopy. *Physiol Meas*. 1998;19:235-245.
29. Brandstrup B, Svensen C, Engquist A. Hemorrhage and surgery cause a contraction of the extracellular space needing replacement—evidence and implications. *Surgery*. 2006;139:419-432.
30. Nadler SB, Hidalgo JU, Bloch T. Prediction of blood volume in normal human adults. *Surgery*. 1962;51:224-232.
31. Fouad-Tarazi F, Calcatti J, Christian R, Armstrong R, Depaul M. Blood volume measurement as a tool in diagnosing syncope. *Am J Med Sci*. 2007;334:53-56.
32. Sear JW. Kidney dysfunction in the postoperative period. *Br J Anaesth*. 2005;95:20-32.
33. Levin AR, Gardner DG, Samson WK. Natriuretic peptides. *N Engl J Med*. 1998;339:321-328.
34. Conte G, Bellizzi V, Cianciaruso B, et al. Physiologic role and diuretic efficacy of atrial natriuretic peptide in health and chronic renal disease. *Kidney Int*. 1997;51:S28-S32.
35. Laragh JH. The endocrine control of blood volume, blood pressure and sodium balance: atrial hormone and renin system interactions. *J Hypertens*. 1986;4:S143-S156.
36. Haljamae H. Anatomy of the interstitial tissue. *Lymphology*. 1978;11:128-132.
37. Starling EH. On the absorption of fluids from the connective tissue spaces. *Journal of Physiology*. 1896;19:312-326.
38. Chappell D, Jacob M, Hofmann-Kiefer K, et al. Hydrocortisone preserves the vascular barrier by protecting the endothelial glycocalyx. *Anesthesiology*. 2007;107:776-784.
39. Chappell D, Westphal M, Jacob M. The impact of the glycocalyx on microcirculatory oxygen distribution in critical illness. *Curr Opin Anaesth*. 2009;22:155-162.
40. Rehm M, Bruegger D, Christ F, et al. Shedding of the endothelial glycocalyx in patients undergoing major vascular surgery with global and regional ischemia. *Circulation*. 2007;116:1896-1906.
41. Bruegger D, Jacob M, Rehm M, et al. Atrial natriuretic peptide induces shedding of endothelial glycocalyx in coronary vascular bed of guinea pig hearts. *Am J Physiol Heart Circ Physiol*. 2005;289: H1993-H1999.
42. Svensen C, Clifton B, Brauer K, et al. Sepsis produced by Pseudomonas Bacteremia does not alter volume expansion after 0.9% saline infusion in sheep. *Anesth Analg*. 2005;101:832-845.
43. Brauer K, Brauer L, Prough DS, et al. Hypoproteinemia does not alter plasma volume expansion in response to a 0.9% saline bolus in awake sheep. *Crit Care Med*. 2010;38:1-5.
44. Nicholson JP, Wolmarans MR, Park GR. The role of albumin in critical illness. *Br J Anaesth*. 2000;85:599-610.
45. Chan STF, Kapadia CR, Johnson AW, Radcliffe AG, Dudley HAF. Extracellular fluid volume expansion and third space sequestration at the site of small bowel anastomoses. *Br J Surg*. 1983;70:36-39.
46. Berson SA, Yalow RS. Critique of extracellular space measurements with small ions: Na24 and Br82 spaces. *Science*. 1955;121:34-36.
47. Anderson RW, Simmons RL, Collins JA, et al. Plasma volume and sulfate spaces in acute combat casualties. *Surg Gynecol Obstet*. 1969;128:719-724.
48. Roth E, Lax LC, Maloney JV. Ringer's lactate solution and extracellular fluid volume in the surgical patient: a critical analysis. *Ann Surg*. 1969;169:149-164.
49. Dillon J, Lynch R, Myers HR, Butcher J, Moyer CA. A bioassay of treatment of hemorrhagic shock. *Arch Surg*. 1966;98:537-561.
50. Ewaldsson C-A, Hahn RG. Kinetics and extravascular retention of acetated Ringer's solution during isoflurane or propofol anesthesia for thyroid surgery. *Anesthesiology*. 2005;103:460-469.
51. Svensen C, Hahn RG. Volume kinetics of Ringer solution, dextran 70, and hypertonic saline in male volunteers. *Anesthesiology*. 1997;87:204-212.
52. Finfer S, Bellomo R, Boyce N, et al. A comparison of albumin and saline for fluid resuscitation in the intensive care unit. *N Engl J Med*. 2004;350:2247-2256.
53. Perel P, Roberts I. Colloids versus crystalloids for fluid resuscitation in critically ill patients. *Cochrane Database Syst Rev*. 2007;4:CD000567.
54. Perel P, Roberts I. Colloids versus crystalloids for fluid resuscitation in critically ill patients. *Cochrane Database Syst Rev*. 2011;3:CD000567.

55. Brunkhorst FM, Engel C, Bloos F, et al. Intensive insulin therapy and pentastarch resuscitation in severe sepsis. *N Engl J Med.* 2008;358:125-139.

56. Lamke LO, Nilsson GE, Reithner HL. Water loss by evaporation from the abdominal cavity during surgery. *Acta Chir Scand.* 1977; 143:279-284.

57. Lamke LO, Liljedahl SO. Plasma volume changes after infusion of various plasma expanders. *Resuscitation.* 1976;5:93-102.

58. Jacob M, Rehm M, Orth V, et al. Exact measurement of the volume effect of 6% hydroxyethyl starch 130/0.4 (Voluven) during acute preoperative normovolemic hemodilution. *Anaesthesist.* 2003;52: 896-904.

59. Klein HG, Spahn DR, Carson JL. Red blood cell transfusion in clinical practice. *Lancet.* 2007;370:415-426.

60. Ince C, Sinaasappel M. Microcirculatory oxygenation and shunting in sepsis and shock. *Crit Care Med.* 1999;27:1369-1377.

61. Shoemaker WC, Appel PL, Kram HB, Waxman K, Lee TS. Prospective trial of supranormal values of survivors as therapeutic goals in high-risk surgical patients. *Chest.* 1988;94:1176-1186.

62. Boyd O, Grounds RM, Bennett ED. A randomized clinical trial of the effect of deliberate perioperative increase of oxygen delivery on mortality in high-risk surgical patients. *J Am Med Assoc.* 1993;270: 2699-2707.

63. Guest JF, Boyd O, Hart WM, Grounds RM, Bennett ED. A cost analysis of a treatment policy of a deliberate perioperative increase in oxygen delivery in high risk surgical patients. *Intens Care Med.* 1997;23:85-90.

64. Hayes MA, Timmins AC, Yau EHS, et al. Elevation of systemic oxygen delivery in the treatment of critically ill patients. *N Engl J Med.* 1994;330:1717-1722.

65. Kern JW, Shoemaker WC. Meta-analysis of hemodynamic optimization in high-risk patients. *Crit Care Med.* 2002;30:1686-1692.

66. Balogh Z, McKinley BA, Cocanour CS, et al. Patients with impending abdominal compartment syndrome do not respond to early volume loading. *Am J Surg.* 2003;186:602-607.

67. Thiel SW, Kollef MH, Isakow W. Non-invasive stroke volume measurement and passive leg raising predict volume responsiveness in medical ICU patients: an observational cohort study. *Crit Care.* 2009;13:R111.

68. Nixon JV, Murray RG, Leonard PD, Mitchell JH, Blomqvist CG. Effect of large variations in preload on left ventricular performance characteristics in normal subjects. *Circulation.* 1982;65:698-703.

69. Kastrup M, Markewitz A, Spies C, et al. Current practice of hemodynamic monitoring and vasopressor and inotropic therapy in postoperative cardiac surgery patients in Germany: results from a postal survey. *Acta Anaesthesiol Scand.* 2007;51:347-358.

70. Weil MH, Henning RJ. New concepts in the diagnosis and fluid treatment of circulatory shock. Thirteenth annual Becton, Dickinson and Company Oscar Schwidetsky Memorial Lecture. *Anesth Analg.* 1979;58:124-132.

71. Marik PE, Baram M, Vahid B. Does central venous pressure predict fluid responsiveness? A systematic review of the literature and the tale of seven mares. *Chest.* 2008;134:172-178.

72. Swan HJC, Ganz W, Forrester JS, et al. Catheterization of the heart in man with use of a flow-directed balloon-tipped catheter. *N Engl J Med.* 1970;283:447-451.

73. Michard F, Teboul J. Predicting fluid responsiveness in ICU patients: a critical analysis of the evidence. *Chest.* 2002;121:2000-2008.

74. Osman D, Ridel C, Ray P, et al. Cardiac filling pressures are not appropriate to predict hemodynamic response to volume challenge. *Crit Care Med.* 2007;35:64-68.

75. Sandham JD, Hull RD, Brant RF. The pulmonary artery catheter takes a great fall. *Crit Care Med.* 1998;26:1288-1289.

76. Sandham JD, Hull RD, Brant RF, et al. A randomized, controlled trial of the use of pulmonary-artery catheters in high-risk surgical patients. *N Eng J Med.* 2003;348:5-13.

77. Diebel LN, Wilson RF, Tagett MG, Kline RA. End-diastolic volume. A better indicator of preload in the critically ill. *Arch Surg.* 1992;127:817-821.

78. Belloni L, Pisano A, Natale A, et al. Assessment of fluid-responsiveness parameters for off-pump coronary artery bypass surgery: a comparison among LiDCO, transesophageal echocardiography, and pulmonary artery catheter. *J Cardiothorac Vasc Anesth.* 2008;22:243-248.

79. Hofer CK, Muller SM, Furrer L, et al. Stroke volume and pulse pressure variation for prediction of fluid responsiveness in patients undergoing off-pump coronary artery bypass grafting. *Chest.* 2005; 128:848-854.

80. Wiesenack C, Fiegl C, Keyser A, Prasser C, Keyl C. Assessment of fluid responsiveness in mechanically ventilated cardiac surgical patients. *Eur J Anaesthesiol.* 2005;22:658-665.

81. Michard F, Teboul JL. Using heart-lung interactions to assess fluid responsiveness during mechanical ventilation. *Crit Care.* 2000;4: 282-289.

82. Cannesson M, Desebbe O, Rosamel P, et al. Pleth variability index to monitor the respiratory variations in the pulse oximeter plethysmographic waveform amplitude and predict fluid responsiveness in the operating theatre. *Br J Anaesth.* 2008;101:200-206.

83. Norberg Å, Hahn R, Li H, et al. Population volume kinetics of crystalloid infusions in the awake vs isoflurane anesthetized state in healthy volunteers. *Anesthesiology.* 2007;107:24-32.

84. Gan TJ, Soppitt A, Maroof M, et al. Goal-directed intraoperative fluid administration reduces length of hospital stay after major surgery. *Anesthesiology.* 2002;97:820-826.

85. Noblett SE, Snowden CP, Shenton BK, Horgan AF. Randomized clinical trial assessing the effect of Doppler-optimized fluid management on outcome after elective colorectal resection. *Br J Surg.* 2006;93:1069-1076.

86. Sinclair S, James S, Singer M. Intraoperative intravascular volume optimisation and length of hospital stay after repair of proximal femoral fracture: randomised controlled trial. *Br Med J.* 1997; 315:909-912.

87. Wakeling H, MvFall M, Jenkins C, et al. Intraoperative oesophageal Doppler guided fluid management shortens postoperative hospital stay after major bowel surgery. *Br J Anaesth.* 2005; 95:634-642.

88. Bundgaard-Nielsen M, Holte K, Secher NH, Kehlet H. Monitoring of peri-operative fluid administration by individualized goal-directed therapy. *Acta Anaesth Scand.* 2007;51:331-340.

89. Heringlake M, Garbers C, Kabler JH, et al. Preoperative cerebral oxygen saturation and clinical outcomes in cardiac surgery. *Anesthesiology.* 2011;114:58-69.

90. Hahn RG. Volume kinetics for infusion fluids. *Anesthesiology.* 2009;113:470-481.

91. Hahn RG, Drobin D. Urinary excretion as an input variable in volume kinetic analysis of Ringer's solution. *Br J Anaesth.* 1998;80: 183-188.

92. Gabrielsson J, Weiner D. *Pharmacokinetic and Pharmacodynamic Data Analysis: Concepts and Applications.* 3rd ed. Stockholm: Swedish Pharmaceutical Press; 2000.

93. Guyton AC, Hall JE. *Textbook of Medical Physiology.* 9th ed. Philadelphia: WB Saunders; 1996.

94. Rodhe P, Drobin D, Hahn RG, et al. Modelling of peripheral fluid accumulation after a crystalloid bolus in female volunteers—a mathematical study. *Computat Math Method Med.* 2010;25:1-11.

95. Svensen C, Olsson J, Rodhe P, et al. Arteriovenous differences in plasma dilution and the kinetics of lactated Ringer's solution. *Anesth Analg.* 2009;108:128-133.

96. Drobin D. A single-model solution for volume kinetic analysis of isotonic fluid infusions. *Acta Anaesthesiol Scand.* 2006;50:1074-1080.

97. Svensen C, Drobin D, Olsson J, Hahn RG. Stability of the interstitial matrix after crystalloid fluid loading studied by volume kinetic analysis. *Br J Anaesth.* 1999;82:496-502.

98. Drobin D, Hahn RG. Kinetics of isotonic and hypertonic plasma expanders. *Anesthesiology.* 2002;96:1371-1380.

99. Sjöstrand F, Edsberg L, Hahn RG. Volume kinetics of glucose solutions given by intravenous infusions. *Br J Anaesth.* 2001; 87:1-10.

100. Connolly C, Kramer G, Hahn RG, et al. Isoflurane but not mechanical ventilation promotes third-space fluid losses during crystalloid volume loading. *Anesthesiology.* 2003;98:670-681.

101. Drobin D, Hahn RG. Volume kinetics of Ringer's solution in hypovolemic volunteers. *Anesthesiology.* 1999;90:81-91.

102. Ewaldsson C-A, Hahn RG. Volume kinetics if Ringer's solution during induction of spinal anaesthesia. *Br J Anaes.* 2001;87:406-414.

103. Drobin D, Hahn RG. Distribution and elimination of crystalloid fluid in pre-eclampsia. *Clin Sci (Lond).* 2004;106:307-313.

104. Hahn R, Brauer LP, Rodhe P, Svensen C, Prough DS. Isoflurane inhibits transcapillary compensatory volume expansion. *Anesth Analg.* 2006;103:350-358.

105. Svensen C, Olsson J, Hahn R. Intravascular fluid administration and hemodynamic performance during open abdominal surgery. *Anesth Analg*. 2006;103:671-676.

106. Hahn RG, Svensen C. Plasma dilution and the rate of infusion of Ringer's solution. *Br J Anaesth*. 1997;79:64-67.

107. Stevens SA, Lakin WD, Penar PL. Modeling steady-state intracranial pressures in supine, head-down tilt and microgravity conditions. *Aviat Space Environ Med*. 2005;76:329-338.

108. Maines BH, Brennen CE. Lumped parameter model for computing the minimum pressure during mechanical heart valve closure. *J Biomech Eng*. 2005;127:648-655.

109. Cavalcanti S, Di Marco LY. Numerical simulation of the hemodynamic response to hemodialysis-induced hypovolemia. *Artif Organs*. 1999;23:1063-1073.

110. Gyenge CC, Bowen BD, Reed RK, Bert JL. Transport of fluid and solutes in the body. I. Formulation of a mathematical model. *Am J Physiol*. 1999;277:H1215-H1227.

111. Rawson RE, Dispensa ME, Goldstein RE, Nicholson KW, Vidal NK. A simulation for teaching the basic and clinical science of fluid therapy. *Adv Physiol Educ*. 2009;33:202-208.

112. Ikeda N, Marumo F, Shirataka M, Sato T. A model of overall regulation of body fluids. *Ann Biomed Eng*. 1979;7:135-166.

113. Healey MA, Davis RE, Liu FC, Loomis WH. Lactated ringer's is superior to normal saline in a model of massive hemorrhage and resuscitation. *J Trauma*. 1998;45:894-899.

114. Bulger EM, Jurkovich GJ, Nathens AB, et al. Hypertonic resuscitation of hypovolemic shock after blunt trauma: a randomized controlled trial. *Arch Surg*. 2008;143:139-148.

115. Bulger EM, May S, Kerby JD, et al. Out-of-hospital hypertonic resuscitation after traumatic hypovolemic shock: a randomized, placebo controlled trial. *Ann Surg*. 2011;253:431-441.

116. Ringer S. Regarding the action of the hydrate of soda, hydrate of ammonia, and the hydrate of potash on the ventricle of the frog's heart. *J Physiol*. 1882;3:195-202.

117. Kuze S, Naruse T, Ito Y, Nakamaru K. Comparative study of intravenous administration of Ringer's lactate, Ringer's acetate and 5% glucose containing these Ringer's solutions in human being. *J Anesth*. 1990;4:155-161.

118. Ahlborg G, Hagenfeldt L, Wahren J. Influence of lactate infusion on glucose and FFA metabolism in man. *Scand J Clin Lab Invest*. 1976;36:193-201.

119. ATLS. *Advanced Trauma Life Support for Doctors: Student Course Manual*. Chicago: American College of Surgeons; 2008.

120. Jacob M, Chappell D, Conzen P, Finsterer U, Rehm M. Blood volume is normal after pre-operative overnight fasting. *Acta Anaesth Scand*. 2008;52:522-529.

121. Svensen C, Hjelmqvist H, Hahn RG. Volume kinetics of Ringer solution in endotoxinaemia in conscious rabbits. *J Endotoxin Re*. 1997;4:425-430.

122. Sjostrand F, Hahn RG. Volume kinetics of glucose 2.5% solution during laparoscopic cholecystectomy. *Br J Anaesth*. 2004;92:485-492.

123. Van den Berghe G, Wouters P, Weekers F, et al. Intensive insulin therapy in the critically ill. *N Engl J Med*. 2001;345:1359-1367.

124. Mesotten D, Van den Berghe G. Glycemic targets and approaches to management of the patient with critical illness. *Curr Diabet Rep*. 2012;12:101-107.

125. Wilkes MM, Navickis RJ, Sibbald WJ. Albumin versus hydroxyethyl starch in cardiopulmonary bypass surgery: a meta-analysis of postoperative bleeding. *Ann Thorac Surg*. 2001;72:527-533.

126. Sinclair S, James SA, Singer M. Intraoperative intravascular volume optimisation and length of hospital stay after repair of proximal femur fracture: randomised controlled trial. *Br Med J*. 1997;315:909-912.

127. Reinhart K, Hartog CS. Hydroxyethyl starch in patients with trauma. *Br J Anaesth*. 2012;108:321-322.

128. Perner A, Haase N, Guttormsen A, et al. Hydroxyethyl Starch 130/0.4 versus Ringer's Acetate in Severe Sepsis. *N Engl J Med*. 2012;367:124-134.

129. Myburgh JA, Finfer S, Bellomo R, et al. Hydroxyethyl Starch or Saline for Fluid Resuscitation in Intensive Care. *N Engl J Med*. 2012 October 17. [Epub ahead of print]

130. Dyer RA, Farina Z, Joubert IA, et al. Crystalloid preload versus rapid crystalloid administration after induction of spinal anaesthesia (coload) for elective caesarean section. *Anaesth Intensive Care*. 2004;32:351-357.

131. Brandstrup B. Fluid therapy for the surgical patient. *Best Pract Res Clin Anaesthesiol*. 2006;20:265-283.

132. Rawlinson A, Kang P, Evans J, Khanna A. A systematic review of enhanced recovery protocols in colorectal surgery. *Ann R Coll Surg Engl*. 2011;93:583-588.

ELECTROLYTES AND DIURETICS

Christer Svensén

Appropriate electrolyte levels are essential for human health. The major electrolytes, sodium (Na^+), potassium (K^+), calcium (Ca^{2+}), phosphate (PO_4^{3-}) and magnesium (Mg^{2+}), are critical to basic physiologic functions including action potential generation, cardiac rhythm control, muscle contraction, and energy storage, among others. Electrolytes, most notably Mg^{2+}, are also important cofactors that are vital for the proper function of many crucial enzyme systems including enzymes involved in DNA and protein synthesis, and energy metabolism. Because appropriate electrolyte concentrations are so critical in human physiology, sophisticated homeostatic mechanisms maintain their concentrations within a narrow range.

When pathologic states alter electrolyte concentrations, severe physiologic aberrations can result despite these homeostatic mechanisms. Therapies to increase or decrease electrolyte concentrations are thus important in modern medicine, especially in critical care. Sometimes electrolyte supplementation is necessary; in this context, an electrolyte intravenous solution or oral preparation can be viewed as a drug.

In this chapter, the physiologic role, the most common pathologic alterations, and the appropriate therapies, including the use of electrolytes as drugs, are discussed for each major electrolyte. The physiology and therapeutic considerations related to diuretics, a group of drugs that play an important role in perioperative medicine and that have a pronounced influence on electrolyte homeostasis, are also discussed.

ELECTROLYTES

Sodium

PHYSIOLOGIC ROLE

Sodium ion (Na^+) is the principal extracellular cation and solute, and is essential for generation of action potentials in nervous and cardiac tissue. Pathologic increases or decreases in *total body* Na^+ are associated with corresponding increases or decreases of extracellular volume (ECV) and plasma volume (PV). Disorders of Na^+ *concentration* (i.e., hyponatremia and hypernatremia) usually result from relative excesses or deficits, respectively, of water. Regulation of total body Na^+ and plasma Na^+ concentration ($[Na^+]$) is accomplished primarily by the endocrine and renal systems (Table 34-1). Secretion of aldosterone and antinatriuretic peptide (ANP) control *total body* Na⁺. Antidiuretic hormone (ADH) is secreted in response to increased osmolality or decreased blood pressure, and primarily regulates [Na⁺].

HYPONATREMIA

Hyponatremia, defined as [Na⁺] <135 mEq/L or mM, is the most common electrolyte disturbance in hospitalized patients with a prevalence reaching 30% and can be associated with a high mortality.[1-5] In the majority of hyponatremic hospitalized patients, total body Na⁺ is normal or increased. The most

common clinical associations with hyponatremia include the postoperative state, acute intracranial disease, malignant disease, medications, and acute pulmonary disease.

The signs and symptoms of hyponatremia depend on both the rate and severity of the decrease in plasma [Na⁺]. Symptoms that can accompany severe hyponatremia ([Na⁺] <120 mM) include loss of appetite, nausea, vomiting, cramps, weakness, altered level of consciousness, coma, and seizures. Acute central nervous system (CNS) manifestations relate to brain swelling. Because the blood-brain barrier is poorly permeable to Na⁺ but freely permeable to water, a rapid decrease in plasma [Na⁺] promptly increases both extracellular and intracellular brain water. Because the brain rapidly compensates for changes in osmolality, acute hyponatremia produces more severe symptoms than chronic hyponatremia. The symptoms of chronic hyponatremia probably relate to depletion of brain electrolytes. Once brain volume has compensated for hyponatremia, rapid increases in [Na⁺] can lead to abrupt brain dehydration (Figure 34-1).[4]

Hyponatremia can be classified as true hypoosmotic hyponatremia, pseudohyponatremia, and syndrome of inappropriate secretion of antidiuretic hormone (SIADH) (Tables 34-2, 34-3, and 34-4). Pseudohyponatremia is an artifact associated with the use of flame photometry, now an obsolete technique, to measure plasma [Na⁺] in severely hyperproteinemic or hyperlipidemic patients. The current analytic method, direct potentiometry, directly measures [Na⁺] and is uninfluenced by plasma components such as proteins and lipids.

Hyponatremia can be isotonic (P_{osm} 280-295 mOsm/kg), hypotonic (P_{osm} < 280 mOsm/kg), or hypertonic (P_{osm} >

Table 34-1. Regulation of Electrolytes

ELECTROLYTE	REGULATED BY
Sodium	Aldosterone
	Atrial natriuretic peptide (ANP)
	[Na⁺] altered by ADH
Potassium	Aldosterone
	Epinephrine
	Insulin
	Intrinsic renal mechanisms
Calcium	PTH
	Vitamin D
Phosphorus	Primarily renal mechanisms
	Minor: PTH
Magnesium	Primarily renal mechanisms
	Minor: PTH, vitamin D

ADH, Antidiuretic hormone; *PTH,* parathyroid hormone.

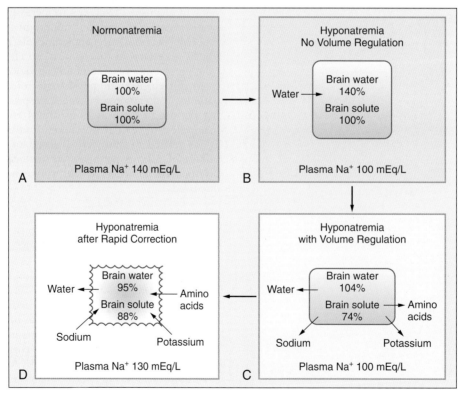

Figure 34-1 Brain water and solute concentrations in hyponatremia. If normal plasma sodium (Na⁺) concentration **(A)** suddenly decreases, the theoretical increase in brain water is proportional to the decrease in plasma Na⁺ **(B)**. However, because of adaptive loss of cerebral intracellular solute, cerebral edema is minimized in chronic hyponatremia **(C)**. Once adaptation occurs, a rapid return of plasma Na⁺ concentration toward normal results in brain dehydration **(D)**.

Table 34-2. Causes of True Hypo-Osmotic Hyponatremia

Hypovolemia
  Renal losses (urinary sodium >20 mEq/L)
    Diuretic therapy
    Mineralocorticoid deficiency
    Cerebral salt wasting syndrome (e.g., subarachnoid hemorrhage)
    Renal disease
    Renal tubular acidosis (bicarbonaturia with renal tubular acidosis
      and metabolic alkalosis)
    Renal tubular defect (salt wasting nephropathy)
  External losses (urinary sodium <20 mEq/L)
    Gastrointestinal disease—vomiting, diarrhea, gastric suctioning
    Skin losses—burns, sweating, cystic fibrosis
    Pancreatitis
    Trauma
Hypervolemia
  Renal causes (urinary sodium >20 mEq/L)
    Renal failure
  Other causes (urinary sodium <20 mEq/L)
    Congestive heart failure
    Hepatic cirrhosis
    Nephrotic syndrome
    Pregnancy
Euvolemia (Urinary Sodium >20 mEq/L)
  Glucocorticoid deficiency
  Hypothyroidism
  Syndrome of inappropriate antidiuretic hormone
  Reset osmostat—psychosis, malnutrition

Table 34-3. Causes of Pseudohyponatremia

Normal Plasma Osmolality
  Hyperlipidemia
  Hyperproteinemia
  Transurethral resection of prostate, hysteroscopy
Increased Plasma Osmolality
  Hyperglycemia
  Mannitol administration

Table 34-4. Causes of Syndrome of Inappropriate Secretion of Antidiuretic Hormone (SIADH)

Malignancy
  Lung (especially small cell carcinoma)
  Central nervous system
  Pancreas
Pulmonary
  Pneumonia
  Tuberculosis
  Fungal
  Abscess
Neurologic
  Infection
  Trauma
  Cerebrovascular accident
Drugs
  Amitriptyline
  Chlorpropamide
  Cyclophosphamide
  Desmopressin
  Morphine
  Nicotine
  Nonsteroidal antiinflammatory drugs (NSAIDs)
  Oxytocin
  Selective serotonin reuptake inhibitors
  Vincristine

295 mOsm/kg). Calculated plasma osmolality is determined by the following formula:

$$P_{osm} = 2.0 \times [Na^+] + Glucose/18 + BUN/2.8 \quad [1]$$

where serum $[Na^+]$ is measured in mM, and blood glucose and urea (blood urea nitrogen; BUN) are expressed as mg/dL. There are other minor solutes such as Ca^{2+}, Mg^{2+}, and K^+ that make small contributions to plasma osmolality. Considering plasma is 93% water and Na^+ is not completely dissociated into solution, these factors tend to cancel out.

Patients with disorders such as hypoproteinemia or hyperlipidemia that cause increased osmolality and pseudohyponatremia have an abnormal osmolality gap. These disorders highlight the importance of measuring plasma osmolality in hyponatremic patients. Hyponatremia with a normal or high serum osmolality results from the presence of a nonsodium solute, such as glucose or mannitol, that holds water within the extracellular space and results in dilutional hyponatremia. The presence of a nonsodium solute resulting in "factitious" hyponatremia can be inferred if measured osmolality exceeds calculated osmolality by more than 10 mOsm/kg. For example, plasma $[Na^+]$ decreases approximately 2.4 M for each 100 mg/dL rise in glucose concentration, with perhaps even greater decreases for glucose concentrations greater than 400 mg/dL.[5]

In anesthesia practice, a common cause of hyponatremia associated with a normal osmolality is the absorption of large volumes of sodium-free irrigating solutions (containing mannitol, glycine, or sorbitol as the solute) during transurethral resection of the prostate (TURP).[6] Neurologic symptoms are minimal if mannitol is employed because the agent does not cross the blood-brain barrier and is excreted with water in the urine. In contrast, as glycine or sorbitol is metabolized, hypoosmolality can gradually develop and cerebral edema can appear as a late complication. Consequently hypoosmolality is more important in generating symptoms than hyponatremia per se.[6] The problem of excessive fluid absorption during TURP can be monitored by using small amounts of alcohol in the irrigating fluid; the level of alcohol can be detected in expired air as a quantitative measure of irrigating fluid absorption.[7] True hyponatremia with a normal or elevated serum osmolality also can accompany renal insufficiency. BUN, included in the calculation of total osmolality, distributes throughout both ECV and intracellular volume (ICV). Calculation of *effective* osmolality (2 $[Na^+]$ + glucose/18) excludes the contribution of urea to tonicity and demonstrates true hypotonicity.

True hyponatremia (Table 34-5; Figure 34-2) with low serum osmolality can be associated with a high, low, or normal total body Na^+ and PV. Therefore hyponatremia with hyposmolality is evaluated by assessing total body Na^+ content, BUN, serum creatinine (SCr), urinary osmolality, and urinary $[Na^+]$. Hyponatremia with increased total body Na^+ is characteristic of edematous states, such as congestive heart failure, cirrhosis, nephrosis, and renal failure.[8] Aquaporin 2, the vasopressin-regulated water channel, is upregulated in experimental congestive heart failure and cirrhosis, and decreased by chronic vasopressin stimulation.[9,10] In patients with renal insufficiency, reduced urinary diluting capacity can lead to hyponatremia if excess free water is given.

The underlying mechanism of hypovolemic hyponatremia is secretion of ADH in response to volume contraction with ongoing oral or intravenous intake of hypotonic fluid.[11]

Table 34-5. Classification of Hypotonic Hyponatremia by Volume Status

HYPOVOLEMIC		EUVOLEMIC ($FE_{Na} < 1\%$, $U_{Na} > 20$ mEq/L)	HYPERVOLEMIC ($U_{Na} < 20$ mEq/L)
Extrarenal Sodium Loss ($FE_{Na} < 1\%$, $U_{Na} < 20$ mEq/L)	Renal Sodium Loss ($FE_{Na} > 2\%$, $U_{Na} > 20$ mEq/L)		
Dehydration	Diuretics	Glucocorticoid deficiency	CHF
Diarrhea	Osmotic diuresis	SIADH	Liver disease
Vomiting	Salt-losing nephropathy	Hypothyroidism	Nephrotic syndrome
Gastrointestinal suctioning	Mineralocorticoid deficiency	Psychogenic polydipsia (>15 L/day)	Pregnancy
Skin losses		Beer potomania/malnutrition	
Trauma		(alcoholism, anorexia)	
Pancreatitis			

FE_{Na}, Fractional excretion of sodium; U_{Na}, urine sodium.

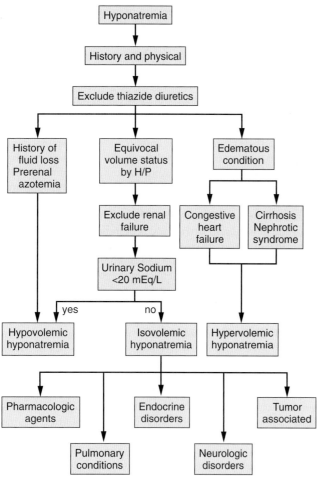

Figure 34-2 Decision tree for evaluation of hyponatremia. *H/P*, History and physical.

Angiotensin II also decreases renal free water clearance. Thiazide diuretics, unlike loop diuretics, promote hypovolemic hyponatremia by interfering with urinary dilution in the distal tubule of the nephron.[11] Hypovolemic hyponatremia associated with a urinary [Na+] greater than 20 mM suggests mineralocorticoid deficiency, especially if serum [K+], BUN, and SCr are increased.[11]

The cerebral salt-wasting syndrome is an often severe, symptomatic salt-losing diathesis that appears to be mediated by brain natriuretic peptide (BNP) and is independent of

SIADH.[12] Patients at risk include those with cerebral lesions due to trauma, subarachnoid hemorrhage, tumors, and infection.[13]

Euvolemic hyponatremia most commonly is associated with nonosmotic vasopressin secretion, such as glucocorticoid deficiency, hypothyroidism, thiazide-induced hyponatremia, SIADH, and reset osmostat syndrome. Total body Na+ and ECV are relatively normal and edema is rarely evident. SIADH can be idiopathic but also is associated with CNS or pulmonary diseases (see Table 34-4). Euvolemic hyponatremia is usually associated with exogenous ADH administration, pharmacologic potentiation of ADH action, drugs that mimic the action of ADH in the renal tubules, or excessive ectopic ADH secretion. Tissues from some small-cell lung cancers, duodenal cancers, and pancreatic cancers increase ADH production in response to osmotic stimulation.[14]

At least 4% of postoperative patients develop plasma [Na+] less than 130 mM. Although neurologic manifestations usually do not accompany postoperative hyponatremia, signs of hypervolemia are occasionally present.[15] Much less frequently postoperative hyponatremia is accompanied by mental status changes, seizures, and transtentorial herniation, attributable in part to intravenous administration of hypotonic fluids, secretion of ADH, and other factors, including drugs and altered renal function, that influence perioperative water balance.[1] Menstruating women are particularly vulnerable to brain damage secondary to postoperative hyponatremia.[16] Smaller patients change plasma [Na+] more in response to similar volumes of hypotonic fluids. Based on a report of apparent postoperative SIADH in a 30-kg 10-year-old girl, it has been suggested that children receive no sodium-free water perioperatively.[17,18] Postoperative hyponatremia can develop even with infusion of isotonic fluids if ADH is persistently increased. Twenty-four hours after surgery, mean plasma [Na+] in patients undergoing uncomplicated gynecologic surgery decreased from 140 to 136 mM.[19] Although the patients retained Na+ perioperatively, they retained proportionately more water (an average of 1.1 L of electrolyte-free water). Careful postoperative attention to fluid and electrolyte balance can minimize the occurrence of symptomatic hyponatremia.

If both [Na+] and measured osmolality are below the normal range, hyponatremia is further evaluated by first assessing volume status using physical findings and laboratory data (see Figure 34-2 and Table 34-5). In hypovolemic patients or edematous patients, the ratio of BUN to SCr should be greater than 20:1. Urinary [Na+] is generally less than 20 mM in edematous states and volume depletion, and more than 20 mM in hyponatremia secondary to renal salt wasting or renal failure with water retention.

Criteria for the diagnosis of SIADH include hypotonic hyponatremia, urinary osmolality greater than 100 to 150 mOsm/kg, absence of ECV depletion, normal thyroid and adrenal function, and normal cardiac, hepatic, and renal function. Urinary [Na$^+$] should be greater than 20 mM unless fluids have been restricted. The diagnosis of SIADH is inaccurately applied to functionally hypovolemic postoperative patients, in whom, by definition, ADH secretion would be "appropriate."[18]

Treatment of hyponatremia associated with normal or high serum osmolality requires reduction of the elevated concentrations of the responsible solute. Uremic patients are treated by free water restriction or dialysis. Treatment of edematous (hypervolemic) patients necessitates restriction of both sodium and water. Therapy is directed toward improving cardiac output and renal perfusion and using diuretics to inhibit Na$^+$ reabsorption. In hypovolemic, hyponatremic patients, intravascular volume must be restored, usually by infusion of 0.9% saline, and excessive Na$^+$ losses must be curtailed. Correction of hypovolemia usually results in removal of the stimulus for ADH release accompanied by a rapid water diuresis.

The cornerstone of SIADH management is free water restriction and elimination of precipitating causes. Water restriction, sufficient to decrease total body water (TBW) by 0.5 to 1.0 L/day, decreases ECV even if excessive ADH secretion continues. The resultant reduction in glomerular filtration rate (GFR) enhances proximal tubular reabsorption of salt and water, thereby decreasing free water reabsorption, and stimulating aldosterone secretion. As long as free water losses (i.e., renal, skin, gastrointestinal) exceed free water intake, serum [Na$^+$] will increase. During treatment of hyponatremia, increases in plasma [Na$^+$] are determined both by the composition of the infused fluid and by the rate of renal free water excretion. Free water excretion can be increased by administering furosemide. However, the correction of hyponatremia continues to generate controversy.[20-22] When plasma [Na$^+$] is less than 130 mM or hyponatremia is present together with cerebral symptoms, it is recommended to immediately administer one or more intravenous boluses of 2 mL/kg of 3% NaCl or corresponding amounts of hypertonic saline 7.5%.[1] This should result in a prompt response and should be followed by boluses every 5 to 10 minutes as needed. Symptoms should disappear when plasma [Na$^+$] has risen by 4 to 6 mM.

This approach differs from a previously advocated focus on a separation between acute or chronic causes for hyponatremia. Apart from the fact that this can be very difficult to distinguish based on history and physical examination, when seriously symptomatic the problem must be addressed expeditiously. When cerebral function has been restored there is an inadvertent risk of overcorrection with the risk of osmotic demyelination. Of course there are no prospective studies identifying the optimal rate for correction of hyponatremia. Goals can be set to 8 mM in 24 hours, 14 mM in 48 hours and 16 mM in 72 hours.[1,20] A formula for predicting changes of plasma [Na$^+$] is shown:

$$[Na^+]_2 = \frac{[Na^+]_1 \times TBW + \Delta(Na^+ + K^+)}{TBW + \Delta TBW} \qquad [2]$$

where [Na$^+$]$_1$ is the initial plasma [Na$^+$] and [Na$^+$]$_2$ is the concentration in plasma [Na$^+$] that results from the change in the external balances of water (TBW + ΔTBW) and cations [Δ(Na$^+$ + K$^+$)]. Treatment should be interrupted or slowed when symptoms improve. Frequent determinations of [Na$^+$] are important to prevent too rapid correction.[1] It is also important to insert a bladder catheter for closely tracking production of urine, which should be analyzed to determine [Na$^+$] and [K$^+$].

Although delayed correction of hyponatremia can result in neurologic injury, inappropriately rapid correction can result in abrupt brain dehydration (see Figure 34-1), permanent neurologic sequelae, cerebral hemorrhage, or congestive heart failure. The symptoms of the syndrome vary from mild (transient behavioral disturbances or seizures) to severe (including pseudobulbar palsy and quadriparesis).[23] The principal determinants of neurologic injury appear to be the magnitude and chronicity of hyponatremia and the rate of correction. The syndrome is more likely when hyponatremia has persisted for more than 48 hours. Most patients in whom the syndrome is fatal have undergone correction of plasma [Na$^+$] of more than 20 mM/day. Even a moderate decrease in [Na$^+$] in pigs can cause significant brain edema.[24] Other risk factors for development of the syndrome include alcoholism, poor nutritional status, liver disease, burns, and hypokalemia.

For patients who require long-term pharmacologic therapy of hyponatremia, demeclocycline is the drug of choice.[25] Although better tolerated than lithium, demeclocycline can induce nephrotoxicity, a particular concern in patients with hepatic dysfunction. Hemodialysis is occasionally necessary in severely hyponatremic patients who cannot be adequately managed with drugs or hypertonic saline. Once hyponatremia has improved, careful fluid restriction is necessary to avoid recurrence.

Vasopressin receptor antagonists (AVP antagonists) are a relatively new class of drugs that exert their effects by inhibiting one of three subtypes of vasopressin receptors. Vasopressin receptors V$_{1A}$ and V$_{1B}$ act via the inositol trisphosphate (IP$_3$) pathway to increase cytosolic Ca^{2+} as a second messenger, while V$_2$ receptors act via the adenylyl cyclase pathway to increase cyclic adenosine monophosphate (cAMP) as a second messenger. V$_{1A}$ activation produces vasoconstriction, platelet aggregation, inotropic stimulation, and myocardial protein synthesis. V$_{1B}$ activation leads to pituitary adrenocorticotrophic hormone secretion. V$_2$ activation causes antidiuretic effects by activity on the renal collecting ducts. The ideal treatment would increase free water clearance and increase serum [Na$^+$]. Conivaptan is a dual antagonist of V$_{1A}$ and V$_2$ receptors used for euvolemic or hypervolemic hyponatremia. Tolvaptan is an orally active, nonpeptide, selective V$_2$ receptor antagonist. It increases free water clearance, decreases urine osmolality, and increases [Na$^+$], and can be used for hyponatremic patients with heart failure and SIADH that resists water restriction.[26]

HYPERNATREMIA

Hypernatremia ([Na$^+$] >150 mM) indicates an absolute or relative water deficit. The condition can exist in several forms categorized in terms of the adequacy of intravascular volume.

Hypovolemic hypernatremia (water deficit > Na$^+$ deficit). Adipsic hypernatremia is secondary to decreased thirst.

This can be behavioral or, rarely, secondary to damage to the hypothalamic thirst centers. Hypovolemia can result from extrarenal losses (e.g., diarrhea, vomiting, fistulas, and significant burns) and renal losses (e.g., osmotic diuretics, diuretics, postobstructive diuresis, and intrinsic renal disease).

Hypervolemic hypernatremia (Na⁺ gain > water gain). Hypernatremia with hypervolemia is often iatrogenic (e.g., administration of excessive hypertonic saline or sodium bicarbonate) or accidental (e.g., ingestion of seawater or high salt content infant formula because of an error in formula preparation). Less common pathologic causes include excess mineralocorticoid (i.e., Cushing disease or syndrome).

Euvolemic hypernatremia (Na⁺ gain without volume change). Hypernatremia with normal volume status can be divided into causes stemming from extrarenal water losses and renal water losses. A common pathologic condition resulting in excessive renal losses of free water is diabetes insipidus (DI; both central and nephrogenic). Although rare, extrarenal loss of free water sufficient to produce hypernatremia can result from excessive insensible fluid loss such as with prolonged hyperventilation.

Normally, even slight increases in tonicity or [Na⁺] stimulate thirst and ADH secretion. Therefore severe, persistent hypernatremia occurs only in patients who cannot respond to thirst by voluntary ingestion of fluid such as obtunded patients, anesthetized patients, and infants.

Hypernatremia produces neurologic symptoms (including stupor, coma, and seizures), hypovolemia, renal insufficiency (occasionally progressing to renal failure), and decreased urinary concentrating ability.[27,28] Because hypernatremia frequently results from DI or osmotically induced losses of Na⁺ and water, many patients are hypovolemic or bear the stigmata of renal disease. Postoperative neurosurgical patients who have undergone pituitary surgery are at particular risk for development of transient or prolonged DI. Polyuria can be present for only a few days within the first week of surgery, can be permanent, or can demonstrate a triphasic sequence: early DI, return of urinary concentrating ability, then recurrent DI.

The clinical consequences of hypernatremia are most serious at the extremes of age and when hypernatremia develops abruptly. Older patients are at increased risk for hypernatremia because of decreased renal concentrating ability and thirst.[29] Brain shrinkage secondary to rapidly developing hypernatremia can damage delicate cerebral vessels, leading to subdural hematoma, subcortical parenchymal hemorrhage, subarachnoid hemorrhage, and venous thrombosis. Polyuria can cause bladder distention, hydronephrosis, and permanent renal damage.[30] At the cellular level, restoration of cell volume occurs remarkably quickly after normal tonicity is restored.[31] Although the mortality of hypernatremia is 40% to 55%, it is unclear whether hypernatremia is the cause or a marker of severe associated disease. Surprisingly, if plasma [Na⁺] is initially normal, moderate acute increases in plasma [Na⁺] do not appear to precipitate osmotic demyelination (which is much more likely in the setting of correcting hyponatremia). However, larger accidental increases in plasma [Na⁺] have produced severe consequences in children. In experimental animals, acute severe hypernatremia (acute increase from 146 to 170 mM) caused neuronal damage at 24 hours, suggestive of early osmotic demyelination.[32]

By definition, hypernatremia indicates an absolute or relative water deficit and is always associated with hypertonicity. Hypernatremia can be generated by hypotonic fluid loss, as in burns, GI losses, diuretic therapy, osmotic diuresis, renal disease, mineralocorticoid excess or deficiency, and iatrogenic causes, or can be generated by isolated water loss, as in central or nephrogenic DI. The acquired form of nephrogenic DI is more common and usually less severe than the congenital form. As chronic renal failure advances, most patients have defective concentrating ability resulting in resistance to ADH with hypotonic urine. Because hypovolemia accompanies most pathologic water loss, signs of hypoperfusion also can be present. In many patients, preceding the development of hypernatremia, an increased volume of hypotonic urine suggests an abnormality in water balance. Although uncommon as a cause of hypernatremia, isolated Na⁺ gain occasionally occurs in patients who receive large quantities of Na⁺, such as treatment of metabolic acidosis with 8.4% sodium bicarbonate, in which [Na⁺] is approximately 1000 mM, or perioperative or prehospital treatment with hypertonic saline resuscitation solutions. In large randomized trials in the prehospital area, harmful effects of transiently increased [Na⁺] have not been seen.[33]

Plasma [Na⁺] does not reflect total body Na⁺, which must be estimated separately based on signs of the adequacy of ECV. In polyuric hypernatremic patients, the differential diagnostic decision is between solute (osmotic) diuresis and DI. Measurement of urinary Na⁺ and osmolality can help differentiate the various causes. Urinary osmolality less than 150 mOsm/kg in the setting of hypertonicity and polyuria is diagnostic of DI.

Treatment of hypernatremia produced by water loss consists of repletion of water and correction of associated deficits in total body Na⁺ and other electrolytes (Table 34-6). Common errors in treating hypernatremia include excessively rapid correction, failure to appreciate the magnitude of the water deficit, and failure to account for ongoing maintenance requirements and continued fluid losses. The first step in treating hypernatremia is to estimate the TBW deficit, which can be accomplished using the measured plasma [Na⁺] and the equation:

$$\text{TBW deficit} = 0.6 \times \text{body weight (kg)} \times \left(\frac{[\text{Na}^+] - 140}{140} \right) \quad [3]$$

where 140 is the middle of the normal range for [Na⁺].

Table 34-6. Hypernatremia: Acute Treatment

Sodium Depletion (Hypovolemia)
  Hypovolemia correction (0.9% saline)
  Hypernatremia correction (hypotonic fluids)
Sodium Overload (Hypervolemia)
  Enhance sodium removal (loop diuretics, dialysis)
  Replace water deficit (hypotonic fluids)
Normal Total Body Sodium (Euvolemia)
  Replace water deficit (hypotonic fluids)
  Control diabetes insipidus
    Central diabetes insipidus:
      DDAVP, 10-20 µg intranasally; 2-4 µg SC
      Aqueous vasopressin, 5 U every 2-4 hr IM or SC
    Nephrogenic diabetes insipidus:
      Restrict sodium, water intake
      Thiazide diuretics

IM, Intramuscularly; *SC,* subcutaneously.

Hypernatremia must be corrected slowly because of the risk of neurologic sequelae such as seizures or cerebral edema (see Figure 34-1).[34] At the cellular level, restoration of cell volume occurs remarkably quickly after tonicity is altered; as a consequence, acute treatment of hypertonicity can result in overshooting the original, normal tonic cell volume.[34] The water deficit should be replaced over 24 to 48 hours, and plasma [Na$^+$] should not be reduced by more than 1 to 2 mM/hr. Reversible underlying causes should be treated. Hypovolemia should be corrected promptly with 0.9% saline. Although the [Na$^+$] of 0.9% saline is 154 mEq/L, the solution is effective in treating volume deficits and will reduce [Na$^+$] that exceeds 154 mEq/L. Once hypovolemia is corrected, water can be replaced orally or with intravenous hypotonic fluids depending on the ability of the patient to tolerate oral hydration. In the occasional sodium-overloaded patient, Na$^+$ excretion can be accelerated using loop diuretics or dialysis.

The management of hypernatremia secondary to DI varies according to whether the etiology is central or nephrogenic. The two most suitable agents for correcting central DI (an ADH deficiency syndrome) are desmopressin (DDAVP) and aqueous vasopressin. DDAVP, given subcutaneously in a dose of 1 to 4 μg or intranasally in a dose of 5 to 20 μg every 12 to 24 hours, is effective in the vast majority of patients. It is less likely than vasopressin to produce vasoconstriction and abdominal cramping.[35] Incomplete ADH deficits (partial DI) often are effectively managed with pharmacologic agents that stimulate ADH release or enhance the renal response to ADH. Chlorpromazine, which potentates the renal effects of vasopressin, and carbamazepine, which enhances vasopressin secretion, have been used to treat partial central DI, but are associated with clinically important side effects. In nephrogenic DI, salt and water restriction or thiazide diuretics induce contraction of ECV, thereby enhancing fluid reabsorption in the proximal tubules. When less filtrate passes through the collecting ducts, less water is excreted.

Potassium

PHYSIOLOGIC ROLE

Potassium ion (K$^+$) is perhaps the most frequently supplemented electrolyte.[36] Potassium plays an important role in cell membrane physiology, especially in maintaining resting membrane potential and in generating action potentials in the nervous system and heart. Potassium is actively transported into cells by the Na$^+$,K$^+$-ATPase (Na$^+$ pump), which maintains intracellular potassium concentration [K$^+$] at least 30-fold greater than extracellular [K$^+$]. Intracellular K$^+$ concentration is normally 150 mM, while the extracellular concentration is only 3.5 to 5 mM. Serum [K$^+$] measures about 0.5 mM higher than plasma [K$^+$] due to cell lysis during clotting. Total body K$^+$ in a 70-kg adult is approximately 4256 mEq, of which 4200 mEq is intracellular; of the 56 mEq in the ECV, only 12 mEq is located in the PV. Common causes of renal K$^+$ losses are listed in Table 34-7. The ratio of intracellular to extracellular [K$^+$] contributes to the resting potential difference across cell membranes and therefore to the integrity of cardiac and neuromuscular transmission. Extracellular [K$^+$] is determined by catecholamines, the renin-angiotensin-aldosterone system, glucose and insulin, as well as direct release from exercising or injured muscle.[36] The primary

Table 34-7. Causes of Renal Potassium Loss

DRUGS	BICARBONATURIA
Diuretics	**Distal Renal Tubular Acidosis**
Thiazide diuretics	**Treatment of Proximal Renal**
Loop diuretics	**Tubular Acidosis**
Osmotic diuretics	**Correction Phase of Metabolic**
Antibiotics	**Alkalosis**
Penicillin and penicillin	**Magnesium Deficiency**
analogues	**Other Less Common Causes**
Amphotericin B	Cisplatin
Aminoglycosides	Carbonic anhydrase inhibitors
Hormones	Leukemia
Aldosterone	Diuretic phase of acute tubular
Glucocorticoid-excess states	necrosis
	Intrinsic Renal Transport
	Defects
	Barter syndrome
	Gitelman syndrome

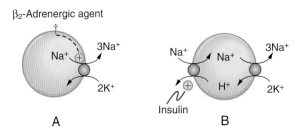

Figure 34-3 Extracellular signals that shift potassium into cells. **A,** β$_2$ adrenergic agents. **B,** Insulin.

mechanism that maintains K$^+$ inside cells is the transport of three Na$^+$ ions out of the cell for every two K$^+$ ions transported in by the Na$^+$ pump.[37] Both insulin and β-adrenergic agonists promote K$^+$ entry into cells (Figure 34-3).[37] In contrast, α-adrenergic agonists impair cellular K$^+$ uptake.[38] Metabolic acidosis tends to shift K$^+$ out of cells, while metabolic alkalosis favors movement into cells.

Usual K$^+$ intake is 50 to 150 mEq/day. Freely filtered at the glomerulus, most K$^+$ excretion is urinary with some fecal elimination. Most filtered K$^+$ is reabsorbed; excretion is usually approximately equal to daily intake. As long as GFR is greater than 8 mL/kg, dietary K$^+$ intake, unless greater than normal, can be excreted. Assuming plasma [K$^+$] of 4 mM and normal GFR of 180 L/day, 720 mEq of K$^+$ is filtered daily, of which 85% to 90% is reabsorbed in the proximal convoluted tubule and loop of Henle. The remaining 10% to 15% reaches the distal convoluted tubule, which is the major site at which K$^+$ excretion is regulated. Excretion of K$^+$ ions is a function of open K$^+$ channels and the electrical driving force in the cortical collecting duct.[37]

The two most important regulators of K$^+$ excretion are plasma [K$^+$] and aldosterone, although there is some evidence to suggest involvement of the CNS and of an enteric reflex mediated by potassium-rich meals. Potassium secretion into the distal convoluted tubules and cortical collecting ducts is increased by hyperkalemia, aldosterone, alkalemia, increased delivery of Na$^+$ to the distal tubule and collecting duct, high urinary flow rates, and the presence in luminal fluid of non-reabsorbable anions such as carbenicillin, phosphates, and sulfates. As Na$^+$ reabsorption increases, the electrical driving force opposing reabsorption of K^+ is increased. Aldosterone increases Na^+ reabsorption by inducing opening of the epithelial Na^+ channel; potassium-sparing diuretics (amiloride and triamterene) and trimethoprim block the epithelial Na^+ channel, thereby increasing K^+ reabsorption.[39] Magnesium depletion contributes to renal K^+ wasting.

HYPOKALEMIA

Uncommon among healthy persons, hypokalemia ($[K^+]$ <3 mM) is a frequent complication of treatment with diuretic drugs (see Diuretics) and occasionally complicates other diseases and treatment regimens. As a general rule, a chronic decrement of 1 mM in plasma $[K^+]$ corresponds to a total body deficit of approximately 200 to 300 mEq. In uncomplicated hypokalemia, the K^+ deficit exceeds 300 mEq if plasma $[K^+]$ is <3 mM and 700 mEq if plasma $[K^+]$ is <2 mM. Plasma $[K^+]$ poorly reflects total body K^+; hypokalemia can occur with normal, low, or high total body K^+.

Hypokalemia causes muscle weakness and, when severe, even paralysis. With chronic K^+ loss, the ratio of intracellular to extracellular $[K^+]$ remains relatively stable; in contrast, acute redistribution of K^+ from the extracellular to the intracellular space substantially changes resting membrane potential.

Cardiac rhythm disturbances are among the most dangerous complications of K^+ deficiency. Acute hypokalemia causes hyperpolarization of cardiac cells that can lead to ventricular escape activity, reentrant phenomena, ectopic tachycardias, and delayed conduction. In patients taking digoxin, hypokalemia increases toxicity by increasing myocardial digoxin binding and pharmacologic effectiveness. Hypokalemia contributes to systemic hypertension, especially when combined with a high-sodium diet.[40] In diabetic patients, hypokalemia impairs insulin secretion and end-organ sensitivity to insulin. Although no clear threshold has been defined for a level of hypokalemia below which safe conduct of anesthesia is compromised, $[K^+]$ less than 3.5 mM has been associated with increased incidence of perioperative dysrhythmias, especially atrial fibrillation/flutter, in cardiac surgery patients.[41]

Potassium depletion also induces defects in renal concentrating ability, resulting in polyuria and a reduction in GFR. Potassium replacement improves GFR, although the concentrating deficit might not improve for several months after treatment. If hypokalemia is sufficiently prolonged, chronic renal interstitial damage can occur. In experimental animals, hypokalemia is associated with intrarenal vasoconstriction and a pattern of renal injury similar to that produced by ischemia. Hypokalemia can result from chronic depletion of total body K^+ or from acute redistribution of K^+ from the ECV to the ICV. Redistribution of K^+ into cells occurs when the activity of the Na^+ pump is acutely increased by hyperkalemia or increased intracellular concentration of Na^+, as well as by insulin, carbohydrate loading (which stimulates release of endogenous insulin), β_2-adrenergic agonists, or aldosterone.[37] Both metabolic and respiratory alkalosis lead to decreases in plasma $[K^+]$.[37]

Causes of chronic hypokalemia include those etiologies associated with renal K^+ conservation (extrarenal K^+ losses; low urinary $[K^+]$) and those with renal K^+ wasting.[37] Low urinary $[K^+]$ suggests inadequate dietary intake or extrarenal depletion (in the absence of recent diuretic use). Diuretic-induced urinary K^+ losses are frequently associated with

hypokalemia secondary to increased aldosterone secretion, alkalemia, and increased renal tubular flow. Aldosterone does not cause renal K^+ wasting unless Na^+ is present; that is, aldosterone primarily controls Na^+ reabsorption, not K^+ excretion. Renal tubular damage due to nephrotoxins such as aminoglycosides or amphotericin B can also cause renal K^+ wasting.

Initial evaluation of hypokalemia includes a medical history (diarrhea, vomiting, diuretic, or laxative use), physical examination (hypertension, Cushingoid features, and edema), measurement of serum electrolytes (Mg^{2+}), arterial pH assessment, and evaluation of the electrocardiogram (ECG). A majority of trauma patients develop hypokalemia that returns to normal within 24 hours without specific therapy. Measurement of 24-hour urinary excretion of Na^+ and K^+ can distinguish extrarenal from renal causes. Magnesium deficiency, associated with aminoglycoside and cisplatin therapy, can generate hypokalemia that is resistant to replacement therapy. Plasma renin and aldosterone levels can be helpful in the differential diagnosis. Characteristic electrocardiographic changes associated with hypokalemia include flat or inverted T waves, prominent U waves, and ST segment depression.[42]

The treatment of hypokalemia consists of K^+ repletion, correction of alkalemia, and removal of offending drugs (Table 34-8). Hypokalemia secondary only to acute redistribution might not require treatment. There is no urgent need for K^+ replacement therapy in mild to moderate hypokalemia (3 to 3.5 mM) in asymptomatic patients. If total body K^+ is decreased, oral K^+ supplementation is preferable to intravenous replacement. Potassium is usually replaced as the chloride salt because coexisting chloride deficiency can limit ability of the kidney to conserve K^+.

Potassium repletion must be performed cautiously usually at a rate ≤10-20 mEq/hr because the magnitude of K^+ deficits is unpredictable. Plasma $[K^+]$ and the ECG must be monitored during rapid repletion (10-20 mEq/hr) to avoid hyperkalemic complications.[43] Particular care should be taken in patients with concurrent acidemia, type IV renal tubular acidosis, diabetes mellitus, or those receiving nonsteroidal anti-inflammatory agents, angiotensin-converting enzyme (ACE) inhibitors, or β blockers, all of which delay movement of extracellular K^+ into cells.

In patients with life-threatening dysrhythmias secondary to hypokalemia, serum $[K^+]$ must be rapidly increased. Assuming that PV in a 70-kg adult is 3 L, administration of 6 mEq of potassium over a minute will increase serum $[K^+]$ by no more than 2 mM because redistribution into interstitial fluid will decrease the quantity remaining in plasma.[37]

Table 34-8. Hypokalemia: Treatment

Correct Precipitating Factors
Increased pH
Decreased Mg^{2+}
Drugs
Mild Hypokalemia ($[K^+]$ >2 mEq/L)
Intravenous KCl infusion ≤10 mEq/hr
Severe Hypokalemia ($[K^+]$ ≤2 mEq/L, Paralysis or ECG Changes)
Intravenous KCl infusion ≤40 mEq/hr
Continuous ECG monitoring
If life-threatening, 5-6 mEq bolus

ECG, Electrocardiogram.

Hypokalemia associated with hyperaldosteronemia (e.g., primary aldosteronism, Cushing syndrome) usually responds favorably to reduced Na^+ intake and increased K^+ intake. Hypomagnesemia, if present, aggravates the effects of hypokalemia, impairs K^+ conservation, and should be treated. Potassium supplements or potassium-sparing diuretics should be given cautiously to patients who have diabetes mellitus or renal insufficiency, which limit compensation for acute hyperkalemia. In patients, such as those who have diabetic ketoacidosis, who are both hypokalemic and acidemic, K^+ administration should precede correction of acidosis to avoid a precipitous decrease in plasma $[K^+]$ as pH increases.

HYPERKALEMIA

The most lethal manifestations of hyperkalemia ($[K^+]$ >5 mM) involve the cardiac conduction system and include dysrhythmias, conduction abnormalities, and cardiac arrest. In anesthesia practice, the classic example of hyperkalemic cardiac toxicity is associated with the administration of succinylcholine to paraplegic, quadriplegic, or severely burned patients.[44] If plasma $[K^+]$ is less than 6 mM, cardiac effects are negligible. As $[K^+]$ increases further, the ECG shows tall peaked T waves, especially in the precordial leads. With further increases, the PR interval becomes prolonged, followed by a decrease in the amplitude of the P wave. Finally, the QRS complex widens into a pattern resembling a sine wave as a prelude to cardiac standstill.[44] Hyperkalemic cardiotoxicity is enhanced by hyponatremia, hypocalcemia, or acidosis. Because progression to fatal cardiotoxicity is unpredictable and often swift, the presence of hyperkalemic electrocardiographic changes mandates immediate therapy. The life-threatening cardiac effects usually require more urgent treatment than other manifestations of hyperkalemia. However, ascending muscle weakness appears when plasma $[K^+]$ approaches 7 mM and can progress to flaccid paralysis, inability to phonate, and respiratory arrest.

The most important diagnostic issues are history, emphasizing recent drug therapy, and assessment of renal function. If hyponatremia is also present, adrenal function should be evaluated. Although the ECG can provide the first suggestion of hyperkalemia in some patients, and despite the well-described effects of hyperkalemia on cardiac conduction and rhythm, the ECG is an insensitive and nonspecific method of detecting hyperkalemia.[45]

Hyperkalemia can occur with normal, high, or low total body K^+ stores. Deficiency of aldosterone, a major regulator of K^+ excretion, leads to hyperkalemia in adrenal insufficiency and hyporeninemic hypoaldosteronism, a state associated with diabetes mellitus, renal insufficiency, and advanced age. Because the kidneys excrete K^+, severe renal insufficiency commonly causes hyperkalemia. Patients with chronic renal insufficiency can maintain normal plasma $[K^+]$ despite markedly decreased GFR because urinary K^+ excretion depends on tubular secretion rather than glomerular filtration when GFR exceeds 8 mL/min.

Drugs are now the most common cause of hyperkalemia, especially in older patients. Drugs that can limit K^+ excretion include nonsteroidal antiinflammatory drugs, ACE inhibitors, cyclosporin, and potassium-sparing diuretics such as triamterene. Drug-induced hyperkalemia most commonly occurs in patients with other predisposing factors, such as diabetes mellitus, renal insufficiency, advanced age, or hyporeninemic

hypoaldosteronism. ACE inhibitors are particularly likely to produce hyperkalemia in patients who have congestive heart failure.[46]

In patients with normal total body K^+, hyperkalemia can accompany a sudden shift of K^+ from the ICV to the ECV because of acidemia, increased catabolism, or rhabdomyolysis. Metabolic acidosis and respiratory acidosis can also cause an increase in plasma $[K^+]$. However, organic acidosis (lactic acidosis, ketoacidosis) has little effect on $[K^+]$, whereas mineral acids cause significant cellular shifts. In response to increased hydrogen ion activity because of addition of acids, K^+ will increase if the anion remains in the extracellular volume.[37] Neither lactate nor ketoacids remain in the extracellular fluid. Therefore hyperkalemia in these circumstances reflects tissue injury or lack of insulin.[37] Pseudohyperkalemia, which occurs when K^+ is released from cells in blood collection tubes, can be diagnosed by comparing serum and plasma K^+ levels from the same blood sample. Hyperkalemia usually accompanies malignant hyperthermia.

The treatment of hyperkalemia is aimed at eliminating the cause, reversing membrane hyperexcitability, and removing K^+ from the body.[37] Emergent management of severe hyperkalemia is shown in Table 34-9. Hyperkalemia is best treated with insulin plus glucose, β agonists (see Figure 34-3), and furosemide.[36] Mineralocorticoid deficiency can be treated with 9-α-fludrocortisone (0.025-0.10 mg/day). Hyperkalemia secondary to digitalis intoxication can be resistant to therapy because attempts to shift K^+ from the ECV to the ICV are often ineffective. In this situation, use of digoxin-specific antibodies has been successful.

Membrane hyperexcitability can be antagonized by translocating K^+ from the ECV to the ICV, removing excess K^+, or (transiently) by infusing calcium chloride to depress the membrane threshold potential. Pending definitive treatment, rapid infusion of calcium chloride (1 g over 3 minutes, or 2-3 ampules of 10% calcium gluconate over 5 minutes) can stabilize cardiac rhythm. Calcium should be given cautiously if digitalis intoxication is likely. Acute alkalinization using sodium bicarbonate (50-100 mEq over 5-10 minutes in a 70-kg adult) transiently promotes movement of K^+ from the ECV to the ICV. Bicarbonate can be administered even if pH exceeds 7.4; however, it should not be administered to patients with congestive cardiac failure or hypernatremia. When used alone, bicarbonate is relatively ineffective and is no longer favored. Insulin, in a dose-dependent fashion, causes cellular uptake of K^+ by increasing the activity of the Na^+ pump. Insulin increases cellular uptake of K^+ best when high insulin

Table 34-9. Severe Hyperkalemia*: Treatment

Reverse Membrane Effects
 Calcium (10 mL of 10% calcium chloride IV over 10 min)
Transfer Extracellular K^+ into Cells
 Glucose and insulin ($D_{10}W$ + 5-10 U regular insulin per 25-50 g glucose)
 Sodium bicarbonate (50-100 mEq over 5-10 min)
 $β_2$ agonists
Remove Potassium from Body
 Diuretics, proximal or loop
 Potassium-exchange resins (sodium polystyrene sulfonate)
 Hemodialysis
Monitor ECG and Serum $[K^+]$

*Potassium concentration ($[K^+]$) >7 mEq/L or electrocardiographic changes.

levels are achieved by intravenous injection of 5 to 10 U of regular insulin, accompanied by 50 mL of 50% glucose.[46] β_2-adrenergic agonists such as salbutamol and albuterol also increase K^+ uptake by skeletal muscle and reduce plasma $[K^+]$, an action that can explain hypokalemia with severe acute illness.

Potassium can also be removed from the body by the renal or gastrointestinal routes. Furosemide promotes kaliuresis in a dose-dependent fashion. Sodium polystyrene sulfonate resin (Kayexalate), which exchanges Na^+ for K^+, can be given orally (30 g) or as a retention enema (50 g in 200 mL of 20% sorbitol). However, Na^+ overload and hypervolemia are potential risks. Rarely, when temporizing measures are insufficient, emergency hemodialysis can remove 25 to 50 mEq/hr. Peritoneal dialysis is less efficient.

Calcium

PHYSIOLOGIC ROLE

Calcium is a divalent cation found primarily in the extracellular fluid. The free calcium concentration $[Ca^{2+}]$ in ECV is approximately 1 mM, whereas the free $[Ca^{2+}]$ in the ICV approximates 100 nM, a gradient of 10,000 to 1. Circulating Ca^{2+} consists of a protein-bound fraction (40%), a chelated fraction (10%), and an ionized fraction (50%), which is the physiologically active and homeostatically regulated component.[47] Acute acidemia increases and acute alkalemia decreases ionized Ca^{2+}. Because mathematical formulas that "correct" total Ca^{2+} measurements for albumin concentration are inaccurate in critically ill patients, ionized Ca^{2+} should be directly measured.

In general, Ca^{2+} is essential for all movement that occurs in mammalian systems. Essential for normal excitation-contraction coupling, Ca^{2+} is also necessary for proper function of muscle tissue, swallowing, mitosis, neurotransmitter and hormone release, enzyme secretion, and hormonal secretion. cAMP and phosphoinositides, which are major second messengers regulating cellular metabolism, function primarily through the regulation of Ca^{2+} movement. Activation of numerous intracellular enzyme systems requires Ca^{2+}. Calcium is important both for generation of cardiac pacemaker activity and for generation of the cardiac action potential for which it is the primary ion responsible for the plateau phase of the action potential. Calcium also plays vital functions in membrane and bone structure.

Serum $[Ca^{2+}]$ is regulated by multiple factors (Figure 34-4) including a Ca^{2+} receptor and several hormones. Parathyroid hormone (PTH) and calcitriol, the most important

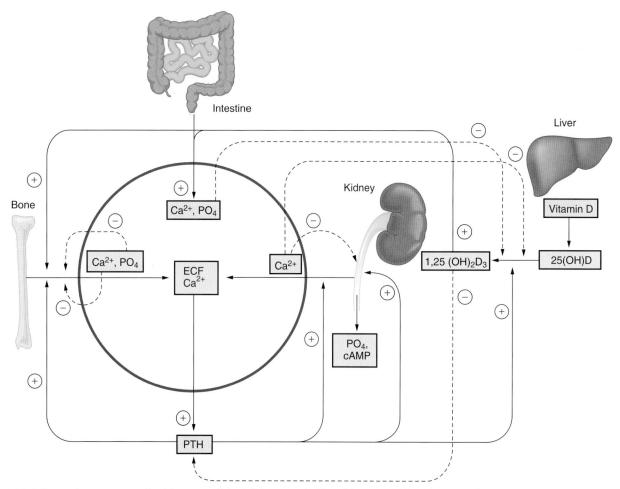

Figure 34-4 The regulatory system maintaining extracellular Ca^{2+} homeostasis. The solid arrows and lines delineate effects of parathyroid hormone and 1,25 $(OH)_2D_3$ on their target tissues; dashed arrows and lines show examples of how extracellular Ca^{2+} or phosphate ions act directly on tissues regulating mineral ion metabolism. *Ca²⁺,* Calcium; *ECF,* extracellular fluid; *PO₄,* phosphate; *PTH,* parathyroid hormone; *1,25 (OH)₂D₃,* 1,25 dihydroxyvitamin D; *25(OH)D,* 25-hydroxyvitamin D; negative signs indicate inhibitory actions and plus signs indicate stimulatory effects.

neurohumoral mediators of serum $[Ca^{2+}]$, mobilize Ca^{2+} from bone, increase renal tubular reabsorption of Ca^{2+}, and enhance intestinal absorption of Ca^{2+}.[48] Vitamin D, after ingestion or cutaneous manufacture under the stimulus of ultraviolet light, is 25-hydroxylated to calcidiol in the liver and then is 1-hydroxylated to calcitriol, the active metabolite, in the kidney. Even in the absence of dietary Ca^{2+} intake, PTH and vitamin D can maintain a normal circulating $[Ca^{2+}]$ by mobilizing Ca^{2+} from bone.

HYPOCALCEMIA

Hypocalcemia occurs frequently in critical care, affecting 80% to 90% of patients. Hypocalcemia is associated with increased mortality in this population.[36] Hypocalcemia (ionized $[Ca^{2+}]$ <4 mg/dL or <1 mM) occurs as a result of failure of PTH or calcitriol action or because of Ca^{2+} chelation or precipitation, not because of Ca^{2+} deficiency alone. PTH deficiency can result from surgical damage or removal of the parathyroid glands or from suppression of the parathyroid glands by severe hypomagnesia or hypermagnesemia. Burns, sepsis, and pancreatitis can suppress parathyroid function and interfere with vitamin D action. Vitamin D deficiency can result from lack of dietary vitamin D or vitamin D malabsorption in patients with low sunlight exposure.

Hyperphosphatemia-induced hypocalcemia can occur as a consequence of overzealous phosphate therapy, from cell lysis secondary to chemotherapy, or as a result of cellular destruction from rhabdomyolysis. Precipitation of $CaHPO_4$ complexes occurs with hyperphosphatemia. However, ionized $[Ca^{2+}]$ only decreases approximately 0.019 mM for each 1 mM increase in phosphate concentration. In massive transfusion, citrate can produce hypocalcemia by chelating Ca^{2+}; however, decreases are usually transient and produce no cardiovascular effects. A healthy, normothermic adult who has intact hepatic and renal function can metabolize the citrate present in 20 units of blood per hour without becoming hypocalcemic. However, when citrate clearance is decreased (e.g., by hepatic or renal disease or hypothermia) and when blood transfusion rates are rapid (e.g., >2 mL/kg/min), hypocalcemia and cardiovascular compromise can occur. Alkalemia resulting from hyperventilation or sodium bicarbonate injection can acutely decrease $[Ca^{2+}]$. Furthermore, resuscitation induced hemodilution is an important causative factor of early hypocalcemia in trauma patients.[36] This is an iatrogenic rather than adaptive complication of treatment and can have deleterious effects on blood coagulation and cardiovascular function.

The hallmark of hypocalcemia is increased neuronal membrane irritability and tetany (Table 34-10). Early symptoms include sensations of numbness and tingling involving fingers, toes, and the circumoral region. In frank tetany, tonic contraction of respiratory muscles can lead to laryngospasm, bronchospasm, or respiratory arrest. Smooth muscle spasm can result in abdominal cramping and urinary frequency. Mental status alterations include irritability, depression, psychosis, and dementia. Hypocalcemia can impair cardiovascular function and has been associated with heart failure, hypotension, dysrhythmias, insensitivity to digitalis, and impaired β-adrenergic action.

Reduced *ionized* serum Ca^{2+} occurs in as many as 88% of critically ill patients, 66% of less severely ill intensive care unit (ICU) patients, and 26% of hospitalized non-ICU patients.[49]

Table 34-10. Hypocalcemia: Clinical Manifestations

Cardiovascular	Respiratory
Dysrhythmias	Apnea
Digitalis insensitivity	Laryngeal spasm
ECG changes	Bronchospasm
Heart failure	**Psychiatric**
Hypotension	Anxiety
Neuromuscular	Dementia
Tetany	Depression
Muscle spasm	Psychosis
Papilledema	
Seizures	
Weakness	
Fatigue	

ECG, Electrocardiographic.

Table 34-11. Hypocalcemia: Acute Treatment

Administer Calcium
  IV: 10 mL 10% calcium gluconate* over 10 min, followed by elemental calcium 0.3-2 mg/kg/hr
  Oral: 50-100 mg elemental calcium every 6 hr
Administer Vitamin D
  Ergocalciferol, 1200 µg/day ($T_{1/2}$ = 30 days)
  Dihydrotachysterol, 200-400 µg/day ($T_{1/2}$ = 7 days)
  1,25-dihydroxycholecalciferol, 0.25-1 µg/day ($T_{1/2}$ = 1 day)
Monitor Electrocardiogram

*Calcium gluconate contains 93 mg elemental calcium per 10-mL vial; $T_{1/2}$, half-life.

Patients at particular risk include patients following multiple trauma and cardiopulmonary bypass. In most patients, ionized hypocalcemia is clinically mild ($[Ca^{2+}]$ 0.8-1 mM).

Initial diagnostic evaluation should concentrate on history and physical examination, laboratory evaluation of renal function, and measurement of serum phosphate concentration. Latent hypocalcemia can be diagnosed by tapping on the facial nerve to elicit the Chvostek sign or by inflating a sphygmomanometer to 20 mmHg above systolic pressure, which produces radial and ulnar nerve ischemia and causes carpal spasm known as the Trousseau sign.

The differential diagnosis of hypocalcemia can be approached by addressing four issues: age of the patient, serum phosphate concentration, general clinical status, and duration of hypocalcemia.[50] High phosphate concentrations suggest renal failure or hypoparathyroidism. In renal insufficiency, reduced phosphorus excretion results in hyperphosphatemia, which downregulates the 1α-hydroxylase responsible for renal conversion of calcidiol to calcitriol. This, in combination with decreased production of calcitriol secondary to reduced renal mass, causes reduced intestinal absorption of Ca^{2+} and hypocalcemia.[48] Low or normal phosphate concentrations imply vitamin D or Mg^{2+} deficiency. An otherwise healthy patient with chronic hypocalcemia probably is hypoparathyroid. Chronically ill adults with hypocalcemia often have disorders such as malabsorption, osteomalacia, or osteoblastic metastases.

The definitive treatment of hypocalcemia necessitates identification and treatment of the underlying cause (Table 34-11). Symptomatic hypocalcemia usually occurs when serum ionized $[Ca^{2+}]$ is <0.7 mM. The clinician should carefully consider whether mild, asymptomatic ionized hypocalcemia requires therapy, particularly in ischemic and septic states in which experimental evidence suggests that Ca^{2+} can increase cellular damage.

Unnecessary offending drugs should be discontinued. Hypocalcemia resulting from hypomagnesemia or hyperphosphatemia is treated by repletion of Mg^{2+} or removal of phosphate. Treatment of a patient with tetany and hyperphosphatemia requires coordination of therapy to avoid the consequences of metastatic soft tissue calcification.[51] Potassium and other electrolytes should be measured and abnormalities corrected. Hyperkalemia and hypomagnesemia potentiate hypocalcemia-induced cardiac and neuromuscular irritability. In contrast, hypokalemia protects against hypocalcemic tetany; therefore correction of hypokalemia without correction of hypocalcemia can provoke tetany.

Mild, ionized hypocalcemia should not be overtreated. For instance, in most patients after cardiac surgery, administration of Ca^{2+} only increases blood pressure and actually attenuates the β-adrenergic effects of epinephrine.[52] In normocalcemic dogs, calcium chloride primarily acts as a peripheral vasoconstrictor, with transient reduction of myocardial contractility; in hypocalcemic dogs, Ca^{2+} infusion significantly improves contractile performance and blood pressure.[53] Therefore Ca^{2+} infusions should be of limited value in surgical patients unless there is evidence of hypocalcemia.[53] Calcium salts appear to confer no benefit to patients already receiving inotropic or vasoactive agents.

The cornerstone of therapy for confirmed, symptomatic, ionized hypocalcemia ($[Ca^{2+}] <0.7$ mM) is Ca^{2+} administration. In patients who have severe hypocalcemia or hypocalcemic symptoms, Ca^{2+} should be administered intravenously. In emergency situations in an average-sized adult, the "rule of 10s" advises infusion of 10 mL of 10% calcium gluconate (93 mg elemental calcium) over 10 minutes, followed by a continuous infusion of elemental calcium of 0.3-2 mg/kg/hr (i.e., 3-16 mL/hr of 10% calcium gluconate for a 70-kg adult). Calcium salts should be diluted in 50 to 100 mL D5W (to limit venous irritation and thrombosis), should not be mixed with bicarbonate (to prevent precipitation), and must be given cautiously to digitalized patients because Ca^{2+} increases the toxicity of digoxin. Continuous ECG monitoring during initial therapy will detect cardiotoxicity (e.g., heart block, ventricular fibrillation). During Ca^{2+} replacement, serum Ca^{2+}, Mg^{2+}, phosphate, K^+, and creatinine should be monitored. Once the ionized $[Ca^{2+}]$ is stable in the range of 4 to 5 mg/dL (1-1.25 mM), oral calcium supplements can substitute for parenteral therapy. Urinary Ca^{2+} should be monitored in an attempt to avoid hypercalciuria (>5 mg/kg/day) and urinary tract stone formation.

When supplementation fails to maintain serum Ca^{2+} within the normal range, or if hypercalciuria develops, vitamin D can be added. Although the principal effect of vitamin D is to increase enteric Ca^{2+} absorption, osseous Ca^{2+} resorption is also enhanced. When rapid changes in dosage are anticipated or an immediate effect is required (e.g., postoperative hypoparathyroidism), shorter-acting calciferols such as dihydrotachysterol are preferable. Because the effect of vitamin D is not regulated, the dosages of Ca^{2+} and vitamin D should be adjusted to raise serum Ca^{2+} into the low normal range.

Adverse reactions to Ca^{2+} and vitamin D include hypercalcemia and hypercalciuria. If hypercalcemia develops, Ca^{2+} and vitamin D should be discontinued and appropriate therapy

given. The toxic effects of vitamin D metabolites persist in proportion to their biologic half-lives (ergocalciferol, 20-60 days; dihydrotachysterol, 5-15 days; calcitriol, 2-10 days). Glucocorticoids antagonize the toxic effects of vitamin D metabolites.

HYPERCALCEMIA

Although ionized $[Ca^{2+}]$ most accurately demonstrates hypercalcemia (ionized $[Ca^{2+}]$ >1.5 mM or total serum $[Ca^{2+}]$ >10.5 mg/dL), hypercalcemia customarily is defined in terms of total serum $[Ca^{2+}]$. In hypoalbuminemic patients, total serum $[Ca^{2+}]$ can be estimated by assuming an increase of 0.8 mg/dL for every 1 g/dL of albumin concentration below 4 g/dL. Patients with total serum $[Ca^{2+}]$ less than 11.5 mg/dL are usually asymptomatic. Patients with moderate hypercalcemia (total serum $[Ca^{2+}]$ 11.5-13 mg/dL) can show symptoms of lethargy, anorexia, nausea, and polyuria. Severe hypercalcemia (total serum $[Ca^{2+}]$ >13 mg/dL) is associated with more severe neuromyopathic symptoms, including muscle weakness, depression, impaired memory, emotional lability, lethargy, stupor, and coma. The cardiovascular effects of hypercalcemia include hypertension, arrhythmias, heart block, cardiac arrest, and digitalis sensitivity. Skeletal disease occurs secondary to direct osteolysis or humoral bone resorption.

Hypercalcemia impairs urinary concentrating ability and renal excretory capacity for Ca^{2+} by irreversibly precipitating Ca^{2+} salts within the renal parenchyma and by reducing renal blood flow and glomerular filtration rate. In response to hypovolemia, renal tubular reabsorption of Na^+ enhances renal Ca^{2+} reabsorption. Effective treatment of severe hypercalcemia is necessary to prevent progressive dehydration and renal failure leading to further increases in total serum $[Ca^{2+}]$, because volume depletion exacerbates hypercalcemia.[54] Hypercalcemia occurs when Ca^{2+} enters the ECV more rapidly than the kidneys can excrete the excess. Clinically, hypercalcemia most commonly results from an excess of bone resorption over bone formation, usually secondary to malignant disease, hyperparathyroidism, hypocalciuric hypercalcemia, thyrotoxicosis, immobilization, and granulomatous diseases. Granulomatous diseases produce hypercalciuria and hypercalcemia due to conversion by granulomatous tissue of calcidiol to calcitriol.[55]

Malignancy can produce hypercalcemia either through bone destruction or secretion by malignant tissue of hormones that promote hypercalcemia.[56] Although weakness, weight loss, and anemia associated with primary hyperparathyroidism might suggest malignancy, these can result simply from the primary disease process. Hypercalcemia associated with granulomatous diseases (e.g., sarcoidosis) results from the production of calcitriol by granulomatous tissue. To compensate for increased gut absorption or bone resorption of Ca^{2+}, renal excretion can readily increase from 100 to more than 400 mg/day. Factors that promote hypercalcemia might be offset by coexisting disorders such as pancreatitis, sepsis, or hyperphosphatemia that cause hypocalcemia.

Although definitive treatment of hypercalcemia requires correction of underlying causes, temporizing therapy can be necessary to avoid complications and to relieve symptoms. Total serum $[Ca^{2+}]$ exceeding 14 mg/dL represents a medical emergency. General supportive treatment includes hydration, correction of associated electrolyte abnormalities, removal of offending drugs, dietary Ca^{2+} restriction, and increased physical activity. Because anorexia and antagonism by Ca^{2+} of ADH action invariably lead to Na^+ and water depletion, infusion of 0.9% saline will dilute serum Ca^{2+}, promote renal excretion, and can reduce total serum $[Ca^{2+}]$ by 1.5 to 3 mg/dL. Urinary output should be maintained at 200 to 300 mL/hr. As GFR increases, Na^+ increases Ca^{2+} excretion by competing with Ca^{2+} for reabsorption in the proximal renal tubules and loop of Henle.

Furosemide further enhances Ca^{2+} excretion by increasing tubular Na^+. Patients who have renal impairment require higher doses of furosemide. During saline infusion and forced diuresis, careful monitoring of cardiopulmonary status and electrolytes, especially Mg^{2+} and K^+, is required. Intensive diuresis and saline administration can achieve net Ca^{2+} excretion of 2000 to 4000 mg per 24 hours, a rate eight times greater than saline alone but still somewhat less than the rate of removal achieved by hemodialysis (6000 mg per 8 hours). Patients treated with phosphates should be well hydrated.

Bone resorption, the primary cause of hypercalcemia, can be minimized by increasing physical activity and initiating drug therapy. Bisphosphonates, currently the first-line therapy for acute hypercalcemia, inhibit osteoclast function and viability. Bisphosphonates are the principal drugs for the management of hypercalcemia mediated by osteoclastic bone resorption.[57] Pamidronate, unlike earlier bisphosphonates, does not appear to worsen renal insufficiency. More recently released biphosphonates include alendronate, risedronate, and zoledronic acid. Risedronate has been associated with fewer nonvertebral fractures than alendronate.[58] Zoledronic acid has the most rapid onset of action among the biphosphonates and prolongs the duration before relapse of hypercalcemia; however, it has been associated with compromised renal function.[59]

Other osteoclast-inhibiting agents used to treat hypercalcemia include mithramycin and calcitonin.[60] Mithramycin, a cytotoxic agent, lowers serum Ca^{2+} primarily by inhibiting bone resorption, probably because of toxicity to osteoclasts. The hypocalcemic effect, usually seen within 12 to 24 hours following a single intravenous dose of 25 μg/kg, peaks at 48 to 72 hours and persists for 5 to 7 days. Major toxic effects of mithramycin, more likely to occur in patients with renal insufficiency, include thrombocytopenia, nephrotoxicity, and hepatotoxicity. Calcitonin lowers serum Ca^{2+} within 24 to 48 hours and is more effective when combined with glucocorticoids.[59] Usually calcitonin reduces total serum $[Ca^{2+}]$ by only 1 to 2 mg/dL. Although calcitonin is relatively nontoxic, more than 25% of patients do not respond. Thus calcitonin is unsuitable as a first-line drug during life-threatening hypercalcemia.

Hydrocortisone is effective in treating hypercalcemic patients with lymphatic malignancies, vitamin D or A intoxication, and diseases associated with production by tumor or granulomas of $1,25(OH)_2D$ or osteoclast-activating factor. Glucocorticoids rarely improve hypercalcemia secondary to malignancy or hyperparathyroidism. In the future, Ca^{2+} receptor agonists could become treatments of choice for suppressing primary and secondary hyperparathyroidism. Currently undergoing initial clinical trials, these agents also reduce inorganic phosphate concentration and the calcium × phosphate product.[61]

Phosphates lower serum Ca^{2+} by causing deposition of Ca^{2+} in bone and soft tissue. Because the risk of extraskeletal calcification of organs such as the kidney and myocardium is less if phosphates are given orally, the intravenous route should be reserved for patients with life-threatening hypercalcemia or patients in whom other measures have failed.

Phosphate

PHYSIOLOGIC ROLE

Phosphorus, in the form of inorganic phosphate (PO_4^{3-}; P_i), is distributed in similar concentrations throughout intracellular and extracellular fluid. Of total body phosphorus, 90% exists in bone, 10% is intracellular and less than 1% is found in the extracellular fluid. Phosphate circulates as the free ion (55%), complexed ion (33%), and in a protein-bound form (12%). Plasma levels vary widely: normal total P_i ranges from 2.7 to 4.5 mg/dL in adults.

Control of P_i is achieved by altered renal excretion and redistribution of body compartments. Absorption occurs in the duodenum and jejunum and is largely unregulated. Phosphate reabsorption in the kidney is primarily regulated by PTH, dietary intake, and insulin-like growth factor.[62] Phosphate is freely filtered at the glomerulus and its concentration in the glomerular ultrafiltrate is similar to that of plasma. Filtered phosphate is then reabsorbed in the proximal tubule where it is cotransported with Na^+ by passive cotransport.[62,63] Cotransport is regulated by phosphorus intake and PTH.[64] Phosphate excretion is increased by volume expansion and decreased by respiratory alkalosis.

Phosphates provide the primary energy bond in adenosine triphosphate (ATP) and creatine phosphate. Therefore severe phosphate depletion results in cellular energy depletion. Phosphorus is an essential element of second-messenger systems, including cAMP and phosphoinositides, and a major component of nucleic acids, phospholipids, and cell membranes. As part of 2,3-diphosphoglycerate, phosphate promotes release of oxygen from hemoglobin. Phosphorus also functions in protein phosphorylation and acts as a urinary buffer.

HYPOPHOSPHATEMIA

Hypophosphatemia is characterized by low levels of phosphate-containing cellular components, including ATP, 2,3-diphosphoglycerate, and membrane phospholipids. Serious life-threatening organ dysfunction can occur when serum $[P_i]$ falls below 1 mg/dL. Neurologic manifestations of hypophosphatemia include paresthesias, myopathy, encephalopathy, delirium, seizures, and coma.[65] Hematologic abnormalities include dysfunction of erythrocytes, platelets, and leukocytes. Because hypophosphatemia limits the chemotactic, phagocytic, and bactericidal activity of granulocytes, associated immune dysfunction contributes to the susceptibility of hypophosphatemic patients to sepsis. Muscle weakness and malaise are common. Respiratory muscle failure and myocardial dysfunction are potential problems of particular concern to anesthesiologists. Rhabdomyolysis is a complication of severe hypophosphatemia.[66]

Common in postoperative and traumatized patients, hypophosphatemia ($[P_i]$ <2.5 mg/dL) is caused by three primary abnormalities in P_i homeostasis: an intracellular shift of P_i, an increase in renal P_i loss, and a decrease in gastrointestinal P_i absorption. Carbohydrate-induced hypophosphatemia (refeeding syndrome), mediated by insulin-induced cellular P_i

uptake, is the type most commonly encountered in hospitalized patients.[67] Hypophosphatemia also occurs as catabolic patients become anabolic, and during medical management of diabetic ketoacidosis. Acute alkalemia, which can reduce serum $[P_i]$ to 1 to 2 mg/dL, increases intracellular consumption of P_i by increasing the rate of glycolysis. Hyperventilation significantly reduces $[P_i]$ and, importantly, the effect is progressive after cessation of hyperventilation.[68] Acute correction of respiratory acidemia can also result in severe hypophosphatemia. Respiratory alkalosis probably explains the hypophosphatemia associated with gram-negative bacteremia and salicylate poisoning. Excessive renal loss of P_i explains the hypophosphatemia associated with hyperparathyroidism, hypomagnesemia, hypothermia, diuretic therapy, and renal tubular defects in P_i absorption. Excess gastrointestinal loss of P_i is most commonly secondary to the use of P_i-binding antacids or to malabsorption syndromes.

Measurement of urinary $[P_i]$ aids in differentiation of hypophosphatemia due to renal losses from that due to excessive gastrointestinal losses or redistribution of P_i into cells. Extrarenal causes of hypophosphatemia cause avid renal tubular P_i reabsorption, reducing urinary excretion to less than 100 mg/day.

Patients who have severe (<1 mg/dL) or symptomatic hypophosphatemia require intravenous phosphate administration.[64,68] In chronically hypophosphatemic patients, 0.2 to 0.68 mmol/kg (5-16 mg/kg elemental phosphorus) should be infused over 12 hours. For moderately hypophosphatemic adult patients suffering from critical illness, the use of 15 mmol boluses (465 mg) mixed with 100 mL of 0.9% sodium chloride and given over a 2-hour period safely repletes phosphate.[69] The dosage is then adjusted as indicated by serum $[P_i]$ because the cumulative deficit cannot be predicted accurately. Oral therapy can be substituted for parenteral P_i once the serum $[P_i]$ exceeds 2 mg/dL. Continued therapy with P_i supplements is required for 5 to 10 days in order to replenish body stores.

Phosphate should be administered cautiously to hypocalcemic patients because of the risk of precipitating more severe hypocalcemia. In hypercalcemic patients, P_i can cause soft tissue calcification. Phosphorus must be given cautiously to patients with renal insufficiency because of impaired excretory ability. During treatment, close monitoring of serum P_i, Ca^{2+}, Mg^{2+}, and K^+ is essential to avoid complications.

HYPERPHOSPHATEMIA

The clinical features of hyperphosphatemia ($[P_i]$ >5 mg/dL) relate primarily to the development of hypocalcemia and ectopic calcification. Hyperphosphatemia is caused by three basic mechanisms: inadequate renal excretion, increased movement of P_i out of cells, and increased P_i or vitamin D intake. Rapid cell lysis from chemotherapy, rhabdomyolysis, and sepsis can cause hyperphosphatemia, especially when renal function is impaired. Renal failure is the most common cause of hyperphosphatemia.[65] Renal excretion of P_i remains adequate until the GFR falls below 20 to 25 mL/min.

Measurements of BUN, creatinine, GFR, and urinary P_i are helpful in the differential diagnosis of hyperphosphatemia. Normal renal function accompanied by high P_i excretion (>1500 mg/day) indicates an oversupply of P_i. An elevated BUN, elevated creatinine, and low GFR suggest impaired

renal excretion of P_i. Normal renal function and P_i excretion less than 1500 mg/day suggest increased P_i reabsorption (i.e., hypoparathyroidism).

Hyperphosphatemia is corrected by eliminating the cause of the P_i elevation and correcting the associated hypocalcemia. Calcium supplementation of hypocalcemic patients should be delayed until serum phosphate has fallen below 2 mM (6 mg/dL).[55] Serum $[P_i]$ is reduced by restricting intake, increasing urinary excretion with saline and acetazolamide (500 mg every 6 hours), and increasing gastrointestinal losses by enteric administration of aluminum hydroxide (30-45 mL every 6 hours). Aluminum hydroxide absorbs P_i secreted into the bowel lumen and increases P_i loss even if none is ingested. Hemodialysis and peritoneal dialysis are effective in removing P_i in patients who have renal failure.

Magnesium

PHYSIOLOGIC ROLE

Magnesium is a physiologically important, multifunctional, divalent cation located primarily in the intracellular space (intracellular Mg^{2+} ~ 2400 mg; extracellular Mg^{2+} ~ 280 mg). Approximately 50% of Mg^{2+} is located in bone, 25% is found in muscle, and less than 1% of total body Mg^{2+} circulates in plasma. Of the normal circulating total $[Mg^{2+}]$ (1.5-1.9 mEq/L or 0.75 to 0.95 mM or 1.7 to 2.2 mg/dL), there are three components: protein-bound (30%), chelated (15%), and ionized (55%), of which only ionized Mg^{2+} is active.[70]

Magnesium is necessary for enzymatic reactions involving DNA and protein synthesis, energy metabolism, glucose utilization, and fatty acid synthesis and breakdown.[71,72] As a primary regulator or cofactor in many enzyme systems, Mg^{2+} is important for the regulation of the Na^+ pump, Ca-ATPase enzymes, adenylyl cyclase, proton pumps, and slow Ca^{2+} channels. Magnesium has been called an endogenous Ca^{2+} antagonist, because modulation of slow Ca^{2+} channels contributes to maintenance of normal vascular tone, prevention of vasospasm, and perhaps to prevention of Ca^{2+} overload in many tissues. Because Mg^{2+} partially regulates PTH secretion and is important for maintenance of end-organ sensitivity to both PTH and vitamin D, abnormalities in ionized Mg^{2+} concentration ($[Mg^{2+}]$) can result in abnormal Ca^{2+} metabolism. Magnesium functions in K^+ metabolism primarily through regulating the Na^+ pump, which controls K^+ entry into cells, especially in potassium-depleted states, and controls reabsorption of K^+ by the renal tubules. In addition, Mg^{2+} functions as a regulator of membrane excitability and serves as a structural component in both cell membranes and the skeleton.

Because Mg^{2+} stabilizes axonal membranes, hypomagnesemia decreases the threshold of axonal stimulation and increases nerve conduction velocity. Magnesium also influences release of acetylcholine at the neuromuscular junction by competitively inhibiting the entry of Ca^{2+} into the presynaptic nerve terminals. The concentration of Ca^{2+} required to trigger Ca^{2+}-induced Ca^{2+} release and the rate at which Ca^{2+} is released from the sarcoplasmic reticulum are inversely related to the ambient Mg^{2+} concentration. Thus the net effect of hypomagnesemia is muscle that contracts more in response to stimuli and is tetany prone.

Magnesium is widely available in foods and is absorbed through the gastrointestinal tract, although dietary consumption appears to have decreased over several decades.[72] The distal tubule is the major site of Mg^{2+} regulation. Plasma $[Mg^{2+}]$ regulates Mg^{2+} reabsorption through the Ca^{2+}/Mg^{2+}-sensing receptor, located on the capillary side of cells in the thick ascending limb.[73] While both Mg^{2+} and P_i are primarily regulated by intrinsic renal mechanisms, PTH exerts a greater effect on renal loss of P_i.[71]

Magnesium has been used to help manage an impressive array of clinical problems in patients who are not hypomagnesemic.[74] Therapeutic hypermagnesemia is used to treat patients with premature labor, preeclampsia, and eclampsia. Because Mg^{2+} blocks the release of catecholamines from adrenergic nerve terminals and the adrenal glands, it has been used to reduce the effects of catecholamine excess in patients with tetanus and pheochromocytoma. Magnesium administration can influence dysrhythmias by direct effects on myocardial membranes, by altering cellular K^+ and Na^+ concentrations, by inhibiting cellular Ca^{2+} entry, by improving myocardial oxygen supply and demand, by prolonging the effective refractory period, by depressing conduction, by antagonizing catecholamine action on the conducting system, and by preventing vasospasm. Administration of Mg^{2+} reduces the incidence of dysrhythmias after myocardial infarction and in patients with congestive heart failure.[75] In humans with ischemic myocardium, Mg^{2+} prevents ischemic increases in action potential duration and membrane repolarization. After acute myocardial infarction, intravenous Mg^{2+} decreased short-term mortality.[76] In addition, Mg^{2+} can be useful as treatment for torsades de pointes, even in normomagnesemic patients.[77]

HYPOMAGNESEMIA

The clinical features of hypomagnesemia ($[Mg^{2+}]$ <1.8 mg/dL), like those of hypocalcemia, are characterized by increased neuronal irritability and tetany.[78] Symptoms are rare when serum $[Mg^{2+}]$ is 1.5 to 1.7 mg/dL; in most symptomatic patients serum $[Mg^{2+}]$ is less than 1.2 mg/dL. Patients frequently complain of weakness, lethargy, muscle spasms, paresthesias, and depression. When severe, hypomagnesemia can induce seizures, confusion, and coma. Cardiovascular abnormalities include coronary artery spasm, cardiac failure, dysrhythmias, and hypotension. Severe hypomagnesemia can reduce the response of adenylyl cyclase to stimulation of the PTH receptor.[79] Hypomagnesemia can aggravate digoxin toxicity and congestive heart failure.

Rarely resulting from inadequate dietary intake, hypomagnesemia most commonly is caused by inadequate gastrointestinal absorption, excessive losses, or failure of renal conservation. Excessive Mg^{2+} loss is associated with prolonged nasogastric suctioning, gastrointestinal or biliary fistulas, and intestinal drains. Inability of the renal tubules to conserve Mg^{2+} complicates a variety of systemic and renal diseases, although advanced renal disease with decreased GFR can lead to Mg^{2+} retention. Polyuria, whether secondary to ECV expansion or to pharmacologic or pathologic diuresis, can result in excessive urinary Mg^{2+} excretion. Various drugs, including aminoglycosides, cis-platinum, cardiac glycosides, and diuretics, enhance urinary Mg^{2+} excretion. Intracellular shifts of Mg^{2+} as a result of thyroid hormone or insulin administration can also decrease serum $[Mg^{2+}]$.

Because the Na^+ pump is Mg^{2+}-dependent, hypomagnesemia increases myocardial sensitivity to digitalis preparations and can cause hypokalemia as a result of renal K^+ wasting.

Attempts to correct K^+ deficits with K^+ replacement therapy alone might not be successful without simultaneous Mg^{2+} therapy. Magnesium is important in the regulation of K^+ channels. The interrelationships of Mg^{2+} and K^+ in cardiac tissue have probably the greatest clinical relevance in terms of arrhythmias, digoxin toxicity, and myocardial infarction. Both severe hypomagnesemia and hypermagnesemia suppress PTH secretion and can cause hypocalcemia. Severe hypomagnesemia can also impair end-organ response to PTH.

Hypomagnesemia is associated with hypokalemia, hyponatremia, hypophosphatemia, and hypocalcemia. The reported prevalence of hypomagnesemia in hospitalized and critically ill patients varies from 11% to 61%, with the variability attributable to differences in measurement technique.[80] Recent development of a specific electrode to measure ionized $[Mg^{2+}]$ has demonstrated an association between hypomagnesemia, use of diuretics and development of sepsis.[80] Patients who develop hypomagnesemia while in intensive care have an increased mortality.[80] Of alcoholic patients admitted to the hospital, 30% are hypomagnesemic.[81] Serum $[Mg^{2+}]$ might not reflect intracellular $[Mg^{2+}]$. Peripheral lymphocyte $[Mg^{2+}]$ correlates well with skeletal and cardiac Mg^{2+} content.

Measurement of 24-hour urinary Mg^{2+} excretion is useful in separating renal from nonrenal causes of hypomagnesemia. Normal kidneys can reduce Mg^{2+} excretion to less than 1 to 2 mEq/day in response to depletion. Hypomagnesemia accompanied by high urinary excretion (>3-4 mEq/day) suggests a renal etiology. In the Mg^{2+}-loading test, urinary Mg^{2+} excretion is measured for 24 hours after an intravenous load.

Magnesium deficiency is treated by administration of Mg^{2+} supplements (Table 34-12). One gram of magnesium sulfate provides approximately 4 mmol (8 mEq, or 98 mg) of elemental magnesium. Mild deficiencies can be treated with diet alone. Replacement must be added to daily requirements (0.3 to 0.4 mEq/kg/day). Symptomatic or severe hypomagnesemia ($[Mg^{2+}]$ <1 mg/dL) should be treated with parenteral Mg^{2+} 1-2 g (8-16 mEq) of magnesium sulfate as an intravenous bolus over the first hour, followed by a continuous infusion of 2 to 4 mEq/hr. Therapy should be guided subsequently by serum $[Mg^{2+}]$. The rate of infusion should not exceed 1 mEq/min, even in emergency situations, and continuous cardiac monitoring is necessary to detect cardiotoxicity. Because Mg^{2+} antagonizes Ca^{2+}, blood pressure and cardiac function should be monitored, although blood pressure and cardiac output usually change little during Mg^{2+} infusion. Treatment of hypomagnesemia during cardiopulmonary bypass was found to decrease the incidence of postoperative ventricular tachycardia from 30% to 7% and increase the frequency of continuous sinus rhythm from 5% to 34%.[82]

During repletion, patellar reflexes should be monitored frequently and Mg^{2+} withheld if they become suppressed. Patients who have renal insufficiency have a diminished ability to excrete Mg^{2+} and require careful monitoring. Repletion of systemic Mg^{2+} stores usually requires 5 to 7 days of therapy,

Table 34-12. Hypophosphatemia: Acute Treatment

Parenteral phosphate, 0.2 mM-0.68 mmol/kg (5-16 mg/kg) over 12 hr
Potassium phosphate (93 mg/ml phosphate)
Sodium phosphate (93 mg/ml phosphate)

after which daily maintenance doses should be provided. Magnesium can be given orally, usually in a dose of 60 to 90 mEq/day of magnesium oxide. Hypocalcemic, hypomagnesemic patients should receive Mg^{2+} as the chloride salt, because sulfate can chelate Ca^{2+} and further reduce serum $[Ca^{2+}]$.

HYPERMAGNESEMIA

Most cases of hypermagnesemia ($[Mg^{2+}] >2.5$ mg/dL) are iatrogenic, resulting from administration of Mg^{2+} in antacids, enemas, or parenteral nutrition, especially to patients with impaired renal function. Other rarer causes of mild hypermagnesemia are hypothyroidism, Addison disease, lithium intoxication, and familial hypocalciuric hypercalcemia. Hypermagnesemia is rarely detected in routine electrolyte determinations.[78,83,84] Hypermagnesemia antagonizes the release and effect of acetylcholine at the neuromuscular junction. The result is depressed skeletal muscle function and neuromuscular blockade. Magnesium potentiates the action of nondepolarizing muscle relaxants and decreases K^+ release in response to succinylcholine.[78]

The neuromuscular and cardiac toxicity of hypermagnesemia can be acutely, but transiently, antagonized by giving intravenous Ca^{2+} (5-10 mEq) to buy time while more definitive therapy is instituted.[78] All Mg^{2+}-containing preparations must be stopped. Urinary excretion of Mg^{2+} can be increased by expanding ECV and inducing diuresis with a combination of saline and furosemide. In emergency situations and in patients with renal failure, Mg^{2+} can be removed by dialysis.

DIURETICS

The most prominent property of diuretics is that they reduce reabsorption of sodium chloride at different sites in the nephron, thereby increasing urinary Na^+ and water losses. This makes them useful in treatment of a variety of conditions such as edematous states, hypertension, heart failure, renal dysfunction, hypercalcemia, nephrolithiasis, glaucoma, and mountain sickness. Their efficacy, safety, and optimal dosing are however based on small and underpowered trials.[85,86] They can be divided into three major classes depending on which site at which they impair Na^+ reabsorption. Loop diuretics act in the thick ascending limb of the loop of Henle, thiazide type diuretics in the distal tubule and connecting segment and potassium sparing diuretics in the aldosterone-sensitive principal cells in the cortical collecting tubule.

It is important to understand the general mechanism behind Na^+ reabsorption (Figure 34-5). Each of the Na^+ transporting cells contain Na^+ pumps in the basolateral membrane.[87] These pumps have two major functions. They return reabsorbed Na^+ to the systemic circulation and maintain intracellular $[Na^+]$ concentration at low levels. This is important because otherwise no Na^+ transport occurs. Each of the major nephron segments has a unique Na^+ entry mechanism and the inhibition of this step is the major mechanism by which each of the different classes of diuretics acts. Approximately two thirds of filtered Na^+ is reabsorbed in the proximal tubuli by primary and secondary active transport.

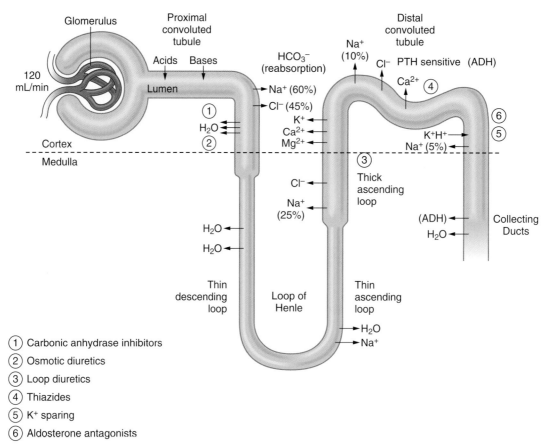

Figure 34-5 Sites of action of diuretics at various locations in the nephron.

Proximal Convoluted Tubule—Carbonic Anhydrase Inhibitors

Acetazolamide and dorzolamide inhibit the activity of carbonic anhydrase, which plays an important role in proximal bicarbonate, Na^+ and Cl^- reabsorption. These agents thus produce NaCl and $NaHCO_3$ loss. The net diuresis is however small because most of the excess fluid is reclaimed at more distal segments, particularly at the loop of Henle. The diuretic action is also attenuated by the metabolic acidosis that is the result of the loss of bicarbonate (Figure 34-6).

The major uses of these diuretics are for edematous states and metabolic alkalosis.[88,89] Clinical uses are glaucoma (decrease of aqueous humor which lowers the intraocular pressure), acute mountain sickness (lowers the incidence of pulmonary as well as cerebral edema), metabolic alkalosis (such as caused by thiazide diuretics), and elimination of acidic drugs. Adverse effects are acidosis, bicarbonaturia, hypokalemia, paresthesias, and renal stones (hypercalciuria, phosphaturia).

Ascending Loop of Henle—Loop Diuretics

Fluid entering the loop of Henle is isotonic (osmolarity 300 mOsm/L) but the volume is only a third of the volume originally filtered into Bowman's capsule. The loop of Henle acts as a countercurrent multiplier (see Figure 35-5) and as such creates a medullary interstitial osmolar gradient. The descending limb of the loop of Henle is permeable to water. Water diffuses into the hyperosmolar medullary interstitium. The osmolarity can reach a maximum of 1200 mOsm/L at the tip of the medullary interstitium in antidiuresis. The ascending limb (where loop diuretics work) is impermeable to water. NaCl is pumped from the tubule into the interstitium in the ascending limb. The tubular osmolarity decreases and

fluid that leaves the loop is hypotonic. The collecting duct is impermeable to water without ADH.

The loop diuretics—furosemide, torsemide, bumetanide, and ethacrynic acid—can lead to excretion of 20% to 25% of filtered Na^+ when given in large doses.[90,91] They act principally in the medullary and cortical aspects of the thick ascending limb and the macula densa cells in the early distal tubule. The loop diuretics compete for the Cl^- site, thereby diminishing net reabsorption.[92,93] Sodium reabsorbed via the $Na^+/K^+/2Cl^-$ transporter is transported back into the blood by the Na^+ pump and by a Na^+/Cl^- cotransporter, the excess Cl^- returning to blood via passive diffusion. High intracellular $[K^+]$ results in its back diffusion across the luminal membrane providing a positive potential that drives reabsorption of both Mg^{2+} and Ca^{2+} (Figure 34-7). Inhibition of this mechanism thus increases urinary Na^+, K^+, Ca^{2+}, Mg^+, and Cl^- losses.

The clinical uses of loop diuretics include acute pulmonary edema, acute renal failure, anion overdose, heart failure, hypercalcemia, hypertension, and refractory edemas.

Adverse effects are allergies, alkalosis, hypocalcemia, hypokalemia, hypomagnesemia, hyperuricemia, hypovolemia, and ototoxicity (ethacrynic acid > furosemide).

Distal Convoluted Tubule—Thiazides

Hydrochlorothiazide, indapamide, and metolazone are organic acids that are both filtered and secreted and inhibit the Na^+/Cl^- transporter on the luminal membrane on the distal convoluted tubule. Normally, the Na^+ that is brought in by the Na^+/Cl^- cotransporter is exchanged for K^+ that returns to blood via back diffusion. Chloride also returns to blood by such a mechanism, while Ca^{2+} returns by a Ca^{2+}/Na^+ antiporter. If the Na^+/Cl^- cotransporter is inhibited by thiazides, hypokalemia and alkalosis occur. Hypercalcemia can

Proximal Convoluted Tubule

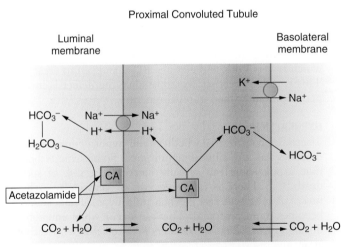

Thick Ascending Loop

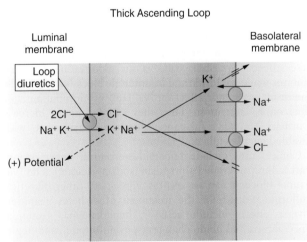

Figure 34-6 Actions of carbonic anhydrase inhibitors on the proximal convoluted tubule. Carbonic anhydrase inhibitors like acetazolamide inhibit the reabsorption of bicarbonate. Intracellular carbonic anhydrase normally catalyzes the conversion of carbon dioxide to bicarbonate, that is transported across the basolateral membrane, and protons, that are transported across the luminal membrane by the Na^+/H^+ exchanger. Here the protons react with tubular bicarbonate to form carbon dioxide, which is reabsorbed. Inhibition of luminal carbonic anhydrase reduces this reaction resulting in bicarbonate excretion and diuresis. *CA,* Carbonic anhydrase. Acetazolamide is a carbonic anhydrase inhibitor.

Figure 34-7 Actions of loop diuretics on the thick ascending loop of Henle. Loop diuretics are secreted into the tubular fluid by proximal tubule cells. In the thick ascending limb of the loop of Henle, they inhibit the $Na^+/K^+/Cl^-$ symporter that is driven by the Na^+ gradient. These cell have a high capacity for Na^+ reabsorption, so inhibition of this symporter has a large effect on NaCl reabsorption and causes a large diuresis that cannot be compensated for by more distal tubule cells.

Distal Tubule

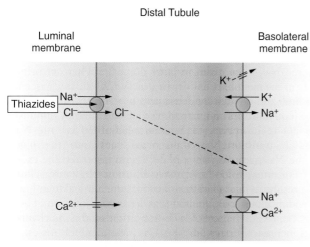

Figure 34-8 Actions of thiazides on the distal convoluted tubule. Thaizide diuretics, which are secreted into the tubular fluid by proximal tubular cells, inhibit the Na^+/Cl^- symporter driven by the Na^+ gradient. This blocks reabsorption of NaCl, producing a diuresis. The Cl^- then leaves the cell via a chloride channel. Passive ion leak is indicated by the parallel lines.

occur due to increased activity of the Na^+/Ca^{2+} antiporter (Figure 34-8).

Clinical uses of thiazides are hypertension and heart failure. Their effects are improved by Na^+ restriction and attenuated by low GFR. Adverse effects are allergies, alkalosis, hypokalemia, hyperuricemia, hypovolemia, hyperglycemia, hyperlipidemia, hypercalcemia, and sexual dysfunction.

Collecting Ducts—Potassium Sparing Diuretics

Spironolactone, amiloride, and triamterene are weak diuretics that act at the level of the collecting tubules and ducts. Most K^+ is secreted in the collecting ducts. In the normal situation, aldosterone exerts its mineralocorticoid action via interaction with specific receptors, increasing insertion of Na^+ channels on the luminal membrane thereby increasing activity of Na^+/K^+ and H^+ exchangers. Na^+ diffuses through the channels increasing intracellular positive charge, and thereby extrusion of K^+ into the lumen. The potassium-sparing diuretics prevent these effects. Spironolactone is an aldosterone receptor inhibitor while amiloride and triamterene block Na^+ channels. The result is a minor effect on Na^+ reabsorption but a major effect on K^+ retention. Thus they cause a minor increase in urinary Na^+ but a substantial decrease in urinary K^+ with possible hyperkalemia and acidosis.

Clinical uses include hyperaldosteronism, hypertension, heart failure, and female hirsutism (spironolactone). The Na^+ channel blockers can be used as adjuncts to other diuretics. Amiloride is used for the treatment of diabetes insipidus. Adverse effects include acidosis, hyperkalemia, azotemia, gynecomastia and libido changes (spironolactone), and nephrolithiasis (triamterene).

Osmotic Diuretics

Mannitol is a non-reabsorbable sugar that acts as an osmotic diuretic, inhibiting water reabsorption in the proximal convoluted tubule (main site), the thin descending loop of Henle, and the collecting ducts.[94,95] Mannitol produces a profound water diuresis in which water is lost in excess of electrolytes.

However, retention of the hypertonic mannitol can induce further volume expansion. This can potentially cause pulmonary edema in patients with heart failure. Major clinical uses include early stages of oliguria, early phases of brain edema, and postischemic acute renal failure. It is also commonly used in neurosurgical anesthesia to provide good operating conditions (see Chapter 8).

Diuretics in Heart Failure

In acute decompensated heart failure, there are no differences between low and high furosemide dose strategies in outcome. Because a high-dose strategy brings more relief of dyspnea, diuresis, and weight loss and a transient worsening of renal function without evidence of worse clinical outcome at 60 days, this regimen might be more beneficial.[96] The action of drugs producing diuresis and natriuresis in patients with heart failure is illustrated in Figure 34-9 (see Chapter 23).

Adverse Effects of Diuretics

At high doses, diuretics produce adverse effects such as hypotension, hypovolemia, electrolyte abnormalities, renal dysfunction, and neurohumoral activation. They can also contribute to longer hospitalization and higher mortality.[97] Major fluid and electrolyte disturbances can occur within the first 2 to 3 weeks of diuretic administration, which is due to attainment and maintenance of new steady-state requirements.[98] Maximum diuresis always occurs with the first dose; as soon as fluid loss occurs, activation of Na^+ retaining mechanisms takes place.[99]

VOLUME DEPLETION
Although the duration of Na^+ loss is limited, some patients have a large initial response of volume loss, particularly in patients with hypertension. In patients who remain edematous, the circulatory volume can be depleted and tissue perfusion reduced.

AZOTEMIA
If circulating volume is depleted, renal perfusion can fall, which lowers GFR and elevates BUN and serum creatinine. This is called prerenal azotemia since the defect is in renal perfusion rather than in renal function.[100]

HYPOKALEMIA
There is a controversy whether mild hypokalemia caused by diuretics has any clinical significance. Some experts believe that hypokalemia can actually increase the risk of sudden death.[101,102] There is increased risk of ventricular arrhythmia.[103] A pertinent risk is when mild hypokalemia suddenly becomes more profound. This can occur when epinephrine during a stress situation transfers K^+ into cells via β_2-receptor agonism.

HYPONATREMIA
This is a common side effect in edematous patients with heart failure or cirrhosis. Volume loss enhances the release of ADH and thereby causes dilution of Na^+. This is almost solely due to thiazide diuretics, which do not impair concentration ability. Other diuretics reduce the medullary osmolar gradient and concentrating ability.

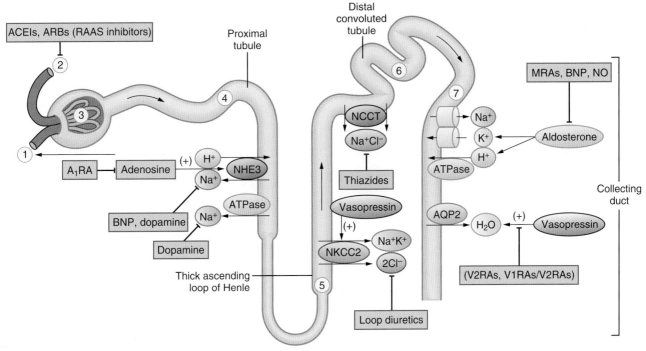

Figure 34-9 Sites of action of drugs producing diuresis and natriuresis.[104] Adenosine produces afferent arteriolar vasoconstriction and increases Na[+] reabsorption in the proximal tubule. Aldosterone stimulates Na[+] and K[+] channels and Na[+],K[+]-ATPase activity in the collecting tubules. Vasopressin stimulates the activity of the Na[+]/K[+]/2 Cl[−] cotransporter NKCC2 (also known as SLC12A1) and aquaporin2 (AQP2). ① Afferent arteriolar vasodilatation. ② Efferent arteriolar vasodilation. ③ Increase in glomerular filtration rate. ④ Inhibition of Na[+] reabsorption in the proximal tubule. ⑤ Thick ascending loop of Henle. ⑥ Distal tubule. ⑦ Collecting ducts. Drugs that act at these sites are shown in colored boxes. *A₁RA,* Adenosine A₁ receptor antagonist; *ACEI,* angiotensin converting enzyme inhibitor; *ARB,* angiotensin II type 1 receptor blocker; *ATPase,* Na[+],K[+]-ATPase; *BNP,* brain natriuretic peptide; *MRA,* mineralocorticoid receptor antagonist; *NCCT,* Na[+]/Cl[−] cotransporter; *NHE3,* Na[+]/H[+] exchanger 3 (also known as SLC9A3); *NO,* nitric oxide; *RAAS,* renin-angiotensin-aldosterone system; *V1RA/V2RA,* vasopressin receptor antagonist.

EMERGING DEVELOPMENTS

Electrolytes are major contributors to basic physiologic functions. Knowledge about electrolytes is therefore essential. In recent years there are new approaches to the treatment of hyponatremia. Prompt bolus treatment of symptomatic hyponatremia with hypertonic saline is crucial. The underlying disorder must be addressed. Furthermore, new and interesting insights have been made regarding treatment for heart failure.[104]

KEY POINTS

- The major electrolytes (sodium, potassium, calcium, phosphate, and magnesium) are critical to basic physiologic functions, including action potential generation, cardiac rhythm control, muscle contraction, and energy storage.
- Hyponatremia is the most common electrolyte disorder in hospitalized patients; it is sometimes associated with severe symptoms and even death, especially when the hyponatremia is corrected too rapidly.
- New approaches differ from the previously advocated focus on separation between acute or chronic causes for hyponatremia. When seriously symptomatic, hyponatremia must be addressed expeditiously.
- Hypernatremia is categorized in terms of the adequacy of intravascular volume. It is treated first with volume resuscitation when needed followed by repletion of the free water deficit, and by addressing the underlying cause (e.g., diabetes insipidus, iatrogenic causes).
- No clear threshold has been defined for a level of hypokalemia below which safe conduct of anesthesia is compromised. There is no urgent need for K[+] replacement therapy in mild to moderate hypokalemia (3 to 3.5 mEq/L) in asymptomatic patients.
- Drugs are now the most common causes of hyperkalemia (e.g., nonsteroidal antiinflammatory drugs, ACE inhibitors, cyclosporin, and potassium-sparing diuretics) that occurs most commonly in patients with predisposing comorbidities (e.g., diabetes mellitus, renal insufficiency). In anesthesia practice, hyperkalemic cardiac toxicity is associated with the administration of succinylcholine to patients with upper motor neuron lesions or severe burns.
- The definitive treatment of hypocalcemia necessitates identification and treatment of the underlying cause. Symptomatic hypocalcemia usually occurs when serum ionized [Ca[2+]] is less than 0.7 mM. The clinician should carefully consider whether mild, asymptomatic ionized hypocalcemia requires therapy, particularly in ischemic and septic states in which experimental evidence suggests that Ca[2+] can increase cellular damage.
- Carbohydrate-induced hypophosphatemia (refeeding syndrome), mediated by insulin-induced cellular

Continued

Key References

Ayus JC, Armstrong DL, Arieff AI. Effects of hypernatraemia in the central nervous system and its therapy in rats and rabbits. *J Physiol*. 1996;492:243-255. An interesting study in animals showing the effect of untreated hypernatremia that results in brain lesions, myelinolysis, and cellular necrosis. (Ref. 32)

Brooks MJ, Melnik G. The refeeding syndrome: an approach to understanding its complications and preventing its occurrence. *Pharmacotherapy*. 1995;15:713-726. The refeeding syndrome should be characterized as a syndrome of generalized fluid and electrolyte imbalance. Recommended electrolyte supplementation and laboratory monitoring can help prevent the disorder in susceptible patients. (Ref. 67)

Overgaard-Steensen C. Initial approach to the hyponatremic patient. *Acta Anaesthesiol Scand*. 2010;55:139-148. This paper presents a practical and unified approach based on a literature study of the physiology of plasma Na^+, the brain's response, and clinical and experimental studies of hyponatremia. (Ref. 1)

Tamargo J, Lopez-Sendon J. Novel therapeutic targets for the treatment of heart failure. *Nat Rev Drug Discov*. 2011;10:536-555. Despite considerable therapeutic advances, heart failure remains refractory to treatment in many patients. In recent years, new potential targets that are involved in the pathogenesis of heart failure have been identified. Several drugs targeting these mechanisms are in phase 2 and phase 3 trials. (Ref. 104)

Wahr JA, Parks R, Boisvert D, et al. Preoperative serum potassium levels and perioperative outcomes in cardiac surgery patients. Multicenter Study of Perioperative Ischemia Research Group. *J Am Med Assoc*. 1999;281:2203-2210. Prospective, observational, case-control study of data collected from 24 diverse U.S. medical centers. Perioperative arrhythmia and the need for CPR increased as preoperative serum potassium level decreased below 3.5 mmol/L. (Ref. 41)

Weisinger JR, Bellorin-Font E. Magnesium and phosphorus. *Lancet*. 1998;352:391-396. A summary of new findings regarding alterations of magnesium and phosphorus metabolism are reviewed for the clinician. (Ref. 70)

References

1. Overgaard-Steensen C. Initial approach to the hyponatremic patient. *Acta Anaesthesiol Scand*. 2010;55:139-148.
2. Upadhyay A, Jaber BL, Madias NE. Epidemiology of hyponatremia. *Semin Nephrol*. 2009;29:227-238.
3. Tierney WM, Martin DK, Greenlee MC, Zerbe RL, McDonald CJ. The prognosis of hyponatremia at hospital admission. *J Gen Intern Med*. 1986;1:380-385.
4. Ayus JC, Achinger SG, Arieff A. Brain cell volume regulation in hyponatremia: role of sex, age, vasopressin, and hypoxia. *Am J Physiol Renal Physiol*. 2008;295:F619-F624.
5. Kashyap AS. Hyperglycemia-induced hyponatremia: is it time to correct the correction factor? *Arch Intern Med*. 1999;159:2745-2746.
6. Gravenstein D. Transurethral resection of the prostate (TURP) syndrome: a review of the pathophysiology and management. *Anesth Analg*. 1997;84:438-446.
7. Hjertberg H. The use of ethanol as a marker to detect and quantify the absorption of irrigation fluid during transurethral resection of the prostate. *Scand J Urol Nephrol Suppl*. 1996;178:1-64.
8. Chatterjee K. Hyponatremia in heart failure. *J Intens Care Med*. 2009;24:347-351.
9. Xu DL, Martin PY, Ohara M, et al. Upregulation of aquaporin-2 water channel expression in chronic heart failure rat. *J Clin Invest*. 1997;99:1500-1505.
10. Fujita N, Ishikawa SE, Sasaki S, et al. Role of water channel AQP-CD in water retention in SIADH and cirrhotic rats. *Am J Physiol*. 1995;269:F926-F931.
11. Kumar S, Berl T. Sodium. *Lancet*. 1998;352:220-228.
12. Berendes E, Walter M, Cullen P, et al. Secretion of brain natriuretic peptide in patients with aneurysmal subarachnoid haemorrhage. *Lancet*. 1997;349:245-249.
13. Yamaki T, Tano-oka A, Takahashi A, et al. Cerebral salt wasting syndrome distinct from the syndrome of inappropriate secretion of antidiuretic hormone (SIADH). *Acta Neurochir*. 1992;115:156-162.
14. Kim JK, Summer SN, Wood WM, Schrier RW. Osmotic and non-osmotic regulation of arginine vasopressin (AVP) release, mRNA, and promoter activity in small cell lung carcinoma (SCLC) cells. *Molecular and cellular endocrinology*. 1996;123:179-186.
15. Chung HM, Kluge R, Schrier RW, Anderson RJ. Postoperative hyponatremia. A prospective study. *Arch Intern Med*. 1986;146:333-336.
16. Ayus JC, Arieff AI. Brain damage and postoperative hyponatremia: the role of gender. *Neurology*. 1996;46:323-328.
17. Gomola A, Cabrol S, Murat I. Severe hyponatraemia after plastic surgery in a girl with cleft palate, medial facial hypoplasia and growth retardation. *Paediatr Anaesth*. 1998;8:69-71.
18. Arieff AI. Postoperative hyponatraemic encephalopathy following elective surgery in children. *Paediatr Anaesth*. 1998;8:1-4.
19. Steele A, Gowrishankar M, Abrahamson S, et al. Postoperative hyponatremia despite near-isotonic saline infusion: a phenomenon of desalination. *Ann Intern Med*. 1997;126:20-25.
20. Sterns RH, Nigwekar SU, Hix JK. The treatment of hyponatremia. *Semin Nephrol*. 2009;29:282-299.
21. Verbalis JG, Goldsmith SR, Greenberg A, Schrier RW, Sterns RH. Hyponatremia treatment guidelines 2007: expert panel recommendations. *Am J Med*. 2007;120:S1-S21.
22. Hoorn EJ, Lindemans J, Zietse R. Development of severe hyponatraemia in hospitalized patients: treatment-related risk factors and inadequate management. *Nephrol Dial Transplant*. 2006;21:70-76.
23. Brown WD. Osmotic demyelination disorders: central pontine and extrapontine myelinolysis. *Curr Opin Neurol*. 2000;13:691-697.
24. Overgaard-Steensen C, Stodkilde-Jorgensen H, Larsson A, et al. Regional differences in osmotic behavior in brain during acute hyponatremia: an in vivo MRI-study of brain and skeletal muscle in pigs. *Am J Physiol Regul Integr Comp Physiol*. 2010;299:R521-R532.
25. Kumar S, Beri T. Sodium. *Lancet*. 1998;352:220-228.
26. Ferguson-Myrthil N. Novel agents for the treatment of hyponatremia: a review of conivaptan and tolvaptan. *Cardiol Rev*. 2010;18:313-321.
27. Ober KP. Endocrine crises. Diabetes insipidus. *Crit Care Clin*. 1991;7:109-125.
28. Bagshaw SM, Townsend DR, McDermid RC. Disorders of sodium and water balance in hospitalized patients. *Can J Anaesth*. 2009;56:151-167.
29. Rowe JW, Shock NW, DeFronzo RA. The influence of age on the renal response to water deprivation in man. *Nephron*. 1976;17:270-278.
30. Joelsson-Alm E, Nyman CR, Lindholm C, Ulfvarson J, Svensén C. Perioperative bladder distension—a prospective study. *Scand J Urol Nephrol*. 2009;43:58-62.
31. McManus ML, Churchwell KB, Strange K. Regulation of cell volume in health and disease. *N Engl J Med*. 1995;333:1260-1266. 32. Ayus JC, Armstrong DL, Arieff AI. Effects of hypernatraemia in the central nervous system and its therapy in rats and rabbits. *J Physiol*. 1996;492:243-255.
33. Mattox KL, Maningas PA, Moore EE, et al. Prehospital hypertonic saline/dextran infusion for post-traumatic hypotension. The U.S. Multicenter Trial. *Ann Surg*. 1991;213:482-491.

34. Adrogue HJ, Madias NE. Hypernatremia. *N Engl J Med.* 2000;342:1493-1499.

35. Chanson P, Jedynak CP, Dabrowski G, et al. Ultralow doses of vasopressin in the management of diabetes insipidus. *Crit Care Med.* 1987;15:44-46.

36. Sedlacek M, Schoolwerth AC, Remillard BD. Electrolyte disturbances in the intensive care unit. *Semin Dial.* 2006;19:496-501.

37. Halperin ML, Kamel KS. Potassium. *Lancet.* 1998;352:135-140.

38. Rose BD, Post TW. *Clinical Physiology of Acid-Base and Electrolyte Disorders.* New York: McGraw-Hill; 2001.

39. Rossier BC. 1996 Homer Smith Award Lecture. Cum grano salis: the epithelial sodium channel and the control of blood pressure. *J Am Soc Nephrol.* 1997;8:980-992.

40. Weiner ID, Wingo CS. Hypokalemia–consequences, causes, and correction. *J Am Soc Nephrol.* 1997;8:1179-1188.

41. Wahr JA, Parks R, Boisvert D, et al. Preoperative serum potassium levels and perioperative outcomes in cardiac surgery patients. Multicenter Study of Perioperative Ischemia Research Group. *J Am Med Assoc.* 1999;281:2203-2210.

42. Osadchii OE. Mechanisms of hypokalemia-induced ventricular arrhythmogenicity. *Fundam Clin Pharmacol.* 2010;24:547-559.

43. Gennari FJ. Hypokalemia. *N Engl J Med.* 1998;339:451-458.

44. Kuvin JT. Electrocardiographic changes of hyperkalemia. *N Engl J Med.* 1998;338:662.

45. Wrenn KD, Slovis CM, Slovis BS. The ability of physicians to predict hyperkalemia from the ECG. *Ann Emerg Med.* 1991;20:1229-1232.

46. Kim HJ, Han SW. Therapeutic approach to hyperkalemia. *Nephron.* 2002;92:33-40.

47. Zaloga GP, Chernow B. Hypocalcemia in critical illness. *J Am Med Assoc.* 1986;256:1924-1929.

48. Bushinsky DA, Monk RD. Electrolyte quintet: Calcium. *Lancet.* 1998;352:306-311.

49. Zivin JR, Gooley T, Zager RA, Ryan MJ. Hypocalcemia: a pervasive metabolic abnormality in the critically ill. *Am J Kidney Dis.* 2001;37:689-698.

50. Guise TA, Mundy GR. Clinical review 69: Evaluation of hypocalcemia in children and adults. *J Clin Endocrinol Metab.* 1995;80:1473-1478.

51. Sutters M, Gaboury CL, Bennett WM. Severe hyperphosphatemia and hypocalcemia: a dilemma in patient management. *J Am Soc Nephrol.* 1996;7:2056-2061.

52. Zaloga GP, Strickland RA, Butterworth JF IV, et al. Calcium attenuates epinephrine's adrenergic effects in postoperative heart surgery patients. *Circulation.* 1990;81:196-200.

53. Mathru M, Rooney MW, Goldberg SA, Hirsch L. Separation of myocardial versus peripheral effects of calcium administration in normocalcemic and hypocalcemic states using pressure volume (conductance) relationships. *Anesth Analg.* 1993;77:250-255.

54. Bilezikian JP. Clinical review 51: Management of hypercalcemia. *J Clin Endocrinol Metab.* 1993;77:1445-1449.

55. Bushinsky DA, Monk RD. Calcium. *Lancet.* 1998;352:306-311.

56. Mundy GR, Guise TA. Hypercalcemia of malignancy. *Am J Med.* 1997;103:134-145.

57. Berenson JR, Lichtenstein A, Porter L, et al. Efficacy of pamidronate in reducing skeletal events in patients with advanced multiple myeloma. *N Engl J Med.* 1996;334:488-493.

58. Watts NB, Worley K, Solis A, Doyle J, Sheer R. Comparison of risedronate to alendronate and calcitonin for early reduction of nonvertebral fracture risk: results from a managed care administrative claims database. *J Manag Care Pharm.* 2004;10:142-151.

59. Ariyan CE, Sosa JA. Assessment and management of patients with abnormal calcium. *Crit Care Med.* 2004;32:S146-S154.

60. Chan FKW, Koberle LMC, Thys-Jacobs S, Bilezikian JP. Differential diagnosis, causes, and management of hypercalcemia. *Curr Probl Surg.* 1997;34:449-523.

61. Urena P, Frazao JM. Calcimimetic agents: review and perspectives. *Kidney Int Suppl.* 2003:S91-S96.

62. Murer H, Werner A, Reshkin S, Wuarin F, Biber J. Cellular mechanisms in proximal tubular reabsorption of inorganic phosphate. *Am J Physiol.* 1991;260:C885-C899.

63. Murer H, Markovich D, Biber J. Renal and small intestinal sodium-dependent symporters of phosphate and sulphate. *J Exp Biol.* 1994;196:167-181.

64. Peppers MP, Geheb M, Desai T. Endocrine crises. Hypophosphatemia and hyperphosphatemia. *Crit Care Clin.* 1991;7:201-214.

65. Peppers MP, Geheb M, Desai T. Hypophosphatemia and hyperphosphatemia. *Crit Care Clin.* 1991;7:201-214.

66. Knochel JP. Hypophosphatemia and rhabdomyolysis. *Am J Med.* 1992;92:455-457.

67. Brooks MJ, Melnik G. The refeeding syndrome: an approach to understanding its complications and preventing its occurrence. *Pharmacotherapy.* 1995;15:713-726.

68. Paleologos M, Stone E, Braude S. Persistent, progressive hypophosphataemia after voluntary hyperventilation. *Clin Sci (Lond).* 2000;98:619-625.

69. Rosen GH, Boullata JI, O'Rangers EA, Enow NB, Shin B. Intravenous phosphate repletion regimen for critically ill patients with moderate hypophosphatemia. *Crit Care Med.* 1995;23:1204-1210.

70. Weisinger JR, Bellorin-Font E. Magnesium and phosphorus. *Lancet.* 1998;352:391-396.

71. Whang R, Hampton EM, Whang DD. Magnesium homeostasis and clinical disorders of magnesium deficiency. *Annals Pharmacother.* 1997;28:220-226.

72. Gums JG. Magnesium in cardiovascular and other disorders. *Am J Health Syst Pharm.* 2004;61:1569-1576.

73. Quamme GA. Renal magnesium handling: new insights in understanding old problems. *Kidney Int.* 1997;52:1180-1195.

74. McLean RM. Magnesium and its therapeutic uses: a review. *Am J Med.* 1994;96:63-76.

75. Sueta CA, Clarke SW, Dunlap SH, et al. Effect of acute magnesium administration on the frequency of ventricular arrhythmia in patients with heart failure. *Circulation.* 1994;89:660-666.

76. Teo KK, Yusuf S, Collins R, Held PH, Peto R. Effects of intravenous magnesium in suspected acute myocardial infarction: overview of randomised trials. *Brit Med J.* 1991;303:1499-1503.

77. Tzivoni D, Banai S, Schuger C, et al. Treatment of torsade de pointes with magnesium sulfate. *Circulation.* 1988;77:392-397.

78. Topf JM, Murray PT. Hypomagnesemia and hypermagnesemia. *Rev Endocr Metab Disord.* 2003;4:195-206.

79. Abbott LG, Rude RK. Clinical manifestations of magnesium deficiency. *Miner Electrolyte Metab.* 1993;19:314-322.

80. Soliman HM, Mercan D, Lobo SS, Melot C, Vincent JL. Development of ionized hypomagnesemia is associated with higher mortality rates. *Crit Care Med.* 2003;31:1082-1087.

81. Elisaf M, Merkouropoulos M, Tsianos EV, Siamopoulos KC. Pathogenetic mechanisms of hypomagnesemia in alcoholic patients. *J Trace Elem Med Biol.* 1995;9:210-214.

82. Wilkes NJ, Mallett SV, Peachey T, Di Salvo C, Walesby R. Correction of ionized plasma magnesium during cardiopulmonary bypass reduces the risk of postoperative cardiac arrhythmia. *Anesthesia and Analgesia.* 2002;95:828-834.

83. Whang R, Ryder KW. Frequency of hypomagnesemia and hypermagnesemia. Requested vs routine. *J Am Med Assoc.* 1990;263:3063-3064.

84. Wong ET, Rude RK, Singer FR, et al. A high prevalence of hypomagnesemia and hypermagnesemia in hospitalized patients. *Am J Clin Pathol.* 1983;79:348-352.

85. Dickstein K, Vardas PE, Auricchio A, et al. 2010 Focused update of ESC guidelines on device therapy in heart failure: an update of the 2008 ESC guidelines for the diagnosis and treatment of acute and chronic heart failure and the 2007 ESC guidelines for cardiac and resynchronization therapy. Developed with the special contribution of the Heart Failure Association and the European Heart Rhythm Association. *Europace.* 2010;12:1526-1536.

86. Hunt SA, Abraham WT, Chin MH, et al. 2009 Focused update incorporated into the ACC/AHA 2005 Guidelines for the Diagnosis and Management of Heart Failure in Adults: A Report of the American College of Cardiology Foundation/American Heart Association Task Force on Practice Guidelines Developed in Collaboration With the International Society for Heart and Lung Transplantation. *J Am Coll Cardiol.* 2009;53:e1-e90.

87. Katz AI. Distribution and function of classes of ATPases along the nephron. *Kidney Int.* 1986;29:21-31.

88. Leaf A, Schwartz WB, Relman AS. Oral administration of a potent carbonic anhydrase inhibitor (Diamox). I. Changes in electrolyte and acid-base balance. *N Engl J Med.* 1954;250:759-764.

89. Preisig PA, Toto RD, Alpern RJ. Carbonic anhydrase inhibitors. *Ren Physiol.* 1987;10:136-159.

90. Rose BD. Diuretics. *Kidney Int.* 1991;39:336-352.

91. Stanton BA, Kaissling B. Adaptation of distal tubule and collecting duct to increased Na delivery. II. Na+ and K+ transport. *Am J Physiol*. 1988;255:F1269-F1275.
92. O'Grady SM, Palfrey HC, Field M. Characteristics and functions of Na-K-Cl cotransport in epithelial tissues. *Am J Physiol*. 1987;253:C177-C192.
93. Amsler K, Kinne R. Photoinactivation of sodium-potassium-chloride cotransport in LLC-PK1/Cl 4 cells by bumetanide. *Am J Physiol*. 1986;250:C799-C806.
94. Seely JF, Dirks JH. Micropuncture study of hypertonic mannitol diuresis in the proximal and distal tubule of the dog kidney. *J Clin Invest*. 1969;48:2330-2340.
95. Mathisen O, Raeder M, Kiil F. Mechanism of osmotic diuresis. *Kidney Int*. 1981;19:431-437.
96. Felker GM, O'Connor CM, Braunwald E. Loop diuretics in acute decompensated heart failure: necessary? Evil? A necessary evil? *Circ Heart Fail*. 2009;2:56-62.
97. Maronde RF, Milgrom M, Vlachakis ND, Chan L. Response of thiazide-induced hypokalemia to amiloride. *J Am Med Assoc*. 1983;249:237-241.
98. Rudy DW, Voelker JR, Greene PK, Esparza FA, Brater DC. Loop diuretics for chronic renal insufficiency: a continuous infusion is more efficacious than bolus therapy. *Ann Intern Med*. 1991;115:360-366.
99. Felker GM, Lee KL, Bull DA, et al. Diuretic strategies in patients with acute decompensated heart failure. *N Engl J Med*. 2011;364:797-805.
100. Dossetor JB. Creatininemia versus uremia. The relative significance of blood urea nitrogen and serum creatinine concentrations in azotemia. *Ann Intern Med*. 1966;65:1287-1299.
101. Kuller LH, Hulley SB, Cohen JD, Neaton J. Unexpected effects of treating hypertension in men with electrocardiographic abnormalities: a critical analysis. *Circulation*. 1986;73:114-123.
102. Siscovick DS, Raghunathan TE, Psaty BM, et al. Diuretic therapy for hypertension and the risk of primary cardiac arrest. *N Engl J Med*. 1994;330:1852-1857.
103. Cohen JD, Neaton JD, Prineas RJ, Daniels KA. Diuretics, serum potassium and ventricular arrhythmias in the Multiple Risk Factor Intervention Trial. *Am J Cardiol*. 1987;60:548-554.
104. Tamargo J, Lopez-Sendon J. Novel therapeutic targets for the treatment of heart failure. *Nat Rev Drug Discov*. 2011;10:536-555.

Chapter 35

BLOOD AND COAGULATION

Jerrold H. Levy, Roman M. Sniecinski, and Linda J. Demma

Hemostasis involves vascular, cellular, and plasma components that interact to stop bleeding.[1] Vascular effects include vasoconstriction, expression of procoagulant factors such as tissue factor, and loss of normal anticoagulation pathways due to endothelial and tissue injury.[2,3] Coagulation and clot formation occur by cellular and humoral factors that interact together with local and systemic factors. Hemostasis in surgical patients is influenced by a number of factors that are unique to the perioperative environment. Surgery produces complex alterations and defects in hemostatic mechanisms, particularly in trauma, cardiac surgery with or without cardiopulmonary bypass, major orthopedic surgery, and neurosurgery.[4] In many patients, multiple quantitative and qualitative hemostatic abnormalities develop as part of surgery, tissue injury, and complex underlying medical conditions. The increasing use of multiple anticoagulation agents to treat cardiovascular disease contributes to a perioperative hemostatic defect due to tissue injury associated with surgery.[2] Further massive bleeding can produce an acquired hemostatic defect called massive transfusion coagulopathy that is characterized by tissue injury, dilutional hemostatic changes, hypothermia, acidosis, and multiorgan dysfunction, all of which can contribute to coagulopathy and the potential for bleeding.[5]

Managing hemostatic dysfunction and bleeding perioperatively requires an understanding of underlying hemostatic mechanisms. Tissue injury and the stress response activate fibrinolysis that can further contribute to coagulopathy and bleeding. This chapter reviews the basis of normal hemostasis, the procoagulant and anticoagulant changes that occur in surgical patients, as well as perioperative coagulation testing and treatment of bleeding.

NORMAL HEMOSTATIC MECHANISMS

Complex interactions between coagulation proteins, platelets, and the vascular endothelium maintain normal hemostasis (Figure 35-1). The vascular endothelium plays a major role in preventing clotting; it presents an important anticoagulation interface with circulating blood. Multiple substances are released to prevent activation of both cellular and humoral components of hemostasis. Understanding hemostasis and coagulation and therapy of coagulopathy and perioperative

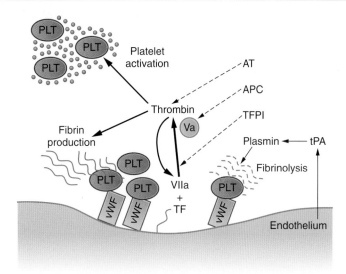

Figure 35-1 Schematic summary of procoagulant and anticoagulant processes. Initial plug formation begins with von Willebrand factor (vWF) binding to collagen at the site of injury, which acts as a bridge for platelets to adhere. At the same time, exposed tissue factor (TF) at the site of injury binds with small amounts of circulating activated factor VII (VIIa) to produce thrombin via the tissue factor (extrinsic) pathway. Thrombin activates a positive feedback loop by producing more of itself, cleaves fibrinogen to insoluble fibrin, and activates platelets that release more procoagulant and inflammatory factors. The process is kept in check by anticoagulant forces. Away from the site of injury, antithrombin (AT) inhibits thrombin. Additionally, activated protein C (APC) destroys factor V (Va—needed for the tissue factor pathway), and tissue factor pathway inhibitor (TFPI) destroys TF-FVIIa complexes. The endothelium releases tissue plasminogen activator (tPA) that cleaves plasminogen into plasmin to initiate fibrinolysis.

bleeding in the current era requires knowledge of the multiple interactions that occur between molecular and cellular components of the coagulation cascade.

Hemostasis protects the individual from massive bleeding secondary to minor trauma. In pathologic states, life-threatening bleeding can occur or thrombosis can occlude the vascular tree. Hemostasis is regulated by a number of factors, including (1) vascular extracellular matrix and alterations in endothelial reactivity, (2) platelets, (3) coagulation proteins, (4) inhibitors of coagulation, and (5) fibrinolysis. These involve tissue factor release, generation of factor VIIa, platelet activation, and multiple cellular and humoral amplification pathways.[2,4,6] Prostacyclin (PGI₂), tissue plasminogen activator (tPA), heparan sulfate, antithrombin III, protein C, and endothelium-derived relaxing factor (EDRF) are normally expressed or secreted to inhibit platelet activation, fibrin formation, and to provide vascular patency. However, if a blood vessel is cut or damaged, tissue factor and other promoters of coagulation are released or exposed to provide a thrombotic surface. Exposure of subendothelial vascular basement membrane activates platelets, and expression of tissue factor also activates thrombin generation and signals other inflammatory pathways.[4]

Platelet activation is an important mechanism for initiation of the coagulation cascade. Receptors on platelets bind to the damaged blood vessel by forming a bridge with von Willebrand factor (vWF) to initiate platelet adhesion. Once platelets adhere, they undergo surface receptor changes that cause platelets to aggregate. Once platelets aggregate, they expose factors on their surface that provide a substrate for activation of the coagulation cascade and formation of the early hemostatic plug. Platelets play vital roles in maintaining vascular hemostasis. Any abnormality in platelet number or function poses significant risk for perioperative coagulopathy.

HYPERCOAGULABILITY

Normal hemostasis is a balance between procoagulant and anticoagulant mechanisms. The coagulation system ensures that bleeding does not continue indefinitely following vascular injury, but is balanced by thromboresistant forces involving anticoagulant proteins to control clot formation and fibrinolytic proteins to remove clot once vascular injury has been repaired. A proper balance between these systems must be maintained to ensure the fluid nature of blood, yet be readily activated when pathologic activation occurs.[7] Thus fluidity of the blood is maintained by counterbalances within the coagulation and fibrinolytic systems.

In surgical patients, especially postoperatively, there is potential for a hypercoagulable state. Hypercoagulability, also known as *thrombophilia* or a *prothrombotic state*, is a condition in which blood clots more readily than normal. It results from a shift of the normal equilibrium of procoagulant and anticoagulant forces in favor of coagulation.[7,8] Although arterial and venous thrombi were once thought to represent distinct problems, patients with hypercoagulability can be at risk for both, and it has been suggested that hypercoagulability represents a spectrum of disease rather than separate clinical entities.[9-11] In the perioperative environment, clinicians are usually aware and concerned about the risk of bleeding; however, hypercoagulability is also a potential cause of postoperative adverse outcomes that is often overlooked.[7,12,13]

Risk factors for hypercoagulability can be inherited or acquired, and are caused by either increasing procoagulant activity and/or decreasing anticoagulant or fibrinolytic ativity.[7,14] About 80% of patients with venous thromboembolism (VTE) have an underlying risk factor.[15] Because of this increased risk, hypercoagulable patients often receive prophylactic anticoagulation therapy.[16,17]

Inherited Risk Factors

Most patients with inherited risk factors for hypercoagulability are at risk to develop venous thromboembolic events early in life.[18] One of the most common risk factors is inherited antithrombin deficiency.[7] Other conditions, for example the prothrombin G20210A mutation, are continually being discovered.[2,8,19] Inherited risk factors can enhance procoagulant effects, reduce natural anticoagulation, impair fibrinolysis, or have other potential effects.[7] Figure 35-2 presents an overview of the interaction of coagulation and fibrinolytic pathways, and illustrates how different inherited risk factors modify hemostasis.

Increased Procoagulant Effects

The most common inherited risk factors for VTE are factor V Leiden, present in approximately 5% of the population, and the prothrombin G20210A mutation, present in approximately 2% of Caucasians.[20,21] In the factor V Leiden gene mutation, an amino acid replacement modifies activated

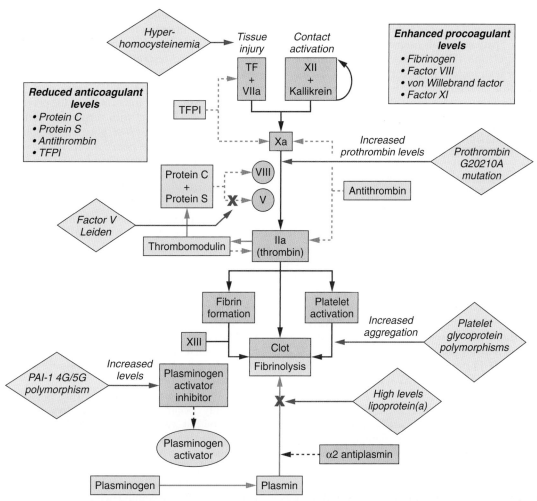

Figure 35-2 Inherited risk factors for hypercoagulability. Procoagulant forces *(red)* and natural anticoagulant/fibrinolytic forces *(green)* are shown. *Dashed lines* indicated an inhibitory effect. Inherited risk factors are presented in diamond shapes with lettering and arrows indicating the mechanism for the hypercoagulable effect. "X" denotes a specific block in a pathway. See text for full details. *PAI,* Plasminogen activator inhibitor; *TF,* tissue factor; *TFPI,* tissue factor pathway inhibitor. *(Modified with permission from Sniecinski RM, Hursting MJ, Paidas MJ, et al. Etiology and assessment of hypercoagulability with lessons from heparin-induced thrombocytopenia. Anesth Analg. 2010;112:46-58.)*

procoagulant factor V so that it is no longer inactivated or inhibited by activated protein C. In patients with factor V Leiden, thrombotic risk is increased approximately threefold in heterozygotes, 18-fold in homozygotes, and ninefold overall compared to individuals without the mutation.[7] Patients heterozygous for the prothrombin G20210A mutation have higher plasma levels of prothrombin, the precursor for thrombin, and approximately threefold greater risk for VTE; homozygous individuals for the G20210A mutation are rare.[7,22,23] Whether factor V Leiden and prothrombin G20210A carriers have increased risk for arterial thrombosis is less clear.[24]

Other common procoagulant effects include fibrinogen abnormalities caused by increased levels or structural variants that are either more or less susceptible to clot formation, known as *dysfibrinogenemia*. Fibrinogen is an increasingly important target for therapeutic interventions in bleeding and coagulopathy. Likewise, patients with the highest plasma fibrinogen concentration have approximately twofold increased risk for arterial thrombosis, and stroke patients with fibrinogen levels of 450 mg/dL or greater have poorer functional outcomes.[25,26] Hyperfibrinogenemia also increases the

risk for VTE.[27,28] Dysfibrinogenemias can also cause hypercoagulability if the resulting fibrin molecules fail to inhibit thrombin or are less susceptible to cleavage by plasmin.[29,30] Elevated coagulation factor levels, including vWF and factor VIII, can occur in patients with unexplained VTE, and increased factor VIII levels are a risk factor for arterial vascular events.[31-33]

Reduction of Natural Anticoagulant Factors

Two important circulating anticoagulants are protein C and protein S. These are vitamin K–dependent proteins that inhibit the activated procoagulant factors V and VIII.[7] Inherited qualitative or quantitative deficiencies of protein C and protein S increase the risk for VTE by 5- to 10-fold.[34] Antithrombin (antithrombin III) is a serine protease inhibitor that avidly binds to thrombin; this interaction is facilitated by heparin and is the mechanism for its anticoagulant action. Heparin and related glycosaminoglycans are normally present on endothelial surfaces or administered therapeutically. Heterozygous antithrombin deficiency is associated with approximately 50% of normal levels. Acquired anti-thrombin deficiency can also occur following heparin administration or in patients with sepsis or disseminated intravascular coagulation (DIC).[35] Patients with antithrombin deficiency are at an increased risk for thrombotic events.[36] Homozygous antithrombin deficiency is likely always fatal in the newborn or in utero, and is exceedingly rare.[37]

Fibrinolysis Modulation

Lipoprotein(a) is a plasma lipoprotein that has structural similarities to plasminogen and inhibits fibrinolysis. Levels are influenced by genetic factors, and increased levels are associated with VTE and cardiovascular disease.[7] Other important serine protease inhibitors that regulate fibrinolysis include plasminogen activator inhibitor-1 (PAI-1). A specific polymorphism (4G/5G) correlates with higher plasma levels.[38] The 4G allele is associated with an increased risk of VTE but only when combined with another genetic risk factor for thromboembolic complications.[39] Abnormalities in tPA, another important regulator of fibrinolysis, are associated with a twofold to threefold increased risk of myocardial infarction and thrombotic stroke.[7] Inherited deficiencies of plasminogen and polymorphisms affecting plasma levels of thrombin-activatable fibrinolysis inhibitor are reported, but their associations with thrombotic risk remain unclear.[7]

Other Inherited Conditions

Increased levels of homocysteine are thought to produce endothelial dysfunction, and could have variable effects on arterial or venous thrombosis and potentially other vascular ischemic events.[7] Hyperhomocystinemia can also be acquired in individuals with folic acid deficiency, and folate therapy was once thought to reduce ischemic cardiovascular disease. Other important polymorphisms exist for regulatory glycoproteins on platelets. Lack of the Ib/IX or vWF receptor results in Bernard Soulier disease. Common deficiencies include abnormalities of the IIb/IIIa receptor that binds fibrinogen and allows platelet cross linking, known as Glanzmann's thrombasthenia. Patients with these platelet glycoprotein genetic variants can still have ischemic cardiovascular disease despite their relative platelet dysfunction, although some reports suggest reduced cardiovascular risk.[12,40]

Acquired Risk Factors

Acquired risk factors are usually transient, yet can confer higher thrombotic risk than genetic disorders. Like inherited factors, some acquired conditions enhance procoagulant effects (e.g., heparin-induced thrombocytopenia) while others decrease levels of natural anticoagulants (e.g., antiphospholipid antibodies). However, most acquired risk factors are multifactorial and have mechanisms that remain to be fully characterized. We have grouped the acquired risk factors into three broad categories: disease states, patient related, and pharmacologic causes (Figure 35-3).

DISEASE STATES ASSOCIATED WITH HYPERCOAGULABILITY

Antiphospholipid antibodies, including lupus anticoagulants, anticardiolipin antibody, and anti-β2-glycoprotein-1 antibody are associated with increased risk of thrombosis.[7] Patients with lupus anticoagulants are actually hypercoagulable despite increased prothrombin times, and have increased risk for both arterial and venous thrombosis, and miscarriage.[7] Multiple mechanisms are responsible for increased thrombotic risk with antiphospholipid antibodies and are thought to be due to decreased thrombomodulin expression, increased tissue factor expression, and impairment of the protein C anticoagulant pathway.[41] Patients with thrombosis (arterial or venous) or repeated pregnancy loss plus antiphospholipid antibody detected on at least two occasions at least 12 weeks apart meet diagnostic criteria for antiphospholipid syndrome.[42] Patients with known antiphospholipid antibodies are at risk for recurrent thrombotic events and require ongoing anticoagulation, usually with warfarin.[7]

Other important factors that contribute to hypercoagulability include renal and hepatic dysfunction, although these are commonly considered risks for bleeding. Severe hepatic dysfunction and cirrhosis lead to decreased synthetic capabilities and decreased levels of anticoagulant factors including antithrombin, protein C, protein S, and plasminogen.[7] Endothelial dysfunction, especially with renal failure, and often pulmonary and portal vascular dysfunction also occur. This in turn increases platelet activation and is an important cause of hypercoagulability.[7] In nephrotic syndrome, fibrinogen levels are increased and antithrombin levels are low, increasing the potential for thrombosis.[7]

Another important clinical setting is blood stasis, which commonly occurs with postoperative immobility or low cardiac output associated with heart failure—important risk factors for hypercoagulability. While a low-flow state is a component of Virchow's triad, it alone does not create thrombosis. The importance of Virchow's other two factors, vessel wall abnormalities and dysfunctional blood constituents, are now becoming clear at the molecular level.[7] Metabolic syndrome characterized by abdominal obesity, hypertension, elevated glucose, and increased cholesterol levels is associated with endothelial dysfunction and increased platelet aggregation.[43] Cancer can have multiple causes for hypercoagulability, including cells that release microparticles to promote fibrin deposition.[44] Advanced age is associated with procoagulant changes including vascular dysfunction, increased fibrinogen levels, increased factor VII, impaired fibrinolytic activity, and increased platelet aggregation.[7] Many of these factors can be additive with complex interactions that are not well understood. Routine VTE prophylaxis is therefore an important part of perioperative management.

HEPARIN-INDUCED THROMBOCYTOPENIA

Heparin-induced thrombocytopenia (HIT) is an important antibody-mediated prothrombotic complication of heparin therapy that occurs in 0.5% to 5% of patients treated with heparin for at least 5 days.[17,45] HIT is characterized by an otherwise unexplained drop in platelet count by 50% or more, often to less than 150,000/μL and frequently accompanied by thrombosis, plus the presence of HIT antibodies.[45] When HIT is suspected, treatment should be initiated even before laboratory confirmation.[17,45]

Pathogenesis and Frequency

HIT is mediated by antibodies to a complex of heparin and platelet factor 4 (PF4). Antibodies recognize antigenic sites

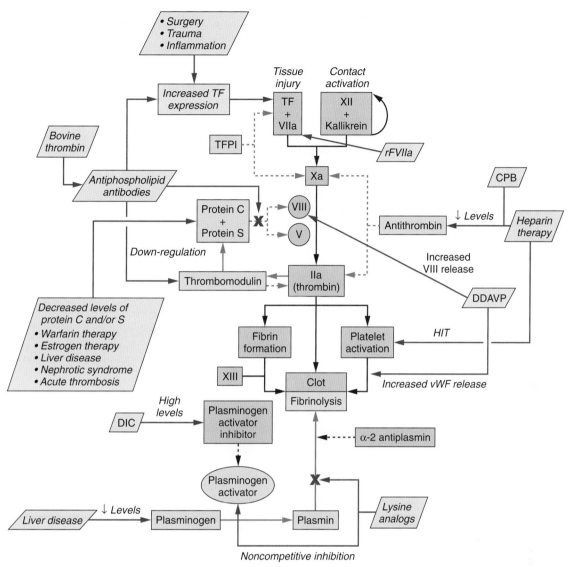

Figure 35-3 Acquired risk factors for hypercoagulability. Procoagulant forces *(red)* and natural anticoagulant/fibrinolytic forces *(green)* are diagrammed. Dashed lines indicate an inhibitory effect. Acquired risk factors are presented in diamond shapes with lettering and arrows indicating the mechanism for the hypercoagulable effect. "X" denotes a specific block in a pathway. Note that some acquired risk factors have multiple effects; see text for full details. *CPB,* Cardiopulmonary bypass; *DDAVP,* desmopressin; *DIC,* disseminated intravascular coagulation; *TF,* tissue factor; *TFPI,* tissue factor pathway inhibitor. *(Modified with permission from Sniecinski RM, Hursting MJ, Paidas MJ, et al. Etiology and assessment of hypercoagulability with lessons from heparin-induced thrombocytopenia.* Anesth Analg. *2010;112:46-58.)*

newly exposed on PF4 when it is conformationally modified by binding to heparin. Platelets are activated by the Fc domain of the IgG in the heparin-PF4 immune complexes, and release microparticles that promote thrombin formation and thrombosis. Thrombocytopenia, excessive thrombin generation, and a prothrombotic state ensue. Antibody-mediated endothelial injury and tissue factor production further increase the prothrombotic state.[45]

Up to 7% to 50% of heparin-treated patients generate heparin-PF4 antibodies, especially following cardiovascular surgery. HIT antibodies circulate with a median half-life of approximately 90 days. The presence and level of HIT antibodies, regardless of thrombocytopenia, are associated with increased morbidity or mortality in various clinical settings. Clinical HIT occurs in 1% to 5% of patients administered unfractionated heparin and less than 1% of

patients administered low molecular weight heparin. Cardiac transplant and neurosurgery patients (11% and 15%, respectively), as well as orthopedic patients, are at increased risk of HIT.[45]

HIT increases the risk of thrombosis including deep VTE, pulmonary embolism, myocardial infarction, stroke, and limb artery occlusion requiring amputation. The overall risk for thrombosis in patients with HIT is 38% to 76%. Other risk factors for HIT-related thrombosis include female gender, malignancy, higher titer heparin-PF4 antibodies, and more severe thrombocytopenia. Other complications include skin lesions at heparin injection sites, DIC, warfarin-associated venous limb ischemia, and acute systemic reactions following heparin bolus. Although counterintuitive, bleeding is rare even in the presence of severe thrombocytopenia.[45]

Diagnosis

HIT should be suspected whenever the platelet count drops by 50%, or new thrombosis occurs in a patient 5 to 14 days after the start of heparin therapy. Other causes of thrombocytopenia (e.g., sepsis, mechanical destruction with an intraaortic balloon pump, or another drug-induced thrombocytopenia) should be excluded. In "rapid onset" HIT, the platelet count begins to drop minutes to hours after heparin exposure, usually due to heparin-PF4 antibodies from a previous heparin exposure, within the prior 3 months. HIT should also be suspected if acute systemic reactions, such as hypotension, pulmonary hypertension, and/or tachycardia, occur 2 to 30 minutes after intravenous heparin bolus. This can be observed intraoperatively and can present as anaphylaxis, usually accompanied by acute thrombocytopenia.[17,45,46] HIT can also occur days to weeks after stopping heparin ("delayed onset HIT"), and should be considered if a recently hospitalized, heparin-treated patient presents with thrombosis.[45]

For suspected HIT, laboratory testing for heparin-PF4 antibody is recommended. Because of the high thrombotic risk early in HIT, treatment should not be withheld while awaiting laboratory results.[45]

Treatment

The recommended treatment for strongly suspected or confirmed HIT, with or without complicating thrombosis, is stopping heparin and initiating a nonheparin alternative anticoagulant such as a direct thrombin inhibitor (e.g., lepirudin, argatroban, desirudin, or bivalirudin). Other heparin sources such as catheter flushes and heparin-coated devices should be eliminated; a sign on the patient's bed and/or chart stating "No heparin: HIT" helps prevent inadvertent heparin exposure. Different direct thrombin inhibitors are approved in the United States for use in HIT patients without initial thrombosis (argatroban), in HIT patients with thrombosis (lepirudin, argatroban), and in patients with or at risk of HIT undergoing percutaneous coronary intervention (PCI) (argatroban, bivalirudin). Desirudin is another agent available for thromboembolism prophylaxis. Recent evidence-based guidelines from the American College of Chest Physicians (ACCP) for the use of these alternative anticoagulants in patients with HIT in noninterventional and interventional settings have been reported.[17] Alternative nonheparin anticoagulant strategies are required in HIT patients who need intraoperative anticoagulation. If heparin use is unavoidable or planned, the heparin exposure should be limited to the surgery itself, with alternative anticoagulation used preoperatively and postoperatively. If cardiac surgery is required, prospective studies have evaluated bivalirudin as the most investigated and useful alternative.[17]

HYPOCOAGULABILITY: PERIOPERATIVE BLEEDING

Bleeding in surgical patients is a common and multifactorial problem. Surgery-induced tissue injury with both large vessel bleeding and microvascular bleeding can occur. Patients often have acquired defects that can be complicated by the surgical insult, or coagulation abnormalities that occur due to antiplatelet or anticoagulant drug use or massive blood loss. Major coagulation abnormalities occur perioperatively and are influenced by multiple factors including type of surgery,

Table 35-1. Coagulopathic States Associated with Increased Risk for Bleeding

Hemophilia
Inherited platelet disorders
von Willebrand disease
Liver failure
Renal failure (uremia)
Disseminated intravascular coagulation
Dilutional coagulopathy
Anticoagulant and antiplatelet therapy
Other coagulation disorders (factor deficiencies)

Table 35-2. Risk Factors for Bleeding in Surgical Patients

Advanced age
Small body size or preoperative anemia (low red cell volume)
Antiplatelet or antithrombotic drugs
Preexisting coagulopathy
Prolonged operation including prolonged cardiopulmonary bypass time
Emergency operation
Comorbidities: heart failure, chronic obstructive pulmonary disease, hypertension, peripheral vascular disease, renal failure, liver failure

cardiopulmonary bypass, and preexisting abnormalities. Coagulopathic states and risk factors predisposing to surgical bleeding are listed in Tables 35-1 and 35-2.

Patients with atherosclerotic cardiovascular disease often receive anticoagulation and/or antiplatelet therapies that interfere with hemostasis (see Chapter 37).[47-51] Patients can also receive prophylactic anticoagulation therapy for atrial fibrillation, VTE prophylaxis, or prosthetic valves. Surgical patients have acquired changes in hemostasis that contribute to postoperative bleeding, including activation of coagulation, fibrinolytic, and inflammatory pathways.[47,48,52,53] Trauma and obstetric patients can also develop massive hemorrhage.[4,54,55] Therapies that prevent clot from forming in pathologic states also interfere with normal hemostasis, an important mechanism protecting patients from exsanguination during surgery.

Risk Factors for Bleeding

Perioperative bleeding with increased transfusion requirements is caused by patient-related, procedure-related, and process-related factors.[56] Most studies do not distinguish between red blood cell (RBC) and hemostatic factor transfusion. Important indicators of high-risk for bleeding and transfusion requirements include (1) advanced age, (2) low preoperative RBC volume (preoperative anemia or small body size), (3) preoperative antiplatelet or antithrombotic treatment, (4) reoperation or complex procedures, (5) emergency operations, and (6) noncardiac patient comorbidities (see Table 35-2).[56]

PATIENT-RELATED CAUSES OF BLEEDING

Risk for bleeding is increased by acquired or congenital coagulopathies including hemophilia, complex procedures (e.g., multilevel spine surgery, combined valve/coronary revascularization, aortic dissection, and major aortic surgery), repeat cardiac and orthopedic procedures, and sepsis with thrombocytopenia. Certain patients have an accentuated response to antiplatelet drugs. Thrombocytopenia from whatever cause (defined as platelet count <50,000/µL) leads to a high risk of excessive bleeding; however, this also depends on platelet function, which is variable and difficult to measure. Anemia also contributes to bleeding in complex ways. Congenital or acquired qualitative platelet defects increase bleeding risk (see earlier).

COMMON INHERITED HEMOSTATIC DISORDERS

There are multiple disorders of hemostasis not involving platelets that are classified by whether they increase or decrease coagulation. Procoagulant disorders (see earlier) are complex, in that some disorders may have both hemorrhagic and thrombotic manifestations. Other disorders also produce bleeding disorders (see Table 35-1). Hemophilia and von Willebrand disease (vWD) are the most common.

Hemophilia A is X-linked coagulopathy due to factor VIII deficiency. It represents the most common form of hemophilia, present in about 1 in 5000 to 10,000 men; hemophilia B, a factor IX deficiency, occurs in approximately 20,000 to 34,000 men. Hemophilia is a recessive, sex-linked X chromosome disorder that occurs more commonly in men than women because men have a single X chromosome. There has been significant progress in hemostatic therapy with the development of highly purified, virally inactive plasma-derived and recombinant factor VIII (FVIII) and factor IX (FIX). These products have also facilitated perioperative management of these patients when they require surgery. Patients with hemophilia who are treated with factors can develop antibody inhibitors, and the advent of factor concentrates and the activated factors (e.g., recombinant factor VIIa) has greatly facilitated management. The perioperative management of these patients requires involvement of a hematologist familiar with the specific guidelines established for these patients. Guidelines for the management of hemophilia are available at www.wfh.org.

vWD and its acquired form is a rare bleeding disorder that can lead to unforeseen bleeding in surgical patients.[57] It is classified as (1) partial quantitative deficiency (type I), (2) qualitative deficiency (type II), or (3) total deficiency (type III). Qualitative vWD type II is further divided into four variants based on the characteristics of the involved von Willebrand protein factor (vWF). Each form of vWD corresponds to specific mechanisms, with corresponding clinical features and therapeutic requirements. Type I can be responsive to desmopressin therapy, while qualitative and quantitative deficiencies might require replacement therapy. vWF is a glycoprotein that allows platelet adhesion to subendothelial collagen and platelet aggregation under high shear stress associated with arterial flow. It acts as a carrier for coagulation factor VIII (FVIII) in the plasma.[57]

There is also an acquired form of vWD that can present due to reduced synthesis, increased removal, or generation of subunits/multimers with reduced activity. With inherited vWD, patients have a lifelong history of bleeding episodes, while the acquired form can present with acute or refractory bleeding episodes perioperatively. Patients with aortic stenosis and ventricular assist devices often develop acquired forms

of vWD. Typically, no family history of bleeding is noted, however, acquired vWD presents as the hereditary form with mucocutaneous and increased perioperative bleeding.[58]

Laboratory evaluation of vWD is based on measurement of vWF activity and antigens as well as multimeric analysis of vWF. Treatment options include desmopressin, factor VIII/vWF concentrates, high-dose intravenous immunoglobulin, cryoprecipitate, and plasma exchange. Because the half-life of vWF is reduced in acquired forms, high doses of factor VIII/vWF concentrate administered at frequent intervals can be necessary during bleeding episodes. In cases unresponsiveness to standard therapy, recombinant activated factor VIIa (rFVIIa) might be an alternative option. The most effective therapy is treating the underlying disease.[58]

PHYSICIAN-RELATED FACTORS

Surgical technique is an important factor influencing perioperative bleeding and blood transfusion.[59] Multiple factors influence perioperative bleeding risk, including differences in surgical technique and operating time. Differences in threshold for transfusion therapy and surgical reexploration of excessive postoperative hemorrhage also contribute to variability in transfusion practices. Transfusion algorithms and practices vary regionally and between centers.[56,60,61]

PROCEDURE-RELATED FACTORS

Procedure-related factors increase risk for both bleeding and perioperative morbidity and mortality. Repeat procedures have higher transfusion rates, and the type and urgency of operation are independent predictors for transfusion. Cardiopulmonary bypass impairs platelet function and coagulation. Complex, long procedures including aortic surgery, major oncologic surgery, bilateral internal mammary artery grafts, aortic valve replacement with pulmonary autograft (Ross procedure), ventricular assist devices, and artificial hearts are examples of complex surgeries associated with high risk of bleeding.[56] Although off-pump cardiac surgery can be associated with an overall reduction in transfusion requirements, with extensive surgery, blood loss, and hemodilution, these patients are also at risk for bleeding.[62,63] Repeat procedures and long operating times due to surgical complexity increase the risk of bleeding from multiple causes, including hypothermia.

PHARMACOLOGIC FACTORS

Preoperative prophylactic antiplatelet and anticoagulant treatment is associated with increased perioperative bleeding and transfusion. Preoperative antiplatelet regimens must be managed for maximum cardioprotective benefit, while minimizing risk of hemorrhage.[56,64] Clopidogrel and aspirin therapy result in higher postoperative bleeding, more transfused blood products, and higher rate of reexploration for mediastinal hemorrhage during emergency coronary artery bypass grafting.[65-67] Current guidelines recommend stopping adenosine diphosphate (ADP) receptor-inhibitors (i.e., clopidogrel and prasugrel) 5 to 7 days before cardiac operations if possible. Patients undergoing operations less than 5 days after discontinuation of ADP inhibitors risk increased bleeding and transfusions and possibly worse long-term outcomes.[64,68] Newer anticoagulation agents, including dabigatran, rivaroxaban, and apixaban should be stopped, as recommended by prescribing information.[69]

Disorders of Hemostasis: Disseminated Intravascular Coagulation

DIC occurs following pathologic inflammatory states such as sepsis or tissue injury.[35,70] Excessive activation known as DIC occurs when normal anticoagulation mechanisms both in plasma and on vascular endothelium are incapable of modulating or inhibiting the excessive thrombin formation. The pathologic hallmark of DIC is microvascular fibrin deposition and thrombotic microangiopathy. Platelet activation and sequestration, and a consumptive coagulopathy deplete platelets and hemostatic factors. Patients with DIC have a complex coagulopathic state characterized by thrombocytopenia, consumptive coagulopathy, and hypofibrinogenemia.

THROMBOCYTOPENIA

Thrombocytopenia is a diagnostic feature of DIC. Platelet counts of less than 100,000/μL occur in 50% to 60% of patients, and of less than 50,000/μL in 10% to 15% of patients. However, there are multiple perioperative causes of thrombocytopenia. Dilutional thrombocytopenia is common following resuscitation of major bleeding following trauma and surgery. Intracranial bleeding in DIC occurs in only 0.3% to 0.5% of patients. Thrombocytopenia is also an independent predictor of intensive care unit (ICU) mortality (relative risk 1.9-4.2).[70] Thrombocytopenia lasting more than 4 days in the ICU or a 50% reduction of platelet counts during ICU stay is associated with a fourfold to sixfold increase in mortality. HIT can also contribute.

COAGULOPATHY

Reduction in coagulation factor is another hallmark of DIC. Impaired synthesis due to hepatic dysfunction or vitamin K deficiency, and consumption of coagulation proteins with bleeding can also contribute to DIC. Coagulation factor levels correlate with DIC severity. This manifests by prolonged prothrombin time (PT) or activated partial thromboplastin time (aPTT). Increased PT or aPTT occurs in 14% to 28% of ICU patients, but is part of the diagnostic criteria in DIC. Factor VIII levels can be increased in patients with DIC. In DIC and similar syndromes, insufficiency of the von Willebrand cleaving protease ADAMTS-13 can occur. This enzyme normally cleaves the prothrombotic ultralarge von Willebrand multimers in plasma that facilitate platelet–vessel wall interactions and contribute to development of thrombotic microangiopathy and organ dysfunction.[35]

FIBRINOGEN CONSUMPTION

Fibrinogen levels have been suggested for the diagnosis of DIC. However, fibrinogen is an acute phase reactant, and levels can vary depending on the starting level. Despite consumption, plasma levels can remain normal, in part depending on the starting level that often is not available. Low fibrinogen levels indicate severe DIC.[35] Following plasmin-mediated lysis of the cross-linked γ-chain of fibrinogen, a fragment called D-dimer is liberated, the measurement of which reflects degradation of cross-linked fibrin. D-dimer levels are increased in DIC, but also following VTE, recent trauma or surgery, and commonly in ICU patients. Other assays for fibrin degradation products have also been used in evaluating DIC. D-dimer levels are also influenced by hepatic and renal function.[35]

REDUCTIONS IN COAGULATION INHIBITORS

Plasma levels of antithrombin, protein C, and other circulating coagulation inhibitors can be useful in evaluating DIC. These are commonly abnormal following cardiac surgery, in critically ill patients, and in 90% of patients with DIC. Antithrombin might be an important predictor for outcomes in sepsis and DIC. Protein C levels can also decrease in DIC, and is a therapeutic target with activated protein C (Xigris), an agent withdrawn from the market due to lack of efficacy. Protein C is activated by thrombin. The endothelial protein thrombomodulin binds to thrombin to modulate its effect, but also activates protein C. Protein C has pleiotropic effects, but inhibits factors V and VIII and functions as an anticoagulant. Thrombomodulin also activates thrombin activatable fibrinolysis inhibitor. In sepsis and DIC, the protein C system is defective due to multiple causes and represents a therapeutic target.[35] Tissue factor pathway inhibitor (TFPI), another serine protease inhibitor, inhibits TF–factor VIIa complex and factor Xa, a key initiator of hemostasis. TFPI is reduced in DIC, and TFPI has been studied as a therapeutic target in sepsis.[35]

FIBRINOLYSIS INDICATORS

Release of tPA and urokinase-type plasminogen activator occurs in DIC. These plasminogen activators generate plasmin, which is balanced by increases in plasminogen activator inhibitor (PAI-1). In DIC increased D-dimer levels occur as a manifestation of increased fibrinolytic activity. However, fibrinolysis is unable to counteract the concomitant coagulation activation. Fibrin degradation products including D-dimers suggest both clot formation and fibrinolytic activity. Other methods to monitor fibrinolytic activity include measuring plasminogen and α_2-antiplasmin levels. However, in DIC these proteins can also be consumed. Plasmin generation can be determined in part by measuring plasmin–α_2-antiplasmin (PAP) complexes that can be increased in DIC.[35]

HEMOSTATIC TESTING

Hemostatic testing is often used preoperatively to identify patients at risk for bleeding and to better define the specific defect producing bleeding. Platelet dysfunction due to dilutional coagulopathy is a major cause of bleeding following massive transfusion, following cardiac surgery, or due to concurrent use of antiplatelet agents. Hemostatic testing facilitates a rational approach to pharmacologic and transfusion-based therapy. However, most platelet function tests available for point-of-care (POC) testing or as laboratory-based testing have not been suitably validated in surgical patients and non-POC testing is not readily available. Dilutional thrombocytopenia can also affect test results. Better tests of platelet dysfunction are needed to allow more accurate diagnosis of the underlying disorder, particularly in high risk surgical patients.

Standard hemostatic testing is routinely used in surgical patients to evaluate hemostasis (PT, aPTT, platelet count, fibrinogen level, and platelet function testing). Despite the lack of studies supporting the absolute utility of hemostatic function tests in the perioperative management of surgical patients, multiple studies have shown that using algorithms based on POC coagulation tests can reduce bleeding and

Table 35-3. Perioperative Coagulation Tests for Surgical Patients: Prothrombin Time

Typical normal range is 11-13 seconds
International normalized ratio (INR) = $(PT_{test}/PT_{normal})^{ISI}$, where ISI is the International Sensitivity Index (a quality control measure for the tissue factor used)
Overview
Assesses the extrinsic and common coagulation pathways
Primarily used to monitor long-term use of anticoagulant therapy through the INR, evaluate liver function, evaluate coagulation disorders
Method
Prothombin time (PT) is the time it takes for clot to form after recalcification and thromboplastin is added to citrated plasma.
Important Notes
The normal range for the laboratory in which PT is tested should be used in the interpretation.

Table 35-4. Perioperative Coagulation Tests for Surgical Patients: Activated Partial Thromboplastin Time

Typical normal range is 25-38 seconds
Overview
Assesses the intrinsic and common coagulation pathways
The best single screening test for coagulation disorders; when properly performed, activated partial thromboplastin time (aPTT) is abnormal in 90% of patients with coagulation disorders.
Used to monitor heparin therapy, screen for hemophilia A and B, detect clotting inhibitors.
Method
aPTT is the time it takes for clot to form after recalcification and addition of phospholipid and an activator of the intrinsic coagulation system to citrated plasma.
Important Notes
The normal range for each laboratory should be used in the interpretation.
Reagents are variably sensitive to the effects of lupus anticoagulant. If sensitive, a false-positive aPTT elevation can result from this cross-reactivity rather than from a bleeding tendency.

Table 35-5. Perioperative Coagulation Tests for Surgical Patients: Fibrinogen

Typical normal range is 2-4 g/L
Overview
Fibrinogen, or factor I, is a glycoprotein synthesized in the liver. It is cleaved by thrombin to produce fibrin monomer, the basis of clot formation.
Decreased levels of fibrinogen can indicate disseminated intravascular coagulation, liver disease, or dilutional coagulopathy.
Method
Fibrinogen can be assessed both quantitatively, using immunologic methods, and qualitatively, with clotting assays similar to one-stage assay methods used for other clotting factors.

Table 35-6. Perioperative Coagulation Tests for Surgical Patients: Platelet Aggregation Studies

Typical normal range is >65% aggregation in response to the platelet activators adenosine diphosphate, epinephrine, collagen, ristocetin, and arachidonic acid.
Overview
Platelet aggregation studies are used to classify qualitative platelet abnormalities.
Abnormalities can be in adhesion, release, or aggregation.
Method
Platelet aggregation is stimulated by introducing activators in vitro.
Aggregation is measured using a turbidimeter and expressed graphically by wave patterns.
Important Notes
Platelet aggregation studies are rarely useful in evaluating acquired bleeding disorders.

transfusion requirements after cardiac surgery. Transfusion algorithms can prevent or reduce the empirical administration of hemostatic factors to guide intraoperative transfusion.[71] A summary of the standard hemostatic tests and their utility is provided in Tables 35-3 through 35-6.

Point-of-Care Coagulation Testing

POC coagulation monitors that evaluate viscoelastic properties of whole blood include thrombelastography (TEG), rotation thromboelastometry (ROTEM), and Sonoclot analysis.[72] These systems measure multiple aspects of the clotting process, including hemostatic factor and platelet interactions, fibrin formation, clot retraction, and fibrinolysis (see Chapter 36). The tests are routinely evaluated in whole blood, allowing potential evaluation of platelet function, although fibrinogen highly influences these tests. This type of hemostatic testing is increasingly used in managing patients following trauma and massive hemorrhage or other major surgery.

When viscoelastic testing is normal, surgical bleeding should be considered; however, these tests can also be used to guide transfusional procoagulant therapies.

Transfusion Algorithms

Most studies demonstrate that transfusion algorithms based on coagulation testing reduce the need for platelets, fresh frozen plasma, or cryoprecipitate. Indeed, any test that prevents empirical administration likely will reduce transfusions. Most transfusion algorithms suggest transfusion when bleeding is accompanied by a PT or aPTT greater than 1.5 times normal value, thrombocytopenia with a platelet count less than 50,000-100,000/μL, or fibrinogen concentration less than 100 mg/dL (or 1 g/L). Because most laboratory testing is slow, POC testing, TEG, ROTEM, or platelet function testing has been the focus of these studies.[73] While thromboelastographic-based algorithms can reduce blood product use, the POC machines are not widely available. Prospective algorithms using platelet function data have also been reported. However, platelet function testing is problematic in that most tests need a relatively higher number of platelets to work and it is unclear whether they are applicable to the platelet dysfunction encountered following cardiopulmonary bypass.

Ideally, surgical patients should receive transfusions based on laboratory-guided algorithms, and the possible benefits of POC testing should be tested against this standard. Battlefield trauma can cause massive bleeding and massive transfusion coagulopathy, defined as 10 or more units of RBC transfusions in a 24-hour period. With life-threatening bleeding, multiple blood volumes might be replaced before hemostatic test results are available. Therefore transfusion protocols often use fixed doses of component therapies that include fresh frozen plasma and platelets following transfusion of a defined number of RBCs, often in an attempt to mimic the transfusion of fresh whole blood.[74] This battlefield transfusion protocol has been demonstrated to improve survival.[75,76] Perioperative blood transfusion and blood conservation guidelines have been defined in certain patient populations and usually include a multimodal approach to blood conservation (see Chapter 36).[56]

BLOOD CONSERVATION

Blood conservation is often discussed in many perioperative settings, but not actively practiced, in part due to the additional work involved. Pharmacologic management of hemostasis in patients undergoing surgery represents an important therapeutic approach in the management of complex surgical patients and for blood conservation. Because surgery represents a major consumer of blood products and because agents can be administered prophylactically, pharmacologic approaches are an important aspect of blood conservation. Unfortunately, many studies have reviewed issues related to RBC use and not hemostatic factor use.

Of the major preoperative patient risk factors for transfusion, low RBC mass due to small body size or from preoperative anemia is important. Additional important considerations for perioperative blood conservation are preoperative treatment of anemia, especially for elective surgery. A low starting RBC volume, calculated by hematocrit multiplied by estimated blood volume, correlates with bleeding and the need for allogeneic RBC transfusion. Blood conservation guidelines should reduce hemodilution and conserve red cells. The judicious use of preoperative erythropoietin and supplemental iron can increase RBC mass, but this requires interventions weeks before surgery. Minimizing extracorporeal circuits with circuits that require reduced priming volumes may be useful in cardiopulmonary bypass. Additional strategies before surgical intervention include normovolemic hemodilution, salvage of RBCs from the operative field, and use of pharmacologic agents that reduce bleeding. In cardiac surgical patients, additional considerations include modified ultrafiltration. Multimodal interventions provide the best opportunity to reduce bleeding and the need for allogenic transfusion.

An important aspect of preoperative risk evaluation is the management of preoperative therapies that interfere with normal hemostasis. Surgical patients are increasingly receiving both antiplatelet agents and anticoagulation for perioperative thromboprophylaxis and as therapy for ischemic cardiovascular disease (see Chapter 37). As a result, patients often present for surgery with an acquired hemostatic imbalance because of preexisting anticoagulation. These agents should be discontinued before surgery, including the thienopyridines, drugs that inhibit P2Y12 receptor binding. For

Table 35-7. Management of Patients with Hemophilia for Elective Surgery

Surgical procedures should be performed in coordination with a team experienced in the management of hemophilia.
Procedures should take place in a center with adequate laboratory support for reliable monitoring of clotting factor levels.
Preoperative assessment should include inhibitor screening.
Surgery should be scheduled early in the week and early in the day for optimal laboratory and blood bank support, if needed.
Availability of sufficient quantities of clotting factor concentrates should be ensured before undertaking major surgery.
The dosage and duration of clotting factor concentrate coverage depends on the type of surgery performed.

Modified from Srivastava A, Brewer AK, Mauser-Bunschoten EP, Key NS, Kitchen S, Llinas A, Ludlam CA, Mahlangu JN, Mulder K, Poon MC, Street A; Treatment Guidelines Working Group The World Federation Of Hemophilia. Haemophilia. 2012 Jul 6. doi: 10.1111/j.1365-2516.2012.02909.x. [Epub ahead of print].

drugs like clopidogrel, there is variability in patient response to their use; however, newer P2Y12 inhibitors such as prasugrel are more potent than clopidogrel and have a much lower incidence of resistance. Specific laboratory assays that include POC testing, such as VerifyNow, might help identify patients who can safely undergo urgent operations.

Managing blood resources with a multidisciplinary team of anesthesiologists, blood bankers, surgeons, and intensivists should be considered when developing blood conservation strategies.[47] Patients with known coagulopathies or hereditary deficiencies should be optimized preoperatively as suggested in Table 35-7. Most studies suggest that developing a transfusion algorithm that all team members agree with, and the use of laboratory and/or POC testing to guide transfusion decisions are important aspects of blood conservation.

MASSIVE TRANSFUSION

Massive transfusion can be defined as the acute replacement of more than one blood volume or more than 10 units of RBCs within several hours. The transfusion of four or more red cell units within 1 hour when ongoing need is foreseeable, or replacing 50% of the total blood volume within 3 hours, might be more appropriate in the acute clinical setting.[77,78] The most common clinical situation leading to massive transfusion is extensive trauma; however, it also occurs in nontrauma settings during surgical procedures causing large blood loss, especially after cardiothoracic surgery. Extensive information has come from experience in the Iraq war. Blood transfusion is the main therapy option for treating acute hemorrhage, and in trauma patients the ideal solution is fresh whole blood. However, this is not widely available. The etiology of coagulopathy during massive transfusion is complex, involving dilution of factors, hypothermia, tissue hypoperfusion/ischemia, acidosis, and potential DIC. Treatment of the coagulopathy includes volume replacement, normothermia, resolution of acid-base abnormalities, and blood component therapy. Because of fibrinolysis, antifibrinolytic drugs should be considered if present. The role of off-label use of recombinant activated factor VII (rFVIIa) to manage bleeding that cannot be controlled by conventional measures is still evolving.

KEY POINTS

- Hemostasis is a complex process that involves interactions between vascular components with blood cellular and plasma components.
- Coagulopathy in surgical patients can result from consumption/loss of coagulation components, drug effects, surgical trauma, and preexisting hemostatic defects.
- The growing use of anticoagulants and antiplatelet agents poses potential problems in the perioperative period.
- Both congenital and acquired forms of hypercoagulability can occur in surgical patients.
- HIT is a hypercoagulable state complicating anticoagulation therapy and is a major risk factor for adverse events.
- Acquired hemostatic disorders due to anticoagulation agents are common perioperative considerations requiring factor therapy.
- Inherited bleeding disorders such as hemophilia and vWD require specific perioperative management.
- DIC is a severe consumptive hemostatic disorder that can occur in diverse settings.
- The etiology of coagulopathy associated with massive transfusion is complex, and involves dilution of factors, hypothermia, tissue hypoperfusion, acidosis, and possible DIC.
- Although transfusion therapies remain important, blood conservation has gained priority to minimize adverse effects.
- Laboratory testing coupled with objective algorithms are important approaches to reduce transfusion of banked blood products.

Key References

Aird WC. Phenotypic heterogeneity of the endothelium: I. Structure, function, and mechanisms. *Circ Res.* 2007;100:158-173. Aird WC. Phenotypic heterogeneity of the endothelium: II. Representative vascular beds. *Circ Res.* 2007;100:174-190. A two-part review of endothelial cells, the vascular tree, properties of endothelium, and hemostatic interactions as described by a hematologist/vascular biologists who have made many contributions to this area. (Refs. 54 and 55)

Hoffman M, Monroe DM 3rd. A cell-based model of hemostasis. *Thromb Haemost.* 2001;85:958-965. An important description of a novel model to describe hemostatic function not using standard intrinsic and extrinsic coagulation pathways, but rather the complex cellular and protein interactions that more likely occur in vivo. (Ref. 1)

Levy JH, Dutton RP, Hemphill JC 3rd, et al. Multidisciplinary approach to the challenge of hemostasis. *Anesth Analg.* 2010;110:354-364. A multidisciplinary review by experts in anesthesiology, blood banking, hematology, critical care, and surgery of hemostasis and management of the bleeding patient across different clinical settings, with a focus on perioperative considerations. This review focuses on advances in hemostasis research and need for a multidisciplinary approach to improve patient care and develop management strategies. (Ref. 47)

Levy JH, Key NS, Azran MS. Novel oral anticoagulants: implications in the perioperative setting. *Anesthesiology.* 2010;113:726-745. With the increasing use of new and older anticoagulation agents, this review describes clinical studies, pharmacokinetics,

and pharmacodynamics of new anticoagulation agents and current management strategies for perioperative consideration of patients receiving them. (Ref. 69)

Sniecinski RM, Hursting MJ, Paidas MJ, et al. Etiology and assessment of hypercoagulability with lessons from heparin-induced thrombocytopenia. *Anesth Analg.* 2010;112:46-58. A recent review of hemostatic interactions based on a multidisciplinary approach. This review describes common hypercoagulability issues and perioperative considerations. (Ref. 7)

Warkentin TE, Greinacher A, Koster A, et al. Treatment and prevention of heparin-induced thrombocytopenia: American College of Chest Physicians evidence-based clinical practice guidelines (8th edition). *Chest.* 2008;133:340S-380S. Management of HIT using evidence-based medicine. (Ref. 17)

References

1. Hoffman M, Monroe DM, 3rd. A cell-based model of hemostasis. *Thromb Haemost.* 2001;85:958-965.
2. Sniecinski RM, Levy JH. Bleeding and management of coagulopathy. *J Thorac Cardiovasc Surg* 2011;142:662-7.
3. Levy JH, Tanaka KA, Steiner ME. Evaluation and management of bleeding during cardiac surgery. *Curr Hematol Rep.* 2005;4:368-372.
4. Tanaka KA, Key NS, Levy JH. Blood coagulation: hemostasis and thrombin regulation. *Anesth Analg.* 2009;108:1433-1446.
5. Shaz BH, Dente CJ, Harris RS, MacLeod JB, Hillyer CD. Transfusion management of trauma patients. *Anesth Analg.* 2009;108:1760-1768.
6. Mackman N. The role of tissue factor and factor VIIa in hemostasis. *Anesth Analg.* 2009;108:1447-1452.
7. Sniecinski RM, Hursting MJ, Paidas MJ, Levy JH. Etiology and assessment of hypercoagulability with lessons from heparin-induced thrombocytopenia. *Anesth Analg.* 2010;112:46-58.
8. Martinelli I, Bucciarelli P, Mannucci PM. Thrombotic risk factors: basic pathophysiology. *Crit Care Med.* 2010;38: S3-S9.
9. Franchini M, Mannucci PM. Venous and arterial thrombosis: different sides of the same coin? *Eur J Intern Med.* 2008;19:476-481.
10. Lowe GD. Common risk factors for both arterial and venous thrombosis. *Br J Haematol.* 2008;140:488-495.
11. Lowe GD. Arterial disease and venous thrombosis: are they related, and if so, what should we do about it? *J Thromb Haemost.* 2006;4:1882-1885.
12. Chan MY, Andreotti F, Becker RC. Hypercoagulable states in cardiovascular disease. *Circulation.* 2008;118:2286-2297.
13. Kfoury E, Taher A, Saghieh S, Otrock ZK, Mahfouz R. The impact of inherited thrombophilia on surgery: a factor to consider before transplantation? *Mol Biol Rep.* 2009;36:1041-1051.
14. Mannucci PM. Laboratory detection of inherited thrombophilia: a historical perspective. *Semin Thromb Hemost.* 2005;31:5-10.
15. Whitlatch NL, Ortel TL. Thrombophilias: when should we test and how does it help? *Semin Respir Crit Care Med.* 2008;29:25-39.
16. Geerts WH, Bergqvist D, Pineo GF, et al. Prevention of venous thromboembolism: American College of Chest Physicians Evidence-Based Clinical Practice Guidelines (8th Edition). *Chest.* 2008;133:381S-453S.
17. Warkentin TE, Greinacher A, Koster A, Lincoff AM. Treatment and prevention of heparin-induced thrombocytopenia: American College of Chest Physicians Evidence-Based Clinical Practice Guidelines (8th Edition). *Chest.* 2008;133:340S-380S.
18. Parker RI. Thrombosis in the pediatric population. *Crit Care Med.* 2010;38: S71-S75.
19. Bezemer ID, Bare LA, Doggen CJ, et al. Gene variants associated with deep vein thrombosis. *J Am Med Assoc.* 2008;299:1306-1314.
20. De Stefano V, Chiusolo P, Paciaroni K, Leone G. Epidemiology of factor V Leiden: clinical implications. *Semin Thromb Hemost.* 1998;24:367-379.
21. Rosendaal FR, Doggen CJ, Zivelin A, et al. Geographic distribution of the 20210 G to A prothrombin variant. *Thromb Haemost.* 1998;79:706-708.
22. Poort SR, Rosendaal FR, Reitsma PH, Bertina RM. A common genetic variation in the 3′-untranslated region of the prothrombin

gene is associated with elevated plasma prothrombin levels and an increase in venous thrombosis. *Blood.* 1996;88:3698-3703.

23. Gohil R, Peck G, Sharma P. The genetics of venous thromboembolism. A meta-analysis involving approximately 120,000 cases and 180,000 controls. *Thromb Haemost.* 2009;102:360-370.

24. Ye Z, Liu EH, Higgins JP, et al. Seven haemostatic gene polymorphisms in coronary disease: meta-analysis of 66,155 cases and 91,307 controls. *Lancet.* 2006;367:651-658.

25. Maresca G, Di Blasio A, Marchioli R, Di Minno G. Measuring plasma fibrinogen to predict stroke and myocardial infarction: an update. *Arterioscler Thromb Vasc Biol.* 1999;19:1368-1377.

26. del Zoppo GJ, Levy DE, Wasiewski WW, et al. Hyperfibrinogenemia and functional outcome from acute ischemic stroke. *Stroke.* 2009;40:1687-1691.

27. van Hylckama Vlieg A, Rosendaal FR. High levels of fibrinogen are associated with the risk of deep venous thrombosis mainly in the elderly. *J Thromb Haemost.* 2003;1:2677-2678.

28. Tsai AW, Cushman M, Rosamond WD, Heckbert SR, Polak JF, Folsom AR. Cardiovascular risk factors and venous thromboembolism incidence: the longitudinal investigation of thromboembolism etiology. *Arch Intern Med.* 2002;162:1182-1189.

29. Martinez J. Congenital dysfibrinogenemia. *Curr Opin Hematol.* 1997;4:357-365.

30. Mosesson MW. Dysfibrinogenemia and thrombosis. *Semin Thromb Hemost.* 1999;25:311-319.

31. O'Donnell J, Tuddenham EG, Manning R, Kemball-Cook G, Johnson D, Laffan M. High prevalence of elevated factor VIII levels in patients referred for thrombophilia screening: role of increased synthesis and relationship to the acute phase reaction. *Thromb Haemost.* 1997;77:825-828.

32. O'Donnell J, Mumford AD, Manning RA, Laffan M. Elevation of FVIII: C in venous thromboembolism is persistent and independent of the acute phase response. *Thromb Haemost.* 2000;83:10-13.

33. Bank I, van de Poel MH, Coppens M, et al. Absolute annual incidences of first events of venous thromboembolism and arterial vascular events in individuals with elevated FVIII:C. A prospective family cohort study. *Thromb Haemost.* 2007;98:1040-1044.

34. Rosendaal FR, Reitsma PH. Genetics of venous thrombosis. *J Thromb Haemost.* 2009;7(Suppl 1):301-304.

35. Levi M, Meijers JC. DIC: which laboratory tests are most useful. *Blood Rev.* 2011;25:33-37.

36. Patnaik MM, Moll S. Inherited antithrombin deficiency: a review. *Haemophilia.* 2008;14:1229-1239.

37. Moll S. Thrombophilias–practical implications and testing caveats. *J Thromb Thrombolysis.* 2006;21:7-15.

38. Tsantes AE, Nikolopoulos GK, Bagos PG, Bonovas S, Kopterides P, Vaiopoulos G. The effect of the plasminogen activator inhibitor-1 4G/5G polymorphism on the thrombotic risk. *Thromb Res.* 2008;122:736-742.

39. van der Bom JG, de Knijff P, Haverkate F, et al. Tissue plasminogen activator and risk of myocardial infarction. The Rotterdam Study. *Circulation.* 1997;95:2623-2627.

40. Franchini M, Veneri D, Salvagno GL, Manzato F, Lippi G. Inherited thrombophilia. *Crit Rev Clin Lab Sci.* 2006;43:249-290.

41. Todorova M, Baleva M. Some recent insights into the prothrombogenic mechanisms of antiphospholipid antibodies. *Curr Med Chem.* 2007;14:811-826.

42. Miyakis S, Lockshin MD, Atsumi T, et al. International consensus statement on an update of the classification criteria for definite antiphospholipid syndrome (APS). *J Thromb Haemost.* 2006;4:295-306.

43. Franchini M, Targher G, Montagnana M, Lippi G. The metabolic syndrome and the risk of arterial and venous thrombosis. *Thromb Res.* 2008;122:727-735.

44. Prandoni P, Falanga A, Piccioli A. Cancer and venous thromboembolism. *Lancet Oncol.* 2005;6:401-410.

45. Levy JH, Tanaka KA, Hursting MJ. Reducing thrombotic complications in the perioperative setting: an update on heparin-induced thrombocytopenia. *Anesth Analg.* 2007;105:570-582.

46. Levy JH, Adkinson NF Jr. Anaphylaxis during cardiac surgery: implications for clinicians. *Anesth Analg.* 2008;106:392-403.

47. Levy JH, Dutton RP, Hemphill JC, 3rd, et al. Multidisciplinary approach to the challenge of hemostasis. *Anesth Analg.* 2010;110:354-364.

48. Levy JH, Dutton RP, Hemphill JC 3rd, et al. Multidisciplinary approach to the challenge of hemostasis. *Anesth Analg* 2010;110:354-64.

49. Steinhubl SR, Schneider DJ, Berger PB, Becker RC. Determining the efficacy of antiplatelet therapies for the individual: lessons from clinical trials. *J Thromb Thrombolysis* 2007;26:8-13.

50. Weitz JI, Hirsh J, Samama MM. New antithrombotic drugs: American College of Chest Physicians Evidence-Based Clinical Practice Guidelines (8th Edition). *Chest.* 2008;133:234S-256S.

51. Mannucci PM, Levi M. Prevention and treatment of major blood loss. *N Engl J Med.* 2007;356:2301-2311.

52. Lawson JH, Murphy MP. Challenges for providing effective hemostasis in surgery and trauma. *Semin Hematol.* 2004;41:55-64.

53. Achneck HE, Sileshi B, Lawson JH. Review of the biology of bleeding and clotting in the surgical patient. *Vascular.* 2008;16(Suppl 1):S6-S13.

54. Aird WC. Phenotypic heterogeneity of the endothelium: II. Representative vascular beds. *Circ Res.* 2007;100:174-190.

55. Aird WC. Phenotypic heterogeneity of the endothelium: I. Structure, function, and mechanisms. *Circ Res.* 2007;100:158-173.

56. Ferraris VA, Ferraris SP, Saha SP, et al. Perioperative blood transfusion and blood conservation in cardiac surgery: the Society of Thoracic Surgeons and the Society of Cardiovascular Anesthesiologists clinical practice guideline. *Ann Thorac Surg.* 2007;83:S27-S86.

57. Mannucci PM. Treatment of von Willebrand's disease. *N Engl J Med.* 2004;351:683-694.

58. Lison S, Dietrich W, Spannagl M. Unexpected bleeding in the operating room: the role of acquired von Willebrand disease. *Anesth Analg* 2012;114:73-81.

59. Ott E, Mazer CD, Tudor IC, et al. Coronary artery bypass graft surgery—care globalization: the impact of national care on fatal and nonfatal outcome. *J Thorac Cardiovasc Surg.* 2007;133:1242-1251.

60. Stover EP, Siegel LC, Parks R, et al. Variability in transfusion practice for coronary artery bypass surgery persists despite national consensus guidelines: a 24-institution study. Institutions of the Multicenter Study of Perioperative Ischemia Research Group. *Anesthesiology.* 1998;88:327-333.

61. Johnson RG, Thurer RL, Kruskall MS, et al. Comparison of two transfusion strategies after elective operations for myocardial revascularization. *J Thorac Cardiovasc Surg.* 1992;104:307-314.

62. Wijeysundera DN, Beattie WS, Djaiani G, et al. Off-pump coronary artery surgery for reducing mortality and morbidity: meta-analysis of randomized and observational studies. *J Am Coll Cardiol.* 2005;46:872-882.

63. Cheng DC, Bainbridge D, Martin JE, Novick RJ. Does off-pump coronary artery bypass reduce mortality, morbidity, and resource utilization when compared with conventional coronary artery bypass? A meta-analysis of randomized trials. *Anesthesiology.* 2005;102:188-203.

64. Hall R, Mazer CD. Antiplatelet drugs: a review of their pharmacology and management in the perioperative period. *Anesth Analg.* 2011;112:292-318.

65. Yende S, Wunderink RG. Effect of clopidogrel on bleeding after coronary artery bypass surgery. *Crit Care Med.* 2001;29:2271-2275.

66. Hongo RH, Ley J, Dick SE, Yee RR. The effect of clopidogrel in combination with aspirin when given before coronary artery bypass grafting. *J Am Coll Cardiol.* 2002;40:231-237.

67. Ray JG, Deniz S, Olivieri A, et al. Increased blood product use among coronary artery bypass patients prescribed preoperative aspirin and clopidogrel. *BMC Cardiovasc Disord.* 2003;3:3.

68. Braunwald E, Antman EM, Beasley JW, et al. ACC/AHA 2002 guideline update for the management of patients with unstable angina and non-ST-segment elevation myocardial infarction—summary article: a report of the American College of Cardiology/American Heart Association task force on practice guidelines (Committee on the Management of Patients With Unstable Angina). *J Am Coll Cardiol.* 2002;40:1366-1374.

69. Levy JH, Key NS, Azran MS. Novel oral anticoagulants: implications in the perioperative setting. *Anesthesiology.* 2010;113:726-745.

70. Levi M, Toh CH, Thachil J, Watson HG. Guidelines for the diagnosis and management of disseminated intravascular coagulation. British Committee for Standards in Haematology. *Br J Haematol.* 2009;145:24-33.

71. Avidan MS, Alcock EL, Da Fonseca J, et al. Comparison of structured use of routine laboratory tests or near-patient assessment with clinical judgement in the management of bleeding after cardiac surgery. *Br J Anaesth*. 2004;92:178-186.

72. Ganter MT, Hofer CK. Coagulation monitoring: current techniques and clinical use of viscoelastic point-of-care coagulation devices. *Anesth Analg*. 2008;106:1366-1375.

73. Steiner ME, Despotis GJ. Transfusion algorithms and how they apply to blood conservation: the high-risk cardiac surgical patient. *Hematol Oncol Clin North Am*. 2007;21:177-184.

74. Stainsby D, MacLennan S, Thomas D, Isaac J, Hamilton PJ. Guidelines on the management of massive blood loss. *Br J Haematol*. 2006;135:634-641.

75. Dente CJ, Shaz BH, Nicholas JM, et al. Improvements in early mortality and coagulopathy are sustained better in patients with blunt trauma after institution of a massive transfusion protocol in a civilian level I trauma center. *J Trauma*. 2009;66:1616-1624.

76. Holcomb JB, Wade CE, Michalek JE, et al. Increased plasma and platelet to red blood cell ratios improves outcome in 466 massively transfused civilian trauma patients. *Ann Surg*. 2008;248:447-458.

77. Hardy JF, de Moerloose P, Samama CM. Massive transfusion and coagulopathy: pathophysiology and implications for clinical management. *Can J Anaesth*. 2006;53: S40-S58.

78. Karkouti K, O'Farrell R, Yau TM, Beattie WS. Prediction of massive blood transfusion in cardiac surgery. *Can J Anaesth*. 2006;53:781-794.

Chapter 36

TRANSFUSION AND COAGULATION THERAPY

Kenichi Tanaka

HISTORICAL CONSIDERATIONS

The observation that blood circulates in a closed vascular system by Harvey in 1628 was pivotal in the practice of blood transfusion.[1] Because blood was recognized as vital to sustaining life, Denis in Paris and Lower in Oxford attempted xeno-transfusion (animal blood to humans) with little success in the 17th century. The first documented transfusion of human blood was made in 1818 by Blundell, an obstetrician in London, who recognized the need for transfusion in women suffering from postpartum hemorrhage. His results were not reproducible due to the lack of knowledge of blood types and anticoagulants.

Major advances were made in the beginning of 20th century when Landsteiner identified blood groups A, B, and C (later renamed group O). Storage and distribution of donated blood became possible after sodium citrate was added as an anticoagulant during World War I. The infrastructure of the modern blood banking system was established by World War II, and use of fresh whole blood transfusion saved many wounded soldiers, although hepatitis transmission was not uncommon. During World War II, Cohn and colleagues developed the cold ethanol method to separate albumin, γ-globulin, and fibrinogen from plasma, which became the basic principle for commercial plasma fractionation.

In the late 1970s and early 1980s, pooling of random donor plasma to manufacture factor (F) VIII concentrates without effective donor screening or virus inactivation steps led to transfusion-related transmission of viruses, particularly human immunodeficiency virus (HIV) and hepatitis C to a large number of hemophiliac patients worldwide. Since the mid-1980s, many precautions for bloodborne pathogens have been implemented, including vapor heat treatment and nanofiltration, and recombinant coagulation factors became available in the 1990s. The risk of infectious transmission also fueled efforts to develop synthetic oxygen carriers.[2,3] Over the years, clinicians have recognized the importance and potential harms of blood component therapies. The rational and cost-effective uses of blood components are now the subject of published transfusion guidelines.[4-7]

HEMOGLOBIN AND PLATELET REPLACEMENT

Packed Red Blood Cells

Circulating red blood cells (RBCs) are anuclear, hemoglobin-carrying cells of about 7 to 8 μm in diameter. The biconcave and discoid shape of RBCs confers advantages in increasing surface area for gas exchange and flexibility in passing through capillaries. On average, RBCs remain in circulation for 120 days. Senescent or abnormal RBCs are eliminated by the spleen. The synthesis of RBCs (erythropoiesis) is regulated by erythropoietin, which is elevated in anemia and hypoxia. Erythropoiesis is also affected by the availability of iron, an integral component of hemoglobin.

Packed RBCs are prepared by separating most plasma components of donated whole blood by centrifugation. One unit of RBCs collected in anticoagulant-preservative solution is about 300 mL with a hematocrit of 50% to 70%. Dextrose is added to maintain glucose metabolism, and adenine and phosphate allow synthesis of adenosine triphosphate. Additive solutions (adenine, glucose, mannitol, sodium chloride) are also used to extend shelf life up to 42 days (Table 36-1).[8] Depending on the storage solution, RBCs have a shelf life of 28 to 42 days at 1°C to 6°C. During storage, intracellular 2,3-DPG is reduced to less than 10% of normal at 5 weeks such that release of oxygen from hemoglobin is significantly impaired (Figure 36-1).

CLINICAL USES

Transfusion of RBCs is indicated to restore the oxygen-carrying capacity in patients with severe anemia or major blood loss. There is no absolute level of hemoglobin that indicates a threshold for transfusion ("transfusion trigger"); underlying clinical conditions and laboratory data for each patient should be considered. Acute anemia is less well tolerated compared to chronic anemia in which peripheral oxygen delivery is compensated by elevated 2,3-DPG levels in RBCs and higher cardiac output (see Figure 36-1). In patients with moderate to severe cardiovascular dysfunction, anemia might not be well tolerated. The extent and duration of clinical bleeding are also important criteria for transfusion in major trauma and surgery. According to the American Society of Anesthesiologists (ASA) guidelines for blood component therapy, transfusion of RBCs is almost always indicated for hemoglobin less than 6 g/dL, whereas it is rarely indicated for hemoglobin greater than 10 g/dL. For hemoglobin between 6 g/dL and 10 g/dL, transfusion should be considered if complications due to inadequate oxygenation are anticipated.[4]

ABO and Rh blood group–specific packed RBCs should be administered whenever possible (Figure 36-2). In case of life-threatening hemorrhage without time for formal cross-matching, either Rh-positive or Rh-negative group O RBCs can be transfused in principle. In Rh-negative women of

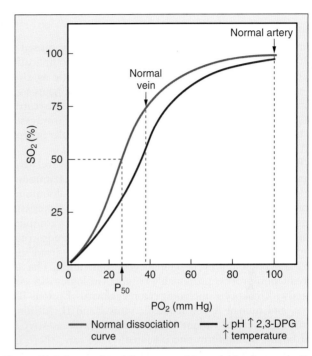

Figure 36-1 Oxygen-dissociation curve of hemoglobin at normal pH is shown in blue. The dissociation of oxygen from hemoglobin can be increased (in *purple*) by acidosis, elevated 2,3-DPG (diphosphoglycerate), or higher temperature. Conversely, the curve can be shifted to left by alkalosis, low 2,3-DPG, or hypothermia. The P_{50}, or partial pressure of oxygen (PO_2) when hemoglobin saturation (SO^2) is 50%, is about 26.6 mmHg.

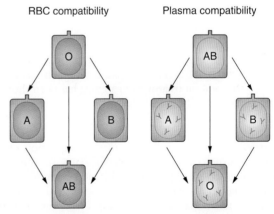

Figure 36-2 ABO compatibility. For RBC transfusion, the recipient can receive the same blood type or blood group(s) specified by the *arrow(s)*. Blood group O recipients can be only transfused with group O blood whereas group AB recipients can be transfused with either O, A, B, or AB group RBCs. Rh-positive or Rh-negative RBCs can be transfused in an Rh-positive recipient, and Rh-negative RBCs should be given to an Rh-negative recipient. For plasma product transfusion, the recipient can receive the same plasma type or plasma group(s) specified by the arrow(s). Blood group AB recipient can be only transfused with group AB plasma whereas type O recipient can be transfused with either O, A, B, or AB group plasma. Rh types are not considered for plasma product transfusion. *Orange symbol,* anti-B antibody; *green symbol,* anti-A antibody.

Table 36-1. Blood Component Volumes and Stability

COMPONENT	VOLUME	SHELF LIFE	STORAGE TEMPERATURE
Red blood cells	220-340 mL	42 days	1°C-6°C
Apheresis platelets	250-300 mL	5 days	20°C-24°C
Random donor platelets	50-70 mL	5 days	20°C-24°C
Plasma*	200-250 mL	1 year	<−18°C
Cryoprecipitate	10-15 mL	1 year	<−18°C

*Plasma frozen within 8 hours is called FFP, and plasma frozen between 8 and 24 hours of collection is called FP24.

childbearing age, Rh-negative group O RBCs should be preferred for reducing the risk of alloantibody (anti-D) development, which can cause anemia in an Rh-positive fetus. Transfusion of mismatched RBCs, typically related to ABO, can induce IgM antibody-mediated acute hemolysis, but in less serious mismatches of minor antigens such as Rh, Kell, and Duffy, survival of transfused RBCs is shortened.

SIDE EFFECTS

Acute hemolytic transfusion reactions are usually caused by ABO incompatibility. This potentially fatal complication occurs in about 1 in 30,000 transfusions. As little as 20 to 30 mL of incompatible RBCs can cause agitation, nausea and vomiting, dyspnea, fever, flushing, hypotension, tachycardia, and hemoglobinuria. Two major complications of intravascular hemolysis include renal failure from acute tubular necrosis and disseminated intravascular coagulation (DIC).

Febrile nonhemolytic transfusion reaction is relatively common (0.1%-1% of RBC transfusions). Other immunologic complications of transfusion include HLA alloimmunization, graft-versus-host disease, and immunosuppression triggered by donor leukocytes.[9] The risk of these complications can be partially reduced by use of leukocyte adsorption (leukoreduction) filters at blood collection, and γ-irradiation after collection to prevent lymphocyte proliferation. The leukoreduction process presumably reduces virologic risks associated with leukocytes including cytomegalovirus, Epstein-Barr virus, and human T-cell leukemia virus I and II. Although transfusion-related variant Creutzfeldt-Jakob diseases (vCJD and bovine spongiform encephalopathy) are rare, there is a theoretical advantage in leukodepletion to prevent prion transmission.[10]

Erythropoietin

Erythropoietin is a hormone produced in the kidney in response to hypoxemia as seen in chronic pulmonary disease and at high altitudes. The primary indication for recombinant erythropoietin is anemia associated with chronic renal insufficiency. Other indications for erythropoietin include treatment of anemia related to the antiviral zidovudine in HIV-infected patients, and of chemotherapy-induced anemia in patients with metastatic, nonmyeloid malignancies. Preoperative erythropoietin treatment of anemia has been shown to reduce allogeneic RBC transfusion.[11]

SIDE EFFECTS

Erythropoietin therapy induces a marked expansion of erythroid cells, which can result in iron deficiency, so iron should be supplemented as appropriate. Target hemoglobin levels should not be set above 13 g/dL because the risk for cardiovascular events and stroke is increased. Hypertension can be worsened by erythropoietin, especially in patients with chronic renal failure. Erythropoietin therapy can adversely affect the survival of cancer patients, and progression or recurrence of certain tumors.

Blood Substitutes

The limited availability of blood and infection risks are the driving forces in developing oxygen-carrying blood substitutes. Two major classes of substitutes are hemoglobin-based

oxygen carriers (HBOC) and perfluorocarbon (PFC) emulsions. Bovine-derived hemoglobin glutamer-200 (Oxyglobin) is currently approved for canine anemia in the United States. In South Africa, bovine hemoglobin glutamer-250 (Hemopure) is approved for the treatment of human anemia. Free hemoglobin solutions have a higher affinity for oxygen than RBCs (P50 of 12-14 mmHg for HBOC vs. 27 mmHg for RBCs).[12,13] The modification of hemoglobin by pyridoxal phosphate increases P50 to 32 mmHg, improving release of oxygen.[3] Potential benefits of HBOCs include sparing allogeneic RBC transfusion in anemia, trauma, and major surgery, and reduction of transfusion-related infection and other complications. However, the vasoconstrictive property of HBOC, due to scavenging of nitric oxide, remains a major concern.[2,3]

PFC emulsions consist of halogen-substituted hydrocarbons that enhance plasma oxygen solubility. Hydrophobic PFC molecules are dissolved in plasma using emulsifiers. Unlike hemoglobin, the oxygen-carrying capacity of PFC is directly proportional to oxygen partial pressure.[2] Febrile reactions or flulike symptoms can occur in that PFC emulsion is taken up by the reticuloendothelial system. PFC is not clinically available at present, but potential perioperative uses include acute lung injury, and acute normovolemic hemodilution to spare RBCs from extracorporeal circuits.

Platelet Concentrates

Platelets are anuclear, granulated cells about 2 to 4 μm in diameter derived from bone marrow megakaryocytes. Normal half-life of platelets is 7 to 10 days. There are 150 to 350 × 10^9/L platelets in circulation, but their concentration near arterial vessel walls is significantly higher due to the margination of platelets by larger RBCs.[14] Platelets rapidly respond to disruption of normal endothelium, contributing to the initial arrest of bleeding (primary hemostasis), and the support of localized thrombin generation and fibrin formation (secondary hemostasis or coagulation) (Figure 36-3).[15] Procoagulant activity of platelets can increase the risk of vascular occlusion of atheromatous lesions (see Chapter 37).

Since the first platelet transfusion in the 1950s, platelet concentrate remains the mainstay therapy for thrombocytopenia.[16] Platelet concentrates are prepared by centrifugation of citrated whole blood within 8 hours of collection. After separating RBCs from platelet-rich plasma, further centrifugation yields one unit of platelet concentrate and plasma. Each unit of platelets, referred to as "random-donor platelets," contains 5.5 × 10^{10} platelets in 50 to 70 mL of plasma. Four to eight random-donor units are pooled to increase platelet count by 15 to 30 × 10^9/L in the adult. In order to decrease multiple donor exposures, single donor platelet apheresis is increasingly used. During the apheresis procedure, donor blood is placed in the extracorporeal circuit and centrifuged to separate platelets. One platelet apheresis unit contains 30 to 50 × 10^{10} platelets in 250 to 300 mL of plasma.

Platelet concentrates are agitated and stored at room temperature (20°C to 24°C) for up to 5 days (see Table 36-1).

CLINICAL USES

Platelet transfusion is used to prevent or treat bleeding due to platelet dysfunction or thrombocytopenia. Hereditary platelet dysfunction is rare, but adhesion defects in Bernard-Soulier syndrome (GPIb/IX deficiency), aggregation defects

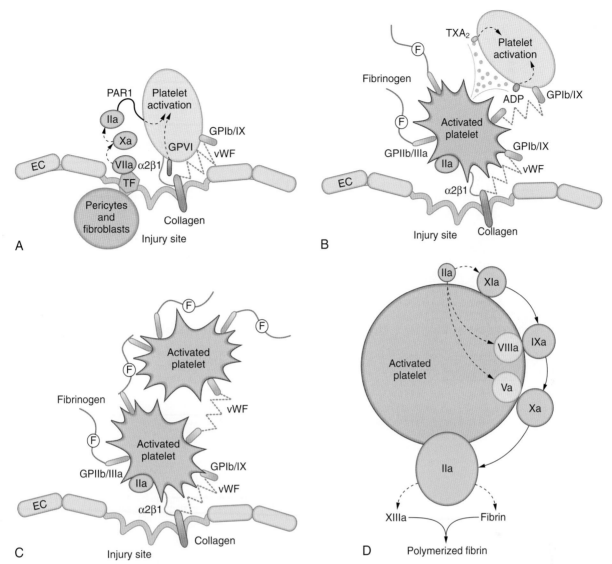

Figure 36-3 Clot formation at vascular injury site. At the injury site, platelets adhere to subendothelial collagen via interactions between von Willebrand factor (vWF) and the platelet-surface glycoprotein (GP) receptor GPIb/IX. Platelet integrin receptor $\alpha_2\beta_1$ reinforces binding to collagen. Trace amounts of thrombin are generated during the initiation phase of coagulation by factor Xa (FXa) via interactions between circulating FVIIa and tissue factor (TF) expressed on subendothelial pericytes and fibroblasts **(A).** Platelets activated by collagen and thrombin release adenosine-5'-diphosphate (ADP) and thromboxane A_2 (TXA_2), which activate platelets in the vicinity **(B).** Activated platelets express GPIIb/IIIa and capture fibrinogen (F) **(C).** On the activated platelet surface, thrombin-mediated feedback activation of FXI, FVIII, and FV results in the propagation phase of thrombin generation. Sustained activation of prothrombin is feasible via formation of tenase (IXa-VIIIa) and prothrombinase (Xa-Va). Polymerization of fibrin is achieved by thrombin-activated FXIII during the propagation phase **(D).** *(Modified with permission from Bolliger D, Gorlinger K, Tanaka KA. Pathophysiology and treatment of coagulopathy in massive hemorrhage and hemodilution.* Anesthesiology. *2010;113:1205-1219.)*

in Glanzmann's thrombasthenia (GPIIb/IIIa deficiency), and a secretion defect in Hermansky-Pudlak syndrome (lack of dense granules) are prototypical hemorrhagic conditions resulting from decreased primary hemostasis.[17] Platelet dysfunction in the perioperative patient is usually due to antiplatelet therapy (see Chapter 38). Platelet transfusion may be required even with a normal platelet count if platelet dysfunction due to acetylsalicylic acid (aspirin), thienopyridines, or GPIIb/IIIa inhibitors is clinically suggested or identified by platelet aggregometry. For thrombocytopenia associated with bone marrow disorders, the threshold for platelet transfusion is 10×10^9/L, which is usually sufficient to maintain vascular integrity.[18] In trauma or major surgery, platelet transfusion is empirically administered to maintain platelet counts above 50×10^9/L, although the hemostatic threshold for platelet

count remains to be established.[4-7] A platelet count of 50×10^9/L is reached after loss of twice the blood volume in an average sized adult.[19] Although a fixed ratio (1:1:1) transfusion of RBC, fresh frozen plasma (FFP), and pooled platelet units has been suggested to improve acute survival in severely injured patients with massive bleeding, hemostatic efficacy of platelet transfusion is difficult to validate without platelet function testing.[20,21] The timing and amount of platelet transfusion can be individualized by point-of-care laboratory tests (platelet count or thromboelastometry/graphy; Figure 36-4).[22,23]

SIDE EFFECTS

The risk of bacterial contamination is higher with platelet concentrates than with other blood components because they

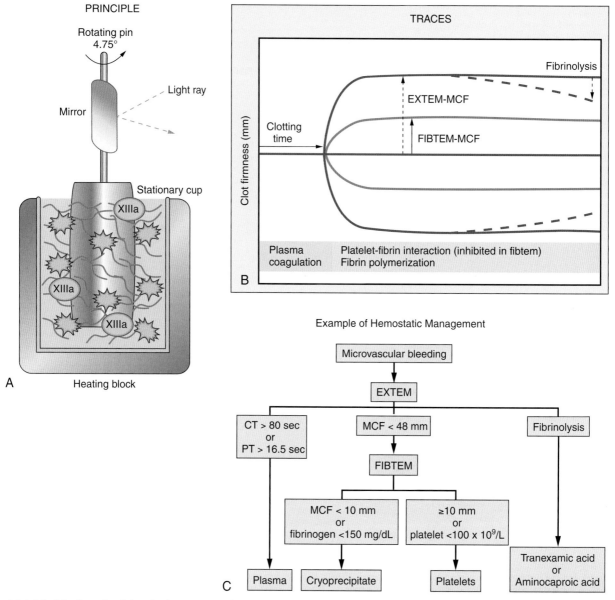

Figure 36-4 Principle of rotational thromboelastometry. **A,** The rotational thromboelastometry (ROTEM) instrument has a rotating pin immersed in the sample blood. Viscoelastic changes due to fibrin polymerization are detected optically. **B,** Blood samples can be activated by tissue factor (EXTEM) or ellagic acid (INTEM). The initial lagtime of coagulation (clotting time; CT) reflects procoagulant reactions to generate thrombin in plasma. Thrombin-mediated activation of platelets (pink oval), FXIII (blue oval), and fibrin (blue line) result in increased linkage (viscoelasticity) between the pin and cup *(A)*. When cytochalasin D is added, platelet-fibrin interactions are inhibited, and fibrinogen levels can be estimated (FIBTEM). **C,** In the event of microvascular bleeding in surgery, an algorithm such as this example can be used to standardize hemostatic therapy (see references 22 and 23).

are stored at room temperature. An immunoassay kit is available to test for aerobic or anaerobic gram-positive and gram-negative bacteria (sensitivity, 10^3-10^5 colony formation units/mL). Alloimmunizations after platelet transfusion can result in antibodies against HLA class I antigens and platelet-specific antigens. Problems due to platelet alloimmunization include refractoriness to platelet transfusion, and posttransfusion purpura. For those who require frequent platelet transfusions, the use of leukoreduced, HLA-matched, and ABO-compatible platelet units should be considered to reduce the risk of platelet alloimmunization.[24] The hemolysis of RBCs can be caused by anti-A or anti-B antibody present in the donor plasma of platelet concentrates. This typically occurs after group O platelet transfusion in non–group O

recipient.[25] The incidence of severe hemolysis is estimated to be in the range of 1 in 6600 (apheresis platelet transfusion) to 1 in 9000 (non–ABO-identical platelet transfusions).

Other potential complications of platelet transfusion in surgical patients include transfusion-associated lung injury (TRALI) and thrombotic complications.[26]

PLASMA AND COAGULATION FACTORS

Fresh Frozen Plasma

FFP is a unit of plasma separated from whole blood (~500 mL) or apheresis donations, and frozen at −18°C within 8 hours of collection. FP24 is an FDA-approved plasma product frozen between 8 and 24 hours of collection. Each unit is approximately 200 to 250 mL and contains all components of donor plasma, including procoagulant and anticoagulant factors, albumin, and immunoglobulins. The recovery of coagulation factors after each plasma unit is about 2% to 3% in the adult, but can vary with donors, clinical hemorrhage, and/or consumption. Plasma products can be stored frozen up to 12 months. Thawed plasma can be kept at 1°C to 6°C and used within 5 days since coagulation factors including the most labile FV and FVIII remain adequate for this period.[27] Donor plasma should be compatible with recipients' ABO types (see Figure 36-2), but Rh types do not need to be considered. Blood group AB plasma can be used as the universal donor for emergency.

CLINICAL USES
Plasma transfusion is mainly indicated for the treatment of complex coagulopathies in which multiple coagulation factors and inhibitors are depleted. For congenital factor deficiency, plasma transfusion should be considered only if recombinant or plasma-derived factor concentrate is not available (Table 36-2). Plasma products can be transfused prophylactically before invasive procedures when risk of bleeding is high. When the international normalized ratio (INR) is less than 1.5, excessive bleeding is unlikely.[28,29] Plasma transfusion is used to treat bleeding conditions when prothrombin time (PT) is greater than 1.5 times the midpoint of the normal range, or activated partial thromboplastin time (aPTT) is greater than 1.5 times the upper limit of normal.[30] The usual dose is 5 to 8 mL/kg, but up to 10 to 30 mL/kg might be necessary to keep coagulation factors above 50% of normal.[31,32] Plasma products need to be administered early rather than late to avoid fluid overload in cases of massive hemorrhage.[33] Early plasma transfusions using a 1:1 ratio of FFP:RBC improved early survival in military and civilian trauma,[34-37] but some retrospective data suggest no benefit of increased plasma transfusion, and increased risk of multiorgan failure.[38-40] The guidelines of the American Association of Blood Banks and the European task force recommend early plasma transfusion without a specific FFP:RBC ratio.[7,30] The rational use of plasma is facilitated by rapid point-of-care coagulation monitors (see Figure 36-4), and by adopting safer transfusion protocols and products (e.g., lyophilized plasma-derived or recombinant protein concentrates).[41]

For congenital factor deficiencies, plasma-derived or recombinant factor concentrates are often available, and are preferable to plasma transfusion in terms of safety and efficacy (Table 36-3). Plasma can be used as a replacement fluid (plasma exchange) in patients undergoing a therapeutic apheresis procedure.[42] It is the first-line therapy to reduce mortality from thrombotic thrombocytopenia purpura by providing metalloprotease (ADAMTS13) that cleaves high-molecular von Willebrand factor (vWF).[43] For acute reversal of vitamin K antagonist (e.g., warfarin) therapy, FFP is used in conjunction with vitamin K. Plasma-derived, virus-inactivated prothrombin complex concentrate (PCC) is an alternative therapy for this indication as described below.[6]

Table 36-2. Plasma Concentrations and Half-Lives of Coagulation Factors

	CONCENTRATION (μM)	HALF-LIFE (Hr)	AVAILABLE CONCENTRATE(S)
Fibrinogen	7.6	72-120	pd-fibrinogen, cryoprecipitate
Prothrombin	1.4	72	PCC, FEIBA
Factor V	0.03	36	None
Factor VII	0.01	3-6	pd-FVII, r-FVIIa, PCC*, FEIBA
Factor VIII	0.00003	12	pd-FVIII, r-FVIII
Factor IX	0.09	24	pd-FIX, r-FIX, FEIBA
FX	0.17	40	pd-FX, PCC, FEIBA
Factor XI	0.03	80	pd-FXI
Factor XIII	0.03	120-200	pd-FXIII, r-FXIII, cryoprecipitate
vWF	0.03	10-24	pd-vWF, r-vWF, cryoprecipitate
Protein C	0.08	10	pd-Protein C, PCC*
Protein S	0.14	42.5	PCC*
Antithrombin	2.6	48-72	pd-antithrombin, r-antithrombin

Adapted with permission from Bolliger D, Gorlinger K, Tanaka KA. Pathophysiology and treatment of coagulopathy in massive hemorrhage and hemodilution. *Anesthesiology.* 2010;113:1205-1219.
FEIBA, Factor eight inhibitor bypassing activity; *PCC,* prothrombin complex concentrate (*some PCC products contain minimal levels of FVII, protein C and S; see Table 36-3); *pd,* plasma-derived; *r,* recombinant; *vWF,* von Willebrand factor.

Table 36-3. Contents of Commercial Prothrombin Complex Concentrates in North America

PRODUCT	MANUFACTURER	FACTOR II %	FACTOR VII %	FACTOR IX %	FACTOR X %	PROTEIN C U/mL	PROTEIN S U/mL	ANTITHROMBIN U/mL	HEPARIN U/mL
Bebulin	Baxter	120	13	100	139	Present	Present	Not on label	<0.15 U per IU of FIX
Beriplex	CSL Behring	111	57	100	150	15-45	13-26	0.2-1.5	0.4-2.0
Octaplex	Octapharma	98	66	100	96	7-32	7-32	Not on label	Not on label
Profilnine	Grifols	148	11	100	64	Not on label	Not on label	Not on label	Not contained

Each PCC vial is labeled according to the FIX content in international units (IU). The contents of other procoagulant factors are shown relative to FIX (e.g., one 500-IU vial of Bebulin contains 65 IU of FVII and 600 IU of FII).

SIDE EFFECTS

Allergic reactions to plasma are the most common complications occurring in 1% to 3% of all transfusions. The risk of fluid overload due to a large volume of plasma transfusion should be considered in patients with a limited cardiovascular reserve. Hypocalcemia can result from citrate accumulation after plasma transfusion, and is treated with calcium chloride. Risk of viral transmission has been significantly reduced since the 1990s by implementing nucleic acid testing for human immunodeficiency virus and hepatitis C virus. Use of pathogen-inactivated plasma (solvent-detergent or methylene blue-treated plasma) might further reduce viral transmission risks.[44]

TRALI is a serious complication of plasma transfusion. It is causally associated with anti-HLA antibodies. Multiparous females are often sensitized to HLA antigens, and thus the incidence of TRALI has gone down after many blood centers started to produce the majority of plasma products from male donors.[45]

Albumin

Albumin is a 69-kDa protein synthesized in the liver and present in plasma at 3 to 5 g/dL (~60% of plasma protein). Plasma-derived pasteurized (60°C for 10 hours) fractions are available in iso-oncotic (5%) or hyperoncotic (25%) solutions. Albumin exerts oncotic activity (colloid osmotic pressure) to retain intravascular water. The oncotic pressure of 5% albumin is equivalent to plasma. Albumin also serves to carry poorly water-soluble molecules (e.g., apoprotein, bilirudin, transferrin). Indications for albumin use include fluid replacement for hypovolemic shock, priming for extracorporeal circuits, and plasma exchange therapy. In acute liver failure, albumin can be used to restore oncotic pressure. The intravascular retention of albumin is affected by increased vascular permeability (e.g., first 24 hours of thermal injury) and excretion (e.g., nephrotic syndrome). Albumin does not affect hepatic or renal function.

Synthetic Colloids

Synthetic colloid solutions include hydroxyethyl starches (HES) in which rapid degradation by α-amylase is prevented by hydroxyethylation of glucose subunits (Figure 36-5). The molar replacement ratio indicates the proportion of glucose molecules replaced with hydroxyethyl units (e.g., 0.4 = 40% replacement). The C2/C6 ratio indicates the number of hydroxyethyl units at C2 relative to C6. HES with higher molar replacement and C2/C6 ratios is retained longer due to slower metabolism (Table 36-4). HES is excreted by the kidney after degradation.

Differences between albumin and HES in efficacy and safety are controversial. HES products are available in iso-oncotic (6%) or hyperoncotic (10%) solutions. The 6% HES solutions with the average molecular weight of 600 to 670 kDa (Hespan, Hextend) are most commonly used, but low molecular weight HES (130 kDa, Voluven) has recently become available in the United States.[46] HES products are as effective as albumin as fluid replacements, but large doses of HES (particularly Hespan) can adversely affect coagulation (fibrin polymerization) and exacerbate renal dysfunction in sepsis.[47,48] Excess HES can falsely elevate turbidimetric fibrinogen measurements.[49]

Cryoprecipitate

Cryoprecipitate is prepared from thawing FFP at 1°C to 6°C. The cold-insoluble precipitate contains FVIII, vWF, FXIII, fibrinogen, and fibronectin. The precipitate is resuspended in a small amount of plasma (~15 mL) and is stored at −18°C up to 12 months. Cryoprecipitate was the first concentrated source of FVIII and used to be called cryoprecipitated antihemophilic factor. Plasma-derived or recombinant factor concentrate has largely replaced the use of cryoprecipitate in congenital deficiency of FVIII, vWF, FXIII, or fibrinogen.[50]

Table 36-4. Synthetic Hydroxyethyl Starch Colloid Solutions

TYPE OF HES	600/0.7	670/0.75	260/0.45	130/0.4
Product name	Hespan	Hextend	Pentaspan	Voluven
Concentration	6%	6%	10%	6%
Solvent	Saline	LR	Saline	Saline
Oncotic pressure (mmHg)	25-30	25-30	55-60	36
Mean molecular mass (kDa)	600	670	260	130
Molar substitution	0.7	0.75	0.45	0.4
C2/C6 ratio	5	4.5	6	9
Maximum daily dose (mL/kg)	20	20	20	33

LR, Lactated Ringer's.

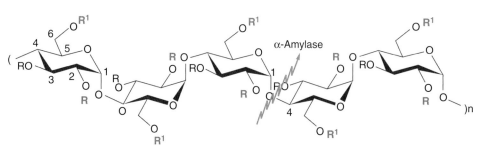

Figure 36-5 Hydroxyethyl substitution of hydroxyethyl starch (HES). The structural formula of HES poly(0-2-hydroxyethyl)starch. R, −H, −CH₂CH₂OH; R¹, −H, CH₂CH₂OH or glucose unit. Enzymatic cleavage site of α-amylase *(yellow arrow)* is at C1 and C4 atoms. Hydroxyethyl groups at position C2 inhibit the access of α-amylase to the substrate more effectively than those at C6. HES products with high C2/C6 ratios are more slowly degraded. *(Reprinted with permission from Kozek-Langenecker SA. Effects of hydroxyethyl starch solutions on hemostasis. Anesthesiology. 2005;103:654-660.)*

CLINICAL USES

Cryoprecipitate is used to manage bleeding due to acquired hypofibrinogenemia (<100-150 mg/dL). Each unit contains 150 to 250 mg of fibrinogen; 5 to 10 units are thawed and pooled before infusion. Each unit of cryoprecipitate increases plasma fibrinogen by approximately 100 mg/dL per 5-kg body weight. The volume of cryoprecipitate required to increase fibrinogen levels is far less than that of FFP. However, it takes longer to thaw and pool multiple units of cryoprecipitate, whereas thawed FFP is more readily available for transfusion. In many European countries, cryoprecipitate is no longer available, and plasma-derived, pasteurized fibrinogen concentrate is used.[51] It is feasible to rapidly treat hypofibrinogenemia with the fibrinogen concentrate because no thawing and blood type matching are required, and it can be infused at a low volume (1 g of fibrinogen per 50 mL after reconstitution).

The minimal level of plasma fibrinogen to minimize perioperative bleeding has not been well established.[52] International guidelines previously recommended a minimal fibrinogen of 80 to 100 mg/dL, similar to management of congenital afibrinogenemia.[5,31] More recently, higher fibrinogen levels (150-200 mg/dL) are recommended in European guidelines for perioperative transfusion based on clinical data supporting fibrinogen above 200 mg/dL in postpartum hemorrhage, coronary bypass grafting, aortic replacement, and cystectomy.[6,7,53-58] Plasma fibrinogen levels can be estimated by the modified Clauss method or platelet-inhibited thromboelastometry/graphy (see Figure 36-4).[59,60]

SIDE EFFECTS

The exposure to multiple donors from pooled cryoprecipitate units is a major concern since no viral inactivation procedure is clinically available.[61] Use of pasteurized plasma-derived fibrinogen concentrates is strongly recommended for patients with congenital afibrinogenemia or dysfibrinogenemia. Cryoprecipitate contains some plasma, but the risk of TRALI is unknown. Risk of thrombotic complications is unknown, but is potentially of concern because cryoprecipitate rapidly increases plasma fibrinogen, FVIII, FXIII, and vWF (ADAMTS13 is minimal in cryoprecipitate units).[62]

Recombinant Factor VIIa

Recombinant activated factor VIIa (rFVIIa) is an activated form of human FVII produced in hamster kidney cells. Its hemostatic activity is mainly mediated by tissue factor-dependent activation of FX and subsequent thrombin generation. Use of rFVIIa is clinically indicated for prophylaxis or treatment of bleeding in hemophiliacs who develop neutralizing antibodies to FVIII or FIX and with congenital FVII deficiency.

Off-label use of rFVIIa is common after major bleeding in trauma and surgery, but efficacy and safety of rFVIIa outside of congenital factor deficiency has not been established.[63] It is not uncommon to observe multifactorial coagulopathy in addition to hypothermia and acidosis in nonhemophiliac patients who developed profuse bleeding after trauma or surgery. The use of rFVIIa should be considered only after replenishing plasma proteins (particularly prothrombin and fibrinogen), and optimizing body temperature and pH.

CLINICAL USES

The recommended initial dose of rFVIIa for hemophiliacs with inhibitors is 90 to 120 μg/kg, but higher doses of 200 to 400 μg/kg have been used without major thrombosis. In refractory bleeding, combination therapy with factor eight inhibitor bypassing activity (FEIBA), an activated PCC, has been suggested.[64]

In nonhemophiliacs, the initial dose of rFVIIa is lower (20-70 μg/kg).[63] In randomized trauma trials, the efficacy of higher initial doses (200 μg/kg) was limited to a small reduction in RBC use with no effect on 30-day mortality.[65,66] In a randomized trial in intracerebral hemorrhage, rFVIIa at 80 μg/kg reduced hematoma expansion but led to increased arterial thrombosis.[67] Similarly, in a study of bleeding after cardiac surgery there were fewer reoperations and decreased allogeneic blood use with rFVIIa at 40 μg/kg and 80 μg/kg, but with increased adverse events including stroke.[68]

SIDE EFFECTS

Thrombotic complications after rFVIIa are infrequent in hemophilia, but these risks appear to be increased in nonhemophiliacs undergoing surgery.[69] In an analysis of 35 published randomized clinical studies, the incidence of arterial thromboembolic events, but not venous thrombosis, was increased by 1.7-fold with rFVIIa therapy.[70] Higher rFVIIa dose (>80 μg/kg), age, and coronary artery disease were contributing factors to thrombosis.

Prothrombin Complex Concentrate

PCC is a sterile, lyophilized concentrate of factors II, VII, IX, and X and protein C and S. Before development of FIX concentrates, PCC with low amounts of FVII (3-factor PCC) was used to treat hemophilia B. The content of PCC is thus standardized to the amount of FIX in each vial (each vial contains at least 500 IU of FIX) (see Table 36-3). Advantages of PCC include rapid availability, small volume of infusion, and avoidance of complications such as ABO incompatibility and TRALI associated with FFP. PCC containing clinically relevant FVII levels (4-factor PCC) is available for acute reversal of vitamin K antagonists in Europe and Canada (currently in clinical trials in the United States).[71] PCCs increase thrombin generation by interacting with negatively charged phospholipids on activated platelets at the vascular injury site.[72] Commercial PCCs are fractionated from pooled plasma and undergo viral inactivation using vapor-heat or solvent/detergent-treatment and nanofiltration.

CLINICAL USES

PCC can be rapidly reconstituted with sterile water (20 mL per 500 IU) without the need for thawing and blood type matching. Dosing depends on the extent of anticoagulation. A high initial dose of 30 to 50 IU/kg (maximum, 5000 IU) is used in life-threatening bleeding associated with anticoagulation including intracranial hemorrhage and retroperitoneal bleeding. A lower dose of 20 to 25 IU/kg is used for soft tissue bleeding, epistaxis, and hematuria. Subsequent doses are based on PT/INR measurements. In acute bleeding, the major advantage of PCC is that procoagulant FII, FVII, FIX, and FX can be rapidly (<30 minutes; Figure 36-6) increased by 40% to 80% without dilution of RBCs and platelets.[73,74] The vicious cycle of hematoma formation, tissue edema, and

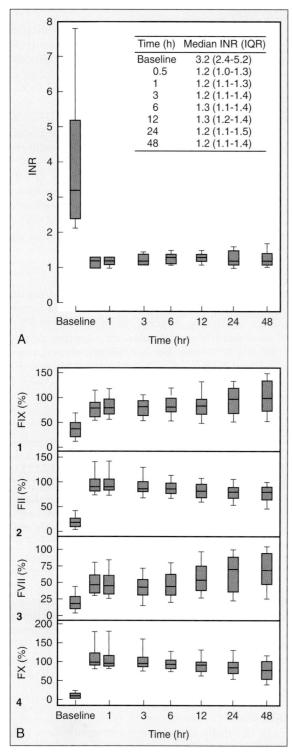

Time (h)	Median INR (IQR)
Baseline	3.2 (2.4-5.2)
0.5	1.2 (1.0-1.3)
1	1.2 (1.1-1.3)
3	1.2 (1.1-1.4)
6	1.3 (1.1-1.4)
12	1.3 (1.2-1.4)
24	1.2 (1.1-1.5)
48	1.2 (1.1-1.4)

Figure 36-6 Time course of international normalized ratio and vitamin K–dependent procoagulant factors after reversal of oral anticoagulation with PCC. **A,** The changes in international normalized ratio (INR) during acute oral anticoagulant reversal with PCC are shown. **B,** Time course of plasma levels of (1) FIX, (2) FII, (3) FVII, and (4) FX after PCC therapy. Levels are shown as a percent of normal. Boxes span the interquartile range (IQR). Horizontal lines bisecting the boxes indicate median values and lower and upper error bars the 10th and 90th percentiles, respectively. (*Data from Pabinger I, Brenner B, Kalina U, et al. Prothrombin complex concentrate (Beriplex P/N) for emergency anticoagulation reversal: a prospective multinational clinical trial. J Thromb Haemost. 2008;6:622-631.*)

rebleeding can be prevented by prompt reestablishment of hemostasis.[75] Adjunctive vitamin K is recommended to sustain PT/INR because plasma FVII falls quickly after a dose of PCC due to its short half-life.[73] The incidence of thrombotic complications after PCCs for acute reversal of anticoagulation is about 0.9% to 2%.[76]

There is a paucity of data on PCC for treatment of coagulopathy in trauma, major surgery, and hepatic dysfunction. In small retrospective studies, PCC was effective in achieving hemostasis in postcardiac surgical patients who were refractory to platelets, FFP, and cryoprecipitate.[77,78] The use of PCC after initial treatment with fibrinogen concentrate in trauma patients reduced the need for FFP without affecting survival.[41]

SIDE EFFECTS

Use of PCC is generally safe for acute reversal of anticoagulation, but thrombogenicity is a concern in the setting of massive hemorrhage and hemodilution. Prothrombotic risks might be increased with anticoagulant deficiency associated with hepatic cirrhosis or severe hemodilution.[79,80] PCC should not be administered to patients with DIC.[6]

Current antiviral protocols for factor concentrates are not effective against prions (e.g., vCJD) or non–lipid-enveloped, heat-resistant viruses (e.g., parvovirus B19), but these risks are considered to be low.[81]

Antithrombin Concentrate

Antithrombin (AT) is a serine protease inhibitor with a molecular weight of 58 kDa. Normal plasma AT is about 150 μg/mL (2.6 μM). Anticoagulant activity of AT is potentiated by endothelial surface heparan sulfate or exogenously administered heparin. In congenital AT deficiency, AT is 40% to 60% of normal, resulting in prolonged half-life of FXa and thrombin (Figure 36-7).[82] The incidence of venous thromboembolism is increased in congenital AT deficiency during pregnancy and after major trauma or surgery. Replacement of AT using plasma-derived (Thrombate III) and recombinant AT concentrate (Atryn) are indicated to prevent thrombotic complications in congenital deficiency. Recombinant AT is produced in transgenic goats, and has different glycosylation and a shorter half-life (11 hours vs. 2.5 days). Whether the cost of higher doses is justified by the improved viral safety of recombinant AT is unknown.

Acquired AT deficiency is frequently observed following treatment with intravenous heparin for more than 4 to 5 days. In cardiac surgical patients with heparin insensitivity (activated clotting time <400 seconds), plasma-derived or recombinant AT concentrates restore plasma AT activity effectively without the need for additional heparin or FFP.[83,84] AT concentrates are less likely to decrease hematocrit and platelet count compared to FFP. Both plasma-derived and recombinant AT concentrates contain trace amounts of heparin, and so should not be used in patients with heparin-induced thrombocytopenia (HIT).[6]

Protein C Concentrate

Protein C is a vitamin K–dependent factor similar to prothrombin, FVII, FIX, and FX. Protein C activation by thrombin is limited in the presence of fibrinogen, FV, FVIII, and

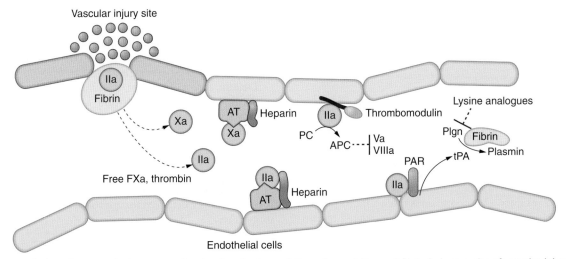

Figure 36-7 Regulation of procoagulant responses. Local and systemic regulation of coagulation and fibrinolysis at a site of vascular injury is shown. Hemostasis is established as fibrin is polymerized by thrombin (IIa) and activated FXIII. When thrombin or FXa is released (i.e., free thrombin) into the systemic circulation during hemostatic activation, antithrombin (AT) and thrombomodulin of intact endothelium bind to thrombin and reduce its procoagulant activity. Thrombomodulin-bound thrombin activates protein C (APC), which inactivates coagulation factors Va and VIIIa. Thrombin also causes the release of tissue plasminogen activator (tPA) from endothelium, which promotes plasminogen (Plgn) conversion to plasmin on the fibrin surface. Broken lines indicated inhibitory action of respective protease inhibitors. *PAR*, Protease-activated receptor (thrombin receptor on endothelium). *(Adapted with permission from Ide M, Bolliger D, Taketomi T, et al. Lessons from the aprotinin saga: current perspective on antifibrinolytic therapy in cardiac surgery. J Anesth. 2010;24:96-106.)*

platelets at a vascular injury site, but is more efficiently activated by thrombin bound to thrombomodulin expressed on the endothelium (see Figure 36-7). Elevated systemic thrombin activity thus increases protein C activation as observed in thrombophilia, sepsis, and traumatic injury.[85-87] Activated protein C with protein S downregulates activated FV and FVIII and exerts antiinflammatory and cytoprotective functions by modulating endothelial protein C receptor and protease-activated receptor-1 (PAR-1, thrombin receptor).[88] Antiinflammatory effects of activated protein C (recombinant) might be beneficial in patients with severe sepsis (APACHE score >25), but serious bleeding is the major side effect.[89]

Homozygous protein C deficiency in newborns manifests as purpura fulminans with thrombosis in small vessels causing skin necrosis.[90] Incidence of venous thromboembolism is eightfold to 10-fold higher in individuals with heterozygous protein C deficiency.[91]

Lyophilized protein C concentrate (Ceprotin) is available for prevention and treatment of purpura fulminans and venous thrombosis in the North America. The initial dose for acute thrombosis is 100 to 120 IU/kg, followed by maintenance doses of 45 to 60 IU/kg every 6 to 12 hours. The infectious risk of plasma-derived protein C is low due to viral inactivation steps, including polysorbate-80, vapor-heat, and ion exchange chromatography. Precautions for use include bleeding, sodium overload, rare allergic reactions, and heparin-induced thrombocytopenia due to trace amounts of heparin.

PHARMACOLOGIC AND TOPICAL AGENTS

Lysine Analogues

The lysine analogues ε-aminocaproic acid (EACA) and tranexamic acid (TXA) prevent plasminogen from binding to fibrin by occupying the plasminogen lysine-binding site (see Figure 36-7). By preventing colocalization of tissue plasminogen activator and plasminogen on fibrin, plasmin activation, and subsequent fibrin degradation are inhibited. Both EACA and TXA have a low molecular weight (131 Da and 157 Da, respectively) in contrast to the bovine plasmin inhibitor aprotinin (6512 Da). Reduced perioperative blood loss has been reported in cardiac, hepatic, and orthopedic surgeries, although most studies are underpowered to demonstrate safety.[92] The use of aprotinin has been on hold from the market after higher 30-day morbidity and mortality was reported compared with lysine analogues.[93,94]

CLINICAL USES

The approved indication of lysine analogues is to reduce bleeding in hemophilia patients.[95] EACA is administered orally or intravenously for bleeding associated with fibrinolysis with an initial dose of 5 g in adults. In hemophiliacs having dental extraction, TXA is given at a dose of 10 mg/kg three to four times a day.

In cardiac surgery with cardiopulmonary bypass, the loading dose of intravenous EACA and TXA is 50 mg/kg and 10-15 mg/kg, respectively, after systemic anticoagulation. Continuous infusion of EACA and TXA is commonly used at 15 mg/kg/hr for EACA and 7.5 mg/kg/hr for TXA until the end of surgery. In trauma patients, TXA (1 g loading, followed by 1 g over 8 hours) improved mortality without increasing cardiovascular complications.[96]

SIDE EFFECTS

Systemic thrombosis is uncommon with EACA or TXA, but they should not be used in patients with DIC.[6] Lysine analogues are mainly excreted by the kidney, and dosage should be reduced based on serum creatinine level. EACA and TXA are eliminated by hemofiltration or dialysis. With renal or ureteral bleeding, lysine analogues can increase the risk of ureteral obstruction due to clot formation. Prolonged infusion of TXA is associated with seizures. Presumably this is due to TXA crossing the blood-brain barrier and antagonizing GABA receptors.[97]

Desmopressin

Desmopressin (1-desamino-8-D-arginine vasopressin) is a synthetic vasopressin analogue with antidiuretic activity. In mild to moderate von Willebrand disease and hemophilia A, intravenous desmopressin (0.3-0.4 µg/kg) increases plasma vWF and FVIII by twofold to threefold within 60 to 90 minutes. Increased vWF might improve platelet adhesion to sites of vascular injury. Desmopressin is often administered to patients with preexisting platelet dysfunction related to antiplatelet drugs and uremia. Desmopressin appears to reduce blood loss, but most studies failed to demonstrate reduced RBC transfusion in nonhemophilic surgical patients.[98] Inconsistent efficacy could be related to simultaneous release of tPA and tachyphylaxis or exhaustion of stored vWF-FVIII in high-stress situations.

SIDE EFFECTS

Rapid intravenous administration of desmopressin causes flushing and mild hypotension via vasopressin V_2 receptor stimulation. Vascular occlusion due to elevated vWF is rare in von Willebrand disease and hemophilia A, but could be a concern in surgical patients with preexisting cardiovascular disease.[98]

Topical Hemostatic Agents

Topical hemostatic agents are useful in controlling minor bleeding from bone (bone wax, Ostene) or small capillaries and venules (e.g., topical thrombin).[99] Bovine thrombin has been clinically used for a long time, but is associated with major immunologic reactions including immunization against endogenous prothrombin, thrombin, FV, and cardiolipin. Acquired FV deficiency due to bovine thrombin exposure can result in serious bleeding.[100] Plasma-derived thrombin (Evithrom) or recombinant thrombin (Recothrom) are preferred to bovine thrombin (Thrombin–JMI) as a topical agent.

Oxidized cellulose (Surgicel) induces local hemolysis of RBCs by lowering pH, and provides a physical matrix for coagulation. Disadvantages include inactivation of natural clotting enzymes such as thrombin and potential for inflammation and delayed wound healing. Microfibrillar collagen (Avitene) increases local platelet adhesion and activation, leading to hemostasis within 5 minutes. The collagen particles do not cause much swelling and are reabsorbed within 8 weeks. It should be cautioned that microfibrillar collagen can pass through red blood cell salvage system filters. Platelet gel (Vitagel) combines microfibrillar collagen and thrombin with the patient's own platelet and plasma (fibrinogen), but requires centrifugation for preparation.

Fibrin sealants (Tisseel, Crosseal, Evicel) are effective for venous oozing from raw surfaces. They are supplied with separate vials of fibrinogen, thrombin, and calcium chloride that are mixed at the wound by a dual-syringe applicator. Hemostasis results from topical fibrin formation. A patch sponge (Tachosil) impregnated with lyophilized human fibrinogen and thrombin is also available for treatment of raw

surface bleeding. To prevent viral transmission from the human plasma, fibrinogen and thrombin are treated with solvent-detergent, nanofiltration, or vapor-heat. Recombinant aprotinin (Tisseel) and tranexamic acid (Crosseal) are added for improved clot stability.

Gelatin forms (Gelfoam, Gelfilm, Surgiform) provide a physical matrix for clot formation, and are effective in bleeding from small capillaries and venules. Another gelatin-based sealant (FloSeal) is a mixture of human thrombin and bovine-derived gelatin-based matrix. Thrombin generates fibrin from blood fibrinogen, and the gelatin particles expand to tamponade bleeding. Gelatin matrix is reabsorbed after 6 to 8 weeks.

These topical agents are generally safe and useful adjuncts for hemostasis when used for appropriate indications and anatomic sites.[99]

SPECIAL CONSIDERATIONS

Liver Failure

Patients with liver failure often develop abnormal hemostasis because most coagulation factors and inhibitors are synthesized by hepatocytes. Hemophilia A and B can be cured by liver transplantation.[101] The liver is also the major site for clearance of activated coagulation factors and plasminogen activators. The extent of coagulopathy varies with the type and stage of liver and biliary tract disease.[102,103] PT/INR has been used to estimate the outcome of liver disease because decreased levels of prothrombin, FV, FVII, and FX reflect severity of liver disease.[104] Coagulopathy in end-stage liver disease is often viewed as a hemorrhagic condition, but recent clinical data indicate that the hypocoagulable state coexists with a potentially prothrombotic state due to generalized decreases in both procoagulant and anticoagulant proteins.[102,103]

Jehovah's Witnesses

Devout Jehovah's Witnesses do not accept transfusion of "primary components" including red blood cells, white blood cells, platelets, and plasma. The use of immunoglobulins, albumin, and plasma-derived FVIII and FIX ("hemophiliac preparations" per religious leaders) have been allowed since 1978. The policy on blood transfusion was changed recently, and acceptance of fractionated products of "primary components" was left to the individual believer (Table 36-5). In

Table 36-5. Primary Components and Fractionated Products for Jehovah's Witnesses

PRIMARY COMPONENTS	FRACTIONATED PRODUCTS OF PRIMARY COMPONENTS
Not Acceptable	**Up to the Individual Believer**
Red blood cells	Hemoglobin-based oxygen carrier
White blood cells	Interleukins, Interferons
Platelets	Platelet gels
Plasma	Albumin, immunoglobins, coagulation factor/inhibitor concentrates, recombinant human proteins, topical hemostatics

addition to recombinant proteins such as erythropoietin and rFVIIa, plasma-derived factor concentrates (see Table 36-2) can be acceptable to Jehovah's Witnesses.[105]

EMERGING DEVELOPMENTS

Improved pathogen detection in donors and pathogen reduction treatments should allow increasingly safer supplies of allogeneic blood products.[106]

The duration and resources (e.g., culture medium) required for autologous cell production remain major hurdles in filling clinical needs. Better understanding and technologies related to hematopoietic progenitors, embryonic stem cells, and pluripotent stem cells have recently enabled in vitro production of functional RBCs in terms of deformability, enzyme content, and oxygen-carrying capacity.[107] In time, cultured autologous RBCs and platelets could become valid transfusion resources for those with rare antigens and multiple alloantibodies.

In addition to cellular components, human stem cell technology can be applied to produce structured tissue sheets (e.g., hepatocytes).[108] Deficient coagulation factors and inhibitors can be replaced by implanted hepatocellular tissue sheets.[109]

Clinical application of nanoparticles (diameter <100 nm) holds some promise. For example, biodegradable GPIb-conjugated nanoparticles might be used to compensate for impaired platelet function.[110]

Novel recombinant coagulation proteins or synthetic chemicals are being developed for bleeding disorders. Examples of such molecules are modified recombinant FVIIa with prolonged half-life and improved potency for hemophilia, and a synthetic 700 Da plasmin inhibitor for perioperative antifibrinolytic therapy.[111,112]

activity of thrombin, fibrinogen, and FXIII) can be assessed.
- Early administration of FFP along with RBCs in major hemorrhage has recently gained popularity at civilian trauma centers. This approach theoretically prevents excessive factor dilution, and can improve hemostasis and early survival. Potential concerns regarding more plasma use include increased acute lung injury, immunomodulation, and volume overload.
- For certain hereditary deficiencies of coagulation factors or inhibitors, plasma-derived or recombinant concentrates are available, and are preferable for safety (e.g., reduced risk of viral transmission) and efficacy. Use of factor concentrates in acquired factor deficiency is generally considered as off-label, but there are some supportive data available for certain indications (e.g., PCCs for vitamin K antagonist reversal and fibrinogen for dilutional coagulopathy).
- Topical hemostatic agents are frequently used by surgeons, and can be potentially useful to reduce blood loss. The proper indications and sites should be considered to reduce untoward complications (e.g., tissue swelling, necrosis, intravascular absorption).

Key References

Bolliger D, Gorlinger K, Tanaka KA. Pathophysiology and treatment of coagulopathy in massive hemorrhage and hemodilution. *Anesthesiology.* 2010;113:1205-1219. Reviews the pathogenesis of hemodilution-induced coagulopathy with a focus on component-based hemostatic therapies. Significant consumption and loss of fibrinogen is common in major trauma and surgical patients. The minimal fibrinogen level was previously set at 80 to 100 mg/dL, similar to hereditary fibrinogen deficiency. However, recent clinical data suggest improved hemostasis at higher fibrinogen levels, and many revised guidelines adopted 150 to 200 mg/dL as a threshold fibrinogen level. Hemodilution also affects anticoagulant factors (e.g., antithrombin), and reduced thrombin inhibition can paradoxically increase thrombotic complications in bleeding patients. (Ref. 52)
Goodnough LT, Brecher ME, Kanter MH, et al. First of two parts—blood transfusion. *N Engl J Med.* 1999;340:438-447; Goodnough LT, Brecher ME, Kanter MH, et al. Transfusion medicine. Second of two parts—blood conservation. *N Engl J Med.* 1999;340:525-533. Reviews trends in transfusion medicine including indications for therapy, immunomodulation, infectious risks, and the feasibility and efficacy of blood conservation techniques (autologous donation, erythropoietin, acute normovolemic hemodilution) in a two-part article. (Refs. 12 and13)
Lisman T, Porte RJ. Rebalanced hemostasis in patients with liver disease: evidence and clinical consequences. *Blood.* 2010;116:878-885. Coagulation abnormalities cannot be predicted by prolonged PT values. The liver is the site for synthesis and degradation of many procoagulant and anticoagulant as well as profibrinolytic and antifibrinolytic factors. The balance of hemostasis and bleeding is delicate in patients with liver disease due to concomitant changes in both procoagulant and anticoagulant pathways. (Ref. 103)
Nuttall GA, Oliver WC, Santrach PJ, et al. Efficacy of a simple intraoperative transfusion algorithm for nonerythrocyte component utilization after cardiopulmonary bypass. *Anesthesiology.* 2001;94:773-781. Investigates the algorithm for non-RBC transfusion based on laboratory coagulation test during cardiac surgery. In this prospective randomized study, 92 patients (11%) developed microvascular bleeding, and 51 of 92 were randomized to receive empirical care. The algorithm-based therapy, which

---

KEY POINTS

- Transfusion of blood components can be life saving, but there are a number of potentially serious complications. ABO incompatible transfusion and TRALI are two of the most common causes of death after blood transfusion. The proper identifications of the donor unit and the patient and careful risk-benefit assessments are essential before each component transfusion.
- Transfusion of RBC concentrates should be determined, not only by threshold hemoglobin values but also by the rate/extent of hemorrhage, clinical conditions (e.g., reduced cardiovascular reserve), and the risk-benefit ratio.
- Hemodilution can be extensive in major trauma and surgery, and affects both procoagulant and anticoagulant factors. Reduced plasma levels of fibrinogen and factor XIII early during hemodilution result in fragile clot formation, which is susceptible to fibrinolysis. Fibrinogen can be replaced more efficiently by cryoprecipitate (or plasma-derived fibrinogen) than by FFP.
- Plasma-based PT and aPTT are frequently used to evaluate coagulopathy, but are not predictive of perioperative bleeding risks. Thromboelastography/metry is a useful adjunct to PT/aPTT and platelet count because the stability of fibrin polymerization (i.e.,

was given to 41 of 92 patients, consisted of threshold values for platelet (count below 102 × 10⁹/L, or thromboelastography-amplitude <48 mm), plasma (PT > 16.6 sec or aPTT > 57 sec), and cryoprecipitate (fibrinogen <144 mg/dL). The algorithm group had significantly less blood loss and lower rates of platelet and plasma transfusion. (Ref. 22)

Pabinger I, Brenner B, Kalina U, et al. Prothrombin complex concentrate (Beriplex P/N) for emergency anticoagulation reversal: a prospective multinational clinical trial. *J Thromb Haemost.* 2008;6:622-631. Prospectively studies 43 patients for emergency oral anticoagulation reversal using 25, 35, or 50 IU/kg PCC for baseline INR of 2 to 3.9, 4 to 6, or greater than 6, respectively. Vitamin K was administered to 88% of subjects prior to PCC dosing. The median INR of 3.2 was decreased to 1.2 in 30 minutes after PCC therapy, and maintained in the range of 1.1 to 1.5 for 48 hours. Plasma levels were FII, FVII, FIX, FX, protein C and protein S were rapidly restored and maintained above 50% for 48 hours. (Ref. 74)

Slichter SJ. Relationship between platelet count and bleeding risk in thrombocytopenic patients. *Transfus Med Rev.* 2004;18:153-167. A comprehensive review on platelet transfusion, largely based on clinical trials in chronic thrombocytopenia. Clinically available platelet concentrates, indications, and potential side effects (e.g., alloimmunization) are discussed. Threshold platelet concentration to prevent spontaneous bleeding (maintenance of vascular integrity) is surprisingly low (~7 × 10⁹/L), and platelet transfusion is used to maintain the level above 10 × 10⁹/L. In most invasive procedures, the minimal platelet count is presumed to be 50 × 10⁹/L, but the site/extent of vascular injury and the presence of antiplatelet agents should also be considered. (Ref. 18)

Roback JD, Caldwell S, Carson J, et al. Evidence-based practice guidelines for plasma transfusion. *Transfusion.* 2010;50:1227-1239. Evidence-based guidelines for plasma transfusion. The panel recommended the use of plasma in patients requiring massive transfusion. However, the panel was unable to agree on increasing the transfusion ratio of plasma to RBC above 1:3 during massive transfusion or on the use of plasma in surgical patients without massive transfusion. (Ref. 30)

References

1. Counts RB. A history of transfusion medicine. In: Spiess BD, Spence RK, Shander A, eds. *Perioperative Transfusion Medicine.* Baltimore: Lippincott Williams & Wilkins; 1997:3-12.
2. Spahn DR. Blood substitutes. Artificial oxygen carriers: perfluorocarbon emulsions. *Crit Care.* 1999;3:R93-R97.
3. Jahr JS, Walker V, Manoochehri K. Blood substitutes as pharmacotherapies in clinical practice. *Curr Opin Anaesthesiol.* 2007;20:325-330.
4. Therapies TFoP-oBTaA. Practice guidelines for perioperative blood transfusion and adjuvant therapies. *Anesthesiology.* 2006;105:198-208.
5. Spahn DR, Cerny V, Coats TJ, et al. Management of bleeding following major trauma: a European guideline. *Crit Care.* 2007;11:R17.
6. Association GM. Cross-sectional guidelines for therapy with blood components and plasma derivatives. 4th revised edition. *Transfus Med Hemother.* 2009;36:419-436.
7. Rossaint R, Bouillon B, Cerny V, et al. Management of bleeding following major trauma: an updated European guideline. *Crit Care.* 2010;14:R52.
8. Harris SB, Hillyer CD. Blood manufacturing: component preparation, storage, and transportation. In: Hillyer CD, ed. *Blood Banking and Transfusion Medicine: Basic Principles and Practice.* 2nd ed. Philadelphia: Churchill-Livingstone, Elsevier; 2007:185-187.
9. Blumberg N, Heal JM. Blood transfusion immunomodulation: the silent epidemic. *Arch Pathol Lab Med.* 1998;122:117-119.
10. Murphy MF. New variant Creutzfeldt-Jakob disease (nvCJD): the risk of transmission by blood transfusion and the potential benefit of leukocyte-reduction of blood components. *Transfus Med Rev.* 1999;13:75-83.
11. Goldberg MA, McCutchen JW, Jove M, et al. A safety and efficacy comparison study of two dosing regimens of epoetin alfa in patients undergoing major orthopedic surgery. *Am J Orthop (Belle Mead NJ).* 1996;25:544-552.
12. Goodnough LT, Brecher ME, Kanter MH, AuBuchon JP. Transfusion medicine. First of two parts—blood transfusion. *N Engl J Med.* 1999;340:438-447.
13. Goodnough LT, Brecher ME, Kanter MH, AuBuchon JP. Transfusion medicine. Second of two parts—blood conservation. *N Engl J Med.* 1999;340:525-533.
14. Aarts PA, van den Broek SA, Prins GW, Kuiken GD, Sixma JJ, Heethaar RM. Blood platelets are concentrated near the wall and red blood cells, in the center in flowing blood. *Arteriosclerosis.* 1988;8:819-824.
15. Tanaka KA, Key NS, Levy JH. Blood coagulation: hemostasis and thrombin regulation. *Anesth Analg.* 2009;108:1433-1446.
16. Stroncek DF, Rebulla P. Platelet transfusions. *Lancet.* 2007;370:427-438.
17. George JN. Platelets. *Lancet.* 2000;355:1531-1539.
18. Slichter SJ. Relationship between platelet count and bleeding risk in thrombocytopenic patients. *Transfus Med Rev.* 2004;18:153-167.
19. Hiippala ST, Myllyla GJ, Vahtera EM. Hemostatic factors and replacement of major blood loss with plasma-poor red cell concentrates. *Anesth Analg.* 1995;81:360-365.
20. Sihler KC, Napolitano LM. Massive transfusion: new insights. *Chest.* 2009;136:1654-1667.
21. Sperry JL, Ochoa JB, Gunn SR, et al. An FFP:PRBC transfusion ratio >/= 1:1.5 is associated with a lower risk of mortality after massive transfusion. *J Trauma.* 2008;65:986-993.
22. Nuttall GA, Oliver WC, Santrach PJ, et al. Efficacy of a simple intraoperative transfusion algorithm for nonerythrocyte component utilization after cardiopulmonary bypass. *Anesthesiology.* 2001;94:773-781.
23. Kozek-Langenecker S. Management of massive operative blood loss. *Minerva Anestesiol.* 2007;73:401-415.
24. Slichter SJ. Evidence-based platelet transfusion guidelines. *Hematology.* 2007;2007:172-178.
25. Fung MK, Downes KA, Shulman IA. Transfusion of platelets containing ABO-incompatible plasma: a survey of 3156 North American laboratories. *Arch Pathol Lab Med.* 2007;131:909-916.
26. Spiess BD, Royston D, Levy JH, et al. Platelet transfusions during coronary artery bypass graft surgery are associated with serious adverse outcomes. *Transfusion.* 2004;44:1143-1148.
27. Downes KA, Wilson E, Yomtovian R, Sarode R. Serial measurement of clotting factors in thawed plasma stored for 5 days. *Transfusion.* 2001;41:570.
28. Stanworth SJ, Brunskill SJ, Hyde CJ, McClelland DB, Murphy MF. Is fresh frozen plasma clinically effective? A systematic review of randomized controlled trials. *Br J Haematol.* 2004;126:139-152.
29. Segal JB, Dzik WH. Paucity of studies to support that abnormal coagulation test results predict bleeding in the setting of invasive procedures: an evidence-based review. *Transfusion.* 2005;45:1413-1425.
30. Roback JD, Caldwell S, Carson J, et al. Evidence-based practice guidelines for plasma transfusion. *Transfusion.* 2010;50:1227-1239.
31. O'Shaughnessy DF, Atterbury C, Bolton Maggs P, et al, British Committee for Standards in Haematology BTTF. Guidelines for the use of fresh-frozen plasma, cryoprecipitate and cryosupernatant. *Br J Haematol.* 2004;126:11-28.
32. Chowdhury P, Saayman AG, Paulus U, Findlay GP, Collins PW. Efficacy of standard dose and 30 mL/kg fresh frozen plasma in correcting laboratory parameters of haemostasis in critically ill patients. *Br J Haematol.* 2004;125:69-73.
33. Hiippala S. Replacement of massive blood loss. *Vox Sang.* 1998;74(Suppl 2):399-407.
34. Gonzalez EA, Moore FA, Holcomb JB, et al. Fresh frozen plasma should be given earlier to patients requiring massive transfusion. *J Trauma.* 2007;62:112-119.
35. Maegele M, Lefering R, Paffrath T, Tjardes T, Simanski C, Bouillon B. Red-blood-cell to plasma ratios transfused during massive transfusion are associated with mortality in severe multiple injury: a retrospective analysis from the Trauma Registry of the Deutsche Gesellschaft fur Unfallchirurgie. *Vox Sang.* 2008;95:112-119.
36. Riskin DJ, Tsai TC, Riskin L, et al. Massive transfusion protocols: the role of aggressive resuscitation versus product ratio in mortality reduction. *J Am Coll Surg.* 2009;209:198-205.

37. Shaz BH, Dente CJ, Nicholas J, et al. Increased number of coagulation products in relationship to red blood cell products transfused improves mortality in trauma patients. *Transfusion*. 2010;50:493-500.

38. Scalea TM, Bochicchio KM, Lumpkins K, et al. Early aggressive use of fresh frozen plasma does not improve outcome in critically injured trauma patients. *Ann Surg*. 2008;248:578-584.

39. Snyder CW, Weinberg JA, McGwin Jr G, et al. The relationship of blood product ratio to mortality: survival benefit or survival bias? *J Trauma*. 2009;66:358-364.

40. Watson GA, Sperry JL, Rosengart MR, et al. Fresh frozen plasma is independently associated with a higher risk of multiple organ failure and acute respiratory distress syndrome. *J Trauma*. 2009; 67:221-230.

41. Schochl H, Nienaber U, Hofer G, et al. Goal-directed coagulation management of major trauma patients using thromboelastometry (ROTEM)-guided administration of fibrinogen concentrate and prothrombin complex concentrate. *Crit Care*. 2010;14:R55.

42. Shehata N, Kouroukis C, Kelton JG. A review of randomized controlled trials using therapeutic apheresis. *Transfus Med Rev*. 2002;16:200-229.

43. Fontana S, Kremer Hovinga JA, Lammle B, Mansouri Taleghani B. Treatment of thrombotic thrombocytopenic purpura. *Vox Sang*. 2006;90:245-254.

44. Pamphilon D. Viral inactivation of fresh frozen plasma. *Br J Haematol*. 2000;109:680-693.

45. Triulzi DJ. Transfusion-related acute lung injury: current concepts for the clinician. *Anesth Analg*. 2009;108:770-776.

46. Westphal M, James MF, Kozek-Langenecker S, Stocker R, Guidet B, Van Aken H. Hydroxyethyl starches: different products–different effects. *Anesthesiology*. 2009;111:187-202.

47. Kozek-Langenecker SA. Effects of hydroxyethyl starch solutions on hemostasis. *Anesthesiology*. 2005;103:654-660.

48. Delaney AP, Dan A, McCaffrey J, Finfer S. The role of albumin as a resuscitation fluid for patients with sepsis: a systematic review and meta-analysis. *Crit Care Med*. 2011;39:386-391.

49. Fenger-Eriksen C, Moore GW, Rangarajan S, Ingerslev J, Sorensen B. Fibrinogen estimates are influenced by methods of measurement and hemodilution with colloid plasma expanders. *Transfusion*. 2010;50:2571-2576.

50. Key NS, Negrier C. Coagulation factor concentrates: past, present, and future. *Lancet*. 2007;370:439-448.

51. Sorensen B, Bevan D. A critical evaluation of cryoprecipitate for replacement of fibrinogen. *Br J Haematol*. 2010;149:834-843.

52. Bolliger D, Gorlinger K, Tanaka KA. Pathophysiology and treatment of coagulopathy in massive hemorrhage and hemodilution. *Anesthesiology*. 2010;113:1205-1219.

53. Charbit B, Mandelbrot L, Samain E, et al. The decrease of fibrinogen is an early predictor of the severity of postpartum hemorrhage. *J Thromb Haemost*. 2007;5:266-273.

54. Blome M, Isgro F, Kiessling AH, et al. Relationship between factor XIII activity, fibrinogen, haemostasis screening tests and postoperative bleeding in cardiopulmonary bypass surgery. *Thromb Haemost*. 2005;93:1101-1107.

55. Bolliger D, Szlam F, Molinaro RJ, Rahe-Meyer N, Levy JH, Tanaka KA. Finding the optimal concentration range for fibrinogen replacement after severe haemodilution: an in vitro model. *Br J Anaesth*. 2009;102:793-799.

56. Karlsson M, Ternstrom L, Hyllner M, et al. Prophylactic fibrinogen infusion reduces bleeding after coronary artery bypass surgery. A prospective randomised pilot study. *Thromb Haemost*. 2009;102:137-144.

57. Rahe-Meyer N, Pichlmaier M, Haverich A, et al. Bleeding management with fibrinogen concentrate targeting a high-normal plasma fibrinogen level: a pilot study. *British Journal of Anaesthesia*. 2009; 102:785-792.

58. Fenger-Eriksen C, Jensen TM, Kristensen BS, et al. Fibrinogen substitution improves whole blood clot firmness after dilution with hydroxyethyl starch in bleeding patients undergoing radical cystectomy: a randomized, placebo-controlled clinical trial. *J Thromb Haemost*. 2009;7:795-802.

59. Lang T, Toller W, Gutl M, et al. Different effects of abciximab and cytochalasin D on clot strength in thrombelastography. *J Thromb Haemost*. 2004;2:147-153.

60. Manco-Johnson MJ, Dimichele D, Castaman G, et al. Pharmacokinetics and safety of fibrinogen concentrate. *J Thromb Haemost*. 2009;7:2064-2069.

61. Groner A. Reply. Pereira A. Cryoprecipitate versus commercial fibrinogen concentrate in patients who occasionally require a therapeutic supply of fibrinogen: risk comparison in the case of an emerging transfusion-transmitted infection. *Haematologica*. 2007;92: 846-849. Author reply: *Haematologica*. 2008;93:e24-e27.

62. Stanworth SJ. The evidence-based use of FFP and cryoprecipitate for abnormalities of coagulation tests and clinical coagulopathy. *Hematology Am Soc Hematol Educ Program*. 2007:179-186.

63. Hardy JF, Belisle S, Van der Linden P. Efficacy and safety of recombinant activated factor VII to control bleeding in nonhemophiliac patients: a review of 17 randomized controlled trials. *Ann Thorac Surg*. 2008;86:1038-1048.

64. Key NS, Christie B, Henderson N, Nelsestuen GL. Possible synergy between recombinant factor VIIa and prothrombin complex concentrate in hemophilia therapy. *Thromb Haemost*. 2002;88: 60-65.

65. Boffard KD, Riou B, Warren B, et al. Recombinant factor VIIa as adjunctive therapy for bleeding control in severely injured trauma patients: two parallel randomized, placebo-controlled, double-blind clinical trials. *J Trauma*. 2005;59:8-18.

66. Hauser CJ, Boffard K, Dutton R, et al. Results of the CONTROL trial: efficacy and safety of recombinant activated Factor VII in the management of refractory traumatic hemorrhage. *J Trauma*. 2010;69:489-500.

67. Mayer SA, Brun NC, Begtrup K, et al. Efficacy and safety of recombinant activated factor VII for acute intracerebral hemorrhage. *N Engl J Med*. 2008;358:2127-2137.

68. Gill R, Herbertson M, Vuylsteke A, et al. Safety and efficacy of recombinant activated factor VII: a randomized placebo-controlled trial in the setting of bleeding after cardiac surgery. *Circulation*. 2009;120:21-27.

69. O'Connell KA, Wood JJ, Wise RP, Lozier JN, Braun MM. Thromboembolic adverse events after use of recombinant human coagulation factor VIIa. *J Am Med Assoc*. 2006;295:293-298.

70. Levi M, Levy JH, Andersen HF, Truloff D. Safety of recombinant activated factor VII in randomized clinical trials. *N Engl J Med*. 2010;363:1791-1800.

71. Holland L, Warkentin TE, Refaai M, Crowther MA, Johnston MA, Sarode R. Suboptimal effect of a three-factor prothrombin complex concentrate (Profilnine-SD) in correcting supratherapeutic international normalized ratio due to warfarin overdose. *Transfusion*. 2009;49:1171-1177.

72. Tanaka KA, Szlam F, Dickneite G, Levy JH. Effects of prothrombin complex concentrate and recombinant activated factor VII on vitamin K antagonist induced anticoagulation. *Thrombosis Research*. 2008;122:117-123.

73. Riess HB, Meier-Hellmann A, Motsch J, Elias M, Kursten FW, Dempfle CE. Prothrombin complex concentrate (Octaplex) in patients requiring immediate reversal of oral anticoagulation. *Thromb Res*. 2007;121:9-16.

74. Pabinger I, Brenner B, Kalina U, Knaub S, Nagy A, Ostermann H. Prothrombin complex concentrate (Beriplex P/N) for emergency anticoagulation reversal: a prospective multinational clinical trial. *J Thromb Haemost*. 2008;6:622-631.

75. Mayer SA, Rincon F. Ultra-early hemostatic therapy for acute intracerebral hemorrhage. *Semin Hematol*. 2006;43:S70-S76.

76. Leissinger CA, Blatt PM, Hoots WK, Ewenstein B. Role of prothrombin complex concentrates in reversing warfarin anticoagulation: a review of the literature. *Am J Hematol*. 2008;83:137-143.

77. Stuklis RG, O'Shaughnessy DF, Ohri SK. Novel approach to bleeding in patients undergoing cardiac surgery with liver dysfunction. *Eur J Cardiothorac Surg*. 2001;19:219-220.

78. Bruce D, Nokes TJ. Prothrombin complex concentrate (Beriplex P/N) in severe bleeding: experience in a large tertiary hospital. *Crit Care*. 2008;12:R105.

79. Dusel CH, Grundmann C, Eich S, Seitz R, Konig H. Identification of prothrombin as a major thrombogenic agent in prothrombin complex concentrates. *Blood Coag Fibrin*. 2004;15:405-411.

80. Sniecinski RM, Chen EP, Tanaka KA. Reduced levels of fibrin (Antithrombin I) and anithrombin III underlie coagulopathy following complex cardiac surgery. *Blood Coag Fibrin*. 2008;19: 178-179.

81. Kleinman SH, Glynn SA, Lee TH, et al. A linked donor-recipient study to evaluate parvovirus B19 transmission by blood component transfusion. *Blood*. 2009;114:3677-3683.

82. Bauer KA, Rosenberg RD. Congenital antithrombin III deficiency: insights into the pathogenesis of the hypercoagulable state and its management using markers of hemostatic system activation. *American Journal of Medicine*. 1989;87:39S-43S.

83. Williams MR, D'Ambra AB, Beck JR, et al. A randomized trial of antithrombin concentrate for treatment of heparin resistance. *Ann Thorac Surg*. 2000;70:873-877.

84. Avidan MS, Levy JH, Scholz J, et al. A phase III, double-blind, placebo-controlled, multicenter study on the efficacy of recombinant human antithrombin in heparin-resistant patients scheduled to undergo cardiac surgery necessitating cardiopulmonary bypass. *Anesthesiology*. 2005;102:276-284.

85. Nicolaes GAF, Dahlback B. Factor V and thrombotic disease: description of a janus-faced protein. *Arteriosclerosis, Thrombosis & Vascular Biology*. 2002;22:530-538.

86. Liaw PCY, Esmon CT, Kahnamoui K, et al. Patients with severe sepsis vary markedly in their ability to generate activated protein C. *Blood*. 2004;104:3958-3964.

87. Cohen MJ, Bir N, Rahn P, et al. Protein C depletion early after trauma increases the risk of ventilator-associated pneumonia. *J Trauma*. 2009;67:1176-1181.

88. Riewald M, Petrovan RJ, Donner A, Mueller BM, Ruf W. Activation of endothelial cell protease activated receptor 1 by the protein C pathway. *Science*. 2002;296:1880-1882.

89. Bernard GR, Vincent JL, Laterre PF, et al, Recombinant human protein CWEiSSsg. Efficacy and safety of recombinant human activated protein C for severe sepsis. [comment]. *N Engl J Med*. 2001;344:699-709.

90. Griffin JH, Evatt B, Zimmerman TS, Kleiss AJ, Wideman C. Deficiency of protein C in congenital thrombotic disease. *J Clin Invest*. 1981;68:1370-1373.

91. Franchini M, Veneri D, Salvagno GL, Manzato F, Lippi G. Inherited thrombophilia. *Crit Rev Clin Lab Sci*. 2006;43:249-290.

92. Henry DA, Carless PA, Moxey AJ, et al. Anti-fibrinolytic use for minimising perioperative allogeneic blood transfusion. *Cochrane Database Syst Rev*. 2007:CD001886.

93. Fergusson DA, Hebert PC, Mazer CD, et al. A comparison of aprotinin and lysine analogues in high-risk cardiac surgery. [see comment]. *N Engl J Med*. 2008;358:2319-2331.

94. Ide M, Bolliger D, Taketomi T, Tanaka KA. Lessons from the aprotinin saga: current perspective on antifibrinolytic therapy in cardiac surgery. *J Anesth*. 2010;24:96-106.

95. Hvas AM, Sorensen HT, Norengaard L, Christiansen K, Ingerslev J, Sorensen B. Tranexamic acid combined with recombinant factor VIII increases clot resistance to accelerated fibrinolysis in severe hemophilia A. *J Thromb Haemost*. 2007;5:2408-2414.

96. Shakur H, Roberts R, Bautista R, et al. Effects of tranexamic acid on death, vascular occlusive events, and blood transfusion in trauma patients with significant haemorrhage (CRASH-2): a randomised, placebo-controlled trial. *Lancet*. 2010;376:23-32.

97. Furtmuller R, Schlag MG, Berger M, et al. Tranexamic acid, a widely used antifibrinolytic agent, causes convulsions by a gamma-aminobutyric acid(A) receptor antagonistic effect. *J Pharmacol Exp Ther*. 2002;301:168-173.

98. Carless PA, Henry DA, Moxey AJ, et al. Desmopressin for minimising perioperative allogeneic blood transfusion. *Cochrane Database Syst Rev*. 2004:CD001884.

99. Achneck HE, Sileshi B, Jamiolkowski RM, Albala DM, Shapiro ML, Lawson JH. A comprehensive review of topical hemostatic agents: efficacy and recommendations for use. *Ann Surg*. 2010; 251:217-228.

100. Ortel TL, Mercer MC, Thames EH, Moore KD, Lawson JH. Immunologic impact and clinical outcomes after surgical exposure to bovine thrombin. *Ann Surg*. 2001;233:88-96.

101. Wilde J, Teixeira P, Bramhall SR, Gunson B, Mutimer D, Mirza DF. Liver transplantation in haemophilia. *Br J Haematol*. 2002;117: 952-956.

102. Tripodi A, Salerno F, Chantarangkul V, et al. Evidence of normal thrombin generation in cirrhosis despite abnormal conventional coagulation tests. *Hepatology*. 2005;41:553-558.

103. Lisman T, Porte RJ. Rebalanced hemostasis in patients with liver disease: evidence and clinical consequences. *Blood*. 2010;116:878-885.

104. Tripodi A, Chantarangkul V, Primignani M, et al. The international normalized ratio calibrated for cirrhosis (INR(liver)) normalizes prothrombin time results for model for end-stage liver disease calculation. *Hepatology*. 2007;46:520-527.

105. Bolliger D, Sreeram G, Duncan A, et al. Prophylactic use of factor IX concentrate in a Jehovah's Witness patient. *Ann Thorac Surg*. 2009;88:1666-1668.

106. Neisser-Svae A, Bailey A, Gregori L, et al. Prion removal effect of a specific affinity ligand introduced into the manufacturing process of the pharmaceutical quality solvent/detergent (S/D)-treated plasma OctaplasLG. *Vox Sang*. 2009;97:226-233.

107. Giarratana MC, Rouard H, Dumont A, et al. Proof of principle for transfusion of in vitro-generated red blood cells. *Blood*. 2011;118: 5071-5079.

108. Ohashi K, Yokoyama T, Yamato M, et al. Engineering functional two- and three-dimensional liver systems in vivo using hepatic tissue sheets. *Nat Med*. 2007;13:880-885.

109. Ohashi K, Waugh JM, Dake MD, et al. Liver tissue engineering at extrahepatic sites in mice as a potential new therapy for genetic liver diseases. *Hepatology*. 2005;41:132-140.

110. Lin A, Sabnis A, Kona S, et al. Shear-regulated uptake of nanoparticles by endothelial cells and development of endothelial-targeting nanoparticles. *J Biomed Mater Res A*. 2010;93:833-842.

111. Persson E, Bolt G, Steenstrup TD, Ezban M. Recombinant coagulation factor VIIa—from molecular to clinical aspects of a versatile haemostatic agent. *Thromb Res*. 2010;125:483-489.

112. Dietrich W, Nicklisch S, Koster A, Spannagl M, Giersiefen H, van de Locht A. CU-2010—a novel small molecule protease inhibitor with antifibrinolytic and anticoagulant properties. *Anesthesiology*. 2009;110:123-130.

Chapter 37

ANTICOAGULANT AND ANTIPLATELET THERAPY

David Royston

Arterial and venous thrombosis are major causes of morbidity and mortality. Venous thromboembolism (VTE) is the leading cause of preventable in-hospital mortality. Deep vein thrombosis (DVT) leading to VTE causes as many as 300,000 deaths annually in the United States and approximately 300,000 within the European Union as well.[1,2]

Arterial thrombosis is the most common cause of myocardial infarction (MI), ischemic stroke, and limb gangrene. Arterial thrombi, which typically form under high shear conditions, consist of platelet aggregates held together by small amounts of fibrin. Because of the predominance of platelets, strategies to inhibit arterial thrombogenesis focus mainly on drugs that block platelet function, but include anticoagulants for prevention of cardioembolic events in patients with atrial fibrillation or mechanical heart valves.

DVT can lead to pulmonary thromboembolism (PE), which can be fatal, and to postphlebitic syndrome. Venous thrombi, which form under low shear, are composed mainly of fibrin and trapped red cells, with relatively few platelets. With the predominance of fibrin in venous thrombi, anticoagulants are the agents of choice for the prevention and treatment of DVT and VTE.

The incidence of VTE is about 20% higher in men than in women and increases with age in both sexes. Asian and Hispanic populations have a lower risk of VTE, whereas Caucasians and African Americans have a 2.5-fold higher risk.

NORMAL PLATELET FUNCTION AND HEMOSTASIS

A brief overview of the hemostatic system is provided herein as background for consideration of antiplatelet and anticoagulant drugs; further detail is provided in Chapters 35 and 36. The initial response of the hemostatic system to tissue or endothelial injury is to produce a platelet plug (primary hemostasis). Platelets have multiple surface receptors, which when stimulated produce a shape change involving the energy-dependent actin-myosin system. Principal among these receptors are the glycoprotein Ib (GpIb) receptor, which binds to von Willebrand factor (vWF). This factor is expressed on the abluminal side of endothelial cells and is thus exposed if there is endothelial injury. The GpIb receptor is expressed at all times. There are also receptors for adenosine diphosphate (ADP), thrombin, and thromboxane A_2. These receptors principally allow a feedback amplification pathway to enhance the generation of the primary hemostatic plug.

With the shape change, the surface of the platelet also changes with expression of a second binding site, the glycoprotein IIb/IIIa (GpIIb/IIIa) receptor. GpIIb/IIIa receptors bind fibrinogen to provide bridging between adjacent platelets. In addition, the surface of the platelet becomes electronegatively charged and expresses binding sites for factor V, an essential cofactor in the generation of thrombin.

MECHANISMS OF THROMBIN AND FIBRIN GENERATION

The coagulation phase of hemostasis involves generation by thrombin of fibrin, which binds and stabilizes the weak platelet hemostatic plug. Thrombin is highly specific in cleaving fibrinogen at only two arginine sites. The active site of thrombin is surrounded by negatively charged amino acid residues and away from this are positively charged exosites. This arrangement allows the very specific alignment and cleavage of fibrinogen (Figure 37-1).

There are no covalent bonds holding platelets together during the formation of the primary hemostatic plug. If left in this state, the platelet plug disintegrates in a few hours, resulting in late bleeding. The process of blood coagulation, with soluble factors in the blood entering into a cascade of protease activation that leads to the formation of fibrin, is localized to the site where the original platelet plug was formed. This localization is achieved by two methods. First, the chain of reactions that leads to conversion of fibrinogen to fibrin is restricted to a surface, such as platelet phospholipids. Second, a series of inhibitors constrains the reaction to the site of injury and platelet deposition.

Historically the blood coagulation system is divided into two initiating pathways: the tissue factor (extrinsic) pathway and the contact factor (intrinsic) pathway. These pathways meet in a final common pathway whereby factor Xa converts prothrombin to thrombin, which then cleaves fibrinogen to fibrin. The prothrombin time (PT) is a plasma and test tube test of the integrity of the extrinsic pathway, and the activated clotting time (ACT) or activated partial thromboplastin time (aPTT) are tests of the intrinsic system for blood and plasma, respectively.

This model based on the concept of a waterfall or cascade is an over-simplification of the coagulation system, as proteins from each pathway influence one another. It is probably more correct to think of the coagulation system as an interactive network with carefully placed amplifiers and restraints.

Fibrin formation is a process of initiation and amplification. The specific properties of platelets and the coagulation system cooperate to ensure that fibrin formation occurs only at the localized site where it is required to initiate wound repair. This is achieved by a number of physicochemical means:

1. The surface of resting platelets contains acidic phospholipids such as phosphatidylserine that have their negatively charged pole directed inward. During irreversible shape change, this pole is flipped to the outside of the platelet to provide a negatively charged outer surface.
2. The coagulation system relies primarily on soluble factors synthesized in the liver that circulate in the plasma in an inactive, zymogen form and become active after proteolytic cleavage. Apart from factor XIII, which is a transglutaminase, all active factors are serine proteases related to the digestive enzyme trypsin. Other factors in the coagulation process, such as tissue factor, factor V, factor VIII, and high molecular weight kininogen (HK) act as cofactors.

Factors VII, IX, X, and prothrombin contain carboxylated glutamic acid residues at their N-terminal regions. Vitamin K acts as a cofactor for the enzyme that carboxylates glutamic acid, forming gamma-carboxy glutamic acid, with a resultant higher density of negative charges. This charged area interacts at the organizing surface of the platelet with ionized Ca^{2+}, acting as a bridge with the negative surface charge on the activated platelet.

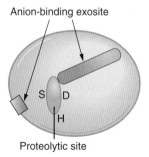

Anion-binding exosite

Proteolytic site

Figure 37-1 Thrombin structure. The thrombin active site (shown in *green*) is surrounded by a ring of negative charge and contains three conserved amino acid residues (serine 195 *[S]*, aspartic acid 102 *[D]*, and histidine 57 *[H]*). Fibrinogen interacts with the negatively charged ring around the active site as well as with the active site itself. Fibrinogen also interacts with the positively charged exosite shown on the right (anion-binding exosite), which is likely important in both orienting fibrinogen correctly within the active site and maintaining a strong bond between enzyme and substrate. Upon recognition of the correct substrate sequence, the hydroxyl of Ser195 cleaves the postarginine peptide bond. The anion-binding site on the right will also bind hirudin-like proteins. The anion-binding exosite to the left binds to glycosaminoglycans (heparan and chondroitin) and to heparin.

INDIRECT INHIBITORS OF THROMBIN GENERATION

Historical Considerations

Heparin, one of the oldest anticoagulant drugs currently still in widespread clinical use, was discovered in 1916 by a second-year medical student, Jay McLean, and Professor Howell at Johns Hopkins University. McLean was investigating procoagulant preparations when he isolated a fat-soluble phosphatide anticoagulant in canine liver for which Howell coined the term *heparin* (from *hepar*, Greek for liver). In the early 1920s, Howell isolated a water-soluble polysaccharide anticoagulant, which was also termed *heparin*, although it was distinct from the phosphatide preparations previously isolated.

Research on heparin continued into the 1930s. Jorpes described the structure of heparin in 1935, which made it possible for the Swedish company Vitrum AB to launch the first heparin product for intravenous use in 1936. Best perfected a technique for producing safe, nontoxic heparin that could be administered in a salt solution. The first human trials of heparin began in 1935, and by 1937 it was clear that heparin was a safe, easily available, and effective anticoagulant. The U.S. Food and Drug Administration (FDA) first approved heparin products in the 1940s.

Heparins

Heparins are available as unfractionated heparin (UFH) and low molecular weight heparins (LMWHs), which are chemical modifications of unfractionated heparin. The pharmacology of both has been extensively reviewed.[3-7]

UNFRACTIONATED HEPARIN

UFH is a naturally occurring glycosaminoglycan. It is a negatively charged sulfated polysaccharide formed from alternating residues of D-glucosamine and L-iduronic acid. Heparin is mostly located in lung, intestine, and liver in mammals. Standard preparations are derived from either porcine intestine or bovine lung and prepared as calcium or sodium salts. The number and sequence of the saccharides are variable, producing a heterogeneous collection of polysaccharides. Molecular weights range from 3000 to 30,000 Da, with a mean of 15,000 Da representing 40 to 50 saccharides in length. There is no apparent difference between any of the available forms of UFH with respect to pharmacology or anticoagulant profile.[4]

MECHANISM OF ACTION

Numerous physiologic actions have been proposed for heparin. Heparin has a direct antiinflammatory action in humans and a wide spectrum of interactions with various enzymes, hormones, biogenic amines, and plasma proteins. The role of heparin as an antiinflammatory agent is strengthened when one considers that heparin alone has no effects on coagulation and is found in lower orders of the animal kingdom, such as molluscs, which lack a coagulation system.

Heparin alone has no anticoagulant activity but requires a plasma cofactor, originally designated antithrombin III, and now simply called *antithrombin* or *AT*. AT has a low level of intrinsic anticoagulant activity, mediated by an arginine center that binds to the catalytic serine of proteases of the coagulation cascade. The arginine provides a strong positive charge to facilitate binding.

Binding of heparin to AT is highly specific via a pentasaccharide sequence found in about one third of molecules and is reversible. Binding of heparin and subsequent anticoagulant activity depend on saccharide chain length (Figure 37-2). The binding of AT to thrombin is suicidal to the thrombin-antithrombin (T-AT) complex but the heparin molecule is able to dissociate from this complex unchanged. Inhibition of thrombin activation also prevents feedback by thrombin on factors V and VIII, which normally amplifies the clotting cascade.

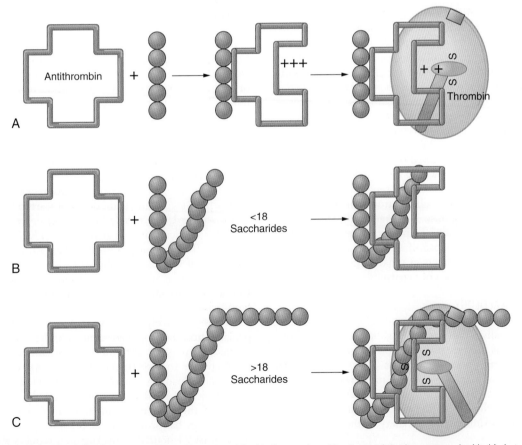

Figure 37-2 Effects of heparin chain length on antithrombin (AT) and its binding to thrombin. In panel **A**, the pentasaccharide binds to AT to induce a conformational change, but the arginine-derived electropositivity (+++) remains to reduce affinity for thrombin. With increasing saccharide chain length contributing more anionic charge, this effect is reduced, as shown in panel **B**. The most avid reaction with thrombin requires heparin binding, not only to AT but also to thrombin itself, at the anionic binding site that normally binds glycosaminoglycans (shown as a lavender box) to form a ternary complex. Only heparin moieties with more than 18 saccharides are able to do this, as shown in panel **C**.

In contrast, inhibition of factors IXa, Xa, and XIIa requires only that heparin bind AT to form the heparin-AT complex.[4] This explains why LMWHs and the synthetic pentasaccharide fondaparinux act as inhibitors of factor Xa but not necessarily of thrombin.

Heparin has actions in addition to anticoagulant effects mediated via AT. At high blood levels (>4 IU/mL) heparin is capable of binding heparin cofactor II, potentiating its inactivation of bound activated thrombin.[8] This action does not require the specific AT binding site but does require heparins of greater than 7200 Da or 24 saccharide units in length. The clinical importance of this action is unclear, but it might account for the need for higher doses of heparin to inhibit clot-bound thrombin. Much higher levels of heparin are needed to prevent the extension of venous thrombosis compared to those required to inhibit initiation of thrombosis.[3,4]

Heparin also stimulates release of tissue factor plasma inhibitor (TFPI), which binds and neutralizes the tissue factor–VIIa complex, reducing prothrombinase production via the extrinsic pathway. Plasma concentrations of TFPI rise two- to six-fold following injection of UFH and LMWH.

Heparin also impairs platelet aggregation mediated by vWF and collagen, and inhibits platelet function by direct binding to platelets. The higher molecular weight heparins interfere most with platelet function.[9] These actions might contribute to heparin-induced hemorrhage by a mechanism separate from its anticoagulant actions.

METABOLISM AND ELIMINATION

Elimination of heparin is nonlinear and occurs by two separate processes. The rapid saturable phase of heparin clearance is thought to be due to cellular degradation. Macrophages internalize heparin, then depolymerize and desulfate it; saturation occurs when all receptors have been utilized and further clearance depends on new receptor synthesis. This process accounts for the poor bioavailability after low-dose subcutaneous injection, in that the slow rate of absorption barely exceeds the capacity of cellular degradation. Significant plasma levels can only be achieved once these cellular receptors have been saturated following a loading dose. The slower phase of heparin elimination is due to renal excretion. As the dose of heparin is increased, elimination half-life increases and the anticoagulant response is exaggerated. At a dose of 25 U/kg the half-life is about 30 minutes, increasing to about 150 minutes with a bolus dose of 400 U/kg. There are no consistent reports of the effects of renal or hepatic dysfunction on the pharmacokinetics of heparin.[3,4]

CLINICAL PHARMACOLOGY

Pharmacokinetics and Pharmacodynamics

Heparins are usually administered by subcutaneous or intravenous injection as they are poorly absorbed from the gastrointestinal tract and cause hematomas after intramuscular injection. Intravenous injection is the preferred route for a rapid anticoagulant effect; however, similar levels of anticoagulation can be achieved by the subcutaneous route with a delayed time to maximum effect.[4] Safety of the two routes is comparable.

There is great variability in plasma concentration of heparin in relation to dose. After intravenous injection, more than 50% of heparin circulates bound to plasma proteins, including platelet factor 4, histidine-rich glycoprotein,

vitronectin, fibronectin, and vWF. The first three of these neutralize heparin activity and its bioavailability. Increased levels of these proteins might account for heparin resistance sometimes seen in malignancy and inflammatory disorders.[3] Plasma levels also decline rapidly due to redistribution and uptake by endothelial cells and macrophages.

Therapeutic Effects

Heparin is given to reduce thrombin generation and activity and therefore 'anticoagulate' the patient. The therapeutic target dose depends on the indication. For example, the degree of anticoagulation required to prevent thrombosis in a hemodialysis system is not as great as that required in cardiopulmonary bypass. Typically effectiveness of the dose is assessed at regular intervals using a coagulation test initiated by contact activation. The plasma version of this is the activated partial thromboplastin time (aPTT), which measures the effect of heparin on thrombin and factors IXa and Xa. The therapeutic range most commonly quoted is aPTT between 1.5 and 2.5 times the control value. However, commercially available kits for measurement of aPTT differ in their sensitivity to heparins. The whole blood version of the aPTT usually used when higher doses are administered is the Automated or Activated Coagulation Time (ACT). This is the standard of care used in cardiac surgical practice; typically ACT is maintained above 400-480 seconds. As there is a marked variation in response between individuals to the anticoagulant effect of a fixed dose of unfractionated heparin, regular monitoring of anticoagulation is routine.

CLINICAL USE

For thromboembolic prophylaxis, UFH is administered either as "low dose" (5000 U subcutaneously 8 or 12 hourly) or "adjusted dose" (3500 U 8 or 12 hourly adjusted to maintain aPTT about 3 to 5 seconds above control). For treatment of established thromboembolic disease, full therapeutic doses of heparin are used either by intravenous infusion or subcutaneous injection following an intravenous loading dose. Long-term heparin therapy is only used during pregnancy (unlike warfarin, neither UFH nor LMWH are able to cross the placenta) and for recurrent thromboembolic complications whilst taking adequate doses of warfarin.

Low-dose UFH is safe and effective prophylactic treatment for surgical patients at risk for VTE. Low-dose subcutaneous UFH produces a greater than 50% reduction in the incidence of venous thrombosis, and fatal and nonfatal PE.[10] Although this is associated with an increased incidence of wound hematoma, there was no increase in major or fatal hemorrhage.

Whilst relatively low doses of heparin are sufficient to provide thromboprophylaxis, much higher concentrations are needed to prevent thrombus propagation. Recommended regimens for the treatment of DVT with UFH include an intravenous loading dose of 5000 to 10,000 U then a continuous infusion of 1300 U per hour, adjusted to maintain aPTT 1.5 to 2.5 times control. This should be continued until warfarin therapy has prolonged the PT into the therapeutic range for at least 24 hours.[11] This regimen reduces the recurrence of venous thrombosis and mortality from PE. The most common reason for failure of treatment is inadequate anticoagulation, particularly within the first 24 hours, which is overcome by the large intravenous loading dose.[11] These treatment protocols have been compared with twice-daily subcutaneous LMWHs without laboratory assessment, which is safer and more effective, with significant and important reductions in recurrence of thrombosis and major hemorrhage.[12]

ADVERSE EFFECTS
Until 2008, the standard of heparin potency was different between heparins marketed in North America, which used the United States Pharmacopeia (USP) standard and that of the World Health Organization's International Standard or International Unit. In 2008, the USP adopted new manufacturing controls for heparin, which included a modification to the reference standard for heparin unit dose. These changes were precipitated by a number of cases of severe hypotension, sometimes leading to death, reported in association with administration of heparin manufactured in China. In March 2008, the FDA identified "oversulfated chondroitin sulfate" (OSCS) as a contaminant in the heparin originating from China. This contaminant mimics heparin activity and behaved like UFH in standard USP tests. In vitro and in vivo studies showed that OSCS directly activates the kinin-kallikrein pathway in human plasma, which can lead to generation of bradykinin, a potent vasodilator.[13] In addition, OSCS induced generation of C3a and C5a, potent anaphylatoxins derived from complement proteins. Screening of plasma samples from various species indicated that swine and humans are sensitive to the effects of OSCS in a similar manner. OSCS-containing heparin and synthetically derived OSCS induce hypotension associated with kallikrein activation when administered by intravenous infusion in swine. Adopting the WHO IU standards and introducing other safeguards should allow early detection of this contaminant.

The new standardized heparin now has a different strength that results in about a 10% reduction in "anticoagulant" potency compared to the previous USP standard. The current WHO standard has a potency of 122 IU/mg heparin. The reduced potency should have no clinical effect in that dosing regimens are tailored to individual patient needs.

Hemorrhage
Although hemorrhage is rare in patients on prophylactic doses of either UFH or LMWHs, it is a frequent complication of therapeutic heparin therapy. With comparable doses, risks are similar using either continuous intravenous or subcutaneous route of administration.[3,4] Many patient factors increase the risk of hemorrhage, including length of treatment, presence of cardiac, hepatic or renal dysfunction, aspirin or other antiplatelet drug therapy and recent surgery, trauma, or invasive procedures. Approximately 30% of patients who suffer anticoagulant-related hemorrhage are found to have previously undiagnosed predisposing lesions, particularly of the gastrointestinal and genitourinary tracts. The incidence of major bleeding in anticoagulated patients has been estimated as approximately 5%. The estimated daily frequency of fatal, major, and all types of hemorrhage in patients receiving therapeutic anticoagulation is 0.05%, 0.8%, and 2%, respectively. This is approximately twice the level expected in the absence of anticoagulation.[14]

Thrombocytopenia
Heparin-induced thrombocytopenia (HIT) is a relatively common complication with an incidence of 1.1% and 2.3% of patients receiving therapeutic doses of intravenous porcine and bovine heparin, respectively. Affected patients are generally receiving high doses of UFH, but rare cases have been attributed to low-dose subcutaneous heparin prophylaxis or to flushing lines with heparin. The risk of HIT is less with LMWH than with UFH, perhaps due to the lesser interaction with platelets. Two distinct clinical syndromes have been described.[15] Type I involves mild thrombocytopenia with platelet count rarely less than 100×10^9/L that occurs during the first few days of treatment and usually recovers rapidly even if heparin is continued. Patients are normally asymptomatic and no specific treatment is required. The underlying mechanism probably involves the action of heparin as a mild platelet aggregator.

Type II HIT is characterized by a delayed onset of severe, progressive thrombocytopenia with platelet counts less than 100×10^9/L and often $<50 \times 10^9$/L. Platelet count does not recover unless heparin therapy is stopped and recurs promptly if heparin is restarted. Recovery of platelet count usually occurs within a week but can occasionally be prolonged. An immune mechanism has been suggested in which heparin binds to platelet factor 4 to stimulate production of an IgG antibody. This antibody binds the heparin-platelet factor 4 complex, which is capable of binding to platelets to produce two separate effects. First, the immune complexes coat platelets and increase their removal from the circulation by the reticuloendothelial system. Second, the immune complexes activate platelets and the coagulation cascade, leading to a hypercoagulable state.[15] Hemorrhage is uncommon and resistance to anticoagulation can occur due to heparin-induced release of platelet factor 4. A high index of suspicion is necessary, because only immediate withdrawal of heparin reduces mortality and morbidity. A clinical score system (4 T's) as an aid (Table 37-1) has been validated in clinical practice.[16] The most serious complication associated with type II HIT is new thromboembolic events due to platelet-rich thrombi that continue to form until the heparin is withdrawn. Arterial and venous thrombosis occur either alone or together, and multiple sites are often involved. In patients receiving therapeutic doses of porcine heparin, 0.4% exhibited manifestations of thrombosis, most commonly lower limb thrombosis, thrombotic cerebrovascular events, or acute myocardial infarction.

MISCELLANEOUS
Heparin administration can cause anaphylactic reactions, osteoporosis following long-term high dose therapy, suppression of aldosterone synthesis, delayed transient alopecia, priapism, and rebound hyperlipidemia on withdrawal of heparin.

Low Molecular Weight Heparin

BASIC PHARMACOLOGY
Structure Activity
LMWHs are produced from UFH by depolymerization. The resulting marked changes in the properties of LMWHs leads to their clinical advantages over UFH.[5,6] LMWHs have mean molecular weights of 4000 to 6500 Da, although the range is 2000 to 10,000 Da. The production methods used and source of UFH lead to significant variations between different commercial preparations (Table 37-2). LMWHs differ in the distribution of their fragment molecular weights, potency (anti-Xa, antithrombin, and anticoagulant activities), and

Table 37-1. Scoring System for Diagnosing Type II Heparin-Induced Thrombocytopenia (HIT)*

4 T'S	2 POINTS	1 POINT	0 POINT
Thrombocytopenia	Platelet count fall >50% and platelet nadir >20 × 10⁹/L	Platelet count fall 30%-50% or platelet nadir 10-19 × 10⁹/L	Platelet count fall <30% or platelet nadir <10 × 10⁹/L
Timing of platelet count fall	Clear onset between days 5 and 10 or platelet fall 1 day or less (prior heparin exposure within 30 days)	Consistent with days 5-10 fall, but not clear (e.g., missing platelet counts); onset after day 10 or fall 1 day or less (prior heparin exposure 30-100 days ago)	Platelet count fall <4 days without recent exposure
Thrombosis or other sequelae	New thrombosis (confirmed); skin necrosis; acute systemic reaction postintravenous unfractionated heparin bolus	Progressive or recurrent thrombosis; nonnecrotizing (erythematous) skin lesions; suspected thrombosis (not proven)	None
Other causes for thrombocytopenia	None apparent	Possible	Definite

*With a total score of 6-8, the probability is high (>80%), intermediate with a score of 4-5, and low (<5%) with a score of 0-3.[16]

Table 37-2. Preparations of Low Molecular Weight Heparin

PREPARATION	METHOD OF PRODUCTION	AVERAGE MOLECULAR MASS (DA)	2000-6000 DALTONS (%)
Nadroparin	Nitrous acid depolymerization and fractionation	4200	85
Enoxaparin	Benzoylation followed by alkaline depolymerization	3900	75
Dalteparin	Nitrous acid depolymerization and gel filtration	5700	80
Tinzaparin	Depolymerization with heparinase	6000	64
Certoparin	Depolymerization with isoamylnitrate	5100	63
Ardeparin	Peroxidative cleavage	6000	
Reviparin	Nitrous acid depolymerization and chromatographic separation	4000	

Table 37-3. Properties of Various Low Molecular Weight Heparins Compared to Unfractionated Heparin

PREPARATION	POTENCY Anti-Xa Activity (Unit/mg)	Anti-Xa to IIa Ratio	HALF-LIFE (MIN)	BIOAVAILABILITY (%)
Unfractionated Heparin		1	30-150	10-20
Nadroparin	95	3.6:1	132-162	89
Enoxaparin	105	3.8:1	129-180	91
Dalteparin	130	2.7:1	119-139	87
Tinzaparin	83	1.9:1	111	90
Certoparin	88	2.0:1	240	90
Ardeparin	100	1.9:1	200	90
Reviparin	130	3.6:1	180	90

consequently in their biodynamic patterns, recommended doses, and efficacy/safety ratio (Table 37-3).[7]

MECHANISM OF ACTION

The molecular weight profiles of LMWHs vary significantly, so their anticoagulant properties are not identical.[17] The exact mechanisms underlying the anticoagulant effects of LMWH remain uncertain. The proportion of LMWH containing the critical pentasaccharide responsible for binding AT is less than in the parent UFH.[5,6] The reduced amounts of this pentasaccharide in LMWH results in less inhibition of thrombin via AT in vitro. However, the heparin-AT complex is able to inhibit Xa and this action remains intact in LMWH. Although LMWHs have a weak anti-IIa action, their high bioavailability and long half-life mean that the anti-Xa action is four times greater than for UFH. Potency of LMWHs is further increased by their resistance to inactivation by platelet factor 4 and by lack of protein binding. Like UFH, the main action of LMWHs is to prevent formation of prothrombinase and amplification of the coagulation cascade.

METABOLISM AND ELIMINATION

LMWHs do not bind to endothelial cells or macrophages, and so are not subject to the rapid uptake that UFH suffers. Similar to UFH they are partially metabolized by desulfation and depolymerization. The affinity of plasma proteins for LMWHs is much less than for UFH so that only 10% is protein bound. This increased bioavailability ensures a more predictable anticoagulant action. LMWHs have nearly complete bioavailability at all doses when given by subcutaneous injection, compared with 40% for low-dose subcutaneous UFH. Urinary excretion of anti-Xa activity for enoxaparin, dalteparin, and nadroparin, all given at doses for prevention of venous thrombosis, is between 3% and 10% of the injected dose. However, these LMWHs differ in the extent of their nonrenal clearance, resulting in different apparent elimination half-life values and relative apparent bioavailability. When given at thromboprophylactic doses, LMWHs do not significantly cross the placenta. Although clearance of LMWH depends on renal excretion, producing a half-life two to four times as long as for UFH, effects of renal dysfunction are not clinically apparent for creatinine clearance greater than 15 mL/min.

CLINICAL PHARMACOLOGY

LMWHs are as safe and effective as UFH in placebo controlled and comparative trials. Metaanalysis of these trials suggests low-dose LMWHs are slightly superior to low-dose UFH, particularly in reducing the incidence of PE.[18] LMWHs given as prophylaxis cause an increase in wound hematomas but no change in the incidence of hemorrhage. In contrast, a significant reduction in major hemorrhage is seen when LMWHs are used to treat established thrombosis.[6,11]

Pharmacokinetics

Because LMWHs are mainly administered subcutaneously, compared to UFH they are almost completely absorbed and, in contrast to UFH, exhibit linear pharmacokinetics with proportionality between anti-Xa (and anti-IIa in some cases), plasma activity and dose, and stationary distribution volume and clearance processes when the dosage is increased. Unlike UFH, their distribution volume is close to the blood volume.

Pharmacodynamics

Because of differences between LMWHs, the clinical profile of a given LMWH cannot be extrapolated to another or generalized to the whole LMWH family. These differences also lead to major problems in providing a reference standard to assess potency. This has a huge impact on licensing generic versions of the currently marketed drugs.

ADVERSE EFFECTS

The principal adverse effect of LMWH is hemorrhage. Unlike UFH there is no antidote such as protamine. Protamine reduces some anticoagulant effects of LMWH but is itself a drug with significant side effects. LMWHs have a high incidence of cross-reaction with the heparin-dependent antibody found in HIT. This can be monitored using a platelet aggregation test. If no cross-reaction occurs, successful anticoagulation can be safely undertaken with LMWH.

Pentasaccharide

BASIC PHARMACOLOGY
Structure Activity and Mechanism of Action

Fondaparinux is a synthetic preparation of the pentasaccharide sequence found in heparin manufactured to a high degree of purity and uniformity. The antithrombotic activity of fondaparinux is the result of AT-mediated selective inhibition of factor Xa. By selectively binding to AT, fondaparinux potentiates (about 300 times) the innate neutralization of factor Xa by AT. Fondaparinux does not interact with AT to inactivate thrombin and has no known effect on platelet function. At the recommended dose, fondaparinux does not affect fibrinolytic activity or bleeding time.

METABOLISM AND ELIMINATION

In healthy individuals with normal kidney function up to 75 years of age, about 80% of a single subcutaneous dose is eliminated in urine as unchanged drug in 72 hours with an elimination half-life of 17 to 21 hours. Since the majority of the administered dose is eliminated unchanged, metabolism of fondaparinux has not been investigated.

CLINICAL PHARMACOLOGY
Pharmacokinetics

Fondaparinux administered by subcutaneous injection is rapidly and completely absorbed (absolute bioavailability is 100%). In healthy adults, fondaparinux is highly (about 94%) and specifically bound to AT, and is thus mainly confined to the blood volume. This is reflected in the apparent volume of distribution of 7 to 11 L. It does not bind significantly to other plasma proteins (including platelet factor 4) or red blood cells.

Pharmacodynamics

Anti-Xa activity is used to define the pharmacology of this agent. As with LMWH there is a need for a standard against which to calibrate this activity and this standard is unique to fondaparinux. Anti-Xa activity increases with increasing drug concentration, reaching maximum values in 2 to 3 hours.

Therapeutic Effects

Fondaparinux is licensed for VTE prevention in high-risk orthopedic surgery patients and in some countries for general surgical or medical patients. It also is licensed for treatment of acute DVT when administered in conjunction with a vitamin K antagonist. Fondaparinux appears more effective than LMWH for VTE prophylaxis in high-risk orthopedic patients.[19,20] It is as effective and safe as LMWH for prophylaxis in general surgical patients, and as heparin or LMWH for initial VTE treatment.[19,21-23]

SPECIAL POPULATIONS
Renal Impairment

Fondaparinux elimination is prolonged in patients with renal impairment in that the major route of elimination is urinary excretion of unchanged drug. In patients undergoing prophylaxis following elective hip surgery or hip fracture surgery, the clearance of fondaparinux is 25% lower in patients with mild renal impairment (creatinine clearance [CrCl] 50 to 80 mL/min), 40% lower in patients with moderate renal impairment (CrCl 30 to 50 mL/min), and 55% lower in patients with severe renal impairment (CrCl < 30 mL/min) compared to patients with normal renal function.

Hepatic Impairment

In patients with moderate hepatic impairment (Child-Pugh category B), small changes in pharmacokinetics but not pharmacodynamic parameters such as aPTT, PT/international normalized ratio (INR), and AT have been observed. Based on these data, no dosage adjustment is recommended for hepatic impairment. However, a higher incidence of hemorrhage has been noted in subjects with moderate hepatic impairment than in normal subjects.

Age and Frailty

Fondaparinux elimination is prolonged in patients older than 75 years with total clearance 25% lower compared to patients younger than 65 years. Total clearance is also decreased by 30% in patients weighing less than 50 kg.

EMERGING DEVELOPMENTS

Idraparinux is a second-generation pentasaccharide with greater half life (about 80 hours) than fondaparinux, achieved by replacing the sulfated groups on the pentasaccharide with other groups. It was as effective as a standard regimen of LMWH followed by an oral vitamin K antagonist in patients with DVT but not in those with pulmonary embolus.[24] A study comparing idraparinux with a vitamin K antagonist to prevent stroke in patients with atrial fibrillation (AMADEUS) was stopped early due to excess bleeding in the idraparinux arm[25] of the study. Primarily due to the risk of bleeding in patients undergoing long-term therapy, development of this agent was halted. However, the molecule has been modified further to add a biotin moiety to the pentasaccharide. This idrabiotaparinux is rapidly (<10 min) removed from the circulation following intravenous injection of avidin, an egg-derived biotin-binding protein with low antigenicity. Idrabiotaparinux is in clinical trials and should be available clinically in the next 2 to 3 years.

Vitamin K Antagonists

HISTORICAL CONSIDERATIONS

In the early 1920s, there was an outbreak of a previously unrecognized hemorrhagic cattle disease in the northern United States and Canada. A Canadian veterinary pathologist determined that the cattle were ingesting moldy sweet clover that functioned as a potent anticoagulant. In 1933, Link, working at the University of Wisconsin, isolated and characterized the hemorrhagic agent as 3,3'-methylenebis-(4-hydroxycoumarin), later named *dicoumarol*.

Over the next few years, numerous similar chemicals were found to have the same anticoagulant properties. The first drug in the class to be widely commercialized was dicoumarol itself, patented in 1941 and later used as a pharmaceutical. Link continued working on developing more potent coumarin-based anticoagulants for use as rodent poisons, resulting in warfarin in 1948. The name warfarin stems from the acronym WARF, for Wisconsin Alumni Research Foundation + the ending -arin indicating its link with coumarin. Studies on the use of warfarin as a therapeutic anticoagulant found it to be generally superior to dicoumarol, and in 1954 it was approved for medical use in humans. The exact mechanism of action remained unknown until it was demonstrated in 1978 that warfarin inhibits epoxide reductase and hence interferes with vitamin K metabolism.

BASIC PHARMACOLOGY

Mechanism of Action

Warfarin inhibits vitamin K–dependent synthesis of biologically active forms of clotting factors II, VII, IX, and X, as well as the regulatory factors protein C and protein S. The precursors of these factors require carboxylation of specific glutamic acid residues to allow the coagulation factors to bind to phospholipid surfaces such as that of the activated platelet. The enzyme that carries out carboxylation of glutamic acid is γ-glutamyl carboxylase. The carboxylation reaction proceeds only if this enzyme is able to convert reduced vitamin K (vitamin K hydroquinone) to vitamin K epoxide. The vitamin K epoxide is in turn recycled back to vitamin K and vitamin K hydroquinone by another enzyme, vitamin K epoxide reductase (VKOR; Figure 37-3). Warfarin inhibits epoxide reductase (specifically the VKORC1 subunit), thereby diminishing available vitamin K and vitamin K hydroquinone, which inhibits carboxylation activity of glutamyl carboxylase.

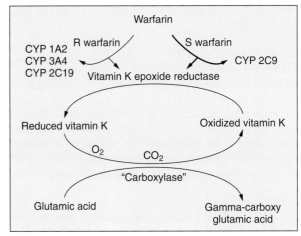

Figure 37-3 Mechanism of action of the vitamin K antagonist warfarin. The glutamate residues of certain coagulation factors require carboxylation by γ-glutamyl carboxylase (carboxylase) to achieve full activity. The carboxylation reaction proceeds only if the reduced form of vitamin K is available as a cosubstrate for conversion to vitamin K epoxide (oxidized vitamin K). The vitamin K epoxide is in turn recycled back to reduced vitamin K by vitamin K epoxide reductase. Warfarin inhibits the epoxide reductase thereby blocking the carboxylase reaction. Also shown are the principal cytochrome P450 enzymes in the metabolic pathways of the two enantiomers of warfarin. The S enantiomer is clinically and functionally most important and is metabolized by CYP 2C9.

Coagulation factors not carboxylated are incapable of binding to surface phospholipids and are thus biologically inactive.

METABOLISM

Warfarin consists of a racemic mixture of two active enantiomers—R and S forms. S-warfarin has five times the potency of the R-isomer with respect to vitamin K antagonism. The enantiomers of warfarin are differentially metabolized by human cytochrome P450 (CYP). R-warfarin is metabolized primarily by CYP 1A2 to 6- and 8-hydroxywarfarin, by CYP 3A4 to 10-hydroxywarfarin, and by carbonyl reductase to diastereoisomeric alcohols. S-warfarin is metabolized primarily by CYP 2C9 to 7-hydroxywarfarin (see Figure 37-3). The efficacy of warfarin is affected primarily when metabolism of S-warfarin is altered. Potential warfarin-drug interactions occur with any of a very wide range of drugs that are metabolized by these CYP isoforms; a large number of such interactions have been reported (Table 37-4).

CLINICAL PHARMACOLOGY

Pharmacokinetics

Warfarin has a long half-life (~35 hours) and therefore needs only be given once a day. It takes several days for warfarin to produce a therapeutic effect since it affects only newly synthesized but not circulating coagulation factors. This also means that it remains effective for several days after administration is stopped. Loading doses of warfarin of more than 5 mg produce a rapid decline in carboxyglutamyl factor VII (half-life 5-7 hours), resulting in an initial prolongation of the INR, but full antithrombotic effect does not occur until a significant reduction in prothrombin activity occurs (half-life about 60 hours) days later. Initiation of warfarin therapy can promote clot formation temporarily because anticoagulant protein C and protein S are also dependent on vitamin K activity. Warfarin causes reduced protein C levels (half-life 14 hours). In addition, reduced levels of protein S (half-life

Table 37-4. Warfarin Drug Interactions

DRUGS THAT CHANGE PLASMA CONCENTRATION OF WARFARIN	ADDITIVE ANTICOAGULANT EFFECT WITH NO CHANGE IN PLASMA CONCENTRATION	UNKNOWN MECHANISMS
Prolong Prothrombin Time/Increase Bleeding Risk	Inhibit vitamin K cycle	Ketoconazole/fluconazole
Inhibit S isomer clearance	Acetaminophen	Tamoxifen
Metronidazole	Antibiotics inhibiting gut vitamin K	Phenytoin
Sulphinpyrazone	Altered diet	Erythromycin
Trimethoprim		
Disulfiram	Inhibit coagulation and/or platelet function	
Inhibit R isomer clearance	Heparin	
Cimetidine	Aspirin/clopidogrel	
Omeprazole		
Ciprofloxacin		
Metronidazole		
Inhibit both S and R isomer clearance		
Amiodarone		
Reduce Prothrombin Time/Decrease Bleeding Risk		
Reduced absorption		Penicillins
Cholestyramine		
Increased metabolism		
Barbiturates		
Rifampicin		
Griseofulvin		
Carbamazepine		
St. John's Wort		

42 hours) lead to a reduction in activity of protein C (for which it is the cofactor) and therefore reduced inactivation of factor Va and factor VIIIa. The hemostasis system then becomes temporarily biased toward thrombus formation. Thus it is beneficial to coadminister heparin with initiation of warfarin therapy for 4 to 5 days until the full effect of warfarin has been achieved.

Pharmacodynamics

The effect of warfarin on blood coagulation is measured using an in vitro coagulation test, either the PT or the better standardized International Normalized Ratio (INR). Mathematically, INR = (PR)ISI, where PR is the prothrombin ratio (PT divided by the laboratory control PT) and ISI is the international sensitivity index of the thromboplastin reagent. Use of the INR eliminates variation in PT results between laboratories caused by differences in thromboplastin reagents.

There is little correlation between warfarin dose, serum concentration, and therapeutic effect between patients, necessitating individualized dosing guided by therapeutic monitoring of PT or INR. The pharmacokinetic and pharmacodynamic properties of warfarin as well as its narrow therapeutic index make it particularly susceptible to interactions with other drugs (see Table 37-4). This necessitates increased PT monitoring and warfarin dosing adjustments to maintain safe and effective anticoagulation.

THERAPEUTIC EFFECTS

Warfarin is used in a number of chronic thrombotic and thromboembolic prone conditions. Some of these, together with the recommended INR range for effective therapy or prophylaxis, are listed in Table 37-5.

ADVERSE EFFECTS

Hemorrhage

The only common side effect of warfarin is hemorrhage. The risk of severe bleeding is small but definite (a median annual

Table 37-5. Recommended International Normalized Ratio Targets, Warfarin Therapy and Prophylaxis

INDICATION	INR
Treatment of venous thrombosis. 6 weeks for calf vein and 3-6 months for proximal deep vein thrombosis	2.0-3.0
Treatment of pulmonary embolism for at least 6 months	2.0-3.0
Prevention of systemic embolism	2.0-3.0
Tissue heart valves	2.0-3.0
To prevent systemic embolism after acute myocardial infarction	2.0-3.0
To prevent recurrent myocardial infarction	2.5-3.5
Valvular heart disease	2.0-3.0
Atrial fibrillation. Older than age 75 years, consider lower range (1.5-2.5) due to increased risk of intracranial bleed	2.0-3.0
Bileaflet mechanical valve in aortic position	2.0-3.0
Mechanical prosthetic valves with cage	2.5-3.5
Systemic recurrent emboli	2.5-3.5

rate of 0.9% to 2.7% has been reported). Any benefit needs to outweigh this significant risk when warfarin is considered as a therapeutic measure. Risk of bleeding is augmented if the INR is out of range (due to accidental or deliberate overdose, or to drug interactions). This can cause hemoptysis, excessive bruising, bleeding from nose or gums, or blood in urine or stool. Risk of bleeding is increased when warfarin is combined with antiplatelet drugs such as clopidogrel, aspirin, or other nonsteroidal antiinflammatory drugs. The risk is also increased in older patients, those prone to falls, and those with trauma or undergoing procedures.

Warfarin Necrosis

A rare but serious complication is warfarin necrosis, which occurs more frequently shortly after commencing treatment in patients with a deficiency of protein C. Protein C requires vitamin K–dependent carboxylation for its activity. Because warfarin initially decreases protein C levels faster than the coagulation factors, it can paradoxically increase coagulation when treatment is first begun, leading to thrombosis typically manifesting as skin necrosis and peripheral gangrene.

Osteoporosis

Several studies have demonstrated a link between warfarin use and osteoporosis-related fracture. A retrospective study of Medicare recipients showed that warfarin use for more than 1 year was linked with a 60% increased risk of osteoporosis-related fracture in men; there was no association in women.[26] The mechanism was thought to be a combination of reduced intake of vitamin K, which is necessary for bone health, and inhibition by warfarin of vitamin K–mediated carboxylation of certain bone proteins, rendering them nonfunctional.

DRUG INTERACTIONS

Warfarin has become the archetypical drug associated with drug interactions and pharmacogenetic effects (see Chapters 4-6). Hundreds of drugs can increase the risk of hemorrhage in patients receiving warfarin, including some nonprescription drugs widely perceived as innocuous. Patients receiving warfarin are typically older and take other medications concomitantly, increasing the chances for drug interactions.

Major interactions occur that modify bleeding risk with warfarin:

- *Interference with platelet function:* Platelet aggregation is a crucial first step in primary hemostasis (see Chapter 35). Drugs that impair platelet function, especially acetylsalicylic acid (aspirin) and clopidogrel, increase the risk of major hemorrhage in patients taking warfarin without elevating the INR. Selective serotonin reuptake inhibitors can inhibit platelet aggregation by depleting platelet serotonin. They also inhibit CYP 2C9 and coadministration with warfarin increases the risk of major bleeding.
- *Injury to gastrointestinal mucosa:* Nonsteroidal antiinflammatory drugs cause dose- and duration-dependent gastrointestinal erosions in a substantial proportion of patients. Most of these erosions are asymptomatic, but the risk of hemorrhage increases with concomitant use of warfarin, even with therapeutic INR.
- *Altered gut vitamin K availability:* Many fruits and vegetables are rich in vitamin K and increase available vitamin K. Most important in this regard are leafy greens such as broccoli, Brussels sprouts, kale, and spinach. The response to warfarin also depends on synthesis of vitamin K_2 (menaquinone) by intestinal microflora. Many antibiotics alter the balance of gut flora, thereby enhancing the effect of warfarin. This response is highly variable. In addition, some antibiotics also inhibit metabolism of warfarin by CYP enzymes. These antibiotics include cotrimoxazole and metronidazole and, to a lesser extent, the macrolides and fluoroquinolones (see Table 37-4).
- *Interference with warfarin metabolism:* Many drugs modify warfarin activity through inhibition or enhancement of CYP metabolic pathways (see Table 37-4).
- *Interruption of the vitamin K cycle:* Some patients experience a rapid and dramatic rise in the INR following standard doses of acetaminophen. Recent evidence suggests that this interaction is caused by N-acetyl (p)-benzoquinoneimine,

the highly reactive acetaminophen metabolite that is responsible for hepatic injury following overdose that also inhibits vitamin K–dependent carboxylase activity.

PHARMACOGENETICS

Warfarin effect is determined partially by genetic factors. Three single nucleotide polymorphisms (SNPs), two in the *CYP2C9* gene and one in the *VKORC1* gene, play key roles in determining the effect of warfarin therapy. The normal variant of the *CYP2C9* gene is *1(star 1) and the two SNPs *2 and *3. The prevalence of each variant varies by race; 10% and 6% of Caucasians carry the *2 and *3 variants, respectively, but both variants are rare (<2%) in those of African or Asian descent. CYP 2C9*1 metabolizes warfarin normally, CYP2 C9*2 reduces warfarin metabolism by 30%, and CYP 2C9*3 reduces warfarin metabolism by 90%.

In the *VKORC1* SNP, the common G allele is replaced by the A allele. Because people with an A allele (or the "A haplotype") produce less VKORC1 than do those with the G allele (or the "non–A haplotype"), lower warfarin doses are needed to inhibit VKORC1 and to produce an anticoagulant effect in carriers of the A allele. The prevalence of these variants also varies by race, with 37% of Caucasians and 14% of Africans carrying the A allele.

Carriers of *CYP 2C9*2* and *CYP 2C9*3* require, on average, a 19% and 33% reduction, respectively, per allele in warfarin dose compared to those who carry the *1 allele. Carriers of the *VKORC1* A allele require, on average, a 28% reduction in warfarin dose compared to the G allele.

Compared to *VKORC1*, the *CYP 2C9* polymorphisms do not influence time to effective INR but do shorten the time taken to achieve INR greater than 4.

Major drug interactions come from the use of other drugs that use the same CYP pathways for their metabolism or that induce increased enzyme expression, leading to numerous potentially adverse drug interactions. More than 600 drugs reportedly interact with warfarin. The most common and most significant are listed in Table 37-4.

SPECIAL POPULATIONS

Pregnancy

Warfarin is contraindicated in pregnancy because it crosses the placenta and can cause bleeding in the fetus. Coumarin (e.g., warfarin) is also teratogenic.

DIRECT THROMBIN INHIBITORS

Intravenous Direct Thrombin Inhibitors

HISTORICAL PERSPECTIVE

In the 1980s and early 1990s there was considerable interest in developing protease inhibitors to control both inflammatory and hemostatic processes. Many of these products were based on biomolecules found in the mouthparts of the medicinal leech. For the antiinflammatory pathway a powerful antielastase called *eglin-c* was investigated. Control of the hemostasis focused on modifications to the direct thrombin inhibitor hirudin to produce a series of hirudin analogues or hirulogs. There was also interest in developing modifications to an agent called PPACK (D-Phe-Pro-Arg-chlormethylketone) to inhibit thrombin and other proteases.

BASIC PHARMACOLOGY
Structure Activity and Mechanism of Action

The hirudin-like molecules are made by recombinant technology in cultured yeast cells. Lepirudin is identical to natural hirudin except for the substitution of a leucine residue for isoleucine at the N-terminus and the absence of sulfation of tyrosine 63 of the 65 amino acid residue molecule. Desirudin is identical to hirudin but omits the sulfate on the tyrosine residue. Bivalirudin has a unique structure with a dodecapeptide attached to the active binding site moiety by four glycine residues (Figure 37-4). This structure together with the recombinant hirudins (Figure 37-5, left panel) binds to both the active site and an exosite-binding site. For this reason they are termed *bivalent direct thrombin inhibitors*.

Argatroban is also a synthetic compound derived from arginine but is attached only to the active enzymatic site of thrombin and is termed a monovalent inhibitor (see Figure 37-5, right panel). All of these compounds inhibit both free and bound thrombin, and none are affected by platelet factor 4.

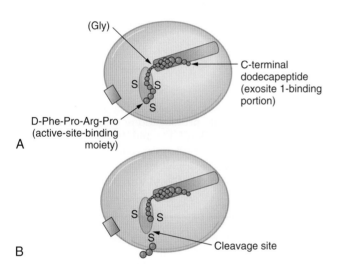

Figure 37-4 Mechanism of bivalirudin. **A,** the binding of bivalirudin to thrombin is shown. Pink circles represent amino acid residues of the inhibitor. Binding of the C-terminal dodecapeptide is at the anion-binding site used by fibrinogen *(brown area)*, and the 4 amino acid residue D-Phe-Pro-Arg-Pro binds in the active site *(tourquoise oval)*. **B** shows the effect of thrombin to cleave the Pro-Arg bond of the active site binding moiety to inactivate the direct thrombin inhibition.

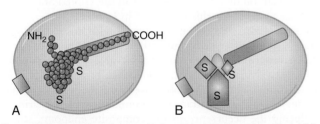

Figure 37-5 Mechanism of monovalent and bivalent direct thrombin inhibitors. **A** shows the binding of a bivalent hirudin like molecule to both the active proteolytic site of the thrombin molecule and also an anionic exosite *(brown area)* similar to that of bivalirudin. Pink circles represent amino acid residues of the inhibitor. Because binding is at two sites, these agents are collectively termed *bivalent direct thrombin inhibitors*. **B** shows chloromethylketone agent binding to active site *(tourquoise oval)* only (*pink trapezoids* represent halide and aliphatic groups and the *pink pentagon* is a ketone moiety in this molecule). Agents such as argatroban are included in this category of single site or monovalent direct thrombin inhibitors.

CLINICAL PHARMACOLOGY

These medications are indicated for the treatment and prevention of thrombosis in patients with heparin-induced thrombocytopenia.[27] Desirudin is approved in Europe for prevention of DVT/PE after hip replacement. Bivalirudin is also licensed for use during percutaneous coronary intervention/angioplasty procedures.

Pharmacokinetics

Table 37-6 outlines the basic pharmacokinetic profile of each drug. The excretion of the recombinant hirudins is affected by renal function, whereas argatroban is entirely metabolized by the liver. While impaired liver function is not a contraindication to the use of argatroban, the dose should be lowered and full reversal of anticoagulant effects might require more than 4 hours. Bivalirudin has renal excretion but also a unique metabolic elimination process. Thrombin can cleave the Pro-Arg bond of the active site binding moiety to metabolize bivalirudin (see Figure 37-4). This improves the safety of use of bivalirudin in patients with impaired renal function such as the elderly.

Pharmacodynamics

The anticoagulant effect of thrombin inhibitors is monitored by the aPTT or ACT (see Table 37-6); coagulation time increases in a dose-dependent manner. Argatroban also prolongs the PT in a dose-dependent manner. This has implications for assessing anticoagulation when transferring patients to long-term anticoagulation with vitamin K antagonists. The manufacturers recommend no loading dose of warfarin, but starting with a dose near the anticipated maintenance dose. The individual effects of argatroban and a vitamin K antagonist on the INR can be calculated using a nomogram.

ADVERSE EFFECTS

The major adverse effect of direct thrombin inhibitors is hemorrhage. Hemorrhagic complications, particularly when combined with thrombolytic or antiplatelet agents, can be life threatening. There is no antidote to any of these agents, so the antithrombin effect cannot be reversed pharmacologically.

In addition, the recombinant hirudins are associated with allergic/anaphylactic reactions that limit their use. Allergy to bivalirudin and argatroban is rare.

Oral Direct Thrombin Inhibitors

The first oral direct thrombin inhibitor licensed for human use was ximelagatran, a prodrug administered twice daily. It was licensed in certain European and South American countries for prophylaxis against DVT following knee and hip replacement, and has also shown efficacy in atrial fibrillation and acute coronary syndromes. Subsequent postmarketing surveillance showed that about 56% of patients given the drug had elevation of hepatic enzymes, even after withdrawal. This led to its withdrawal from the market. The only oral direct thrombin inhibitor currently available is dabigatran.

BASIC PHARMACOLOGY
Structure Activity and Mechanism of Action

Dabigatran is a competitive direct thrombin inhibitor. It is orally administered as the prodrug dabigatran etexilate. The

Table 37-6. Basic Pharmacokinetics, Monitoring Method, and Excretion for Intravenous Direct Thrombin Inhibitors*

DRUG	ADMINISTRATION	HALF-LIFE	DOSING SCHEDULE	MONITORING	RENAL EXCRETION	DOSE REDUCTIONS
Desirudin	Intravenous and subcutaneous	2-3 hours after intravenous injection	15 mg twice daily	aPTT of 1.5 times control. Stop drug if >2 times control	40%-50%	3-fold reduction with creatinine clearance 30-49 mL/min 9-fold reduction with creatinine clearance <30 mL/min
Lepirudin	Intravenous	1.3 hours in health men 2 hours in both healthy females and older than 70 yr 2 days with creatinine clearance <15 mL/min	Load of 0.4 mg/kg followed by continuous infusion of 0.15 mg/kg/hr	aPTT 1.5-2.5 times control	45%-50%	Creatinine clearance <60 mL/min or plasma creatinine >1.5 mg/dL (124 µmol/L)
Bivalirudin	Intravenous	25 minutes Coagulation tests within normal limits after 2 hours	0.75 mg/kg bolus then 1.75 mg/kg/hr		25%-50%	Creatinine clearance <30 mL/min infusion rate to 1 mg/kg/min
Argatroban	Intravenous	Coagulation tests are within normal limits 4 hours after discontinuing infusion	2 µg/kg/min increasing to 10 µg/kg/min based on raising aPTT 2- to 3-fold	aPTT, ACT	None	Hepatic failure/impairment

*Also shown are the conditions for reductions in dose in patients with renal or hepatic failure.
aPTT, Activated partial thromboplastin time; *ACT,* activated clotting time; *NR,* None reported.

active drug inhibits both free and clot-bound thrombin and thrombin-induced platelet activation.

CLINICAL PHARMACOLOGY
Pharmacokinetics and Pharmacodynamics
Dabigatran has a predictable pharmacokinetic and pharmacodynamic profile, allowing for a fixed-dose regimen. Peak plasma concentrations are reached 2 hours after oral administration in healthy volunteers, with no unexpected accumulation upon multiple dosing. This is followed by a rapid distribution and elimination phase and a terminal phase, with associated estimated half-lives of 8 to 10 hours and 14 to 17 hours with single and multiple dose administrations, respectively. Dabigatran exhibits linear pharmacokinetic characteristics with dose-proportional increases observed in maximum plasma concentration and area under the curve.

Excretion is predominantly renal as unchanged drug. The dose should be reduced from 150 mg twice daily to 75 mg twice daily if the estimated creatinine clearance is 30 to 50 mL/min.

Dabigatran is not metabolized by CYP isoenzymes. Concomitant use with P-glycoprotein inducers (e.g., rifampin) reduces exposure to dabigatran and should generally be avoided. Administration with the P-glycoprotein inhibitors ketoconazole, verapamil, amiodarone, quinidine, and clarithromycin does not require dose adjustments.

The formulation is highly acidic and was associated with an increased incidence of gastritis in the RE-LY study.[28] Of more importance, bioavailability of the drug after oral administration is only 6% to 7%. This is increased to about 75% if the capsule is chewed before swallowing, so patients should be warned to swallow the capsule whole.

Time curves for aPTT, INR, thrombin time (TT), and ecarin clotting time (ECT) parallel plasma concentration–time curves with values increasing rapidly in a dose-dependent

manner. At the highest dose of 400 mg administered three times daily, maximum prolongations over baseline of 3.1 (aPTT), 3.5 (INR), 29 (TT), and 9.5-fold (ECT) were observed.[29] Dabigatran undergoes conjugation with glucuronic acid to form pharmacologically active conjugates that account for approximately 20% of total dabigatran in plasma.

THERAPEUTIC EFFECTS
Dabigatran has been investigated for prevention of VTE after knee and hip replacement and prevention of stroke in patients with chronic atrial fibrillation. When data from various studies (RE-NOVATE, RE-MODEL, RE-MOBILIZE) were combined, dabigatran was found to be noninferior to enoxaparin using the efficacy endpoint of VTE, which had a 3% to 4% incidence in each treatment arm.[30] The safety endpoint of major bleeding also did not show a difference between the two treatments, at about 1% to 1.5% of patients. Because there was no efficacy benefit, the drug was not initially licensed for prevention of VTE by the FDA in the United States, but did get a license for this indication in Europe.

The RE-LY study compared two blinded doses of dabigatran (110 mg twice daily and 150 mg twice daily) with open-label warfarin (dosed to target INR of 2 to 3) in patients with nonvalvular, persistent, paroxysmal, or permanent atrial fibrillation.[28] The primary objective of this study was to determine whether dabigatran was noninferior to warfarin in reducing the occurrence of the composite endpoint, stroke (ischemic and hemorrhagic) and systemic embolism. Dabigatran at a dose of 110 mg was associated with rates of stroke and systemic embolism similar to those associated with warfarin, as well as lower rates of major hemorrhage. Dabigatran administered at a dose of 150 mg was associated with lower rates of stroke and systemic embolism but similar rates of major hemorrhage at 3.11%. These data led to dabigatran being licensed in the United States, Europe, and other countries for use as an alternate to vitamin K antagonists for prevention of stroke with atrial fibrillation. Regulatory authorities are reviewing postmarketing surveillance data following reports of 260 deaths due to hemorrhage.

SPECIAL SITUATIONS AND ADVERSE EVENTS

As with other anticoagulants, the major risk is for bleeding, which can be life threatening, particularly with major trauma. There is no specific antidote to dabigatran. It is recommended to discontinue dabigatran 1 to 2 days (CrCl ≥ 50 mL/min) or 3 to 5 days (CrCl < 50 mL/min) before invasive or surgical procedures because of the increased risk for bleeding. If surgery cannot be delayed, there is an increased risk for bleeding. Bleeding risk can be assessed by the ecarin clotting time (ECT), a laboratory test used to monitor anticoagulation during treatment with hirudin, which is a better marker of the anticoagulant activity of dabigatran than aPTT, PT/INR, or TT. If ECT is not available, the aPTT provides the next best approximation of dabigatran anticoagulant activity.

Inhibitors of Activated Factor X

HISTORICAL PERSPECTIVE

Factor Xa is at the convergence of the extrinsic and intrinsic pathways leading to thrombin activation. The crystal structure of human factor Xa reveals an active site divided into four subpockets (S1-4). The S1 subpocket is the major determinant of selectivity and binding of inhibitors. The first generation of oral factor Xa inhibitors was based on dibasic inhibitors binding to both the primary specificity pocket and a putative cation-binding site. The high basicity of these compounds limited oral bioavailability. Recent efforts have focused on development of nonpeptide inhibitors of low basicity by screening and rational design.

BASIC PHARMACOLOGY

Structure-Activity and Mechanism of Action

Due to shortcomings of vitamin K antagonists as the only form of oral anticoagulant (Table 37-7) and the critical role of factor Xa in the coagulation cascade, factor Xa has become an important target for anticoagulant development. These novel agents bind to and inhibit factor Xa directly without a requirement for AT. The major advantage of direct factor Xa inhibitors is their small size and resultant ability to inactivate circulating, as well as bound, forms of factor Xa. Inhibition is

produced by stoichiometric binding of one molecule of factor Xa inhibitor to one molecule of factor Xa. In theory, the capacity to inhibit factor Xa within the prothrombinase complex, as well as clot-bound factor Xa, suggests more powerful control over thrombus formation and progression and, therefore, potentially greater clinical efficacy. It also seems rational to inhibit the system at this point, because inhibition of one factor Xa moiety can lead to a 50-fold reduction in thrombin production.

Inhibitors of activated factor Xa generally bind in an L-shaped conformation involving the anionic S1 pocket and the aromatic S4 pocket. Typically, a fairly rigid linker group bridges these two interaction sites.

Apixaban, betrixaban, edoxaban, and rivaroxaban are the most advanced in clinical development. Both apixaban and rivaroxaban have licensed indications in Europe and the latter in the United States. Edoxaban is licensed in Japan only for thromboprophylaxis after major orthopedic surgery.

Rivaroxaban (BAY-59-7939) is an oral, direct, reversible, competitive, rapid, and dose-dependent inhibitor of factor Xa. Rivaroxaban inhibits factor Xa with more than 10,000-fold greater selectivity than other biologically relevant serine proteases, such as thrombin, trypsin, plasmin, factor VIIa, factor IXa, urokinase, and activated protein C.

Apixaban is a follow-up compound of the oral direct factor Xa inhibitor razaxaban. Apixaban is a highly selective and potent ($K_i = 0.8$ nM) inhibitor of both free and prothrombinase bound factor Xa.

CLINICAL PHARMACOLOGY

Pharmacokinetics and Pharmacodynamics

The relative pharmacokinetic profiles for the four most clinically advanced factor Xa antagonists are shown in Table 37-8.

Table 37-7. Limitations and Clinical Consequences of Vitamin K Antagonists

LIMITATION	CONSEQUENCE
Slow onset	Overlap with parenteral anticoagulation
Genetic variation in metabolism	Variable dose requirements
Multiple food and drug interactions	Frequent coagulation monitoring
Narrow therapeutic index	Frequent coagulation monitoring

Table 37-8. Basic Pharmacology of Orally Active Factor Xa Inhibitors

DRUG	ENZYME ANTAGONIZED	PRODRUG	BIOAVAILABILITY	HALF-LIFE	DOSING SCHEDULE	METABOLISM	RENAL EXCRETION	DOSE REDUCTION CRITERIA
Rivaroxaban	Xa	No	90%	9 hr 12-16 hr, age older than 75 years	Once daily	CYP 3A4	35%	Age older than 75 years Caution if creatinine clearance <49 mL/min
Apixaban	Xa	No	50%-80%	12 hr	Once daily	CYP 3A4	25%	NR
Edoxaban	Xa	No	45%	9-11 hr	Once daily	NR	35%	NR
Betrixaban	Xa	No	45%-50%	20 hr	Once daily	NR	5%	NR

NR, None recorded

The most striking difference between the agents is the very low renal clearance of betrixaban. This should lead to a more consistent effect without dose adjustments in older patients and those with impaired renal function, compared for example with rivaroxaban. Betrixaban is also unique in that the pharmaceutical company developing the drug was also developing a specific antidote. All of the agents have protein binding of about 90%, meaning they will be difficult to remove by dialysis. Despite the potential benefits of betrixaban over the other agents, development has been suspended.

All these agents induce a prolongation of coagulation time by 2 to 3 hours following ingestion, with increases in PT and aPTT by approximately 20%.

THERAPEUTIC EFFECTS

A large number of phase 2/3 studies of a number of oral factor Xa inhibitors are underway. The targets for these studies are typically short-term thromboprophylaxis to prevent DVT/VTE when the comparator is a LMWH. The second short-term indication is treatment of acute coronary syndrome. Longer-term thromboprophylaxis studies center around stroke prevention in patients with atrial fibrillation and prevention of thrombosis in prosthetic heart valves. For the latter studies the comparator is a vitamin K antagonist or aspirin.

Results of the studies published thus far have not been universally successful for this class of compound, in part because of the design of the studies and also due to increased bleeding. It may be that this class of compound will be of benefit to replace vitamin K antagonists, but there could be safety issues when the drug is combined with antiplatelet therapy.[31]

ADVERSE EFFECTS AND SPECIAL SITUATIONS

The obvious adverse event with any anticoagulant agent is hemorrhage. Spontaneous hemorrhage while taking these compounds appears not to be a problem in the absence of antiplatelet therapy. The safety of these agents with urgent surgery or trauma is unknown, and only rivaroxaban has been formally licensed for use in Europe. It should be noted that the prescribing information for this drug states that epidural hematoma has been reported during rivaroxaban therapy.

ANTIPLATELET AGENTS

Examination of histologic sections from postmortem material shows that the major component of the occlusive thrombus in arterial disease is the platelet.

Because acute arterial occlusion leading to MI or stroke is a leading cause of death worldwide, it is not surprising that considerable effort has been made to develop drugs to modify platelet function and reduce these cardiovascular events. In the past, aspirin was the mainstay of therapy. With increasing knowledge of the mechanisms of action of platelet activation, more recent therapies have concentrated on specific receptor inhibition.

Platelets can be activated in a number of ways. The major targets for pharmacologic intervention have been inhibition of cyclooxygenase with aspirin and phosphodiesterase with dipyridamole. More recent pharmacologic interventions have been to inhibit receptors at the platelet surface. In particular there is considerable interest in inhibition of purinergic receptors and those binding fibrinogen (the GpIIb/IIIa receptor). Agents that inhibit vWF binding to the glycoprotein Ib receptor are in early clinical development. Inhibitors of the protease-activated receptor 1 (PAR-1 or thrombin receptor) on the platelet surface are more advanced. The targets and agents in clinical use or development are shown in Figure 37-6.

Oral Agents

ASPIRIN
Historical Considerations
Acetylsalicylic acid (ASA) is a derivative of salicylic acid that works by inhibiting the enzyme prostaglandin H-synthase also known as *cyclooxygenase* (COX).

The history of ASA as an analgesic can be traced back to the time of Hippocrates (who lived between 460 BC and 377 BC), who recorded pain relief treatments, including the use of powder made from the bark and leaves of the willow tree to treat headaches, pains, and fevers. By 1829, the salicin in willow plants was identified as analgesic and this was later converted to salicylic acid.

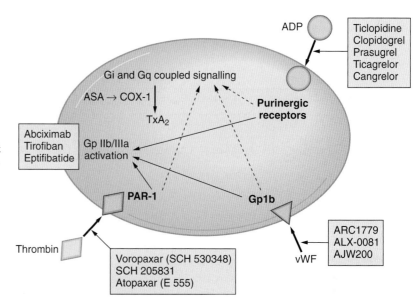

Figure 37-6 Sites of action of various agents that inhibit platelet function or activation. See text for further details.

In 1853, Gerhardt neutralized salicylic acid by buffering it with sodium (sodium salicylate) and acetyl chloride, creating acetylsalicylic acid, but he did not market it. In 1899, Hoffmann working for the German company Bayer rediscovered Gerhardt's formula and convinced Bayer to market the drug. Aspirin was patented in1900; the name *Aspirin* comes from "A" in acetyl chloride, "spir" in *Spiraea ulmaria* (the plant the salicylic acid came from), and "in," which was a familiar name ending for medicines.

Basic Pharmacology

MECHANISM OF ACTION. Prostaglandin H-synthase 1 and 2 (also known as COX 1 and 2) catalyze the conversion of arachidonic acid to prostaglandin H_2 (PGH_2). Human platelets and vascular endothelial cells convert PGH_2 primarily to thromboxane A_2 (TXA_2) and prostaglandin I_2 (PGI_2).[32] TXA_2 induces platelet aggregation and vasoconstriction, whereas PGI_2 inhibits platelet aggregation and induces vasodilatation. Platelet TXA_2 synthesis is reduced by about 98% following ASA administration. Whereas TXA_2 is largely a COX-1–derived product (mostly from platelets) and thus highly sensitive to aspirin inhibition, vascular PGI_2 can derive both from COX-1 and, to a greater extent even under physiologic conditions, from COX-2. COX-2–mediated PGI_2 production occurs mainly in response to shear stress and is insensitive to aspirin inhibition at conventional antiplatelet doses.

The molecular mechanism of permanent inactivation of COX activity by aspirin is as a consequence of acetylation of a serine residue (Ser529 in human COX-1, Ser516 in human COX-2) that results in a lack of access of the substrate to the catalytic site.[32] Acetylation of the COX-2 site is inhibited in cells with a raised oxidative state, including nucleated cells such as the endothelium. Additionally, nucleated cells rapidly resynthesize COX-2.

Inhibition of COX-1–dependent platelet function can be achieved with low doses of ASA given once daily. Inhibition of COX-2–dependent inflammatory processes requires larger doses of aspirin and a much shorter dosing interval. Thus there is an approximately 100-fold variation in daily doses of aspirin when used as an antiinflammatory rather than as an antiplatelet agent.

Clinical Pharmacology

PHARMACOKINETICS. ASA is rapidly absorbed in the stomach and upper intestine. Peak plasma levels occur 30 to 40 minutes after ingestion, and inhibition of platelet function is evident by 1 hour. In contrast, it can take 3 to 4 hours to reach peak plasma levels after administration of enteric-coated aspirin. The oral bioavailability of regular aspirin tablets is approximately 40% to 50% over a wide range of doses and is less for enteric-coated tablets.[33] Lower bioavailability of some enteric-coated preparations and poor absorption from the higher pH environment of the small intestine can result in inadequate platelet inhibition.

PHARMACODYNAMICS. The plasma concentration of ASA decays with a half-life of 15 to 20 minutes. Despite rapid clearance from the circulation, its platelet-inhibitory effect lasts for the life span of the platelet because it irreversibly inactivates platelet COX-1.[34,35] Aspirin also acetylates the enzyme in megakaryocytes before new platelets are released into the circulation.[36] The mean life span of human platelets is 5 to 10 days, so 10% to 20% of circulating platelets are replaced daily.[37] Bleeding times, implying normal primary hemostasis, require about 20% to 30% of normal platelet numbers/function. This suggests that cessation of ASA ingestion for 48 hours will result in a return to normal hemostatic activity.

Numerous studies have shown a risk reduction of about 15% to 20% for myocardial ischemia and stroke, with doses starting at about 60 mg ASA daily.[38-40] Some patients are resistant to usual doses, as manifested by incomplete inhibition of platelet aggregation and/or ongoing TXA_2 production. Such patients might be more prone to recurrent cardiovascular events.[41] One approach to this phenomenon would be to increase the dose of ASA, but this has potential problems. There is no substantive evidence for greater efficacy with greater dosage, but there is evidence for increasing morbidity as dose increases. In particular, bleeding is dose-dependent in patients treated for stroke and with acute coronary syndrome.[42] A retrospective subgroup analysis of the relationship between the aspirin dose and risk of major bleeding found a dose of 100 mg/day to have the lowest rate of major or life-threatening bleeding complications.[43] Bleeding risks increased with increasing ASA dose with or without clopidogrel. Approximately 300 mg/day produce fewer gastrointestinal side effects than 1200 mg/day, and 30 mg/day produces fewer side effects than 300 mg/day.[44,45]

In summary, the antiplatelet effect of ASA at low doses, the lack of dose-response relationship in clinical studies evaluating its antithrombotic effects, and the dose dependence of its side effects all support the use of as low a dose as has been found to be effective in the treatment of various thromboembolic disorders (Table 37-9). Use of the lowest effective dose (50-100 mg/day for long-term treatment) is currently the most appropriate strategy to maximize efficacy and minimize toxicity.[46]

ASA has been studied in a wide range of diseases ranging from preeclampsia to bowel cancer, usually at doses of 50 to 100 mg/day. The mechanisms of action for the observed benefits in these conditions remain to be elucidated.

DIPYRIDAMOLE

Basic Pharmacology

MECHANISM OF ACTION. Dipyridamole is a pyrimidopyrimidine derivative with vasodilator and antiplatelet properties. The mechanism of action of dipyridamole as an antiplatelet agent involves increased intracellular cyclic adenosine

Table 37-9. Lowest Effective Daily Dose of Aspirin to Reduce the Risk of Thrombotic Events by Condition

DISORDER	LOWEST EFFECTIVE DAILY DOSE (MG)
Transient ischemic attack or ischemic stroke*	50
Men at high cardiovascular risk	50
Hypertension	75
Stable angina	75
Unstable angina*	75
Severe carotid artery stenosis*	75
Polycythemia vera	100
Acute myocardial infarction	160
Acute ischemic stroke*	160

*Higher doses have been studied but did not show added benefit.

monophosphate (cAMP), which inhibits the platelet shape change. Increased cAMP concentration is due to one or both of two mechanisms: inhibition of phosphodiesterase and blockade of uptake of adenosine (which acts at adenosine A_2 receptors to stimulate platelet adenylyl cyclase and thus increase cAMP).

Clinical Pharmacology
PHARMACOKINETICS. Following an oral dose of dipyridamole tablets, the average time to peak concentration is about 75 minutes. The decline in plasma concentration fits a two-compartment model with an α half-life (initial decline following peak concentration) of 40 minutes and a β half-life of 10 hours. This is consistent with the twice-daily regimen used in recent clinical studies.

Absorption of dipyridamole from conventional formulations is quite variable and can result in low systemic bioavailability. A modified-release formulation of dipyridamole with improved bioavailability has been developed. Dipyridamole is highly bound to plasma proteins, and is metabolized in the liver where it is conjugated to a glucuronide and excreted in the bile. It is subject to enterohepatic recirculation.

PHARMACODYNAMICS AND THERAPEUTIC EFFECTS. Early clinical trials questioned the efficacy of dipyridamole, alone or in combination with ASA, probably due to variability in bioavailability. Recent studies have suggested significant benefit with the new formulation. Addition of modified-release dipyridamole 200 mg twice daily to ASA 25 mg twice daily was associated with a 22% relative risk reduction of major vascular events compared with ASA alone.[47] In a study of ASA (30-325 mg/day) with or without dipyridamole (200 mg twice

daily) in patients within 6 months of a transient ischemic attack (TIA) or minor stroke showed 20% reduction of a composite of major vascular events by the combined treatment.[48] The fixed combination of modified-release dipyridamole and low-dose ASA has been approved for stroke prevention.

Platelet Receptor Inhibitors

PURINERGIC RECEPTORS
There are three known subtypes of ADP receptors on platelets: $P2X_1$, $P2Y_1$, and $P2Y_{12}$ (Figure 37-7). The $P2Y_{12}$ receptor (previously known as $P2T_{AC}$, P_{2T}, and $P2Y_{cyc}$) is abundantly expressed on human platelets and on smooth muscle. ADP is released from damaged vessels, red blood cells, and platelets stimulated by other agonists. ADP binds to the $P2Y_1$ receptor to initiate platelet aggregation and to the $P2Y_{12}$ receptor, which amplifies platelet aggregation. Sustained ADP-induced platelet aggregation requires coactivation of $P2Y_1$ and $P2Y_{12}$ receptors. The $P2Y_{12}$ receptor acts by inhibiting adenylyl cyclase via a G_i protein and potentiates dense granule secretion, procoagulant activity, and platelet aggregation. Without continued $P2Y_{12}$ activation, aggregated platelets disaggregate. Inhibition of the $P2Y_{12}$ receptor became a recent focus of clinical drug development and licensing.

THIENOPYRIDINES
Basic Pharmacology
Thienopyridines selectively inhibit ADP-induced platelet aggregation with no direct effects on arachidonic acid metabolism. Although thienopyridines also can inhibit platelet

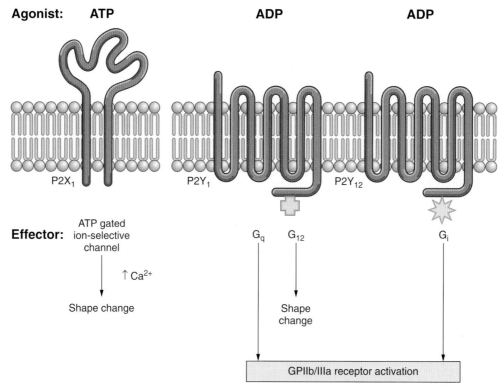

Figure 37-7 Three types of purinergic receptors expressed on platelets and their mechanisms of platelet activation. The two seven-transmembrane receptors act through G-protein mechanisms. The $P2Y_1$ receptor initiates platelet aggregation and the $P2Y_{12}$ receptor amplifies and completes the aggregation process. Continued stimulation of $P2Y_{12}$ receptors is needed to prevent platelet disaggregation.

aggregation induced by collagen and thrombin, these inhibitory effects are abolished by increasing the agonist concentration and therefore are likely to reflect blockade of ADP-mediated amplification of the platelet response to other agonists.

The thienopyridines do not act directly, but are administered as prodrugs requiring hepatic transformation. Clopidogrel is metabolized into 2-oxo-clopidogrel through a CYP-dependent pathway (Figure 37-8). The most important of these clinically is CYP 2C19. Prasugrel is not detected in plasma following oral administration. It is rapidly hydrolyzed by esterase in the intestine to a thiolactone, which is then converted to the active metabolite by a single step, primarily by CYP 3A4 and CYP 2B6, and to a lesser extent by CYP 2C9 and CYP 2C19. The active metabolite of prasugrel is metabolized to two inactive compounds by S-methylation or

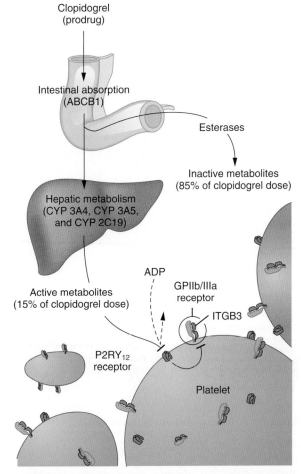

Figure 37-8 Role of metabolism in activation of the prodrug clopidogrel. Intestinal absorption of the prodrug clopidogrel is limited by an intestinal efflux pump P-glycoprotein (ABCB1). The majority of the prodrug is metabolized into inactive metabolites by ubiquitous esterases. The minority is bioactivated by various cytochrome P450 (CYP) isoforms into active metabolites. These metabolites irreversibly antagonize the adenosine diphosphate (ADP) receptor, which in turn inactivates the fibrinogen receptor (the glycoprotein [GP] IIb/IIIa receptor) involved in platelet aggregation. Many of these genes are subject to genetic polymorphisms that can affect drug response and result in nonresponders. *(Modified from Simon T, Verstuyft C, Mary-Krause M, et al; French Registry of Acute ST-Elevation and Non-ST-Elevation Myocardial Infarction (FAST-MI) Investigators. Genetic determinants of response to clopidogrel and cardiovascular events. N Engl J Med. 2009;360:363-375.)*

conjugation with cysteine. The major inactive metabolites are highly bound to plasma proteins. Clopidogrel is also metabolized by esterases to produce an inactive carboxylic acid derivative designated as SR 26334, which is thought to represent more than 80% of circulating metabolites.

The active metabolites of both clopidogrel and prasugrel couple through a covalent disulfide bond to P2Y12 receptors rendering the receptor unresponsive to ADP. Because the bond is covalent it is essentially irreversible; thus platelets exposed to the active thiol are affected for the remainder of their lifespan (about 7-10 days). Return of global platelet function requires the generation of a new platelet pool.

The relevance of the CYP system in producing the active metabolite is discussed below in the sections on drug interactions and pharmacogenetics.

Clinical Pharmacology

PHARMACOKINETICS. Following oral administration, about 80% of prasugrel and about 50% of clopidogrel is absorbed; this is not affected by food ingestion.[49]

Metabolism of both drugs is rapid, with peak plasma concentrations of the active metabolite occurring approximately 30 minutes after dosing. For prasugrel and clopidogrel, repeat daily doses do not lead to accumulation of the active metabolite, which has an elimination half-life of about 7 hours in both cases. Both drugs are highly protein bound (>95%).

Approximately 70% of the prasugrel dose is excreted in urine and 30% in feces as inactive metabolites. The corresponding figures for clopidogrel are about 50% by each route.

With both drugs the recommendation is to give a loading dose followed by a once daily maintenance dose: a 300 mg load and 75 mg/day for clopidogrel and for prasugrel 60 mg and 10 mg/day, respectively.

PHARMACODYNAMICS. Dose-dependent inhibition of platelet aggregation occurs about 2 hours following ingestion. With prasugrel, platelet inhibition reaches about 50% 1 hour after a loading dose of 60 mg. Steady-state inhibition of about 70% occurs after 3 to 5 days with a maintenance dose of 10 mg/day. Platelet aggregation returns to baseline over 5 to 9 days, reflecting production of new platelets. With clopidogrel at a dose of 75 mg once daily, platelet inhibition reaches a steady-state of 40% to 60% after 3 to 7 days. Platelet aggregation and bleeding time return to baseline about 5 days after stopping therapy.

Because both thienopyridines are prodrugs, their pharmacodynamic effects could be affected by alterations in metabolism. This apparently is only the case with clopidogrel, in that prasugrel has not been shown to have significant metabolic drug interactions.

Therapeutic Effects

Both clopidogrel and prasugrel are indicated in patients with acute coronary syndromes. This includes patients with unstable angina or non-ST-elevation myocardial infarction (NSTEMI) and patients with ST-elevation myocardial infarction (STEMI) when managed with primary or delayed percutaneous coronary intervention (PCI).

Clopidogrel reduces the rate of a combined endpoint of cardiovascular death, MI, or stroke, as well as the rate of a combined endpoint of cardiovascular death, MI, stroke, or refractory ischemia. Compared with clopidogrel, prasugrel reduces the rate of a combined endpoint of cardiovascular death, nonfatal MI, or nonfatal stroke.[50] The difference between treatments was driven predominantly by the incidence of MI, with no difference in stroke and little difference in cardiovascular death. Prasugrel is also indicated to reduce the rate of thrombotic cardiovascular events (including stent thrombosis) in patients with acute coronary syndrome (ACS) who are to be managed with PCI. As discussed later, the U.S. FDA allowed a license for use of prasugrel only after a considerable debate and inclusion of black box warnings.

Adverse Outcomes

The principal adverse outcome related to the use of thienopyridines is bleeding.[51] The CURE study showed similar rates for nonfatal and major hemorrhage but highlighted dose-dependent effects of ASA on rates for bleeding, and also an effect of age in both clopidogrel-treated and placebo groups (Table 37-10).

In the TRITON TIMI38 study, bleeding rates with prasugrel were markedly higher than with clopidogrel. Major bleeding was reported in 11.3% of prasugrel-treated patients compared with 3.6% in clopidogrel-treated patients, with differences in rates of fatal bleeding (0.9% to 0%), need for reoperation (3.8% to 0.5%), and requirement for red cell transfusion of at least 5 units (6.6% to 2.2%). As expected, there was also an effect of time on the rates of bleeding after stopping the drugs. Patients having surgery within 3 days of stopping the study medication had rates of major/minor bleeding of 26.7% for prasugrel and 5% for clopidogrel. This rate fell to 11.3% and 3.4%, respectively, for patients having surgery 4 to 7 days after stopping study medications. These issues resulted in the FDA making a black box warning for prasugrel.

Drug Interactions

The major interactions with clopidogrel involve drugs that modify the CYP 2C19 and CYP 3A4 isoenzymes. An example of the former is the proton pump inhibitor omeprazole, which reduces platelet ADP response. The CYP 3A4 and 3A5 isozymes metabolize clopidogrel more rapidly than other CYP enzymes and are most abundant in the liver. Atorvastatin and other CYP 3A4 inhibitors reduce platelet inhibition and a CYP 3A4 activator enhances this inhibition when coadministered with clopidogrel.[52] Despite these known interactions, there is no evidence that this is clinically relevant, as shown by a lack of a statistically discernible effect on cardiovascular outcomes.[40]

Pharmacogenetics

In contrast to the lack of clinically obvious adverse outcomes from drug interactions, there is a considerable interest in polymorphisms of CYP 2C19. Among clopidogrel-treated subjects in TRITON-TIMI 38, carriers of the *2 variant had a relative increase of 53% in the risk of death from cardiovascular causes, MI, or stroke compared with noncarriers (12.1% vs. 8.0%); and an increase by a factor of 3 in the risk of stent thrombosis (2.6% vs. 8%).[53] These observations resulted in the FDA requiring a black box warning for clopidogrel. A parallel study of prasugrel found no effect of this polymorphism on pharmacodynamic or clinical outcomes.[54]

Specific Populations

TIA OR STROKE. Prasugrel is contraindicated in patients with a history of prior TIA or stroke.[55] Patients with a history of TIA or ischemic stroke (>3 months before enrollment) had a higher rate of stroke when taking prasugrel (6.5%; of which 4.2% cases were thrombotic stroke and 2.3% were intracranial hemorrhage) than when taking clopidogrel (1.2%; all thrombotic). Prasugrel is not recommended for patients 75 years of age or older due to an increased incidence of fatal and intracranial bleeding, except in higher risk situations such as diabetes mellitus or history of previous MI. The mean exposure to the prasugrel active metabolite is approximately 30% to 40% higher in subjects with a body weight of less than 60 kg than in those weighing 60 kg or more. While not contraindicated in this group, a higher rate of bleeding can be anticipated. There are no published age or weight limitations with clopidogrel.

RENAL IMPAIRMENT. Patients with renal dysfunction are considered to be more prone to bleeding when receiving antithrombotic drugs. In a post hoc analysis of data from the CURE trial, cardiovascular death, MI, and stroke combined and bleeding occurred more frequently in the lowest glomerular filtration rate tercile.[56] This observation is not reflected in the effects of renal function on drug activity. For patients with end-stage or severe chronic renal failure (estimated creatinine clearance <15 mL/min), exposure to the active prasugrel metabolite was *reduced* to about half that in healthy controls. Similarly for clopidogrel in these patients, platelet inhibition was about half that anticipated following administration of 75 mg daily at only 25%. The reason for opposed effects on pharmacodynamic endpoints and patient outcomes is unclear.

Adenosine Diphosphate Analogues

TICAGRELOR
Basic Pharmacology
Ticagrelor is the first of a new chemical class of antiplatelet agents, the cyclopentyltriazolopyrimidines. Similar to the thienopyridines, ticagrelor is an oral $P2Y_{12}$ receptor antagonist that exerts antiplatelet effects by blocking ADP. In contrast to the other antiplatelet drugs, ticagrelor has a binding site different from ADP, making it an allosteric antagonist, and the block is reversible. Unlike the thienopyridines, ticagrelor is not a prodrug and therefore does not require metabolic activation in order to inhibit platelets. These properties give ticagrelor several theoretical advantages over clopidogrel. Since ticagrelor does not require metabolic activation, it avoids the variability seen with the CYP system and therefore

Table 37-10. Effect of Aspirin Dose and Age on Bleeding Event Rates

TREATMENT GROUP	ASPIRIN DOSE		
	<100 mg/day	100-200 mg/day	>200 mg/day
Clopidogrel	2.6%	3.5%	4.9%
Placebo	2.0%	2.3%	4.0%
Age	<65 yr	65-75 yr	>75 yr
Clopidogrel	2.5%	4.1%	5.9%
Placebo	2.1%	3.1%	3.6%

Data from the Clopidogrel in Unstable angina to prevent Recurrent Events (CURE) study.

produces a more consistent antiplatelet effect. However, the parent drug is metabolized, principally by CYP 3A to about 10 metabolites. The major metabolite, AR-C124910XX, formed by O-deethylation, is as active as ticagrelor in inhibiting ADP-induced platelet aggregation.

Clinical Pharmacology

PHARMACOKINETICS. Ticagrelor is about 36% bioavailable after oral administration and is rapidly absorbed with a maximum plasma concentration at 1.5 hours. Both ticagrelor and AR-C124910XX are highly (>95%) protein bound. Total clearance is about 25 L/hour with an apparent half-life of 8 to 12 hours.

Pharmacodynamics and Therapeutic Effects

Inhibition of platelet activity (IPA) using ADP-stimulated platelet aggregation showed 88% platelet inhibition with ticagrelor in the ONSET/OFFSET study.[57] Ticagrelor inhibited platelets to a greater extent than did clopidogrel at 30 minutes mean IPA, 40% compared to approximately 5%, respectively, and at 2 hours, mean IPA, approximately 90% compared to approximately 40%, respectively. Other measures of platelet function showed more rapid and robust IPA (typically 3- to 5-fold greater effectiveness) for ticagrelor compared to clopidogrel, and that the rate of recovery following withdrawal of therapy was more rapid with ticagrelor than clopidogrel.

The two drugs were also studied in a head to head comparison in the PLATO study. The primary endpoint, death from vascular causes, MI, or stroke, occurred significantly less often in the ticagrelor group than in the clopidogrel group (9.8% compared to 11.7% at 12 months). This difference was apparent as early as 30 days after the start of treatment. In patients who went on to have coronary artery bypass graft surgery (CABG), there was an early (at 1 month) difference in cardiovascular death, which continued out to 1-year follow-up (7.9% with clopidogrel compared to 4.1%). This striking benefit was unrelated to excess bleeding in either group.[58] These data have led to licensing of ticagrelor for use in acute coronary syndrome in Europe but not in the United States.

Adverse Effects

BLEEDING. In the PLATO study, the two treatment groups did not differ significantly in the rates of CABG-related major bleeding (11.6% and 11.2%), even though ticagrelor was only withheld for 24 to 72 hours before surgery while clopidogrel was withheld for 5 days. However, there was a higher rate of non–CABG-related major bleeding. The prescribing information has been amended to suggest this drug be withheld for 5 days before surgery or invasive procedure.

ADENOSINE-RELATED ADVERSE EFFECTS. Ticagrelor is metabolized to adenosine and administration is associated with related effects. Particular patients receiving ticagrelor had significantly more episodes of dyspnea (10%-20%) and ventricular pauses lasting more than 3 seconds (6%). However, with ticagrelor most of the episodes of dyspnea were minor, and only 1% of patients in the ticagrelor group stopped therapy because of this adverse event. Even so, these events suggest that close monitoring of patients taking ticagrelor is necessary during their early exposure.

Drug Interactions

Inhibitors of CYP 3A4 such as ketoconazole and drugs that are metabolized by CYP 3A4, for example simvastatin, are associated with increased plasma levels. Conversely, CYP 3A4 inducers, for example rifampicin and possibly St. John's wort, are associated with reduced ticagrelor plasma concentrations.

Ticagrelor inhibits P-glycoprotein, leading to increased plasma levels of digoxin, cyclosporin, and other substrates. P-glycoprotein inhibitors do not significantly influence ticagrelor and AR-C124910XX levels.

Special Populations

Plasma concentrations of ticagrelor are slightly increased (12%-23%) in older patients, women, patients of Asian ethnicity, and patients with mild hepatic impairment. The pharmacodynamics of ticagrelor are not materially affected in patients with severe renal impairment. The drug has not been tested in patients with severe hepatic impairment.

Unique Features

Consistent with its reversible mode of action, ticagrelor acts more quickly and is effective for a shorter time than clopidogrel. This means it has to be taken twice instead of once a day, which is a disadvantage with respect to compliance, but its effects are more quickly reversible, which can be useful before surgery or if side effects occur. The compliance issue has relevance to patients with stents in situ, because the effects of missing doses of ticagrelor will increase the risk for in stent thrombosis.

CANGRELOR
Basic Pharmacology

Cangrelor is an intravenous $P2Y_{12}$ purinoreceptor antagonist.[59] Manipulation of the chemical structure of ATP resulted in a novel class of compounds known as purinoreceptor modulators. Cangrelor inhibits platelet aggregation by inhibition of the $P2Y_{12}$ receptor, leading to an increase in cAMP. In addition this compound increases intra-platelet cAMP by an additional mechanism that is thought to act via a Gs signaling pathway.

Clinical Pharmacology

PHARMACOKINETICS. Cangrelor has a short half-life (2-6 minutes) and plasma clearance (50 L/hr). Steady-state inhibition of ADP-induced platelet aggregation is achieved within 30 minutes of infusion of cangrelor titrated up to 4 μg/kg/min in healthy volunteers. Return of baseline platelet aggregation was reestablished in 70% of volunteers within 1 hour of infusion termination.

PHARMACODYNAMICS. Cangrelor produces concentration-dependent inhibition of thrombin receptor-activating, peptide-induced aggregation in human platelets, indicating competitive antagonism. Furthermore, cangrelor acts directly at the $P2Y_{12}$ receptor without need for conversion in the liver to an active metabolite. Plasma concentrations of cangrelor are unaffected by severe renal or hepatic impairment.

Cangrelor was studied in two large-scale phase 3 studies that were both ended early following a decision by the interim analysis review committee that the study would not demonstrate the "persuasive" clinical efficacy needed for regulatory approval.

Table 37-11. Basic Pharmacology and Safety Aspects of Available Purinergic Receptor Antagonists*

	CLOPIDOGREL	PRASUGREL	CANGRELOR	TICAGRELOR
Chemical structure	Thienopyridine	Thienopyridine	ADP analogue	Cyclopentyltriazolopyridine (ADP analogue)
Prodrug	Yes	Yes	No	No
Administration	Oral	Oral	Intravenous	Oral
Time to peak effect	Dose dependent	2 hour	30 min	2 hr
Platelet inhibition with ADP stimulus 2 hr following loading dose	40%-50%	70%-90%	90%-100%	80%-90%
Half-life	6 hr	8 hr	1.5 to 3 min	6-12 hr
Time to steady-state platelet inhibition	4-5 days	2-4 days	30 min	2-3 days
Reversible	No	No	Yes	Yes
Time to recovery of platelet aggregation	5 days	7 days	60-90 min	24-48 hr
Safety with prior CVA	Yes	No	NA	Yes
Non-CABG bleeding		Increased risk		Increased risk
CABG bleeding		Increased risk		Reduced risk

*The risk of CABG and non-CABG related bleeding is in comparison to standard dose clopidogrel therapy.
CABG, Coronary artery bypass graft; *CVA*, cerebrovascular accident; *NA*, not available.

Table 37-12. Basic Pharmacology of Noncompetitive (Monoclonal Antibody) and Two Competitive Inhibitors of the Glycoprotein IIb/IIIa Receptor

COMPOUND	CHEMISTRY	PLASMA HALF-LIFE	BIOLOGIC HALF-LIFE	CLEARANCE MECHANISM
Abciximab	Monoclonal antibody	10 min	12-24 hr	Reticuloendothelial system
Tirofiban	Peptidomimetic	2 hr	4-8 hr	Renal
Eptifibatide	Polypeptide	2.5 hr	4-6 hr	Renal

Table 37-11 compares and contrasts the basic pharmacology and safety data for available purinergic receptor antagonists.

Glycoprotein IIb/IIIa Antagonists

BASIC PHARMACOLOGY

GpIIb/IIIa is a member of a family of adhesive receptors (integrins) composed of α and β transmembrane proteins. GpIIb/IIIa itself is composed of αIIb and β3 units and is specific for platelets. There are an estimated 50,000 to 80,000 GpIIb/IIIa receptors on the surface of each platelet. Internal stores of GpIIb/IIIa can be mobilized to join the existing surface receptors and further increase the overall surface expression. Platelet activation results in a change in the shape of the receptor, which greatly increases its normal low affinity for fibrinogen and vWF.

Two types of GpIIb/IIIa receptor antagonists are available[60]: noncompetitive (monoclonal antibodies) and competitive (a peptide and a peptidomimetic).

Abciximab is a chimeric mouse-human antibody modified from an original murine monoclonal antibody to reduce its immunogenicity. The ability of abciximab to bind to the vitronectin receptor and the leukocyte receptor (MAC-1) might also contribute to the anti-inflammatory properties of this drug. It is taken up by the reticular endothelial system where it is degraded by proteolysis.

Eptifibatide is a cyclic heptapeptide containing six amino acids and one mercaptopropionyl (des-amino cysteinyl) residue. Tirofiban is a non-peptide peptidomimetic. Both agents mimic the arginine-glycine-aspartate (RGD) sequences on fibrinogen. They contain either the RGD sequence itself or a similar sequence. The therapeutic efficacy of these drugs depends on maintaining plasma levels high enough to compete with fibrinogen for GpIIb/IIIa. Neither agent is significantly metabolized and both are renally excreted. Neither tirofiban nor eptifibatide react with the vitronectin or MAC-1 receptor.

CLINICAL PHARMACOLOGY

Pharmacokinetics

Comparator data for the three available agents are listed in Table 37-12. All three drugs are administered as a bolus followed by a continuous intravenous infusion. Following bolus administration of abciximab, free plasma concentrations decrease very rapidly, with an initial half-life of less than 10 minutes and a second phase half-life of about 30 minutes, probably related to rapid binding to platelet GpIIb/IIIa receptors and uptake by the reticuloendothelial system. High receptor affinity results in a long biologic half-life of 12 to 24 hours. Platelet function generally recovers over the course of 48 hours, although abciximab remains in the circulation for 15 days or more in a platelet-bound state. Abciximab can redistribute from the originally bound platelet to newly produced platelets, thus prolonging the antiplatelet effect. GpIIb/IIIa receptor occupancy by abciximab exceeds 30% at 8 days and 10% at 15 days, with residual binding documented as late as 21 days after therapy.

Intravenous administration of a 0.25 mg/kg bolus followed by continuous infusion of 10 µg/min produces relatively constant free plasma concentrations throughout the infusion. At the termination of the infusion period, free plasma concentrations fall rapidly for approximately 6 hours then decline at a slower rate. Skin bleeding time recovers with 12 hours of stopping the infusion.

Tirofiban has a half-life of approximately 2 hours. It is cleared from the plasma largely by renal excretion, with about 65% of an administered dose appearing in urine and about 25% in feces, both largely as unchanged tirofiban. Tirofiban is not highly bound to plasma proteins; the unbound fraction in human plasma is 35%.

The pharmacokinetics of eptifibatide are linear and dose related. Plasma elimination half-life is approximately 2.5 hours. Administration of a single 180 μg/kg bolus combined with an infusion produces an early peak level, followed by a small decline before attaining steady-state (4-6 hours). The extent of eptifibatide binding to human plasma protein is about 25%. In healthy subjects, renal clearance accounts for approximately 50% of total body clearance, with the majority of the drug excreted in the urine as eptifibatide, deaminated eptifibatide, and other, more polar metabolites. No major metabolites have been detected in human plasma.

Pharmacodynamics

The most commonly used method for assessing the pharmacodynamic effects of the various GpIIb/IIIa antagonists is platelet aggregometry. Administration of these agents alone does not prolong PT or aPTT.

Intravenous administration in humans of a single bolus dose of abciximab of 0.25 mg/kg followed by a continuous infusion of 10 μg/min produced sustained high-grade GpIIb/IIIa receptor blockade (>80%) and inhibition of platelet function.[61] Although low levels of GpIIb/IIIa receptor blockade are present for more than 10 days following cessation of the infusion, platelet function typically returns to normal over a period of 24 to 48 hours.

Tirofiban inhibits ex vivo ADP-induced platelet aggregation and prolongs bleeding time. Following a loading dose of 0.4 μg/kg over 30 minutes, platelet aggregation was inhibited by more than 90% and bleeding time was prolonged about threefold. Following discontinuation of an infusion of tirofiban, ex vivo platelet aggregation returns to near baseline in approximately 90% of patients in 4 to 8 hours.[62]

In clinical trials, eptifibatide inhibits ex vivo platelet aggregation induced by ADP and other agonists in a dose- and concentration-dependent manner.[63] The effect of eptifibatide was observed immediately after administration. Platelet aggregation is inhibited by about 85% after bolus injection and more than 90% during the steady-state infusion. Platelet aggregation returns to less than 50% inhibition 4 hours after discontinuing the infusion, and bleeding time returns to baseline within 6 hours of discontinuing the drug.

Therapeutic Effects

The benefit of GpIIb/IIIa inhibitors is mainly limited to high-risk patients with unstable angina or NSTEMI.[64] The most notable conditions where benefit is shown are in troponin-positive patients, whether or not they undergo revascularization and those with diabetes mellitus. The TARGET trial provides the only direct comparison of a small molecule (tirofiban) agent versus abciximab, and this trial demonstrated superiority for abciximab in reducing ischemic endpoints. For diabetic patients, abciximab is the only GpIIb/IIIa inhibitor observed to provide a significant survival advantage in patients undergoing PCI with angioplasty or stent placement and thus is singled out as the agent of choice for use in diabetic patients undergoing stent implantation. Abciximab also has the greatest weight of data supporting safety of use in patients with severe renal insufficiency, likely due to its non–renal mode of metabolism and elimination.

Current ACC/AHA guidelines recommend a platelet GpIIb/IIIa antagonist in patients with moderate- to high-risk ACS in whom catheterization and PCI are planned (class I, level A). Patients receiving bolus plus infusion of abciximab have a significant (35%-50%) reduction in the composite endpoint of death, nonfatal MI, refractory ischemia, or urgent revascularization within 30 days. Treatment benefits are observed within hours following intervention and are sustained through 6 to 12 months. Eptifibatide or tirofiban should be administered in patients with high-risk ACS in whom an invasive management strategy is not planned (class IIa, level A). In contrast to the data for abciximab, treatment with eptifibatide in the IMPACT II study showed a treatment effect over 30 days that was lost at 6-month follow-up. Similarly in the RESTORE study, the early treatment effect to prevent restenosis after angioplasty with tirofiban was lost at 6-month follow-up. An evidence-based approach would thus favor abciximab as the standard GpIIb/IIIa inhibitor for administration during PCI, especially in patients with ACS accompanied by high-risk features, including diabetes mellitus.

Adverse Effects

BLEEDING. As with all anticoagulant and antiplatelet agents, bleeding is a risk. The main concern is when these agents are given with anticoagulants, especially heparin. With abciximab, the incidence of bleeding decreases to only about 2% when used with low-dose heparin (70 U/kg) and further studies have reported major bleeding rates that are at least as low, if not lower, than that due to heparin alone. With tirofiban, the addition of heparin does not significantly alter inhibition of platelet aggregation, but does increase the average bleeding time, as well as the number of patients with bleeding times prolonged to more than 30 minutes. The principal site for bleeding is the femoral artery puncture site used for vascular access. To reduce the risk of bleeding, manufacturers recommend stopping the heparin 3 to 4 hours before withdrawal of these cannulae.

THROMBOCYTOPENIA. Thrombocytopenia can occur with all the GpIIb/IIIa receptor antagonists, with some variability related to the agent administered, dosage, duration of treatment, and the various drugs coadministered. Incidence of thrombocytopenia ranges from 1.1% to 5.6%. An immune mechanism is believed to be responsible. Binding of the antagonist to GpIIb/IIIa receptors might lead to exposure of ligand-induced binding sites to preexisting or induced antibodies. Another possible mechanism for thrombocytopenia is drug-induced activation of platelets. Thrombocytopenia induced by these mechanisms occurs within the first 24 hours of administration. All patients receiving parenteral GpIIb/IIIa antagonists should be monitored within 24 hours of initiation of therapy for development of thrombocytopenia and the drug discontinued if this occurs.

Special Populations and Contraindications

Treatment with GpIIb/IIIa receptor antagonists is contraindicated in patients with severe hypertension (systolic blood pressure >200 mmHg or diastolic blood pressure >110 mmHg) not adequately controlled on antihypertensive therapy, major surgery or history of major trauma within the preceding 4 to 6 weeks, history of stroke within 30 days or any history of hemorrhagic stroke (for tirofiban and eptifibatide), increased to 2 years before the use of abciximab, or a history of intra-cranial hemorrhage, intracranial neoplasm, arteriovenous malformation, or aneurysm.

For abciximab, additional contraindications are administration of oral anticoagulants within 7 days unless PT is less than or equal to 1.2 times control, use of intravenous dextran before percutaneous coronary intervention, or intent to use it during intervention, or presumed or documented history of vasculitis.

Tirofiban is also contraindicated with a history, symptoms, or findings suggestive of aortic dissection or pericarditis. As both tirofiban and eptifibatide are principally cleared by the kidney, both should have the dose of the maintenance infusion reduced to half with an estimated creatinine clearance less than 50 mL/min. Both are also contraindicated in patients receiving long-term renal dialysis, as is abciximab, but in this case because of a lack of safety data in this population.

Special Populations and Unique Features

Apart from patients with renal disease, there are no groups of patients in whom these drugs are associated with a relative increase in adverse effects.

Administration of abciximab can result in the formation of human antichimeric antibodies (HACA) that could potentially cause allergic or hypersensitivity reactions (including anaphylaxis), thrombocytopenia, or diminished benefit upon readministration. Readministration might be associated with an increased incidence and severity of thrombocytopenia.

EMERGING DEVELOPMENTS

In addition to a number of novel anticoagulants under development for the treatment of VTE discussed above,65 there are also emerging developments in antiplatelet therapy.

Protease Activated Receptor-1 (Thrombin Receptor)

Platelets have a specific surface G protein–coupled receptor known as *protease activated receptor-1* (PAR-1) receptor for thrombin. The extracellular portion is a long polypeptide, which has an arginine residue at position 41, and a serine at 42. Thrombin cleaves this peptide at this position, resulting in a hexapeptide SFLLRN at the N-terminal end. This is the tethered ligand for the stimulation of the receptor (Figure 37-9). Compounds have been developed that inhibit the ligand-binding site on PAR-1. Because the proteolytic activity of thrombin to cleave fibrinogen is not inhibited, coagulation should be unaffected.

Two compounds are at an advanced stage of trials in humans. Atopaxar (E5555) is a benzimidazole derivative that can be given orally on a once per day dose schedule. More than 90% inhibition of platelet activation to the synthetic thrombin receptor agonist peptide (TRAP) is achieved with no inhibition of responses to ADP or collagen. Phase 2 studies

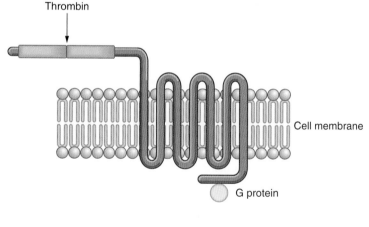

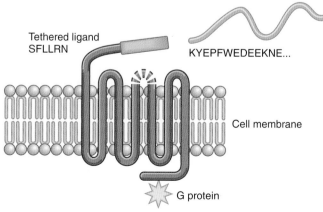

Figure 37-9 Mechanism of activation of the thrombin receptor. Thrombin cleaves the side chain of the thrombin receptor (protease activated receptor-1; PAR-1), a seven-transmembrane receptor, at arginine 41. The new six N-terminal amino acid residues (SFLLRN) act as a tethered ligand for the receptor. Inhibition of this interaction prevents platelet activation by thrombin but not the normal action of thrombin to cleave fibrinogen to form stable clot.

in patients with acute coronary syndromes (LANCELOT and J–LANCELOT) were not powered to investigate efficacy but were targeted on the safety aspect of bleeding.[66] While there was no difference between treatment and placebo, the safety data did show an increased proportion of treated patients with abnormal liver function and with a prolonged QTc interval.

Himbacine is a tetracyclic piperidine alkaloid isolated from the bark of Australian magnolia trees and has a strong anti-muscarinic activity. A modification of himbacine designated as SCH 530348 (now named Voropaxar) is orally active at a once-daily dose of 2.5 mg to produce 80% inhibition of platelet activation by TRAP without any muscarinic activity. Phase 2 studies in patients with nonurgent PCIs suggest appropriate safety and tolerability.[67]

Preliminary analysis of the data from two major clinical trials showed a significantly increased incidence of hemorrhagic stroke in patients allocated to the study medication. The status of development of both these compounds is currently unclear.

KEY POINTS

- Arterial and venous occlusion with thrombus is a major factor in mortality and morbidity.
- Improvements in physical chemistry have allowed the configuration of the chemistry and activity of many receptors associated with the coagulation network and platelet function to inhibit coagulation and platelet aggregation.
- Until recently the mainstay of anticoagulant therapy was heparin and the vitamin K antagonists, and the mainstay for platelet inhibition was acetylsalicylic acid.
- Understanding the receptor structure and function of platelets and the active proteolytic sites of coagulation proteins has allowed the rational development of novel drugs to modify or inhibit thrombogenesis and coagulation.
- However, the new direct oral anticoagulant drugs and new platelet inhibiting agents increase bleeding risk associated with surgery and invasive procedures, and have no validated antagonists.
- In the case of the new oral anticoagulants there is no ability to monitor their effect using simple standard laboratory assays, and antiplatelet activity can be measured only by highly specific, uncommon, and expensive methods.
- Most importantly, pharmacokinetics and pharmacodynamics of anticoagulant and antiplatelet drugs can differ significantly between patients depending on such factors as renal function, age, and frailty.

Key References

Collaborative meta-analysis of randomised trials of antiplatelet therapy for prevention of death, myocardial infarction, and stroke in high risk patients. *Br Med J*. 2002;324:71-86. Collated data from controlled trials to show that therapy with antiplatelet agents, and especially aspirin, was able to reduce mortality and morbidity associated with high shear stress arterial occlusions found in patients with myocardial infarction and stroke. This

observation paved the way for further drug development in this area. (Ref. 38)

Tapson VF. Acute pulmonary embolism. N Engl J Med. 2008;358(10):1037-1052. A review of low sheer stress venous thrombosis and thromboembolism. The article highlights risk factors for venous thrombosis that are being included in standard perioperative risk-management strategies. (Ref. 1)

Patrono C, Baigent C, Hirsh J, et al. Antiplatelet drugs: American College of Chest Physicians evidence-based clinical practice guidelines, 8th ed. *Chest*. 2008;133:199S-233S. Consensus evidence-based document outlining the best practice use of antiplatelet agents in the prevention and treatment of MI and ischemia. (Ref. 40)

Weitz JI. Emerging anticoagulants for the treatment of venous thromboembolism. *Thromb Haemost*. 2006;96:274-284. Reviews the pharmacology of newer anticoagulant agents outlining their potential strengths and weaknesses, and their use in the management of venous thrombosis and thromboembolism. (Ref. 65)

References

1. Tapson VF. Acute pulmonary embolism. *N Engl J Med*. 2008; 358:1037-1052.
2. Cohen AT, Agnelli G, Anderson FA, et al. Venous thromboembolism (VTE) in Europe. The number of VTE events and associated morbidity and mortality. *Thromb Haemost*. 2007;98:756-764.
3. Hirsh J. Heparin. *N Engl J Med*. 1991;324:1565-1574.
4. Hirsh J, Dalen JE, Deykin D, Poller L. Heparin: mechanism of action, pharmacokinetics, dosing considerations, monitoring, efficacy, and safety. *Chest*. 1992;102(4 Suppl):337s-351s.
5. Hirsh J, Levine MN. Low molecular weight heparin. *Blood*. 1992;79:1-17.
6. Hirsh J, Levine MN. Low molecular weight heparin: laboratory properties and clinical evaluation. A review. *Eur J Surg Suppl*. 1994;571:9-22.
7. Frydman A. Low-molecular-weight heparins: an overview of their pharmacodynamics, pharmacokinetics and metabolism in humans. *Haemostasis*. 1996;26(Suppl 2):24-38.
8. Tollefsen DM, Majerus DW, Blank MK. Heparin cofactor II. Purification and properties of a heparin-dependent inhibitor of thrombin in human plasma. *J Biol Chem*. 1982;257:2162-2169.
9. Salzman EW, Rosenberg RD, Smith MH, Lindon JN, Favreau L. Effect of heparin and heparin fractions on platelet aggregation. *J Clin Invest*. 1980;65:64-73.
10. Gallus AS. Anticoagulants in the prevention of venous thromboembolism. *Baillieres Clin Haematol*. 1990;3:651-684.
11. Litin SC, Gastineau DA. Current concepts in anticoagulant therapy. *Mayo Clin Proc*. 1995;70:266-272.
12. Green D, Hirsh J, Heit J, Prins M, Davidson B, Lensing AW. Low molecular weight heparin: a critical analysis of clinical trials. *Pharmacol Rev*. 1994;46:89-109.
13. Kishimoto TK, Viswanathan K, Ganguly T, et al. Contaminated heparin associated with adverse clinical events and activation of the contact system. *N Engl J Med*. 2008;358:2457-2467.
14. Landefeld CS, Beyth RJ. Anticoagulant-related bleeding: clinical epidemiology, prediction, and prevention [see comments]. *Am J Med*. 1993;95:315-328.
15. Linkins LA, Warkentin TE. The approach to heparin-induced thrombocytopenia. *Semin Respir Crit Care Med*. 2008;29:66-74.
16. Lo GK, Juhl D, Warkentin TE, Sigouin CS, Eichler P, Greinacher A. Evaluation of pretest clinical score (4 T's) for the diagnosis of heparin-induced thrombocytopenia in two clinical settings. *J Thromb Haemost*. 2006;4:759-765.
17. Fareed J, Walenga JM, Hoppensteadt D, Huan X, Racanelli A. Comparative study on the in vitro and in vivo activities of seven low-molecular-weight heparins *Haemostasis*. 1988;18(Suppl 3):3-15.
18. Nurmohamed MT, Rosendaal FR, Buller HR, et al. Low-molecular-weight heparin versus standard heparin in general and orthopaedic surgery: a meta-analysis. *Lancet*. 1992;340:152-156.
19. Turpie AG, Bauer KA, Eriksson BI, Lassen MR. Fondaparinux vs enoxaparin for the prevention of venous thromboembolism in major orthopedic surgery: a meta-analysis of 4 randomized double-blind studies. *Arch Intern Med*. 2002;162:1833-1840.

20. Turpie AG, Bauer KA, Eriksson BI, Lassen MR. Superiority of fondaparinux over enoxaparin in preventing venous thromboembolism in major orthopedic surgery using different efficacy end points. *Chest.* 2004;126:501-508.

21. Buller HR, Davidson BL, Decousus H, et al. Subcutaneous fondaparinux versus intravenous unfractionated heparin in the initial treatment of pulmonary embolism. *N Engl J Med.* 2003;349:1695-1702.

22. Buller HR, Davidson BL, Decousus H, et al. Fondaparinux or enoxaparin for the initial treatment of symptomatic deep venous thrombosis: a randomized trial. *Ann Intern Med.* 2004;140:867-873.

23. Agnelli G, Bergqvist D, Cohen AT, Gallus AS, Gent M. Randomized clinical trial of postoperative fondaparinux versus perioperative dalteparin for prevention of venous thromboembolism in high-risk abdominal surgery. *Br J Surg.* 2005;92:1212-1220.

24. van Gogh Investigators, Buller HR, Cohen AT, Davidson B, et al. Idraparinux versus standard therapy for venous thromboembolic disease. *N Engl J Med.* 2007;357(11):1094-1104.

25. Amadeus Investigators, Bousser MG, Bouthier J, Büller HR, et al. Comparison of *idraparinux* with vitamin K antagonists for prevention of thromboembolism in patients with atrial fibrillation: a randomised, open-label, non-inferiority trial. *Lancet.* 2008;371(9609):315-321.

26. Gage BF, Birman-Deych E, Radford MJ, Nilasena DS, Binder EF. Risk of osteoporotic fracture in elderly patients taking warfarin: results from the National Registry of Atrial Fibrillation 2. *Arch Intern Med.* 2006;166(2):241-246.

27. Lee CJ, Ansell JE. Direct Thrombin Inhibitors. *Br J Clin Pharmacol.* 2011;72(4):718.

28. Connolly SJ, Ezekowitz MD, Yusuf S, et al. Dabigatran versus warfarin in patients with atrial fibrillation. *N Engl J Med.* 2009;361:1139-1151.

29. Stangier J, Rathgen K, Stähle H, Gansser D, Roth W. The pharmacokinetics, pharmacodynamics and tolerability of *dabigatran* etexilate, a new oral direct thrombin inhibitor, in healthy male subjects. *Br J Clin Pharmacol.* 2007;64(3):292-303.

30. Friedman RJ, Dahl OE, Rosencher N, et al; RE-MOBILIZE, RE-MODEL, RE-NOVATE Steering Committees. Dabigatran versus enoxaparin for prevention of venous thromboembolism after hip or knee arthroplasty: a pooled analysis of three trials. *Thromb Res.* 2010;126(3):175-182.

31. Alexander JH, Lopes RD, James S, et al. APPRAISE-2 Investigators. Apixaban with antiplatelet therapy after acute coronary syndrome. *N Engl J Med.* 2011;365(8):699-708.

32. Majerus PW. Arachidonate metabolism in vascular disorders. *J Clin Invest.* 1983;72:1521-1525.

33. Pedersen AK, FitzGerald GA. Dose-related kinetics of aspirin. Presystemic acetylation of platelet cyclooxygenase. *N Engl J Med.* 1984;311:1206-1211.

34. Roth GJ, Majerus PW. The mechanism of the effect of aspirin on human platelets. I. Acetylation of a particulate fraction protein. *J Clin Invest.* 1975;56:624-632.

35. Roth GJ, Stanford N, Majerus PW. Acetylation of prostaglandin synthase by aspirin. *Proc Natl Acad Sci U S A.* 1975;72:3073-3076.

36. Demers LM, Budin RE, Shaikh BS. The effects of aspirin on megakaryocyte prostaglandin production. *Proc Soc Exp Biol Med.* 1980;163:24-29.

37. Najean Y, Ardaillou N, Dresch C. Platelet lifespan. *Annu Rev Med.* 1969;20:47-62.

38. Collaborative meta-analysis of randomised trials of antiplatelet therapy for prevention of death, myocardial infarction, and stroke in high risk patients. *Br Med J.* 2002;324:71-86.

39. Tran H, Anand SS. Oral antiplatelet therapy in cerebrovascular disease, coronary artery disease, and peripheral arterial disease. *J Am Med Assoc.* 2004;292:1867-1874.

40. Patrono C, Baigent C, Hirsh J, Roth G. Antiplatelet drugs: American College of Chest Physicians evidence-based clinical practice guidelines. 8th ed. *Chest.* 2008;133:199S-233S.

41. Hankey GJ, Eikelboom JW. Aspirin resistance. *Lancet.* 2006;367:606-617.

42. Slattery J, Warlow CP, Shorrock CJ, Langman MJ. Risks of gastrointestinal bleeding during secondary prevention of vascular events with aspirin—analysis of gastrointestinal bleeding during the UK-TIA trial. *Gut.* 1995;37:509-511.

43. Peters RJ, Mehta SR, Fox KA, et al. Effects of aspirin dose when used alone or in combination with clopidogrel in patients with acute coronary syndromes: observations from the Clopidogrel in Unstable angina to prevent Recurrent Events (CURE) study. *Circulation.* 2003;108:1682-1687.

44. Farrell B, Godwin J, Richards S, Warlow C. The United Kingdom transient ischaemic attack (UK-TIA) aspirin trial: final results. *J Neurol Neurosurg Psychiatry.* 1991;54:1044-1054.

45. Dutch TIA Trial Study Group. A comparison of two doses of aspirin (30 mg vs. 283 mg a day) in patients after a transient ischemic attack or minor ischemic stroke. *N Engl J Med.* 1991;325:1261-1266.

46. Patrono C, Garcia Rodriguez LA, Landolfi R, Baigent C. Low-dose aspirin for the prevention of atherothrombosis. *N Engl J Med.* 2005;353:2373-2383.

47. Diener HC, Cunha L, Forbes C, Sivenius J, Smets P, Lowenthal A. European Stroke Prevention Study. 2. Dipyridamole and acetylsalicylic acid in the secondary prevention of stroke. *J Neurol Sci.* 1996;143(1-2):1-13.

48. Dengler R, Diener HC, Schwartz A, et al; EARLY Investigators. Early treatment with aspirin plus extended-release dipyridamole for transient ischaemic attack or ischaemic stroke within 24 h of symptom onset (EARLY trial): a randomised, open-label, blinded-endpoint trial. *Lancet Neurol.* 2010;9(2):159-166. Epub 2010 Jan 7.

49. Achar S. Pharmacokinetics, drug metabolism, and safety of prasugrel and clopidogrel. *Postgrad Med.* 2011;123(1):73-79.

50. Montalescot G, Wiviott SD, Braunwald E, et al. Prasugrel compared with clopidogrel in patients undergoing percutaneous coronary intervention for ST-elevation myocardial infarction (TRITON-TIMI 38): double-blind, randomised controlled trial. *Lancet.* 2009;373:723-731.

51. Quinlan DJ, Eikelboom JW, Goodman SG, et al. Implications of variability in definition and reporting of major bleeding in randomized *trials* of oral P2Y12 inhibitors for acute coronary syndromes. *Eur Heart J.* 2011;32(18):2256-2265.

52. Lau WC, Waskell LA, Watkins PB, et al. Atorvastatin reduces the ability of clopidogrel to inhibit platelet aggregation: a new drug-drug interaction. *Circulation.* 2003;107:32-37.

53. Mega JL, Close SL, Wiviott SD, et al. Cytochrome P-450 polymorphisms and response to clopidogrel. *N Engl J Med.* 2009;360:354-362.

54. Mega JL, Close SL, Wiviott SD, et al. Cytochrome P450 genetic polymorphisms and the response to prasugrel: relationship to pharmacokinetic, pharmacodynamic, and clinical outcomes. *Circulation.* 2009;119:2553-2560.

55. Alexopoulos D, Xanthopoulou I, Mylona P, et al. Prevalence of contraindications and conditions for precaution for prasugrel administration in a real world acute coronary syndrome population. *J Thromb Thrombolysis.* 2011;32(3):328-333.

56. Keltai M, Tonelli M, Mann JF, et al. Renal function and outcomes in acute coronary syndrome: impact of clopidogrel. *Eur J Cardiovasc Prev Rehabil.* 2007;14:312-318.

57. Gurbel PA, Bliden KP, Butler K, et al. Randomized double-blind assessment of the ONSET and OFFSET of the antiplatelet effects of ticagrelor versus clopidogrel in patients with stable coronary artery disease: the ONSET/OFFSET study. *Circulation.* 2009;120(25):2577-2585.

58. Held C, Asenblad N, Bassand JP. Ticagrelor versus clopidogrel in patients with acute coronary syndromes undergoing coronary artery bypass surgery: results from the PLATO (Platelet Inhibition and Patient Outcomes) trial. *J Am Coll Cardiol.* 2011;57:672-684.

59. Yousuf O, Bhatt DL. The evolution of antiplatelet therapy in cardiovascular disease. *Nat Rev Cardiol.* 2011;8(10):547-559.

60. Schneider DJ. Anti-platelet therapy: glycoprotein IIb-IIIa antagonists. *Br J Clin Pharmacol.* 2011;72(4):672-682.

61. Saucedo JF, Lui HK, Garza L, Guerra GJ, Jacoski MV, Jennings LK. Comparative pharmacodynamic evaluation of eptifibatide and *abciximab* in patients with non-ST-segment elevation acute coronary syndromes: the TAM2 study. *J Thromb Thrombolysis.* 2004;18(2):67-74.

62. Solinas E, Gobbi G, Dangas G, et al. Comparison of the effects of pretreatment with tirofiban, clopidogrel or both on the inhibition of platelet aggregation and activation in patients with acute coronary syndromes. *J Thromb Thrombolysis.* 2009;27(1):36-43.

63. Saucedo JF, Lui HK, Garza L, Guerra GJ, Jacoski MV, Jennings LK. Comparative pharmacodynamic evaluation of *eptifibatide* and

abciximab in patients with non-ST-segment elevation acute coronary syndromes: the TAM2 study. *J Thromb Thrombolysis*. 2004;18(2):67-74.

64. Friedland S, Eisenberg MJ, Shimony A. Meta-analysis of randomized controlled *trials* of intracoronary versus intravenous administration of glycoprotein IIb/IIIa inhibitors during percutaneous coronary intervention for acute coronary syndrome. *Am J Cardiol*. 2011;108(9):1244-1251.

65. Weitz JI. Emerging anticoagulants for the treatment of venous thromboembolism. *Thromb Haemost*. 2006;96:274-284.

66. Goto S, Ogawa H, Takeuchi M, Flather MD, Bhatt DL; J-LANCELOT (Japanese-Lesson from Antagonizing the Cellular Effect of Thrombin) Investigators. Double-blind, placebo-controlled Phase II studies of the protease-activated receptor 1 antagonist E5555 (atopaxar) in Japanese patients with acute coronary syndrome or high-risk coronary artery disease.

67. Becker RC, Moliterno DJ, Jennings LK, et al. Safety and tolerability of SCH 530348 in patients undergoing non-urgent percutaneous coronary intervention: a randomised, double-blind, placebo-controlled phase II study. *Lancet*. 2009;373:919-928.

INDEX

Page numbers followed by f indicate figures; t, tables.